THE OPHTHALMIC ASSISTANT

a guide for ophthalmic medical personnel

the OPHTHALMIC ASSISTANT

a guide for ophthalmic medical personnel

HAROLD A. STEIN, MD, MSc (Ophth), FRCS (C)

Professor of Ophthalmology, University of Toronto, Toronto, Ontario;
Attending Ophthalmologist, Scarborough General Hospital, Scarborough, Ontario;
Attending Ophthalmologist, Mount Sinai Hospital, Toronto, Ontario;
Past President,
Joint Commission on Allied Health Personnel in Ophthalmology, St. Paul, Minnesota;
Past President, Contact Lens Association of Ophthalmologists, New Orleans, Louisiana;
Past President,
Canadian Ophthalmological Society, Ottawa, Canada;
Director, Professional Continuing Education
Centennial College of Applied Arts, Toronto, Ontario

BERNARD J. SLATT, MD, FRCS (C)

Associate Professor of Ophthalmology, University of Toronto, Toronto, Ontario;
Attending Ophthalmologist, Scarborough General Hospital, Scarborough, Ontario;
Attending Ophthalmologist, Mount Sinai Hospital, Toronto, Ontario

RAYMOND M. STEIN, MD, FRCS (C)

Chief, Department of Ophthalmology, Scarborough General Hospital, Scarborough, Ontario;
Assistant Professor of Ophthalmology, University of Toronto, Toronto, Ontario;
Attending Ophthalmologist, Mount Sinai Hospital, Toronto, Ontario;
Past Commissioner, Joint Commission of Allied Health Personnel in Ophthalmology,
St. Paul, Minnesota

SIXTH EDITION

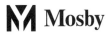 Mosby

St. Louis Baltimore Berlin Boston Carlsbad Chicago London Madrid
Naples New York Philadelphia Sydney Tokyo Toronto

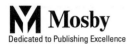 **Mosby**
Dedicated to Publishing Excellence

Editor: Laurel Craven
Managing Editor: Kathy Falk
Developmental Editor: Dana Battaglia
Project Manager: Gayle May Morris
Production Editor: Lisa Marcus
Manufacturing Supervisor: Betty Richmond
Design Manager: Susan Lane
Cover Design: GW Graphics

SIXTH EDITION

Copyright © 1994 by Mosby–Year Book, Inc.

Previous editions copyrighted 1968, 1971, 1976, 1983, 1988

Printed in the United States of America
Composition by Graphic World Inc.
Color insert by Color Dot Graphics
Printing/binding by R.R. Donnelley

Mosby–Year Book, Inc.
11830 Westline Industrial Drive
St. Louis, MO 63146

International Standard Book Number 0-8151-7560-4

93 94 95 96 97 / 9 8 7 6 5 4 3 2 1

Contributors

Howard S. Barnebey, MD

Clinical Assistant Professor of Ophthalmology
Department of Ophthalmology
University of Washington
Seattle, Washington

Bernard R. Blais, MD, FACS

Clinical Professor, Uniformed Services
University of Health Sciences
Force Medical Officer, Military Sealift Command
Washington, D.C.

David L. Guyton, MD

Associate Professor
Johns Hopkins University School of Medicine
The Wilmer Eye Institute
Baltimore, Maryland

Alex V. Levin, MD, FAAP, FAAO, FRCSC

Assistant Professor
Pediatrics and Ophthalmology
University of Toronto
Hospital for Sick Children
Toronto, Ontario, Canada

Csaba L. Martonyi, CRA, FOPS

Associate Professor
Director of Ophthalmic Photography
W.K. Kellogg Eye Center
Department of Ophthalmology
University of Michigan Medical School
Ann Arbor, Michigan

Gerard E. Meltzer, MD

Assistant Clinical Professor
Department of Ophthalmology
University of Colorado Health Sciences Center
Denver, Colorado

Richard P. Mills, MD

Professor and Vice Chairman
Department of Ophthalmology
University of Washington Medical Center
Seattle, Washington

E. Rand Simpson, MD

Associate Professor
Ophthalmology
University of Toronto
Toronto, Ontario, Canada

Foreword

An ophthalmologist who does not work with an ophthalmic assistant is a person who does his own scheduling, answers his own phone, does surgery alone, does his own visual field examination and does his own diagnostic workup of the patients. I have not heard of such a person in years. We sometimes forget how many assistants we have and how vitally important they are to us and our patients. In this sixth edition of *The Ophthalmic Assistant,* Harold Stein, Bernard Slatt, and Raymond Stein demonstrate their superb ability to write in an easy-to-read style. Their knowledge and understanding of the variety of information ophthalmic assistants need to know to perform their tasks comfortably, capably, and appropriately is impressive. Complete ophthalmologic care can best be provided when all team members are secure in their knowledge of ocular problems and clear in their role and responsibility.

The desire of the authors to ensure that ophthalmic assistants — from the operating room nurse to the office receptionist — have a fundamental background in disease processes is achieved herein. This text contains basic information on everything from testing vision to certain surgical procedures, with an emphasis throughout on technical considerations.

This text is of value to all those associated with ophthalmologists — from the billing personnel in the front office to the "detail" people in the pharmaceutical and instrumentation industries. Most of all, the assistant who works day-to-day with the ophthalmologist to assist in providing patient care will gain — as will our patients — by reading and discussing this book with the ophthalmologist. Applying the valuable information contained in this text to their invaluable responsibilities is in the best interest of patient care.

Previous editions of *The Ophthalmic Assistant* have been used as the standard text by ophthalmic assistants the world over, and this enhanced edition will be the new standard.

Bruce E. Spivey, M.D.

President, CEO, Northwestern Health Care Network; Attending Ophthalmologist, Northwestern Memorial Hospital; Clinical Professor of Ophthalmology, Northwestern University, Chicago, Illinois

Preface

This book has been written expressly for ancillary ophthalmic workers who assist the ophthalmologist in the day-to-day care of eye patients. Many ophthalmic assistants and technicians have had no opportunity for formal training and have learned their duties on the job. Experience alone may become a highly repetitious teacher. To paraphrase Sir William Osler, experience without knowledge is to sail an uncharted course, but knowledge without experience is never to go to sea at all. This book, originally published in 1968, has grown in size by over 50%. We have tried to include not only new skill but background information. This book is designed to help fill the vacuum in our community by providing a training basis for ancillary ophthalmic personnel and meeting the needs for a reference source. We have purposely avoided controversial subjects and highly specialized technical areas because of the varying degrees of training of ophthalmic assistants and technicians. Rather, the emphasis has been placed on illustrations and photographs to illuminate and clarify ophthalmic technology and to foster interest wherever possible.

The role of the ophthalmic assistant is to provide reliable and competent eye care before and following regular visits to offices, clinics, and hospitals. These individuals must be familiar with procedures regarding sterility, the nature of emergency patients, and the technical aspects of ophthalmology. With this knowledge the ophthalmic assistant can increase efficiency and ensure that all details of diagnostic workup and regimen are understood and carried out by the patient. Although emphasis is on the paramedical functions of the ophthalmic assistant and not the secretarial aspects, we recognize that in a small office both positions may have to be carried out by the same individual.

In this sixth edition we have attempted to keep pace with the ever-expanding new developments in the field of ophthalmology. New chapters have been introduced, old chapters updated, and some sections entirely eliminated. We have tried to keep to the original concept: to provide a concise up-to-date review of the field of ophthalmology that is readable, interesting, and illustrated.

Over the years we have broadened the scope of the textbook to provide not only practical technical information but also background information on ophthalmic disease processes and surgical procedures. We have sections for the hospital ophthalmic assistant who aids in the operating room and for the nurse who aids in the surgical and postoperative care of patients after surgery. We continue to include material of interest to those individuals working for optical and associated pharmaceutical companies. We have added and updated material for contact lens technicians, with a more detailed review to be found in our companion book, *Fitting Guide for Hard and Soft Contact Lenses,* third edition, published by Mosby–Year Book. A companion book, *Ophthalmic Terminology,* third edition, published by Mosby–Year Book, serves to expand the limited glossary and is designed as a vocabulary builder.

While the main thrust of this book is toward the ophthalmic assistant, we hope the clarity, organization, and readability of the book will attract others in the ophthalmic community.

The sixth edition has seen the incorporation of a new chapter on the expanding interest in refractive surgery as well as a new section on computerized corneal topography. These two areas have absorbed great clinical interest. This edition has also seen an expansion of disease processes of commonly seen eye disorders. We have included a new chapter on pediatric ophthalmology by Dr. Alex Levin of the Sick Children's Hospital and an excellent update on strabismus by Dr. Stephen Kraft. Also, Anne Jackson gave a very thorough review of the chapter on CPR.

We have included in the sixth edition a color atlas of common eye diseases and disorders, from our book *Primer in Ophthalmology,* so the reader can have a clear color picture of these disorders. As in past editions we are also indebted to a loyal friend, Mr. Norman Deer, and Laurie Stein, who have been responsible for the artwork and photography and to

Ms. Jill Klintworth for secretarial help. We are also indebted to our colleagues Mr. Keith Harrison, Ms. Lynn Maund and Ms. Alice Gelinas, all of whom have given generously of their time and help in reviewing sections for this edition.

Individuals who have helped with previous editions are listed alphabetically in the acknowledgments.

Harold A. Stein
Bernard J. Slatt
Raymond M. Stein

Acknowledgments
for aid as reviewers in previous editions

Bud Appleton

Richard Augustine

Howard Barneby

Tony Benson

Bernard Blais

†Maxwell Bochner

Albert Cheskes

Penny Cook

John Crawford

Norman Deer

Katherine Delmer

†Saul Fainstein

John Fowler

Therese Fredette

Ivan Gareau

Alice Gelinas

Paul Graczyk

Desmond Grant

Mark Grieve

Darll Guthmiller

David Guyton

G. Peter Halberg

Keith Harrison

William Hunter

John Hymers

Anne Jackson

Jerome Kazdan

Edna Kelly

D'Arcy Kingsmill

Jill Klintworth

Steven Kraft

Laurette LaRocque

Les Landecker

Sze Kong Luke

Bernice Mandelcorn

Theodore Martens

Lynn Maund

Gerard Meltzer

Richard Mills

Donald Morin

†Kenneth Ogle

John Parker

Thomas Pashby

Charles Pavlin

Karen Quam

Paula Quigley

Robert Rosen

†Barnet Sakler

Abraham Schlossman

Rand Simpson

Anne Skryzpnik

Laurie Stein

Kenneth Swanson

Spencer Thornton

Kenneth Woodward

†Deceased.

Contents

PART ONE

Basic sciences

CHAPTER I

Anatomy of the eye

- Surface anatomy
- Tear film
- Cornea
- Sclera
- Uvea
- Angle structures
- Lens
- Vitreous
- Retina
- Optic nerve
- Visual pathway
- Ocular muscles

Although the eye is commonly referred to as the *globe,* it is not really a true sphere. It is composed of two spheres with different radii, one set into the other (Figs. 1-1 and 1-2). The front, or anterior, sphere, which is the smaller and more curved of the two, is called the *cornea.* The cornea is the window of the eye because it is a completely transparent structure. It is the more curved of the two spheres and sets into the other as a watch glass sets into the frame of a watch. The posterior sphere is a white opaque fibrous shell called the *sclera.* The cornea and the sclera are relatively nondistensible structures that encase the eye and form a protective covering for all the delicate structures within.

In terms of size the eye measures approximately 24 mm in all its main diameters in the normal adult.

SURFACE ANATOMY

The eye itself is covered externally by the eyelids, which are movable folds protecting the eye from injury and excessive light. The lids serve to swab the eye and spread a film of tears over the cornea, thereby preventing evaporation from the surface of the eye. The upper eyelid extends to the eyebrow, which separates it from the forehead, whereas the lower eyelid usually passes without any line of demarcation into the skin of the cheek. The upper eyelid is the more mobile of the two, and when it is open, it covers about 1 mm of the cornea. A muscle that elevates the lid, the *levator palpebrae superioris,* is always active, contracting to keep the eyelid open. During sleep the eyelid closes by relaxation of this muscle. The lower lid lies at the lower border of the cornea when the eye is open, and it rises slightly when it shuts.

Normally, when the eyes are open, a triangular space is visible on either side of the cornea. These triangular spaces, formed by the junction of the upper and lower lids, are called the *canthi* (Fig. 1-3). These canthi are denoted by the terms *medial* and

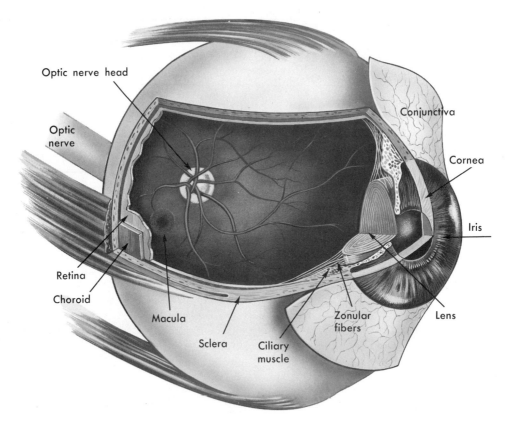

Fig. 1-1 Cutaway section of the eye.

lateral, the former being closer to the nasal bridge. Most eyes are practically the same size; therefore, when we speak of the eyes appearing large or small, we usually refer not to the actual size but to the portion of the eyeball visible on external examination, which in turn depends on the size of the palpebral fissure. The shape of the fissure also determines its appearance. In Orientals, a fold of skin extends from the upper lid to the lower lid and covers the medial fissure, giving the eye its characteristic obliquity. In the medial fissure there are two fleshy mounds: the deeper one, called the *plica semilunaris,* and the superficial one, called the *caruncle* (Fig. 1-4). The caruncle is modified skin that contains sweat and oil glands. Occasionally it also contains fine cilia, or hairs. When the eyes are open,

the palpebral fissures measure about 30 mm in width and 15 mm in height.

The free margin of each lid is about 2 mm broad and has an anterior and a posterior border. From the anterior, or front, border are the eyelashes, which are hairs arranged in two or three rows. The upper eyelid lashes are longer and more numerous than the lower, and they tend to curl upward. The lashes are longest and most curled in childhood. The posterior border of the lid margin is sharp and tightly abuts against the front surface of the globe. By depressing the lower lid, one can see a thin gray line that separates the two borders of the lid. This line, called the *gray line,* is used in many surgical procedures to split the upper and lower lids into two portions. Also visible on both lids are the tiny openings that

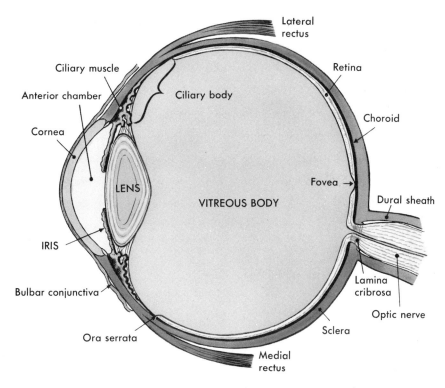

Fig. 1-2 The eye cut in horizontal section.

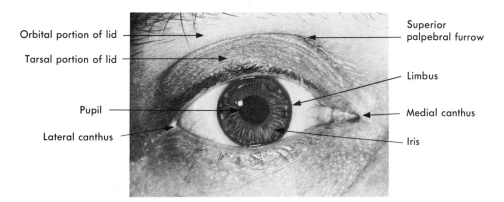

Fig. 1-3 Surface anatomy of the eye.

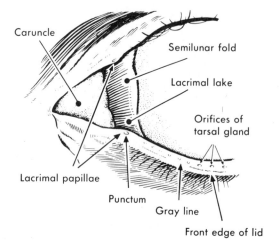

Fig. 1-4 Inner canthus, showing the semilunar fold and the caruncle. Normally the punctum is not visible unless the lower lid is depressed.

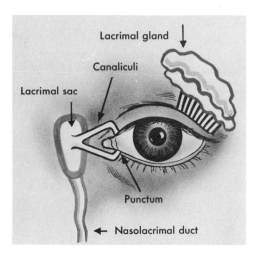

Fig. 1-5 Lacrimal apparatus. Tears produced by the lacrimal gland are drained through the punctum, lacrimal sac, and nasolacrimal duct into the nose.

are the orifices of the sweat- and oil-secreting glands. The largest oil-secreting glands, which are embedded in the posterior connective tissue substance of the lids (called the *tarsus*), are called the *meibomian glands*. The lacrimal gland is located above and lateral to the globe. Tears are produced by the lacrimal gland and travel through fine channels referred to as *ducts* to empty onto the conjunctival surface. On the medial aspect of the lower lid where the lashes cease is a small *papilla*. At the apex of this papilla is a tiny opening called the *punctum* (see Fig. 1-4). The punctum leads, by means of a small canal, through the lower lid to the *lacrimal sac* (Fig. 1-5), which eventually drains into the nose. Tears are carried to the punctum by the pumping action of the lids, and there they are drained effectively from the eye by means of tiny channels that drain the punctum. A similar but smaller opening is found in the upper lid almost directly above it. The punctum normally cannot be seen by looking directly at the eye. It can be seen only by depressing the lower lid or everting the upper lid. The muscle underlying the eyelid skin is the *orbicularis oculi*, which is roughly circular. When it contracts, it closes the eye.

The portions of the eye that are normally visible in the palpebral fissures are the cornea and sclera. Because the cornea is transparent, what is seen on looking at the cornea is the underlying *iris* and the black opening in the center of the iris, called the *pupil*. The sclera forms the white of the eye and is covered by a mucous membrane called the *conjunctiva*. The conjunctiva extends from the junction of the cornea and sclera and terminates at the inner portion of the lid margin (Fig. 1-6). The conjunctiva that covers the eye itself is referred to as the *bulbar conjunctiva*, whereas the portion that lines the inner surface of the upper and lower lids is called the *palpebral portion*. The *junctional bay* created when the two portions of the conjunctiva meet is referred to as the *fornix*. The lower fornix can easily be viewed by depressing the lower lid.

The conjunctiva has almost invisible blood vessels. The role of the conjunctiva is to defend and repair the cornea in the event of scratches, wounds, or infections. The blood vessels that are present dilate and leak nutrients, antibodies, and leukocytes into the tears that then wash over the avascular corneal surface. The conjunctiva also secretes mucus and oil, both of which help to keep the cornea moist and clean and to reduce friction when the lids blink over the cornea. The conjunctival mucous film over the ocular surface catches microorganisms. This mucous net then condenses into a ball and is carried to the nasal canthus where it dries and rolls onto the

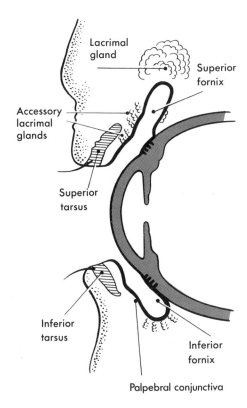

Fig. 1-6 Vertical section of the eyelids and conjunctiva. The lids act as a protective curtain for the eye. Only a small portion of the eye is actually exposed.

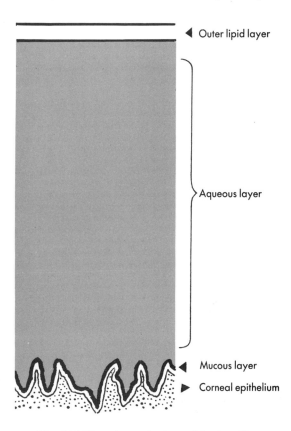

Fig. 1-7 Three-layer structure of the tear film.

skin. The conjunctiva also helps to resurface the cornea with epithelial cells should the entire corneal surface be scraped or burned.

TEAR FILM

The tear film is composed of three layers (Fig. 1-7). The outermost layer consists of a lipid or fatty layer, mostly cholesterol esters, and is extremely thin. This layer is secreted by the meibomian glands. It acts to prevent evaporation of the underlying aqueous layer. The central layer is chiefly aqueous, with some dissolved salts as well as glucose, urea, proteins, and lysozyme. This layer is secreted by the lacrimal glands. The third layer is a very thin mucous layer lying over the surface of conjunctiva and cornea. This layer is secreted by specific cells of the conjunctiva referred to as *goblet cells*. This mucous

layer is important in the stability of the tear film. Tear film abnormalities may arise in association with a number of clinical problems in elderly persons and in particular problems related to contact lenses.

CORNEA

The cornea is a clear, transparent structure, with a brilliant, shiny surface. It has a convex surface that acts as a powerful lens. Most of the refraction of the eye takes place not through the crystalline lens of the eye but through the cornea.

The cornea is relatively large at birth and almost attains its adult size during the first and second years. Although the eyeball as a whole increases a little less than three times in volume from birth to maturity, the corneal segment plays a small role in this part, being fully developed by 2 years of age.

The cornea is thicker at its periphery (1 mm) than at the center (0.5 mm). It can be divided into five distinct portions (Fig. 1-8): the epithelium, Bowman's layer, the stroma, Descemet's membrane, and the endothelium.

The epithelium, which is the part of the cornea usually injured by superficial abrasions or small foreign bodies, regenerates rapidly and heals without leaving a scar. Injury to the deeper structures nearly always results in formation of an opacity in the cornea.

The junction of the cornea and sclera is demarcated by a gray, semitransparent area referred to as the *limbus*. This transitional zone is only 1 mm wide and marks the point of insertion of the conjunctiva. The cornea, which contains no blood vessels, is completely nourished by three sources: a plexus of fine capillaries at the limbus, the tear film, and the aqueous humor.

SCLERA

The opaque sclera forms the posterior five sixths of the protective coat of the eye. Its anterior portion is visible and constitutes the white of the eye. In chil-dren the sclera is thin, and therefore it appears bluish because the underlying pigmented structures are visible through it. In old age it may become yellowish because of the deposition of fat. Attached to the sclera are all the extraocular muscles. Through the sclera pass the nerves and the blood vessels that penetrate into the interior of the eye. At its most posterior portion, the site of attachment of the *optic nerve*, the sclera becomes a thin, sievelike structure called the *lamina cribrosa*. It is through this sieve that the retinal fibers leave the eye to form the optic nerve. The episcleral tissue is a loose connective and elastic tissue that covers the sclera and unites it with the conjunctiva above. Unlike the sclera the episcleral tissue is highly vascular.

UVEA

The uveal tract consists of three structures: *iris, ciliary body,* and *choroid*.

Iris

The iris is the most anterior structure of the uveal tract. It is perforated at its center by a circular aperture called the *pupil*. The surface of the iris has many ridges and furrows on its anterior surface. Contraction of the iris, which occurs in response to bright light, is accomplished by the activity of a flat, washerlike muscle buried in its substance just surrounding the pupillary opening. This muscle is called the *sphincter pupillae*. Expansion or dilation of the pupil is facilitated by relaxation of the sphincter muscle and by activation of the dilator muscle of the iris found at its peripheral circumference. Expansion and contraction of the iris, like an accordion, form circular pleat lines or furrows visible on its surface. In addition to these ridges and furrows on the surface of the iris, numerous white zigzag lines are formed by the blood vessels of the iris. Between the iris and the cornea is a clear fluid called the *aqueous humor*. This fluid occupies the space called the *anterior chamber* of the eye.

Ciliary body

The ciliary body is in direct continuity with the iris and is adherent to the sclera. Directly posterior to the iris, the ciliary body is plump and thrown into

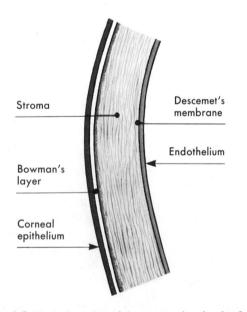

Stroma

Descemet's membrane

Endothelium

Bowman's layer

Corneal epithelium

Fig. 1-8 Vertical section of the cornea showing its five layers.

numerous folds referred to as the *ciliary processes*. This portion of the ciliary body is only about 2.5 mm in length and is responsible for the major production of aqueous fluid. The equator of the lens is only 0.5 mm from the ciliary processes and is suspended by fine, ligamentous fibers known as the *zonular fibers* of the lens. The posterior portion of the ciliary body is flat. Most of the zonular fibers of the lens originate from the ciliary body. The ciliary body in general is triangular, with its shortest side anterior. The anterior side of the triangle in its inner part enters into the formation of the angle of the anterior chamber. From its middle portion the iris takes root.

On the outer side of the triangle is the ciliary muscle, which lies against the sclera. Contraction of the ciliary muscle releases the tension of the zonular fibers, controlling the size and shape of the lens. This in turn allows the anterior surface of the lens to bulge forward and increase its power. Therefore the ciliary muscle directly controls the focusing ability of the eye. In children this muscle is extremely active and the lens is easily deformed, which accounts for its powerful range of accommodation, or focusing abilities. The ciliary muscle declines in power with age. After the age of 40 years, its power becomes weaker and the lens is less able to change shape, so that focusing at near point, or accommodating, becomes difficult. This condition is commonly referred to as *presbyopia*.

Choroid

The choroid is in direct continuity with the iris and ciliary body and lies between the retina and sclera (see Fig. 1-2). The choroid is primarily a vascular structure, and its prime function is to provide nourishment for the outer layers of the retina.

ANGLE STRUCTURES

The angle structures are formed by the tissues posterior to the cornea and anterior to the iris, the aqueous humor intervening (Fig. 1-9). Included in the angle structures are (1) the root of the iris, (2) a portion of the anterior surface of the ciliary body, (3) a spur from the sclera, (4) the canal of Schlemm, and (5) the corneoscleral trabeculum.

Aqueous humor leaves the eye by filtering through the crevices of the trabecular meshwork. The trabecular meshwork consists of tiny pores through which aqueous humor travels until it reaches Schlemm's canal. From Schlemm's canal the aqueous humor leaves the eye through the aqueous veins that penetrate the sclera. Obstruction within the trabecular meshwork or the angle structures, by iris or scar tissue, results in raised intraocular pressure and glaucoma.

LENS

The lens of the eye is a transparent biconvex structure situated between the iris and the vitreous (Fig. 1-10). Only that portion of the lens not covered by iris tissue (that is, only that portion directly behind the pupillary space) is visible. The center of the anterior surface of the lens, known as its anterior pole, is only about 3 mm from the back surface of the cornea. The diameter of the lens is about 9 to 10 mm. Its peripheral margin, called the *equator,* lies about 0.5 mm from the ciliary processes. It is attached to the ciliary processes and to the posterior portion of the ciliary body by means of fine suspensory ligaments referred to as the *zonular fibers* (Fig. 1-11).

The lens is surrounded by a capsule, which is a transparent, highly elastic envelope. The lens material within this elastic bag is rather soft and puttylike in infants. With age it tends to grow harder, especially toward the center of the lens. The harder central portion of the lens found in adults 30 years of age or older is called the *nucleus* of the lens, and the outer lens fibers form the lens cortex. The harder nucleus is a product of the normal developmental growth of the lens. As new lens fibers are produced, the older fibers are pushed more toward the center and are compressed in a concentric fashion. It is this constant lamination of lens fibers over a period of years that eventually produces the nucleus.

VITREOUS

The vitreous is a jellylike structure, thick and viscous, that occupies the vitreous chamber in the posterior concavity of the globe. Actually, it fills the largest cavity of the eye, occupying two thirds of its volume. It is surrounded in the main by retina.

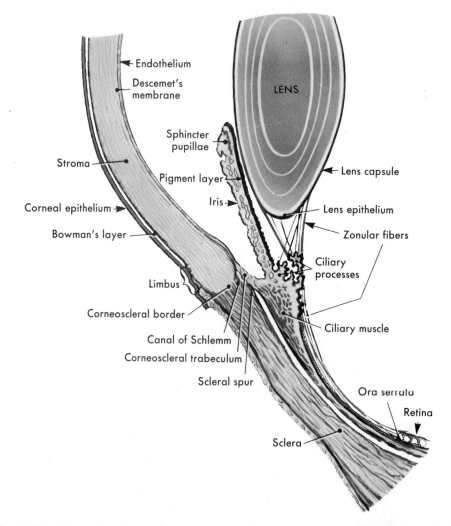

Endothelium

Descemet's
membrane

Sphincter
pupillae

Stroma

Pigment layer

Iris

Corneal epithelium

Bowman's layer

LENS

Lens capsule

Lens epithelium

Zonular fibers

Ciliary
processes

Limbus

Corneoscleral border

Canal of Schlemm

Corneoscleral trabeculum

Scleral spur

Ciliary muscle

Ora serrata

Retina

Sclera

Fig. 1-9 Angle structures of the eye. The angle is formed between the iris and the back surface of the cornea, with aqueous humor of the anterior chamber interposed. The angle structures include corneoscleral trabeculum, Schlemm's canal, scleral spur, a small extension of the ciliary muscle, and the root of the iris.

Anteriorly it forms a slight depression behind the lens and is attached to it around the circumference of this depression. Normally the vitreous is quite transparent.

The vitreous is not simply an inert jelly. Within the body of the vitreous, fine collagen fibers criscross in a scaffolding manner. The resulting matrix is filled with a viscous mucopolysaccharide, hyaluronic acid.

Vitreous is almost 99% water. Hyaluronic acid is a great shock absorber and can compress slowly and rebound slowly. This is important in injuries to the eye from such things as a fast-moving squash ball.

The envelope that surrounds the vitreous is primarily a condensate of the jell and is anchored to the more forward part of the retina, the *ora serrata*

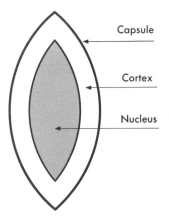

Fig. 1-10 Crystalline lens.

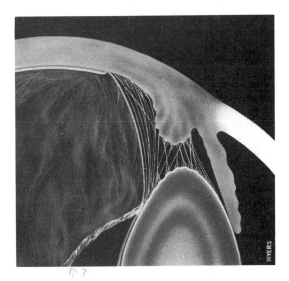

Fig. 1-11 Distribution of zonular fibers. Zonular lamella forms external layer of lens capsule consisting of anterior insertion 1 mm from equator and posterior insertion 1.5 mm from equator. (From Jaffe NS: *The vitreous in clinical ophthalmology,* St Louis, 1969, Mosby.)

at the head of the optic nerve along the major retinal blood vessels. If the vitreous shrinks, the resulting tension on its anchors can produce a tear in the retina. This may permit the adjacent vitreous to enter between the choroid and retina and produce a retinal detachment.

With age some of the collagen fibers of the vit-reous often break away from the main structure. These may condense into strands and float freely in the watery sections of the vitreous. Patients often see floating specks or webs that move as their eyes move and that are mildly annoying but usually harmless. These often disappear in time.

RETINA

The retina, which contains all the sensory receptors for the transmission of light, is really part of the brain. The retinal receptors are divided into two main populations—the *rods* and the *cones*. The rods function best in dim light; the cones function best under daylight conditions. The cones are far fewer in number than the rods, numbering 6 million, whereas the rods number 125 million. Cones enable us to see small visual angles with great acuity. Vision with rods is relatively poor. Color vision is totally dependent on the integrity of the cones. The cones form a concentrated area in the retina known as the *fovea,* which lies in the center of the *macula lutea.* Damage to this area can severely reduce the ability to see directly ahead. The rods are distributed in the periphery of the retina (not in the macula). Damage to these structures results in night blindness but with retention of good visual acuity for straight-ahead objects.

The junction of the peripheral of the retina and the ciliary body is called the *ora serrata.* In the extreme periphery of the retina there are no cones and only a few rods. The retina is firmly attached to the choroid at the ora serrata. This is the reason that retinal detachments never extend beyond the ora serrata. The other site of firm attachment of the retina is at the circumference of the optic nerve. The posterior layer of the retina, called the *pigment epithelium,* is firmly secured to the choroid. Retinal detachment occurs as a result of cleavage between its anterior layers and the posterior pigment layer.

OPTIC NERVE

The optic nerve is located at the posterior portion of the globe and transmits visual impulses from the retina to the brain itself. Only the head of the optic nerve, called the *optic disc,* can be seen by ophthalmoscopic examination (Fig. 1-12). The optic nerve

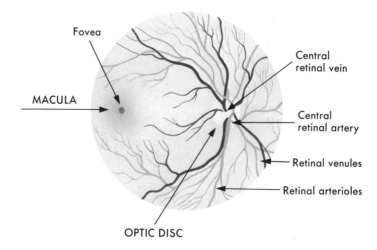

Fig. 1-12 Normal fundus. Note that the central retinal vein emerges from the optic disc lateral to the central retinal artery.

contains no sensory receptors itself, and therefore its position corresponds to the normal blind spot of the eye. Branching out from the surface of the optic disc are the *retinal arterioles* and *veins,* which divide soon after leaving the optic disc and extend out on the surface of the retina to supply the inner one third with nutrients. As the optic disc enters the globe, it goes through a fibrous, sievelike structure, visible on ophthalmoscopic examination, called the *lamina cribrosa*. When the lamina cribrosa is prominent, it forms the base of a depression in the disc called the *physiologic cup*. The optic nerve consists of 1 million axons arising from the ganglion cells of the retina. The nerve emerges from the back of the eye through a small circular opening; it extends for 25 to 30 mm and travels within the muscle cone to enter the bony optic foramen, where it travels for 4 to 9 mm to pass into the intracranial cavity and joins its fellow optic nerve to form the optic chiasm.

VISUAL PATHWAY

As the retinal fibers leave the optic nerves, half of them cross to the opposite side (Fig. 1-13). The fibers that cross are derived from the retinal receptors nasal to the macula. The structure so formed by the mutual crossing of nasal fibers by both optic nerves is the *optic chiasm*. From the optic chiasm the nasal

fibers emanating from the nasal half of the retina of one eye intermingle with the fibers derived from the temporal sector of the retina of the opposite eye, forming a band called the *optic tract*. Fibers in the optic tract continue toward a cell station in the brain called the *lateral geniculate body,* so named because this body in the brain is shaped like a knee (Latin *genu*). The geniculate body is a relay station. From here, fibers spread out in a fan-shaped manner and extend to the parietal and temporal lobe of the brain. They continue to their final destination, the posterior portion of the brain called the "occipital" lobe in an area denoted as the *visual striate area*. It is in this area of the brain that conscious recognition of visual impulses takes place.

OCULAR MUSCLES

The globe is moved by six ocular muscles: the *medial, lateral, superior,* and *inferior rectus muscles* and the *superior* and *inferior oblique muscles* (Fig. 1-14). The medial rectus muscle moves the eye toward the nose, or *adducts* the eye. The lateral rectus muscle moves the eye horizontally to the outer side, or *abducts* the eye. The superior rectus muscle elevates the eye primarily, whereas the inferior rectus muscle depresses the eye. The rectus muscles are inserted very close to the limbus, the

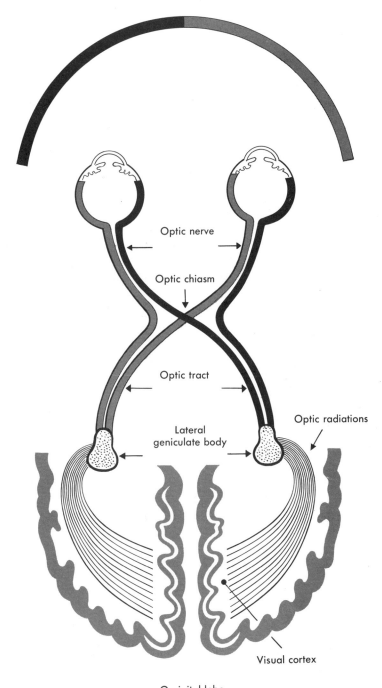

Fig. 1-13 Visual pathway. One half the visual field from each eye is projected to one side of the brain. Thus visual impulses from the right visual field of each eye will be transmitted to the left occipital lobe.

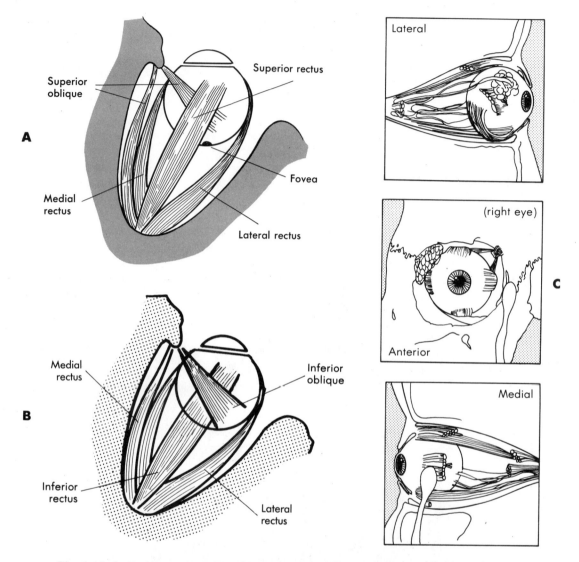

Fig. 1-14 A, Ocular muscles of the right eye viewed from above. Only the oblique muscles are inserted behind the center of rotation of the eye. All the rectus muscles are inserted in front of the center of rotation of the eye near the limbus, where they are easily accessible for muscle surgery. **B,** Ocular muscles of the right eye viewed from below. **C,** The right eye viewed laterally, anteriorly, and medially.

medial rectus lying approximately 5.5 mm and the lateral rectus approximately 7 mm from the limbus. The rectus muscles normally are not visible inasmuch as they are covered with conjunctiva and subconjunctival tissue. Because they lie on the surface of the globe, they are readily accessible for muscle surgery. The superior oblique muscle functions pri-

marily as an intorter by rotating the vertical and horizontal axis of the eye toward the nose; it also functions to depress the eye. The inferior oblique muscle acts to extort the eye and also serves to elevate the eye. The oblique muscles are inserted behind the equator of the globe.

In the lid the *levator palpebrae superioris muscle*

serves to elevate the lid, whereas the *orbicularis oculi muscle* closes the eye during winking, blinking, or forced lid closure. If the levator muscle is weak or absent, the lid droops and ptosis results.

SUMMARY

A brief sketch of the anatomy of the eye and its surrounding structures has been presented. Each of these structures, when diseased, gives rise to problems, depending on their anatomic location and function. Because many diagnoses made in ophthalmology are formulated from anatomic terminology, familiarity with these structures is essential before any understanding of patients' problems can be realized. The foundation of any course in medicine is based on anatomy. The ophthalmic assistant is advised to learn this section well and utilize it as a foundation for further reading.

QUESTIONS FOR REVIEW AND THOUGHT

The questions that follow, as well as those following the chapters in the rest of this book, are designed for review of the material. They are intended to sharpen your understanding by testing your knowledge of the material and stimulating you to think. Answers to some of the questions at the end of each chapter may be found in other parts of this book or, in some cases, only in other sources.

1. Draw a horizontal section of the eye with attached muscles, and label as many parts as you can without referring to the text.
2. Outline the production and flow of tears.
3. Name the five layers of the cornea.
4. How does the iris contract and expand?
5. Discuss the functions of the rods and cones.
6. Draw the pathway of fibers from the optic nerve to the visual cortex.
7. What is the limbus?
8. How many ocular muscles are attached to the eye? Name them.
9. Describe the muscles that open and close the eye.
10. Describe the macula.
11. What is the ora serrata?
12. At what age is the cornea fully formed? At what age is the rest of the eyeball fully formed?
13. Describe the vitreous.

SELF-EVALUATION QUESTIONS

True-false statements

Directions: Indicate whether the statement is true (T) or false (F).

T or F   1. The main function of the sclera is to keep out light.
T or F   2. If the epithelium of the cornea is damaged, a fine scar will appear.
T or F   3. Aqueous humor leaves the eye by filtering through the trabecular meshwork.

Missing words

Directions: Write in the missing word in the following sentences.

4. The transparent lens of the eye is attached to the ciliary body by fine suspensory ligaments called _____.

5. The retina consists of rods and cones. The _____ function best in daylight.
6. The head of the optic nerve is called the _____.

Choice-completion questions

Directions: Select the one best answer in each case.

7. The meibomian glands are:
   a. In the ciliary body
   b. In the tarsus
   c. In the hair follicles
   d. Associated with the lacrimal glands
   e. In the conjunctiva
8. The vitreous body comprises:
   a. The pigment structure of the eye
   b. The aqueous-forming part of the eye
   c. The sensory structure of the eye
   d. Two thirds of the volume of the eye
   e. The heat-absorbing portion of the eye
9. The orbicularis oculi is the muscle that:
   a. Dilates the pupil
   b. Affects accommodation
   c. Closes the eyelids
   d. Opens the lids
   e. Constricts the pupil

ANSWERS, NOTES, AND EXPLANATIONS

1. **False.** The main function of the sclera is protective. The sclera is a fibrous coat that is firm and prevents injury from outside the eye and prevents rupture when there is increased intraocular pressure to the globe. This is the chief function of this fibrous membrane. The sclera has an opaque white appearance, in contrast to the transparent cornea, because of the greater water content of the sclera and the fact that the collagen fibers are not as uniformly oriented. In some situations, however, the sclera may become exposed and dehydrated and it can become transparent.

2. **False.** The epithelium may be removed partially or completely from the cornea, and it has an amazing ability to regenerate completely and cover over the other layers of the cornea without leaving a scar. Only if the injury involves the deeper layers of the cornea, such as Bowman's membrane, stroma, or through-and-through lacerations of the cornea, will an opacity form because of the development of scar formation.

3. **True.** Water, electrolytes, and nonelectrolytes enter and leave the eye by diffusion from the ciliary body and by secretion from the epithelium of the ciliary process. From the posterior chamber, the fluid then passes through the pupil into the anterior chamber and out through the filtering trabecular meshwork. From here it passes into Schlemm's canal where about 30 collector channels conduct the fluid to about 12 aqueous veins out into the venous system.

4. **Zonular fibers.** These fine suspensory ligaments are composed of numerous fibrils arising from the surface of the ciliary body and inserting into the lens equator. Normally the ciliary muscle is relaxed and consequently the zonular fibers are taut, which reduces the anteroposterior diameter of the lens to its minimal dimension. However, when the ciliary muscle contracts to focus light from a near object, the tension is released on the zonular fibers, and the lens of the eye assumes

a thicker shape, with a corresponding greater refractive power. This is what occurs with the act known as *accommodation*.

5. **Cones.** The cones are used during daylight to allow detailed vision and color perception. They predominate in the macular area and receive visual images, partially analyze them, and submit this modified information to the brain. If these cones are damaged, the central vision is affected, and the patient will have difficulty reading and discerning small objects in the distance.

6. **Optic disc.** The optic disc is seen with an ophthalmoscope and represents the head of the optic nerve as the nerve bundle fibers pass from the eye back toward the brain. The optic disc corresponds to the normal blind spot of the eye and represents about 1 million axons, which arise from the ganglion cells of the retina. The optic nerve then travels about 25 to 30 mm in the orbit within the muscle cone to enter the bony optic foramen and then the cranial cavity.

7. **b. In the tarsus.** The meibomian glands lie in the tarsus and secrete sebaceous material, which creates an oily layer on the surface of the tear film. This oily layer helps prevent evaporation of the normal tear layer. When these glands become obstructed, they give rise to a condition known as *meibomianitis* and produce internal hordeolum or chalazion.

8. **d. Two thirds of the volume of the eye.** The vitreous is a structure that occupies the largest cavity of the eye, over two thirds of its volume. Normally the vitreous is quite transparent and jellylike. However, it changes with age and becomes more fluidlike and less jellylike in high degrees of myopia.

9. **c. Closes the eyelids.** The main function of the orbicularis oculi muscle is to close the eyelid. An accessory function is to evacuate the tear sac so as to continue the pumping action and removal of tears from the conjunctival sac. This muscle is innervated by the seventh cranial nerve so that when this nerve is paralyzed the eye will fail to close. During intraocular surgery a facial block often is given to paralyze this nerve.

CHAPTER 2

Physiology of the eye

- Alignment of the eyes
- Looking straight ahead, or fixation
- Locking images, or fusion
- Eye movements
- Looking toward a close object
- Seeing in depth
- Focusing at near point, or accommodation
- Transparent pathway for light
- Retinal images
- Intraocular pressure
- Tears
- Color vision

Physiology of the eye dcals with the function of the eye, its capacities and limitations. The actual perception of light takes place in a well-delineated area called the *field of vision*. What is not seen beyond these boundaries is catalogued and stored in our visual memory center, so that we are not uncomfortable or handicapped by this imposition. Most eyes cannot form a sharp image on the retina without an internal adjustment made by focusing or by some external appliance such as lenses placed before them. There is a limit to how much detail the eye can resolve, its magnifying abilities being only ×15, considerably less than most microscopes. The spectrum of light that is sensitive to our retinal receptors is confined to specific wavelengths of light; the world of ultraviolet and infrared is invisible to ordinary perception.

Despite these limitations the human eye is an extremely versatile instrument capable of seeing both in daylight and in dim light, registering colors, appreciating depth, and exercising rapid focusing adjustments. This chapter deals with the mechanisms that enable the eye to carry out these tasks.

ALIGNMENT OF THE EYES

In human beings the two eyes work as though they were one, both projecting to the same point in space and fusing their images so that a single mental impression is obtained by this collaboration. Without this delicate balance we would "see double" because two images would be formed by the independent action of each eye. In other words, stereopsis would be lost inasmuch as this faculty is totally dependent on the eyes' seeing in unison. The ability of the eyes to fuse two images into a single one is called *binocular vision*.

Binocular vision depends on an exquisite balance of motor and sensory function. The eyes must be parallel when looking straight ahead, and they must be able to maintain this alignment when gazing in other positions. Each impulse that directs an eye to move in one direction must be equally received by the other eye. Further, the contraction of an eye muscle pulling the eye in one direction must be accompanied by an equivalent amount of relaxation of its opponent muscle. Without perfectly harmonious eye movement, binocular vision would be impossible because eyes that do not move together do not see together.

Each eye must have good vision because a clear image and a fuzzy image cannot be fused. The fuzzy image usually is ignored by the brain (suppression). Each macula must have its projection straight ahead, so that the line of vision from each eye intersects at one point in space. Also, the field of vision from each eye must overlap (Fig. 2-1). Although we can see more with two eyes than with one, this difference is not great (about 35 degrees), because most of the field of vision from one eye overlaps the field from the other eye. Overlapping visual fields act as a locking device, forging our peripheral vision in place and thereby ensuring central fusion.

LOOKING STRAIGHT AHEAD, OR FIXATION

Fixation involves the simple task of looking straight ahead toward an object in space. Fixation requires stability of the eyes and good monocular function. If the eyes are constantly moving, such as occurs with congenital nystagmus, the eyes can make only scanning motions around an object and never adequately see it in detail. Needless to say, if the ability to fixate becomes compromised by constant eye movements, then the visual acuity of the affected eyes is reduced. If the macula is damaged, fixation is difficult because anything viewed directly ahead becomes enshrouded in relative darkness.

Fixation can be reduced without organic changes in the macula. Children with strabismus often are found to have poor vision in the turned eye. If a child has crossed eyes, we would think that double vision would occur inasmuch as the two eyes would not be directed to the same point in space (Fig. 2-2). Children, however, have a wonderful faculty for completely ignoring the image in the turned eye to avoid confusion. It is this constant habit of actively suppressing the image in the turned eye that eventually leads to loss of vision, or *amblyopia*. In some of these children, in whom the suppression mechanism has become profound and the resultant vision very poor, foveal function becomes so depressed that a new point just outside the fovea is used. Such an eye no longer can see straight ahead, and the fixation pattern is described as *eccentric*.

LOCKING IMAGES, OR FUSION

Fusion is the power exerted by both eyes to keep the position of the eyes aligned so that both foveae project to the same point in space. Because fusion is a binocular act, it is easily disrupted by covering one eye. The eye under cover drifts to its fusion-free position. The amount of movement that the eye makes is a measure of the latent muscular imbalance kept in check by fusion, or the amount of heterophoria. *Heterophoria*, then, may be defined as the position the eyes assume when fusion is disrupted. The eye under cover may drift in, called *esophoria*, or may drift out, called *exophoria*. The eye also may drift up and down; this position is called *hyperphoria*. Fusion also may be disrupted by placing a Maddox rod before one eye. The Maddox rod changes the size and shape of the image presented to the eye under cover so that fusion becomes impossible.

The power of fusion is measurable by prisms (see Chapter 3). For example, a 4-diopter prism is placed

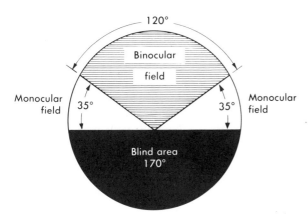

Fig. 2-1 Field of vision. Binocular field of vision (120 degrees) represents the overlapping field of vision from each eye.

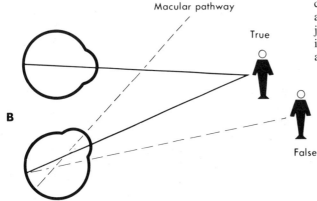

Fig. 2-2 A, Binocular vision (both eyes the same figure). **B,** One eye is turned in, resulting in double vision. In this case the figure is received by the macula of one eye and a point nasal to the macula of the turned eye. The projection of this nasal point results in the person seeing two images instead of one of the same figure. This is an example of uncrossed diplopia, as seen in eso deviations.

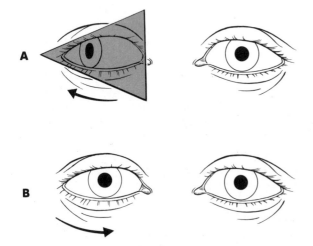

Fig. 2-3 A, The prism displaces the image toward its apex, and the eye moves outward because of the fusional reflex. **B,** When the prism is removed, the eye returns to its original position because of the fusional reflex.

with the base toward the nose of an observer looking at a small letter placed 16 inches from the eye. The prism will displace the image before that eye in a direction toward its apex, and the eye moves outward to follow it because of the power exerted by the fusional reflex (Fig. 2-3, *A*). Now the prism is removed, and the uncovered eye returns to its original position in response to the fusional reflex (Fig. 2-3, *B*). Normally, 20- to 40-prism diopters can be exercised by fusional convergence. The amount of fusion exercised with respect to divergence is less, being only 10- to 20-prism diopters. This is measured by using base-out prisms. Vertical imbalances are difficult to overcome because our eyes can overcome only about 2- to 4-prism diopters.

EYE MOVEMENTS

The primary position of the eyes is the straight-ahead position as they look at a point just below the horizon with the head held erect. Movement of the eye from the primary position to a secondary position occurs when the eyes are moved either horizontally or vertically. If the eyes are directed in an oblique position (up and in or down and in), they are said to be in a tertiary position.

The movement of one eye from one position to another in one direction is called a *duction*. In duction the fellow eye is either covered or patched. The movement of two eyes in the same direction is called a *version* (dextro-, levo-, sursum-, and deorsum-) (Fig. 2-4):

Eyes right: dextroversion
Eyes left: levoversion
Eyes up: sursumversion
Eyes down: deorsumversion

An outline of the functions of the extraocular muscles is given in Table 2-1. The medial and lateral rectus muscles have only one action—to move the eye horizontally. The other four muscles of the eye have auxiliary functions. When these secondary roles are used—assisting the lateral or medial rectus muscles to abduct or adduct—they are called *synergists* (Fig. 2-5).

The main function of the oblique muscles is to

Table 2-1	Actions of extraocular muscles	
Muscle	**Prime action**	**Secondary action**
Medial rectus	Turns eye inward toward nose, or adducts eye	None
Lateral rectus	Turns eye outward toward temples, or abducts eye	None
Superior rectus	Elevates eye	Intortion Adduction
Inferior rectus	Depresses eye	Extortion Adduction
Superior oblique	Intorts eye	Depression Abduction
Inferior oblique	Extorts eye	Elevation Abduction

rotate the globe either inward *(intorsion)* or outward *(extorsion)*. Intorsion occurs when the eye rotates on its long axis so that the 12 o'clock position on the cornea moves toward the nose. For example, if a point on the cornea of the right eye moves inward from 12 to 1 o'clock, then intorsion is said to occur because of the primary action of the right superior

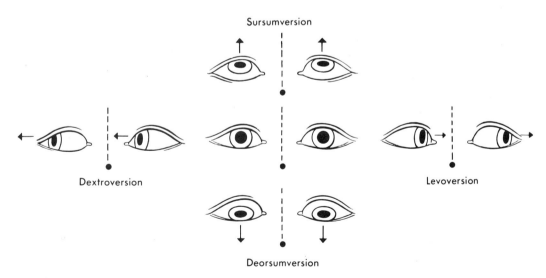

Sursumversion

Dextroversion

Levoversion

Deorsumversion

Fig. 2-4 Version movements of the eyes. These are movements formed by both eyes working together.

Right eye   **Left eye**

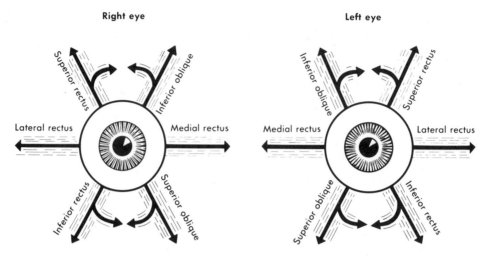

Fig. 2-5 Action of the extraocular muscles. The arrows reveal that the superior and inferior rectus muscles function best as an elevator and a depressor, respectively, when the eye is abducted. The inferior and superior oblique muscles function best as an elevator and depressor, respectively, when the eye is adducted.

oblique muscle or secondary action of the right superior rectus muscle. Similarly, if the point on the right cornea moves outward from 12 to 11 o'clock, then extorsion is said to occur because of the primary action of the right inferior oblique muscle or secondary action of the right inferior rectus muscle.

Control centers for eye movements

The eyes move in response to our own volition, or they can move in a passive manner, such as in following a slow-moving target. Volitional eye movements usually are rapid, starting at high speeds and ending just as abruptly. Such movements occur with reading when words or phrases are quickly scanned, with an abrupt halt coming at the end of a section or a line. These voluntary eye movements are controlled from centers in the frontal lobe of the brain.

Whereas voluntary eye movements tend to be short and choppy, following or pursuit eye movements are rather slow, smooth, and gliding. The velocity of a following movement depends entirely on the speed of the object the eye is tracking. If the fovea is fixed on a moving target with an angular velocity (less than 30 degrees per second), the eye

follows the target almost exactly. With greater speeds, following movement becomes difficult, and the smooth, gliding movement is replaced with an irregular, jerky movement. Pursuit movements are controlled from centers in the occipital lobe of the brain.

LOOKING TOWARD A CLOSE OBJECT

Vergence is the term applied to simultaneous ocular movements in which the eyes are directed to an object in the midline in front of the face. The term usually is applied to *convergence,* in which the eyes rotate inward toward each other, or to *divergence,* in which they rotate outward simultaneously (Fig. 2-6).

Convergence is invariably accompanied by narrowing, or constriction, of the pupils and by accommodation. The triad of convergence, pupillary constriction, and accommodation often is called the *accommodative reflex,* although in the true sense these movements are merely associated reactions (a synkinesis) rather than a true reflex. Each component of the triad facilitates fixation at near. The constriction of the pupil is the attempt by the eye to form a pinhole camera device so that a clearer image is seen.

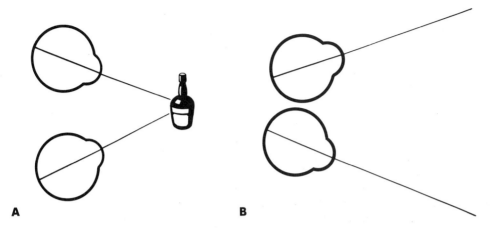

Fig. 2-6 A, Convergence. The eye is turned in toward the midline plane. **B,** Divergence. The eye is turned out, away from the midline plane.

Accommodation enables the object to be focused on the retina; convergence brings the eye inward toward the object of regard.

SEEING IN DEPTH

The ability to see in depth enables us to travel comfortably in space. Without it, we could not judge distances, estimate the size of objects beyond us, or avoid bumping into things. Without depth perception even the simplest of tasks would be difficult. We would be unable to reach accurately for our morning coffee, and passing a car on the highway would be tantamount to suicide. Fortunately, everyone has some depth perception, whether the person has one eye or two. Those with only one eye learn to estimate depth with monocular clues (Figs. 2-7 and 2-8). They know that the speck in the distance that becomes a huge train standing beside them in the station has not grown larger but has merely come closer. Other clues besides the size of the object also assist. The train tracks spread from a point and become parallel, the color of the train changes from a misty blue-gray to dark green, the sound increases, and when the train is alongside, one can feel the heat. There are many monocular clues that facilitate depth perception. They include the following:

1. Magnification. Well-recognized objects, if they become larger, are deemed to be nearer.

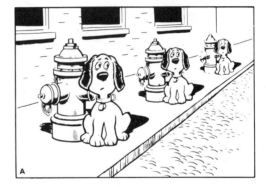

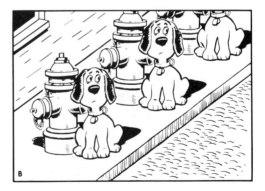

Fig. 2-7 A, Artist has drawn the picture with proper depth perspective. Monocular clues include decrease in size of dogs and confluence of lines toward a point. **B,** Artist has ignored the usual monocular clues so that our appreciation of depth and size is erroneous. The second dog appears larger than the first, although both are the same size.

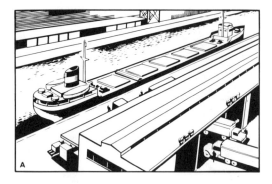

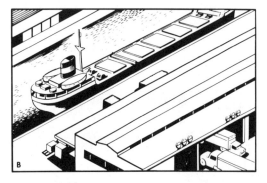

Fig. 2-8 A, The scene is drawn using normal monocular clues of distance, thereby giving it perspective. **B,** The same scene is drawn without regard to the normal impressions of distance. Therefore the scene loses its perspective.

2. Confluence of parallel lines to a point—for example, railway tracks.
3. Interposition of shadows.
4. Blue-gray mistiness of objects at a great distance.
5. Parallax. If two objects situated at different points in space are aligned and the head of the observer is moved in one direction, the nearer object will appear to move in the opposite direction.

A monocular person, however, if removed from familiar surroundings, would have great difficulty in judging distances because of a lack of any intrinsic depth-perception mechanism. For example, a one-eyed pilot would create a hazard because of the difficulty he or she would experience in maneuvering in space without the normal monocular clues.

Stereopsis is a higher quality of binocular vision. Each eye views an object at a slightly different angle, so that fusion of images occurs by combining slightly dissimilar images. It is the combination of these angular views that yields stereopsis. The same method is used in photography in making three-dimensional pictures. The stereoscopic picture is taken at slightly different angles and later viewed that way.

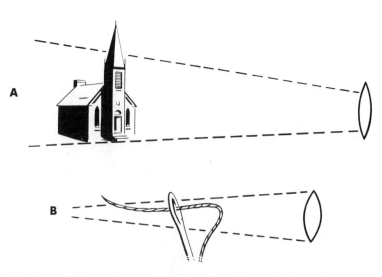

Fig. 2-9 A, Crystalline lens of the eye is thin for distant objects. **B,** Crystalline lens accommodates for near objects by becoming thicker. This increases its effective power.

FOCUSING AT NEAR, OR ACCOMMODATION

Any object can be moved from a distance to about 20 feet in front of an observer and still be seen clearly without accommodation. This distance is called the *range of focus*. As the object is brought closer than 20 feet, however, the eye must continuously readjust to keep the image of the object clearly focused on the retina. This readjustment requires an increase in the power of the eye and is brought about by an automatic change in the shape of the lens in response to a blurred image (Fig. 2-9). This zoom-lens mechanism in the eye is very active in children; they are able to see a small letter in clear focus only 7 cm from the eye, whereas an adult of 55 years can focus no closer than 55 cm. The *range of accommodation* is the distance in which an object can be carried toward an eye and be kept in focus. The power of accommodation of an eye is the dioptric equivalent of this distance. By age 75 years this power is zero.

Both the range and the power of accommodation are measured quite easily. When the full spectacle correction is worn, it is merely the closest point at which an accommodative target (such as a small letter) can be seen clearly. It usually is equal in both eyes. The range of accommodation is measured in centimeters, whereas the power is converted to diopters (Table 2-2).

Table 2-2   Accommodation and near point of the normal eye

Age	Near point in centimeters	Available accommodation in diopters
10	7	14
20	9	11
30	12	8
40	22	4.5
45	28	3.5
50	40	2.5
55	55	1.75
60	100	1
65	133	0.75
70	400	0.25
75	Infinity	0 .

This stimulus for accommodation is a blurred image on the retina. As an object is moved closer to the eye, the rays of light entering the pupil must be continuously converged. This change in focusing power of the eyes is brought about by active contraction of the ciliary muscle. The contraction of this muscle causes the zonular fibers of the lens to relax, which in turn allows the lens of the eye to change its shape (Fig. 2-10). In the child and the young adult, the lens can be molded, and it increases its power by becoming thicker and increasing the curvature of its anterior space. In an adult the ability of the ciliary muscle to effectively contract declines with age, and the lens becomes harder and less malleable with advancing years.

The decline in accommodation with age, called *presbyopia,* is remedied with reading glasses or bifocals. It usually becomes apparent by the age of 45 years.

TRANSPARENT PATHWAY FOR LIGHT

For light to effectively stimulate retinal receptors, clear media for transmission are necessary. One of the prime functions of the eye is maintenance of the transparent pathway for light (Fig. 2-11).

The *cornea* is the window through which light rays pass on their way to the retina. It is a five-layered transparent structure whose cells and collagen fibers are so arranged that light can pass through it with a minimum of diffraction and internal reflection. The cornea is transparent because its fibrils are arranged in a parallel manner and are tightly packed and separated by less than a wavelength of light. When the cornea is swollen, this arrangement is distorted and the cornea becomes hazy. The cornea contains no opaque substances, such as blood vessels, that would mar its clarity. It receives its nourishment from perilimbal vessels, the tear film, and the aqueous humor. The cornea is kept shiny and lubricated by tears that keep its surface moist and fill out any irregularities in its superficial epithelium.

The tears are composed of three main layers. The outermost oily, or lipid, layer comes from the meibomian gland and retards evaporation of the aqueous or watery layer. Aqueous water makes up the middle

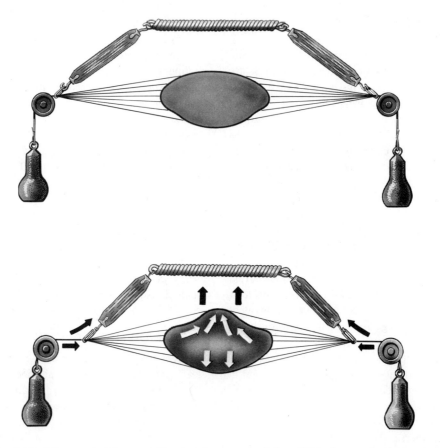

Fig. 2-10 Adjustment of the crystalline lens by accommodation. When the zonular ligaments are relaxed, the inherent elasticity of the lens causes it to increase in thickness and therefore increase in power. (Redrawn from Krug WFS: *Functional neuro-anatomy,* New York, 1953, The Blakiston Co.)

layer and arises from the main lacrimal and the accessory lacrimal glands in the conjunctiva. It is filled with inorganic matter, salts, and varying amounts of mucin. This functions to keep the cornea moist. The innermost layer of the tears is mucin, which arises from the goblet cells of the conjunctiva and fills in the tiny irregularities of the corneal epithelium, thereby producing a mirrorlike finish to the cornea.

The most important factor in maintaining corneal transparency is the ability of the cornea to keep itself relatively dehydrated. If a section of cornea is placed in isotonic saline solution, it becomes hydrated, opaque, and edematous. On the other hand, if the sclera is dehydrated, it becomes transparent.

The cornea has an active, pumplike mechanism located in the corneal epithelium and endothelium that enables it to keep itself relatively dehydrated. Damage to the corneal epithelium or endothelium results in the cornea's becoming hydrated and swollen. Swelling of the cornea, be it localized or diffuse, always results in a loss of transparency. If the swelling (that is, corneal edema) is located centrally, then vision will be blurred. In acute angle-closure glaucoma, the sudden rise in intraocular pressure causes epithelial edema. The individual droplets in the epithelium break up white light to its colored spectral components, and the patient complains of seeing colored halos around lights. The rainbow we see

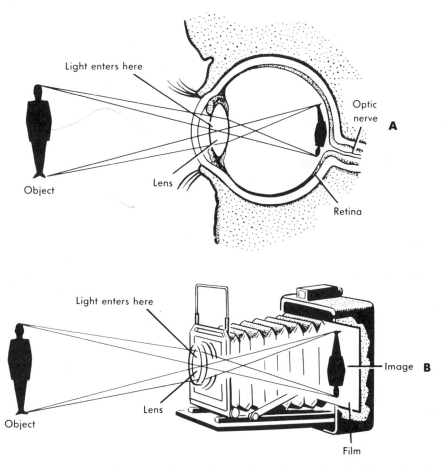

Fig. 2-11 The eye is like a camera. Light must have a clear pathway to be clearly focused on the sensory receptors of the retina or the film of a camera.

after a storm is similarly explained. It is merely the effect of suspended water droplets in air breaking up white light.

Transparency also is aided by the ability of the corneal epithelium to rapidly regenerate. The corneal epithelium, by sliding over defects and regenerating its cells, can cover a large abrasion within 24 hours, and without leaving a scar. If Bowman's layer or the corneal stroma is damaged, repair takes much longer and a permanent scar forms.

The *aqueous humor* found between the lens and the cornea is a clear, colorless, watery fluid. It is formed by active secretion from the ciliary processes and to a lesser extent by diffusion from the vessels of the iris. The aqueous humor is in constant circulation, flowing from the posterior chamber through the pupil to the anterior chamber, where it leaves the inner eye proper through the trabecular meshwork, Schlemm's canal, and the aqueous veins (Fig. 2-12). If the exit of aqueous humor from the eye is blocked, the volume of fluid within the eye increases; because the coats of the eye are relatively nondistensible, the pressure within the eye also increases.

As light travels through the eye, the next structure it encounters is the *iris,* with its central round opening called the *pupil.* The iris is the shutter mechanism of the eye, controlling the amount of light entering the eye in the interest of clear vision. If the amount

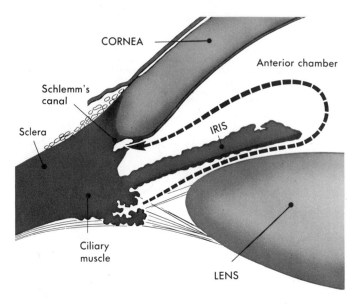

Fig. 2-12 Flow of aqueous humor. Aqueous humor is produced largely by the ciliary processes in the posterior chamber; it flows into the anterior chamber and leaves the eye through Schlemm's canal.

of available light is excessive, the pupil constricts by the action of the sphincter muscle of the iris to reduce excessive light or glare. If the illumination is poor, then the pupil dilates to increase the amount of light entering the eye. Other factors also control the size of the pupil. Emotional arousal (for example, fear, anxiety, or erotic stimulation) tends to dilate the pupils. Pain in the body dilates the pupil. The pupils generally are large in the young, the blue-eyed, and the myopic, and they tend to be smaller in the brown-eyed and in older persons. The pupils normally are round in shape and equal in size. If a light is directed to one eye, both pupils constrict. The constriction of the pupil on the side toward which light is directed is called the *direct light reflex,* whereas the pupillary response in the fellow eye is called the *consensual light reflex.*

As light passes through the pupil, the next structure it encounters is the *lens.* The lens of the eye is a biconvex structure, completely surrounded by a capsule. It has only a single layer of epithelial cells under its anterior capsule, which does not significantly interfere with its transparency. Like the cornea it contains no opaque tissue such as blood vessels,

nerve fibers, or connective tissue. It is nourished solely by the aqueous humor that bathes it.

Lens material in a child is very soft and puttylike in consistency. With age, however, the lens becomes harder, especially centrally. As new lens fibers form, they envelop the previously existing fibers, compressing them and pushing them into a compact unit toward the center. Thus growth of the lens is not accompanied by an increase in size after puberty but by a compression and tight lamination of the older fibers. The central hard portion, called the *nucleus,* usually becomes well-formed by the age of 30 years.

There are two main parts of the lens: the dense center, or nucleus, and the surrounding cortex. This arrangement offers an optical advantage in making the total refractive power of the lens greater than if the index of refraction were uniform throughout.

The *vitreous body* is located directly behind the lens and occupies two thirds of the entire volume of the eye. It is a transparent gel, that is, a viscous fluid midway in composition between a solid and a liquid. Functionally and metabolically the vitreous is relatively inactive. If the lens and cornea are compared with the lenses of a camera, the vitreous body

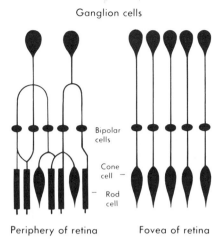

Fig. 2-13 Rods and cones of the retina.

is the space before the film. Frequently with age the gel breaks down in part, becoming liquid. This degeneration of the vitreous gives rise to the often-heard complaint of seeing spots before the eyes.

Once light has left the vitreous, the last great transparent structure of the eye, it finally strikes the retina, which contains all the receptors sensitive to light.

The *retinal receptors* are divided into two different populations of cells—the rods and the cones (Fig. 2-13). The rods are far more numerous (approximately 125 million) than the cones (approximately 6 million) and function best in dim illumination (scotopic vision). Without rods, night blindness occurs. Individuals affected by a disorder involving a selective loss of rod cells can see very well during the day as long as the illumination is high; however, under conditions of poor illumination, as in movie theaters or darkrooms, they are totally unable to adapt and behave as though blind. The cones function best in daylight (photopic vision) and mediate straight-ahead vision and color vision. A selective loss of cone cells results in a loss of visual acuity and an inability to perceive colors. This duplicity of function among the retinal receptors is easily demonstrated by entering a darkroom illuminated only by a red light. The rods are relatively insensitive to red and therefore do not lose their

function with this type of lighting. At first everything appears quite dark, then hazy, and finally the definite shapes of objects at the sides come into view as the rods begin to function. The total duration for dark adaptation to be completed is about 30 minutes. Darkrooms (for example, photography darkrooms and x-ray rooms) usually are equipped with a red light because it allows the cones to function and straight-ahead vision to be preserved while enabling the rods to become adapted to the dark.

The process of dark adaptation requires a neural change in the rod cells that is rapid and a chemical change in the outer segments of the rod cells that is slow (at least 30 minutes). The chemical change is a complex process that requires the synthesis of the rod pigment called *rhodopsin*. Rhodopsin, or visual purple, forms under conditions of dark adaptation and is destroyed by light. Therefore it is continuously being used and restored. One of the main components of rhodopsin is vitamin A, found in carrots and other vegetables. Vitamin A deficiency causes night blindness, but the corollary that an excess of vitamin A will help the eyes is not true. The cones also contain a pigment called *iodopsin*.

Because the fovea contains no rods, but only a concentration of specialized cones, it is found that when the eye is fully dark-adapted, there is a central loss of vision. Although visual acuity is not as good in this state, the perception of light is enhanced because the rods have a lower threshold for light sensitivity than do the cones. Visual information in the form of light strikes the photoreceptors, and this sets off a chain of events that leads to the process of seeing. Impulses from the photoreceptors are carried to the bipolar cells and then in turn to the ganglion cells. The site of connections between cells is called the *synaptic zone*. The information from the ganglion cells then travels via axons through the optic nerves, the chiasm, and the optic tract to synapse with cells in the lateral geniculate body. Impulses are then carried by axons to the occipital cortex for the processing of the information.

RETINAL IMAGES

Retinal images, once formed, persist for a very short period of time. They are called *positive afterimages*.

Normally one is not aware of this persistence of retinal images because the eyes take up a new gaze that obliterates the former afterimage. In making movies, sensation of motion or flow is produced only when the film speed of the camera is sufficiently fast to enable fusion of the images produced by the moving frames on the film. If the camera is slowed, flickering occurs because there is a time gap between the afterimage of the first sequence and that of the next.

Negative afterimages also occur. This is commonly witnessed as a dark spot appearing before the eyes after one has been photographed with the use of a flashbulb. The high-intensity light exhausts the retinal receptors, and they become unresponsive to further light stimulation for seconds after. Negative afterimages are employed in a test for strabismus to determine the direction of fixation. High-intensity flashes placed in a vertical or horizontal position will produce a dark line of the same dimension as a flash. This line can be drawn by the patient. If fixation is central and straight ahead, the reproduction is exact. If the fixation pattern is eccentric, then the picture drawn will be decentered by an amount equal to the degree of eccentric fixation.

INTRAOCULAR PRESSURE

The normal intraocular pressure is between 13 and 19 mm Hg. These numbers are derived by measurements obtained with use of a tonometer and indicate the pressure in the eye that will not normally cause damage to the intraocular contents. Individual eyes respond to intraocular pressures differently. Some can tolerate pressures in the high 20s, and some will have damage to the optic nerve with lower pressures.

Transient and physiologic variations occur in the intraocular pressure. With respiration, these variations in intraocular pressure can amount to 4 mm Hg, whereas changes of 1 to 2 mm Hg occur with each pulsation of the central retinal artery. The changes with pulse beat are nicely demonstrated on tonographic recordings, which always show a sawtooth type of graph in rhythm with the beats of the pulse. Throughout the day the intraocular pressure can vary as much as 3 to 4 mm Hg, the maximum

pressure being found around 6 AM. In a glaucomatous eye the fluctuations in diurnal pressures can be 6 to 8 mm Hg per day or even greater.

The pressure in the eye depends largely on the amount of aqueous humor secreted into the eye (1 to 2 cu mm per minute) and the ease by which it leaves. The flow of aqueous into the eye varies with the general hydration of the body. In dehydrated states, the amount of aqueous produced will decrease, and so will the pressure within the eye. On the other hand, if large quantities of fluid are quickly ingested, the amount of aqueous secreted will increase. Forced hydration is used in the water-drinking test inasmuch as a rise of 8 mm Hg or more 45 minutes after drinking 1 liter of water is suggestive of glaucoma. The drug acetazolamide (Diamox), used in the treatment of glaucoma, acts by reducing the volume of aqueous produced.

The rate of fluid exit from the eye, or its facility of outflow, is the most important single factor regulating the intraocular pressure. Glaucoma rarely is due to an increase in aqueous production but invariably is linked to a decrease in the facility of outflow.

There are three primary methods of occluding the outflow channels of the eye. In open-angle glaucoma (the most common type) the diameter of the openings of the trabecular meshwork becomes narrowed, thereby increasing the resistance of fluid flow (Fig. 2-14). This situation is analogous to a drainage system in which the final common drain tube is suddenly reduced to a tube of only one half its diameter at the very end. The amount of water leaving the system should be very small, and the pressure in the tube in front of the narrowing would be very high.

In secondary glaucoma the trabecular meshwork becomes blocked. The obstructing matter can be in the meshwork and may consist of red blood cells with hyphemas, tumor cells, pigment, and debris. In addition, the obstructing matter may cover the meshwork itself in the form of scar tissue or in anterior synechiae between the iris and the angle structures. These adhesions, which are commonly formed after a severe iritis, an episode of angle-closure glaucoma, or a central retinal vein occlusion, produce a severe and intractable glaucomatous state.

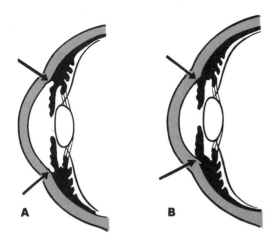

Fig. 2-14 Glaucoma. **A,** Open-angle glaucoma. The obstruction to aqueous flow lies in the trabecular meshwork. **B,** Closed-angle glaucoma. The trabecular meshwork is covered by the root of the iris.

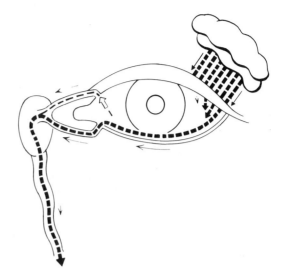

Fig. 2-15 Flow of tears. Note that most of the tears flow through the lower punctum.

Another method of occluding the outflow channels occurs with pupillary block, as typified in primary angle-closure glaucoma. In eyes predisposed to this condition, the angle formed by the root of the iris and the angle structures is quite narrow. If the pupil in such an eye is dilated, the iris tissue, which folds up like an accordion on dilation, abuts against the angle structures and partially blocks it. In addition, the aqueous humor in the posterior chamber has difficulty in circulating through the anterior chamber. Therefore the pressure in the posterior chamber increases and bows the iris to a more forward position, obstructing even further the already compromised exit channels of the eye. This process occurs quite suddenly, and the eye does not have the chance to accommodate itself to the high intraocular pressures reached. As a result the eye becomes red, the cornea edematous, the pupil fixed and dilated, and the patient complains of considerable pain. Angle-closure glaucoma constitutes an ocular emergency and is relieved by a peripheral iridectomy, where a small portion of the peripheral iris is removed to facilitate transfer of fluid between chambers. This procedure can be performed in the operating room; it is more commonly performed in the office with the use of either the argon or neodynium YAG lasers.

TEARS

The surface of the eye is kept moist by tears formed by the lacrimal gland and the accessory lacrimal glands located in the superior and inferior fornices. Evaporation is minimized by a thin film of oil secreted by the meibomian glands over the layer of tears. Tears function to keep the globes moist and to fill in the interstices between the corneal epithelial cells, thus providing a smooth, regular corneal refractive surface.

Only 0.5 to 1 ml of tears is produced during the day; minimal tears are produced at night. About 50% of the tears are lost through evaporation; the rest are carried to the superior and inferior puncta on the medial aspect of the upper and lower lids and are drained through the nasal lacrimal duct into the inferior meatus of the nose (Fig. 2-15).

Tears contain an antibacterial enzyme, called *lysozyme,* which is mainly effective against nonpathogenic bacteria by dissolving their outer coating.

Tear formation occurs as a result of psychic stimuli and reflex stimuli. Reflex stimuli involve uncomfortable retinal stimulation by bright lights or irritation of the cornea, conjunctiva, and nasal mucosa. The amount of tear production is measured by the

Schirmer test. This test is performed by simply placing a strip of filter paper 5 mm wide into the lower fornix for 5 minutes; more than 10 mm of wetting indicates normal function.

COLOR VISION

The cones of the human eye are believed to contain three different photosensitive pigments in their outer segments. These pigments act by absorbing light of certain definite wavelengths according to their period of vibration. The pigments of the cones are sensitive to red, green, and blue, the three primary colors of light. (This is not to be confused with the three primary colors of red, blue, and yellow, as found in the paint mixing field and used by artists.) Other colors are formed by mixtures of these pigments.

Color depends on *hue, saturation,* and *brightness.* An object will have a particular hue because it reflects or transmits light of a certain wavelength. The addition of black to a given hue produces the various *shades.* Saturation is an index of the purity of a hue. The brightness of an object depends on the light intensity. Today we can experiment with all these aspects of color by turning various knobs of a color television set to achieve the variations of hue, saturation, and brightness.

Color vision defects are believed to arise from a deficiency or absence of one or more visual pigments. Clinically, persons with abnormal color vision fall into three major categories. The *trichromat* possesses all three cone pigments and has normal color vision. Those of us who have been tested and found normal belong to this category. The *anomalous trichromat* has a partial deficiency of one of the three cone pigments. This person may have (1) *protanomaly*—deficiency in sensitivity to the first color (red), as well as poor red-green and blue-green discrimination; (2) *deuteranomaly*—deficiency of one pigment mediating green, as well as poor green-purple and red-purple discrimination; or (3) *tritanomaly*—deficiency of the cone pigment for blue, as well as blue-green and yellow-green insensitivity. The *dichromat* has a complete deficiency in one cone pigment but preserves the remaining two cone pigments. This person may have (1) protanopia, in which red is absent, (2) deuteranopia, in which green is absent, or (3) tritanopia, in which blue is absent. The *monochromat* has only one cone pigment.

The degree of color deficiency is determined by a series of plates or charts. The most common test used is the Ishihara color plate test in which the ability to trace patterns on a multicolored chart is measured.

The milder deficiencies (anomalous trichromasy) are by far the most common, with red and green deficiency predominating. This type of color deficiency has a sex-linked recessive mode of inheritance and affects approximately 8% to 10% of all males and less than 1% of females.

QUESTIONS FOR REVIEW AND THOUGHT

1. What keeps the cornea transparent?
2. What are the fixation and following reflexes?
3. What is amblyopia? What are the causes of amblyopia?
4. What muscles are involved in torsions? In the case of paralysis of the muscles that pull the eye horizontally and vertically, how do you test the function of the superior oblique muscle?
5. What is the accommodation reflex?
6. What are the clues that give a one-eyed person some appreciation of depth?
7. What structures in the human eye have no blood supply?
8. Describe the composition of the aqueous humor.
9. What would the visual acuity be in a person (1) with rods only and (2) with cones only?
10. What are positive and negative afterimages? Why are surgical sheets in operating rooms green?
11. Why is intraocular pressure higher than the pressure in the surrounding orbital tissue? What happens to the ocular structures when the pressure is too high and when it is too low?

12. What are the functions of tears?
13. What is the composition of the tear film?
14. What happens to an eye where there is absence of tear production?
15. What are the primary colors?
16. Can a person who is totally color blind see?
17. The intraocular pressure will vary during the day. What are the usual high and low periods in the normal person?
18. What visual functions are necessary to have binocular depth perception?
19. What happens to vision when the pupil is artificially dilated? Why?
20. What is the purpose of a normal pupillary response that involves constriction?
21. What is the function of blinking?

SELF-EVALUATION QUESTIONS

True-false statements

Directions: Indicate whether the statement is true (T) or false (F).

T or F   1. Color vision should be tested binocularly.
T or F   2. Loss of accommodation is due to failure of the ciliary muscle.
T or F   3. Tear production is increased during the night.

Missing words

Directions: Write in the missing word in the following sentences.
4. When an object is viewed up close, three reactions occur: The eyes converge, the eye accommodates, and the pupils _____.
5. The muscle that moves the eye up and in is called the _____.
6. The rod pigment _____ or visual purple has as its main component vitamin A.

Choice-completion questions

Directions: Select the one best answer in each case.
7. The pupil is not affected by which one of the following?
   a. Pain
   b. Light
   c. Accommodation
   d. Mydriatics
   e. Congenital color blindness
8. Night vision originates in the:
   a. Rods
   b. Cones
   c. Choroid
   d. Macula
   e. Fovea
9. The most powerful refracting surface of the eye is the:
   a. Front surface of the cornea
   b. Back surface of the cornea
   c. Front surface of the lens
   d. Back surface of the lens
   e. Combined refractive index of the aqueous and vitreous

ANSWERS, NOTES, AND EXPLANATIONS

1. **False.** Color vision should be tested separately with each eye. Although sex-linked color defects are present binocularly, certain acquired defects can occur with color vision that will produce color deficiencies in one eye only. Such conditions as optic neuritis may be responsible for a monocular type of acquired color defect, and this would be missed if the examiner were testing binocular color vision.

2. **False.** Loss of accommodation is due to a gradual hardening of the lens substance beginning with the nucleus so that it is more resistant to changes in shape. Stimulus for accommodation is due to a blurred image, which causes the individual to contract the ciliary muscle and so relax the tension of the zonular fibers. This in turn allows the normal lens to assume a more spherical shape and increase its dioptric power. As the lens nucleus hardens with age, however, the lens is no longer as moldable and consequently is not able to bring the rays of light from a near object to focus onto the retina.

3. **False.** Tear production is decreased during the night and becomes almost nonexistent. There is, however, a compensatory lack of evaporation of tears during the sleep mechanism when the eyelids are closed. This provides adequate moisture for the cornea. The absence of tear production at night has important physiologic consequences in the development of an extended-wear contact lens of the soft variety, which is dependent on hydration.

4. **Constrict.** The pupils constrict during this triad in an effort to form a pinhole camera device so that a clear image is seen. This triad of pupillary constriction, convergence, and accommodation often is called the *accommodative reflex*.

5. **Inferior oblique.** The inferior oblique muscle moves the eye up and in. The other action is a torsional action in turning the eye outward, or extorsion.

6. **Rhodopsin.** Rhodopsin or visual purple forms with dark adaptation and is destroyed by light. It is continually being used and restored. Its main component is vitamin A, found in carrots and other vegetables.

7. **e. Congenital color blindness.** *Pain* causes dilation of the pupil. *Light* produces a constriction of the pupil. *Accommodation* produces a synkinesis of convergence and pupillary constriction along with accommodation. *Mydriatics* are drops that produce dilation of the pupil. *Color blindness*, however, does not result in pupillary abnormalities.

8. **a. Rods.** There are approximately 125 million rods present in the extramacular area of the retina. These rods function best in dim light and are responsible for what is called *scotopic vision*. It is the adjustment after we enter a dark movie theater that permits us to walk up the aisles with some degree of accuracy. Pilots during World War II soon learned they had to become night-adapted for bombing missions at night. Rods are relatively insensitive to red and therefore do not lose their function with this type of lighting. Thus red goggles were the chosen method for airline pilots and those in a number of other occupations that require rod adaptation for night vision. About 30 minutes are required for dark adaptation to occur. The use of red glasses, dark rooms, and x-ray rooms permit persons to maintain full cone function while the rods become dark-adapted.

9. **a. Front surface of the cornea.** This surface contributes about two thirds of the refracting power to bend the rays of light coming from a distant object. The lens of the eye contributes to the remaining one third of the refracting power of the eye. The refracting power of the cornea is equivalent to a 43.00-diopter lens.

CHAPTER 3 Optics

- Physical optics
- Geometric optics
- Spherical aberration
- Chromatic aberration
- Cylinders
- Transposition
- Practical aspects of optics
- Optical illusions

The study of optics can be divided into three parts: *physical, geometric,* and *physiologic.* Physical optics is primarily concerned with the nature and properties of *light* itself. Geometric optics is that branch of optics in which the laws of geometry can be used to design lenses that include spectacles, optical instruments, telescopes, microscopes, cameras, and so forth. Physiologic optics deals with the mechanism of vision and the physiology and psychology of seeing. We deal here primarily with physical and geometric optics.

PHYSICAL OPTICS

What is light? Our ancestors pondered and theorized about the nature of light. One theory proposed that light was wavelike and spread like ripples across a still pond (Fig. 3-1). Another theory held that light was a flight of particles similar to the shooting out of droplets of water from the nozzle of a hose (Fig. 3-2). In most recent times scientists have believed that there is truth in both theories—that light can be transmitted both as particles and as waves.

How does light travel? Light, which is basically that aspect of radiant energy to which the eye responds as a visual experience, is called *luminous*

radiation. The light waves travel in a specific direction. The movement of these waves is in an up-and-down motion perpendicular to the direction in which they travel (Fig. 3-3). These same light waves are capable of producing vision in human beings and lower animals by stimulating the very sensitive photoreceptors in the retina.

Nature of the world visible to humans. Human beings are continuously bombarded by electromagnetic energy—including waves from radio transmitters, infrared rays from heat lamps, and ultraviolet rays from the sun and quartz lamps—without receiving any visual sensation as a result of being in contact with these sources. It is only a portion of this *electromagnetic spectrum* that determines the visible world. The wavelengths of some of the waves of the electromagnetic spectrum are extremely short; for example, cosmic rays are only about 4 trillionths of a centimeter in length. Other wavelengths, such as those of radio waves, may be as long as 2 to 3 miles. The rays of wavelengths to which the eye responds lie in about the middle of this spectrum, namely from 400 to 800 nm. Fig. 3-4, an illustration of the electromagnetic spectrum, indicates the range of wavelengths for various parts of the spectrum.

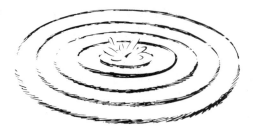

Fig. 3-1 Light travels in a wave motion as demonstrated by ripples in a still pond when a stone is thrown.

Speed of light. Light travels at a speed of 186,000 miles per second. It is many times faster than sound, as is evident by the fact that we see a lightning flash much sooner than we hear the thunder that follows. Each *wavelength* is the distance from the crest of one wave to that of the next, whereas the *frequency* is the number of wavelengths passing a given point in 1 second. The product of these two quantities is equal to the velocity of the electromagnetic radiation.

The speed of light in air is greater than that in

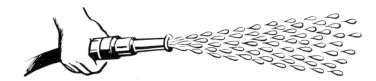

Fig. 3-2 One theory is that light behaves as water droplets shooting out of a hose.

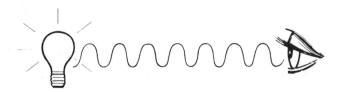

Fig. 3-3 Light travels not in a straight line but in a wave motion.

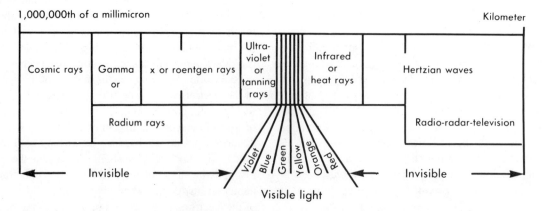

Fig. 3-4 Electromagnetic spectrum.

other transparent media. For example, the speed of light in ordinary glass is only about two thirds of the speed in air. However, we designate the wavelength of light in terms of its speed in air.

How do we measure intensity of a light source? Light intensity is measured in terms of candles, a standard dating from preelectricity times. The light from a single candle falling on a surface at a distance of 1 foot illuminates the surface with an illumination of one candle per square foot. This is the unit of measurement of light. If we hold a candle near a book in order to read, we soon find that as we move the candle away from the book, there is a distance at which the illumination is insufficient to permit us to read. The illumination of light on a surface is inversely proportional to its distance from the light source (Fig. 3-5). The luminance of an object depends on the light reflected, and the equivalent visual sensation is one of brightness. An illumination of 10 footcandles is sufficient for ordinary indoor tasks; 30 footcandles is adequate for sewing and reading, although we often choose a reading lamp that will give us as much as 50 footcandles (Table 3-1).

Because the original standard candle cannot be easily reproduced, it has been replaced by a group of carbon filament lamps operated at a carefully prescribed voltage and maintained in the vaults of the U.S. Bureau of Standards. In modern usage the amount of illumination, or illuminance, is referred to in terms of lumens per foot rather than candles per foot.

Table 3-1	Recommended minimum footcandles
Auditoriums	15
Waiting rooms	15
Building corridors and stairways	20
Libraries	70
Art galleries	30
Reading rooms	30
Study desks	70
Store interiors	30
School chalkboards	150
Kitchen work surfaces	50
Prolonged sewing	100

Color. The dispersion of white light into its many component colors was first demonstrated by Sir Issac Newton, who allowed a narrow beam of light to pass obliquely through a prism and then intercepted the transmitted light, which appeared as colored bands or as a spectrum on a screen. The colors he found were spread into definite bands that the normal eye identified as red, orange, yellow, green, blue, and violet. The sequence of hues were *always found to be in the same order.* Newton called these bands of color the *spectrum,* and he called the spreading effect caused by the prism *dispersion.* He was the first to show that white light is really a mixture of all colors. We enjoy everyday examples of this phenomenon of light breaking up into its constituent colors. Rainbows, for example, are produced by the dispersion

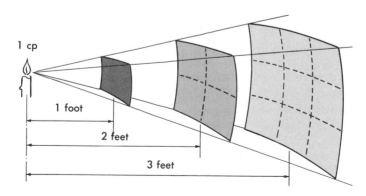

Fig. 3-5 Illumination is inversely proportional to the distance of the surface from the light source. (Modified from Adler FH: *Physiology of the eye,* ed. 4, St Louis, 1965, Mosby.)

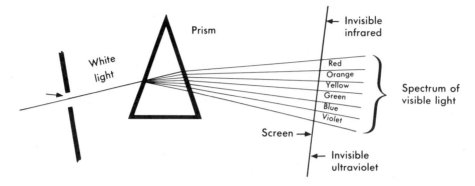

Fig. 3-6 Dispersion of white light into colors by a prism.

of light into its spectral parts by the droplets of rain or mist in the air.

Each wavelength range has a particular color hue. Red, having the longest wavelength, is deviated least by a water droplet or a prism and therefore appears at one end of the spectrum. Violet, which has the shortest wavelength, appears at the other end of the spectrum (Fig. 3-6).

Rays of light and the spectrum. A single ray of light is the path of a single corpuscle of light traveling through a tiny aperture through two successive screens.

A pencil of light is a group of rays that diverges from its point source. It might pass through the aperture of one screen but would not make it through the aperture of the other.

A beam of light is a group of pencils of light. A relatively large aperture is required to admit a beam.

Each filament in an electric bulb has a number of beams and pencils of light. These beams diverge and overlap one another. At close range, they strike an object and create overlapping shadows that are poorly defined. The further the light source, the more parallel are the beams of light. That is why shadows framed from the sun are sharper and more finely etched than those coming from an artificial light source.

Where rays of white light pass through cut glass, they frequently are broken down into lights of varying wavelengths. The longest wavelength is red, followed by orange, yellow, green, blue, and violet:

Red	650-750 nm
Orange	592-650 nm
Yellow	560-592 nm
Green	500-560 nm
Blue	446-500 nm
Violet	400-446 nm

The fragmentation of white light yields the visible spectrum. There are other wavelengths not visible to the eye, including ultraviolet, infrared, x-ray, radio, and electromagnetic.

White light is not regularly broken up unless it travels into and through a different medium such as water droplets or glass. It is important to realize that the various wavelengths travel forward or outward at the same speed. Only their vertical vibrations differ in frequency. Thus the speed of violet light in air is the same as yellow, red, or green, that is, 186,000 miles per second.

When white light enters the eye, all these light waves are moving at the same speed but with a different vibration. These waves fuse with each other, giving the sensation of white, even though they travel through the eye, which has a different index of refraction than air.

Bending of light. For years many people have observed that a straight pole inclined in a clear pond no longer appears straight but appears to be bent at the surface of the water. Fish under the surface of the water appear to someone fishing to be at a different place from where they actually are (Fig. 3-7). This phenomenon is due to *refraction* of light.

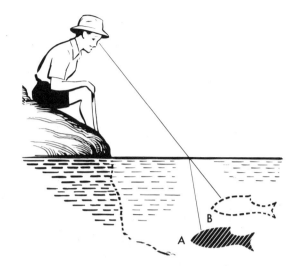

Fig. 3-7 Bending of light upon entering a medium of higher index of refraction. The real fish is at **A**, although the boy sees it at **B**.

If light travels in a straight line, how does one explain this apparent bending of light? Snell discovered the law behind this everyday phenomenon, and it was explained by assuming—and this assumption was later proved by experiment—that light travels at *different speeds in different media*. We have stated that light travels in a vacuum at 186,000 miles per second. However, as it travels through other media, such as water or glass, it travels at a slower velocity. The rate at which light travels through water is 146,000 miles per second. Other media, such as glass and the chambers of the eye, also retard the velocity and alter the direction of light. The ratio of the speed of light in a vacuum to that in a given medium is called the *index of refraction* of that medium. This index, which is a comparison of the speed of light through a particular medium to its speed through air, can be expressed as follows:

$$\text{Index of refraction} = \frac{\text{Speed of light in air}}{\text{Speed of light in substance}}$$

$$\text{For water this index} = \frac{186,000}{140,000} = 1.33$$

Thus the index of refraction of a substance determines the speed of light through it. The index of refraction of the common optical media can be expressed as follows:

Air   = 1.00
Water   = 1.33
Aqueous humor = 1.336
Cornea   = 1.37
Lens cortex   = 1.38
Lens nucleus   = 1.40
PMMA plastic   = 1.52
Crown glass   = 1.49
Flint glass   = 1.65

How light can alter its direction. If rays of light pass from the air through another medium, such as a plate of glass, and pass perpendicularly to the glass, they will be slowed down somewhat but will emerge along the same line on which they entered the medium (Fig. 3-8, *A*). If, however, these rays pass obliquely at any angle to the plate of glass, they will be bent a little at the surface. The oblique rays closest to the glass will enter the glass first, and these rays will be slowed down first on their pathway through the slower medium (Fig. 3-8, *B*).

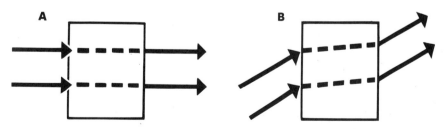

Fig. 3-8 A, Light passing perpendicularly through a plate glass remains unchanged in direction. **B,** Light passing obliquely through a plate glass is displaced laterally but continues in the same direction.

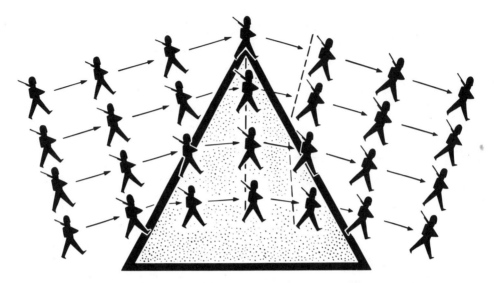

Fig. 3-9 Pathway of the soldiers' march is changed by a sandbar. This is similar to the effect of light striking a glass prism.

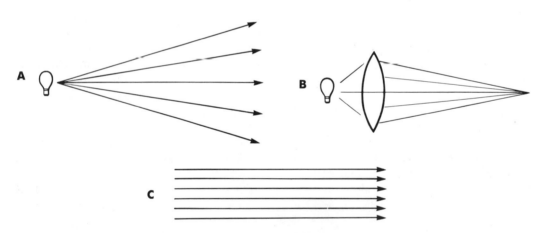

Fig. 3-10 A, Divergence. **B,** Convergence. **C,** Parallel rays.

This effect is similar to the slowing-down effect when a line of soldiers march at an angle toward a deep sandbar (Fig. 3-9). The soldiers who first enter the sandbar will be slowed down first, whereas those at the extreme end will continue at their original speed until they reach the sandbar. This will result in a bend in the straight-line formation. This same effect occurs when a beam of light strikes a glass surface at an oblique angle.

GEOMETRIC OPTICS
Terminology

divergence Rays of light from any luminous point of light will spread out, or diverge (Fig. 3-10, *A*).

convergence When a bundle of rays are brought together, they are said to converge (Fig. 3-10, *B*).

parallel rays Light rays are assumed to be parallel if they emanate from a distant light source, such as the sun (Fig. 3-10, *C*).

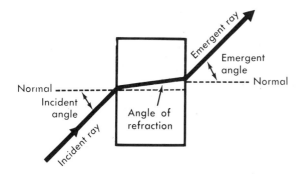

Fig. 3-11 Diagram to show the incident and emergent rays of light through glass.

A ray of light entering a medium is called the *incident ray,* and that ray emerging from the medium is called the *emergent ray.* The angle that the incident ray makes with the perpendicular surface of the new medium is called the *angle of incidence.* The angle the ray makes in the new medium by its change of direction is called the *angle of refraction* (Fig. 3-11).

The relationship between these two angles and the index of refraction of the medium through which the ray of light passes is the basis of *Snell's law,* a fundamental law in optics that governs the refraction of light by a transparent substance. Snell's law states that the

$$\frac{\text{Sine of angle of incidence (i)}}{\text{Sine of angle of refraction (h)}} = \text{Index of refraction}$$

It is on this constant relationship of the incident angle, angle of refraction, and index of refraction of the medium that all lens design depends.

Dispersion

If a spectrum of light travels through a glass with parallel sides, then the deflection of light is such that the emerging rays are parallel to the direction of the original incident rays. The white light may enter a new medium such as glass, be broken up into its spectral components, and then fuse on the way out to a white bundle of rays.

If a ray of light goes through glass whose sides are not parallel, the white light will be broken into its spectral components with the various wavelengths emerging in different directions. This effect is called *dispersion* and results in colored fringes found around anything viewed through prisms or unevenly cut glass. The dispersion value of different types of glass varies, depending on its index of refraction (Fig. 3-12).

Mirrors and reflection

One way of changing the direction of light is to allow light to rebound from a surface and thus be thrown in another direction. This rebounding of light is

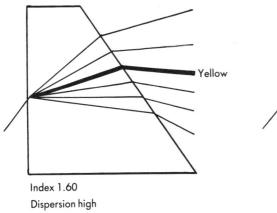

Index 1.60
Dispersion high

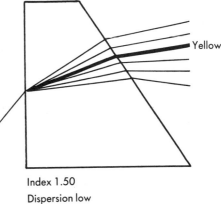

Index 1.50
Dispersion low

Fig. 3-12 Dispersion factor of light through oblique glass with different indexes of refraction.

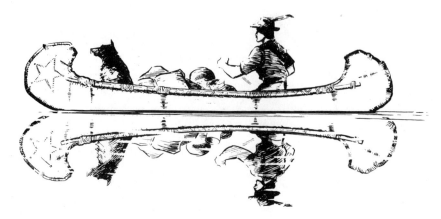

Fig. 3-13 Reflection. A still pond acts as a mirror.

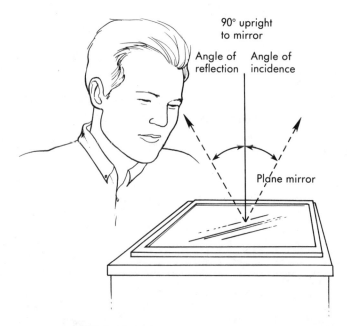

Fig. 3-14 Reflection from plane mirror.

called *reflection,* and certain laws govern its behavior. Mirrors illustrate this phenomenon best. They are primarily silver-coated glass, which allows a minimum transmission of light while reflecting the greater portion of the light. It should be noted that any reflecting surface, such as glass, water, or metal, can reflect light. Because glass and water transmit light primarily, their reflection is secondary. There are many other examples of reflecting surfaces in nature, such as the still pond (Fig. 3-13). Mirrors obey a law that the *angle of incidence equals the angle of reflection* (Fig. 3-14). An analogous situation occurs when a billiard ball strikes the elastic cushion of a billiard table. The angle at which the

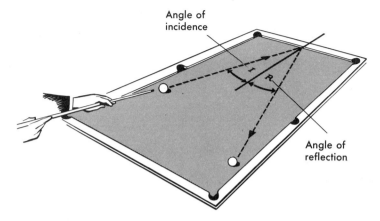

Fig. 3-15 Billiard table. Movement of a billiard ball against the cushion of the table observes the same laws as the reflection of light from mirrors.

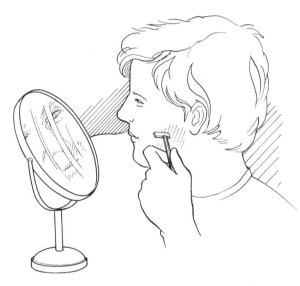

Fig. 3-16 Concave shaving mirror. The image is magnified.

ball strikes the edge of the table is equal to the angle of the caroming ball (Fig. 3-15).

Mirrors may be *curved* or *plane*. Curved mirrors are of two types: *concave* or *convex*. Concave mirrors reflect light in front of them, so that if an object is placed before the focal point of a mirror, its image is magnified. This property is employed to great advantage in the production of mirrors for shaving (Fig. 3-16). Convex mirrors reflect light away from their principal axes, so that if objects are placed before them, the images will appear behind the mirrors in smaller size (Fig. 3-17). One application of this second type of mirror is employed in large stores, in which store managers can observe large areas through small mirrors (Fig. 3-18).

Lenses

Spectacle lenses were invented in about the thirteenth century and telescopes in the seventeenth century. In the past 100 years binoculars, cameras, projectors, periscopes, spectroscopes, and many other optical instruments have been developed with refinements of lens design; all have been dependent on the knowledge human beings have gained concerning the properties of lenses. Lenses originally were made of glass but are now also made of plastic. The main feature of curved lenses is their ability to bend rays of light.

How do lenses bend rays of light? The basic principle of all lenses may be considered best by a discussion of prisms. One may consider a lens as being made up of prisms.

What is a prism? A prism is a triangular piece of glass or plastic with an *apex* and a *base*. Rays of light, entering from air and going through a prism,

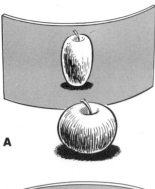

A

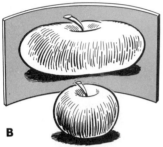

B

Fig. 3-17 A, Reflection from a convex mirror; the image is minified. **B,** Reflection from a concave mirror; the image is magnified.

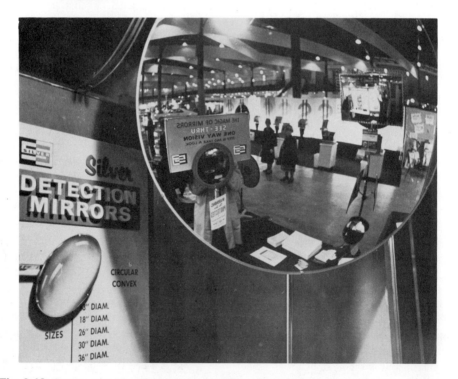

Fig. 3-18 Convex mirrors used to prevent shoplifting. The minified image of the store allows easy scrutiny of a large area. (Courtesy Globe and Mail, Toronto, Ontario.)

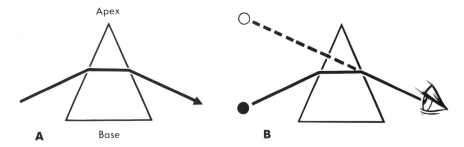

Fig. 3-19 A, Light is deviated by the prism toward its base. **B,** The observer views an object through the prism and the object appears displaced toward its apex.

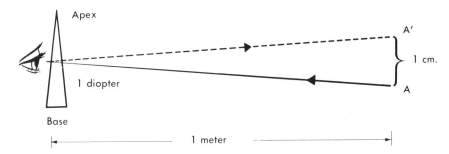

Fig. 3-20 Object at *A* appears to be at *A'* when viewed through a 1.00-diopter prism at 1 meter.

bend toward the base of the prism. This phenomenon is related to the oblique surface of the prism and its medium (Fig. 3-19, *A*).

The magnitude of the prismatic effect depends on the size of the angle of the apex of the prism. Light always is bent in the direction toward the base of a prism. When one looks through a prism, however, the object of regard appears displaced toward its apex (Fig. 3-19, *B*).

How are prisms measured? Prisms employed in ophthalmology are calibrated in diopters. By definition, *1 prism diopter* is that prism which appears to displace an object 1 cm at a distance of 1 meter from the eye (Fig. 3-20). At 0.5 meter, if the object is displaced 1 cm, then the dioptric power of the prism is 2.00 diopters. At 2 meters, if the object is displaced 1 cm, then the dioptric power is 0.50 diopter. This is expressed by the formula:

$$P = C/D$$

where:

P = Prism power
C = Displacement of object in centimeters
D = Distance from prism in meters

The use of prisms. Prisms are used in ophthalmology in the following devices and procedures:

1. Ophthalmic instruments such as gonioscopes and ophthalmoscopes.
2. Measurements of muscle balance of the eye in cases of strabismus. A prism can alter the direction of light so that the projection of the deviating eye is the same as its fellow eye, and in effect it corrects the sensory alignment of the eye without disturbing the motor alignment.
3. Spectacles to correct muscle imbalance, especially those of a vertical nature.
4. Eye exercise for muscular imbalance, such as convergence insufficiency.

Prisms may be used as reflectors or mirrors. A

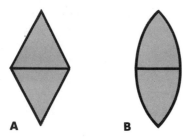

Fig. 3-21 A, Two prisms placed base to base. **B,** A convex lens derived from **A** by smoothing off the middle corners.

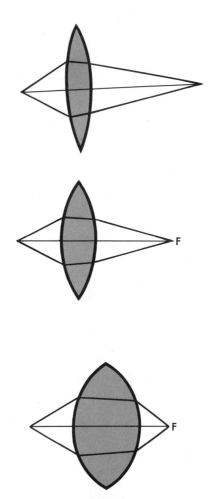

Fig. 3-22 Convex lenses. As the curvature of the lens increases, the closer to the lens is the focal point. Also, the more curved the lens, the greater is its power.

ray of light usually travels through a piece of glass, but there is a critical angle in which light is reflected rather than refracted. Any light rays striking a glass surface at an angle smaller than the critical angle will be refracted through the glass. When light hits the glass at an angle greater than the critical angle, the rays of light will be reflected as though the glass were a silvered mirror.

Convex lenses. A convex lens is a piece of glass in which one or both surfaces of the lens are curved outward. If two prisms are placed base to base (Fig. 3-21, *A*) and the middle corners of the prism are smoothed off, a *convex lens* is created (Fig. 3-21, *B*).

Alteration in the radius, or curvature, of the lens alters its point of convergence, or focal point. A more curved lens will bend rays of light to a shorter focus than will a less curved lens. Lenses are considered as positive lenses, or *plus lenses,* if they converge rays of light to a focus behind the lens (Fig. 3-22).

Concave lenses. A concave lens is a piece of glass in which one or both surfaces of the lens are curved inward. If two prisms are placed apex to apex (Fig. 3-23, *A*) and the straight surfaces of the prisms are then curved, a concave lens is created (Fig. 3-23, *B*).

With a concave lens, the emergent rays of light diverge after refraction and thus cannot be focused behind the lens. If, however, we extend the direction of the rays of light backward, we can draw an imaginary focus in front of the lens. Thus this lens is called a negative lens, or *minus lens* (Fig. 3-24).

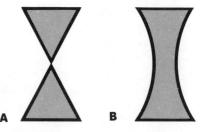

Fig. 3-23 A, Two prisms placed apex to apex. **B,** A concave lens derived from **A.**

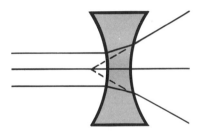

Fig. 3-24 Concave lens demonstrating an imaginary or virtual point of focus in front of the lens.

Up to this point the lenses under dicussion have all been spheres. The convex lenses are *converging lenses,* and the concave lenses are *diverging lenses*. Converging means bringing together and diverging means spreading apart, and that is what these lenses do to rays of light. Variations of the spherical lens

occur when the curvatures of the anterior and the posterior surfaces are not the same (Fig. 3-25).

Focal length. In any lens the ray penetrating through the center of the lens is undeviated, but all rays on either side will converge to or from a point. This central ray, or axial ray, travels along a line called the *principal axis* of the lens. The rays on either side, or *paraxial* rays, converge to a point on this principal axis, which is called the *focal point;* the length of this point from the center of the lens is called the *focal length* (Fig. 3-26).

A lens must be considered in terms of its focal length. The power of a lens is equal to the reciprocal of its focal distance measured in meters. The power is expressed in units called *diopters*.

The formula for conversion of focal length into diopters of lens power is

$$D = 1/F$$

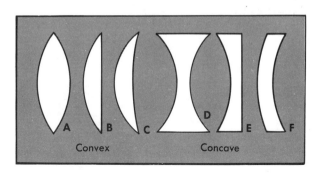

Fig. 3-25 Lens forms: **A,** biconvex; **B,** planoconvex; **C,** convex meniscus; **D,** biconcave; **E,** planoconcave; **F,** concave meniscus.

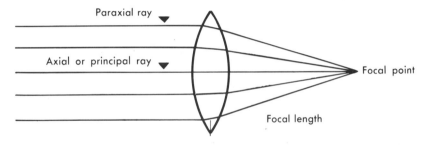

Fig. 3-26 Convergence of rays by a convex lens to a focal point.

where:

   D = Power of lens in diopters
   F = Focal length in meters

For example:

Lens with focal length of 1 m = 1.1 = 1.00 D

Lens with focal length of 2 m = ½ = 0.50 D

Lens with focal length of 4 m = ¼ = 0.25 D

Lens with focal length of ¼ = 1/0.25 = 4.00 D

To clearly capture the image from a convex lens, a screen must be placed at its exact focal point. An example of this is shown in Fig. 3-27.

In a convex lens the focal point always is behind the lens, and therefore convex lenses are considered positive (Fig. 3-28). With concave lenses, however, the focal point always is in front of the lens, erect and virtual. Concave lenses are designated as minus lenses.

Until now we have considered point sources and point focal points. With regard to an object such as a house, each point on the house will have its own focal point in terms of a plus lens system (Fig. 3-29). It also should be noted that the image behind a

convex lens is always real, behind the lens, and inverted. A real image is one that can be captured by a screen or photographic film.

When an object is placed before a positive lens, a sharp image is formed at its focal point.

To determine the focal length and the power of the lens, one must know the distance of the object from the lens and the distance of the image from the lens. The following formula is employed:

$$I/U + 1/V = 1/F$$

where:

   U = Distance of object from lens
   V = Distance of image from lens
   F = Focal length of lens

If any two of these factors are known, then the third can easily be derived.

A simpler alternate method to determine the focal length of a lens is to use the formula

$$U + D = V$$

where:

   U = Distance in centimeters that object is in front of lens

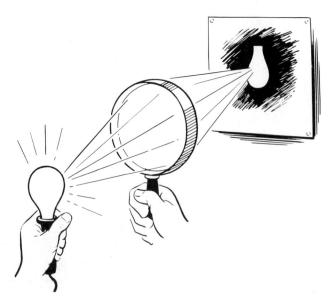

Fig. 3-27 A real inverted image of the light bulb is seen when the screen is placed at the focal point of the convex lens.

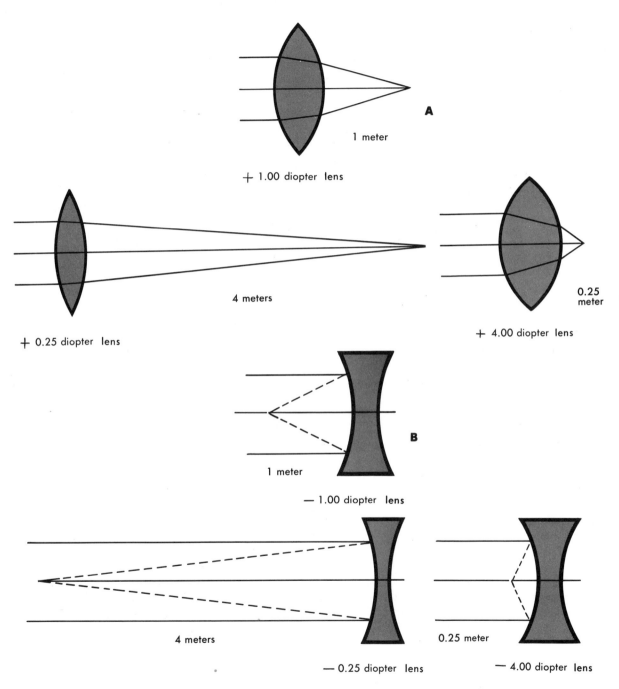

Fig. 3-28 Focal distance varies with the power of the lens. **A,** Plus, or convex, lens: the point focus is behind the lens. **B,** Minus, or concave, lens: the point focus is in front of the lens.

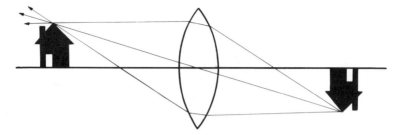

Fig. 3-29 Image of a house through a convex lens is behind the lens, real, and inverted.

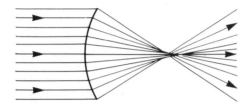

Fig. 3-30 Spherical aberration. The rays of light on refraction by the lens are converged to a meeting area rather than a single focal point.

V = Distance in centimeters that object is behind the lens

D = Dioptric power of the lens

Once one determines the D or dioptric value of the lens, one can use the formula D = 1/F, and if one uses "cm," one can divide the formula D = 100/F(cm) to determine the focal distance in centimeters.

SPHERICAL ABERRATION

Because the periphery of a lens has a different curvature from its center, rays of light striking the lens at its edge do not come to the same focal point as when they strike the lens at its center (Fig. 3-30). To eliminate problems caused by this aberration, grinding techniques have been developed. Spherical aberration becomes a problem only with lenses of high power.

CHROMATIC ABERRATION

We have noted that the edges of spherical lenses act as a prism. However, light, on passing through a prism, is broken down into its spectral components. Therefore color fringes can appear when light passes through a lens. This is particularly noticeable in dealing with lenses of high power. Chromatic aberration can be largely corrected by changes in the shape and index of refraction of the lens. Flint glass has a greater tendency to produce chromatic aberration than does crown glass. This aberration can be corrected by combining two lenses having different indexes of refraction.

If chromatic aberration is excessive, the image formed by the optical system will be fuzzy with colored fringes. There are ways to reduce this color distortion.

1. A light source that has light of only one wavelength (lasers) or a narrow band of wavelengths (sodium vapor lamps) may be employed.

2. A filter may be used to take out all but a few wavelengths. Good camera lenses reduce chromatic aberration with appropriate filters.

3. A doublet lens works, if one lens has a low index of refraction (crown glass) and the other a high index of refraction (flint glass). This combination is called an *anachromatic* lens. The two lenses of equal dispersion value nullify each other, and the chromatic aberration that results is below that of a single lens.

CYLINDERS

A sphere has the same power in all meridians, whereas the cylinder has two principal meridians; one is called the *power* meridian (which has the power of the lens) and the other is called the *axis* (which is only a reference of the cylinder; it has *no power*).

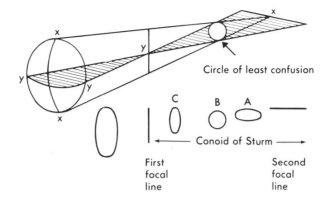

Fig. 3-31 Sturm's conoid. This represents the astigmatic interval between the two focal points of a spherocylindric lens.

Cylinders have the shape of a slice of a pipe or bicycle tire in that they are curved sharply in one direction but not at all in the other direction.

The curvature of a lens in one direction conveys the power of that lens and is called the *meridian* of the lens. The image of a cylinder, however, lies 90 degrees away from the meridian of power. This position is the plane of the *axis* of the lens. Therefore we have two terms: a meridian, which denotes the power of a cylindric lens, and the axis, which denotes the image of the lens, this image being always 90 degrees away from the meridian. Cylindric lenses, as in the trial case, always are denoted by the axis; for example, + 1.00 axis 90 has 1.00 diopter of power at 180 degrees, but it will form an image at 90 degrees.

Spherocylinders are a combination of a sphere and a cylinder. Such a lens system has two radii of curvature, each with its own focal point and image. For example, in Fig. 3-31 the rays of light from meridian X–X focus at X, whereas the rays from Y–Y focus at Y.

The area between the two focal points of a spherocylindric combination assumes a conoid shape, which is called *Sturm's conoid*. This optical effect is illustrated in Fig. 3-31. At *A*, a section of the bundle of converging rays will be in the form of a horizontal ellipse, but later at *C* it will be in the form of a vertical ellipse. At *B*, the bundle forms a circle called the *circle of least confusion*. The circle of

least confusion represents the dioptric average of the spherocylinder. In refraction the conoid of Sturm is "collapsed" so that both the vertical and horizontal foci are placed on the retina. In a situation in which one focus is already on the retina, a simple cylinder will move the other focus back or forward to the retina.

A spherocylindric lens is really two lenses, each with different powers in the two principal meridians, which are 90 degrees apart. The dioptric powers of these two components should be considered separately.

For example, + 7.00 D sph − 1.50 cyl × 90 means that the spherical power is + 7.00, the cylinder is − 1.50 diopters, and its axis is 90 degrees. The power of that cylinder is at right axis to the cylinder. Thus the power in the horizontal meridian is + 5.50 diopters.

TRANSPOSITION

Transposition is the process of changing the prescription from a plus cylinder to a minus cylinder, or from a minus cylinder to a plus cylinder, without changing its refractive value. The rules of transposition are based on the principle that when two cylinders of equal power and like sign are crossed at right angles, they produce the effect of a spherical lens of the same power as one of the cylinders.

The rule for transposition of all compound lenses is as follows: *Add the cylinder power to the sphere power algebraically, change the sign of the cylinder, and change the axis of the cylinder by 90 degrees.* The following are examples of typical transpositions.

Transpose the following prescription to a minus cylinder: +2.00 + 1.00 × 90. Adding +2.00 and +1.00 algebraically, we obtain +3.00 as the new spherical power. Changing the sign of the cylinder to minus and the axis by 90 degrees, we find +3.00 − 1.00 × 180.

Transpose the following prescription to a plus cylinder: +1.00 − 3.00 × 70. Adding +1.00 and −3.00 algebraically, we obtain −2.00 as the spherical power; and changing the sign of the cylinder to plus and the axis by 90 degrees, we find −2.00 + 3.00 × 160.

PRACTICAL ASPECTS OF OPTICS
Fiberoptics

A fiberoptic bundle has a transparent core of material with a high refractive index surrounded by a material of lower refractive index. The core usually is plastic or glass. The rim can be glass or even air. Most fibers are tiny, being only 0.003 to 0.005 inches in diameter.

Light moves along these plastic cores because of total internal reflection. The optical effect is created by the differences in indexes of refraction. Light leaves the pipes at the end of tubing where it is intense and concentrated. Most of the bundles are parallel to one another, the result being a coherent fiberoptic bundle or image conduit. Coherent fibers are used in computer output terminals as well as in many electrooptical devices.

Gonioscopy

The principle of internal reflection is a problem to an observer who has to examine the eye. There are parts of the eye not visible because light cannot get out of the eye. For instance, the angle structures of the anterior chamber are not visible because of total internal reflection.

Light has to get through the cornea for the ex-

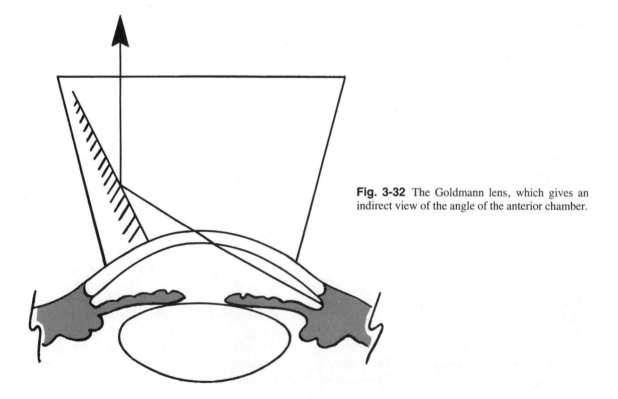

Fig. 3-32 The Goldmann lens, which gives an indirect view of the angle of the anterior chamber.

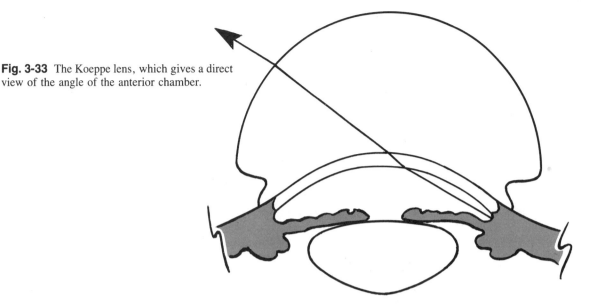

Fig. 3-33 The Koeppe lens, which gives a direct view of the angle of the anterior chamber.

aminer to see the angle structures. At the cornea–air interface, however, an abrupt change from a high to a low index of refraction occurs, which causes total internal reflection exactly like that of the fiberoptic tube.

If a contact lens is applied to the cornea, then light can pass through the cornea into the contact lens, which has a refractive index higher than the refractive index of corneal tissue. Once the light is past the cornea, it can travel to the eyepiece and be seen either through a mirror, as noted in the Goldmann lens (Fig. 3-32), or through simple refraction, as noted in the discussion of the Koeppe lens (Fig. 3-33).

Telescopes

There are two types of telescopes: the astronomic or inverting and the galilean or noninverting.

Astronomic telescope. Both the objective and the eyepiece are of positive power. The primary focus of the eye lens coincides with the secondary focus of the objective lens. They are separated by the distance equal to the sum of their focal lengths. A real image is formed in the focal plane of the objective. The image is inverted, and its size is determined by the power of these lenses. The eye lens acts as a simple magnifier and forms a vertical image at infinity. This telescope, as the name implies, is used in astronomy. Because the stars are so far away, the fact that the image is inverted is not of practical concern.

Galilean telescope. This telescope uses a negative eye lens and positive objective. Again, the two lenses are situated so that their focal points coincide. The focus of the negative lens, however, is on the other side of the lens, so that the two are separated by the difference of the absolute values of their focal length.

The image from this telescope is noninverted because of the negative eyepiece. The erect image has allowed industry to use these basic optical principles to manufacture surgical loops. These consist of a galilean telescope combined with an "add" on the front to allow for close work.

OPTICAL ILLUSIONS

Optics takes us into the fascinating field of optical illusion. In this area, geometric optics are affected by our perceptual senses and our interpretation of what we see. The impression "seeing is believing" is not always true because we are influenced greatly by background effect, as well as the effect of certain lines on each other and their interpretation by the brain. In Fig. 3-34 are examples of some of the illusions that can be created.

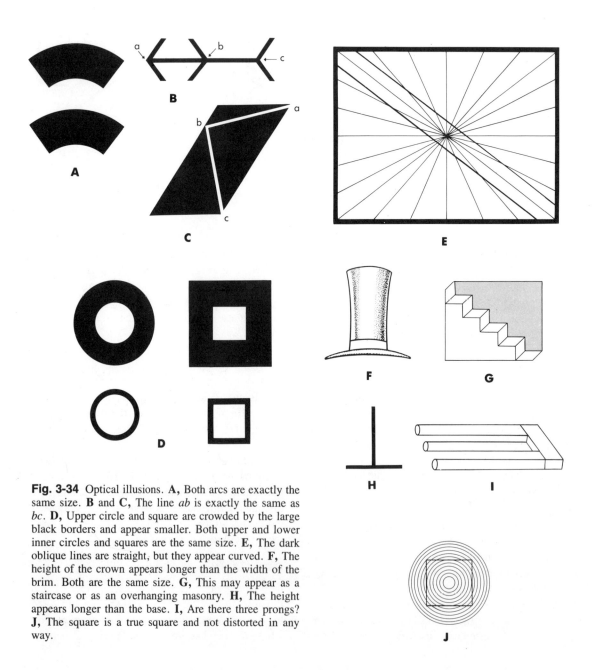

Fig. 3-34 Optical illusions. **A,** Both arcs are exactly the same size. **B** and **C,** The line *ab* is exactly the same as *bc.* **D,** Upper circle and square are crowded by the large black borders and appear smaller. Both upper and lower inner circles and squares are the same size. **E,** The dark oblique lines are straight, but they appear curved. **F,** The height of the crown appears longer than the width of the brim. Both are the same size. **G,** This may appear as a staircase or as an overhanging masonry. **H,** The height appears longer than the base. **I,** Are there three prongs? **J,** The square is a true square and not distorted in any way.

QUESTIONS FOR REVIEW AND THOUGHT

1. How does light travel?
2. What is the cause of the dispersion of white light produced by a prism?
3. Draw a diagram of the electromagnetic spectrum.
4. List the sequence of color hues in the spectrum.
5. What is the law of mirrors?
6. Which type of mirror magnifies, concave or convex?
7. What is a prism?
8. Draw the focal point of a concave lens; of a convex lens.
9. What is a cylinder?
10. What is Sturm's conoid?
11. What aberrations are there with high minus spectacles (greater than 5.00 diopters)?
12. What are aspheric lenses?
13. How do you find the optical center of a lens?
14. Name some common defects found in glass.
15. What is a galilean telescope?
16. When you are looking through a prism, does the image jump to the apex or base?

SELF-EVALUATION QUESTIONS

True-false statements

Directions: Indicate whether the statement is true (T) or false (F).

T or **F**   1. A light entering a prism is deflected toward the apex of the prism.

T or **F**   2. Chromatic aberration occurs when white light enters a new index of refraction and emerges broken into its spectral components.

T or **F**   3. The speed of red light is considerably slower than the speed of white light.

Missing words

Directions: Write in the missing word in the following sentences.

4. Placido's disc uses the front surface of the cornea as a _____.
5. A fiberoptic bundle works by _____ reflection, in which the light strikes the wall of the bundle at an angle greater than the critical angle.
6. Yellow lenses act as _____ filters.

Choice-completion questions

Directions: Select the one best answer in each case.

7. If the mechanical center of a lens is changed by edging, what happens to the optical center?
   a. It remains where it was on the lens
   b. It is displaced toward the edge most shortened
   c. It is displaced according to Prentice's rule
   d. It shifts laterally but never vertically
   e. None of the above

8. Aberrations of a lens include:
   a. Spherical aberration
   b. Astigmatism of oblique pencils
   c. Chromatic aberration
   d. Pincushion and barrel distortion
   e. All of the above
9. Convex mirrors make the size of the image:
   a. Smaller
   b. Larger
   c. Larger if the object is placed within the focal point of the lens
   d. Smaller if the object is placed within the focal point of the lens
   e. None of the above

ANSWERS, NOTES, AND EXPLANATIONS

1. **False.** A prism is a wedge-shaped piece of glass that bends light toward its base because of a change in the direction of light waves. It creates this alteration of direction because of the change in the index of refraction between light traveling in air and light traveling in glass. When light emerges from the prism, it undergoes another change in direction toward the base.

   Although the light is deflected toward the base of the prism, the observer sees it toward the apex. By bringing together images separated in space by a heterotropia of the eyes, prisms are used diagnostically to assess the type and magnitude of a strabismus and to treat diplopia.

2. **True.** Chromatic aberration is seen naturally in rainbows. White light penetrates a suspended droplet of water and is broken up into its spectral components. Clinically, chromatic aberration is seen in patients who have corneal edema. The most common occurrences are in persons with severe or acute glaucoma or those wearing ill-fitting contact lenses. The liberated edema fluid breaks up the intact bundle of white light, and patients complain of seeing halos around lights. Frequently a mucous blob on the cornea will do the same thing, so that not all chromatic aberration occurrences indicate pathologic conditions.

   Some lenses have a higher chromatic aberration than others. For instance, flint glass has a greater tendency to chromatic aberration than does barium.

3. **False.** All the colors, whether they are reds, blues, greens, or oranges, have exactly the same speed of light, which is 186,000 miles per second. A wavelength is the distance from the top of one wave to the top of the next, whereas the frequency is the number of waves passing in one second. Red light may have a longer wavelength than blue, but this indicates only its vertical vibration. All colors, white included, travel at the same speed.

   The velocity of light depends on frequency $\times$ wavelength. When the wavelength is shorter, its frequency is increased so that speed of white versus colored light remains the same.

4. **Mirror.** Placido's disc uses the cornea as a mirror. The disc is used to detect keratoconus. The cone-shaped deformity of the cornea is reflected in the distortion of the annular rings, which appear irregular and oblong on the cornea. Placido's disc is used in a clinical photographic system to give accurate topographic analysis of the central and peripheral sections of the cornea for contact lens fitting. The distance between the rings can be translated into radii of corneal curvature. Reflection from the cornea as a mirror is the basic principle of all keratometers. The image from the keratometer is reflected and brought into focus. A doubling device is used to keep the images aligned. The amount of focusing required to yield sharp corneal images gives the K readings.

5. **Internal.** If light strikes any optical surface at an angle greater than the critical angle, the light, instead of passing through that surface, will be totally reflected.

This principle is well established. Some ophthalmoscopes are based on total reflection by virtue of light striking a prism. In fiberoptic bundles, the light is inside the bundle and cannot escape because the angle of incident light exceeds the critical angle, and the outer coat of the light has a low refractive index. The light emerging from this fiberoptic bundle is compressed, intense, and very high in illumination. It is a pure light because none of it escapes or is broken down to its spectral components.

Fiberoptic illumination has become an integral part of the illuminating systems used in ophthalmic microsurgery. The commercial uses of the fiberoptic system are numerous and include everything from Christmas tree decorations to illuminating systems for space travel.

6. **Haze.** Yellow lenses are basically haze filters. They are used by skiers and hunters to reduce haze and improve definition. They are not useful in night driving, because they reduce the light entering the retina when lack of contrast is already a problem.

7. **a. It remains where it was on the lens.** Obviously, the center of the lens remains where it is, regardless of how the lens is edged. However, high fashion dictates the shape of the frame, and with radical lens designs the optical centers can be shifted in the frame itself and in relation to the eye.

Large frames that contain strong prescriptions, that is, -5.00 diopters or more, frequently slide down the nose with reading. The effect of gravity drops the lens, and the vertex distance of the lens to the eye is changed. With plus lenses it weakens the prescription; with minus lenses it does the reverse. Also, unwanted prism is added with plus lenses, with the opposite occurring with minus lenses.

The optical center and the mechanical center do not coincide. The optical center of a lens is that place of the lens that does not contain unwanted prism. It is the point detected on the lensmeter where the rays of light come into focus. The optical center should be in line with the eye. The mechanical center is the geographic center, and in a perfectly round lens it coincides with the optical center. The optical center concerns us, not the mechanical center.

If the optical center is shifted in the frame, then unwanted prism will occur. If the optical center is shifted outward, and the lens is a plus lens, then base-out prism will be added.

The optical centers of the lenses always should be marked and compared with the interpupillary measurements—the distance from the center of one pupil to the other.

8. **e. All of the above.** *Spherical aberration:* The image from a spherical lens is never a single point because the central and paraaxial rays form more concentrated images than those rays that pass through the periphery of the lens.

The degree of spherical aberration depends on:

(1) The aperture of the system. It is reduced by closing down the size of the aperture.

(2) The precise form of the lenses used. The error can be reduced, making the curvature of the anterior surface greater than the curvature of the posterior surface.

(3) The curvature of the lens. The fault can be diminished by making the peripheral curves less sloped. These are called *aplanatic surfaces.*

Astigmatism of oblique pencils: If light rays strike a lens at an angle instead of perpendicular to it, the image will be distorted in a form similar to that produced by a cylindric lens. Some light rays will strike the lens early and some later. The extra distance has to be traveled by the later rays to strike the lens. Moreover, a flatter section of the lens will be encountered by these rays. The resultant image will be astigmatic, sharp in one direction and fuzzy in the other. If the light rays strike a lens perpendicularly, this type of lens distortion does not occur.

Chromatic aberration: This is discussed in answer 2.

Pincushion and barrel distortion: Distortion occurs when the magnification of the peripheral parts of the lens is different from that of the central area. Pincushion distortion occurs when the peripheral magnification is greater than that of the central magnification. Barrel distortion occurs when the peripheral magnification is less than that of the central magnification.

9. **a. Smaller.** Concave mirrors magnify the image of the object only if it is placed *within* the focal point of the mirror. Cosmetic mirrors always are concave, and the face has to be placed close to the mirror to have its image enlarged and in focus.

Convex mirrors reduce image size. They commonly are used as survey mirrors in retail stores where large areas of the store can be seen with the aid of a convex mirror.

CHAPTER 4

Pharmacology

- General principles
- Complications of locally administered drugs
- Prescription writing
- Autonomic drugs
- Drugs that lower intraocular pressure
- Anesthetics
- Antiallergic and antiinflammatory agents
- Contact lens solutions
- Stains

Pharmacology deals with the basic properties of drugs, their actions, their fate in the human body, and their known side effects. This chapter deals primarily with some of the drugs that act on the eye, either directly by local application or indirectly by systemic absorption.

GENERAL PRINCIPLES
Locally applied medication

Ophthalmic preparations placed directly in the eye are available in solution, suspension, or ointment forms. Solutions usually are instilled in the conjunctival sac and do not interfere with vision. The main disadvantage is that their duration of contact with the eye is short, and therefore they require frequent instillation. Polymers often are added to solutions to enhance contact time. Although ointments remain in contact with the eye for prolonged periods, their tendency to reduce vision by creating a greasy film over the surface of the cornea limits their daily usefulness. Ointments frequently are used for bedtime therapy because of their prolonged contact time; in addition, they are less readily washed out with tears. The also are valuable for use in children who are crying (Table 4-1).

Preparations used in the eye have certain basic requirements regarding tolerance, tonicity, sterility, stability, and penetration.

Tolerance. Eye medications should cause minimal irritation or stinging to the eye. Tolerance of the medication by the eye depends on the solution's having an ideal acid-base balance. The acid-base balance is denoted in terms of its pH.

Solutions that have a pH greater than 7 are alkaline, whereas agents with a pH less than 7 are acid (for example, boric acid solution has a pH of 4.7). Most ophthalmic solutions have a pH that varies from 3.5 to 10.5. Any solution with a pH within this range causes minimal irritation to the eye (Fig. 4-1).

Tonicity. The tonicity of a solution refers to the concentration of the chemical in that solution. Normal saline solution, or a 0.9% sodium chloride equivalent, has a tonicity approximately that of tears and is therefore well tolerated by the eye. Solutions with a high concentration of a chemical, however, are hypertonic and thus can be quite irritating. On the other hand, solutions low in concentration of a chemical (hypotonic solutions), such as water, are equally objectionable in producing irritation to the

Table 4-1	Comparison of characteristics of ophthalmic solutions and ophthalmic ointments	
Characteristics	**Solutions**	**Ointments**
Instillation	Easier	More difficult
Contact time	Shorter	Longer (slower movement through the nasolacrimal drainage)
Irritation on installation	Frequent	Rare
Discharge retention	No	Yes
Skin allergic reactions	Few	More frequent
Blurred vision	No	Yes (film spreads over eye)
Local symptoms (burning, stinging)	More frequent	Less frequent
Readily contaminated (requires preservatives)	Yes	No
Stability a problem with storage	Yes	Less likely

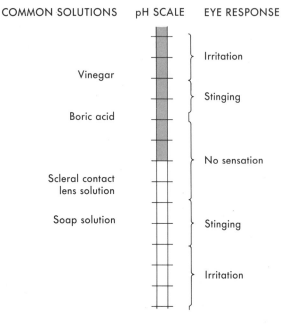

Fig. 4-1 The eye responds by stinging and irritation when the pH varies from 7. (Courtesy J. Krezanowski.)

eye. Ideally, the closer the concentration of the drug to normal tears (0.9% sodium chloride equivalent), the less irritating the drug will be. In some cases in which a high concentration of a locally applied drug is required, this ideal may not be achievable.

Sterility. Solutions must be free from bacterial contamination. This can be achieved either by autoclaving or by passing the solution through bacterial filters. Today most solutions are manufactured sterile by drug companies. To ensure sterility for long periods of time, preservatives usually are added. A good preservative should be well tolerated by the eye, nonallergenic, and inhibit the growth of bacteria and fungi. About 95% of all commercially available ophthalmic products are preserved with (1) benzalkonium chloride, (2) chlorobutanol, or (3) organic mercurials, chiefly thimerosal and phenylmercuric acetate. For eye surgery, however, the preservative drugs usually are eliminated to make the product less irritating to the open tissues. The solutions for eye surgery are available in sterile individual-dose units. For contact lens solutions, these preservatives often

are too toxic to the cornea, and less irritating preservatives are incorporated.

Once a sealed bottle is opened, it is no longer considered sterile. Organisms may enter an open bottle with ease. The most notorious organism found in ophthalmic solutions, including antibiotic drops, is *Pseudomonas aeruginosa,* which can destroy an eye in 48 hours. This organism's predilection for fluorescein solution has led to the development of dry fluorescein-impregnated paper, inasmuch as this organism cannot survive in a dry environment.

Stability. Solutions must be reasonably stable and not deteriorate or lose their effectiveness. Drugs such as phenylephrine hydrochloride (Neo-Synephrine) and epinephrine oxidize in the presence of air and bright light and consequently are often packaged in dark or opaque bottles. Some drugs require a special base to provide stability; for example, diisopropyl flurophosphate (DFP) solution is made up in anhydrous peanut oil because the drug is unstable in water. Eye ointments are prepared in either a petrolatum base or a water-soluble base because these bases have proved to be stable. Drugs such as oxytetracycline (Terramycin) and chloramphenicol (Chloromycetin), which are relatively unstable for any length of time in solution form, have a long shelf life in ointment form and generally are prepared this way.

Penetration. Eye drops penetrate the eye directly through the cornea and into the anterior chamber of the eye. They do not, however, penetrate far behind the crystalline lens and therefore cannot reach the back, or posterior portion, of the eye. The cornea acts as a barrier to many drops by virtue of the lipid content of its epithelium, which functions as a barrier to all medications not soluble in fat. Eye drops also must have water-soluble properties to penetrate the remaining portion of the cornea. Thus agents that penetrate the eye well are those that have both fat- and water-soluble properties.

Drugs penetrate the cornea better if they are instilled directly over its surface. When corneal penetration is of utmost importance, the patient should be asked to look down, and the drop should be placed above so that it will flow over the cornea.

Alternate routes of medication

Subconjunctival injections. Injections may be administered under the conjunctiva. The subconjunctival medication gains access to the eye by absorption into the blood stream by the episcleral and conjunctival vessels. Subconjunctival injections are used primarily in the treatment of intraocular infection.

Continuous-release delivery. The Ocusert permits continuous delivery of medication 24 hours a day for a full 7 days. A small membrane, sandwiching medication, is inserted in the lower conjunctiva by the patient, and it gradually releases its medication. Pilocarpine can be incorporated in the Ocusert and over a 7- to 8-day period steadily releases pilocarpine at a rate of $40/\mu g/hr$. Lacrisert provides a continuous release of hydroxypropyl cellulose for lubrication in patients with dry eyes.

Retrobulbar injections. Drugs may be administered by injecting medication through the skin of the lower lid, the point of the needle emerging behind the eyeball. Retrobulbar injections of a local anesthetic are employed routinely to paralyze the extraocular muscles and anesthetize the eye before commencement of intraocular surgery.

Systemic medication. The term *systemic drugs* refers to those drugs that are taken orally or by injection either subcutaneously (under the skin), intramuscularly (in the muscle), or intravenously (into the vein). When these routes of administration are chosen, it is usually because of some disease in the posterior part of the eye or orbit that cannot be reached by locally applied medication. In particular, conditions such as cellulitis, uveitis, and acute allergic reactions often require systemic medication.

COMPLICATIONS OF LOCALLY ADMINISTERED DRUGS
Allergic reactions

Many ophthalmic preparations can cause contact allergic reactions involving primarily the skin of the lids and the conjunctiva. Because hypersensitivity develops as a result of the patient's exposure to the agent, allergic reactions usually follow repeated application of the medication. Thus a delay in time occurs between the reaction to the use of a particular drug and the development of a state of hypersensitivity. This delay in time can be weeks, months, or years. This period is referred to as the *induction period*. Once the hypersensitivity state is established, further instillation of the agent serves only to aggravate the allergic response. In the skin, allergic reactions may consist of edema, redness, vesiculation, scaling, and oozing, depending on the patient's sensitivity. In the conjunctiva the most common reaction is either marked chemosis, or swelling, or low-grade congestion and redness of the conjunctival tissues. Differentiation should be made between an allergic response and an ocular irritation caused by the drug. Some patients with allergies complain of itchiness. In many cases, however, differentiation between the two can be made only by a smear of the discharge of the conjunctiva that reveals the typical cell of an allergic response, the eosinophil.

One of the most common ophthalmic preparations to cause allergic reactions of the skin of the eyelid

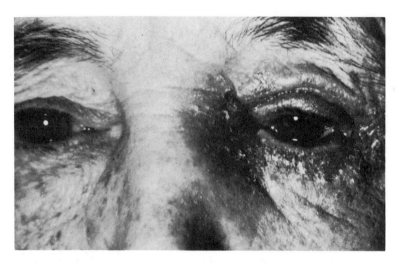

Fig. 4-2 Allergic reaction of the skin and conjunctiva to neomycin.

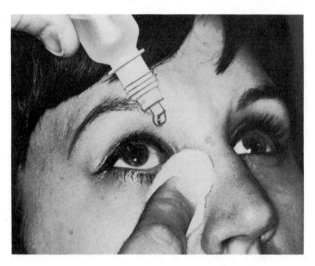

Fig. 4-3 Pressure over tear sac to prevent systemic absorption of medication.

is atropine. Of the antiobiotics, neomycin is most likely to create a hypersensitivity state and induce an allergic response (Fig. 4-2).

Toxic reactions

Some drugs can produce irreversible damage within the eye or cause systemic disturbances within the human body. Echothiophate iodide (Phospholine Iodide), used in glaucoma, can cause cataracts, iris cysts, and retinal detachments. If this drug is absorbed systemically in sufficient quantities, it may cause nausea, vomiting, diarrhea, bladder cramps, and cardiac irregularities. Systemic absorption of eye medication can be reduced by applying a cotton pledget over the lacrimal sac when instilling drops. This will prevent the drops from passing through the nasolacrimal duct to the back of the throat, where they are absorbed (Fig. 4-3).

Discoloration of the eye

Pigmentation of the conjunctiva may occur after the prolonged use of epinephrine, silver nitrate, or silver protein (Argyrol). Epinephrine causes black spots in the lower conjunctival sac. Silver protein produces a slate-silver discoloration of the conjunctiva.

Undesirable side effects

Some side effects may occur that are undesirable. For example, topically applied steroids can (1) raise the intraocular pressure and cause glaucoma, (2) potentiate the growth of viruses, which in herpes simplex infection can cause widespread corneal damage, (3) potentiate the growth of bacteria, and (4) cause delay in wound healing.

Pigmentary changes in the macula with loss of vision may occur in patients using chloroquine, phenothiazines, or indomethacin. Oral contraceptive agents may cause migrainelike syndromes, as well as retinal vascular occlusions. Cataracts can occur after the use of antiglaucoma medication such as echothiophate iodide.

Idiosyncrasy

An idiosyncrasy is a constitutional peculiarity in which an individual reacts in a bizarre fashion to a drug. For example, an unexpected reaction to cocaine may occur, and the person may develop tremors, motor excitability, or convulsions and may even collapse.

Loss of effect by inactivation

Some ophthalmic solutions may lose their potency if not stored properly. For example, epinephrine, if exposed to light and heat, turns brown and loses its effect. Patients receiving ephinephrine derivatives should be warned of this contingency and told to keep their eye drops in a cool, dark place, such as the refrigerator.

Spread of infection

In some offices, hospitals, or clinics, where a single bottle is used for a group of patients, the dropper can easily become contaminated. Consequently, infection may spread from patient to patient. This hazard can be eliminated by using small sterile dispos-

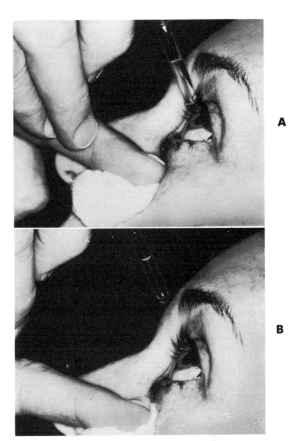

Fig. 4-4 Instillation of eye drops. **A,** Incorrect method. Note contamination of dropper by lashes. **B,** Correct method. Note tip of dropper is held free of globe and lashes.

able bottles of medication or by limiting the use of the eye drops or ointment to one individual. When eye drops are used, care must be exercised that the tip of the eyedropper does not touch the lashes or the eye, so that contamination of the dropper and the eye solution is avoided (Fig. 4-4).

PRESCRIPTION WRITING

Physicians use many symbols for writing prescriptions. These symbols provide a direct communication by the physician to the pharmacist. The use of Latin symbols today is an anachronism; yet several Latin symbols are retained because of tradition and

Table 4-2	Abbreviations and symbols used in prescription writing

Abbreviations or symbols	**Meaning**
℞	take thou
g	gram
h	hour (hora)
q	every
hs	bedtime (hora somni)
qs	quantity sufficient
od	right eye (oculus dexter)
os	left eye (oculus sinister)
ou	both eyes (oculus uterque)
mg	milligram
<	less than
>	greater than
aa	equal parts (ana)
Sol	solution
ung	ointment
ℨ	dram
℥	ounce
tsp	teaspoon
gt, gtt	drop, drops (gutta, guttae)
M	mix (misce)
bid	twice a day (bis in die)
tid	three times a day (ter in die)
qid	four times a day (quater in die)
q 4 h	every 4 hours
ac	before meals (ante cibum)
pc	after meals (post cibum)
non rep	do not repeat (not repetatur)
ad lib	as much as wanted (ad libitum)
ss	half (semis)
aq	water

for brevity (Table 4-2). Following is the format for prescription writing; the setup is shown in Fig. 4-5.

1. The patient's name, address, and date of prescription
2. The name of the drug and the percentage of concentration or the dosage of each unit (the drug usually is written out in full to avoid any confusion)
3. The amount of the drug to be supplied, headed by the symbol M, or Mitte, which signifies the quantity
4. Sig or S—from the Latin *signa,* "to mark," or in English, "label," which indicates to

Dr. John Doe

170 Bloor Street West
Cleveland, Ohio

Name: Miss J. White
Address: 227 Sankta Ave.

℞   Date: Jan. 4

Inscription: Diamox tab.

Subscription: M: 100

Signa: Sig.: Tab. t.i.d.

Signature: John Doe, M.D.

Repeat × 2

Fig. 4-5 Example of a prescription form.

the pharmacist what directions to label on the medicine
5. The signature of the physician
6. Possibly some notation at the bottom of the prescription, for example "may be repeated 2 times"

AUTONOMIC DRUGS

The body contains an involuntary nervous system, which is not under our direct control. This system acts to protect the body, provide nutrition and elimination, and carry on daily regulatory activity. The autonomic nervous system is affected by our emotional behavior. The typical "fear" reaction causes our pupils to dilate, our skin to sweat, and even our hair to stand on end.

The autonomic nervous system is subdivided into the *sympathetic* and *parasympathetic* nervous systems. Drugs that mimic the action of these two opposing types of involuntary nervous systems are said to be *sympathomimetic* and *parasympathomimetic,* respectively. Sympathomimetic drugs such as epinephrine and phenylephrine act directly on the end organ; they are sometimes called *adrenergic agents.* Parasympathomimetic drugs either act on the end

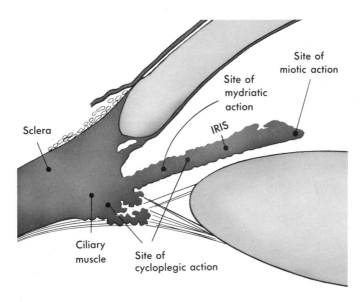

Fig. 4-6 Sites of action of mydriatic, cycloplegic, and miotic agents. Mydriatic drugs act on the dilator muscle of the iris. Cycloplegic drugs act by inhibiting the sphincter muscle of the iris and by paralyzing the ciliary muscle. Miotic drugs act by stimulating the sphincter muscle of the iris, causing the pupil to constrict.

organ in a manner similar to that of acetylcholine or interfere with the action of the enzyme *cholinesterase,* which destroys the acetylcholine normally produced in the tissues. Pilocarpine acts directly on the end organ, whereas eserine, DFP, and echothiophate iodide represent inhibitors of cholinesterase. Some drugs act on the end organ to block the action of the parasympathetic system; they are called *parasympatholytic (cholinergic blocking) agents.* Atropine, homatropine, and cyclopentolate are representative of this group.

Autonomic drugs that affect the eyes are divided into mydriatic, cycloplegic, and miotic agents, which comprise most of the commonly used eye medications.

Mydriatic and cycloplegic agents

Mydriatic drops act on the iris musculature and serve to dilate the pupils. Cycloplegic drops act not only on the iris by dilating the pupil but also on the ciliary body, paralyzing the fine focusing muscles so that the eye is no longer able to accommodate for near vision (Fig. 4-6). Cycloplegic drops are essential in the refraction of children's eyes and for iritis therapy. Mydriatic agents are primarily employed to dilate the pupil for intraocular examinations.

Mydriatic agents. Mydriatic agents with little or no cycloplegic effect are phenylephrine, hydroxyamphetamine, eucatropine, epinephrine, and cocaine.

Phenylephrine hydrochloride (Neo-Synephrine) ranges in strength from 0.25% to 10%. The latter exerts a rapid dilating effect in about 15 minutes and wears off in 1 to 2 hours. Adverse responses with 10% topical phenylephrine have been reported occurring within 20 minutes of the last application of this drug. Some of these patients were treated with a cotton pledget of the drug, some by subconjunctival injection, and others by irrigation of the lacrimal sac. A number of deaths have resulted from myocardial infarction, and some persons have required cardiac and pulmonary resuscitation for treatment of cardiac arrest. Another group of patients had a marked rise in blood pressure, tachycardia (fast heart), or reflex bradycardia (slowing of the heart). The local ocular reaction reported was massive subjunctival hemorrhage.

This drug should be used very cautiously or not at all in patients with heart disease, hypertension, aneurysm, or advanced atherosclerosis. Only the 2.5% solution should be used in elderly persons and in infants. The 10% solution should not be used for irrigation. When the drug is used, a cotton pledget should be held over the lacrimal sac for 1 to 2 minutes. Patients who are taking antidepressants or monoamine oxidase (MAO) inhibitors should be treated with caution. The heart rate may be significantly increased in patients who are taking these drugs.

Phenylephrine is used most commonly as an adjunct to the parasympatholytic drugs—for example, tropicamide (Mydriacyl) and cyclopentolate (Cyclopal)—to dilate the pupil for ophthalmoscopy. Despite these large and serious complications with 10% phenylephrine, no serious adverse effects have been reported with the ophthalmic use of 2.5% phenylephrine hydrochloride.

Hydroxyamphetamine (Paredrine) produces mydriasis slowly, taking 30 to 45 minutes to exert its effect. It is used primarily in Horner's syndrome, a disorder of the sympathetic nervous system that manifests by a unilateral small pupil (miosis) and ptosis. The drug can be used to determine the approximate site of the lesion in the sympathetic pathway.

Epinephrine (Adrenalin) exerts a mild mydriatic effect.

Cocaine is primarily a strong anesthetic agent but also exerts a mild mydriatic effect. It can be used to establish the diagnosis of Horner's syndrome. It allows one to determine whether a small pupil is part of this syndrome or whether it is due to other causes such as a congenital asymmetry of pupil size (physiologic anisocoria).

The drugs that act as pure mydriatic agents exert their effect by stimulating the dilator muscle of the iris.

Cycloplegic agents. Cycloplegic agents act (1) by paralyzing the sphincter muscle of the iris and thereby producing iris dilation and (2) by paralyzing the ciliary muscle, which inactivates accommodation. Examples of cycloplegic agents are atropine, homatropine, hyoscine, cyclopentolate, and tropicamide.

Atropine ranges from 0.5% to 2% in strength and is one of the most powerful cycloplegic and mydriatic agents. After atropine has been instilled in an adult eye, it requires 10 to 14 days for accommodation to return and the pupil to return to its normal size. With children the local effects on the eye are similar, but systemic complications are more common. The side effects of systemic absorption in children consist of rapid pulse, fever, flushing, and mouth dryness. Systemic absorption of atropine can be reduced by applying pressure over the lacrimal sac. Atropine may cause allergic manifestations in the form of an eczematoid rash around the eye and conjunctival injection. Parents should be instructed in the method of giving the drops and in observing for signs of local or systemic toxicity. Adverse reactions should be reported immediately to the ophthalmologist's office so that proper steps can be taken.

Homatropine is a weaker cycloplegic that varies in strength from 2% to 5%. Its effect wears off faster than atropine, and accommodation returns in 1 to 3 days.

Hyoscine (scopolamine) is midway between atropine and homatropine in duration of action. Hyoscine produces fewer allergic responses than atropine and thus is used as a substitute for it.

Cyclopentolate (Cyclogyl, Mydplegic) is available in strengths of 0.5%, 1%, and 2%. It has a rapid onset of effect (30 minutes) and a short duration of action (3 to 6 hours), which make it an ideal agent for office use. Occasionally children can show signs of systemic toxicity not unlike that seen with atropine.

Tropicamide (Mydriacyl), 0.5% to 1%, exerts its effects in 50 to 20 minutes, and wears off in 1 hour. It is a relatively weak agent for paralyzing accommodation and is used primarily for its dilating ability when ophthalmoscopic examination is required.

Cycloplegics are employed in the treatment of iritis to relieve ciliary muscle spasm and produce pupillary dilation. The latter is important in preventing the iris from binding down to the lens to form posterior synechiae. These agents are commonly used to inactivate the ciliary muscle for the purpose of objective refraction (Table 4-3). The eyes

Table 4-3	Routines for common cycloplegic agents	
Drug	**Strength**	**Frequency**
Atropine	Under 2 yr, 0.5%	Under 5 yr, three times daily for 3 days before examination
	Over 2 yr, 1%	
Homatropine	2% to 5%	One drop every 15 min for four applications 1 hr before examination
Cyclopentolate	0.5%, 1%, and 2%	One drop every 5 min for two applications 30 min before examination
Tropicamide	0.5% to 1%	One drop every 5 min for two applications 20 min before examination

of darkly pigmented persons dilate with difficulty and hence require stronger concentrations and repeated instillations to obtain an adequate effect. Drugs such as atropine and homatropine are not used routinely in adult eye refraction because of the prolonged delay in accommodation and pupillary function.

Miotics

Miotics act by stimulating the sphincter muscle of the iris, which in turn causes constriction of the pupil (see Fig. 4-6). These agents are used in (1) the treatment of open-angle glaucoma because they improve the outflow of aqueous humor from the anterior chamber of the eye, (2) angle-closure glaucoma because they withdraw the congestion of iris tissue from the angle structures, (3) the management of convergent strabismus by reducing accommodative effort (used in place of glasses especially for children younger than the age of 2 years), and (4) the treatment of accommodative insufficiency, in which they may play a small role.

Direct-acting miotics. *Pilocarpine nitrate* and *pilocarpine hydrochloride* may range in strength from 0.25% to 10% and have a duration of action of 4 to 6 hours. Pilocarpine is a stable, inexpensive, and reliable drug. The local side effects may consist of (1) ciliary spasm, which may produce a headache, especially in young patients, (2) decreased vision in patients with cataracts inasmuch as the pupil is made smaller, which allows less light to enter the eye, (3) allergic or toxic reactions that involve the lids and conjunctiva. Systemic side effects are uncommon. Pilocarpine is most commonly used in the chronic-care management of open-angle glaucoma and acute-care treatment of angle-closure glaucoma.

Carbachol ranges in strength from 0.75% to 3% and has a slightly longer duration of action than does pilocarpine. It is absorbed poorly through the cornea and usually is prescribed for patients who are allergic to pilocarpine or for those whose condition cannot be adequately controlled by pilocarpine.

Cholinesterase inhibitors. Cholinesterase inhibitors are drugs that inactivate an enzyme in the body called *cholinesterase*. As a result, another chemical, called *acetylcholine,* normally inactivated by cholinesterase, is freely permitted to exert its effects. The effect of acetylcholine is similar to that of the direct-acting miotics.

Eserine (physostigmine) is found in strengths from 0.25% to 0.5%. It is used more frequently in the ointment form because drops are unstable and irritating to the eye. It is a fairly powerful miotic and frequently is combined with pilocarpine in resistant cases of glaucoma. There is a high incidence of allergy to eserine. Combinations of miotics generally are not recommended. However, the combination of pilocarpine and eserine medication sometimes is advocated because these two drugs are able to reinforce each other.

Isoflurophate (Floropryl), or *DFP,* because it is inactivated in water, usually is supplied in either an anhydrous peanut oil or an ointment form. It is an extremely powerful agent employed to control the intraocular pressure if other miotics fail.

Demecarium bromide (Humorsol), 0.25%, has properties similar to DFP and requires similar application.

Echothiophate iodide (Phospholine Iodide), 0.06% to 0.25%, is a powerful and long-acting agent. It has been shown to produce cataracts and iris cysts with prolonged usage. It should be kept refrigerated because it deteriorates at room temperature.

Side effects. The long-acting anticholinesterase agents are the most likely to produce side effects both locally (in the eye) and systemically. *Local effects* include (1) ocular discomfort and pain resulting from ciliary body spasm (most apparent during initial phase of treatment, usually subsiding as treatment continues), (2) induced myopia with blurred vision for distance, (3) cataracts, (4) retinal detachment, and (5) iris cysts. *Systemic effects* include (1) headaches, (2) sweating and salivation, (3) nausea, vomiting, and diarrhea, (4) lethargy and fatigue, and (5) cardiac arrest and fall in blood pressure.

DRUGS THAT LOWER INTRAOCULAR PRESSURE

The introduction of *timolol maleate* (Timoptic) has directed a new program of research toward pharmaceutical agents that do not affect the pupil or accommodation. Timolol is a nonselective beta-adrenergic receptor blocker that acts to decrease the formation of aqueous humor. The drug is available in 0.25% and 0.5% strengths, and dosage ranges from 1 drop daily to 1 drop twice daily with or without other antiglaucomatous medication. Adverse reactions generally are uncommon, but if they are present and significant, they may lead one to discontinue the medication. Ocular side effects include corneal anesthesia, a punctate keratopathy, and an allergic blepharoconjunctivitis. Systemic reactions consist of bronchospasm in those with underlying pulmonary disease, bradycardia, hypotension, central nervous system disturbances (for example, confusion and hallucinations), and gastrointestinal disturbances (for example, nausea and diarrhea). It should be used with caution in patients with known contraindications to systemic use of beta-adrenergic receptor blocking agents, such as patients with obstructive pulmonary disease (for example, asthma and emphysema) and cardiovascular disease (for example, congestive heart failure, bradycardia, heart block, and hypotension). Because of its excellent therapeutic response, its low frequency of application, and its generally uncommon adverse reactions, timolol has gained widespread use in the ophthalmic community.

In an attempt to decrease the systemic side effects so that it can be used in patients with asthma and emphysema, *betaxolol* (Betoptic), a selective β-blocker, was developed. Although fewer pulmonary effects are seen with this drug, they have not been totally eliminated. In addition, the fall in intraocular pressure is not as great with betaxolol as with timolol, a nonselective β-blocker.

A sympathomimetic agent, dipivalyl epinephrine (Propine) is available in a 0.1% concentration for application of 1 drop twice daily. The drug has 17 times greater penetration through the cornea than epinephrine alone; therefore the amount that has to be administered to achieve a similar therapeutic response is significantly less. This reduces the systemic side effects, which may include an elevation in blood pressure, tachycardia, and headache. Ocular side effects may consist of an allergic blepharoconjunctivitis, a punctate keratopathy, and cystoid macular edema. The latter condition is seen in aphakic patients and has been reported to occur in up to 30%. The macular edema is reversible when the medication is discontinued.

The drug armamentarium against glaucoma has been greatly aided by the use of drugs, taken orally or intravenously, that lower the intraocular pressure. Those commonly used are the carbonic anhydrase inhibitors, glycerol, urea, and mannitol.

The *carbonic anhydrase inhibitors* block the formation of aqueous humor and thereby lower the intraocular pressure. Examples include acetazolamide (Diamox), 250-mg tablets; ethoxzolamide (Cardrase, Ethamide), 125-mg tablets; dichlorphenamide (Oratrol, Daranide), 50-mg tablets; and methazolamide (Neptazane), 50-mg tablets. *Side effects* of these drugs are (1) numbness and tingling of the hands, feet, and tongue, (2) drowsiness and fatigue, (3) kidney stones, (4) gastrointestinal upsets (nausea and vomiting), (5) mild skin eruptions, and (6) blood disturbances.

Glycerol is a thick, viscous liquid given in a dosage of 1 to 1.5 ml per kilogram of body weight and is used to lower the intraocular pressure in acute narrow-angle glaucoma and before intraocular surgery. Because of its overly sweet taste, it is mixed with orange juice or lemon juice to make it more palatable. It can cause nausea, vomiting, or headaches.

Urea is a solution administered intravenously in a dosage of 1 to 1.5 g per kilogram of body weight at the rate of 60 drops per minute. It is employed to quickly reduce the intraocular pressure in acute narrow-angle glaucoma. Its main side effect is its tendency to produce phlebitis and sloughing of the skin if the needle penetrates outside the vein and the solution extravasates into the tissue.

Mannitol is administered intravenously in 20% solution, with a total dosage of 2 g per kilogram of body weight given over a period of 30 to 45 minutes. It is used interchangeably with urea. Along with urea and glycerol, mannitol has a large molecular structure that draws fluid out of the eye and other tissues into the vascular tree of the body.

ANESTHETICS
Topical anesthetics

Topical anesthetics in drop or ointment form are applied directly to the eye to abolish corneal sensation. Surface anesthesia of the cornea permits the application of instruments such as the tonometer for the measurement of intraocular pressure. Topical anesthetics also are used to perform surgery on the eye, remove foreign bodies, and facilitate examination with lenses such as the goniolens. Cocaine, the prototype of the group, is a naturally occurring drug. The remainder of topical anesthetics are synthetic. Commonly employed topical anesthetics are proparacaine hydrochloride (Ophthaine, Ophthetic), 0.5%; tetracaine hydrochloride (Pontocaine), 0.5%; cocaine, 2% to 5%; benoxinate hydrochloride (Dorsacaine), 0.4%; and butacaine sulfate (Butyn), 2%. The suffix "-caine" appended to the name of the drug usually indicates that the drug is an anesthetic.

An inflamed eye is much more difficult to anesthetize because the blood vessels carry away the anesthetic. For mild anesthesia, such as tonometry, 1 or 2 drops are sufficient, but to remove a foreign body deeply embedded in the cornea, more drops may be required at 1-minute intervals.

To avoid a self-inflicted corneal abrasion it is important that the patient be cautioned against rubbing the eye for a short period after topical anesthesia.

Side effects. Local anesthetics are capable of producing contact allergy. Some anesthetics, such as butacaine, have fallen into disfavor because of a frequent tendency to produce allergic reactions. Side effects do occur but are minimal with proparacaine and tetracaine, but cocaine has significant side effects, including (1) irregularities in the corneal epithelium, (2) restlessness and delirium, (3) irregular respiration, chills, and fever, (4) convulsions, and (5) cardiovascular disorders. Toxic reactions to cocaine result from central nervous system stimulation and may require the rapid administration of a short-acting sedative to counteract them.

Injectable anesthetics

Local anesthetics by injection are used in ophthalmology to produce (1) anesthesia of the globe, (2) anesthesia of the eyelid, (3) paralysis of the muscles that move the eye and the eyelid, and (4) paralysis of the facial muscles. Commonly used agents are procaine hydrochloride (Novocain), 1% to 4%; lidocaine hydrochloride (Xylocaine), 0.5% to 4%; and prilocaine hydrochloride (Citanest), 1% to 3%. These agents may be combined with epinephrine, which constricts the blood vessels. The purpose of producing vasoconstriction is to reduce the vascularity of tissues and minimize bleeding. These agents also reduce the amount of local anesthetic absorbed by the blood vessels, thereby prolonging the duration of anesthesia. In addition, local anesthetics may be combined with hyaluronidase, which spreads the anesthetic throughout the tissues, thereby producing more prompt and widespread anesthesia.

Side effects. Injectable anesthetic agents may cause (1) depression of blood pressure, (2) depression of respiration, (3) stimulation of the central nervous system, leading to nervousness, dizzy spells, nausea, and convulsions, and (4) depression of the central nervous system, leading to respiratory or circulatory collapse.

Management of toxic side effects

The ophthalmic assistant should be prepared to render assistance to meet the contingency of a reaction to a local anesthetic.

Fainting. The patient who faints should be placed with the head between the knees. A tight collar should be loosened. Smelling salts or spirits of ammonia should be given to help revive the patient. After a fainting spell the patient usually is quite dizzy and unsteady. It is wise to have the patient remain in the office an additional 20 to 30 mintues to regain composure.

Central nervous system stimulation. If tremors or convulsions occur, the ophthalmic assistant should attempt to restrain the patient to avoid self-injury. Again, encumbrances around the neck should be loosened. If the ophthalmologist decides to give the patient diazepam (Valium) to control the reaction, this should be available and ready to use.

Respiratory emergency. A patient who has difficulty in breathing should be watched carefully. If respiration ceases, artificial resuscitation may become necessary. Today, mouth-to-mouth resuscitation is the treatment of choice. *HIV* precautions should be adhered to.

Allergic reaction. Severe allergic reactions or idiosyncrasies to drugs may occur that require immediate specific therapy. This is particularly important to the ophthamologist in view of the increasing number of surgical procedures and fluorescein angiographic examinations being performed in the physician's office. Any patient developing generalized itching, a skin rash, difficulty breathing, and/or a rapid and weak pulse after administration of a drug should be considered as having an allergic reaction. Once an acute allergic reaction is suspected, prompt treatment is indicated: (1) adrenaline injected subcutaneously or intramuscularly, (2) oxygen, (3) corticosteroids injected intravenously, and (4) tracheostomy for laryngeal edema for responding to the aforementioned methods.

The ophthalmic assistant should know where to immediately procure and have available for the ophthalmologist (1) oxygen, (2) epinephrine, (3) diazepam, (4) intravenous cortisone, (5) spirits of ammonia or smelling salts, and (6) syringes with needles.

ANTIALLERGIC AND ANTIINFLAMMATORY AGENTS
Corticosteroids

Corticosteroids are hormones that either are derived from the adrenal gland or are synthetically produced. Cortisone was the first hormone to be isolated. Other steroid preparations are modifications of cortisone, developed to improve and minimize their side effects. For diseases of the eye, steroids are used primarily because they reduce the inflammatory and exudative reaction of diseased tissues. In this regard they are invaluable because they reduce swelling, redness, cellular reaction, and the final stage of tissue repair, scarring.

Steroids may be given topically or systemically (Table 4-4). Topical steroids generally are used for disorders involving the anterior segment of the eye. Systemic steroids are employed for diseases of the posterior segment of the eye and acute allergic reactions of the eyelids (Table 4-5).

Although steroids are useful in a large variety of ocular conditions, they must be administered with good indication, by the proper route (Table 4-6), and under the supervision of a physician. These precautions are necessary because of the sinister complications of these agents both in the eye and in the body (Table 4-7).

If a patient is receiving steroids, the ophthalmic assistant should inquire into his or her medical background. Patients with conditions of diabetes, hypertension, tuberculosis, and peptic ulcers, if given steroids systemically, often will have an exacerbation of their disease.

Table 4-4	Topical steroid preparations
Drug	**Concentration (%)**
Cortisone acetate suspension	0.5
Cortisone acetate ointment	1.5
Hydrocortisone acetate suspension	0.5, 2.5
Hydrocortisone acetate ointment	1.5
Prednisolone acetate	0.12, 1
Prednisolone phosphate	0.5
Dexamethasone phosphate	0.1
Dexamethasone ointment	0.5
Betamethasone solution	0.5

Steroid therapy is used in the following eye diseases:

Contact dermatitis of the eyelids and conjunctiva
Blepharitis
Phlyctenular conjunctivitis and keratitis
Ocular pemphigus
Vernal conjunctivitis
Acne rosacea keratitis
Interstitial keratitis
Sclerosing keratitis
Chemical burns of the cornea and conjunctiva
Marginal corneal ulcers
Iritis
Iridocyclitis
Most forms of posterior uveitis
Sympathetic ophthalmia
Herpes zoster ophthalmicus
Scleritis and episcleritis

Table 4-5   Systemic steroids commonly used and their equivalent dose

Drug	Dose (mg)
Cortisone acetate	25
Hydrocortisone	20
Prednisone	5
Prednisolone	5
Triamcinolone	4
Methylprednisolone	4
Paramethasone	2
Dexamethasone	0.75
Betamethasone	0.5

Table 4-6   Common routes of steroid administration for ocular inflammation

Condition	Route
Conjunctivitis	Topical
Blepharitis	Topical
Episcleritis	Topical
Keratitis	Topical
Scleritis	Topical and systemic
Anterior uveitis	Topical and subconjunctival
Posterior uveitis	Systemic and subconjunctival
Endophthalmitis	Systemic and subconjunctival
Optic neuritis	Systemic
Temporal arteritis	Systemic
Sympathetic ophthalmia	Systemic and topical

Table 4-7   Side effects of steroids

Ocular effects		Systemic effects
From local application	**From prolonged systemic use**	
Glaucoma	Decreased resistance to infection	Water and salt retention
Proliferation of bacteria	Delayed wound healing	Mental disturbance
Overgrowth of fungi	Papilledema	Hypertension
Proliferation of viruses, especially herpes simplex	Edema of face and eyelids	Sweating
Decreased wound healing	Cataracts	Generalized weakness
Cataracts	Glaucoma	Wasting of skeletal muscles
		Demineralization of bone
		Thrombophlebitis
		Delayed wound healing
		Bleeding problems
		Menstrual irregularities
		Acne
		Increased blood glucose level and diabetes mellitus
		Decreased resistance to infection
		Growth retardation in children

Pseudotumor of the orbit
Temporal arteritis
Optic neuritis

Antiinfective preparations

There are three large families of antiinfective preparations: (1) antibiotics, (2) antiviral agents, and (3) antifungal agents.

Antibiotics. Antibiotics are chemical substances that have the capacity to inhibit growth of bacteria and other microorganisms. Some antibiotics act by inhibiting bacterial growth and are called *bacteriostatic agents,* whereas others act by directly killing bacteria and are therefore called *bacteriocidal agents*.

Bacteriocidal agents commonly in use are penicillin, streptomycin, polymyxin B, bacitracin, neomycin, vancomycin, colistin, and ampicillin. Bacteriostatic agents in common use include tetracycline, chloramphenicol, erythromycin, novobiocin, sulfonamides, spiramycin, and amphotericin B.

Ideally an antibiotic should be selected when the organism responsible for the infection is identified and its sensitivity to antibiotics established. However, it is impractical to withhold therapy in all cases until cultures are made and sensitivity is determined. Early treatment is as important as selecting the right drug for the offending agent. Therefore most ophthalmologists employ broad-spectrum antibiotics for treatment of infections about the eyes until cultures and smears have been made and sensitivity has been determined.

Many patients are seen in an ophthalmologist's office with an unresolved bacterial infection of the eye because of indiscriminate use of antibiotics. Often the infective component clears, but a hypersensitivity develops to the very medication the patient is industriously pouring into the eye. The more medication into the eye, the worse the situation becomes. Hypersensitivity reactions from antibiotics most commonly occur in the use of compounds that contain neomycin, but they also result from the use of sulfa derivatives.

Another complication in the treatment of bacterial infection of the eye results from *inadequate dosage* and *infrequency of administration* of antibiotics. Antibiotics are given only occasionally by the systemic route for the treatment of ocular infections inasmuch as greater concentrations of the drug can be achieved topically or subconjunctivally. With topical administration, drops are preferred to ointments because drops do not retain the discharge or interfere with vision. Many infections, however, persist because antibiotic drops are not given frequently enough.

Topical antibiotics chosen for ocular infections are those with a wide spectrum of activity and those that are seldom used systemically. The advantage of these broad-spectrum antibiotics is that they provide complete coverage and minimize the dangers of hypersensitivity reactions. Antibiotics such as neomycin, bacitracin, and polymyxin B frequently are employed because they affect gram-positive and gram-negative bacteria but rarely are used systemically because of their undesirable side effects.

Continuous indiscriminate use of antibiotic drops may lead to the development of resistant strains of bacteria. Also, other strains of bacteria may proliferate if they do not fall within the sensitivity spectrum of the drops employed.

Antibiotics systemically become necessary when the internal or deeper structures of the eye or adjacent tissue are invaded by bacteria. Conditions such as endophthalmitis or orbital cellulitis or chorioretinitis may require judicious use of systemic antibiotics.

Systemic antibiotics, however, can cause serious side effects (Table 4-8). Chloramphenicol (Chloromycetin) can give rise to bone marrow depression, aplastic anemia, and even death. Myasthenia-like syndromes, with induced weakness resembling myasthenia gravis, may occur with streptomycin, neomycin, kanamycin, polymyxin, bacitracin, and colistin. Skin rashes may occur because of allergic reactions to the penicillin group of antibiotics, and on rare occasions, severe serum sickness, angioneurotic edema, and even death may result. Allergy to penicillin can involve as much as 5% of the population.

Sulfonamides have a wide spectrum of activity and are effective against some of the larger viruslike agents as well as bacteria. Hypersensitivity reactions

Table 4-8	Some adverse effects of systemically administered antimicrobial drugs
Drug	**Possible toxic effect**
Ampicillin	Anaphylactic reactions
Chloramphenicol	Bone marrow depression; aplastic anemia
Clindamycin	Pseudomembranous colitis
Erythromycin	Stomatitis; gastrointestinal disturbance
Gentamicin	Hearing defect and kidney damage
Methicillin	Allergic reactions; rarely bone marrow depression and renal damage
Nafcillin	Similar to those of methicillin
Oxacillin	Similar to those of methicillin
Penicillin	Allergic reactions; rash; diarrhea
Sulfisoxazole	Allergic reactions, bone marrow depression
Sulfacetamide	Similiar to those of sulfisoxazole

to sulfa may be quite severe, and patients should be questioned about any previous history of allergy to this drug before its use.

The most commonly used topical sulfonamides are (1) sulfisoxazole (Gantrisin solution, 4%, and Gantrisin ointment) and (2) sulfacetamide sodium (Sulamyd Sodium, 10%, 30%; Bleph, 10%; Isopto Cetamide, 15%; Vasosulf).

Antiviral agents. The first antiviral agent, 5-iodo-2'-deoxyuridine, has been invaluable in the treatment of herpes simplex infections of the cornea. This drug, like the other antivirals, interferes with deoxyribonucleic acid (DNA) synthesis of the virus to produce a virus that cannot function as an infective agent. This drug frequently is referred to as *idoxyuridine (IDU),* or its manufacturing trade names of Herplex or Stoxil may be used.

IDU is used topically for the treatment of herpes simplex and vaccinia keratitis. It is of greatest benefit against the epithelial forms of herpes simplex infections. No serious side effects or contraindications are known in the use of IDU as an ophthalmic solution. This drug is given by instilling 1 drop in the affected eye every hour during the day and every 2 hours during the night until the lesion has cleared. This drug should be stored in a cool place.

Vidarabine (Vira-A) is an antiviral ophthalmic ointment, specifically for herpes simplex. It is useful for early cases of herpes simplex of the cornea and can be used as well in cases of herpes resistant to IDU. It does not appear to have any effect on other viruses.

Trifluorothymidine (TFT), or trifluridine (Viroptic), is an antiviral agent used in the treatment of herpes simplex keratitis. It is available as a 1% solution, and the usual dosing schedule is a frequency of every 2 hours the patient is awake. TFT has been shown to effectively heal 97% of ulcers and to be highly effective in treating diseases resistant to IDU and adenine arabinoside (ara-A), or vidarabine. The drug's characteristics of penetration into the cornea and anterior chamber have been shown to be superior to those of other antivirals; therefore TFT may be the drug of choice in complicated cases.

Acyclovir (Zovirax) is the newest antiviral agent that is administered in an oral form. The drug can be metabolized only in cells that have been infected by the herpes virus, and therefore uninfected human cells will not be affected by the drug. Acyclovir has been shown to be effective in shortening the course of disease in herpes zoster (shingles) and in severe cases of herpes simplex.

Antifungal agents. Fungal infections of the eye are uncommon, but when they occur, they can be devastating, especially when treatment is delayed. Antifungal agents generally act by binding to the fungal cell wall. This leads to changes in permeability that result in death of the organism. The most commonly used antifungal agents include the following four. (1) *Natamycin,* or pimaricin, is available in a 5% suspension. Because this drug penetrates tissues very poorly, it is useful only when applied topically. (2) *Miconazole* (Monistat) is available in a 0.1% to 1.0% solution and can be administered topically, subconjunctivally, or intravenously. (3) *Amphotericin B* also can be administered by the same three routes as miconazole. The drug is highly irritating when used topically and may be toxic to the kidneys when adminstered intravenously.

Use of this drug should be reserved for severe infections or resistant organisms. (4) *Ketoconazole* is available for oral administration. Unlike amphotericin, however, it is generally well tolerated. Significant adverse reactions include liver toxicity.

Decongestants

Decongestants are solutions that shrink the size of the conjunctival blood vessels and in doing so eliminate excess redness of the eye. These solutions are used to provide symptomatic relief of eye irritation and watering caused by hay fever, smog, and smoke and to relieve eye fatigue resulting from driving, excessive reading, and close work.

Some common decongestants are phenylephrine (Zincfrin solution, Prefrin, Neo-Synephrine, Isopto Frin), tetrahydrozoline (Visine), and naphazoline (Vasocon, Privine).

CONTACT LENS SOLUTIONS

With the proliferation of contact lens solutions, three important factors should be considered in choosing a system: safety, efficacy, and cost. Most contact lens solutions contain more than 95% water. The solution formation depends on the addition of preservatives, wetting agents, buffers, surfactants, cleaners, and disinfectants.

Contact lens requirements call for disinfection but not sterilization; although the incidence of eye infection from contact lenses is low relative to millions of wearers, the hazard is always present. Sterilization is the complete destruction of all forms of microbial activity. Disinfection is the destruction of all vegetative bacterial cells but does not include spores. Common contact lens solution preservatives include organomercurials (for example, thimerisal, chlorhexedine, and ethylenediaminetetraacetic acid [EDTA]).

STAINS

Fluorescein is an ocular stain used to show defects or abrasions in the corneal epithelium. The pooling of fluorescein on small corneal defects is best seen by means of ultraviolet or cobalt blue light for illumination. The danger with this agent in solution form is contamination with *Pseudomonas aeruginosa (Bacillus pyocyaneus),* which appears to flourish in fluorescein. Sterile dry fluorostrips are available commercially to prevent this complication. High-molecule fluorescein has been used with soft contact lenses. The high molecule of fluorescein does not penetrate the pore structure of the soft lens and consequently does not ruin the contact lens during examination.

Rose bengal is a red dye that has an affinity for degenerating epithelium. Similar to fluorescein, it will stain areas in which the epithelium has been sloughed off. Unlike fluorescein, however, intact nonviable epithelial cells of the conjunctiva or cornea will stain brightly with rose bengal. The stain is helpful in making the diagnosis of keratoconjunctivitis sicca or other conditions associated with dryness of the conjunctiva and cornea.

QUESTIONS FOR REVIEW AND THOUGHT

1. What is meant by pH? What effect does it have on the patient's acceptance of a drug?
2. How can sterility of a drug be achieved?
3. What is the role of preservatives, and which are the commonly used preservatives?
4. What are the common routes of giving medication to obtain an effect on the eye?
5. What is meant by allergy?
6. How can contamination of eye drops and spread of infection from eye drops in the office or hospital be eliminated?
7. Write out typical prescriptions for phenylephrine eye drops, for acetazolamide tablets, and for atropine ointment.
8. What is the action of cycloplegic drugs? How does it differ from that of mydriatic drugs?

9. List some mydriatic and cycloplegic agents.
10. Name some clinical uses for miotic agents.
11. Name some systemic drugs that lower intraocular pressure.
12. Name some side effects of cortisone therapy.
13. Without referring to the text, list as many clinical uses for cortisone medication to the eyes as you can.
14. What is IDU used for?
15. What is the principal action of decongestants? Why do they "whiten" the eye?
16. Corticosteroids act to suppress inflammation. Name some topical steroid drops.
17. What topical drugs are most prone to create ocular allergies?
18. What are the side effects of giving atropine ointment to children?
19. Which ocular drugs require refrigeration?
20. What are the side effects of pilocarpine?
21. What are some of the side effects of acetazolamide?

SELF-EVALUATION QUESTIONS

True-false statements

Directions: Indicate whether the statement is true (T) or false (F).

T or F 1. Eye drops penetrate the eye directly through the cornea and anterior chamber of the eye.

T or F 2. Topical medication applied directly to the eye may be absorbed into the body system and produce side effects.

T or F 3. Cycloplegic agents paralyze the sphincter muscle of the iris but do not interfere with the ciliary muscle.

Missing words

Directions: Write in the missing word in the following sentences.

4. Echothiophate iodide (Phospholine Iodide), which is used in glaucoma, belongs to the class of _____ inhibitors, which inactivate the enzyme in the body called _____.

5. The pupil dilates poorly with cycloplegics in those patients with darkly pigmented irises and in those persons with any of the following medical conditions: _____.

6. Another name for epinephrine is _____.

Choice-completion questions

Directions: Select the one best answer in each case.

7. The tonicity of an ophthalmic solution refers to the:
   a. Concentration of the chemical in the solution
   b. Acid-base balance as noted by the pH
   c. Sterility as noted by the level of contamination
   d. Stability of the solution
   e. Solubility of fats

8. In which of the following are steroids *not* administered systemically?
   a. Blepharitis
   b. Uveitis
   c. Endophthalmitis
   d. Optic neuritis
   e. Cranial or temporal arteritis

9. Which of the following agents are capable of controlling the herpes simplex organism?
   a. Chloramphenicol
   b. Garamycin
   c. Trifluridine (Viroptic)
   d. Homatropine
   e. Fluorescein

ANSWERS, NOTES, AND EXPLANATIONS

1. **True.** Eye medication in drop form penetrates directly through the cornea by first passing through the epithelium, which acts as a barrier to most medications that are insoluble in fat. The drops must then have water-soluble properties to penetrate the remaining portion of the cornea. Thus agents that penetrate the eye well are those that have both fat- and water-soluble properties. Consequently, manufacturers have designed bases for solutions that will permit the penetration of these drops through the cornea into the anterior chamber of the eye. Eye drops do not, however, penetrate far behind the crystalline lens of the eye and therefore do not reach the posterior portion of the globe.

2. **True.** A small quantity of drops may be absorbed through the conjunctival vessels, but a large portion may pass through the nasal lacrimal duct system and be absorbed by the nasal mucosa directly into the blood stream. The flush that is often produced when atropine is used in small children is a direct result of the systemic absorption of this drug. Pressure over the lacrimal sac with a cotton ball during the instillation of eye drops often will prevent the passage of the drops into the nasal lacrimal system and thus prevent systemic absorption of eye medication.

3. **False.** Cycloplegic agents such as homatropine, atropine, and cyclopentolate paralyze the sphincter muscle of the iris, which dilates the pupil, and the ciliary muscle, which inactivates accommodation. Thus, after using a cycloplegic agent, the patient is not only unable to accommodate for near distance and reading but has a widely dilated pupil that can produce photophobia (light sensitivity) for periods ranging from 1 hour to several days, depending on the medication used.

4. **Cholinesterase.** Cholinesterase inhibitors are a group of drugs that inactivate cholinesterase in the body. As a result, acetylcholine is permitted freely to exert its effects and act directly as a miotic on the iris. It is useful in the management of open-angle glaucoma.

5. **Diabetes, syphilis, or posterior synechiae.** These conditions cause increased vascularity and structural changes in the iris, which impair dilation of the pupil with cycloplegic agents. This effect, however, does not occur in early stages of diabetes but only in the long-standing cases of diabetes associated with retinopathy.

6. **Adrenalin.** Adrenalin, or epinephrine, is a sympathominetic drug that exerts its effect by acting directly on the end organ. In the eye it may exert its effect by dilating the pupil, constricting the blood vessels, and lowering intraocular pressure. If used over a prolonged time in the eye, it is capable of producing a brownish cast in the lacrimal sac.

7. **a. Concentration of the chemical in the solution.** The tonicity of an ophthalmic solution refers to the concentration of the chemical in that solution and its relationship to that of the tears. If the tonicity of the solution is relatively close to that of tears, the ophthalmic drops will be well tolerated by the eye. If, however, there is a high concentration of salts in the solution so that it is "hypertonic," then the drops will be irritating. Similarly, drops that are low in salt concentration, or "hypotonic," such as water, also will produce irritation to the eye.

8. **a. Blepharitis.** Systemic administration of steroids is not without hazard, and its use is confined to those conditions in which the benefits of steroid therapy cannot be achieved by a local topical

route. By systemic administration, the adverse effects may result in water and salt retention, swelling in and about the face and eyelids, mental derangements, hypertension, gastric disturbances, accentuation of diabetes, increased blood glucose level, delayed wound healing, and a number of other medical problems.

9. **Trifluridine (Viroptic).** Trifluridine has been effective in inhibiting the herpes simplex virus by interfering with the early steps of DNA synthesis. It can be used in cases resistant to IDU or vidarabine.

CHAPTER 5   Microbiology

- Clinical indications for smears and cultures
- Taking smears
- Making a stain
- Making a culture
- Other aids to identify organisms

Microbiology is the branch of science that deals with unicellular or small-sized organisms. The common agents that cause eye infections are *bacteria, viruses,* and *fungi*.

In everyday life we are constantly in touch with bacteria. We wash our hands because we have germs on them. We disinfect wounds for the same reason. We cover our sneezes. We wash fruit before eating it and try to keep flies off our food. Our water supply is carefully controlled, and chlorine is added to our swimming pools. We know that refrigeration reduces food spoilage by bacteria. We do hundreds of things daily that would not be necessary if germs did not exist.

The eye is subject to most of the infections that involve the body as a whole, and, in addition, certain infections are peculiar to the eye alone. Despite the fact that invading organisms are everywhere, most eyes with intact epithelium are not very susceptible to this invasion and usually require some alteration in the host tissue for the infection to begin. An altered tissue structure can be seen after trauma, after radiation therapy, from exposure because of inadequate blinking or lid abnormalities, from tear anomalies, or from corneal degenerative changes. Persons with normal ocular and periocular structures may still be susceptible to diseases if their ability to fight against infectious agents is compromised. This can

be seen in patients with diabetes, alcoholism, or acquired immunodeficiency virus (AIDS) and in those taking oral steroids, such as the renal transplant patient. A basic understanding of microbiology is helpful for the ophthalmic assistant, who may be required to take smears, stain the appropriate slide, and take a culture.

A variety of organisms can cause ocular disease to the anterior segment of the eye (see box, p. 80). These infectious agents have a predilection for certain sites of the eye and usually vary in their severity in causing ocular disease. By far the most common infections result from bacterial and viral organisms.

Bacteria are larger than viruses and may easily be seen under magnification by microscope. There are three main forms of bacteria: the round *cocci,* the rod-shaped *bacilli,* and the filamentous or spiral-shaped forms, *spirochetes* (Fig. 5-1). Although the shape can be used to classify the organism, another important differentiating feature is whether the organism stains blue (gram-positive) or pink (gram-negative) with a special stain referred to as *Gram's stain*.

The *coccus* is a round bacterium that arranges itself in a variety of patterns, each with its own characteristic. The staphylococci or pus-producing bacteria are gram-positive organisms that may appear in grapelike clusters or, more commonly, singly

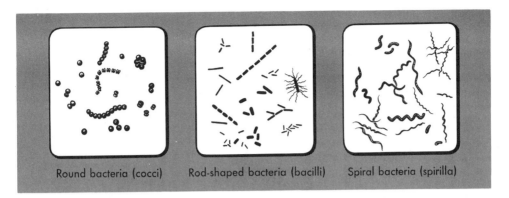

Round bacteria (cocci)   Rod-shaped bacteria (bacilli)   Spiral bacteria (spirilla)

Fig. 5-1 Bacteria.

or in pairs. Staphylococci frequently are present on the skin and give rise to boils and styes. The streptococci are gram-positive cocci that are bullet-shaped and arranged with their flattened ends together in chains. Of the streptococcal organisms, the most common agent to affect the eye is *Streptococcus pneumoniae*. This organism possesses a polysaccharide capsule that can be seen with a special stain called *India ink*. Although the pneumococcus is the common cause of lobar pneumonia, it may be the cause of conjunctivitis, a corneal ulcer, or an infection within the eye referred to as *endophthalmitis*. The gonococcus and meningococcus are gram-negative organisms with a characteristic kidney-bean shape that are capable of significant ocular infection.

The second group of bacteria is the *bacillus*. All the members of this group are rod-shaped, with rods being long or short, plump or slender, curved or straight, or smooth or beaded. Commonly affecting the eye are the gram-negative rods, *Haemophilus influenzae, Haemophilus aegyptius, Moraxella* organisms, the Enterobacteriaceae, and *Pseudomonas aeruginosa*. The *Pseudomonas* organism is the most devastating bacillus and is the most common cause of corneal ulcers in patients wearing contact lenses. Unless treatment is initiated early, the organism can cause significant visual loss. Gram-positive rods that affect the eye include *Corynebacterium diptheriae, Bacillus anthracis, Bacillus cereus,* and *Mycobacterium tuberculosis*.

The third group, the spiral-shaped or *spirochete*

organisms as found in syphilis, comprises small organisms whose diameter is below the range of resolution of the routine microscope. The organism may be observed on a smear with a special technique referred to as *darkfield illumination*.

The positive identification of these organisms by microscopic shape and staining reaction alone is not usually possible, and culture characteristics are often necessary. The ophthalmologist, however, frequently may make a presumptive diagnosis in association with the clinical picture, but the microscopic picture always remains an important aid.

Viruses are the smallest organisms and, unlike bacteria and fungi, penetrate directly into the host cells. Most viruses cannot be seen by our present-day forms of microscopy, and special techniques such as fluorescence microscopy and electron microscopy are necessary for the diagnosis.

To date, numerous viruses have been isolated, and vaccines have been prepared against some of these viruses, such as measles, smallpox, and poliomyelitis. Viruses must live within the cells that they invade and, in doing so, frequently cause considerable damage. The *herpes simplex* virus is perhaps the most common known organism affecting the eye; it invades the corneal epithelium and gives rise to a dendritic or geographic ulcer of the cornea. The virus can be isolated by scraping the ulcer and inoculating any one of a variety of culture systems. In most cases, however, the clinical diagnosis of herpes simplex virus is readily apparent and a scraping is un-

---

ORGANISMS CAUSING DISEASE IN THE ANTERIOR SEGMENT OF THE EYE

BACTERIA
  Cocci
    Gram-positive
      Staphlycoccus
      Streptococcus
    Gram-negative
      Gonococcus
      Meningococcus
  Bacilli
    Gram-negative
      Pseudomonas
      Haemophilus
      Moraxella
    Gram-positive
      Cornebacterium
      Bacillus
      Mycobacterium
  Spirochetes
    Syphilis
VIRUSES
    Herpes simplex
    Herpes zoster
    Adenovirus
FUNGI
    Candida
    Fusarium
    Aspergillus
CHLAMYDIA
    Inclusion conjunctivitis
    Trachoma
PARASITES
    Acanthamoeba

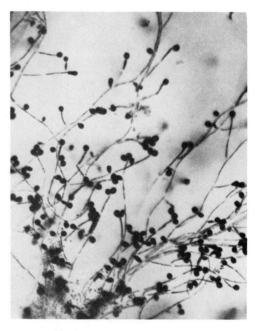

Fig. 5-2 Fungus under high magnification.

All viruses grow intracellularly (within the cell), never on the surface of cells or in the secretions as do most bacteria. See box at left.

Fungal ocular infections, unlike bacterial and viral infections, are uncommon but nevertheless do occur. Everyone is familiar with molds and mildew as fungi. Athlete's foot and ringworm are the two common skin diseases caused by fungi. There are more than 75,000 different fungi on this earth. Some are beneficial, such as the fungus responsible for producing penicillin. Fungal infections are prone to occur in the cornea and in the lacrimal, or tear, sac. Fungi are larger than bacteria and grow either as a mass of branching interlacing filaments (Fig. 5-2) or as rounded yeast forms. They are found on the soil and frequently lodge in the lacrimal sac, where they produce inflammation and obstruction. A typical history is one in which a patient's cornea is scratched by a twig, leaf, or bush, and several days later the eye becomes red and inflamed. One must suspect fungal infection.

Chlamydial organisms deserve a classification of

necessary. One group, the *adenovirus,* may affect the upper respiratory tract, the conjunctiva, and the cornea, causing fever, lymph gland enlargement, conjunctivitis, and keratitis. Varicella-zoster virus is responsible for causing a vesicular eruption on the skin, referred to as *shingles.* Some patients may develop ocular involvement that most commonly manifests as conjunctivitis, keratitis, or iritis. Although the virus can be isolated by culture, the diagnosis is usually evident clinically.

Table 5-1	Cytology in eye scrapings
Finding	**Possible diagnosis**
Polymorphonuclear cells	Bacterial
Mononuclear cells	Viral
Eosinophils	Allergy
Inclusion bodies	Chlamydia
Giant cells	Herpes virus

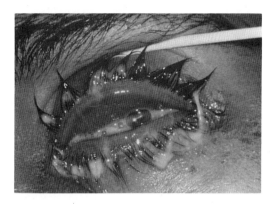

Fig. 5-3 Gonococcal conjunctivitis with a purulent discharge. Smears and a culture should be obtained to confirm one's suspicion that the conjunctivitis is caused by the gonococcal organism.

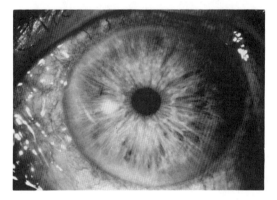

Fig. 5-4 Chlamydial conjunctivitis in an adult, which demonstrates follicles of the bulbar conjunctiva. This may have a chronic course, that is, longer than 1 month, if diagnosed incorrectly or if inappropriately treated.

their own. They are intracellular parasites that are larger than viruses but smaller than most bacteria. In North America the most common chlamydial agent is inclusion keratoconjunctivitis. In other parts of the world, such as North Africa, the Middle East, and South Asia, trachoma remains epidemic and a serious cause of ocular morbidity. Diagnosis of inclusion keratoconjunctivitis can be made by obtaining a scraping of the conjunctiva and looking for inclusion bodies in the cytoplasm of the epithelial cells. In infants the probability of finding inclusion bodies is higher than in adults; therefore the test should be employed in trying to make the diagnosis. A culture or specialized immunofluorescent test also can be used to confirm the diagnosis.

Acanthamoeba is a parasitic organism that can cause significant ocular morbidity. The organism is ubiquitous; it can be found in freshwater, soil, swimming pools, and hot tubs. It is capable of causing keratitis, which can progress depite the best available medication. Contact lens wear is the major risk factor for acquiring this infection. This risk is increased when wearers use homemade saline, rinse lenses with tap water, or swim with contact lenses. Corneal transplantation may be required to restore vision, but unfortunately there is approximately a 30% recurrence rate of the parasite in the graft.

Bacteria, viruses, fungi, chlamydia, and parasites are among the causes of inflammation of various parts of the eye. Various terms are used to denote the specific site of inflammation, as noted in Table 5-1. Each area of the eye is susceptible to attack by a large variety of organisms that have in common a predisposition to attack these specific areas.

CLINICAL INDICATIONS FOR SMEARS AND CULTURES

Smears are obtained and cultures are grown to identify causative organisms of an ocular infection. Although many ocular infections occur in which a clinical diagnosis can be made and smears and cultures are unnecessary, in a number of specific conditions laboratory studies are desirable: (1) acute purulent conjunctivitis (Fig. 5-3), (2) chronic conjunctivitis (Fig. 5-4), (3) conjunctivitis in the newborn infant

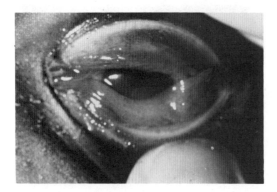

Fig. 5-5 Chlamydial conjunctivitis in a newborn with a mucoid discharge.

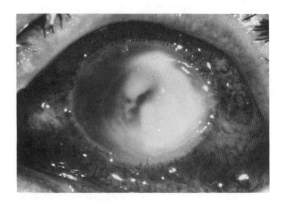

Fig. 5-7 Fungal corneal ulcer, which developed in a patient who had been struck in the eye with a tree branch.

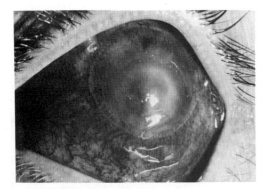

Fig. 5-6 *Pseudomonas* corneal infection developing within 24 hours under a soft contact lens.

Table 5-2	Inflammation of the eye
Part affected	**Condition called**
Lids	Blepharitis
Cornea	Keratitis
Conjunctiva	Conjunctivitis
Tear sac	Dacryocystitis
Uveal tract	Uveitis
Iris	Iritis
Ciliary body	Cyclitis
Iris and ciliary body	Iridocyclitis
Choroid	Choroiditis
Retina	Retinitis
Optic nerve	Optic neuritis
Inner ocular coats	Endophthalmitis
All ocular coats	Panophthalmitis
Orbital tissue surrounding eye	Orbital cellulitis

(Fig. 5-5), and (4) corneal ulcers that possibly have a bacterial, fungal, or parasitic cause (Figs. 5-6 and 5-7). Less commonly infections of the lids, tear passages, intraocular structures (endophthalmitis), or wounds (for example, after surgery or trauma) may result, which require smears and cultures by a variety of specialized techniques.

The conjunctiva is a loose, vascular tissue that reacts to infection by becoming irritated with inflammatory cells and edematous fluid rather than ulceration. Actual organisms may be difficult to find in smears, but the type of inflammatory cells that predominate may give a clue to the type of infection (Table 5-2). The presence of polymorphonuclear leu-

sound very much alike but are quite different. Forkocytes is most characteristic of bacterial infections, mononuclear leukocytes of viral infections, and eosinophils of allergic conditions. Smears are of particular importance in conjunctivitis of the newborn infant. The finding of gram-negative diplococci suggests gonococcus, and the finding of inclusion bodies within the cytoplasm of epithelial cells denotes inclusion keratoconjunctivitis. The presence of giant cells, which are multinucleated epithelial cells, suggests infection by the herpesvirus.

The cornea is one of the few tissues in the body without blood vessels; it commonly reacts to infec-

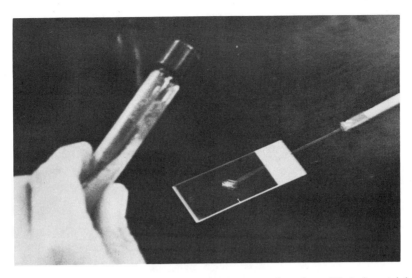

Fig. 5-8 Discharge is spread out evenly and thinly over a dry, clean slide before staining.

tion by ulceration formation. Smears are an important aid to an early diagnosis, particularly in bacterial and fungal ulcers. Results of the smears usually are available within minutes to hours and allow the ophthalmologist to choose antimicrobial agents that generally will be effective against bacterial or fungal oganisms. Culture results usually are available within 1 to 3 days, which allows a modification of the initial antibiotic therapy so as to achieve the best possible clinical response. The etiologic agents of bacterial ulcers vary somewhat with regard to geographic location and patient population. *Pseudomonas* tends to be the most common cause in the southern United States and *Staphylococcus* the most common in Canada and the northern United States. Other groups that account for many of the infections include *Streptococcus, Moraxella,* and the Enterobacteriaceae.

TAKING SMEARS

For rapid diagnosis, smears obtained from infective material are most valuable. A smear is a sample of discharge or infected tissue that is placed on a glass slide (Fig. 5-8). To obtain a good sample of a superficial tissue, a gentle scraping with a platinum spatula may be done. The actual sampling of infected tissues should be performed by the ophthalmologist

or under his or her supervision. All corneal lesions must be sampled by the ophthalmologist because this type of operative procedure has certain hazards. The material for culture and smear is taken from the advancing edge of the corneal lesion with a platinum spatula. The advantage of using such a spatula is that it can be sterilized by passage through an alcohol flame or Bunsen burner, and it cools in a few seconds. The ophthalmic assistant, however, may easily obtain the sample of conjunctival discharge found in the lower fornix in cases of conjunctivitis. The exudate is collected with a small sterile swab or platinum spatula, either from the lower cul-de-sac or from the inner canthus (Fig. 5-9). It is spread as thinly and evenly as possible on the surface of a clean glass slide. The slide can then be stained by a variety of techniques to determine the general category of the infectious agent.

MAKING A STAIN

The routine stains of smears that may be performed by the ophthalmic assistant in the office are *Gram's stain* for bacteria and fungi and the *Giemsa* and *Wright stains* for determining cell structure and the presence of inclusion bodies. Inclusion bodies often are characteristic of certain types of infection. Gram's stain is useful in determining the type of

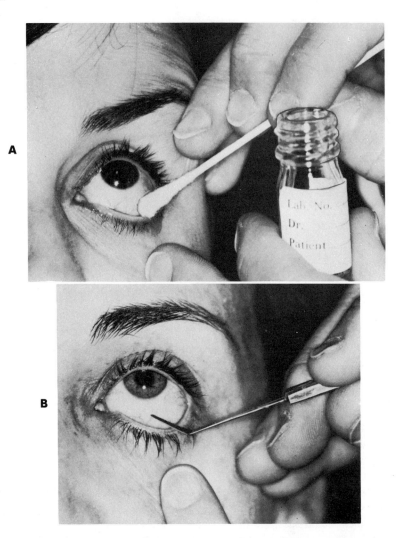

Fig. 5-9 A, Sample of discharge taken by sterile applicator for culture. **B,** Conjunctival sample taken by spatula for smear on glass slide.

agent responsible for the infection, whereas the Wright's and Giemsa stains are useful in determining the cellular response to a particular agent.

The ophthalmic assistant should learn to make Gram's, Giemsa, and Wright's stains. These are the most practical for office use and are performed as follows:

Gram's stain
1. Fix smear by flaming.
2. Cover with gentian violet solution for 1 minute.
3. Wash with water.
4. Cover with Gram's iodine for 1 minute. Pour off solution. Do not wash with water.
5. Decolorize with 95% ethyl alcohol or acetone for 15 to 30 seconds.
6. Wash with water.
7. Counterstain with safranin for 10 to 15 seconds.
8. Wash with water, blot, and dry.

Gram-positive organisms stain dark blue, and gram-negative organisms stain red.

Giemsa stain

1. Dry slide in air.
2. Fix in absolute methyl alcohol for 5 minutes.
3. Immerse slide in Coplin jar containing Giemsa stain (2 ml Giemsa with 50 ml distilled water). A buffer at pH 6.8 may be required. Let stand 1 hour.
4. Decolorize in two changes of 95% ethyl alcohol for 5 seconds each.
5. Air dry.

Wright's stain

1. Dry smear in air.
2. Cover with thin layer of Wright's stain (approximately 10 drops) for 1 minute.
3. Add equal amount of neutral distilled water to the stain on the slide. Allow to remain for 10 minutes. Float resulting scum off the slide.
4. Wash slide with distilled water and dry in air.

MAKING A CULTURE

Cultures are an important aid in diagnosis. When specimens for culture are taken in the physician's office, there is often considerable delay in transporting the specimen to the laboratory. For bacteria and fungi the applicator ends of the swabs used to obtain specimens should be broken off and placed in small bottles containing Stuart's transport medium. In the bacteriology laboratory the swabs are then routinely plated on blood agar culture medium and various other media for particular organisms. If close to a laboratory the ophthalmic assistant may directly plate the swabs on the culture media. In this process the swab is twirled or streaked gently on the plate, and the plate is placed in the incubator for 24 hours at 37° C. If the culture is scanty, the plate is reincubated for another 24 hours. The colonies are best examined during the first 48 hours inasmuch as they may degenerate and not reveal a typical pattern. For viruses, special transport media are available, and preferably specimens should be sent to the viral laboratory in a frozen state.

It usually takes at least 24 hours for bacterial organisms to grow on the culture medium sufficiently to make a positive identification; in the case of fungi and viruses, a few weeks may be required for growth.

The technique used in obtaining cultures is important. For exudates or discharge a sterile swab may be used. It is preferable to moisten the swab first in sterile saline or glucose broth. If a carrier medium is being used, the swab may be moistened in this. The swab should be rolled two or three times over the conjunctiva of the lower fornix while the lid is depressed by the finger. This is a procedure that the ophthalmic assistant can safely perform. A platinum spatula may be used to obtain a sample of superficial tissue cells for culture.

Cultures also are used to determine the sensitivity of the organisms to various drugs, so that effective therapy can be carried out. Disks soaked in antibiotic solution placed on the culture medium will inhibit bacterial growth around them. If the organism is sensitive to a particular drug, an area of "no growth" will be visible about the disk (Fig. 5-10). Many different culture media are employed, but blood agar is the basic medium used in ophthalmology. However, special media that are often used include chocolate agar, thioglycollate broth, Sabouraud's dextrose agar, Löwenstein-Jensen medium, and Thayer-Martin agar. Culture specimens from both eyes should be obtained, even though only one eye is involved. This is done so that comparisons can be made and the normal inhabitants of the conjunctiva will not be interpreted as pathogens. When a culture is taken, it is important to avoid contamination of the applicator by the lashes and lid margin.

OTHER AIDS TO IDENTIFY ORGANISMS

Biopsies have some value in the diagnosis of ocular infections. A biopsy is the removal of a piece of tissue, which is then fixed in formalin and sent to the pathology laboratory or sent in a sterile jar unfixed to the bacteriology laboratory for culture. An example of a condition that is readily diagnosed by a biopsy is the molluscum nodule on the lid margins, which is caused by a large virus.

Skin tests are another diagnostic aid that may be performed in the office or hospital clinic. Various infections (such as tuberculosis), toxoplasmosis, and some fungi produce a skin reaction if the patient has previously been infected.

Serologic tests of the patient's serum are another

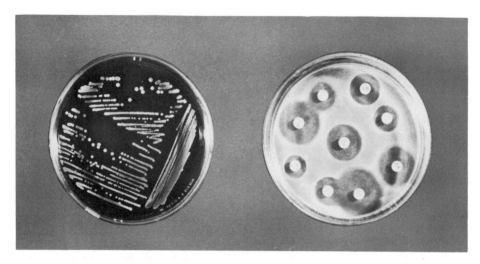

Fig. 5-10 A, Colonies of *Staphylococcus aureus* (pyogenes) on blood agar. **B,** Sensitivity test. Note the clear zone about each disk of antibiotic, indicating inhibition of the staphylococcus by the antibiotic.

diagnostic aid for several forms of infection. They require the taking of blood samples for testing. For example, the diagnosis of syphilis usually is made by various blood tests. The Veneral Disease Research Laboratory (VDRL) test or the rapid plasma reagin (RPR) test is used to determine whether the patient has an active infection. The fluorescent treponemal antibody absorption (FTA-ABS) test is used to determine whether the patient has ever contacted syphilis even if the condition was treated.

SUMMARY

Many known causes of disease of the eye may be attributed to bacteria, viruses, chlamydia, fungi, and parasites. Many of the unknown causes also may someday be ascribed to these organisms as improved techniques in isolating organisms develop. Unfortunately only the exterior portions of the eye are available for routine sampling for identification of organisms. The ophthalmic assistant should be acquainted with the techniques of obtaining cultures and making stains to discover whether abnormal organisms are causing diseases of the eye.

QUESTIONS FOR REVIEW AND THOUGHT

1. Name some common sources of bacteria, viruses, and fungi in your everyday environment.
2. Name some common viral conditions that affect the body.
3. What is the most destructive bacterium that can affect the outer portion of the eye?
4. What is the most common viral condition that affects the cornea?
5. Choroiditis refers to inflammation of the choroid; retinitis refers to inflammation of the retina. If all the coats of the eye are inflamed, what is the term used?
6. Outline a procedure to follow in obtaining a smear and staining it to identify bacteria.

7. Explain how a culture specimen is obtained.
8. Organisms may affect the interior of the eye, making it impossible to obtain smears and cultures. Discuss the value of skin tests.
9. What tests can be used to detect infection in the body?
10. What organisms are regarded as normal inhabitants of the eye?
11. Describe conditions that enhance bacterial growth. Give clinical examples.
12. Describe conditions that enhance viral growth. Give clinical examples.
13. What is the best culture medium for bacterial growth?
14. What is the difference among infection, inflammation, and irritation?
15. What is meant by a bacteriostatic drug? Give an example. What is a bacteriocidal drug? Give an example.
16. What virulent bacterial organisms can survive only in a fluid environment?

SELF-EVALUATION QUESTIONS

True-false statements

Directions: Indicate whether the statement is true (T) or false (F).

T or F 1. A dendritic ulcer of the cornea is classically caused by the herpes simplex virus.
T or F 2. The organisms that infect the eye always can be immediately and positively identified by microscopic shape and staining reaction.
T or F 3. Viruses can be identified by means of light microscopic examination.

Missing words

Directions: Write in the missing word in the following sentences.

4. The _____ and _____ stains are useful in determining the cellular response to a particular agent.
5. Inflammation of the inner ocular coats is called _____.
6. The basic medium used to culture bacteria in ophthalmology is _____.

Choice-completion questions

Directions: Select the one best answer in each case.

7. Conjunctivitis caused by this infectious agent often produces enlargement of the preauricular lymph node.
   a. *Staphylococcus*
   b. *Pneumococcus*
   c. *Haemophilus*
   d. Adenovirus
   e. *Streptococcus*
8. Which of the following is most likely to be responsible for the transmission of epidemic adenovirus keratoconjunctivitis?
   a. Finger-to-eye transmission
   b. Applantation tonometry
   c. Fluorescein solutions
   d. Kissing
   e. All of the above
9. A 30-year old male laborer has a densely infiltrated corneal ulcer 10 days after an abrasion to the central cornea. A hypopyon is present. Which is the most appropriate immediate procedure?

a. Give him an antibiotic drop and tell him to return in 3 days if it has not improved.
b. Presume that the patient has a fungal keratitis, and start him on therapy with an antifungal agent.
c. Make a smear and obtain specimens for culture, and start the appropriate therapy once the laboratory has informed you of the result.
d. Make a smear and take specimens for culture, start antibiotics that are appropriate for gram-negative and gram-positive organisms, and admit him to hospital.
e. Because a hypopyon is present, you should assume the patient has an endophthalmitis, and he should be hospitalized and treated with the full endophthalmitis regimen.

ANSWERS, NOTES, AND EXPLANATIONS

1. **True.** The herpes simplex virus is one of the most common viruses that affects the eye. The virus invades the corneal epithelium and gives rise to a dendritic ulcer, which usually affects the central portion of the cornea. The ulcer is almost always unilateral and may affect any age-group. A history of cold sores about the face can be elicited in approximately 55% of cases. The infection often recurs in the same eye, and the lesion may be precipitated by the following triggering factors:

a. Fever
b. Menstruation
c. Cold
d. Emotion
e. Overexposure to sunlight

Herpesvirus can be cultivated on the chorioallantoic membrane of a developing chick embryo. The virus also has a typical cytopathic effect on HeLa cell cultures.

2. **False.** It is not usually possible to positively identify an organism by means of microscopic shape and staining characteristics, and it often is necessary to obtain a smear and culture the bacteria. A presumptive diagnosis, however, may be made by considering the clinical picture along with the microscopic shape and staining reaction.

3. **False.** Most viruses are the smallest organisms that invade the body. Most cannot be seen by present-day forms of light microscopy, and special techniques such as electron microscopy are necessary for diagnosis.

4. **Wright** and **Giemsa.** The routine stains used to determine cell structure and the presence of inclusion bodies are Wright's and Giemsa stains. These allow the cellular response to a particular agent to be determined. Classically, in acute bacterial conjunctivitis the predominant cells would be polymorphs, in viral conjunctivitis lymphocytes, and in allergic conjunctivitis eosinophils. The detection of inclusion bodies would be of importance in the diagnosis of inclusion conjunctivitis.

   Gram's stain is used mainly for the detection of bacteria.

5. **Endophthalmitis.** Endophthalmitis is a rare condition that usually manifests by a decrease in vision, pain, conjunctival redness, and vitreous haze. In most cases the infection follows a penetrating eye injury or surgery for glaucoma or cataract. In rare instances it is the result of a blood-borne infection. If all three coats of the eye, as well as the vitreous, are involved by the inflammatory process, the condition is called a *panophthalmitis*. It is very difficult to clinically determine whether the patient has an endophthalmitis or a panophthalmitis.

6. **Blood agar.** Cultures are used to determine which infective agent is responsible for a lesion and the sensitivity of the organisms to various drugs. Blood agar is the basic medium used in ophthalmology. Other media used are as follows:

a. Chocolate agar—gonococcus, *Haemophilus influenzae*

b. Blood agar enriched with vitamin K—*Actinomyces israelii*

c. Löwenstein-Jensen—*Mycobacterium tuberculosis*

d. Sabouraud's dextrose agar—fungi

Culture specimens from both eyes should be obtained, even though only one eye is involved. When the specimen is obtained, contamination of the applicator by the lashes and lid margins should be avoided.

7. **Adenovirus.** Viral conjunctivitis is characterized by generalized injection of the conjunctiva, minimal discharge, and profuse tearing. The preauricular lymph node is commonly enlarged in adenovirus infections, and occasionally the patient may have an associated sore throat and fever. Bacterial conjunctivitis is associated with a profuse discharge, which may cause the lids to adhere, and the patient may have difficulty in opening the eyes on awakening. In addition, a history of a sandy, scraping feeling often is obtained. The conjunctiva is diffusely injected, and it is rare for the preauricular lymph node to be enlarged. Answers *a, b, c,* and *e* are all common bacterial causes of conjunctivitis.

In summary, the following table aids in differentiating virus from bacteria:

	Viral	**Bacterial**
Tearing	+ +	−
Discharge	−	+ + + +
Injection	+ +	+ + +
Preauricular node	+ + +	−
Sore throat and fever	+ + +	+

8. **a. Finger-to-eye transmission.** This question emphasizes the fact that medical personnel who touch lids, conjunctiva, and other ocular tissues must wash their hands between patients when patients with ocular infections are examined. The physician's office is the source of many epidemics of adenovirus infection. In many epidemics the spread has been traced to finger-to-eye transmissions; many patients with the infection have not had applanation tonometry.

9. **d.** This patient in all probability has a bacterial corneal ulcer and requires urgent treatment with antibiotics that will be effective against both gram-positive and gram-negative bacteria. Once the organism has been cultured, the antibiotic can be modified appropriately. The presence of the hypopyon does not necessarily imply an endophthalmitis. In all probability it is a "sterile" reaction to the infected corneal ulcer.

PART TWO

Clinical practice

CHAPTER 6

Office efficiency

- How to make patients happy
- The telephone
- Scheduling appointments
- Booking the arriving patient
- The reception room
- Running late
- Making future appointments
- Recall cards
- Filing
- Office equipment
- Personal qualities for improved office efficiency
- Secretarial duties
- Handling the ophthalmologist's schedule
- Handling sales representatives
- Handling mail
- Medical ethics
- In the physician's absence
- Aids in public relations
- Patient surveys
- Publicity
- Advertising

The primary role of the ophthalmic assistant is that of aiding the ophthalmologist in the management of eye patients. Frequently, however, the ophthalmic assistant may be called on to play the role of secretary, bookkeeper, receptionist, or even filing clerk in a busy office. Often the office will not be large enough to require a specialized staff; thus the ophthalmic assistant may have to cover a large number of secretarial duties. In any event, versatility and familiarity with the overall practice of ophthalmology is important, not only in the handling of patients but also in the backup services required, such as completing insurance reports, collecting, billing, and accounting.

HOW TO MAKE PATIENTS HAPPY

Making patients happy is not just good practice; it may even prevent lawsuits. The secret to making patients happy lies in developing good communication skills. Good communication skills start with an attitude of empathy and caring and letting patients know directly and indirectly that they are important. This attitude is reflected not only by what the physician says and does but by what the office staff says and does and how psychologically comfortable the patient is made to feel in the office environment. There are a number of ways in which one can show that the office staff does in fact care.

1. Do not keep patients waiting for long periods of time. One of the key factors affecting patient's overall rating of a practitioner is the time spent waiting in the reception area. Waiting time is a major cause of patient dissatisfaction, and this dissatisfaction increases dramatically when waiting time exceeds 30 minutes. Office schedules cannot always be controlled, especially if emergencies occur. For those physicians who are chronically behind schedule, one should take a close look at how appointments are made and try to prevent snarls in the schedule. If delays are unavoidable, patients should be told why they are waiting and how long the wait may be; this helps minimize the aggravation. In addition, interesting materials should be available to help patients pass the time. These include topical magazines or informed video educational material with television sets in the waiting room.

2. Make patients feel important. The first contact the patient has with a physician's office should be courteous, respectful, and personalized. This can include little gestures of kindess, such as the nurse asking after a recent baby, the receptionist asking for a preferred appointment time, or the physician inquiring after an ailing family member or recalling some details of an earlier conversation.

It is also appropriate for physicians to stand up and shake a patient's hand when first greeting a patient, as well as touching patients in a neutral manner (on the arm, shoulder, or hand) during the course of a consultation. These are gestures that convey empathy, friendliness, and concern. It is critical to convey information in a tone that is neither patronizing nor too technical so that the patient understands what the basic problem is and what is going to be done to help correct it.

The physician should have eye contact with the patient being examined. It is often offensive to elderly persons if the physician directs advice to the younger person who may be accompanying the patient. Patients often are reluctant to ask questions, and it is better to err on the side of too much information rather than insufficient information. Finally, physicians should not make patients feel they are too busy to listen to their problems, because that patient may not only go elsewhere but may be thoroughly dissatisfied and litigious.

3. Create space for comfort. Surprisingly small details, such as how the furniture is arranged, can make a difference in overall patient response. In an eye practice a desk intervening between a patient and the ophthalmologist often serves as a barrier to communication. It is much better to have a direct, closer interaction with the patient. Both intimacy and empathy are given a head start by placing the chairs near each other to eliminate any broad expanse of space between physician and patient.

4. Respect a patient's right to privacy. Any discussions of fees both with the physician or receptionist should be conducted privately so that details of these conversations are not overheard by a room full of strangers.

5. Look the part. People do not respond well to individuals with long hair or those dressed in blue jeans, sports shirts, athletic shoes, and sports socks. To earn patient respect, the physician and staff members should be dressed in conservative attire, the men wearing shirts and ties and the women wearing suits, dresses, blazers, or dress pants.

6. Pay attention to detail. Unclean examining rooms make patients uneasy, especially when evidence from previous examinations is clearly visible. Interruptions during an examination can be particularly annoying. A loud intercom system undermines privacy and is unprofessional. Small conveniences such as a coat rack in the waiting room, along with soothing decor, plants, and art prints, all help create the impression of a pleasant, welcoming environment and a caring physician.

7. Master communication skills. Conversation is an important factor in making or breaking the doctor-patient relationship. Here are a few tips:

a. Be upfront. Give information right at the beginning of the visit and not at the end.

b. Be creative. Use everyday language to explain

what is wrong and how you are planning to correct it.

c. Be personal. Ask questions about the patient's family and his or her social life so that they feel that they have not been forgotten from one visit to the next. Make notes on charts about a patient's interests and concerns for recall at future visits.

d. Be caring. Put a hand on the patient's shoulder or arm to convey empathy.

e. Be prepared. If you have something that needs to be shared with a patient's family, ask them to come in from the waiting room and share the information with them.

f. Solicit patient feedback. Confirm that what you have told the patient has been understood by asking the patient to relay back to you what he or she has understood. This is particularly important for educating patients about care systems for contact lenses. Too often patients leave the office unable to manage their contact lens care systems. Written information will ensure that the message gets across. Handouts are very important and are even more effective if they are personalized.

g. Be human. Patients want human beings looking after them. It is perfectly acceptable to tell patients that you also feel bad when the news you have for them is bad.

8. Be fair in all matters of finance. Charge fairly for your professional services but do not overcharge. Be fair in providing refunds to patients who prove to be unsuited for contact lens wear. Always look at the situation from the standpoint of the patient. Maintain good will at all costs.

THE TELEPHONE

The telephone usually is the first contact the patient makes with the ophthalmologist's office. These calls must be handled in a manner that will reassure the caller, provide confidence in the office, and at the same time protect the physician from unnecessary interruptions. The receptionist who answers the phone must have the wisdom of Solomon to permit access to the physician's services on the basis of priority. Basically two symptoms require immediate

attention—pain and loss of vision. Pain can mean anything from acute glaucoma to a corneal abrasion. Whatever the cause, it requires attention. Loss of vision is more difficult to assess. Sudden loss of vision can be a result of a central retinal artery occlusion and should be seen immediately. Other symptoms to be given top priority include transient loss of vision in one eye (carotid artery disease) or flashes of light (retinal detachment).

The telephone should be operated efficiently. Newer systems include call forwarding, digital punch systems, conference call systems, and music that comes on when the patient is placed on hold. Telephone equipment today provides for on-hold messages. This is an ideal opportunity to improve public relations, as well as add some form of promotion for your practice, for example, an on-hold message such as, "We appreciate that your time is valuable. We will be with you as soon as possible. Thank you for holding." This is an important service for busy lines. An adequate number of telephone lines is needed so that the patient does not spend an excessive amount of time listening to busy signals. The use of physician's lines, "hot" lines, and outgoing unlisted lines are valuable for a busy office.

Frequently called numbers need not be dialed if memory call-through systems are used. In some areas video display units are beginning to appear that make dealing with a caller easier. For example, if the caller has a swollen red eye, that patient will be seen immediately even if there is a language or articulation problem that prevents understanding the patient's complaints.

When the telephone rings, it should be answered at once. The receptionist should not permit the line to ring and ring while completing bookkeeping or other duties. The patient becomes more impatient and difficult to handle with each ring. It is an act of courtesy to permit the caller to hang up the phone first when the conversation is finished. Otherwise, it might seem as if the receptionist is trying to get rid of the patient.

Patience, finesse, and tact are needed to handle many patients on the telephone. The ophthalmic assistant should try to wear a smile at all times. Although callers cannot see the person to whom they

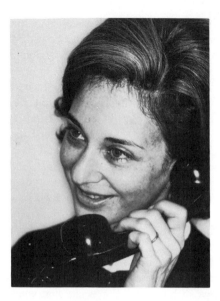

Fig. 6-1 An ophthalmic assistant should be warm and courteous and make the patient feel at ease.

are speaking, they can readily sense an attitude over the telephone. The ophthalmic assistant will be called on to help, advise, and sympathize with many patients. Calls should be screened carefully so that the ophthalmologist may answer nonurgent calls at a convenient hour. Sometimes the physician will want the ophthalmic assistant to take calls from patients reporting on their condition or wishing information, or the physician may personally want to receive all calls from patients (Fig. 6-1).

It is important that all telephone messages be recorded on a pad. Memory should never be trusted; a busy schedule often makes memory very short. It is a good idea to use a telephone message pad with a carbon copy. If the physician wishes a call returned, the assistant has a copy of the name and number. It also is a handy record of incoming messages and telephone numbers.

Risk management

The telephone is an important vehicle for interviews and assessment of the patient's problems. The board of directors of the American Academy of Ophthamology has offered guidelines to reduce litigation risks.

Many patients will telephone with emergency problems. Remember that the caller may be confused, distraught, rude, or even unable to give a clear account of what is occurring. Skillful management by the telephone receptionist may be sight-saving and perhaps even lifesaving. Therefore the staff member should be courteous, compassionate, efficient, and informative in telephone conversations. The ophthalmic assistant should keep the following guidelines in mind:

- Always confer with the physician if you have questions relating to the call.
- Take down the caller's number and promise to call back if in doubt about the correct answer to a question.
- Avoid general medical advice or discussing diagnoses.
- Answer questions in a friendly but noncommittal manner, and refer to the ophthalmologist for definitive answers.
- Do not forget to return the call as soon as possible because the patient often is extremely anxious.
- Try to determine the following:
  —The caller's name, address, and telephone number
  —The essence of the problem
  —When the symptoms first occurred and their duration

The following list includes typical emergencies that require immediate attention:

1. Chemical contact with the eyes and face. Alkali burns are extremely urgent matters. They should have emergency care at the scene of the accident by copious washing before the patient is brought to the ophthalmologist's office. An acceptable measure would be to fill a basin or bucket with tap water and immerse the patient's head into the water with the eyelids open under water.
2. Severe eye, head, or face injury, particularly a perforating eye injury
3. Acute or partial loss of vison
4. Recent onset of pain in or around the eye
5. Postoperative pain, infection, or increased redness or decreased vision
6. Recent bulging of an eye
7. Recent onset of flashing lights, floaters, curtains, or veils across the vision

8. Recent onset of double vision
9. Recent change of pupillary size
10. Recent onset of droopy eyelid
11. Foreign bodies in the eye
12. Urgent consultations requested by other physicians

If the patient has an emergency problem and the physician is unavailable, it is best to advise the patient to see another physician or obtain emergency room care immediately. One outstanding admonition that hangs over the head of every physician is that of "abandonment." One cannot abandon patients and particularly those in the immediate postoperative period. This carries sensitive legal implications.

It is important that one does not release any information regarding a patient without a legally valid written authorization. A caller who identifies himself or herself as a close relative desiring information should be asked to speak to the physician in the patient's presence.

Remember that all recommendations by the American Academy of Ophthalmology are only examples of important considerations. They should be supplemented by instructions by the ophthalmologist and experienced staff members.

Returning telephone calls

Patients' telephone messages should be responded to the same day and within a reasonable period of time, if possible; otherwise the office staff may have to deal with aggravated patients. Waiting until the end of the day to return patients' telephone calls can be a burdensome task; staff members are fatigued, and it may be difficult to reach the patients. In addition, while waiting for their call to be returned, patients have had an opportunity to think about their problems more and they become anxious.

Patients appreciate a quick response. Further, the patient who knows that the call is being made between patient appointments may be less likely to waste time with casual questions. If it appears that the call will take a long time, the staff member can arrange to call the patient back at a later time or encourage the patient to make an appointment to come in to the office.

Telephone manners

A telephone call usually is the first contact a patient has with the ophthalmologist's office. The following rules ensure a good impression.

1. Personality is revealed by voice and language. How you speak and what you say are the two most important factors in handling telephone calls. The voice should be clear, courteous, friendly, and precise. Pronunciation should be clear, with lips placed about half an inch from the mouthpiece. Cultivate an attractive, well-modulated voice, with pleasing inflections. You should try to make your voice attractive, just as you would try to make your appearance attractive. The impression that is created for the person calling depends on the inflection and tone of your voice. The impression you make— good, poor, or indifferent—reflects on the ophthalmologist and the office. You are the ophthalmologist's representative.

2. Use well-selected, appropriate words and phrases (Fig. 6-2). Express yourself with a business-like conciseness in a courteous manner. Use the terms, "please," "thank you," "I am sorry," and other expressions of appreciation and regret with a tone of sincerity, which will be quite obvious to the listener. Do not try to cut the person off with constant interjections. Above all, be understanding.

3. Ask who wishes to speak to the doctor. The doctor may not wish to speak to a brother-in-law or a stockbroker but may be receptive to calls from an industrial nurse.

4. Tell patients that the doctor can best answer a call after hours. There is more time and less disruption of normal service. Make sure the doctor receives all patient calls. It is good public relations to ensure that those calls are returned by the doctor on the same day.

5. The office should have enough lines so that busy signals are kept to a minimum. Use a private line for any outgoing calls and keep these to an absolute minimum. Avoid personal calls.

6. Avoid putting people on hold unless absolutely necessary. If you *must* put someone on hold, explain the situation and ask if the person would like to hold or would prefer that you return the call in a few minutes. If the choice is to hold, thank the person

DO NOT SAY	SAY
When do you want to come in?	Would you prefer a morning or afternoon appointment?
The doctor is booked up until _____ .	The doctor is scheduled at that time. He can see you at _____ .
The doctor is running late.	The doctor was interrupted in his schedule today.
I called to remind you that _____ .	I called to confirm or verify _____ .
Cancellation	Change in schedule
Check-up	Examination
Are you an old patient of Doctor _____ ?	Are you a former or established patient of Doctor _____ ?
You misunderstood.	There was a misunderstanding.
Are you a patient here?	When did we see you last?
Are you on welfare or medicare?	What type of health insurance coverage do you have?
What is your problem?	Can you tell me what your problem is so we can schedule you properly?

Fig. 6-2 Telephone techniques.

for being patient as soon as you return to the line. Remember, courtesy is very important.

7. Be calm and steady, and avoid excitement or abruptness even when the lines become busy. Keep your remarks short. The longer you talk, the more irritable the person on the line or on hold becomes.

8. Try not to abandon the telephone at lunch to an answering service. Rotate the incoming calls among staff members. An answering service should be used sparingly because personnel are not skilled in handling patient questions nor do they have access to the appointment book for schedules.

9. Never repeat personal information you may hear, no matter how unimportant it may seem to you.

10. Do not hesitate to ask for the repetition of words or names if you are in doubt. Many names sound very much alike but are quite different. For-

eign names given by persons with an accent should be repeated or spelled slowly until they are understood. To ensure accuracy, repeat numbers, amounts, addresses, and other important items.

11. Have paper and pencil ready for messages, and obtain accurate and complete information, including correct name, address, and telephone number.

12. Keep a list of frequently called telephone numbers.

13. Sit properly. Poor posture produces fatigue early in the day, and fatigue becomes reflected in your voice.

Office personnel should always remember when answering the telephone that they are important representatives of the ophthalmologist and can assist immensely in the building of a reputation. They must be master psychologists tuned in to the emotional ills and pressures of the public. In many cases a voice is the only contact that the telephone patient has with the office. Therefore the office must be represented with courtesy, dignity, and a spirit of service, with personnel giving clear and complete answers promptly.

SCHEDULING APPOINTMENTS

It is difficult in an ophthalmology office to be on time. With most patients requiring eye drops, it means everyone must wait at least 30 minutes. Therefore waiting patients are always present. If emergencies or difficult cases are added, then the normal waiting time can be extended to 1 hour. Waiting is a tedious chore. No one likes to sit beside a total stranger for prolonged periods of time. Patients become irritated and their tempers grow short. The irritability spreads and affects the entire staff. A hostile patient does not foster good doctor-patient relations.

If waiting is a fact of the office environment, the best way to prevent a potentially disruptive situation is to explain on the patient's arrival that a wait of 30 to 45 minutes may be required to allow for eye drops and a preliminary examination before the patient sees the ophthalmologist. It does not change the reality of waiting, but at least the person knows what to expect and, more important, why the delay. If it is a reasonable explanation, most patients will understand and accept the distress of sitting around. Occasionally a patient will be unreasonable and short-tempered, but one cannot satisfy everybody. The assistant should always forewarn patients about the necessity of waiting for the ophthalmologist and explain why.

The waiting game can produce bitterness on both sides. For the physician, the patient who does not show up for an appointment has kept the clinician waiting. Some physicians charge for missed appointments. A valid case can be made for doing so, because time is the major commodity for the professional. Many patients feel the same way. Who is to say that a physician's time is more important than anyone else's? Some patients have billed their physicians for lost time spent uselessly in a waiting room. Of course, these views represent the extremes of the doctor-patient dispute.

It is difficult to control the size of an ophthalmologic practice and simultaneously retain patient good will. A well-trained ophthalmic assistant can be the solution, in whole or in part, to the ophthalmologist's dilemma. The ophthalmic assistant responsible for telephone appointments acts in the role of doorman to the practice. The assistant is, after all, the first contact the patient has with the office. He or she can attract patients or drive away old ones and discourage new ones from coming.

The ophthalmic assistant may not be primarily responsible for the scheduling of appointments but should act in a supervisory capacity to see that the physician's appointment schedule is not overcrowded. Any appointment system must be formulated to suit the particular working habits and peculiarities of the physician involved. Appointments must be generously spaced and an adequate amount of time allocated for any special procedures that are to be performed. An efficient appointment system makes allowance for the fact that many patients will require eye drops. Special consultations for problem cases will require additional time apportioned to the patient's visit. Emergencies often arise during the course of the day, and blocks of time must be set aside to permit the efficient, smooth handling of these emergencies with minimal disruption of the existing schedule.

The assistant should never rely on memory in recording an appointment. All appointments must be marked in the appointment book, preferably in pencil so that they can be erased in case of cancellation. In making an appointment it is important to spell the name of the patient correctly. The telephone numbers, both home and business, should be obtained in case it is necessary to contact the patient to alter the time of the appointment. The appointment time should be repeated to the patient at least once, so that there is no misunderstanding as to the date and time. Whenever possible, patients should be given the first available appointment time suitable for their needs. Tactful questioning of the patient should reveal who referred the patient, whether it was a physician, an optical house, or another patient. It is a matter of good public relations to note in the appointment book who referred the patient, as a reminder when the patient arrives.

More time should be allowed for first visits inasmuch as the ophthalmologist will require and usually will wish to spend more time examining new patients. When special tests or procedures are anticipated, such as visual fields or minor surgery, they should be noted and suitable time permitted. The appointment book should be marked in advance whenever the physician is attending meetings or conferences so that double bookings do not occur.

BOOKING THE ARRIVING PATIENT

When a patient arrives at the office, certain documentation procedures must be performed to obtain the vital information necessary for the complete charting of the patient.

If the receptionist has a good memory, greeting the patient by name on arrival is good public relations. If not, tact in obtaining vital information is important. Many patients will be reticent about giving their age, particularly in front of other patients. Insurance numbers and statistics on financial affairs must be tactfully handled. If a verbal request for information does not provide sufficient confidentiality, a blank information card on a clipboard can be given to patients to complete while they are seated and then returned to the receptionist

All patients should be given a warm welcome, just as if they were being received into a home. They should feel wanted and comfortable no matter how busy the office situation at the time. Each person should be treated as an individual. Some personal detail that may have been noted previously should be inquired after if the receptionist knows the patient.

Records of patients seen previously will be obtained from the files. If the patient has never been seen, a new record is opened and all the vital information recorded. The name and address must be printed carefully and clearly on each record card in a standard, readily identified area of the card.

Once the day begins with the scheduled appointments, it is important that there be minimal delay in the processing of each patient. Before the patient is seen by the ophthalmologist, politeness, kind words, and a cheerful "hello" will go a long way in promoting good will for the ophthalmologist and the office. The office assistant should always speak to the patients and assure them that they will be seen shortly by the ophthalmologist.

In ophthalmology, because eye drops usually are instilled and the patient must wait a given length of time, a proper flow of patients into different rooms should be planned. The placing of patients into designated rooms by the ophthalmic assistant will ensure proper attention by the ophthalmologist with minimal delay. Patients with sore or painful eyes should be seated in the waiting room in such a position as to avoid facing glaring lights.

THE RECEPTION ROOM*

Once arriving in the office, the patient should not have to wait more than 15 minutes before being shown into an examination room. Those 15 minutes in the reception room should be comfortable and pleasant.

A wide variety of reading material will occupy patients as they wait. Chairs should be spaced so that each person has "elbow" room and does not feel cramped up to the person next to them. As a courtesy to patients who find cigarette smoke irritating, you might post a sign that says "Smoking not permitted in this health care facility."

Many offices have available educational brochures that explain common eye ailments. The reception room is a perfect place to circulate patient information brochures or past newsletters and to dispense information about one's practice. Brochures might contain information on office hours, insurance, emergencies, and new medical developments for eye conditions.

The decor of the reception room should create a bright, cheerful atmosphere. Artwork, photographs, plants, and fresh-cut flowers will assist. Depending on the opthalmologist's wishes, the assistant may choose to have coffee, juice, or water available to patients on request.

RUNNING LATE

No matter how carefully an appointment system is planned, delays and waiting periods will occur in a

---

*Contributed by Robert S. Rosen, M.D., LaMesa, California.

busy ophthalmic practice. Unlike other specialists who can control, to a certain extent, the number of return visits, ophthalmologists, because of the number of emergencies encountered, coupled with demands from referring physicians, have difficulty in adhering to a fixed schedule. Ironically, the qualities that make them run late are the qualities that make them available to patients. When an emergency patient calls, an ophthalmologist says, "Yes, come in and I will take care of you." When a patient talks about ailments (or problems that may be causing the illness), a good doctor will not shove the patient out the door just to stick to a schedule. When confronted with a complicated eye problem requiring extensive testing, a competent ophthalmologist will take the time, no matter how busy, to arrive at the diagnosis that sometimes may be not only sight saving but also lifesaving.

When the ophthalmologist is running late and the waiting patients begin complaining, the ophthalmic assistant should give them a little insight into these facts.

MAKING FUTURE APPOINTMENTS

If a repeat appointment is required within the next 2 to 3 weeks because of iritis, conjunctivitis, glaucoma, or postoperative care, this appointment should be made at a designated time that does not overcrowd an already crowded appointment book. Usually these repeat visits are short and consequently can be scheduled before other regular appointments or integrated into the appointment system by a reserved block of time at the end of the appointment system.

It also is important for working persons that repeat appointment times be given early in the day. A minimal amount of delay is expected in the appointment system at that time because unexpected emergencies tend to occur as the day progresses.

RECALL CARDS*

Recall cards probably are the single most important vehicle an office has to maintain a regular, steady

*Contributed by Robert S. Rosen, M.D., LaMesa, California.

flow of patients. Many patients need to see an ophthalmologist only every 3 months, 6 months, or 12 months. Keeping a record of when they are due for their next examination is a method of ensuring that they receive continuing eye care. It is difficult to provide the quality of eye care necessary if people forget or neglect to check their eyes! A recall card is a friendly reminder inviting them to call the office to schedule an appointment at their earliest convenience.

The best way to establish a recall card system is to set up a tickler file and keep it next to the last person to speak with the patients before they depart from your office. At that time the physician's notes can be read and a recall post card addressed with the month of suggested return on it. It is then filed in the tickler file according to month. At the beginning of each month the recall cards that are in the file for the *following* month should be sent out. Some offices like to follow up the recall card with a personal telephone call. Future appointments may be made as far ahead as 1 to 2 years in an appointment book. It is important to remind these patients by card or by telephone at least 1 to 2 weeks before the appointment. Rescheduling may be required if the date selected is not convenient for the patient.

FILING

Filing is an important aspect of the everyday practice of ophthalmology. If a file is lost or misfiled, not only will a great deal of valuable information be lost but also measurements that may be impossible to obtain again. The ophthalmologist may have to spend considerable time trying to recover some of the information that has been lost. Anyone may remove files from the filing system, but only one person should be delegated the responsibility of refiling. When a file is misplaced, the ophthalmic assistant may be called on to aid in the search for the file. Often the file may have been removed for reports, letters, surgery, and so on.

Most ophthalmic offices have a central filing system, with files placed in alphabetic order. These systems may be further subdivided by an *active drawer*, which includes files of patients who are under active treatment and who will be returning within the next 4 weeks. Some hospitals and offices file their charts under a numeric system. This is more efficient and minimizes lost files, but it requires additional work. Each chart is numbered in order of being opened, and it is filed accordingly. Cross-references are made of all names, in alphabetic order and even double cross-referenced so that any special foster names or married names are indexed. By the alphabetic system of filing, the controversial order of names such as those beginning with Mac and Mc and names such as DeForest are filed according to an agreed-on procedure, which must be known to all. In addition, common names such as Brown, Smith, and Lee should be arranged in the order of the initial of the patient's first name. The numeric filing system eliminates these challenges and minimizes the number of misfiled records.

It has been our practice to separate the financial from the clinical records for each patient seen. With the advent of Medicare, we have found it expedient to change our patient processing routine so that the financial records, including billing and posting, are prepaid at the time of the patient's office visit. The first statement and an account for submission to the insurance company can be given to the patient at this time.

If a computer is going to be used for filing charts, it must have a large memory capacity. The computer must be able to store at least 10 years of data. After 10 years most computers are outdated and have to be replaced anyway.

Laboratory and x-ray reports, along with letters from other physicians, must be appended to the patient's chart and brought to the attention of the ophthalmologist. It is unacceptable simply to file such letters with the chart until the next patient visit without them being seen by the ophthalmologist.

Missed appointments and cancellations should be noted on the patient's chart and brought to the ophthalmologist's attention. Sometimes important litigation hinges on this type of information.

OFFICE EQUIPMENT

Equipment is an important factor in office efficiency. The ophthalmologist or office manager must constantly be on the watch for new business machines that may be of considerable aid in improving office efficiency. These include adding machines, postage meters, and duplicating machines. One also must watch for new ideas in billing procedures and form procedures that will be helpful. Noiseless typewriters and floor and wall coverings that reduce noise should be used. The seats should be arranged to relieve back strain. Stamping and sealing envelopes by machine greatly facilitate the speed of these procedures. The telephone system should be reviewed with the telephone company to ensure that one has the most efficient system available and that proper lines of communication are established between rooms, either through the telephone or an intercom system.

The personal computer, which has now invaded the ophthalmic office, is discussed in detail in Chapter 37.

Ophthalmic equipment is very precise and must be kept in perfect working order. Basic principles to consider include the following:

1. Keep the machines (slit lamp, keratometer) covered when not in use.
2. Standardize regularly such devices as the radioscope, the keratometer, and the lensometer.
3. Learn to maintain the instruments, from changing a bulb in the projector to attaching a topogometer.
4. Make sure maintenance is regularly done for such instruments as the automatic refractor and the pneumotonometer.

PERSONAL QUALITIES FOR IMPROVED OFFICE EFFICIENCY

The attitudes of each of us are based on our likes and dislikes and are expressed in our words, our actions, and our behavior. Some of these attitudes tend to become habits, some of which are helpful and some harmful. They are harmful not only to ourselves and the people we work with but to the patients we greet. The ophthalmic assistant should analyze these attitudes and try to eliminate those that are inappropriate. An attractive personality depends on an expression of physical, mental, social, and moral qualities. Physical qualities give first impressions to people we meet. Our appearance, voice, manner, energy, and bearing portray a first impression to the patient. Social qualities are developed through our everyday contacts with people. To make a favorable impression one must be considerate of others, cooperative, and courteous and show tact, cheerfulness, and kindness. In addition, patience and sympathy must be part of one's personality. These attributes create a pleasant and stimulating atmosphere in the office.

Mental qualities include intelligence, a keen observation, a retentive memory, and an ability to concentrate and apply oneself. The ophthalmic assistant must be orderly, accurate, and careful in conduct, show an ability to answer intelligently and quickly the many questions that patients ask, and above all show a good sense of humor.

Moral qualities are those foundations of character underlying everything else, such as honesty, sincerity, loyalty, and trustworthiness. The ophthalmic as-

sistant should have the courage and determination to do right, regardless of the consequences. These qualities provide an important guideline to the daily behavior of the ophthalmic assistant who works with the public. An assistant can review the effectiveness evaluation to see how he or she rates (see box below).

SECRETARIAL DUTIES

The ophthalmic assistant may be required to compose or type letters to insurance companies, physicians, or suppliers. Although the dictator of the letters is responsible for their clarity, thought, and completeness, the typist must be given credit for their proper setup and form. Margins must be clearly laid out, paragraphs introduced properly, and punctuation correctly placed. The visual setup of the letter is as important as the wording to the impression the

---

RATING EFFECTIVENESS AS AN OPHTHALMIC ASSISTANT

DEPENDABILITY
Trustworthiness in carrying out instructions and assignments
☐ Excellent
☐ Above average
☐ Average
☐ Below average
☐ Unsatisfactory

PRODUCTIVITY
Achievement of satisfactory quantity of work
☐ Excellent
☐ Above average
☐ Average
☐ Below average
☐ Unsatisfactory

ADAPTABILITY
Reception of new ideas and methods; adjustments to changes in work
☐ Excellent
☐ Above average
☐ Average
☐ Below average
☐ Unsatisfactory

COOPERATION
Tact: willingness to assist; agreeable compliance
☐ Excellent
☐ Above average
☐ Average
☐ Below average
☐ Unsatifactory

INDIVIDUALITY
Personal appearance, neatness, behavior on job
☐ Excellent
☐ Above average
☐ Average
☐ Below average
☐ Unsatisfactory

ACCURACY
Exactness, professional skill
☐ Excellent
☐ Above average
☐ Average
☐ Below average
☐ Unsatisfactory

INITIATIVE
Performance in analyzing problems, accepting responsibilities, planning necessary action, and following through
☐ Excellent
☐ Above average
☐ Average
☐ Below average
☐ Unsatisfactory

receiver will have of the office from which the letter has been issued.

As time goes on, many types of forms will become routine and standardized. Even letters will have a standard form of setting up introductory paragraphs and conclusions. The best way of doing things becomes standard. No matter what it may be, there is a best way of doing it, whether it is sealing a letter, putting on a stamp, setting up a letter, or filing a carbon copy. Once these standards are discovered and established, the wasteful and useless movements are eliminated.

HANDLING THE OPHTHALMOLOGIST'S SCHEDULE

Ophthalmologists usually are busy people; consequently, considerable demands are made on their time in the office, in the hospital, and in extra activities. They may be required to fulfill teaching roles and speaking engagements and become involved in community work. From time to time these additional involvements will be made known to the ophthalmic assistant. When they interfere with existing schedules, the assistant should try to ensure that the office and the hospital are organized to accommodate these changes.

The assistant must be sure the appointment book is not overcrowded so that the physician is not constantly harassed by delay in attending meetings or giving lectures. There are times when the ophthalmologist will have to cancel appointments for an emergency, a court case, or an illness. If the physician will be unable to be at the office for an appointment and knows beforehand, the patient should be notified by telephone or letter. Sometimes the appointment may require cancellation by fax. This will be more costly, but it is necessary to prevent putting the patient to the inconvenience of coming to the office.

HANDLING SALES REPRESENTATIVES

Sales representatives from the various drug and optical firms attempt to bring the latest word to the physician on new products and changes in products. Some come only occasionally to the ophthalmologist, and some come frequently. No matter how busy, the ophthalmologist usually prefers to see these salespersons. A few minutes spent with a sales representative may make the ophthalmologist knowledgeable on some new therapeutic tool that may be of service. Sometimes the physician may be too busy to see a salesperson and may wish the ophthalmic assistant to obtain all the pertinent information and to summarize the contents of the individual reports or to obtain summaries and abstracts of these articles. Practical experience can teach the assistant how to make a good abstract and then present it to the ophthalmologist at a more leisurely moment.

The ophthalmic assistant soon will become familiar with the various representatives from the pharmaceutical and optical firms who visit the ophthalmologist. All physicians are interested in receiving firsthand information about their products. One must, however, discriminate between these sales representatives and magazine salespeople, peddlers, and the like. Sales representatives always present cards, are never abusive, and never attempt to get into the physician's office under false pretenses. Accordingly, they should be greeted graciously. When seeing the representatives, the assistant should explain how busy the physician is at the given time and how much of the practitioner's time they may have. The physician is then in a position to close the interview when he or she chooses. If it is inconvenient for the clinician to see a sales representative at the time of his or her call, the caller is entitled to an explanation and should be asked to return at a more convenient time when the physician can allocate a small amount of time.

In addition to these individuals, there may be many callers who take up the physician's time unnecessarily. The ophthalmic assistant may be very useful in graciously handling these callers, talking to them, and diverting them. For example, insurance salespersons and those who sell stocks and bonds can be diverted from office hours to a more convenient time, if the physician wishes to see them. If the caller does not wish to state the nature of business and the ophthalmic assistant knows that the physician does not wish to be disturbed by such visitors, the caller should be asked to write a letter to the clinician about the matter.

HANDLING MAIL

The ophthalmologist should receive mail in an orderly fashion. Personal correspondence is kept together, as is correspondence relating to patients, such as x-ray and laboratory reports and consultation letters. Drug company correspondence is compiled and kept separate from advertisements and medical journals. Such organization expedites the physician's review of the mail. The accounts should be transferred to the personnel primarily responsible for the accounts. Before the ophthalmologist is presented with an insurance form to complete, the record of the patient should be obtained and a certain amount of the form completed by the secretary or ophthalmic assistant.

MEDICAL ETHICS

Physicians are bound by a code of rules and customs to which they are expected to adhere. The background for this code is the hippocratic oath, named after Hippocrates, Greek physician of the fifth century BC. The hippocratic oath is a beautiful and inspiring statement to which physicians are expected to adhere. The hippocratic oath is an oath that was demanded of the young physician about to enter the practice of medicine. This is a composition that dates back to the ancient Greeks. Hippocrates, called "The Father of Medicine," placed medicine on a scientific foundation, freeing it from superstition, philosophy, and religious rites. He gave sound and shrewd descriptions of many diseases and thus raised the ethical standards of medical practice. Today the hippocratic oath serves as a foundation from which the highest standards of medicine are practiced. See box at right.

The principles of medical ethics have been developed over the course of centuries as medicine has evolved. Many of these writings may seem old-fashioned now because they are no longer needed, but others have never varied. Although the hippocratic oath concerns itself only with the relationship between the physician and patient, modern medical ethics also govern the relationship of the physician to the community and to fellow physicians. Even though the overall knowledge and technology of modern medical science are vastly superior to that

---

OATH OF HIPPOCRATES

I swear by Apollo the Physician, by Aesculapius, by Hygeia, by Panacea, and by all the gods and goddesses, calling them to witness that according to my ability and judgement I will in every particular keep this, my Oath and Covenant: To regard him who teaches this art equally with my parents, to share my substance with him and, if he be in need, to relieve his necessities; to regard his offspring equally with my brethren; and to teach them this art if they shall wish to learn it, without fee or stipulation; to impart a knowledge of the art by precept, by lecture, and by every other mode of instruction to my sons, to the sons of my teacher, and to pupils who are bound by stipulation and oath, according to the Law of Medicine, but to no other.

I will follow that regimen which, according to my ability and judgement, shall be for the welfare of the sick, and I will refrain from that which shall be baneful and injurious. If any shall ask of me a drug to produce death, I will not give it, nor will I suggest such counsel. In like manner I will not give a woman a destructive pessary.

With Purity and Holiness will I watch closely my life and my art. I will not cut a person who is suffering from a stone, but will give way to those who are practitioners in this work. Into whatever houses I shall enter, I will go to aid the sick, abstaining from every voluntary act of injustice and corruption, and from lasciviousness with women or men, with freemen and slaves.

Whatever in the life of men I shall see or hear, in my practice or without my practice, which should not be made public, this will I hold in silence, believing that such things should not be spoken.

While I keep this, my Oath, inviolate and unbroken, may it be granted to me to enjoy life and my art, forever honored by all men; but should I by transgression violate it, be mine the reverse.

---

of ancient times, the universal theme of "self-discovery" has not changed since the days of Hippocrates. The ophthalmic assistant should be acquainted with the fundamental rules of medical ethics, because his or her actions will reflect on the ophthalmologist.

One of the principles of medical ethics is strict secrecy, which must be observed regarding all matters pertaining to the patient. It is not ethical to criticize the work of another physician to a patient. If a physician has inadvertently expressed some opinion to the ophthalmic assistant in private, the assistant may, out of loyalty to the ophthalmologist, wish to show superiority to the patient by voicing criticism of the other physician's treatment. This is strictly against medical ethics.

A physician must be careful to avoid exaggerated publicity or connection with any incident that has news value, especially of a sensational kind. When newspaper reporters call at the office for information or a statement by the physician, they should be transferred directly to the ophthalmologist, who is fully cognizant of responsibilities both to the public and to fellow medical colleagues. Discretion in this area belongs solely to the physician.

Each physician has occasion to refer patients to outside agencies for some form of service or for the purchase of optical or medical supplies. Patients often inquire for the name of an individual or organization from whom they may obtain these services. Their confidence in the opinion of their ophthalmologist is an important consideration in deciding whom to consult and where to go. The names, addresses, and telephone numbers of those physicians or optical firms in whom the ophthalmologist has a measure of confidence and to whom he or she might refer patients must therefore be known to the ophthalmic assistant, and must be kept in such a way that the list can be consulted readily. A list should be kept available of such service agencies as the local institute for the blind, diagnostic laboratories, and organizations that deal with the perceptually handicapped child.

IN THE PHYSICIAN'S ABSENCE

The ophthalmic assistant can be of immense help to a physician who presents papers at meetings of medical societies, writes articles or books, or undertakes research work. Physicians who communicate findings to the scientific world usually do extensive writing. The assistant can be of invaluable aid in assembling research or reference material and editing manuscripts. The time when the physician is away from the office for meetings or holidays can be put to good use in this area. The ophthalmic assistant

with a leaning toward writing may prefer this phase of work to all others and be instrumental in obtaining reference materials, in searching cumulative indexes and libraries for material on the pertinent subject, and in assembling these for the attention of the ophthalmologist. This work, whether it is for a lecture, an article, or book, will provide insight into many new facets of ophthalmology.

AIDS IN PUBLIC RELATIONS*

1. At one time or another, every ophthalmic assistant will be confronted with an office full of patients waiting at their appointed times while the ophthalmologist has been delayed. The ophthalmic assistant should attempt to reappoint patients who do not have an urgent problem and those who cannot afford to wait. If reappointments or delays are required, the patient is entitled to an explanation of this inconvenience. Because the physician's day usually is devoted to providing service to others, such explanations can be freely candid. Most patients appreciate the demands constantly made on the physician's time and usually are quite fair in thoughtfully considering these delays. For those patients who prefer to wait in the office, refreshments should be offered if the facilities are available.

2. The waiting room should be kept clean and neat at all times. Magazines without covers should be removed and broken toys removed or repaired.

3. The ophthalmic assistant should always be neat, fresh, and well-groomed. Extreme styles of clothing should be avoided; make-up should never be excessive.

4. Patients should be called from the waiting room with a soft and friendly voice that rings with hospitality. If a patient has poor vision, the tone of voice should remain unchanged. Many people approach the partially sighted as though they had lost their other sensory functions and tend to speak in a loud voice or even shout.

5. Not all patients are blessed with good hearing. The ophthalmic assistant may be required to speak

---

*Portions of this section have been contributed to the sixth edition by Robert S. Rosen, M.D., La Mesa, California.

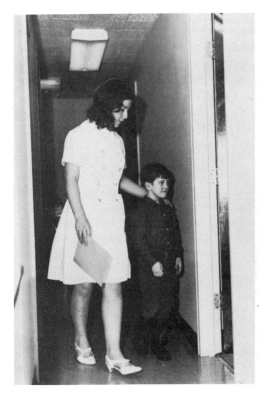

Fig. 6-3 Handling the young child.

in louder tones in communicating to the hard-of-hearing patient.

6. The ophthalmic assistant should attempt to have patients remove overshoes, overcoats, and scarves before entering the ophthalmologist's inner office. This invariably saves time and allows patients to be more comfortable for the examination.

7. Children may be led by the hand to the examining room (Fig. 6-3). A small toy or gift may establish better rapport with the child.

8. Personalizing a practice can be done in many ways. Look around your office. Is everyone wearing a name badge? Do the nurses, assistants, and technicians have cards with their name and title on them so that patients can call directly and ask them questions? When the physician enters the examining room, does the technician introduce the patient to the ophthalmologist?

9. Because of the increasing number of senior citizens who come to ophthalmology offices, more and more physicians are beginning to offer some form of transportation within a certain-mile radius. This is a great service to seniors who might not drive or to surgery patients who are temporarily unable to drive. A limousine or van that seats six to eight people can be used to pick patients up and return them to their homes. When patients call to make an appointment, the assistant can tell them that on Tuesday and Thursday mornings, for example, transportation service is available to those living within a 5-mile radius of the physician's office. Would they like to take advantage of such a service? Scheduling transportation requests *ahead* of time will allow the driver to plan an effective route for picking up patients.

The driver should be a patient, courteous person with an excellent driving record and a personality that will make the passengers feel comfortable and safe.

Advertising a service such as free transportation is bound to increase telephone requests by new patients for further information about your office and its services. At a time when more and more new patients are "shopping" for physicians, a service such as free transportation will draw attention.

10. No matter how minor or short a surgical procedure or hospitalization is according to medical standards, it is of major importance to the patient and should be acknowledged as such by the office personnel. Following up surgical procedures with a call from someone in the office or sending a gift such as a plant to a recuperating patient is an extremely courteous and personal gesture. Often a personal note from the physician will boost the patient's morale beyond anyone's expectations.

Surgical patients always should be given priority scheduling for follow-up appointments, and any questions they may call in with should be answered quickly. *Patients should never feel that the physician or office personnel are ignoring them now that the surgery is over!* Developing a special protocol for handling surgery patients will, in the long run, boost the physician's practice. Patients *love* to talk about their surgeries; let what they say about *your* office be positive and flattering.

11. Keep records of where new patients are com-

Dear _____ ,

    Thank you for referring _____ to our office. We appreciate your confidence in us. We look forward to continuing to serve you and will always make time available for you, your family, and friends.

                         Sincerely,

---

ing from. Have a *tracking* form that you keep next to the appointment book. When new patients call for an appointment, ask them who referred them to the office. If they are responding to an advertisement and your office runs more than one advertisement, ask them *specifically* which ad they read. Enter the information on the tracking form. At the end of the month review the number of new patients and where they came from.

At that time thank-you cards should be sent to current patients who referred new patients to the office. A sample message might read as shown above.

Each of these points contributes to the overall feeling of personalization that is desired in a medical practice. Patient handling is as much a part of medicine as is diagnosis and treatment.

PATIENT SURVEYS

Ultimately the patient is the one to determine just how pleasant, efficient, and effective an office operation is. An office might set a plan into action thinking that the patients will love it and the fact may be that none of the patients have even been aware of its existence!

Feedback from patients can be very valuable, but office personnel must ask for it. Few patients, unless they are angry about something, will voluntarily mention that they had to wait slightly longer than usual the past two or three visits or that the reading material in your reception room is outdated and sloppily tossed about.

Patient information surveys are forms you can devise that contain 10 to 15 questions about how the patient experiences the office—from the time they call to make an appointment to the time they pay

for their service and depart. Questions should be worded positively and be followed by definite choices (Fig. 6-4). For one month, as each patient leaves the office, he or she is handed a survey form together with a stamped return envelope. Office personnel explain to the patients that if they would be so kind as to complete this survey and return it at their earliest convenience, it would provide assistance in maintaining an office that can best serve their needs. Most people will be more than happy to respond. A suggestion is that they do not sign the survey form so that it will remain anonymous and be truly reflective of their opinion. When a substantial number of surveys have been returned, someone in the office tallies the results, which can be discussed at the next office meeting.

PUBLICITY

The major goal of publicity is to stimulate an interest in and public awareness of the physician or the organization. A good public relations program can accomplish many objectives, for example:

- Create an intense interest for a timely event
- Be part of an ongoing promotion
- Promote the physician's image
- Generate good will for the office and physician
- Public relations offers several advantages over other types of promotional tools.

Cost. Advertising and publicity both make use of the media to reach the public, but public relations tends to be less expensive. Both result in publicity. In fact, unlike advertising, publicity coverage is inexpensive. In most cases the only expense for public relations is for paper, postage, mail announcements and, for large users, a public relations firm.

Size of the audience. Public relations can tell the story to thousands of potential patients, possibly millions with the use of mass media. Although the benefit of targeting potentially interested persons may be significant, publicity directed toward the general public results in fast and effective communication.

Credibility. Public relations lends an air of credibility that is missing in advertising. If one is interviewed on the 6:00 o'clock news or quoted in the daily paper, the public tends to perceive the interviewee as an expert. Media attention usually is

PATIENT INFORMATION SURVEY

Dear Patient,

We would like our office to run as effectively as possible so that we can best serve you. To make this happen we need your assistance. Please answer the questions below and mail it back to us in the self-addressed stamped envelope. Thank you.

1. I am treated with courtesy when I call to make an appointment.

✓1	2	3	4
Always	Usually	Occasionally	Never

2. It is easy to make an appointment to see the doctor.

✓1	2	3	4
Always	Usually	Occasionally	Never

3. When I come into the office the doctor sees me on time.

✓1	2	3	4
Always	Usually	Occasionally	Never

4. I am pleased with the selection of reading material in the waiting room.

✓1	2	3	4
Always	Usually	Occasionally	Never

5. The nurses are polite and friendly when they work with me.

✓1	2	3	4
Always	Usually	Occasionally	Never

6. The doctor answers all of my questions completely and thoroughly.

✓1	2	3	4
Always	Usually	Occasionally	Never

7. I am satisfied with the amount of time the doctor spends with me.

✓1	2	3	4
Always	Usually	Occasionally	Never

8. Questions about insurance coverage and/or billing are answered to my satisfaction.

✓1	2	3	4
Always	Usually	Occasionally	Never

9. I would recommend your office to my friends or family.

✓1	2	3	4
Always	Usually	Occasionally	Never

Comments _____ I always enjoy my visits.
Ethel N. McKinney

Fig. 6-4 Patient information survey.

viewed by listeners and viewers as an endorsement of a product, service, or cause.

Impact. Public relations is persuasive. It can shape public opinion, mold personal images, and even reverse negative attitudes.

Versatility. Public relations can be used to place one in a spotlight at almost any time or any place one chooses. By taking advantage of carefully selected media opportunities, one can expand into new areas of practice.

Longevity. Public relations offers longevity and provides a permanent record. A person who has been mentioned in the media can show the clipping to potential clients, quote it in advertising, or use it as a means to gain more publicity.

ADVERTISING

Advertising is seen as a device to ensure that physicians are competitive and that their fees are dictated by the market. Medical advertising should be factual (one cannot claim to be the best cataract surgeon in a given state without being able to prove it) and informative, listing hours of work, the physician's specialty, and practice restrictions. Above all, the advertisement should be *in good taste*. The foes of advertising are upset over the loss of dignity that results from using a commercial vehicle to promote a medical reputation. Good advertising can yield results in months that formerly took years to develop on the basis of word-of-mouth recommendations.

SUMMARY

Office efficiency depends on adaptation to patient needs, as well as skill in combining an effective program for telephone responses, handling of patients in the office, filing and recording data, and providing good public relations through publicity and patient management. The good will that evolves from this combined approach to office efficiency will have a long-lasting effect in ensuring return visits of patients who are pleased with the services provided.

QUESTIONS FOR REVIEW AND THOUGHT

1. Discuss the appointment system in your office (or make up an appointment system) and in particular how you would work emergency appointments into the system.
2. What are some personal qualities of an ophthalmic assistant that greatly enhance his or her ability to get along with people?
3. How may you use your time best when the ophthalmologist is away at meetings or on holidays?
4. How do you handle the small, frightened child? The patient who is almost blind? The patient who is deaf?
5. Mrs. Johnson arrives in intense pain from overwearing her contact lenses. How do you handle this situation?
6. A very important person arrives in the office and in spite of a number of people waiting ahead of him, he insists on being taken next. How do you handle this situation?
7. A drug salesperson arrives who insists on seeing the physician even though the waiting room is crowded. How do you handle this situation?
8. The waiting room is crowded. An angry patient says the doctor is running a factory and begins to be abusive. How do you handle such a person?
9. You are applying for a job as an ophthalmic assistant. The doctor questions your value to him or her. What would you say to indicate that you could improve his or her efficiency (such as seeing more patients more thoroughly)?
10. Write several on-hold messages for callers who are waiting anxiously for the telephone receptionist to return to the line.

SELF-EVALUATION QUESTIONS

Office problems to solve

Office efficiency is promoted through the work of intelligent, responsible people using the faculties of cooperation, creativity, industry, interest, and sensitivity. Problems that may arise in the office often do not have a cut-and-dried solution. Each situation is unique and requires individual attention. The following problems and brief discussions on how to handle them touch on some areas of difficulty that might be encountered. We have put forth some of our ideas, but there are a multitude of others that we encourage you to explore.

Problem 1. A patient calls and demands an immediate appointment because he is having a problem with his eyes. He sounds quite hysterical to you, and the symptoms do not seem to indicate an emergency. What do you do?

Problem 2. The doctor is away for 2 weeks. Shortly after his or her departure, an important letter arrives in the mail and requests a speedy acknowledgment or reply. What should you do?

Problem 3. The doctor has asked you to reschedule some appointments because of a change in his or her surgical schedule. You have been unable to reach a patient by phone, and the appointment is a week away. How should this be handled?

Problem 4. A patient arrives for an appointment, and you are unable to locate her chart. How do you handle this situation?

Problem 5. The doctor is running late in his or her appointments. How would you handle the delay with newly arriving patients?

Problem 6. A sales representative arrives and insists on seeing the doctor even though the waiting room is crowded. How do you handle this situation?

Problem 7. What information should you obtain from patients or referring physicians' offices when they call to make an appointment?

Problem 8. It is sometimes difficult to see our own surroundings objectively. It is an interesting and informative exercise to imagine that you are a patient coming into the ophthalmologist's office for the first time. What is your initial reaction to this office? Is it clean, bright, and pleasant, or stuffy and forbidding? Was your initial contact with the receptionist pleasant? Did you feel relaxed and comfortable with his or her manner, or did he or she seem harassed, overworked, or hostile? Did you find the waiting room to be well-lit, with an interesting assortment of neatly displayed magazines, inviting you to enjoy your wait? Or did you find yourself peering at a tattered 3-month-old periodical in a heated, overcrowded waiting room?

Problem 9. It has been the assumption throughout these questions that you are an employed ophthalmic assistant. Perhaps you are not. Perhaps you are embarking on a search for employment in this field. You will, then, have to prepare a résumé of your skills, experience, and training. You also will have to be prepared for an interview (or several interviews) with ophthalmologists. Consider the initial impression you want to make on him or her and the qualities and abilities you want to convey. Do you present yourself as a dependable, cooperative person who can meet challenges and accept responsibilities? Is your appearance neat and professional? You want to go into an interview feeling good, looking good, and emanating confidence in your ability to do the job and your eagerness for the opportunity to do so. How do you plan on doing this?

ANSWERS, NOTES, AND EXPLANATIONS

Answer 1. There are a few ways to handle this situation. You could tell the patient that you are fully booked and that he can try to reach another physician who might be able to see him on a more immediate basis. You are, however, risking ill-will feelings by turning away this patient. You could inform the patient that he can be placed on a cancellation list and will be notified when an opening becomes available. This means you have taken the responsibility of diagnosing this problem as not urgent. Can a telephone conversation with an upset and frightened patient tell you this?

A third alternative is not to take it upon yourself to diagnose the patient's condition. Take down all the symptoms he is experiencing, get his phone number, pull his chart, and give the message to the doctor. The physician knows his or her patients, as well as possible serious potential problems, and should make the final decision as to what should be done.

Answer 2. The letter should not be left to vegetate for 2 weeks. If the matter is of very pressing importance, then contact the doctor. However, even important correspondence may not be extremely urgent. A courteous and considerate way to handle this would be to send the correspondent a brief note explaining that the doctor is away until a certain date and the letter will be answered promptly on his or her return.

Answer 3. You can make a note to call the patient the following day; the person may be out just for the day. This means that you must not forget to place this call on the next day. However, chances are that the patient has given you only a home number and cannot be reached there during the day. Therefore, if you are relying on this single mode of communication, you will have an irate patient to handle 1 week hence if the person arrives for the appointment.

It is probably best to send a note as soon as you have found it difficult to reach the patient by phone. Rather than leave it another day and waste precious time, post a note advising of the cancelled appointment and provide an alternate date. This is easy and convenient and saves patient anxiety and the feeling of having been overlooked.

Answer 4. You could ask her to sit in the waiting room while you look for the chart. However, if you cannot find it within a reasonable time, you are delaying the patient. If you put her name on a blank chart, you would leave the doctor with an embarrassing problem.

It is best to explain to the patient that you are unable to locate her chart at the moment (this should be said after you have thoroughly searched the various areas where it might be). You should tell her that is will take a bit of time to check the files, and you make up a duplicate chart for today to keep her from being kept waiting. Reassure her that her chart will be located.

Answer 5. It is easiest, but most unwise, to avoid the situation and hope that no one will complain about the delay. This is inconsiderate to the patient who may have another appointment to keep, who must get back to work, or who simply does not appreciate being kept waiting a disproportionate length of time.

One can directly inform an incoming patient that the doctor is running late (because of emergencies, a holdup at the hospital, or whatever the case may be) and, unfortunately, there will be a longer than usual wait. Because the patient is being inconvenienced, offer a choice of waiting or rescheduling the appointment.

Answer 6. Some doctors will see sales representatives when they drop by; others prefer to have the ophthalmic assistant make an appointment for these brief visits or have the representative come at the end of the day.

If the practice is busy, as the crowded waiting room would indicate, it is best to form a consistent policy with sales representatives. The pharmaceutical representative will quickly learn when and how the ophthalmologist is available.

If a representative insists on seeing the doctor, present the doctor with his or her card and let the doctor decide what to do. You will find, however, that the sales representatives who come to your office will be courteous and cooperative. It is up to the ophthalmic assistant to set a mutually accommodating manner for visits to be made with maximum efficiency and minimal time lost.

Answer 7. You will need the patient's full name and phone numbers, home and business. You should ask if the patient has been to the office previously; if not, you should record the person's mailing address. This is needed if you have to change the appointment and the patient cannot be reached by phone.

It is also helpful to know the basic nature of the problem or the reason for the appointment, that is, a postoperative check, a complete eye examination for a driver's licence, a minor surgical procedure, an ocular injury, a contact lens problem, and so on. This information will help you in the scheduling of time for the appointment and in your preparedness for the patient.

When scheduling a consultation appointment, you will need the referring physician's name and, advisably, the nature of the patient's problem. If the patient has undergone any tests related to this particular problem, request that copies be forwarded to you before his appointment date.

Answer 8. Try to go through this mental experiment. Chances are you might see some things you had never before realized existed and that are in need of change or improvement.

Answer 9. This is a personal evaluation and an exercise well worth doing as a method of providing yourself with a self-assessment, as well as learning to put your best foot forward.

CHAPTER 7

History taking

- Organization of a history
- History procedure
- General information
- Chief complaint
- History of present illness
- Past health, medications, and allergies
- Family history
- Tips in history taking

A history is the story of a patient's medical disorder. By means of the history the physician attempts to reconstruct the stages of disease as it has progressed. To elicit a history, the physician must ask questions about the patient's symptoms. Thus a history is really a series of specific questions linked together in an orderly sequence. When a specific problem is identified in the response, specific questions are directed to the problem to elicit more detail. This chapter deals with a method of asking questions so that the patient's chronicle will be orderly, concise, and complete.

Two types of patients are seen in an ophthalmologist's office: the patient who desires a routine ocular examination combined with a refraction and the patient with symptoms of an ocular disorder. Unfortunately it often is impossible to distinguish between the two on the basis of a history. Each patient, then, must be questioned as though one expects to find some ocular disease.

Language problems frequently cause concern for both the ophthalmic assistant and the patient. Appendix 14 gives some commonly asked questions in foreign languages. The help of a translator and particularly a family member is valuable.

ORGANIZATION OF A HISTORY

The history should be subdivided to maintain organization. Many charts have the organization stenciled or printed on them. Regardless of the charting method used, an ophthalmic history should include the following:

Chief complaint
History of present illness
History of past health
    Significant medical illnesses
    Previous eye disorders
    Previous surgery, both ophthalmic and general
Medications currently used and their duration of use
Allergies
    Inhalants
    Contactants
    Ingestants
    Medications
Family history of ocular disorders
    Myopia
    Strabismus
    Glaucoma
    Blindness
Occupation

Type of work

Industrial hazards

Although many complaints are strictly ocular in nature, others are a manifestation of poor general health or emotional problems. Occasionally patients may be taking medication that they do not realize affects the eye and will not reveal this aspect of their history unless specifically asked. For example, a patient with a duodenal ulcer may be given propantheline bromide (Pro-Banthine), an atropine-like drug that inactivates the ciliary muscle. Such a patient would consult the ophthalmologist because of difficulty seeing at near.

HISTORY PROCEDURE

In pursuing a history the ophthalmic assistant should attempt to be precise and pertinent. With some patients an inquiry into previous health can result in a saga of each and every contact they have had with a physician. The patient, who may not know what is important and what is irrelevant, must be guided by questions. Frequently patients will state that they enjoy excellent health but when asked what medications they are taking will respond that they are taking pills for hypertension, injections for diabetes, and iron for anemia. The patient does not connect a general systemic disorder with an ocular problem. Yet all the diseases mentioned have serious and grave consequences within the eye itself.

The ophthalmic assistant should be aware of his or her position to receive privileged information. The covenant that binds the patient and physician and allows private information to be transferred from one to the other also applies to the ophthalmic assistant, who works as an extension of the physician. Patients can be frank in discussing their ailments only when they feel confident that complaints are being aired for analysis, not for public consumption. Information garnered during a history should not be revealed to one's family, friends, or even fellow workers. A seemingly slight betrayal, such as revealing the patient's age, may have disastrous consequences and place the office in an awkward position.

The ophthalmic assistant should not refrain from asking a particular question because it appears to be too private or embarrassing. If the history is con-ducted in a frank and professional manner and the questions are posed with tact and good taste, the patient will reveal even the most private matters, just as he or she would remove a shirt for a chest examination. Above all, patients must have confidence in the professional ethics of the persons who treat them.

Some patients will not reveal the full pertinent history to the ophthalmic assistant. Normally this is not a vote of nonconfidence if the assistant's demeanor and manner of questioning are professional, but it is a failure of the patient to understand completely the importance of history taking. The occasional patient will refuse to speak to anyone except the physician about any eye problems. This is the patient's privilege. These patients should be treated with the same degree of tact and professional air as the others.

The assistant should not attempt to interpret or expand a statement made by the patient, because sorting out the information will waste the ophthalmologist's valuable time, thus negating the intention of the ophthalmic assistant.

The organization of questions is prerequisite to completeness and to a program for efficiency. A routine should be established so that each patient is asked the same basic questions, preferably in the same manner. Of course, the dialogue will differ as the complaints of the patients differ, but the sameness of the structural questionnaire will give a certain firmness to the ophthalmic assistant's approach and also provide an excellent source of data for review or research.

A routine that may be followed in careful history taking is described in the following sections. As with all routines they provide guidelines and should not be rigidly followed.

GENERAL INFORMATION

Included under general information are the essential facts that should appear at the beginning of every chart (Fig. 7-1). These include the patient's name, address, date of birth, work telephone number, and home telephone number. It also is helpful to note the source of referral. If a patient has been referred by a medical doctor, a letter to that physician is

Name:	Norman Deer
Address:	39 Roxborough Road
Telephone:	923-4117
Referred by:	Dr. Peters
Family doctor:	Dr. Peters
Employed by:	Westinghouse
Occupation:	Clerk
Type of insurance	Blue Cross
Insurance No.	464-347-213
Age:	50—Birth date 4/6/1926
Chief complaint:	Difficulty with fine print
History of present illness:	Past 6 months difficulty in reading stock reports. Distance vision fine. No other eye complaints.
Past health:	Diabetes 12-year duration
Medications:	40 units PZI daily
Allergies:	Penicillin, sulfa
Family history:	Glaucoma in mother

Fig. 7-1 Typical history.

necessary. The patient's family physician, even though not the source of referral, should be noted on the chart. At times the ophthalmologist may detect, through the ocular examination, signs of a general medical condition, such as hypertension or diabetes, and will want to write the family physician of these findings despite the fact that a referral was not solicited. For billing purposes the type of insurance plan and policy number should be recorded. Ophthalmic assistants should try to become acquainted with the various insurance plans used in their particular locale. In some instances the wording on a bill may be the sole difference between whether or not the patient receives reimbursement. Certainly, limitations to any particular insurance plan should

be told to the patient. Finally, inquiry should be made into the patient's place and type of employment.

CHIEF COMPLAINT

The chief complaint constitutes the headlines of any ophthalmic history. In a sentence or two the ophthalmic assistant should write down the main reason for which the patient has come to the ophthalmologist for advice and help. In this context the prime question should be direct, simple, and forthright. *How do your eyes trouble you?* Many times the patient responds, "That's what I'm here to find out!" The patient may reply concisely or give a long, rambling account of various symptoms. If the patient cannot provide focused answers on the main issue after repeated questioning, the ophthalmic assistant should record what he or she regards as the most serious problem among the patient's symptoms. Commonly described chief complaints are *pain, loss of vision, eye fatigue,* and *blurred vision for near.* One must then proceed to pin down the specifics of the complaint such as date of onset, cause, and duration.

HISTORY OF PRESENT ILLNESS

After the chief complaint is recorded, the patient should be questioned in greater detail about the main symptoms. When did the problem begin and under what conditions? In other words, what was the patient doing when something was first noted to be amiss? Was the onset slow or rapid in development, and did it affect one or both eyes? Once the onset of the patient's symptoms has been recorded, their development and progress should be noted. What did the patient do after it began? Did the person consult a doctor, a friend, or a pharmacist? Did he or she take any medications internally or place any in the eye? Did the symptoms appear to become worse or abate? Was the problem relieved by taking any medication or stopping a particular activity? In other words, what aggravated it and what made it better? The patient should be asked how long a particular symptom has been present and whether it tends to recur.

To aid the ophthalmic assistant in the dissection of a symptom, the pertinent points regarding the most common ophthalmic complaints are reviewed next.

Loss of vision

Very few patients actually will state that they have lost vision, unless, of course, they have become blind because of some unfortunate tragedy. Most patients complain of blurred vision and state this problem in terms of a limitation of function. Blurred vision may assume many forms.

Blurred vision secondary to an error of refraction. Hazy, foggy, or blurred vision, if it occurs at a particular distance, usually indicates a refraction error. The myope cannot see in the distance, and the hyperope may have difficulty at near. It is the patient with astigmatism who has difficulty seeing both in

the distance and at close range. Even with astigmatism, however, poor visual acuity is not evenly distributed, inasmuch as this type of patient generally will see better at close range because of the magnification afforded by proximity. Most patients with refractive errors have a specific visual disability limited to specific activities.

Blurred vision for close work. A patient whose vision is blurred for close work usually is a presbyope and may complain of an inability to read the stockmarket report or a number in the telephone book.

Blurred vision for distance work. In this instance the patient is not apt to be a young adult for whom a fresh diagnosis of myopia is about to be made. The patient who is in school most often will complain of inability to see the blackboard. The patient who drives an automobile will state that road signs appear to be quite fuzzy, especially at dusk. Occasionally a patient will recognize this problem by noting that the television set appears fuzzy only to him or her. With regard to television, mothers often become very alarmed when their children sit close to a television screen. This is not usually a symptom of myopia because children enjoy sitting close to the screen for two reasons. First, they enjoy the magnification because big things are easier to view, and, second, the closer they are to the screen, the greater is their sense of involvement with the story being told.

Blurred vision secondary to organic disease. The patient with organic disease has difficulty seeing things at all times regardless of the activity. The patient who has a cataract or macular degeneration will be limited in both the distance (driving) and at near (reading). The patient with a cataract sees as though looking through a frosted glass window, and the patient with macular disease finds things missing when looking straight ahead and so must look at them askew.

Loss of central vision. With loss of central vision patients discover that they are unable to see clearly straight ahead but that they have retained peripheral vision (Fig. 7-2). When looking at a face, they may state that the face appears gray or indistinct, whereas the background around the face appears to be clearer. Such a patient commonly sees better in dim illumination. The visual acuity in the affected eye usu-

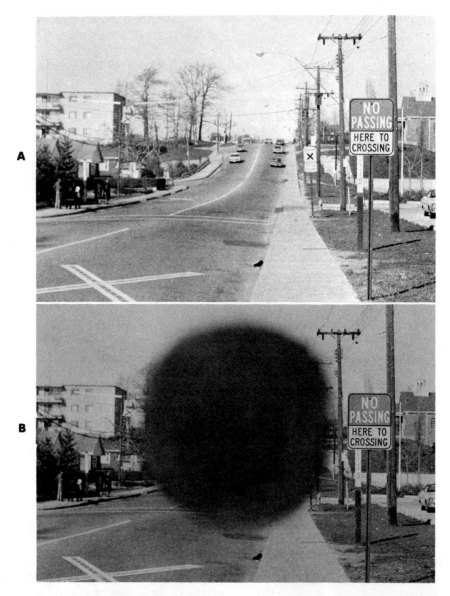

Fig. 7-2 A, The road as it appears to a person with normal central and peripheral fields of vision. **B,** Loss of central field. The central field of vision is indistinct, whereas the peripheral field of vision remains clear.

ally is quite poor. This symptom, if sudden in onset, usually means a disorder of the macula or the optic nerve.

Distorted vision. Distortion of vision is most commonly a sign of macular edema. The patient with this symptom usually complains that objects appear minified and slightly fuzzy and that their contours are curved rather than straight. Visual distortions also are common in patients, such as high myopes, who wear very thick lenses.

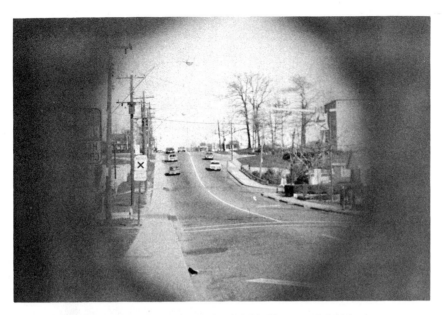

Fig. 7-3 Restricted peripheral visual field. The central field is clear.

Night blindness. The patient with night blindness finds difficulty in seeing things in the early evening, and this difficulty becomes much worse as night falls. Such a patient behaves as though blind in movie theaters, darkrooms, and so forth yet can see quite clearly straight ahead in daylight. Eventually, the patient suffers visual field restrictions, which makes driving and, later, ordinary ambulation quite difficult even during the day (Fig. 7-3). This symptom may be a manifestation of retinitis pigmentosa or vitamin A deficiency.

Transient gray-outs or blur-outs of vision lasting several seconds in one or both eyes. Although this symptom appears to be inconsequential, it often is of great importance. This obscureness of vision may be a symptom of papilledema (swelling of the disc as a result of increased intracranial pressure), carotid insufficiency, or arteriosclerosis.

Inability to see to the right or to the left. This symptom follows a profound field loss in which the patient loses half the field of vision. Such a patient, when reading the visual acuity chart, sees letters on half the chart only and sees them clearly to the 20/20 line of the unaffected side. Usually the patient has difficulty in any visual tasks, such as driving, reading, or even ordinary ambulation (Fig. 7-4). When this occurs on the same side in both eyes, one has to be suspicious of brain involvement of the opposite side.

Ascending veil. The patient may see a dark shadow ascending like a fog arising in the lower field of vision. This symptom frequently is an ominous indicator of a retinal detachment occurring in the superior retinae (Fig. 7-5).

Headaches

Headaches are a headache for all medical personnel. Commonly the patient with a headache has been referred by the family physician, who, unable to find an organic cause for the complaint, has referred the patient to an ophthalmologist for further assessment. Unfortunately most headaches are not caused by a refractive error or a disorder within the eye, and the ophthalmologist must lamely report to the family physician that there appears to be no ocular cause for the patient's headaches. Although the symptom of headache is difficult to evaluate, it must be treated with respect because this complaint may indicate

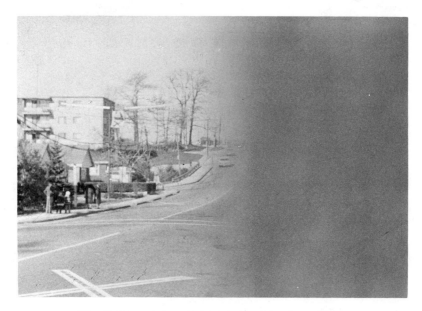

Fig. 7-4 Restriction of vision in the right visual field.

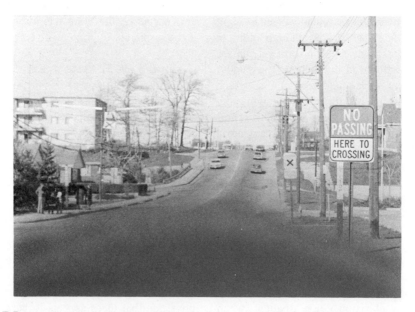

Fig. 7-5 Ascending dark veil from below, which may indicate a retinal detachment from above.

many sinister conditions, such as severe hypertension or brain tumor. Of importance in the assessment of any headaches are the following.

1. *Family history of headaches*. In many of the vascular headaches, such as migraine, a positive family history frequently is obtained.

2. *Onset and duration*.

3. *Severity*.

4. *Associated symptoms*. In this regard the ophthalmic assistant really is searching for other findings associated with the headache. For example, the patient with a migraine headache sometimes sees an aura before the onset of the headache. This aura usually consists of flashing of lines in zigzag formation, extending from the central area to the periphery and lasting approximately 20 minutes. Other important associated symptoms that should be noted are nausea, vomiting, blackouts of vision, fainting spells, weakness of an arm or leg, numbness of the fingertips, and difficulties with coordination.

5. *Relationship of the headache to visual activity*. Do the headaches follow prolonged periods of close work, or do they appear when the patient rises in the morning? Obviously, headaches caused by errors of refraction will not appear at night, during sleep, or on awaking.

6. *Character of the headache and its location*. A notation should be made of the nature of the patient's headache, whether it is vicelike, throbbing, or dull and also of its location, that is, in or above the eyes or in the temple regions.

Asthenopia

Asthenopia is a wastebasket term denoting a number of sensations that accompany uncorrected refractive error and problems in ocular motility. Included in this ocular wastebasket of symptoms are the complaints of (1) general eyestrain, (2) eye fatigue after reading, (3) pulling sensations, (4) inability to focus, (5) heaviness of the lids after reading, (6) sensitivity to sunlight or fluorescent light, (7) tendency to fall asleep after reading one or two pages, and (8) burning, itching, and watering of the eyes with reading.

In addition to refractive errors, these symptoms may be a result of chronic conjunctivitis, allergy, lack of tears, an emotional disorder, or fatigue. The patient with asthenopic complaints is apt to be vague and elusive in describing symptoms. Because the disability tends to be minor, lapses of memory are frequent and the patient often is reduced to repeating that "the eyes just don't feel right" (Table 7-1).

Red eye

The most common cause of a red eye is acute conjunctivitis. The salient features of conjunctivitis are discharge, pain, and blurred vision.

Discharge. The discharge of conjunctivitis can vary from being profuse and watery to being rather scant or purulent. During the day, of course, the discharge tends to drain and is wiped away with handkerchiefs and other tissues, but during the night it tends to accumulate and dry. Thus the patient with conjunctivitis complains that the lids are stuck together in the morning, the lashes being matted together in the dry discharge.

Pain. Normally there is no pain with simple conjunctivitis unless the cornea is involved. A secondary keratitis is a common accompaniment of conjunctivitis, especially if the offending organism is *Staphylococcus aureus*. The patient usually complains of a sandy or scratchy feeling or of having the sensation of a foreign body in the eyes.

Blurred vision. Because the clarity of the optical media is not affected by conjunctivitis, visual loss is not a prominent complaint in this condition. Because of the discharge over the surface of the cornea, however, the vision in the affected eye may be hazy. Occasionally such a patient even complains of seeing halos about lights.

In cases of conjunctivitis it is helpful to gain information regarding the source of the infection. Inquiry should be made into the presence of a similar disorder appearing in relatives or friends. Detection of the source of the infection may be very important, especially in crowded institutions such as orphanages or army barracks, where infection can travel through an entire group. It also is important to ask the patient if treatment has been started either by the family physician or by the patient.

Other causes. The red eye also is a manifestation of *acute iritis* and *acute narrow-angle glaucoma*, although the incidence of these two conditions is far

Table 7-1   Asthenopic symptoms

	Possible causes
SYMPTOMS INDICATING URGENCY	
Pain in the eye	Chemical burn
	Flash burn to cornea
	Keratitis
	Glaucoma
	Iritis
	Temporal arteritis
	Retrobulbar neuritis
Sudden loss of vision	Macular degeneration
	Cortical retinal artery occlusion
	Retinal detachment
	Central retinal vein occlusion
	Retrobulbar neuritis
Transient loss of vision	Carotid artery disease
	Migraine
	Papilledema
	Severe hypertension
Diplopia	Myasthenia gravis
	Thyroid disorders
	Diabetes
	Third nerve palsy from any cause
Ptosis	Third nerve palsy
	Diabetes
	Myasthenia gravis
Flashes of light	Retinal detachment
Trauma	Blow-out fracture of the orbit
	Hyphema
SYMPTOMS REQUIRING PROMPT ATTENTION	
Discharge and matting of the lids in the morning	Conjunctivitis
Red eye	Any external disease of the eye
Swelling of the lids	Bilateral blepharoconjunctivitis
	Acute allergies
	Thyroid disease
Halos around lights	Angle-closure glaucoma
	Cataracts
Blurred vision in the elderly	Macular degeneration
	Cataracts
	Ischemic optic neuropathy
Persistent tearing in one eye	Dacryocystitis
	Blocked tear duct
	Entropion, extropion
	Trichiasis
	Chalazion
	Bell's palsy
Enlarging nodule on the lid	Basal cell carcinoma
Foreign body sensation	Corneal foreign body
	Corneal abrasion
	Herpes simplex keratitis

Table 7-1   Asthenopic symptoms—cont'd

**SIGNIFICANT SYMPTOMS THAT SHOULD BE SEEN
AS SOON AS POSSIBLE**

Gritty feeling	Dry eye syndrome from any cause whatsoever
	Conjunctivitis
	Ocular irritation—dust, wind, ultraviolet lights
Headaches	Often tension
	Hypertension
	Brain tumor
	Migraine, cluster headaches, etc.
Blurred vision for distance in an adult	Diabetes
	Cataract
	Macular edema
Spots before the eye	Retinal tear
	Vitreous detachment
Pain behind the eye	Sinus disease
	Thyroid disorders
	Orbital tumor (rare)
	Aneurysm of the carotid artery (rare)
Eruption on the skin	Atopic allergy
	Seborrhea
	Herpes zoster
	Drug reaction

less than that of acute conjunctivitis. The diagnosis of acute glaucoma can virtually be made over the telephone. The onset of this condition is quite sudden and dramatic, with the entire triad of pain, loss of vision, and congestion of the globe occurring within a matter of 30 minutes. The pain of acute glaucoma, unlike that of conjunctivitis, is quite intense, and the patient may have associated nausea and vomiting. Also, the visual loss is profound, and frequently the vision is reduced to hand movements or counting fingers. The only real distinguishing feature between acute glaucoma and acute iritis, in terms of symptoms, is the difference in the onset of the two conditions. Iritis takes hours or days rather than minutes before it becomes fully developed.

The differential diagnosis of the common causes of an inflamed eye is outlined in Table 7-2.

Double vision, or diplopia

The patient with true diplopia reports seeing two objects instead of one. This symptom occurs when there is an acquired loss of alignment of the eyes, so that each eye does not project to the same place in space. Loss of ocular alignment is a common finding in children with strabismus. Children with stabismus however, do not see double because they are capable of suppressing the vision in one eye to avoid the confusion of double images. Adults are not as adaptable as children and quite disabled by double vision (Fig. 7-6). They have faulty spatial orientation and projection and complain of dizziness, inability to walk straight, and inability to reach accurately toward an object in space. If the diplopia results from the loss of alignment of the eyes, then covering one eye will always eliminate the second image.

Occasionally the patient may have monocular diplopia. With monocular diplopia the double vision persists when one eye is closed. It is important to make this distinction in the history. Binocular double vision always is caused by the development of a weak or paralyzed extraocular muscle. The loss of alignment results from the fact that an opponent muscle carries the eye over to one side. being unopposed

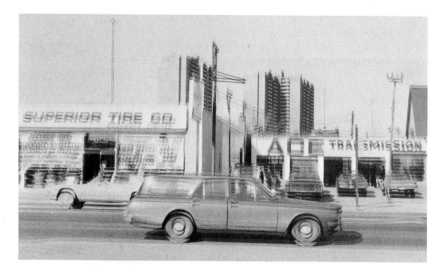

Fig. 7-6 Double vision. The images are just slightly displaced vertically.

Table 7-2 Differential diagnosis of common causes of the inflamed eye

	Acute conjunctivitis	Acute iritis	Acute glaucoma	Corneal trauma or infection
Incidence	Extremely common	Common	Uncommon	Common
Discharge	Moderate to copious	None	None	Watery and/or purulent
Vision	Normal	Slightly blurred	Marked blurring	Usually blurred
Conjunctival injection	Diffuse	Mainly circum-corneal	Diffuse	Diffuse
Pain	None	Moderate	Severe	May be pain or irritation
Cornea	Clear	Usually clear	Steamy	May be corneal abrasion, foreign body, or ulcer due to virus or bacterium
Pupil size	Normal	Small	Large	Normal
Pupillary light response	Normal	Poor	Poor	Normal
Intraocular pressure	Normal	Normal	Elevated	Normal
Smear	Causative organism	No organisms	No organisms	No organisms unless taken directly from cornea in case of bacterial ulcer

From Vaughn D, Cook R, Asbury T: *General ophthalmology,* Los Altos, Calif, 1965, Lange Medical Publications.

by the palsied muscle. For example, if the right lateral rectus muscle becomes paralyzed, the right medial rectus muscle would carry the eye inward toward the nose (esotropia) (Fig. 7-7).

Monocular diplopia is quite uncommon and may be caused by an extra pupil or cataracts, or it may appear in the recovery phase after strabismus repair.

Floating spots and light flashes

Virtually everyone has seen, at some time or another, small spots before the eyes. They may appear singly or in clusters; they may be punctate or linear; they may travel with the movements of the eye or against them. These floaters are most apparent when the illumination is high and when one is gazing at a clear

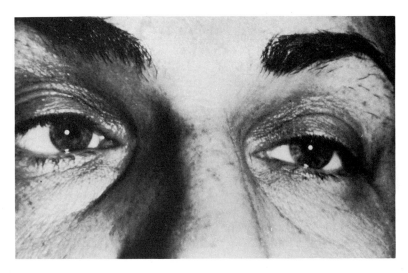

Fig. 7-7 Recent onset of paralysis of right lateral rectus muscle. Right eye has turned in.

surface. The most common situations in which they are seen include looking up at a clear summer sky, gazing against a blank white wall, and reading.

These floaters usually are caused by the formation of small particles in the vitreous body and generally are innocuous. However, floaters may, on occasion, be indicative of a more serious derangement within the eye. They may be caused by cells in the vitreous from an active iridocyclitis, or they may be secondary to a retinal tear, to hemorrhage, or to a detachment.

Tearing

Tearing as an isolated event occurs most commonly as a result of a blockage of the nasolacrimal duct. In infants it results from failure of the duct to become completely canalized. Although tearing most often is a sign of a blocked nasolacrimal duct, it also can be caused by congenital glaucoma, foreign bodies in the cornea, or inturned lashes. Each child with tearing should be assessed carefully.

In adults tearing is a less specific symptom. It may occur as a result of entropion, chronic conjunctivitis, allergy, or obstruction of the nasolacrimal duct. In taking a history of a patient whose primary complaint is tearing, one must note (1) the duration of tearing,

(2) whether it appears to come from one eye or both, and (3) associated findings, such as redness of the eye or discharge.

PAST HEALTH, MEDICATIONS, AND ALLERGIES

Patients should be asked about their general health at present and its status in the past. In particular, diabetes, hypertension, cardiac disorders, and arthritis should be mentioned. Many systemic disorders have ocular manifestations. If a positive history is obtained, the ophthalmologist can direct the examination with greater purpose.

Equally important is obtaining a history of any medications the patient may be taking. Often the patient will not know the name of the medication but will refer, for example, to a green tablet and a yellow tablet, as though the color of the pill or tablet were its identifying mark. When possible the ophthalmic assistant should call the patient's pharmacy to identify the exact name of the medication the patient is taking. If this is not feasible, the patient should be asked the purpose of the medication. Usually most patients are aware of their general function and will state that the pill is for reducing swelling in the legs or relieving high blood pressure.

Inquiry also should be made into the presence or absence of allergies. In general, five types of allergic responses should be inquired about:

1. Allergy to drugs (taken internally or applied topically)
2. Allergy to inhalants (dust, pollens, and so forth)
3. Allergy to contactants (cosmetics, woolens, and so forth)
4. Allergy to ingestants (food allergies)
5. Allergy to injectants (tetanus antiserum)

FAMILY HISTORY

It is helpful if inquiry is made into the familial history of the more common ocular defects. In particular, the presence or absence of such familial diseases as myopia, strabismus, and glaucoma should be asked about. A negative family history does not rule out a genetic familial propensity. Many patients really do not know the ocular status of their relatives, whereas others, being very family proud, are reluctant to confess to any weaknesses in the lineage.

Common familial disorders

Migraine
Retinitis pigmentosa
Retinoblastoma
Color blindness
Nystagmus
Albinism
Sickle cell anemia
Choroideremia
Keratoconus
von Recklinghausen's disease (elephant man's disease; neurofibromatosis)
Marfan's syndrome
Diabetes
Hereditary macular degeneration (Stargardt's disease)

TIPS IN HISTORY TAKING

The ophthalmologic assistant should follow a systematic order in taking an adequate history:

1. Identify the chief reason the patient has sought an eye examination.
2. Identify any secondary reasons or problems the patient has that are referable to the eye.
3. Identify any systemic or general illness the patient presently has and any medication being taken.
4. List past ocular disorders or operations.

5. Determine if the patient is wearing contacts or spectacles, and if so, how old they are and when the last eye examination occurred.
6. Be succinct but also go into detail with any specific ocular problem that arises. General questions, such as time and duration, family involvement, and so on, regarding any abnormality may be important.
7. Record any previous therapy and the response.

SUMMARY

The role of the ophthalmic assistant in obtaining a history will, of course, vary with the attitudes and opinions of the supervising ophthalmologist. Some ophthalmologists prefer to expand on a skeleton history, whereas others prefer to do the entire questioning themselves. Whatever duties are assigned to the ophthalmic assistant, they should be performed as efficiently and expeditiously as possible. Events of a history should be chronicled in breadth rather than in depth. A few short sentences under each heading usually are sufficient to cover an office history. It would be neither appropriate nor efficient for the ophthalmic assistant to spend an hour documenting the patient's complaints. The patient should be left as fresh as possible for examination by the ophthalmologist.

The analysis of the importance of symptoms is a difficult task because a symptom is merely an expression of disordered function. It depends not only on the patient's condition but also on the person's ability to define the trouble with lucidity. Exaggerations, distortions of complaints, irrelevancies, vagaries, and lapses of memory tend to lead the examiner astray. A good historian should not interpret for the patient. If a given history is not precise, a vague statement of the patient's actual complaints should be recorded. The interpretation of the history is the domain of the physician, who will assimilate all the findings from the history, physical examination, and pertinent laboratory investigations to arrive at a final diagnosis.

The ophthalmic assistant, in obtaining a history, should try to combine the qualities of a good police officer and a kindergarten teacher. The patient's interrogation should be directed toward obtaining the facts. The spirit of that interrogation should be calm, sympathetic, and patient. If possible, the ophthalmic assistant should try to make some notation on the chart of a personal nature, such as the patient's interests and hobbies, occupation, recent accomplishments, or recent tragedies. Such notations are helpful to the ophthalmologist in establishing rapport with the patient and setting the mood for the interview.

Of course, on revisits it is quite gratifying to the patient to be recognized as a human being rather than as an eye problem. Office personnel should not forget to ask patients about their gardening, their recent vacation, or the progress of their golf. It is all part of a good history.

QUESTIONS FOR REVIEW AND THOUGHT

1. A patient complains of sudden loss of vision in one eye. Outline a series of questions that will bring out the essential features of the problem.
2. Double vision may indicate a paralysis of one or more muscles of the eye. What factors are important in identifying the seriousness of the condition, and what muscles might be affected?
3. List the factors that will strengthen the professional components of the ophthalmic assistant's behavior.
4. List the various factors necessary to complete a proper insurance claim in your area.
5. A patient complains of seeing small floating objects in his vision. Outline a series of questions that will bring out the highlights of the history.
6. What is eyestrain?
7. For what conditions is the family history important?
8. Outline a useful sequence to follow in obtaining a good history.
9. What common systemic illnesses have an effect on the eye?
10. What medications should be recorded that affect the eye?
11. What color coding is used on miotics and mydriatic eye medications?
12. List and describe the essential elements of a complete problem-oriented medical case history.

SELF-EVALUATION QUESTIONS

True-false statements

Directions: Indicate whether the statement is true (T) or false (F).

T or F 1. History taking is a confidential experience between the patient and the technician who is involved in the questioning.

T or F 2. The most significant question to be asked is "What medications are you taking?"

T or F 3. The patient should be allowed to speak freely of all his or her problems while the technician is getting a history.

Missing words

Directions: Write in the missing word in the following sentences.

4. The most common cause of blurred vision is a _____.
5. Patients who are unable to see in movie theaters or in the evening are said to have _____.
6. An ascending veil in the lower portion of one's vision is an indicator of a possible _____.

Choice-completion questions

Directions: Select the one best answer in each case.

7. Which of the following is not normally considered in the differential diagnosis of an inflamed, red eye?
   a. Acute conjunctivitis
   b. Acute iritis
   c. Acute glaucoma
   d. Keratitis
   e. Dacryocystitis
8. Which of the following is not part of a history?
   a. Chief complaint
   b. History of past health
   c. Family history of eye disease
   d. Visual assessment
   e. Medication currently used

ANSWERS, NOTES, AND EXPLANATIONS

1. **True.** The confidentiality of the patient's symptoms is most important. Although some patients may not care who hears their symptoms, there are many who are quite disturbed by making a public hearing of their problems. In addition, some teen-agers, indigents, public figures, or highly nervous persons require individualized attention to their problems and frequently are offended when their problems become known to others. It may be of no consequence to ask the age of a teen-ager, but asking the age of a woman who has recently gone through menopause when other people are within earshot may evoke a large measure of hostility. Questions such as those that relate to medications taken may be important to the ophthalmologist but must be asked privately of the patient.

2. **False.** The most significant question is, "What is your chief complaint?" It is essential to select efficiently the key problem for which the patient has sought help from an ophthalmologist. Once the essential problem or problems have been identified, then the nature of surrounding involvements can be more effectively detailed. The recording of the history becomes important because if it is clearly itemized, the ophthalmologist can minimize time spent in finding the essential facts and avoid the confusion of a mass of disorganized information. Complaints should be reduced to succinct and compressed expressions related to the character and date of onset.

3. **False.** Allowing a patient to ramble in a disconnected way serves no purpose except to allow the patient to get things "off his chest." The most effective way to get a history is for the examiner to guide the direction of the interview so as to bring out the salient features and to jog the memory of the patient for details pertaining to the relevant complaint. In addition, the interviewer must detail other areas in the interview that the patient normally would not have considered. In this way, one can arrive at an accurate and significant history that will have a meaningful and reliable effect in determining the diagnosis.

4. **Refractive error.** In an ophthalmologist's office the most common thing people complain about is some blurring of vision for either distance or near. For most persons who seek eye attention, it usually is the myopia that leads to the visit, whether the person has been referred by school or the driver's bureau or has just noticed a tendency to squint. In the older age-group it is the presbyope who requires glasses for reading and seeks attention for blurred vision at near. Although numerous causes of organic disease affect loss of vision, these are in the minority in an ophthalmologist's practice, however, they always have to be considered when the eye cannot be refracted to a normal visual acuity or the history suggests more detailed organic loss.

5. **Night blindness.** A number of tests have been developed to determine the levels of light sensitivity and dark adaptation. The term *mesopic acuity* refers to vision under reduced illumination. A number of disease processes affect dark adaptation and produce night blindness. Such conditions as retinitis pigmentosa initially affect the rods that are abundant in the periphery of the eye and are responsible for mesopic vision by gradually obliterating them so that the patient is unable to navigate in the evening, in movie theaters, and in dimly lit rooms. Other diseases that affecting vision under reduced illumination include retinal and choroidal arteriosclerosis, retinal abiotrophies, choroideremia, Oguchi's disease, and hypovitaminosis. The test equipment for dark adaptation and mesopic vision usually is complex and expensive compared with equipment for visual field studies or color discrimination, and consequently it often is unavailable in most practitioner's offices.

6. **Retinal detachment.** When the retina separates from its underlying base, the sensory component is lost and a field of vision that is proportionate to the detached retina becomes diminished. To the patient this manifests as a loss in one or another portion in his or her field of gaze. It may go unnoticed until it begins to affect the macular area of the eye. The patient then responds by complaining of an ascending veil.

7. **e. Dacryocystitis.** This is an inflammation of the lacrimal sac or tear sac and results in a swelling over the tear sac portion. It occasionally will spill bacteria into the conjunctival sac, resulting in a secondary conjunctivitis. It is frequently a painful condition that requires antibiotics, hot compresses, and occasionally surgical intervention for resolution to occur.

8. **d. Visual assessment.** Visual assessment is part of the physical examination of the patient and is part of the objective measurements. The history is related to the person's complaints and past and present health, along with medications and family history. Any objective measurements are part of the physical examination. The diagnosis of any condition depends on both the history and the physical examination.

CHAPTER 8

Preliminary examination

- Vision assessment
- Measurement of glasses
- Accommodation
- Convergence
- Color vision
- Depth perception
- External examination
- Examination of the ocular muscles
- Instillation of eye drops and ointment
- Ophthalmoscopy
- Visual fields

The ophthalmic assistant is of great value when performing preliminary steps in the examination of the patient. A preliminary examination of the eyes trains and alerts the ophthalmic assistant to the numerous variations and abnormalities that occur around the eye and the eyelid. It provides a fascinating change from routine duties and challenges the assistant to sharpen diagnostic acumen and to develop an interest in the many major and minor affections of the eye.

VISION ASSESSMENT

Vision should be assessed both with and without glasses on a standardized chart, and each eye should be tested independently. It has been found that the normal eye can easily distinguish two points separated by an angle of 1 minute to the eye. By convention, most visual acuity charts are constructed so that the sections of a letter subtend 1 minute of arc. Each letter is printed on squares made up of five parts in each direction so that the whole letter to be identified subtends a 5-minute angle to the eye (Fig. 8-1).

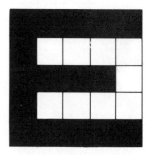

Fig. 8-1 The letter E. Each section of the letter subtends 1 minute of arc. The whole letter subtends 5 minutes of arc.

Visual acuity (VA) is determined by the smallest object that can be clearly seen and distinguished at a distance. The commonly used Snellen charts consist of letters carefully designed to subtend a 5-minute angle to the eye at certain specified distances (Fig. 8-2). Generally speaking, 20 feet, or 6 meters, has been considered a practical distance for assessing vision for distance, and the charts have been calibrated with this in mind (Fig. 8-3). At 20 feet the

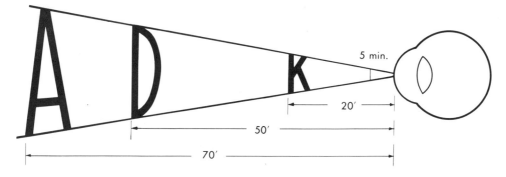

Fig. 8-2 Each letter on the visual acuity chart subtends a 5-minute angle to the eye independent of the distance.

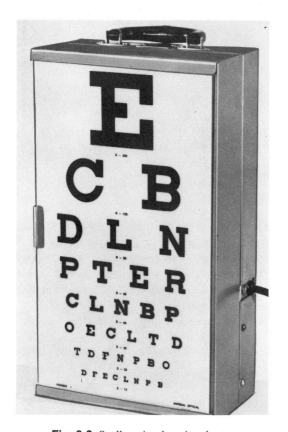

Fig. 8-3 Snellen visual acuity chart.

distant rays of light from an object are practically parallel, and very little effort of accommodation is required. In rooms that are shorter than 20 feet, mirrors may be used to achieve the required distance. Also, charts may be proportionately reduced in size to compensate for a room with a shorter working distance.

The results of vision testing are expressed as a fraction. The numerator denotes the distance the patient is from the chart letters, and the denominator denotes the distance from the chart at which a normal person can see the chart letters. For example, if a person reads the 20/20 line at 20 feet, visual acuity is 20/20 (VA = 20/20). If the person reads the 20/60 line at 20 feet, visual acuity is 20/60 (VA = 20/60). This actually means that the person can see at 20 feet a letter that a normal person can see at 60 feet.

Generally, in the western hemisphere visual acuity charts are designated in feet, whereas in Europe the metric system is used (Table 8-1).

A quiet area should be selected for testing visual acuity. The chart should be placed on a light, uncluttered wall that has no windows nearby. The chart should be fastened at eye level. The recommended illumination on the wall chart is 10 to 30 foot-candles, but many offices use projected types of vision charts or retroilluminated charts (see Fig. 8-3). The general illumination in the room should not be less than one fifth the amount of illumination on the chart.

In assessing vision, the examiner places an oc-

Table 8-1	Conversion table of visual acuity	
	Meters	**Feet**
	6/6	20/20
	6/7	20/25
	6/9	20/30
	6/12	20/40
	6/18	20/60
	6/24	20/80
	6/30	20/100
	6/60	20/200
	6/90	20/300
	6/120	20/400

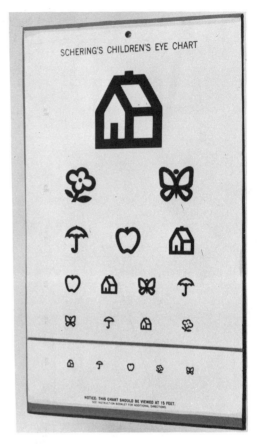

Fig. 8-4 Picture visual acuity chart.

cluder over one of the patient's eyes without exerting any pressure on the eye. The patient is then asked to read the chart. The smallest line of letters identified is noted. Adjacent to the line is a notation such as 20/20 or 20/40. The line read clearly is recorded as 20/20 or whatever the case may be. If one or two letters are missed in the line, this may be recorded. For example, if the patient sees the 20/20 line but misses one letter, visual acuity should be recorded as 20/20 − 1.

If unable to read the largest letter, the patient is asked to walk toward the chart; the distance at which he or she begins to read the large letter is recorded as the numerator. For example, 4/200 indicates that the patient was 4 feet from the 20/200 letter. If it is impossible for the patient to distinguish the large letter, the examiner holds his fingers before the patient's eye in good light and the vision is recorded as the farthest distance at which the fingers can be counted. For example, if the patient can accurately count the number of fingers the examiner is holding up 3 feet away, this is recorded as *counting fingers at 3 feet*. If the patient cannot distinguish fingers, the examiner should wave a hand in front of the eye. If movements of the hand are perceived by the patient, the vision is recorded as *HM*, or *hand movements*. If the patient cannot even detect hand movements, the room is darkened, a test light is shone into the eye from the four quadrants, and the patient is asked to point in the direction of the light. If the

patient can accurately point to light, vision is recorded as *light projection*. If the patient cannot distinguish the position but is able to just detect the light, the visual acuity is recorded as *light perception*. If the patient is unable to detect light at all the vision is recorded as *absent light perception*.

Illiterate persons and preschool children may be tested by charts made up of numbers, pictures (Figs. 8-4 and 8-5), Es (Fig. 8-6), or Landolt's broken rings. In the commonly used E test, the child points in the direction of the E either with a finger (Fig. 8-7) or with a hand-held cutout E. The modern cutout Es are made of plastic. With Landolt's broken-ring test the child merely identifies where the break in the ring occurs (Fig. 8-8).

The New York Association for the Blind has mod-

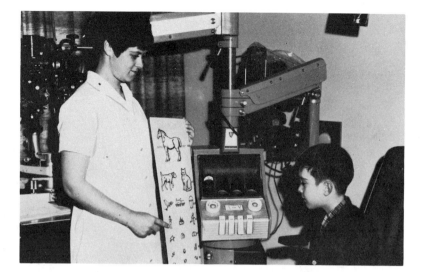

Fig. 8-5 Testing vision with pictures.

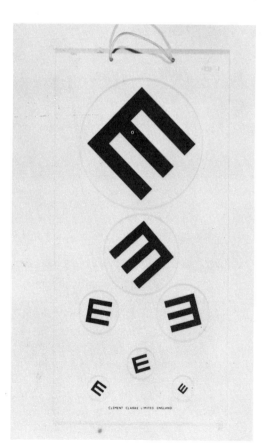

Fig. 8-6 E chart with rotating Es.

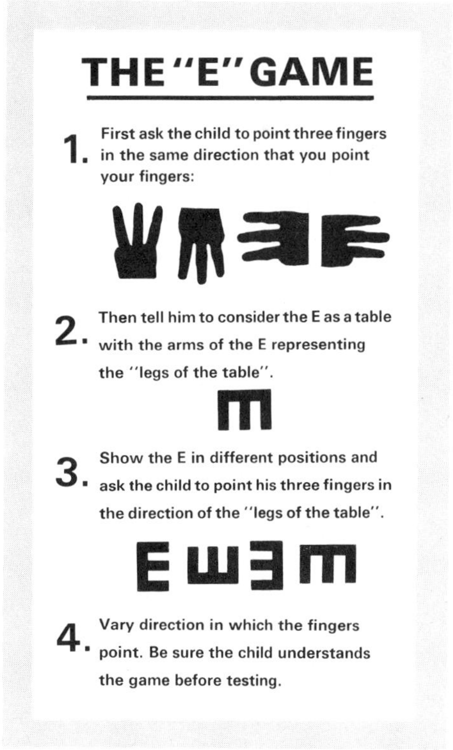

THE "E" GAME

1. First ask the child to point three fingers in the same direction that you point your fingers:

2. Then tell him to consider the E as a table with the arms of the E representing the "legs of the table".

3. Show the E in different positions and ask the child to point his three fingers in the direction of the "legs of the table".

4. Vary direction in which the fingers point. Be sure the child understands the game before testing.

Fig. 8-7

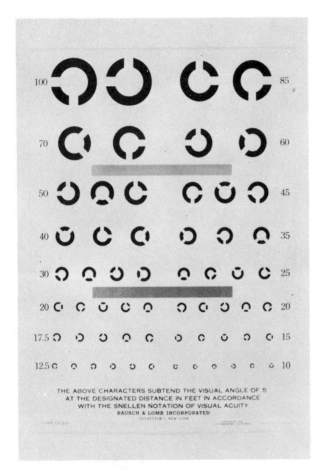

Fig. 8-8 Landolt's broken-ring test.

ified the readily identifiable pictures of the Schering chart into flash cards that can be held 5 or 10 feet from the young child. This distance is more practical for the child, and test results can be readily converted to the 20/20 system. The revised Sheridan-Gardiner Test for young or retarded children is a test in which the child is shown a number of letters at either 20 feet or 10 feet, is given a corresponding key chart and asked to hold the chart and identify the corresponding letter. The letters in the distance are shown in sequence at the proper distance, and the child identifies them by pointing to the key chart.

For near vision the examiner holds the near vision card at normal reading distance, and the child indicates on the key card the letters that he or she can identify.

A miniature toy set may be used to test the young child. The child is asked to match a toy with one held or projected 10 feet away. Young children may also be tested by their ability to see and pick up marbles of varying size on the floor.

It is often difficult to accurately measure visual acuity of young patients, especially preschoolers. Henry F. Allen, MD, has designed a set of four plastic cards to be used as a preschool vision test (Fig. 8-9). The test is a valid index of visual acuity recorded in terms of a 30-foot denominator. It is intended for preschool children, and results have been reliable for children aged 2 and over. It is also useful for retarded older children and for illiterate adults. It can be used for mass screening or for individual testing. No pretraining of younger children is necessary, as is frequently the case with the E game.

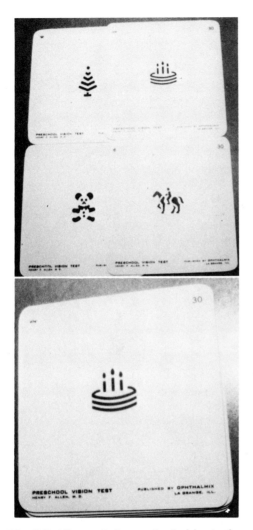

Fig. 8-9 Allen cards for preschool vision testing.

OD = 15 feet: vision = 15/30
OS = 10 feet: vision = 10/30

Comparison of the visual acuity of the child's two eyes is more important than absolute values obtained. Normal children between the ages of 2 and 3 can usually identify the pictures at 12 to 15 feet. Children between ages 3 and 4 can usually identify them at 15 to 20 feet. Adults with good visual acuity can recognize them at distances greater than 30 feet in good light. A difference of 5 feet between a child's two eyes is probable cause for referral.

If the child is shy in the presence of the examiner, it has been found that giving the cards to the mother will often produce adequate responses.

For infants younger than 2 years of age, a gross estimation of visual acuity can be obtained by simply flashing a light into each eye consecutively. If the child is able to fixate on the light centrally and steadily, vision may be assumed to be grossly normal. If the child's fixation is eccentric but steady, the child's vision is probably below normal. If the fixation pattern is unsteady and eccentric, vision is probably extremely poor and the eye defective. An infant should be able to follow a light by the age of 3 months and reach for toys by the age of 4 to 6 months.

When visual acuity is tested, the following points should be noted:

1. Whenever there is doubt about the child's motivation, intelligence, or attention, the E game should be used, because it is unnecessary for the child to make a judgment concerning a visual symbol.

2. A false idea of visual acuity will be obtained if an isolated letter is presented to the patient rather than a line of letters. This is particularly true in persons with amblyopia ex anopsia, who may have 20/40 or 20/50 vision when tested with isolated letters and only 20/200 vision when asked to identify letters in a series.

3. There can be differences in recognition of letters in the same line. The letter *L* is considered the easiest letter in the alphabet to identify, and *B* the most difficult. The letters *T, C, F,* and *E* are progressively more difficult.

The pictures are shown at close range to the seated child with both eyes open, and the child is asked to give a name to each picture. The pictures most eagerly received are most likely to be useful. One eye is then occluded, and the examiner presents the pictures, in sequence, while backing away from the child. The greatest distance at which three of the pictures are accurately recognized by each eye is then recorded as the numerator of a 30-foot denominator. For example:

4. Vision should always be tested with and without the patient's glasses so that a comparison between the two can be made.

5. In children, visual acuity testing should not be prolonged and fatiguing. Children are easily distracted and may fail to respond to conventional visual acuity tests because of loss of interest or short attention span.

6. If the child cannot comprehend the organization of the E game, he or she should receive practice at home. Parents can be given a small E printed on a card or an E cube (Fig. 8-10), or they can cut out the letter E from a piece of cardboard. It is best if a game is made of visual acuity testing. The E can be regarded as a table and the child asked to point a finger in the direction of the legs of the table.

7. In all visual acuity measurements the assistant should note any consistent pattern in the letters missed by the patient. For example, failure to see the nasal or temporal half of the chart may indicate a serious field defect, with loss of vision of half the visual field of each eye.

8. If both eyes are tested together, it is usually found that each eye reinforces the other, so that binocular vision tends to be slightly better than the vision of each eye tested separately.

9. A false visual acuity will be obtained if the patient partially closes an eye, or squints. This causes a decreased pupillary aperture and thus allows only central rays to enter the eye, giving much better vision than the patient would normally have. It is important for the patient to keep the eyes wide open.

10. The patient should be observed during testing to prevent peeking around the occluder. Illiterate patients often say they cannot see rather than admit ignorance. It is important to obtain their confidence and coax them to read a number or illiterate E chart.

11. A video acuity tester, developed at Baylor College of Medicine and available from Codman-Mentor, uses a keyboard microboard processor, which instantly transmits finger input to high-contrast television monitors. These monitors show perfectly spaced letters

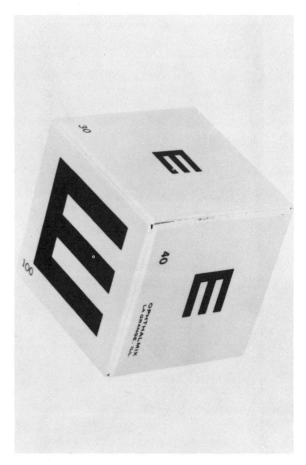

Fig. 8-10 E cube used for practicing the E game at home.

or tumbling Es. There are two screens, one available for the examiner to watch and control, and one for the patient to look at. This apparatus is faster for vision assessment than standard projection charts, and there are zoom capabilities to increase or decrease the size of the letter (Fig. 8-11).

12. New, computerized vision-testing apparatuses are rapidly entering the market. InnoMed's TVA refracting instrument allows the examiner to change the screen by remote control from anywhere in the room. Our experience has shown this to be much faster than standard acuity testing. In addition, there is a glare function test, a contrast test, and a night highway test.

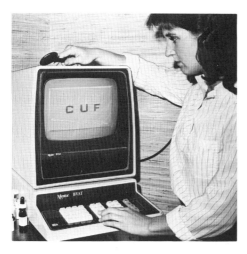

Fig. 8-11 A computerized type of vision-testing apparatus for increased speed in assessing vision.

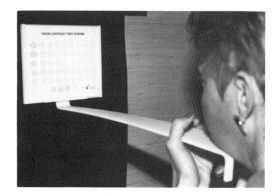

Fig. 8-12 Contrast sensitivity test at near.

Use of pinhole

The pinhole disk, if placed before the eye, eliminates peripheral rays of light, improves contrast, and generally improves vision to almost within normal limits if the patient has a refractive error. The pinhole disk thus serves to differentiate visual loss caused by refractive errors from poor vision resulting from disease of the eye. In the latter condition vision is not improved when a pinhole disk is placed before the eye.

Dynamic visual acuity

Visual acuity measured in an office setting is quite artificial. The eyes are steady, the body is still, and the target is immobile. In real life, as we walk down a street, the eyes are in motion, the body is displaced both forward and vertically, and the object of regard is rarely still. We look at things in action. This type of acuity is sometimes called *kinetic vision* or *dynamic visual acuity.*

Kinetic vision, or moving vision, cannot be measured, but it is known that acceleration reduces acuity. The faster one travels, the worse one's vision becomes. Body displacement spoils good vision. Try reading on a truck with poor shock absorbers. Fast eye movement is also a detriment to seeing clearly. It is impossible to follow a tennis serve traveling at over 100 miles per hour.

Contrast sensitivity

Another aspect of vision that has proven of interest is *contrast gradient visual acuity.* This is a measure of the acuity when hampered by poor contrast. A person can have 20/20 Snellen acuity and complain of poor vision. Snellen acuity measures only an individual's ability to see small, high-contrast images. The visual contrast test can assess the entire spectrum of images and contrast. An individual with cataracts or night blindness may see well in daytime but see poorly at night or on cloudy days when there is little contrast. Vision in the real world can be evaluated more realistically (Fig. 8-12).

Contrast sensitivity testing measures vision that resembles real-life situations more closely than the Snellen Chart. Contrast sensitivity could probably be detected with photographs of real life situations with different variations in their contrast; however, this is not practical and reproducible. Consequently, contrast sensitivity charts or machines are used. The contrast sensitivity chart presents a pattern of stripes of varying contrast, size, and orientation. The patient is asked to describe the orientation of the stripes. If the patient answers several correctly, it is assumed that he or she is able to see these objects at that particular size and contrast. Many sizes and contrasts are presented to determine if the patient has normal or decreased contrast sensitivity.

Contrast sensitivity tests may be presented as a wall chart with grids of varying size and contrast and a recording pad and instruction for analyzing

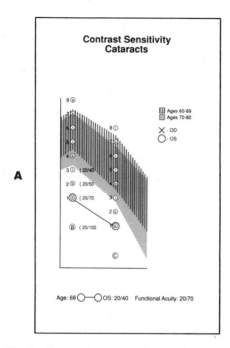

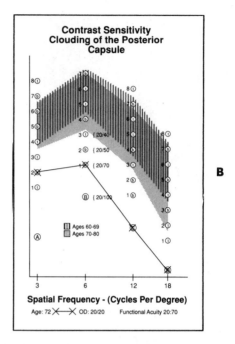

Fig. 8-13 A, This patient's left eye has good visual acuity, 20/40, but the functional acuity in Row B shows the patient to be clearly abnormal, 20/70, due to the cataracts. This patient's results suggest the need for cataract removal. **B,** This patient has clouding of the posterior capsule in his right eye. Although the patient has normal acuity, 20/30, the contrast curve shows the patient to be below normal. Further, the patient's functional acuity in Row B is 20/70. These results suggest the necessity of YAG laser surgery. Data from Maurice John, M.D. (Courtesy Vector Vision, Inc.)

the results. A smaller chart for near vision testing is also available (Fig. 8-13).

In some practices, patients are evaluated for contrast sensitivity before and after fitting contact lenses. If the fit is improper or the lens is improperly designed, the contrast sensitivity may decrease. This may be even more true with bifocal contact lenses. In addition, lenses often spoil with protein accumulation. Protein deposition reduces their contrast sensitivity while providing good Snellen acuity. In addition, contrast sensitivity testing has been found useful to determine improvement in macular degeneration after nutritional supplements. Contrast sensitivity testing has been found useful in evaluating treatment response in patients with glaucoma.

The use of contrast sensitivity tests has become important in refractive surgery. The use of both la-

sers and radial keratotomy to alter the shape of a normal eye so that there is a reduction in myopia must be accompanied by an evaluation. Contrast sensitivity is an important hallmark of the final visual acuity in a person and is much more reliable than Snellen acuity.

Glare testing

Visual acuity may degrade considerably in the presence of bright light. This is particularly true if there are opacities in the media, such as a posterior polar cataract. A number of glare test devices are available on the market (TVA, BAT, Eye Con) that create a dazzle effect and identify the person whose vision is reduced by glare (Fig. 8-16). The BAT test (Fig. 8-14, *B*), developed by Jack Holladay, delivers 3 controlled degrees of light when the eye is viewing

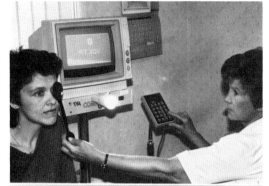

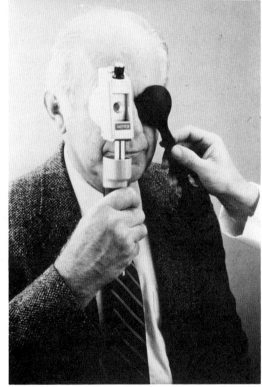

Fig. 8-14 A, The effect of glare on a roadsign is assessed by this programmed vision tester. **B,** Brightness Acuity Tester (BAT) developed by Jack Holladay to test the visual effect of bright sunshine on a patient with cataracts. (Courtest Mentor Co., Boston, Mass.)

a Snellen target. Vision with opacities in the ocular media, cornea, lens, posterior capsule, and vitreous, when under the effect of bright light, will degrade considerably and provide a true visual acuity in ambient lighting.

In glare testing, the patient looks into the machine or at some Snellen letters arranged on a wall chart. The examiner then turns on lights that shine directly into the patient's eyes. The lights have been calibrated to imitate the brightness of headlights coming toward the patient at night, both high and low beams. With the lights on, the patient is instructed to read the letters on the chart. The acuity is measured after glare testing is recorded. With high-beam light, this usually falls off considerably if there are lens opacities present.

The Miller-Nadler glare tester is a device commonly-used to test for visual discrimination during bright daylight conditions. It consists of a tabletop viewing screen and a slide projector with 17 slides of varying sizes of land, dot, sea, rings. The slides are projected onto the viewing screen. With each successive slide, the background is progressively made darker, thus decreasing contrast. The projector screen acts as a glare around the edge of the slide and shines into the patient's eyes. The ability or inability of a patient to detect breaks in rings of smaller size and lower contrast correlates to the loss of functional vision outdoors in bright sunlight.

Macular photostress test

This is a sensitive test for detecting macular dysfunction such as cystoid macular edema, central serous retinopathy, and senile macular degeneration. Under conditions of bright light, these disorders are slow to recover vision. Normal recovery to bright light is 0 to 30 seconds, but it becomes prolonged to over 1 minute in maculopathies.

Potential acuity

Potential acuity meter (PAM). It is often difficult to see behind a dense cataract, or even an early cataract, to give a good estimate of the potential visual acuity of any particular eye. The cataract often partially obscures the fundus so that evidence of optic atrophy, retinal detachment, and macular disease cannot be determined. While B-Scans can sometimes determine retinal detachments, the subtle retinal defects such as macular edema, mucular degeneration, and other vitreoretinal defects are often difficult to determine.

The Guyton-Minkowski potential acuity meter (PAM) is a small apparatus that attaches to a slit lamp. The patient looks into a small aperture in the machine and sees the Snellen acuity chart. The examiner can control the position of the acuity chart, shine it through the pupil, and direct it through particular sections of the patient's crystalline lens. Even patients with mild to moderate cataracts are not totally dense to this light and there are small breaks between opacities. The examiner shines the light through one of these small breaks, and the patient can see it unobstructed by the cataract and can then read down the Snellen chart. This has important prognostic significance for determining what the acuity will be following cataract surgery. It lets the physician know that the retina is intact and gives an estimate of potential acuity.

Interferometer. Interferometry is an apparatus similar to the PAM. Instead of a Snellen chart that is imaged on the retina through breaks in the cataract, the interferometer shines red laser light or white achromatic light directly through the opaque portion of the cataract. The light is not blocked by lens opacity and passes through unchanged. Laser light in a pattern of stripes, either red or white, depending on the type of machine is separated by black stripes of equal size. The width of the stripes can be changed. The patient is asked to name the orientation of each grid as the width is changed to estimate acuity. As the stripes become smaller, it becomes more difficult to detect which way they are pointing. If the patient can name the orientation of several grids with very small-width stripes, it is assumed that the retina can resolve images at that visual level and should approximate good postoperative acuity.

Both the PAM and the interferometer only give an estimate of what the potential acuity is. Patient's acuity may be much better or worse than what was expected.

Near vision testing

Near vision charts are designed to be read at 14 to 16 inches. In patients with accommodative loss, as in patients with early presbyopia, a corrective lens will be required to record the near vision. The near vision is recorded as the smallest type that can be comfortably read at the distance at which the card is held. Test cards are available in a wide variety of forms, such as printed paragraphs, printed words, music, numbers, pictures, and Es (Figs. 8-15 and 8-16).

Near vision for normal individuals may be recorded as 14/14, J2, or N5. The term *14/14* has the same meaning as the Snellen fraction in that the patient is able to read, at 14 inches, small print that is easily seen by a normal individual. The term *J2* refers to the Jaeger system. In the latter part of the nineteenth century Jaeger designed a system of readable print and arbitrarily assigned numbers, beginning J1, to the various sizes. The term *N5* refers to printers' point system; the print ranges in size from N5 to N48.

Near vision in children does not always correspond to the vision taken in the distance. Children can usually read despite significant refractive errors because they can hold reading material close to their eyes and thereby obtain magnification by the powerful range of accommodation.

MEASUREMENT OF GLASSES

Before the refractive status of a patient is evaluated, it is vital to know the previous prescription. The ophthalmic assistant should be very familiar with the technique to neutralize lenses and arrive at the prescription of the glasses the patient is wearing.

The lensmeter is an instrument designed to measure the prescription of an optical lens (Figs. 8-17 and 8-18). (*Lensometer* is the trade name of American Optical Company. All other manufacturers refer to lens-measuring equipment as *lensmeter, Vertometer, Vortexometer, or Focimeter*.) Lenses are made up of either spheres or cylinders, or a combination of both. By using a target area on the lensmeter, one can determine the exact prescription of any lens. All targets have some means of identifying two meridians that are at right angles to each other.

READING CARD--SNELLEN RATING

0.37 M	I walked up the street gazing about, and near the market house I met a boy with bread...	J 2
0.50 M	The difference of money and the greater cheapness I hade him give me three penny worth of any sort...	J 3
0.62 M	of Mr. Read, my future wife's father. She, standing at the door, saw me and thought I made a most awkward appearance, as I certainly did. Then I turned and went down Chestnut Street and a part of Walnut Street. Being filled with one of my rolls, I gave the other two to a woman	J 4
0.75 M	and her child. By this time the street had many clean and well dressed people in it, all walking the same way. I joined them and was led into the great meeting house of the Quakers'. I sat down among them and after looking around a while and hearing nothing said,	J 5
1.00 M	I fell fast asleep. This was the first house I was in, or slept in, in Philadelphia. Looking in the faces of people, I met a young man whose countenance I liked, and asked	J 7
1.25 M	if he would tell me where a stranger could get lodging. "Here," said he, "is one place that entertains strangers."	J 8

The above letters are Snellen sizes at the designated distance in meters, with Jaeger notations at right.

BAUSCH & LOMB INCORPORATED, ROCHESTER 2, N. Y., U. S. A.

71-35-90 PRINTED IN U. S. A.

READING CARD--SNELLEN RATING

15

20

PROP	BELT	HERE	BERG	BURN	LONE	DOLL	DERT	FLUE
DOME	THEU	NEED	FOLE	FRET	FOOL	COLT	PORE	DENE
COSY	HOLT	GILL	LOVE	LEND	WORE	BLEF	DOZY	GLEN

25

HUNT	BOOT	EDGE	HOPE	GOLF	HONE	BELT
BERG	HOWN	COOL	NEED	BOOT	GOLD	TELL
DELL	LOUD	LOST	CUBE	TOOL	FUSS	NUDE

30

SHOP	CHEF	BURN	BONE	FERN	RUBY	ZENO
ZONE	DUET	TENT	CODE	NOTE	SHOE	YULE
SOUL	PORT	SCUD	LUNG	GULL	TREE	VEST

40

DRUG	EDDY	BLUR	TUBE	NOSE
HOSE	BOSS	CLOD	COVE	PONY
LOON	DORY	FELT	SHOT	REEF

The letters subtend an angle of 5' at the designated distance in inches.

BAUSCH & LOMB INCORPORATED, ROCHESTER 2, N. Y., U. S. A.

71-35-90 PRINTED IN U. S. A.

Fig. 8-15 Snellen reading cards.

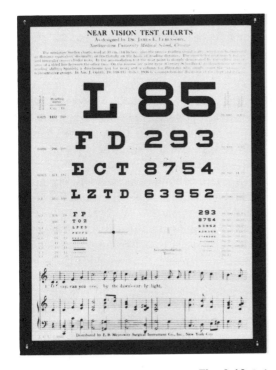

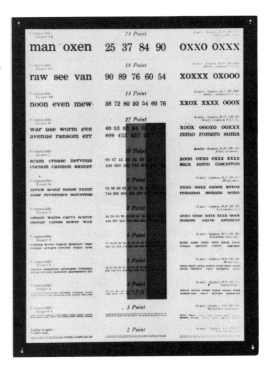

Fig. 8-16 Lebensohn reading chart.

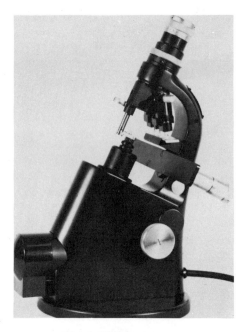

Fig. 8-17 Zeiss lensmeter.

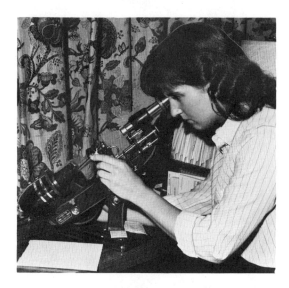

Fig. 8-18 Measurement of spectacles with lensmeter.

There are many types of lensmeters available. Each manufacturer publishes a manual showing how the instrument is used, because the instruments vary in approach. Some work in minus cylinders with plus spheres. Some manual instructions are in plus cylinders for all readings; others are in minus. Therefore the user may be confused when confronted with an unfamiliar instrument.

Although the instruments vary, the eyepiece on all lensmeters (except the projection type) must be adjusted to compensate for the user's refractive error, if any exists, or all readings will be inaccurate. The examiner should follow the procedure below:

1. Turn the power-focusing wheel until the target is *not* visible.
2. Turn the eyepiece fully counterclockwise.
3. Look through the eyepiece and turn it slowly clockwise until the grid or reticule just comes into focus. The correct position is the place where it first comes into focus. If in doubt, repeat.
4. Bring the target into sharp focus. The reading should be zero. If it is not, repeat. If zero cannot be obtained, set the power wheel to

zero, turn the eyepiece counterclockwise to blur the reticule, then clockwise until the target *and* reticule just come into clear focus. Note the number on the scale around the eyepiece for quick, future adjustment.

If the examiner wears distance glasses while making this adjustment of the eyepiece, they should be worn every time the lensmeter is used. If the examiner prefers to use the instrument when not wearing glasses, then the eyepiece adjustment should be made without them. It is important to be consistent.

Lensmeters fall into two categories: (1) those using the American crossed line type target (Fig. 8-19) and (2) those using the European dot type target (Fig. 8-20). Both types are accurate, providing the correct technique is used. The target type, therefore, is a matter of individual choice and of the operator's familiarity with a specific type.

The *American crossed-line type target* consists of solid straight lines at right angles to one another. A single line runs in one direction and three parallel lines run in the opposite direction (see Fig. 8-21). The whole target can be rotated 360 degrees for

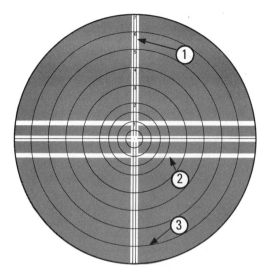

Fig. 8-19 American lensmeter target: *1,* single line; *2,* triple lines; *3,* rings to measure prism in a lens.

determining cylinder axis. To measure a lens with this type of lensmeter it is easiest at the beginning to follow five simple rules:

1. Place the spectacles on the base so that both left and right lenses are resting on the holder. This prevents rotation of the lens and inaccurate axis reading.

2. Focus the single line. Rotate the lines by using the axis wheel so that the single line gives readings closest to zero for both the plus and the minus spheres. This is then marked down as the sphere component.

3. Focus the triple line and record the *difference* from the single line to the triple line. This is the cylinder portion. For example, if the single line is at + 1.00 and the triple line is at + 3.00, the prescription will be + 1.00 + 2.00.

4. Rotate the axis wheel so the target is on axis when the triple lines are continuous. Mark down this axis; this is the axis of the cylinder (for example, + 1.00 + 2.00, axis 90). If the single line and the triple line are in focus at the same time, the lens is a sphere.

5. In determining the reading addition in a bifocal lens, move the lens up to the reading segment and then focus again on the triple lines. The difference from the recording of the last triple

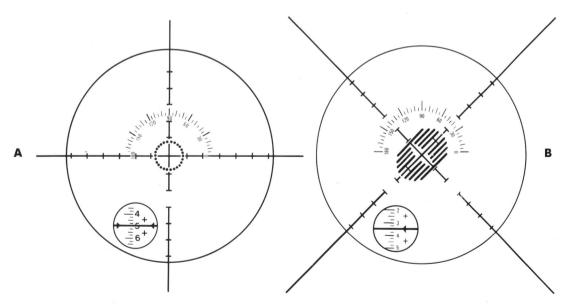

Fig. 8-20 European lensmeter test target. **A,** Test target with spherical lens. **B,** Test target with spherocylinders.

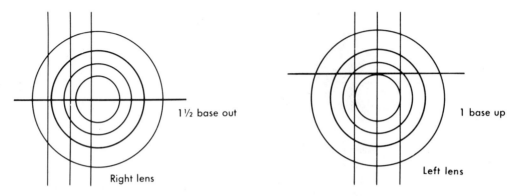

Fig. 8-21 American-made lensmeter target. Neutralization of a lens with a prism incorporated. Note that displacement of the target by the prism is always recorded in terms of the base of the prism.

line to the new triple line in focus will be the reading addition. This is *always* recorded as plus.

If the examiner initially focuses the single line so that it is closest to zero, both the cylinder and the sphere will have the same sign (plus or minus).

In some cases the examiner may wish to record all prescriptions in terms of plus cylinders. In doing so, it is necessary to first bring the single and then the triple line in focus. By rotating the axis wheel, the examiner can arrange that the triple lines come into focus when more plus is introduced, thereby ending up with cylinders recorded as plus.

The *European dot-type target* consists of a circle of dots (or variation thereof) which does not rotate. Instead, a protractor grid rotates in the field of view to determine the cylinder axis. The power of a spherical lens is determined by bringing the dots into sharp focus and then reading the power (see Fig. 8-20).

The power of a toric or cylindric lens is determined as follows:

1. If a lens contains a cylinder, the target will appear as a system of focal lines. These lines will focus in two positions—one perpendicular to the other. First, focus the target so that one of these lines is in focus. The reading closest to zero is marked down as the spherical component (for example, + 1.00).

2. Focus the target so that the second set of lines is now perpendicular to the first reading, and record the *difference* in dioptric powers between the first and second reading. This is the cylinder portion. For example, if the first focal point is at + 1.00 and the second focal point is at + 3.00, then the prescription will be + 1.00 + 2.00.

3. Adjust the cross line so that it is parallel to the focal lines on this second reading. This is the axis of the cylinder (for example, + 1.00 + 2.00, axis 90).

NOTE: It will be impossible with a very weak cylinder to identify a cylindric lens and its axis when the dots are in focus. (When the user is unfamiliar with this instrument, the most common error is that the axis is off by 90 degrees.) There will be no difficulty with stronger cylinders because the dots will smear into distinct lines, and aligning the axis grid offers no problems.

The technique for neutralizing a lens with a weak cylinder is as follows: First, rock the power-focusing wheel on either side of the target's focus point, and note how the individual dots "bloom," or go out of focus. If the blooming is spherical in shape, you have a spherical lens. If the blooming is oval, you have a cylindric lens. While rocking the focusing wheel, rotate the target protractor or reticle to line it up with the direction (axis) of the oval "blooming" or smearing of the circular dots. After establishing the cylindric axis, determine the spherical and cylindric power.

4. In determining the additions in a reading bifocal lens, move the lens up to the reading segment and then focus again on the lines at the second focal point. The difference between the value of the second focal point in the distance prescription, and that found in the reading segment will be the reading addition. This is always recorded as plus.

With *all lensmeters* it is important (1) to center the lens well before reading the prescription and (2) to measure the *prism,* if present. The lens has a prism if the center of the lens does not coincide with the center of the target. There are circles surrounding the central target of the lensmeter to measure the amount of *prism.* The distance between each circle represents 1 prism diopter. It is easy to see at a glance how far the optical center of the lens is displaced in prism diopters from the center of the target. Fig. 8-21 illustrates a prism in a lens with the American type of target.

Universal method of using any lensmeter

There are now many projection instruments that make reading of the lens prescription easier (Fig. 8-22). The following method will work with any lensmeter, standard or projection type, using any type of target:

1. Place the lens to be measured (in frame or otherwise) in the lensmeter on the table, convex side toward you, with the lens surface firmly against the instrument, and with *no tilt.* Tilting a lens will introduce an error that may result in an inaccurate axis and cylinder power. This is a common error made by the inexperienced user in measuring the bifocal segment. Finding the addition of a fused-glass bifocal requires a special technique, which will be covered in detail later.

2. Center the target, then set the power to zero. Move the power wheel from zero to a point well beyond the focus of the target, and then back toward zero to the point where the first target meridian or dots come into focus. Take the reading. This is the *spherical power.*

3. *Continue* rotating the power wheel *in the same direction* (do not reverse direction) to bring the

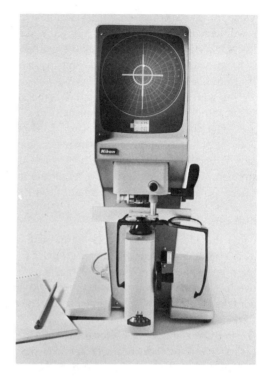

Fig. 8-22 Nikon projection vertexometer.

second meridian into focus. The algebraic difference is the *cylindric power.* The sign of the cylinder will be opposite that of the sphere. Note the *axis* of the second meridian. This may be correct or exactly 90 degrees off.

4. Make this check. If the target line or smeared dots are nearly horizontal, the axis is going to be near zero or 180 degrees. If the target line or smeared dots are nearly vertical, the true reading will be near 90 degrees.

This procedure is the same with all makes of lensmeters, and the user actually has a check on a possible cylinder axis error. The user may be in doubt, however, when the axis is near 45 or 135 degrees, in which case another pair of glasses should be tried (or a cylinder from a trial case) in order to identify which line on the target, or the grid, gives the true axis.

This universal method gives plus cylinder results with minus spheres, and minus cylinder results with plus spheres.

Once the user has mastered the instrument he or she will have no difficulty in modifying the method to work only in plus or only in minus cylinders if this is wished, rather than transposing mathematically from one to the other.

Prism, with the base in any direction, is measured by concentric circles and the displacement of the target. The circles may be in 0.50 or 1.00 prism diopter steps. In addition, some lensmeters have a Risley rotary type prism as an integral part of the instrument; its secondary use is to center the target for accurate axis reading in a prismatic lens.

Addition

To find the addition in spectacle lenses with adds under 3.00 diopters, take the dioptric power of the three lines at the distant portion of the lens. Then move the lens up to the bifocal segment and again record the dioptric power of the three lines. The plus difference is the bifocal addition.

To find the addition of a bifocal lens under 3.00 diopters, the difference in power between the distance and the reading portions must be found. First, the distance power should be found in the conventional manner, holding the lens being tested in the instrument with the rear surface (usually concave) away from the eye. Second, the reading power should be found, holding the lens in the same position—rear surface away from the eye. If the bifocal is less than 3.00 diopters, the above method will produce a correct reading to within 0.06 of a diopter, which is an insignificant error.

For all bifocals over 3.00 diopters, the following is the only procedure that will give accurate results:

1. Check the distance portion in the manner indicated above. This step is identical in checking all lenses and gives an accurate result as to the power of the distance portion.
2. The bifocal must now be reversed in the instrument. Hold its front (usually convex) surface away from the eye, and check the distance portion at a spot about the same distance above the center as the point at which you will check the reading power is below the center. In the case of aspheric surfaces, measure the distance through its optical center.

3. Note the finding made through the distance portion. Now check the power through the reading, again with the convex surface away from the eye. Subtract the power of the distance portion found from the reading power to determine the addition.

When making all readings, the lens must be firmly against the lensmeter stop; its surface at right angles to the axis of the lensmeter. In some lensmeters it is advisable for the operator to hold the lens in position with his or her fingers and not rely on the lens holder.

Automatic lensmeters

Space-age technology has once again simplified the operator portion of arriving at spectacle measurements. Although costly, this technology will save time and improve accuracy in a busy office. The Humphrey Lens Analyzer is an automatic lensmeter that measures in a single operation the sphere, cylinder, axis, and prism of a lens (Fig. 8-23). The values are digitally displayed and can be recorded,

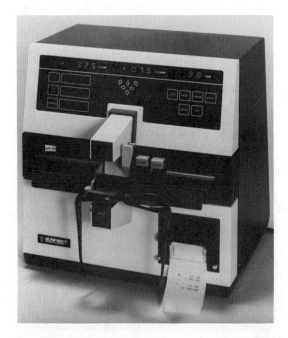

Fig. 8-23 The Lens Analyzer, manufactured by Humphrey Instruments Co.

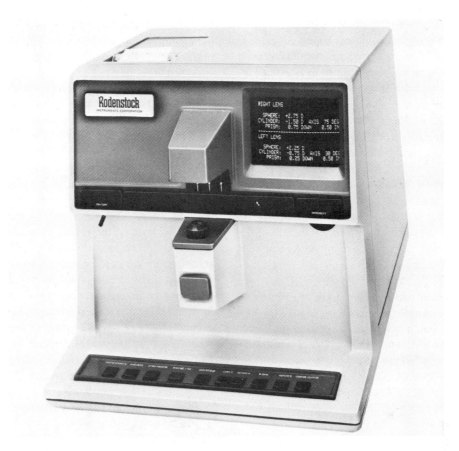

Fig. 8-24 Rodenstock lensmeter, which displays both right and left lenses simultaneously.

if desired, on a paper tape by the built-in printer. This instrument eliminates the focusing and target alignment tasks, which require a fair amount of skill with a conventional lensmeter. It also does the arithmetic tasks of computing cylinder power and of computing the add value of the bifocal segment. The Lens Analyzer has the unique ability to position spectacle lenses at a given interpupillary distance, and then to use prism information collected to compute the net prismatic effect of the spectacle pair. These measurements are made very rapidly. The instrument uses a white light source and a ray trace–type system to make its measurements.

The minicomputer in the Lens Analyzer is used to operate a hard copy printer, to make add computations when bifocals are measured, to change the display cylinder convention, to change roundoff modes, and to make special tests for errors and improper measurements, in addition to its primary mode of calculating and displaying the basic lens values. When a spectacle pair is measured, the printed copy records the lens values for both lenses labeled "left" and "right" with sphere, cylinder axis, and prism shown, plus the net prism for the pair. This automatic lensmeter operates on a standard electric power source.

The MetroLens–II, a lensmeter manufactured by Rodenstock instruments, is a fully automated and accurate measure of ophthalmic and contact lenses. It displays with high accuracy the power of the lenses, rounded off in increments of 0.12 diopter and 0.25 diopter as determined by the operator.

There is a simplified method of centering the lens and making measurements. Both right and left lens measurements can be displayed simultaneously. There is an optional copy printer available (Fig. 8-24).

The Autolensmeter, manufactured by Acuity Systems, similarly is a microprocess computer that provides ophthalmic and contact lens reading with accuracy. Pressing one button provides sphere/cylinder and shows both on a display panel and on printed tape. Pressing another button causes both horizontal and vertical prisms to be displayed. The "add" button automatically computes the additional power on multifocal lenses. The Autolensmeter also simplifies the measurement of progressive power lenses.

Aids in care and use of lensmeter

1. All optical parts of the lensmeter, as well as the spectacle lens, should be kept clean with a soft cloth and lens-cleaning solution.
2. In unusual situations, the spherical power may extend beyond the range of the lensmeter scale. If this occurs, it may be necessary to insert neutralizing or opposite-power lenses in the lensmeter to bring the target into focus. The final figures will be approximate only.
3. Prisms may be detected by counting the number of rings from the center crossmark that the optical center of the lens is displaced. The direction of the base of the prism can be read directly. For example, if the optical center of the lens is displaced two rings temporally from the center of the crossmarks, then the amount of prism present in the lens would be 2.00 prism diopters, base out.
4. If the center of the lens cannot be detected in the field of the target, loose prisms may be required to bring the optical center of the lens to fall within the area of the target. Some lensmeters incorporate the variable-adjusting Risley type prisms (see Chapter 9) for this purpose.

ACCOMMODATION

Accommodation is a mechanism by which the eye internally adjusts to change in the proximity of an object before the eye in order to maintain a clear image on the retina. This change in the total power of the eye is affected by alterations in the radius of curvature and the thickness of the lens of the eye. Increasing the radius of curvature of the anterior face of the lens and increasing its thickness add power to the eye as an optical instrument.

Measurement of amplitude of accommodation

Proximity method. Small print, such as J3 type, is held at a comfortable arm's length and gradually brought closer. The distance at which the patient reports blurring of the letters is measured in *centimeters* and expressed in diopters. To convert the centimeter measurement into diopters, this measurement should be divided into 100. For example, if the patient detects blurring of the print at 20 cm, the range of available accommodation would be from infinity to 20 cm, and the power of accommodation would be 100/20 or 5.00 diopters. It is important that each eye be tested individually and that the patient wear full-distance correction for the test. If the patient is too presbyopic to comfortably hold reading material, an auxiliary lens, such as + 2.50, is added to the patient's correction. The amplitude of accommodation is then measured, and + 2.50 subtracted from the total findings.

Triple line test. In this test two small vertical lines, as found on the Lebensohn chart, are brought toward the patient. The near point is reached when the patient sees three lines instead of two.

Effect of age

The ability of the eye to make these changes in focusing adjustments is greatest in childhood, when the crystalline lens is softest and most malleable. The range of accommodation declines rather precipitously with age as the lens becomes harder. A 10-year-old child has 14.00 diopters of accommodation and a near point of 7 cm, whereas a 40-year-old adult has only 4.50 diopters of accommodation and a near point that has receded to 22 cm (Table 8-2). This means that a 45-year-old man cannot see fine print closer than 22 cm without the assistance of reading glasses.

Table 8-2	Accommodation and near point of the emmetropic eye	

Age	Near point in centimeters	Available accommodation in diopters
10	7	14.00
20	9	11.00
30	12	8.00
40	22	4.50
45	28	3.50
50	40	2.50
55	55	1.75
60	100	1.00
65	133	0.75
70	400	0.25
75	Infinity	0

CONVERGENCE

Convergence is an act by which the eyes are turned toward each other to view an object in the midline plane situated close at hand. It is measured by having the patient look at a small target such as a pin, letter, or toy (Fig. 8-25). The near point of convergence is that point at which fusion can no longer be maintained and one eye deviates outward. The patient may report seeing double at the moment one eye begins to drift outward. The near point of convergence (NPC) is measured in centimeters.

The following points should be kept in mind when measuring convergence:

1. It is a voluntary act that requires the cooperation of the patient and the ability to respond to the test with alertness. If the patient is tired or debilitated at the time of testing, the near point may be unusually remote. If the patient is a distractable, disinterested child, again the near point cannot adequately be measured. For these reasons, the near point of convergence is not regarded as a reliable and completely reproducible test in terms of value.

2. This test requires normal fusion; it cannot be performed if one eye is amblyopic.

COLOR VISION

Defects in color vision may be congenital or acquired. Congenital color defects occur in about 8%

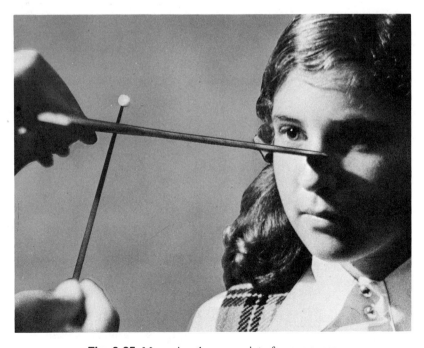

Fig. 8-25 Measuring the near point of convergence.

to 10% of males and in only 0.4% of females. This defect is transmitted through the female and appears predominantly in the male. Acquired color blindness may occur after diseases of the optic nerve or central retina.

Congenital color blindness may be partial or complete. In the completely color-blind patient, the visual acuity is reduced and the patient usually has nystagmus. All colors appear as various shades of gray. Fortunately, this form of color blindness is rare. The partial form is a hereditary disorder transmitted through the female, who usually is unaffected. In the majority of patients, the color deficiency is in the red-green area of the spectrum. With the deficiency in red, this color appears less bright than for the normal individual, and thus mixtures of colors containing red are often confused with other colors. Deficient color vision of the red-green variety may pose problems for sailors, drivers, pilots, and textile designers. Absence of blue color is very uncommon.

Tests for color blindness are multiple and varied and consist of matching colored balls or yarns, the red-green lantern test, and the most popular test, isochromatic plates.

In clinical practice it is sufficient to test with one of the pseudoisochromatic plates. More scientific approaches to color vision testing (such as the Nagel anomaloscope) are available but are not generally useful for routine clinical practice.

Ishihara test plates. (Fig. 8-26). The Ishihara book consists of a series of pseudoisochromatic plates that determine total color blindness and red-green blindness. These plates are viewed by the observer under good illumination. They consist of dotted numbers of one color against a background of another color. If color vision is normal, the dots stand out and the patient can read the appropriate number. A person with normal sight may see one number, whereas the color-blind person viewing the same plate would interpret the dots as forming a completely different number. For patients unable to read numbers, plates are present in the album with colored winding lines that may be traced.

Hardy-Rand-Ritter plates. (Fig. 8-27). This test is no longer manufactured but may still be found in ophthalmic offices. This series of pseudoisochromatic plates includes plates for yellow-blue color blindness as well as red-green color deficiency. The background is a neutral gray on which a series of colored circles, crosses, and triangles are superimposed. These geometric designs are present in higher and lower saturations of color to detect the degree of color vision deficiency. Under proper illumination, the observer is required to detect the geometric designs present on each plate. With this color vision test, not only can a graded diagnosis be made (mild, medium, or severe), but also the yellow-blue defects may be differentiated as well as the red and green.

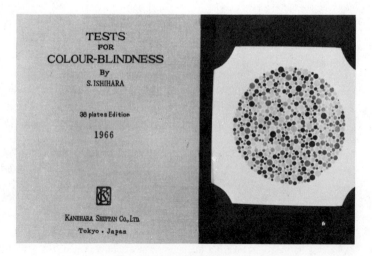

Fig. 8-26 Ishihara's test for color blindness.

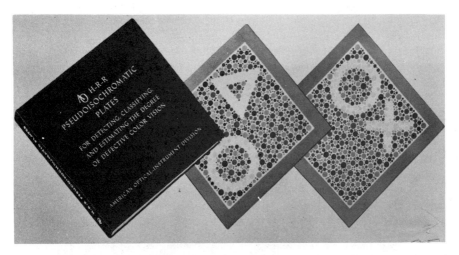

Fig. 8-27 American Optical Hardy-Rand-Ritter test for color blindness.

Although it is possible to memorize the numbers on the round Ishihara plates, this is impossible with the H-R-R-test, because the patient must identify not only what symbols he sees on each plate but also how many and in what quadrant. To ensure against malingering, the plates may be presented right side up, sideways, and upside down. As a result, the malingering patient will have no clues to guide him.

Colormaster. Colormaster is a sophisticated, completely automatic, and programmable computerized form of presenting color sequences of constant hue, saturation, and brightness to an individual. This computer has both clinical and research importance because of its repeatability and reliability.

DEPTH PERCEPTION

Depth perception is the highest quality of binocular vision because it provides the individual with judgment concerning depth, based on the coordinate use of the two eyes together. A prerequisite for depth perception is good vision in each eye, overlapping visual fields, and normal alignment of the eyes in all positions of gaze. Four main tests available are the fly test, the Wirt stereo test, the Worth four-dot test, and the biopter test.

Fly test. The patient is provided with Polaroid lenses and asked to touch the wings of a fly. If the patient has depth perception, the wings will appear to stand out before the picture (Fig. 8-28). This patient will have gross stereopsis of approximately 200 seconds of arc.

Wirt stereo test. Animals in three lines are shown to young school-aged children or even to preschoolers who seem able to grasp the idea of the test (see Fig. 8-28). If all three lines of animals are correctly selected, the patient has stereopsis of approximately 100 seconds of arc.

The raised rings in nine frames are shown to older children, adults, or even to younger children, if possible, depending on the alertness of the child. If all nine groups are correctly selected, it may be assumed that the patient has normal stereopsis of approximately 40 seconds of arc. In this portion of the test, two groups must be missed in succession for the examiner to stop the test. For example, if the patient correctly selects groups 1 through 6 and misses groups 4, 7, and 8, number 6 would be counted as the patient's maximum amount of stereopsis.

Worth four-dot test. In the original Worth four-dot test, one white disk, one red disk, and two green disks are presented to the patient, who is wearing spectacles with a red-free *green* lens before one eye and a green-free *red* lens before the other eye—thus allowing both the patient's eyes to see the white disk. However, the eye covered with the red lens will see, in addition to the white disk, only the red disk. The

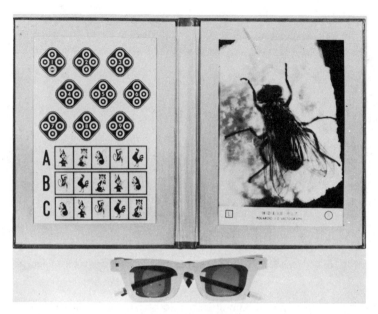

Fig. 8-28 Wirt and fly tests for depth perception.

eye covered with the green lens will see, in addition to the white disk, only the two green disks. The patient is then asked to report the number of disks seen. If four disks are seen, both eyes are functioning. If three disks are seen, then the eye behind the green lens is seeing (the two green and one white), and the eye behind the red lens is suppressing. If two disks are seen, then the eye behind the red lens is seeing and the one behind the green lens is suppressing. If five disks are seen, then another problem is indicated (the eyes are not fusing and muscular imbalance is suspected) (Fig. 8-29).

Variations on this test include the Project-O-Chart slide, wall-mounted internally illuminated tests, or the flashlight form (Fig. 8-30). The symbols shown may be four disks set in a diamond pattern, or a disk, a cross, a triangle, and a square. For children a picture presentation in colors of a clown, a seal, and a ball may be used. In all these tests the red and green spectacles are worn.

Biopter test. This instrument has the fundamentals of a home stereoscopic viewer in which slightly different images are presented to each eye (Fig.

8-31). The sensation of depth is appreciated by the slightly disparate images.

EXTERNAL EXAMINATION

Although the ophthalmic assistant cannot expect to substitute for the trained eye of the ophthalmologist in recognizing abnormalities of the eye and the eyelid, an awareness of abnormal external features, with documentation of such on the record, will aid the ophthalmologist in the recording of these abnormalities, as well as alert him or her to problems that are incidental to the main complaint of the patient. This exercise will also help instill an awareness of and interest in unusual eye problems, whether they are abnormal or pathologic.

The ophthalmic assistant should begin the external examination of the eye by systematically noting the symmetry of the orbits, the lid margins, the conjunctiva, the lacrimal apparatus, the sclera, the cornea, the iris, the pupil, and the lens.

Symmetry of orbits. In *proptosis* (exophthalmos), in which one eye protrudes, the upper lid is often retracted and there is exposed sclera above and below

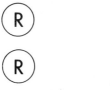

1. Left eye suppression

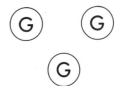

2. Right eye suppression

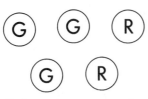

3. Esotropia: no suppression

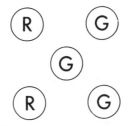

4. Exotropia: no suppression

Fig. 8-29 Worth four dot test. 1 and 2) The suppressing eye, 3 and 4) muscle imblance and no fusion, and 5) normal 4 dot response. R = red lens before right eye, G = green lens before left eye.

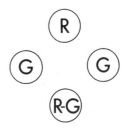

5. Normal 4-dot response: no suppression

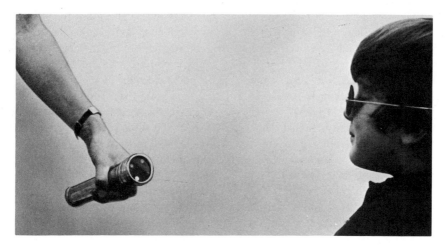

Fig. 8-30 Worth four-dot test to detect suppression.

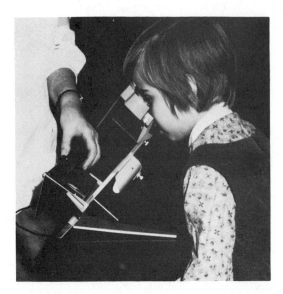

Fig. 8-31 Biopter test for depth perception.

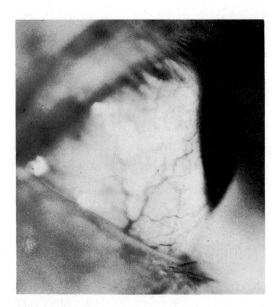

Fig. 8-32 Proptosis of the eye. Note the lid retraction and the exposed sclera above and below the cornea.

the cornea (Fig. 8-32). Another method of determining the presence of proptosis is to stand behind the patient, draw his upper lids upward, and note which eye appears to bulge the most. The ophthalmologist may record the degree of proptosis with an instrument called an exophthalmometer (see Fig. 9-34.)

Eyelids. Cilia, or eyelashes, are hairs on the margins of the lids. They are located in two rows, totalling about 100 to 150 cilia on the upper lid and half that number on the lower lid. The bases of these cilia are surrounded by sebaceous glands (glands of Zeiss). Infections of these glands result in a common sty. The average life of the cilium is from 3 to 5 months, after which it falls out and a new one grows in to take its place. If the cilium is pulled out, the new one replacing it reaches full size in about 2 months. If the cilia are cut short, as is sometimes done preceding surgery on the eye, regrowth is rapid and lashes may appear normal in a few weeks.

Lid margins. The lid margins should be observed for any redness, scaling, or discharge, indicative of *blepharitis*. The position of the lid margin should also be noted. It should be tight against the globe and not sag outward *(ectropion)* or inward *(entro-*

pion). The punctum on the medial aspect of the lower eyelid should not be visible without depressing the lower eyelid. The more common affections of the lid margin are *styes, chalazions,* and *growths.*

Conjunctiva. The bulbar conjunctiva is readily visible. The caruncle is seen as a fleshy mound of tissue at the inner canthus. The palpebral conjunctiva of the lower eyelid is seen by depressing the lower lid while the patient looks toward the ceiling. The palpebral conjunctiva lining the upper eyelid can be seen only by everting the upper lid. Eversion of the upper eyelid is carried out by grasping the lashes of the lid between the thumb and index finger and turning the eyelid over a toothpick or applicator. It is important that the patient be asked to look downward to relax the levator muscle. With eversion of the upper eyelid the tarsal conjunctiva is visible and the meibomian glands running vertically from the lid margin are easily seen. The conjunctiva should be inspected for follicles, discharge, color, and growths such as *pterygium and pinguecula.*

Lacrimal apparatus. The tear film that covers the surface of the eye is composed of the following three layers:

1. A superficial oily layer derived from the mei-

bomian glands and the sebaceous gland of Zeiss. It prevents evaporation of the underlying tear layer.

2. The tear film, which is the middle layer, is secreted by the lacrimal gland and the accessory glands of Frause and Wolfing.

3. The deepest layer is the mucoid layer and is secreted by the goblet cells of the conjunctiva.

The tears are normally carried from lateral to nasal sides along the lid margin. When they reach the opening of the lower lid, the punctum, they drain into the nasolacrimal duct and finally into the nose. Blinking spreads the tear film over the eye but also moves the tears toward the punctum with each blink. Tears contain albumin, globulin fractions, and an antibacterial enzyme called lysozyme. Tear antibodies make up the gamma globulin protein fraction. Tear production may decrease 30% or more in a person over 50 years of age.

The presence of tearing in the absence of any other signs of inflammation should be noted. Distention and chronic inflammation of the lacrimal sac may cause a small, smooth elevation in the lacrimal fossa between the inner canthus and the nose. Pressure inward on this area will cause the contents of the lacrimal sac to be expressed by way of the puncta onto the conjunctiva. It should be noted whether the contents from the lacrimal sac are tears, mucus, or purulent material.

Deficiency of tears is best measured by *Schirmer's test* (Fig. 8-33). In this test a standardized filter paper, 3 mm by 20 mm, is inserted in the unanesthetized lower fornix of each eye at the junction of the middle and nasal third of the lower eyelid margin. With the eyes gently closed, these strips become moistened by the tears. The amount of paper moistened can be measured with a millimeter ruler and recorded.

Normally the lacrimal gland, under the irritation of a piece of filter paper, should produce sufficient tears to wet at least 10 mm of the paper in 5 minutes. This may be slightly less in the elderly. Any tear production less than 10 mm indicates a dryness of the eye and that the condition of *xerosis* may be present. Carefully performed Schirmer's tests often reveal lower secretions of tears, which could cause

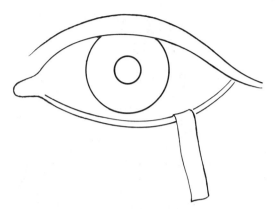

Fig. 8-33 Schirmer's test to detect tear deficiency. A filter paper strip is permitted to remain in contact with the eye for 5 minutes.

minor ocular complaints such as dryness, burning, or a sandy or gritty feeling. This test may also be helpful for wearers of contact lenses to determine whether there are sufficient tears for the comfortable wearing of contact lenses.

A variation of the test is Schirmer's test number two, which is accomplished by placing an anesthetic drop into the conjunctival sac before the Schirmer paper is inserted. The purpose of the topical anesthetic is to eliminate the reflex tearing caused by the paper itself.

Sclera. The normal sclera is visible beneath the conjunctiva as a white, opaque, fibrous structure. Blue discoloration of the sclera may be normal in a very young child because of the sclera's thinness and the underlying prominence of the dark choroid. Blue discoloration in an adult invariably indicates a pathologic condition; it may signify a tumor, a thinness of the sclera with a protrusion of the underlying uvea *(staphyloma),* or a nevus. In the elderly the sclera may appear yellowish because of the presence of fat and other degenerative substances.

Cornea. The cornea is the first and most powerful lens of the optical system of the eye. The radius of curvature of the average cornea that can be measured with the keratometer in the central region is 7.8 mm. The refractive index of the cornea is 1.376, which gives the cornea a power of 48.8 diopters. The concave posterior surface that faces the aqueous

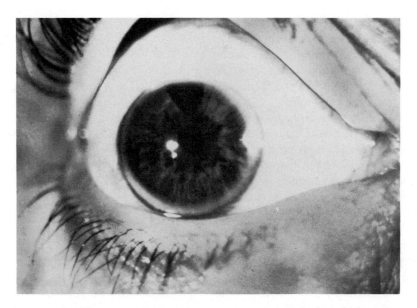

Fig. 8-34 Arcus senilis in a patient with a peripheral iridectomy.

has a power of − 5.8D, which gives the entire cornea a power of 43.00 D or about 70% of the total refractive power of the eye.

The reaction of the cornea to disease is unique. Being avascular, it cannot fend off infection easily. The surface layer of the cornea, the epithelium, is easily disrupted, but fully regenerates when injured. Injury to the epithelium occurs with flash burns, contact lens injuries, abrasions, and superficial corneal foreign bodies. Most infections and injuries usually involve only the corneal epithelium. Bowman's layer shows little resistance to pathologic conditions. It is easily destroyed and never regenerates. Descemet's membrane is quite strong and is highly resistant. The endothelial cells may die and they never regenerate. Neighboring endothelial cells enlarge and fill in the gap of dead cells. Thus the total endothelial cell count in any given area, when viewed by specular microscopy, may drop considerably. If the cornea becomes swollen, it loses its shape and transparency so that loss of vision is common. Total corneal swelling occurs with acute glaucoma, and the cornea may develop a ground-glass appearance.

The normal cornea should be smooth, shiny, and free of irregularities. In children the corneal diameter

should not exceed 11 mm. Corneal enlargement 12 mm or greater is strongly indicative of *congenital glaucoma*. In the elderly a white ring is frequently present near the corneal periphery. This creamy white ring is a result of the deposition of fat and is called *arcus senilis* (Fig. 8-34). The cornea is normally free of blood vessels. If blood vessels are present, they are a pathologic condition and indicate disease. Blood vessels in the cornea are best seen with the slit-lamp microscope but can be appreciated with strong focal illumination and the magnification of an ophthalmic loupe. *Corneal edema* can often be seen with the naked eye because of its characteristic ground-glass appearance. Corneal opacities may be detected by oblique illumination with a small flashlight.

Corneal sensation should be tested with a small wisp of cotton directly applied to the cornea. In this test the patient is instructed to look up. Normally a blink response should occur if the corneal sensation is intact. It is important that the patient does not see the cotton approaching the eye, as the visually-evoked response of seeing a foreign object approach the eye will also cause a blink response. Because of the wide range in individual response, comparison of the corneal reflexes of the two eyes is most useful. Loss of corneal sensitivity follows herpes simplex virus and brain disease involving the fifth nerve.

Use of fluorescein and rose bengal stains. Fluorescein is an ocular stain used to show defects and abrasions in the corneal epithelium. The pooling of fluorescein on small corneal defects is best seen by means of ultraviolet or cobalt blue light for illumination. This causes the fluorescein to fluoresce. There is a danger with fluorescein in solution form. It becomes easily contaminated with *Pseudomonas aeruginosa,* which appears to flourish in fluorescein. Sterile dry fluorostrips in which fluoroscein has been impregnated are available to prevent this complication. The fluorescein strip should be moistened with a drop of saline and applied to the lower fornix. This will cause liquid fluorescein to replace the tear film. The ulcer or denuded epithelium will be visible as a brilliant green.

Rose bengal is a red dye that has an affinity for degenerated epithelium. Similar to fluorescein, it will stain areas in which the epithelium has been sloughed off. However, unlike fluorescein, intact, nonviable epithelial cells of the conjunctiva or cornea will stain brightly with rose bengal. The stain is helpful in diagnosing keratoconjunctivitis sicca or other conditions associated with dryness of the conjunctiva. If the dye stains devitalized epithelium of the nasal bulbar conjunctiva, a diagnosis of keratitis sicca may be made.

Iris. The iris normally is quite clear to inspection. The irides of both eyes are generally the same color. Its color depends on the amount of pigment in the stroma and posterior layer of the iris. A heavily-pigmented iris appears brown, whereas a lightly-pigmented one appears blue. Interestingly enough, there is not any blue pigment in the iris. In the blue iris, the light passes through the nonpigmented stroma, strikes the pigmented epithelial cells on the back of the iris so that light of longer wavelength (red) is absorbed and that of shorter wavelength (blue) is reflected.

A difference in the color between the two irises *(heterochromia)* may be indicative of a congenital abnormality, iris tumor, retained intraocular foreign body (siderosis), or old iritis.

If a light is brought to bear on the iris at close range against the sclera (transillumination), the light may seem to glow in a patchy way in areas where there has been marked pigment loss. This can occur with some forms of glaucoma (pigmentary), after iritis, or with albinism. Freckles on the iris should be noted because iris freckles are frequently associated with intraocular malignant melanomas. Near the root of the iris lies the dilator muscle. When dilation occurs, at a maximum, the pupil may be 9 mm or greater in diameter. When maximally contracted, it may be only 1 mm.

The iris is normally well supported by the underlying lens. Tremulousness of the iris (iridodonesis) usually means the presence of a dislocated lens. Tremulousness of the iris, or undulating movements of the iris structure, is best seen by having the patient look quickly from one point of fixation to another. Near the aperture is a sphincter muscle that constricts the pupil. In the center of the iris, running radially around the pupil and forming a circular web are the blood vessels of the iris. If the lens is absent (aphakia), the iris loses its support, flattens, and deepens the anterior chamber. It may become tremulous.

A defect in the iris is called a *coloboma*. A coloboma, which indicates absence of some portion of the iris, may be the result of previous surgery or a congenital abnormality.

Muddiness of the iris is a term used to express the general loss of clarity of the pattern of the iris. It is caused by inflammatory exudates in the anterior chamber or on its surface. Normally the textured surface of the iris and the white markings of the iris vessels are easily visible (Fig. 8-35).

Anterior chamber. By shining a small penlight from the side, one can make an estimation of the depth of the anterior chamber. If the anterior chamber is shallow, it should be so recorded.

Pupil. The ophthalmic assistant can test pupillary function with no special instrument except a small light. The following points should be noted in the examination of pupillary function.

Pupillary reflexes. For assessment of the *direct light reflex,* the patient should be seated in a dimly illuminated room, with the light evenly distributed

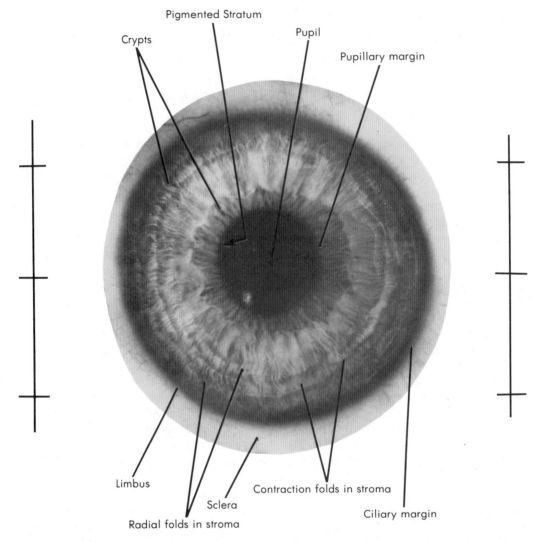

Fig. 8-35 Anatomy of the iris. (Courtesy Eastman Kodak Company, Rochester, N.Y.)

throughout the room. A small light is brought from the side and shone directly into the pupil (Fig. 8-36). The normal direct light response causes constriction of the pupil on that side.

For assessment of the *consensual light reflex,* light is directed into one eye while the second eye is observed. An intact consensual response to light causes constriction of the pupil of the unilluminated eye.

Normally, when an object is viewed close at hand, three associated reactions occur: (1) convergence of the eyes toward the object, (2) accommodation, and (3) pupillary constriction. These three *reactions to near* should not be considered a true reflex, because one may occur without the other. For example, the pupil may be dilated with a mydriatic agent and the patient may still be able to converge his eyes.

The *swinging flashlight test* compares the direct and consensual reflexes in the same eye. The examiner projects the light on the patient's eye and allows the pupil to go through the phases of initial

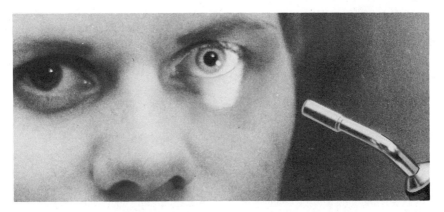

Fig. 8-36 Testing the pupillary light reflex.

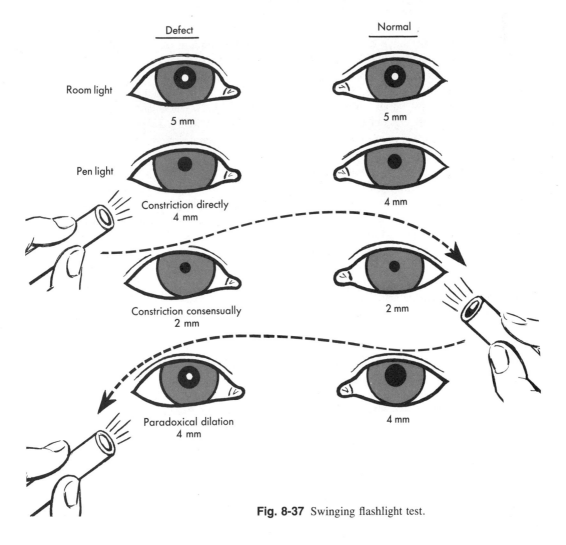

Fig. 8-37 Swinging flashlight test.

constriction to a minimum size and subsequent escape to an intermediate size. At this point the examiner quickly swings the light to the other eye, which will begin at the intermediate size and go through the phases of initial constriction to a minimum size and subsequent escape to an intermediate size. Again as soon as that pupil redilates to the intermediate size, the light is swung to the first eye and a mental note made of the intermediate (starting) size and briskness of the response to light. These characteristics should be exactly the same in both eyes as the light is alternately swung to each eye.

During the swinging flashlight test, if the amount of light information transmitted from one eye is less than that carried by the fellow eye, the following phenomena may be noted when the light is swung from the good eye to the defective eye: immediate dilatation of the pupil, instead of the normal initial constriction. This characterizes an *afferent pupillary defect* or the *Marcus Gunn pupil* (Fig. 8-37).

Size. The size of the pupil varies with age, the color of the iris, and the refractive error. The pupil tends to be largest in blue-eyed young children who are myopic. Conversely, the pupil tends to be smaller in infants and the elderly. The pupils should normally be equal in size. Failure of a large, dilated pupil to constrict to light is most commonly caused by a cycloplegic drug such as atropine. Such a pupil is 7 to 8 mm in diameter, spherical, and immobile when light is shone into the eye. Dilation of a pupil to 5 to 6 mm can result from paralysis of the third cranial nerve. The pupil may also be large, immobile, and unresponsive to the direct application of light because of severe affections of the retina and optic nerve that result in blindness. However, such a pupil can be distinguished from the pupil that is dilated because of paralysis of the third nerve by testing the consensual reaction to light. If the lesion is a result of a third-nerve palsy, the size of the pupil in the affected eye remains unchanged when the light is directed into the fellow eye. If the pupillary dilation is due to disease of the retina or optic nerve, the consensual light reflex produced by shining light into the sound eye will produce a constriction of the pupil in the affected eye.

The pupil may also be dilated and fixed to direct light stimulation and consensual light stimulation after an episode of acute narrow-angle glaucoma. However, this pupil is characteristically oval.

Bilateral constriction of the pupils (miosis) is most commonly caused by glaucoma medication, such as pilocarpine. Small, pinpoint pupils are characteristically found in morphine addicts. Unilateral constriction of the pupil occurs with iritis, interruption of the sympathetic pathways of the eye, and irritative lesions of the cornea.

Psychic influences such as surprise, fear, and pain dilate the pupil markedly. Dim light also dilates the pupil, whereas bright light constricts it. At times the pupil is constantly contracting and dilating—this is called *hippus*.

During sleep, the pupil is constricted. It is such a constant finding that it serves as an aid in differentiating true from simulated sleep.

Any irritation of the cornea or conjunctiva such as an abrasion results in constriction of the pupil.

Shape. The pupil is normally round and regular. Irregularities in the shape of the pupil may result from congenital abnormalities, inflammation of the iris, trauma to the eye, and surgical intervention (Fig. 8-38). Trauma may cause tears of the iris in the form of a wedge-shaped defect, either at the pupillary margin or at its base *(iridodialysis)*. A corneal laceration with prolapse of the iris may result in the drawing up of a segment of the iris to the site of the laceration *(adherent leukoma)*. In severe iritis, the iris may be bound down to the lens by adhesions *(posterior synechiae)*, and irregular changes may occur in the shape of the pupil.

Equality of size. The pupils should be equal in size and react equally to direct light stimulation, consensual light stimulation, and near objects. In the light of an ordinary room, the diameter of the normal adult pupil is between 3 and 5 mm. If the two pupils are unequal in size, the condition is called "anisocoria." Anisocoria may be harmless, but it is never physiologic. Inequality of size may be caused by a tonic pupil *(Adie's syndrome)*. In this condition, which can be mistaken for a partial third-nerve palsy, the pupil responds to light stimulation very slowly. Adie's syndrome is diagnosed by the instillation of 2.5% fresh methacholine solution (Mecholyl) into

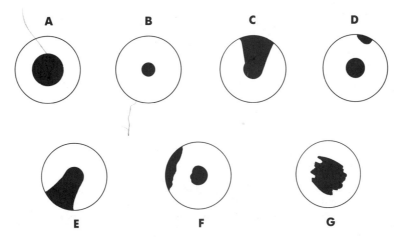

Fig. 8-38 Variations in pupillary size and shape. **A,** Dilated, or mydiatic, pupil. **B,** Constricted, or miotic, pupil. **C,** Full, or sector, iridectomy. **D,** Peripheral iridectomy. **E,** Congenital coloboma of the iris. **F,** Iridodialysis. **G,** Posterior synechiae.

the affected eye, which causes constriction of a tonic pupil, but not of the normal pupil.

Disorders of pupillary function may involve many of the above factors together. For example, the patient with *Argyll Robertson pupils,* one of the classic signs of late syphilis, has pupils that are small, irregular in shape, and nonreactive to either direct or consensual light stimulation but reactive to near stimulation.

Differential diagnosis of a dilated pupil. A dilated pupil may be caused by third-nerve palsy, trauma, Adie's pupil, or acute glaucoma, or it may be drug induced.

Third-nerve palsy. If the dilated pupil is fixed, the cause may be third-nerve palsy. This condition may be associated with ptosis and a motility disturbance, characterized by the eye being deviated out and down. The pupil responds to constricting drops, such as pilocarpine. This is a neurosurgical emergency, and the possibility of an intracranial mass lesion must be ruled out.

Trauma. Damage to the iris sphincter may result from a blunt or penetrating injury. Iris transillumination defects may be visible with the ophthalmoscope or slit lamp, and the pupil may have an irregular shape.

Adie's pupil. In Adie's pupil, the pupil responds better to near stimulation than to light. The condition

is thought to be related to aberrant innervation of the iris by axons that normally stimulate the ciliary body. Absent-knee jerks are usually associated.

Acute glaucoma. The patient may complain of pain and/or nausea and vomiting. The eye is red, vision is diminished, intraocular pressure is elevated, and the pupil is mid-dilated and poorly reactive.

Drug-induced dilation. Iatrogenic or self-contamination may occur with a variety of dilating drops, such as cyclopentolate HCI (Cyclogyl), tropicamide (Mydriacyl), homatropine, scopolamine, and atropine. The pupil is fixed and dilated and, unlike in third-nerve palsy, does not respond to constricting drops.

Differential diagnosis of a constricted pupil. A constricted pupil occurs in Horner's syndrome or iritis and may be drug induced.

Horner's syndrome. Other signs of Horner's syndrome include mild ptosis of the upper lid and retraction of the lower lid. The difference in pupillary size is more notable in dim light, because adrenergic innervation to the iris dilator muscle is diminished.

Iritis. Slit lamp examination shows keratic precipitates and cells in the anterior chamber, and there is a prominent ciliary flush. The intraocular inflammation stimulates pupillary constriction.

Drug-induced constriction. Iatrogenic or self-induced pupillary constriction may be caused by a variety of

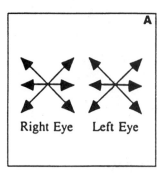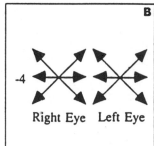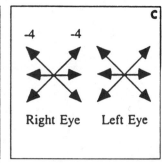

Fig. 8-39 A, Method for examining and recording ocular motility. **B,** Record of sixth nerve palsy of right eye. **C,** Record of right orbital blowout fracture and limited upgaze. (From Stein HA, Slatt BJ, Stein RM: *A primer in ophthalmology, a textbook for students,* St Louis, 1992, Mosby.)

drugs, including pilocarpine, carbachol, and echothiophate iodide (Phospholine Iodide).

Lens. The entire lens is normally not visible without the aid of a slit-lamp microscope. However, an advanced cataract may be seen with the naked eye, because it causes a gray, opaque appearance in the pupillary aperture.

Blinking

Most people blink 15 times per minute. The duration of a blink is approximately 0.3 to 0.4 second. The average period between blinks is about 2.8 seconds in men and just under 4 seconds in women. Spontaneous blinking does not produce a discontinuity of vision in spite of the fact that vision is interrupted during the blink. Continual squeezing of the eyelids together is called "blepharospasm." It occurs as a result of inflammatory diseases of the anterior segment, Parkinson's disease, and stress.

EXAMINATION OF THE OCULAR MUSCLES

There are six extraocular muscles in each eye that are innervated by a total of three nerves. The action of specific muscles can vary, depending on the position of the eye when it is innervated. Table 8-3 shows the general relationships that apply.

The examiner should determine the range of ocular movements in all gaze positions (Fig. 8-39). Limited movement in any gaze position can be documented as −1 minimal, −2 moderate, −3 severe,

Table 8-3	Extraocular muscle innervation	
Innervation	**Muscle**	**Primary action**
3rd nerve	Superior rectus	Up and out
3rd nerve	Medial rectus	In
3rd nerve	Inferior rectus	Down and out
3rd nerve	Inferior oblique	Up and in
4th nerve	Superior oblique	Down and in
6th nerve	Lateral rectus	Out

From Stein HA, Slatt BJ, Stein RM: *A primer in ophthalmology,* St Louis, 1992, Mosby.

or −4 total. For example, a patient with right sixth-nerve palsy can be recorded (see Fig. 8-39, *B*.) Fig. 8-39, *C* shows a record of a blowout fracture to the right orbit with entrapment of the inferior rectus muscle and limitation of upward gaze. Fig. 8-40 illustrates the positions of gaze that may demonstrate weakness of an extraocular muscle.

The corneal light reflex test is a simple practical evaluation of muscle imbalance for patients who cannot cooperate sufficiently for prism cover testing or who have poor fixation. The *Hirschberg method* is the most popular and is based on the premise that 1 mm of corneal light reflection corresponds to 7 degrees or 15 prism diopters of ocular deviation of the visual axis (Fig. 8-41). This is a guestimate method that may be quantitated and refined by the use of prisms, as in the Krismsky method.

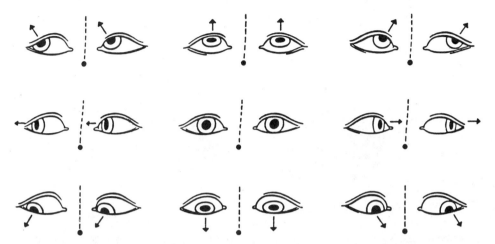

Fig. 8-40 Eye rotations: the primary and eight cardinal positions of gaze that should be tested to detect weakness of an extraocular muscle. (From Stein HA, Slatt BJ, Stein RM: *A primer in ophthalmology, a textbook for students,* St Louis, 1992, Mosby.)

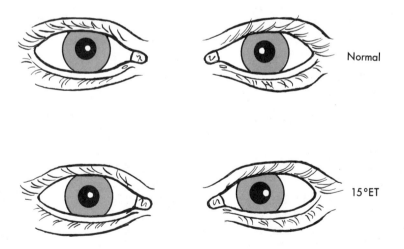

Normal

15°ET

Fig. 8-41 Hirschberg's method of estimating deviation.

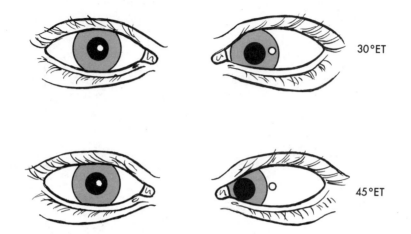

Fig. 8-41, continued.

The alternate cover test is perhaps the most widely employed for the detection and measurement of strabismus, tropia, or phoria. It is reliable, easy to perform, and requires no special equipment. The test is conventionally used at both distance and near, with and without glasses, with the eyes being examined in the primary position. To ensure fixation in very young children, the fixation object should be an interesting and detailed article, such as a brightly-colored toy. Once the examiner is sure that the child is looking at the fixation object, an occluder is interposed in front of one eye. If the left eye is occluded, the following possibilities may ensue:

1. The right eye, which is deviating, may move horizontally (esotropia is a move inward; exotropia is a move outward) or vertically (hypertropia is a move up; hypotropia is a move down), indicating that the child has a manifest strabismus (Fig. 8-42).
2. The right eye may wander slightly, indicating that the fixation of the eye is defective or absent, as may occur with gross amblyopia.
3. There may be no movement of the right eye, indicating that this eye is straight.

The procedure is then repeated, this time covering the right eye without allowing the patient to become binocular during testing. Manifest strabismus is revealed by observation of any movement of the un-covered eye to take up fixation when the occluder is placed before the other eye. Occasionally, a child may be referred who appears to have an ocular deviation, but there is no detectable strabismus. This condition is called *pseudostrabismus*. In most instances, the appearance is caused by the presence of prominent epicanthal folds that extend from the upper lid, cover the inner canthal region, and blend into the medial aspects of the lower lid. This is a false impression of a turn, more noticeable when the child turns the eye to either side. A full discussion of ocular muscle deviations is offered in Chapter 32, Ocular Motility.

INSTILLATION OF EYE DROPS AND OINTMENT

Frequently the assistant is requested to instill various types of liquid medications into the patient's eyes. There are wrong ways and right ways to accomplish this purpose.

All drops, with the exception of topical anesthetics, are placed in the inferior cul de sac with the patient looking up. With the dropper bottle in the right hand, the left forefinger is used to depress the lower lid, making a small pocket of the cul de sac. With the patient's eyes in the elevated position, the dropper bottle is brought over to and close to, but not touching, the cul de sac. One drop is placed

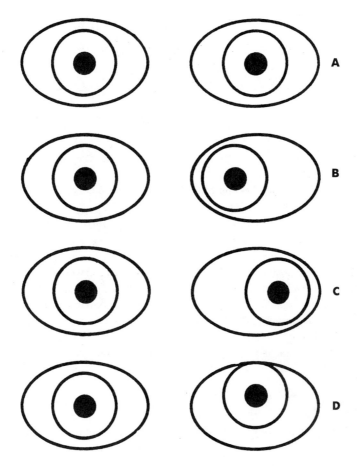

Fig. 8-42 Strabismus. **A,** Eyes are straight. **B,** Esotropia. **C,** Exotropia. **D,** Hypertropia of left eye. (From Stein HA, Slatt BJ, Stein RM: *Ophthalmic terminology,* ed 3, St Louis, 1992, Mosby.)

in the pocket so formed. More than one drop is a waste of solution because the total capacity of the cul de sac is ⅙ of a drop.

Topical anesthetic drops, such as those used when intraocular tension is being measured or before the ophthalmologist removes sutures from the eye, are placed in the eye with the patient looking *down* and with the solution directed to the 12 o'clock position of the sclera near the limbus. With the dropper bottle in the right hand, the upper lid is elevated with the left thumb. While the patient looks down, the right hand with the dropper bottle is placed close to, but not touching, the lashes, and the solution is expressed at the 12 o'clock position of the sclera.

There are two reasons for the different manner of instilling medications into a patient's eye. First, solutions placed in the lower cul de sac with the patient looking up are those medications designed to either dilate the pupils or place a particular medication in contact with the eye for a period of time. Second, when solutions are dropped into the eye, the patient will blink; and when the patient's eyelids close, the cornea goes up underneath the upper lid (Bell's phenomenon). If a topical anesthetic has been placed in the lower cul de sac, as the patient blinks and the cornea travels upward, the maximum amount of topical anesthesia is going to be obtained on the inferior portion of the sclera. However, since the eye is being

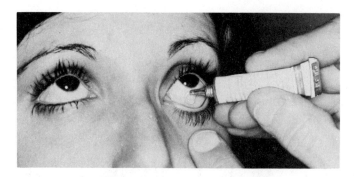

Fig. 8-43 Instillation of ophthalmic ointment.

anesthetized for measurement of intraocular tension, the cornea must be anesthetized. When the patient looks downward as the topical anesthetic is placed in the eye at the 12 o'clock position, the blinking will cause the cornea to travel upward and thus to come into contact with the topical anesthetic just applied, thereby rendering a more complete and well-distributed area of corneal anesthesia. When ointments are required, a small amount (about ¼ inch) is instilled into the lower cul de sac as the patient looks up (Fig. 8-43).

OPHTHALMOSCOPY

There are two types of ophthalmoscopes, direct and indirect. By and large, the indirect ophthalmoscope is used by ophthalmologists and permits binocular vision with depth perception (stereoscopic vision). It also permits a wider field of view of a given area. The image is inverted. It may be used in the operating room without contamination and permits indentation of the sclera and a better view of the periphery of the fundus. It provides more intense illumination and frees the hands for operative manipulation.

However, the direct ophthalmoscope is the one most popular for all practitioners (Fig. 8-44). This permits a greater magnification ($\times 15$). It is easier to use with small or undilated pupils and is mechanically easier to use. This ophthalmoscope was popularized more than 100 years ago by Von Helmholtz. The ophthalmoscope contains a number of spherical lenses that aid the practitioner to focus. However, there are no cylindrical lenses, so that if

the individual has an astigmatic error of refraction, it cannot be compensated for. The direct ophthalmoscope enables the examiner to use the power of the subject's eyes as a magnifying system to see the retina as an erect picture.

The ophthalmoscope, invented by Von Helmholtz in 1851, permitted analysis of the interior of the eye during life. For the first time, this allowed recognition of changes in the eye grounds, providing valuable information in the diagnosis of disease of the general system, as well as of the eye itself.

Ophthalmoscopy is best performed in a dimly-lit room to facilitate pupillary dilation. However, for better inspection of the fundus, the pupil should be dilated with a mydriatic agent such as 2.5% phenylephrine (Table 8-4). This does not inhibit accommodation. With heavily-pigmented irides, a stronger mydriatic agent will be required. Drops such as cyclopentolate (Cyclogyl 1%) or tropicamide (Midriacyl) should be instilled. These drops affect accommodation. When inserting a mydriatic cycloplegic drop, one should be sure that the chamber angles are deep. If not, angle closure glaucoma may be induced.

The examiner stands directly in front of the patient and examines the patient's right eye with the examiner's own right eye, and the left eye in a similar fashion. This permits the examiner to be closer to the patient. Both of the examiner's eyes are kept open. The patient is asked to look at the opposite wall over the shoulder of the examiner. The cornea, anterior chamber, and lens structures are first carefully examined at a distance so that one can explore

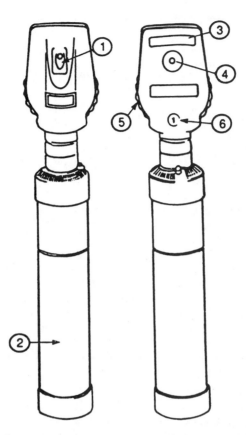

Fig. 8-44 The ophthalmoscope. 1, Mirror that reflects light into the patient's eye with a viewing hole above, through which the examiner looks. It is in this viewing hole that positive or negative lenses can be superimposed to adjust focus. 2, Handle where battery power is supplied. On top of the handle base is a rheostat for light adjustment. 3, Headrest bar, which goes against the examiner's forehead. 4, Viewing hole through which the examiner looks. It is this hole that lenses may superimpose for focus. 5, Focusing wheel. While holding the ophthalmoscope, one's index finger can move this wheel to adjust the lenses in the hole at 4. 6, As the dial wheel (5) is moved, the power of the lens is indicated in this small window. (From Coles WH: *Ophthalmology: a diagnostic text,* Baltimore, 1989, Williams and Wilkins.)

all the medium. Usually the distance is about 15 inches between the patient and the examiner. One gradually approaches the eye of the patient until a red reflex appears. During this period, one will carefully note the cornea, anterior chamber, and lens structures. One then observes a red reflex. This red reflex is a combination of the reflex from the choroidal vasculature and the pigment epithelium. For purposes of orientation, the optic disc is first identified. The color and shape are noted. The disc is an oval structure that represents the site of entrance of the optic nerve. It is usually light pink and may have a central yellowish-white depression called the physiological cup, created by a separation of the nerve fibers. The depression may be large and occupy up to half of the disc. At the base of the cup are grayish spots representing the opening of the lamina cribrosa, the connective tissue layer through which the fibers of the optic nerve pass. The cup size is noted, and the margins of the disc are observed. The mar-

Table 8-4   Drops used in refraction

Drug	Onset of maximum cycloplegia	Duration of activity	Comment
Atropine sulfate 1%	6-24 hr	10-15 days, especially in a blue-eyed child	Not used routinely except for the assessment of accommodative strabismus in children
Scopolamine hydrobromide 1/4%	30-60 min	3-4 days	Used in atropine-allergic patients
Homatropine hydrobromide 1.25% to 5%	1 hr	1-2 days	Requires an hour to take effect and lasts 2 days; not used routinely
Cyclopentolate hydrochloride 1% (Cyclogyl)	10-45 min	12-24 hr	Active in 20-45 minutes; two sets of drops given 5 minutes apart; a good rapid-acting cycloplegic drop for office use
Tropicamide (Mydriacyl) 0.5%	23-30 min	4-10 hr	A good drug for office use with an effect similar to Cyclogyl
Phenylephrine 2.5% (Neosynephrine)	20-30 min (no cycloplegia)	30 min-2 hr	Does not affect accommodation; helpful in presbyopia for fundus examination

From Stein HA, Slatt BJ, Stein RM: *A primer in ophthalmology*, St Louis, 1992, Mosby.

gins of the disc are sharp and distinct, except for the margins of the upper and lower poles, which may be slightly fuzzy. The blood vessels are then examined. From the disc, the retinal arterioles and veins emerge and bifurcate, and extend toward the four quadrants of the retina. The central retinal vein, which is usually found lateral to the central retinal artery, is larger and darker red. The examiner observes for venous pulsation. If venous pulsation is present, it suggests there is no papilledema, because this disappears early. These branch into retinal vesicles and arterioles. The retinoles are darker in color. Retinoles and arterioles will cross over and under each other, but an arteriole will never cross over an arteriole, nor would a retinole ever cross a retinole. Approximately two disc diameters away from the optic disc and slightly below (about 1 mm) its center is the macula, about 5.5 mm in diameter. The macula is a small avascular area that appears darker red than the surrounding fundus. At the center of the macula, there is a glistening oval reflex called the *fovea*. At its

center is the foveola, which has no rod but a high density of cones. This area is a vascular capillary-free zone. This saves the foveola from vessels that obscure visual acuity. Underlying choriocapillaries supply this capillary-free zone. Cilioretinal arteries arising from the ciliary circulation are seen in about 20% of patients and account for the blood supply to the macular region in these individuals. This is an important fact when occlusion of the central retinal artery occurs, in which the cilioretinal artery provides continual nourishment to the macular region and maintains central acuity. In young people, a second reflex, which appears as a glimmering halo, may surround the entire macular region. Each quadrant of the fundus is examined in turn. For the examiner to see as much of the peripheral retina as possible, the patient should be asked to look in the direction of the quadrant under study. The examiner follows out the arterioles in that particular quadrant to the extreme limit. The color of the fundus is usually an even red hue, but it will vary with the general pigmentation of

---

TIPS ON OPHTHALMOSCOPY

1. If the examiner has any significant astigmatic error, he or she should wear corrective glasses.
2. A smaller light spot should be used.
3. The cornea and anterior structures of the eye should be examined from a distance of 1 foot through the sight aperture of the ophthalmoscope. The examiner then moves to within 1 inch of the eye to observe the retina.
4. The patient should be asked to gaze on all quadrants to observe the peripheral retina. Each arteriole is followed out to the periphery.
5. To avoid coming too close to the patient's eye, the examiner may put his or her middle finger forward and rest it against the patient's cheek. This will provide a proprioceptive method of determining how close the examiner is to the patient.

---

the underlying choroid and the general pigmentation of the individual. The background is bright orange-red in persons of fair complexion, whereas it is deeper brick red in darker individuals. Some details of the choroidal vessels may be seen in fair individuals and in the periphery.

Most ophthalmoscopes have two or more beam lights of different sizes. The smaller beam light is particularly useful for viewing the fundus through small pupils, such as those found in glaucoma patients under treatment with pilocarpine. It eliminates some of the glare around the pupil from reflex scattering from the iris. Cobalt blue filters may be present as an aperture disc in the ophthalmoscope. These are used for fluorescein studies of the fundus as well as examination of the cornea with fluorescein strip papers. Ophthalmoscopes sometimes contain a target so the patient can fixate on the center of the grid for viewing the macular area.

VISUAL FIELDS

The ophthalmic assistant can also estimate the visual field. This test is important in a thorough workup of a patient to screen any possible interference in the nerve pathways from the eye to the brain. It is discussed more fully in Chapter 16.

SUMMARY

The ophthalmic assistant will probably learn abbreviations commonly used by the supervising ophthalmologist (Table 8-5). The use of abbreviations is generally to be condemned in public institutions, where the abbreviated word may not be understood by all. However, in private offices it may be helpful and timesaving. The best record and the one that is the easiest to understand is a small sketch of the pathologic condition seen on inspection (Figs. 8-45 and 8-46).

Table 8-5	Symbols commonly used
Symbol	**Meaning**
VA	Visual acuity
od	*Oculus dexter* (right eye)
os	*Oculus sinister* (left eye)
VOD	Vision right eye
VOS	Vision left eye
ou	*Oculi uterque* (both eyes)
RE	Right eye
LE	Left eye
EOM	Extraocular muscles
NPC	Near point of convergence
NPA	Near point of accommodation
℞	Prescription for eyeglasses or drugs
Δ	Prism diopter
D	Diopter
T	Tension

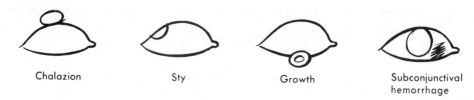

Embedded
foreign body

Fig. 8-45 Diagrammatic recording of external abnormalities.

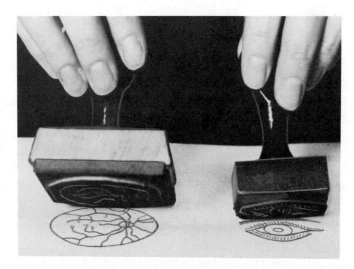

Fig. 8-46 Stamps for illustrating pathologic conditions in the fundus, eye, and eyelid.

QUESTIONS FOR REVIEW AND THOUGHT

1. Discuss what is meant by 20/20 vision; 20/40 vision.
2. Describe a routine to be followed for checking distance vision; for checking near vision.
3. How do you check the vision of an illiterate patient?
4. Describe vision testing in children.
5. If a patient cannot identify the large E on the chart, how can you assess lesser degrees of vision?
6. Describe your method of determining the prescription of a pair of glasses.
7. How do you measure the add on a cataract bifocal?
8. Describe how prisms can be measured on the lensmeter that you work with.
9. Describe a method of measuring the near point of accommodation. What is the importance of this test?
10. Describe a method of measuring the near point of convergence. What is the importance of this test?

11. What are some methods for testing color vision?
12. Describe some rough tests for depth perception. What factors would impair depth perception?
13. Outline a routine for examination of external features of the eyelids and eye.
14. How are the pupillary light reflexes tested?
15. What is Schirmer's test number 1 and number 2? How is each performed?
16. Outline a method of transposing plus cylinders to a minus prescription, using the formula $+ 1.00 + 2.00 \times 90$.
17. Where does the lid margin normally lie on the cornea when the eye is open? How can you tell if it is drooped or retracted?
18. Outline a method of appraising vision in a man with dense cataracts and less than 20/200 vision.
19. What is the normal blink rate? What does increased blink rate usually mean?

SELF-EVALUATION QUESTIONS

True-false statements

Directions: Indicate whether the statement is true (T) or false (F).

T or F   1. In visual acuity recordings, 6/12 is equal to 20/60 vision.
T or F   2. In occlusion nystagmus, the vision is improved when the one eye is occluded.
T or F   3. Shining a light in the eye not being examined is a valid way of doing a pinhole assessment of vision.

Missing words

Directions: Write in the missing word in the following sentences.

4. When neutralizing lenses, the displacement of the target by the prism is always recorded in terms of the _____ of the prism.
5. A 10-year-old boy has 14.00 diopters of accommodation. A 45-year-old man has _____ of accommodation left.
6. Defects in color vision are present predominantly in _____.

Choice-completion questions

Directions: Select the one best answer in each case.

7. The following tests are suitable for color vision testing:
   a. The Worth four-dot test
   b. The Ishihara test plates
   c. The Fly test
   d. All of the above
   e. None of the above
8. Depth perception requires:
   a. Good vision in each eye
   b. Overlapping visual fields
   c. Normal alignment of the eyes
   d. All of the above
   e. None of the above
9. Proptosis is a sign of:
   a. Thyroid disease
   b. Adult glaucoma
   c. Ptosis
   d. Hypertension
   e. All of the above

ANSWERS, NOTES, AND EXPLANATIONS

1. **False.** 6/6 vision in meters is equivalent to 20/20 vision; 6/12 vision in meters is equivalent to 20/40 vision. In Canada and the United States, visual acuity charts are designated in feet, whereas in Europe the metric system is used.

2. **False.** Occlusion nystagmus is a congenital condition in which nystagmus and esotropia may be induced by covering one eye and decreasing vision. The decrease in light sensation is enough to cause the other eye to oscillate. Such children, when given routine vision tests, score poorly because the examiner fails to look for this condition. In such children, the eye that should be occluded can be fogged with a +10.00 diopter lens to allow proper vision in the other eye.

3. **True.** A pinhole disk before the pupil improves vision to normal limits if the loss of vision is due to a refractive error. The pinhole test separates refractive visual loss from pathologic visual loss. With disease, a pinhole over the pupil makes vision worse.

    Shining a light in the other eye causes both pupils to constrict and is a simple way of achieving the pinhole test.

4. **Base.** If the lens has a prism, the center of the lens does not coincide with the center of the target. The displacement measured in circles of expanding radii is a measure of the power of the prism and is recorded as base in, out, up, or down. The distance between each circle represents 1.00 prism diopter.

    With the new automatic devices, prism power is digitally recorded, and the results are instant.

5. **3.50 diopters.** The decline in accommodation is most striking between age 30 and 40 where it drops from 8.00 diopters to 4.50 diopters. It is due to atrophy of ciliary muscle and loss of elasticity of the lens of the eye. Unfortunately, there is no way to halt the process; thus it is inevitable that everyone eventually needs reading glasses, except nearsighted people, who merely take their glasses off.

6. **Boys.** Congenital color defects, red-green being the most common, are transmitted by the female and appear predominantly in the male. In fact 8% to 10% of males are color deficient. Total color blindness is another matter; it is rare and very disabling and causes blindness and nystagmus in children.

7. **b. The Ishihara test plates.** Ishihara test plates are those most commonly used for the detection of color deficiency. Other devices such as the Nagel Anomaloscope are superior in detection of possible defects and in quantifying them. The Ishihara plates however, are inexpensive to purchase so they can be used by every industrial or school nurse. They are simple to use—no expertise is required, and the results are reproducible. It is basically a color vision screener and not an analyzer.

8. **d. All of the above.** Most authorities believe that depth perception cannot be acquired. If there is a congenital strabismus and the eyes are straightened at age 3, that child will not have depth perception. Having poor depth perception may not be of practical importance as there are so many monocular clues to judge distance. Pilots need it in the rare instances that they have to make a visual landing. Athletes, like baseball or tennis players, are also handicapped without depth perception.

9. **a. Thyroid disease.** Protrusion of the eyes is usually measured with the exophthalmometer. When it occurs in one eye, it frequently indicates a retrobulbar mass, the hemangioma being most common. But when it occurs in both eyes, it means thyroid disease until proved otherwise.

    Deposits of fat, hyaluronic acidlike material, and inflammatory cells cause the typical bulging of the eyes.

CHAPTER 9

Understanding ophthalmic equipment

- Equipment used for refraction
- Equipment used to detect muscle imbalance
- Instruments used to determine power of lenses
- Instruments used to examine interior of the eye
- Instruments used to study anterior segment of the eye
- Instruments used to examine angle structures of the eye
- Instruments used to assess the cornea
- Instruments used to measure intraocular pressure (tonometer)
- Special instruments
- Diagnostic ultrasound: a-scan and b-scan
- Radioactive phosphorus
- Electroretinography
- Lasers

Today more than ever before, the ophthalmologist's clinical acumen is enhanced by the many instruments and equipment available that facilitate the determination of refractive errors of the eye, the detection of muscular imbalance, and the magnification and visualization of the interior structures of the eye. This chapter deals with ophthalmic instruments, their purpose and mode of use, and their advantages and limitations.

EQUIPMENT USED FOR REFRACTION

The determination of the refractive error of an eye permits the ophthalmologist to prescribe lenses that enable the patient to obtain the best possible visual acuity.

Projector and projector slides

The projector provides a means of projecting, on a silver screen, test letters and characters that can be used in assessing visual acuity.

It consists of a housing for a bulb, an opening for introduction of different target slides, and a lens system that can be focused on a silver screen. The housing for the bulb is made readily accessible for interchange of bulbs when bulbs darken or burn out. Rheostats may be introduced in the power circuits to lengthen the life of the bulb. The lens system and slides should be kept clean and dust-free.

Projectors that are available provide a means of illuminating (1) a horizontal row of test letters or characters, (2) a vertical row of test letters or characters, (3) a single-test letter or character, and (4) the introduction of red-green to illuminate the letters.

The use of red and green letters is the basis of the duochrome test and a means of "fine-tuning" the refraction. In this test, half the panel is illuminated in red and half the panel in green. Under the duochrome principle green normally is focused in front of the retina, whereas red, having a longer wavelength, is focused behind the retina for the emmetrope. Therefore a patient seeing the letters on the green panel more clearly than those on the red panel is hyperopic, requiring more plus to bring the red wavelengths onto the retina. The patient seeing the letters more clearly on the red panel is myopic, requiring more minus to bring the green onto the retina. The emmetrope sees both equally blurred. The duochrome test provides a means to arrive at the final correcting lens for the refractive error present.

Available projector slides have a large variety of test targets and specialized tests for refraction. Commonly available slides include (1) Snellen test letters, (2) Landolt (split circle) rings, (3) numbers, (4) Es, (5) an astigmatic clock, (6) a picture chart, and (7) a Worth four-dot test.

Projectors may be controlled by remote control units. The use of remote control units is especially important if projectors are installed in inaccessible places or areas that are awkward for the examiner to control.

Trial case and lenses

The trial case is a tray of lenses and accessories used in determining the refractive error of an eye. These lenses are individually marked in the strengths of dioptric power of each lens, as well as in the direction of axis of the cylindric lenses. The trial case consists of (1) a pair of plus spheres ranging from +0.12 to +20.00 diopters, (2) a pair of minus spheres ranging from −0.12 to −20.00 diopters, (3) a pair of plus cylinders ranging from +0.12 to +8.00 diopters, (4) a pair of minus cylinders ranging from −0.12 to −8.00 diopters, and (5) accessory lenses.

These lenses are designed to fit a standard trial frame. Each lens is encircled by a metal rim for protection. Handles are provided with spheres for ease of handling and are optional with cylinders. The choice is governed by the type of trial frames used. Cylinders with handles would be used with the trial frames illustrated in Fig. 9-1 but not with simple types having no revolving cylinder lens carriers. Handles would interfere with the free rotation of the cylinder in the latter type. It should be noted that the cylinder is marked with reference to its axis and not the meridian. Thus the position on the cylinder, as marked on the lens, is the axis of zero

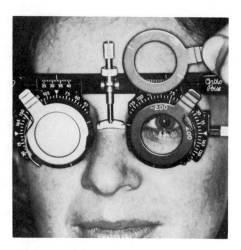

Fig. 9-1 Inserting lenses into the trial frame.

power and will indicate the position of the image on the retina.

Accessory lenses available in a trial case are (1) an occluder lens, (2) a pinhole disk, (3) a stenopeic slit, (4) a Maddox rod lens, (5) prisms ranging from 0.50- to 6.00-prism diopters, and (6) a red glass filter lens.

Use of trial lenses. Trial lenses are not used on a routine basis today because they have been eclipsed by the refractor or phoropter, which offers to the ophthalmologist the speed of exchange of lenses in a completely enclosed housing. The trial lens, however, has a place in the determination of the refractive error of children who are intimidated by the massive bulk of the refractor or whose narrowly set eyes cannot be positioned properly behind the openings in the refractor. Bifocals are prescribed by use of the trial frame with lenses because the patient can best judge a comfortable working and reading distance with the head bent and the eyes lowered in a natural reading position. Trial lenses also are used in refraction of aphakic and high myopic eyes because it is expedient that the correcting lenses and the spectacles the patient receives approximate each other with reference to their distance from the eye itself. Trial lenses must be employed when low visual aids in the form of high plus prescription lenses are used.

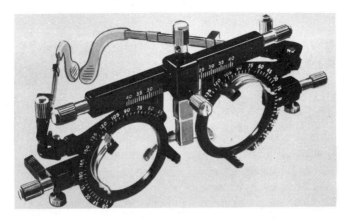

Fig. 9-2 Trial frame.

The trial frame (Fig. 9-2) is essentially a frame capable of holding a group of three or four trial lenses for each eye. It has adjustable ear pieces and an adjustable bridge that alters the interpupillary distance. Some trial frames have an adjustment for tilting the frames toward the reading position. In high minus and high plus prescriptions the proximity of the lens in the frame to the eye (vertex distance) must be measured. This aids the optician in duplicating the prescription. The calibration scale incorporated on the outer side of the frame can be used for this purpose but is really not an accurate method of making this measurement. Modern trial frames have a thumbscrew mechanism on the side of the trial frame to rotate the front lens carrier, which is used to house the cylinder. This enables the cylinder to be rotated to the proper axis.

The front surface of the trial frame is marked off in degrees from 0 to 180 (see Fig. 9-1). By convention, frames are labeled in a counterclockwise direction beginning on the right-hand side of the horizontal meridian.

Refractor or Phoropter

The refractor consists of the entire trial set of lenses mounted on a circular wheel so that each lens can be brought before the aperture of the viewing system by merely turning a dial (Figs. 9-3 and 9-4). In addition to the conventional spheres and cylinders,

accessories are available that may include before each eye a polarizing lens, a pinhole, a Maddox rod, and a working lens for retinoscopy. There are many types of refractors on the market, varying in the number of accessories available and the mode of housing these accessories. Fundamentally, these refractors are of the same design and purpose.

We shall discuss the Bausch & Lomb Phoropter II because it is a typical example of the devices available today. The term *Phoropter* is a trademark of one company whereas all the others are called *refractors*. The terms often are used interchangeably.

Body. The body consists of two disklike casings that house the lenses. The entire instrument is mounted on a pole or a hydraulic stand. A forehead rest is present to ensure that the patient is correctly positioned and that the eyes are as close to the lens system as possible. The knobs at either end on top of the Phoropter adjust the interpupillary distance for the individual patient. If the patient has a head tilt or a vertical muscle imbalance, the Phoropter may have to be tilted so that one aperture is higher than the other. Leveling adjustment knobs are adjacent to the interpupillary distance knobs.

Lenses. For each eye there are large circular discs that contain spheres and cylinders. These lenses may be presented individually or in combination. A large dial on the back surface of the Phoropter introduces spheres in units of 4.00 diopters. A *side wheel* can

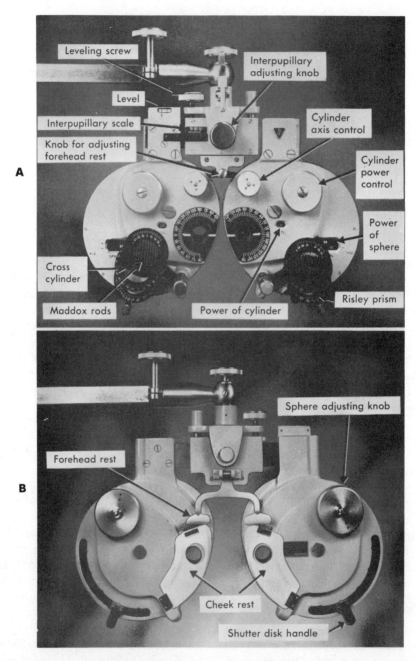

Fig. 9-3 Greens' refractor (older type). **A,** Front view. **B,** Back view. (Courtesy Bausch & Lomb Co, Rochester, New York.)

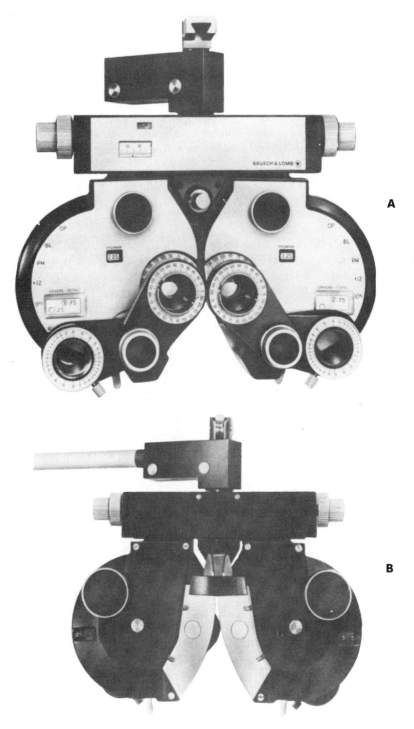

Fig. 9-4 Improved Greens' phoropter II. **A,** Front view. **B,** Back view.

be rotated to introduce spheres in small jumps of 0.25 sphere. The total spherical power is read on the front casing. Plus spheres are recorded in white and minus spheres in red. The range of spherical lenses is from +20.00 diopters to −28.00 diopters.

Phoropters are available in either plus or minus cylinders but never both. Cylinders are introduced by the top knob on the front surface of the Phoropter in units of 0.25 to 2.50. If higher cylinders are required, auxiliary cylinders of 2.50 can be flipped in front of the lens system, extending the range to 5.00. Additional loose auxiliary cylinders may be added to extend the range to 7.50 diopters. Astigmatism may be corrected to 0.12 diopters by introducing an auxiliary cylinder of 0.12 diopters. All cylinders have an axis that is controlled by a small knob, about which the accessories rotate. Markings on the front surface are in degrees from 0 to 180, with individual axis markings in 5 degrees.

Aperture control handle. A small handle on the side of each eye of the Phoropter controls the aperture. By moving the handle up or down, one may introduce the following:
1. An occluder to block out one eye
2. A pinhole disk
3. A +0.12 sphere, which can raise the total spherical power of the combination of lenses by 0.12 diopter
4. A retinoscopy lens, which may be custom-ordered according to the distance at which retinoscopy is performed (the usual retinoscopy lens ranges from +1.00 to +2.00 spheres and is introduced by the control handle for retinoscopy and removed for subjective testing)
5. Prisms, 6.00 diopters base-up before the right eye and 10.00 diopters base-in before the left eye
6. Maddox rods, vertical and horizontal

Auxiliary lenses. Auxiliary lenses include (1) cylinders of 0.12 and 5.00 diopters for each eye (the Phoropter has lenses available in either plus or minus cylinders but not both) and (2) cross cylinders of 0.25, 0.37, and 0.50 for each eye.

Accessory equipment. Accessory equipment includes (1) Risley's prisms to measure muscle im-

balance, (2) a cross cylinder holder, and (3) a reading card holder. The *cross cylinder holder* is geared to follow the cylinder axis control. The cross cylinder is inserted in a double ring of metal, the outer ring being fixed; whereas the inner ring, which holds the cross cylinder, is capable of being flipped or turned to reverse its position. The *reading card holder,* attached to the front of the Phoropter, permits the holding of a reading card at a variable distance from the Phoropter. The reading card holder is a rod, calibrated in inches, centimeters, and diopters, and it is capable of presenting four test cards to the patient.

Aids in care of Phoropter

1. If the lenses are dirty, they should be cleaned with a lint-free swab slightly moistened with either alcohol or ether. Ammonia or ammonia-containing cleansers should not be used. Lenses may be dried with a tissue.

2. Do not put fingers, pens, or pencils in the front aperture to see if a lens is in place, because the marks left are extremely difficult to remove. The rear apertures often are protected by a coverglass.

3. The instrument should not be lubricated, because the design of the instrument is such that no interior oiling is necessary. It may be helpful at times to oil the bearings on which the cross cylinder and the Maddox rod ride.

4. Cleaning material should not be used on the numbers and workings that indicate lens power. These should be cleaned with a dry, soft cloth.

5. The forehead and cheek rests are removable and should be cleaned periodically with cotton moistened in 70% alcohol solution.

6. The instrument should be covered with a plastic cover when not in use.

Retinoscope

The retinoscope is the most valuable instrument in determining the refractive error of an eye (Figs. 9-5 and 9-6). It is useful in determining the total objective refractive error of an eye and may be the only means of assessing refractive error in infants and small children. It also is useful for the objective estimation of the refractive error in illiterate persons,

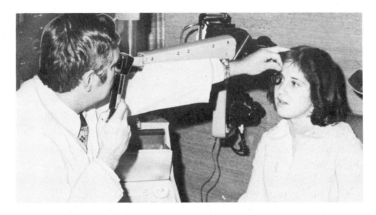

Fig. 9-5 Procedure of retinoscopic examination.

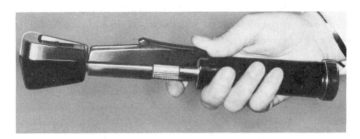

Fig. 9-6 Copeland streak retinoscope.

the mentally retarded, debilitated and uncooperative persons, and patients with speech loss. There are two basic types: (1) the spot retinoscope and (2) the streak retinoscope.

Spot retinoscope. The spot retinoscope is designed so that the refractionist can look down the center of a slightly diverging beam of light through the pupil of the patient's eye. The modern retinoscope has a light source in the handle of the instrument, shining upward, which strikes a mirror set at 45 degrees. The beam is therefore turned through 90 degrees.

The mirror may be semisilvered or may have a hole through its center through which the refractionist can look. Therefore an area of the patient's retina is illuminated, and the refractionist sees this as a red-reflected glow. This is termed a *reflex*.

In the eye with no refractive error the rays of light come to a focus on a point on the retina, and the refractionist sees the whole pupillary area lit with a red glow. This is analogous to an automobile's headlight, in which the whole 6-inch circular diameter of the headlight appears to be illuminated, whereas the source of this illumination is a small filament in the bulb, about 5 mm long, positioned correctly at the point of focus of the optical system of the headlight. Moving the retinoscope away from the pupil will cause the red reflex to be extinguished.

If the patient is myopic, the rays of light from the retinoscope will come to a focus in front of the retina, cross at this point, and illuminate a relatively larger area of the retina behind the focal point. If the light source is moved across the pupil, the rays of light from the retinoscope, pivoting on the focal point, will move the illuminated area on the fundus in an opposite direction to that of the retinoscope. This apparent shift of the illuminated area is termed an *against motion*. The refractionist therefore adds minus lenses before the patient's eyes to move the focal point back onto the retina; when he or she has the correct combination of lenses, the movement of the light across the pupil causes no movement of the reflex—it merely turns *on and off.*

If the patient is hyperopic, the ray of light from the retinoscope, on going through the eye, would focus at a point behind the retina (if the retina does not block the rays of light). Lateral movement of the retinoscope across the pupil causes the area illuminated on the retina (pivoting about the focal point) to move in the same direction as the retinoscope, indicating that the eye is hyperopic, or far-sighted. This shift is termed a *with motion.* The refractionist then adds plus lenses to bring the focusing point up to the retina until the *on and off* light reflex appears without any apparent movement.

In summary, if a retinoscope beam produces a *with motion* of the red reflex, the patient's eye is hyperopic, or farsighted, and needs plus lenses to correct the condition. If the retinoscope beam produces an *against motion,* the patient is myopic, or nearsighted, and needs minus lenses to correct the refractive error.

If the eye is astigmatic, it will exhibit two powers on axes at 90 degrees to one another. The retinoscope is then used, as was just mentioned, to correct the power on one axis and then on the other. A cylindric prescription can be obtained in this manner with use of spheres alone, but generally cylinders are added, as well as the spheres, until the *on and off* reflex is observed on all axes.

All the aforementioned theory depends on the patient's relaxed accommodation—that is, the patient's looking at some object 20 feet away—and on parallel rays of light entering the eye and coming to a focus on the retina. The light source of the retinoscope, held 0.5 meter from the patient during retinoscopy, produces diverging, not parallel, rays of light from the retinoscope. Therefore a +2.00-diopter lens (in the refractor, known as the retinoscopy lens) is put in the trial frame so that the divergent rays from the retinoscope are in fact parallel when they enter the pupil. The power of this lens depends on the working distance of the refractionist; for example, if he or she works at 0.5 meter, this

would be a +2.00-diopter lens. Some refractionists prefer a working distance that requires a +1.50-diopter retinoscopy lens.

The final prescription, taken from the lenses in the trial frame or on the Phoropter, is reduced by the working distance power to determine the distance prescription of the patient.

Streak retinoscope (see Fig. 9-6). The same principles that apply to the spot retinoscope also apply to the streak retinoscope. In the streak retinoscope the light source is a straight-line filament of the bulb. There is a condensing lens between the mirror and the bulb so that the filament itself may be focused onto the patient's eye as a straight line. By means of a movable sleeve that envelops the whole retinoscope, the bulb may be rotated and moved up and down to adjust its focus. Because the light source is a streak of light rather than a cone, if the eye is not emmetropic the area of the retina illuminated becomes a straight line rather than a spot. If astigmatism is present, it is very easy to determine its axis because the streak, playing externally across the patient's face and trial frame with its axis graduation, will not be at the same angle as the streak seen on the retina. The retinoscope streak is rotated until it parallels the streak on the retina, and the axis is thereby established. (See Chapter 10 and Fig. 10-13.)

From this point the procedure is basically the same as with a spot retinoscope, and lenses are added until the reflexes on both axes exhibit no *with* or *against motion* when the streak is passed across the pupil.

Accessories used in refraction

Cross cylinder. The cross cylinder consists of a plus and a minus cylinder set at right angles to each other, with a handle set midway between the two axes (Fig. 9-7). The axis of the plus cylinder marked in white and the axis of the minus cylin-in red. Cross cylinders are available in 0.12-, 0.25-, 0.50-, and 1.00-dioptric strengths.

The cross cylinder is a refining instrument that determines the exact axis of the astigmatic error and the exact power of the cylinder. The method of use is described in Chapter 10.

Pinhole disk. The pinhole disk is a small disk with

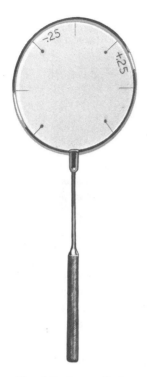

Fig. 9-7 Cross cylinder.

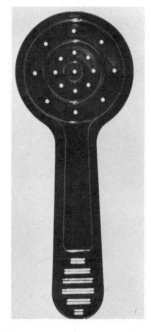

Fig. 9-8 Multiple pinhole disk.

a central small opening that eliminates peripheral rays of light, permitting only the central rays to pass through. The pinhole disk permits the examiner to differentiate poor vision caused by refractive errors from poor vision resulting from disease of the eye. Generally, vision that can be improved with a pinhole disk usually can be improved by spectacle lenses.

A multiple pinhole disk serves the same purpose as the pinhole disk but is an easier device to use because the patient does not have to search for a solitary tiny central hole (Fig. 9-8). The patient is asked to view a small line of print with one eye occluded and with the pinhole disk placed before the other eye. If looking through the pinhole disk improves the patient's visual acuity above the uncorrected vision, the findings are recorded as *vision with PH* (pinhole). Corrective lenses often improve vision to the level obtained with the pinhole disk.

Distometer. The distometer is a caliper used to measure the vertex distance (Fig. 9-9). The vertex

distance is the distance from the cornea of the patient's eye to the back surface of the lens inserted in the trial frame, refractor, or glasses. The distometer consists of a scale in millimeters, an indicator, a movable arm, and a fixed arm.

To use the distometer the fixed arm of the caliper is placed on the closed lid of the eye and the other arm against the back surface of the lens. The separation between the posterior surface of the lens and the eyelid is recorded on the millimeter scale. One millimeter is incorporated in the calibration of the distometer to allow for the thickness of the eyelid to arrive at the true vertex distance. It is important to measure the vertex distance on all high plus or minus lenses; the power of the lens in the trial frame or refractor may change when the lens is moved to a new location in the spectacle frames.

For example, if a +12.00-diopter lens in the trial frame is 10 mm from the cornea, but the correcting lens in the spectacle frame is 13 mm from the cornea, a +11.58 lens will be required at this position to

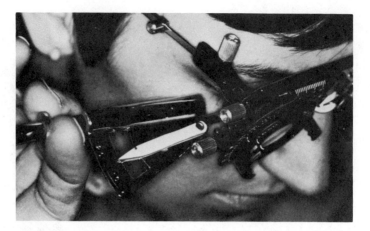

Fig. 9-9 Measuring vertex distance with a distometer.

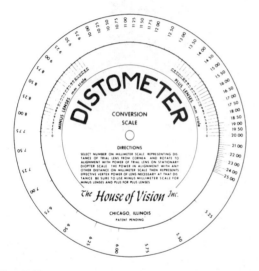

Fig. 9-10 Distometer conversion scale used to calculate change in power of a lens required when converting a prescription from the original trial or phoropter lens to the final spectacle lens.

give the patient the same visual acuity. The vertex measurement by the distometer permits the dispensing optician to calculate the effective power of a lens required in the final prescription when there is disparity between the distance of the position of the trial frame lens to the cornea and the final spectacles. To calculate the change in the power of a lens one may refer to small disk (Fig. 9-10) or vertex conversion tables (see Appendixes 9 and 10).

It should be noted that in such a case if the optician has adjusted the prescription to compensate for this closer vertex distance fitting (an ideal for comfortable vision), the lensmeter reading of the patient's glasses will not correspond with the prescription on the patient's records, either in sphere or in cylinder. The only part of the prescription that will remain the same is the axis.

Halberg and Janelli clips. The Halberg or Janelli trial clip (Fig. 9-11) eliminates the need for measuring the vertex distance. The clip is designed to accommodate two trial case rings (in the case of the Janelli, three case rings), a sphere, and a cylinder. The trial clips are placed on the patient's glasses; by overrefracting, one can arrive at the prescription with proper effective power for that particular frame. This is extremely important in the high minus or high plus prescriptions.

The clips also are useful for small children wearing glasses, where it is not possible to use a conventional trial frame or refractor.

EQUIPMENT USED TO DETECT MUSCLE IMBALANCE
Maddox rod

The Maddox rod is a group of either red or colorless parallel glass rods that together act as a cylinder (Fig. 9-12). The purpose of the Maddox rod is to disassociate the eyes and prevent them from fusing. The Maddox rod accomplishes this by changing the size,

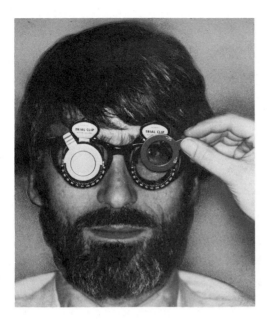

Fig. 9-11 Halberg trial clip used to refract over spectacles.

shape, and color of a point of light to a line, or streak, of light so that fusion is impossible. The relaxed fusion-free position of the eyes can then easily be measured.

The Maddox rod lens is useful in detecting (1) the presence and amount of a heterophoria, which is the fusion-free position of the eyes, and (2) the presence and amount of a heterotropia, which is a manifest deviation of the eyes not held in check by fusion.

The grouped, red cylindric rods of the Maddox lens convert a white point source of light into a red line running perpendicular to the axes of the Maddox rod. In detection of vertical heterophoria the Maddox rod is held before one eye with the rods in a vertical position before the eye. The eye behind the Maddox lens perceives a point source of light as a horizontal red line. If the patient, with both eyes open, sees the red line passing directly through the white point source of light (which is viewed by the other eye), a vertical muscle imbalance is not present. With the Maddox rod lens before the right eye, if the patient sees the red line lower than the point source of light, then the patient has a *right hypertropia* or a *right hyperphoria* (Fig. 9-13). If the red line is above the

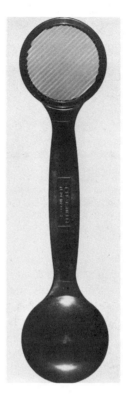

Fig. 9-12 Hand-held Maddox rod combined with occluder.

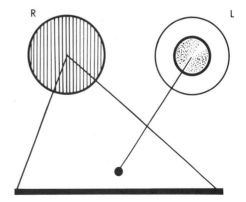

Fig. 9-13 Right hyperphoria or right hypertropia. With the Maddox rod held vertically before the right eye, the horizontal red line appears below the point source of light.

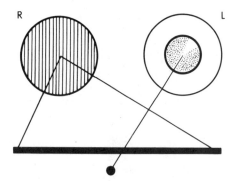

Fig. 9-14 Left hyperphoria or left hypertropia. With the Maddox rod held vertically before the right eye, the horizontal red line appears above the point source of light.

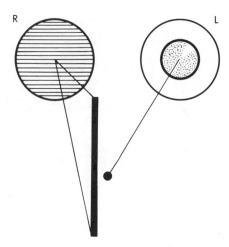

Fig. 9-15 Esophoria or esotropia. With the Maddox rod held horizontally before the right eye, the vertical red line appears on the right side of the point source of light.

point source of light, a *right hypotropia* or a *right hypophoria* is present. By convention, vertical deviations of the eye always are designated in terms of the higher eye, so that in the latter example a right hypotropia would be designated as a *left hypertropia* (Fig. 9-14). The Maddox rod test should be carried out both at near (16 inches) and in the distance (20 feet).

If the Maddox rod is now rotated so that the rods are placed horizontally before the eye, the patient will perceive the red line in the vertical direction. If the Maddox rod is held before the right eye of the patient and the line appears on the right side of the light, then *esophoria* or *esotropia* is present (Fig. 9-15). If the line appears on the left side of the light, then *exophoria* or *exotropia* is said to exist (Fig. 9-16).

The Maddox rod may be employed to detect torsion *cyclophoria* and *cyclotropia*. Torsion is the result of those ocular muscular anomalies that cause the eyes to rotate in a clockwise or counterclockwise fashion. To detect torsion, a red Maddox lens is placed before one eye and a white Maddox lens before the other eye, with the rods of both lenses held in the same direction. If the patient sees that the red line and white lines are not parallel, then torsion is present, as well as *cyclophoria* or *cyclotropia*.

A prism is needed to measure a phoria or a tropia with a Maddox rod. For example, if the patient has

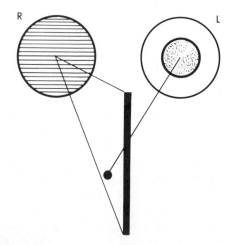

Fig. 9-16 Exophoria or exotropia. With the Maddox rod held horizontally before the right eye, the vertical red line appears on the left side of the point source of light.

a right hypertropia and reports seeing the red line below the point source of light, prisms, base down, are placed before the Maddox rod in increasing strengths until the patient states that the red line runs

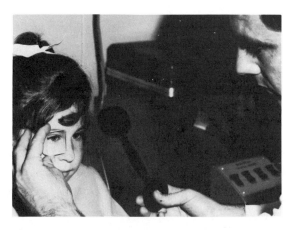

Fig. 9-17 Prism cover test. Hand-held prisms are introduced to neutralize a deviation.

through the light. The amount of prism required to center the red line on the small light is then a measure of the vertical muscle imbalance in prism diopters.

Prisms

A prism is a triangular, or wedge-shaped, piece of plastic or glass that has the property of displacing a bundle of light toward the base of the prism (Fig. 9-17). If the prism is placed before an eye, an object viewed in front of the prism will appear to be displaced toward its apex.

Prisms are employed in measuring the presence and the amount of any tropias or phorias. The tests most commonly used to measure ocular muscle imbalance with prisms are (1) the Krimsky test, (2) the

Maddox rod prism test (discussed previously), and (3) the prism cover test.

In the *Krimsky test* the observer notes the position of the corneal reflexes when a small light is shone into the eyes. The examiner notes where this reflex is centered in the fixating eye. Prisms are then placed before the deviating eye until the position of the reflex in the pupil of the deviating eye is located in the same position as that of the fixating eye. For example, if the patient's right eye is turned in, the light reflex may be found overlying the temporal margin of the pupil, and base-out prisms would be required to displace this reflex to a more central position.

The basis of *prism cover test* is to displace the image of the deviating eye by the use of prisms so that it falls on the macula of that eye. Thus each eye will project to the same point in space, and covering one eye will not require any movement of the other eye to take up fixation. The amount of prism diopters required to achieve this end point is a measure of the deviation (see Fig. 9-17). The mechanics of this test are discussed in the chapter on orthoptics.

Types of prisms available are (1) loose prism, (2) horizontal and vertical prism bars, and (3) Risley's rotary prism.

The *loose,* or *individual, prism* is made of plastic or glass. These prisms are supplied in low powers in standard trial lens sets and in a full range of powers in individual prism boxes (Fig. 9-18).

Horizontal and vertical prism bars (Fig. 9-19) are fused prisms amalgamated into a single bar of grad-

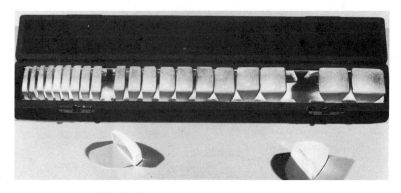

Fig. 9-18 Loose, or individual, prisms set.

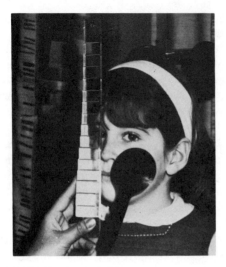

Fig. 9-19 Prism bars used to measure the amplitude or power of fusion.

ually increasing strengths. These prisms may be set in a horizontal direction (base in or out) or in a vertical direction (base up or down). The prism bar is principally employed to measure the amplitude or power of fusion. It sometimes is employed in the cover-uncover test for the measurement of strabismus in children because it permits rapid examination in a patient whose patience and attention may be limited.

Risley's rotary prism (Fig. 9-20) consists of two counterrotating prisms mounted in rings, one in front of the other. These rings are easily rotated in opposite directions by a small thumbscrew. When the two bases are rotated so that they lie behind one another, their effective power is additive. When the apex of one prism is rotated so that it lies behind the base of the other, the effective power is zero. Thus Risley's rotating prism provides a rapid and simple increase in prism power strength so that a deviation may be rapidly adjusted and measured without the delay in introducing individual prisms before the eye.

INSTRUMENTS USED TO DETERMINE POWER OF LENSES

Several instruments are available to assist the ophthalmologist and the ophthalmic assistant in ac-

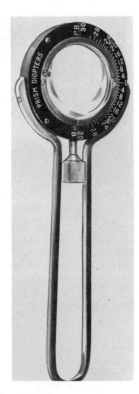

Fig. 9-20 Risley's rotary prism.

curately determining the strength of the lenses the patient has been wearing.

Lensmeter

The lensmeter (for example, Lensometer, Vertometer) is used to determine (1) the dioptric vertex power of a lens, (2) the axis, (3) the optical center of a lens, and (4) the presence of prism and the direction of its base. It consists of an illuminated target, a holder for the glasses to be measured, an adjustable eyepiece, and an optical system designed to focus on an image in the anterior focal plane of the lens to be measured.

To use the lensmeter see the detailed instructions in Chapter 8.

Geneva lens measure

The Geneva lens measures the radius of curvature of the lens surface and records it in diopters. The instrument consists of a dial with a revolving hand and three pins projecting from the instrument. Approximate dioptric power of the lens can be determined by placing the surface of the lens against the pins and then rotating the lens 90 degrees. If the reading on the scale remains constant, no cylinder is present on that side. The algebraic sum of the readings from the front and back surface of the lens represents the dioptric power of the lens (for example, -2.00 sphere on one side and $+6.00$ sphere on the other side is equivalent to a $+4.00$ sphere lens). If the reading is not uniform over the entire surface of the lens, the difference between the lower and higher readings represents the amount of cylinder present. The disadvantage of the Geneva lens is that the gauges are calibrated for crown glass only and are subject to considerable error in determining the axis of the cylinder. The gauge will give incorrect measurements for hard resin (plastic) lenses, for aspheric surfaces, and for invisible progressive bifocals.

INSTRUMENTS USED TO EXAMINE INTERIOR OF THE EYE

Ophthalmologists enjoy the unique privilege of being able to examine, by direct visualization, the interior of a vital organ. They can study the retina, which is a modification of nervous tissue, the head of the optic nerve (optic disc), and the state of the retinal blood vessels, which to a large degree mirror the state of other blood vessels not visible to inspection. Because many systemic and neurologic diseases first manifest by alterations within the eye, the use of the ophthalmoscope and other such devices has assisted in bringing ophthalmologists in closer contact with their medical colleagues in related fields.

Direct ophthalmoscope

The ophthalmoscope was invented more than 100 years ago by Hermann Helmholtz. Helmholtz's work was based on the observations of Ernest Brücke, a well-known Viennese physiologist, who four years previously reported noticing a red light in the pupil of a young man standing in the auditorium of the university as the chandelier light reflected from the student's eye in a direction corresponding to that of his own visual axis. With the popularization of the ophthalmoscope, a wealth of blinding diseases could

be understood, and investigation of their cause and treatment began.

The ophthalmoscope consists fundamentally of a light source, a viewing device, and a reflecting device to channel light into the patient's eye. The reflecting device can be a mirror or a reflecting prism. If the patient and examiner are both emmetropic, then light from the patient's retina will be in focus for the examiner. If, however, either the patient or the examiner is hyperopic or myopic, the spherical lenses must be employed to overcome their refractive error. Because the ophthalmoscope contains no cylindric lenses, astigmatic errors of refraction cannot be compensated for. Thus, if a patient has a large amount of astigmatism, a crystal-clear view of the fundus cannot be obtained. The direct ophthalmoscope enables the examiner to use the power of the subject's eye as a magnifying system to see the retina. Although the field of vision is somewhat restricted compared with that seen with the indirect ophthalmoscope, the magnification is greater, being approximately $\times 15$ for the former and $\times 5$ for the latter (Fig. 9-21).

To facilitate pupillary dilation, ophthalmoscopy is best performed in a dark room. For a better inspection of the fundus, however, the pupils should be dilated with a weak mydriatic agent, such as 2.5% phenylephrine or hydroxyamphetamine hydrobromide (Paredrine). With heavily pigmented irides, a stronger mydriatic agent, such as 10% phenylephrine, should be used but with *caution*. Because there have been deaths recorded from the application of a single drop, 10% phenylephrine should *not* be routinely used. It should not be used in any circumstances with patients who have hypertension or cardiovascular disease. If it is imperative to dilate the pupils of these patients, then cyclopentolate (Cyclogyl) or tropicamide (Mydriacyl) should be employed.

Pupillary dilation with drops usually is performed in all new patients and in those with extremely small pupils. The examiner stands directly in front of the patient and examines the patient's right eye with his or her own right eye and the left eye in similar fashion (Fig. 9-22). The first structure in the fundus noted, for purposes of orientation, is the optic disc. The disc is an oval structure and represents the site of entrance

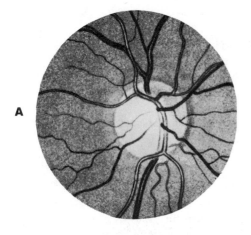

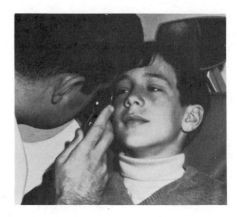

Fig. 9-22 Examination with the direct ophthalmoscope.

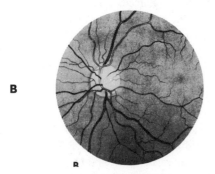

Fig. 9-21 A, Fundus as viewed with the small aperture of the direct ophthalmoscope. Note the magnification obtained but the restrictions in the fields seen. **B,** Fundus as viewed with the indirect ophthalmoscope. Note the larger field of view, reduced magnification, and inverted image.

of the optic nerve (Fig. 9-23). It usually is pink and may have a central white depression, called the *physiologic cup*. The margins of the disc are sharp and distinct except for the margins of the upper and lower poles, which may be slightly fuzzy. From the disc the retinal arterioles and veins emerge and bifurcate; they extend toward the four quadrants of the retina. The retinal vein, which usually is found lateral to the retinal artery, is larger and darker red. Approximately two disc diameters away from the optic disc, and slightly below its center, is the macula. The macula is a small avascular area that appears deeper red than the surrounding fundus. In heavily pigmented persons the macula may have a darker hue than the adjacent fundus. In the center of the macula there is a glistening oval reflex called the *fovea*. In young people a second reflex, which appears as a glimmering halo, may surround the entire macular region. Each quadrant of the fundus is examined in turn. To see as much of the peripheral retina as possible, the examiner should ask the patient to look in the direction of the quadrant under study. The color of the fundus usually is an even red hue, but it will vary with the general pigmentation of the eye, as well as the individual's general pigmentation.

Because the disc of the ophthalmoscope lens permits very close observation of an object, the ophthalmoscope usually examines the lens, the iris, the cornea, and the external eye.

Special devices on the ophthalmoscope

Red-free light. Although a true red-free state cannot be obtained with the yellow-green filters found in many ophthalmoscopes, the filters do, however, serve a purpose. Viewing the fundus with a relatively red-free filter makes the retinal blood vessels appear black and retinal nerve fibers more prominent. The macula stands out against the greenish-gray background of the fundus as a golden-yellow oval patch. The use of red-free light for examining the fundus is particularly valuable for detecting minute superficial hemorrhages, holes in the retina, and early degenerations of the macula.

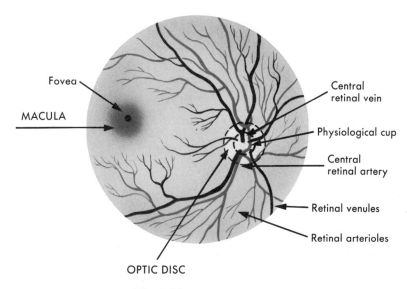

Fovea

MACULA

Central retinal vein

Physiological cup

Central retinal artery

Retinal venules

Retinal arterioles

OPTIC DISC

Fig. 9-23 Fundus of the eye.

Red light. Red filters diminish the contrast between the retinal blood vessels and the retina. However, melanin pigment, which absorbs red rays, contrasts strongly with the surrounding red fundus. Red light illumination therefore is of value in differentiating hemorrhage from pigmented tumors that contain melanin.

Polarized light. Incorporation of two polarizing filters into the optical system, which polarizes the light leaving the ophthalmoscope, minimizes irritating reflections from the patient's cornea. The only problem with the general use of polarized light is that the intensity of the illumination has to be greatly increased to compensate for the filtering effect of the two polarizing filters.

Slit illumination. In the construction of the ophthalmoscope the insertion of a slit or a diaphragm in the course of the illuminating system simply reduces the illumination. For focal high-intensity illumination, better results are attained when the slit is directed from a slit-lamp microscope and the fundus is viewed with a contact or Hruby lens. The use of a slit lamp is valuable in the estimation of the level of various areas of the retina.

Aperture disks. Most ophthalmoscopes have two or more aperture disks of different sizes. The smaller

apertures are particularly useful for viewing the fundus through a small pupil, such as that found in glaucoma patients under treatment.

Cobalt-blue filters. These are used for fluorescein studies of the fundus.

Many types of ophthalmoscopes are available today. Electric-power ophthalmoscopes offer the advantage of illumination that is more controlled and of higher intensity.

Indirect ophthalmoscope

The indirect ophthalmoscope was invented by Dr. C. J. T. Rooter only 1 year after Helmholtz's invention of the direct ophthalmoscope. The indirect ophthalmoscope permits the examiner to see more of the retina in one glance than the direct ophthalmoscope allows. Because of its construction, the instrument also accommodates a larger and brighter light source, which permits the examiner to penetrate moderate cataracts and to see retinal detail. Usually, however, the pupil must be dilated to use this device.

For indirect ophthalmoscopy the patient's eyes must be fully dilated with a mydriatic agent. The examiner holds a convex lens in front of the patient's eye, and through a viewing device attached to the headband of the indirect ophthalmoscope, a *real,*

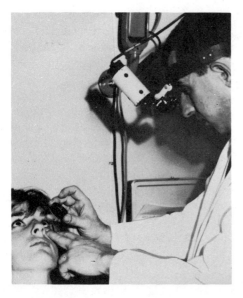

Fig. 9-24 Examination with the indirect ophthalmoscope.

inverted image at the focal point of the hand-held lens can be seen (Fig. 9-24). The size of this aerial image varies with the dioptric strength of the lens employed. The lens most commonly used is a +20.00-diopter lens.

The fundus camera is simply an enclosed indirect ophthalmoscope with a camera back.

Relative merits of direct and indirect ophthalmoscopes

The *direct ophthalmoscope* (1) permits a greater magnification ($\times 15$), (2) is easier to use with small or undilated pupils, and (3) is mechanically easier to use. The *indirect binocular ophthalmoscope* (1) permits binocular vision and depth perception, (2) permits a wider field of view of a given area, (3) is easier to use in the operating room without contamination, (4) permits indentation of the sclera and thus a better view of the periphery of the fundus, (5) provides more intense illumination, and (6) frees the hand for operative manipulation.

Transilluminator

Transillumination is employed when the media are too cloudy to permit inspection of the fundus and

the examiner suspects the presence of an intraocular tumor. The transilluminator consists of a handle and a small, narrow tip that contains a heat-free or insulated high-intensity light source. The beam of the transilluminator is passed over accessible areas of the sclera, and in normal cases a bright red glow comes from the pupil if there are good transmissions from any point where the light is applied. If the light passes over the site of a solid tumor, the brilliance of the glow in the pupillary space will be diminished and an outline of the tumor revealed. The transilluminator also is useful in providing a bright source of illumination for the inspection of the external eye, the lids, and the iris reflex.

INSTRUMENTS USED TO STUDY ANTERIOR SEGMENT OF THE EYE
Slit-lamp microscope

Use of slit lamp. This instrument is used to illuminate and examine under magnification the anterior segment of the eye. The slit-lamp microscope enables the observer to binocularly view the conjunctiva, sclera, cornea, iris, anterior chamber, lens, and anterior portion of the vitreous, and it permits the detection of disease occurring in these areas. The slit lamp is the heart of an ophthalmologic examination. The watch glass on a watch appears relatively clear when viewed from the front; yet when a penlight is directed obliquely at the edge of the watch glass, it brings out scratches and smears that are not easily seen in normal lighting. Similarly, the front surface of the eye and the interior of the eye can be seen more clearly when light is placed obliquely and there is back scattering of the light. Allvar Gullstrand of Stockholm, who won the Nobel Prize in 1911 for his studies on the optics of the eye, realized that a very special system was needed to see structural details in these so-called transparent tissues. Thus the first Gullstrand slit-lamp microscope was developed.

Attachments to the slit-lamp microscope permit examination of the angle structures, ciliary body, and fundus. The attachment of an applanation tonometer permits measurement of the intraocular pressure. Photographic attachments enable photography of the anterior segment of the eye. The slit-lamp microscope is of special importance in conditions, such as dendritic keratitis, corneal foreign body, and early lens changes, that are better diagnosed and treated by having a well-illuminated and highly magnified view of the area.

Design of slit lamp. Slit-lamp microscopes have an illumination system combined with a microscope set on an instrument table fitted with a head and chin rest.

The *illuminating system* is controlled by a transformer with adjustable ranges of voltage to provide intense illumination when required. Good illumination is about 5,000,000 lux units. Controls are placed on the illuminating arm to (1) narrow the beam of light to a narrow slit, (2) vary the length of slit to a small pinpoint of light, (3) introduce color filters to provide a green and a deep cobalt blue to the beam of light, (4) rotate the slit, and (5) adjust the angle between the slit beam and the microscope's line of sight. A Kodak Wratten yellow filter No. 15 may be advantageous when used in conjunction with a cobalt-blue filter to enhance contrast visibility of fluorescein staining of the eye.

The newer slit lamps are designed so that the illuminated slit remains sharply in focus with the microscope at all times. The illuminating system may be shifted to illuminate the eye from any angle and may be altered so that the beam falls to the side of the area to be viewed.

The *instrument table* and *headrest* permit adjustment to make the patient more comfortable. A fixation light usually is attached to the headrest to enable the patient to maintain fixation.

The *microscope* is attached to a movable stage operated by controls to permit focusing. In the new models there is a joy stick type of control. The microscope, along with the illuminating system, is adjustable in both the side-to-side direction and the up-and-down position. The microscope itself is composed of (1) an *eyepiece* (with an extra eyepieces for higher magnification) and (2) an *objective*. The eyepiece is individually adjustable to enable the examiner to neutralize his or her own error of refraction. Without interrupting the examination, the examiner can increase the magnification power of the objective from $\times 6$ to $\times 40$. Some microscopes have

a smaller range of magnification. Some have "zoom" optics. It has been found that a magnification of $\times 15$ is very satisfactory for routine use. Additional magnification may be achieved by changing the eyepiece to that of a higher power.

Types of slit lamps. Several models of slit lamps are available. Each has special features that make it valuable. Available slit lamps include Haag-Streit model 900 (Fig. 9-25), American Optical Campbell, Bausch & Lomb Thorpe, and Carl Zeiss Nikon and Topcon (Fig. 9-26).

Technique of slit-lamp examination. Both the patient and the examiner are seated. The patient places the chin on the chin rest and the forehead against the headrest. The chin rest and the microscope are adjusted so that the beam of light falls on the cornea. The fixation light is adjusted in front of the eye not being examined to position the patient's other eye for the examination. The light is adjusted to a narrow beam and directed from the side onto the cornea. The microscope is set for the low power and the eye is examined. A single-level control on the microscope permits movement and focusing in depth on the cornea and the anterior structures of the eye. Methods of illumination with the slit lamp include direct and indirect illumination, sclerotic scatter, retroillumination, and diffuse illumination. Further details on slit-lamp techniques are illustrated in the chapter on photography (Chapter 33).

Slit-lamp attachments

Hruby lens (Fig. 9-27). The Hruby lens is a -55-diopter lens constructed to permit the examination of the vitreous body and the fundus of the eye under slit-lamp illumination and magnification. The lens is placed before the eye, and the pencil of light is directed through the center of the Hruby lens toward the posterior portion of the eye. The microscope is then focused on the fundus.

Fundus contact lens (Fig. 9-28). This is a hand-held contact lens inserted onto the anesthetized eye. Before the lens is placed in the eye, a drop or two of methyl cellulose is placed on the concave side of the lens. The contact lens permits the examination of the fundus of the eye. In comparison with the Hruby lens, the contact lens eliminates the air interface

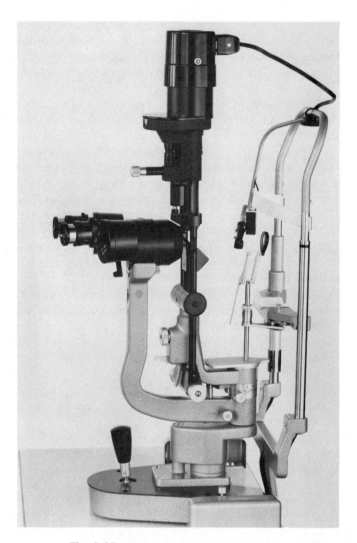

Fig. 9-25 Haag-Streit slit-lamp microscope.

between the lens and the eye and thereby eliminates anomalies of corneal curvature and corneal irregularities.

Pachymeter. Some slit lamps (such as the Haag-Streit model 900) have attachments to measure accurately the thickness of the cornea and the thickness of the anterior chamber. The optical pachymeter is available in two different models: one for measuring the thickness of the cornea and one for estimating the depth of the anterior chamber.

This measuring device consists of two plano glass plates, one above the other edge to edge, which are placed above the right ocular of the slit lamp and which divide the projected beam of light entering the slit lamp equally about a horizontally displaced midway line.

The lower of the two plates is fixed perpendicularly to the optical axis of the objective, but the upper plate can be rotated about a vertical axis by turning the scale segment of the device, thus doubling the

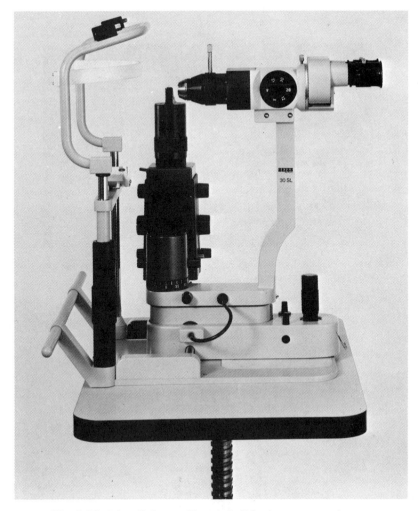

Fig. 9-26 Zeiss slit lamp with endothelial microscope attachment.

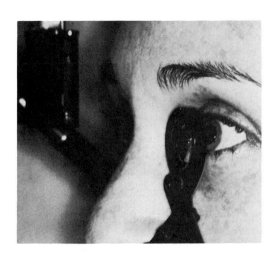

Fig. 9-27 Hruby lens used to examine the fundus under magnification.

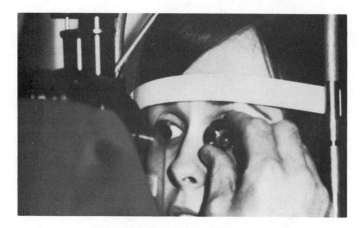

Fig. 9-28 Fundus contact lens.

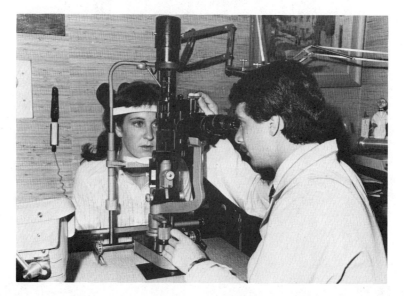

Fig. 9-29 The pachymeter: used to measure the depth of portions of the eye such as the cornea or the anterior chamber.

image. The separation of the two images is dependent on the angle between the fixed and the movable plates (Fig. 9-29).

When observed through the split-image eyepieces, one of the two images in the upper field and one in the lower field, not being needed for the measurement, are displaced prismatically. Thus the measuring points lying in the optical split image can be brought exactly into coincidence.

For measuring corneal thickness, the endothelium and the epithelium are used as measuring points. For measuring the depth of the anterior chamber, the epithelium and the anterior surface of the crystalline lens are the measuring points.

In addition to the optical pachymeter, the ultrasonic pachymeter is gaining more widespread use for the measurement of corneal thickness. Its ease of use and its ready portability make it much simpler

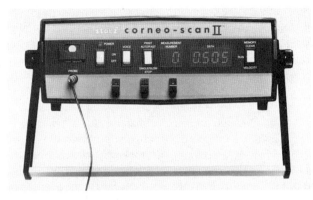

Fig. 9-30 Ultrasound pachymeter used to measure the corneal thickness.

to use. Ultrasonic waves are passed through the cornea to provide a digital readout of the corneal thickness. The head of the pachymeter is either of the solid type or fluid-filled. The probe is applied directly to the cornea. The readouts are given in microns of the thickness of the cornea (Fig. 9-30).

INSTRUMENTS USED TO EXAMINE ANGLE STRUCTURES OF THE EYE
Goniolens

The goniolens is used to examine the ciliary body, the periphery of the retina, and the angle structures. Normally these areas are inaccessible for direct examination. The use of the goniolens is the only method for detecting the presence of angle-closure glaucoma to determine whether the angle is open or closed. The lens is of value in locating preferential surgical sites of drainage in glaucoma and for evaluating the cause of failure after glaucoma surgery. There are two basic types of goniolenses: those using mirrors in their construction to enable the observer to see into the angle and those using the prismatic effect of a very high plus lens to accomplish the same purpose.

The mirror-type goniolens deflects a beam of light into the opposite angle of the anterior chamber (Fig. 9-31). The image of this illuminated angle is reflected along the same course and is visible through the objective lenses of the viewing microscope.

All of the goniolenses available are of the contact-

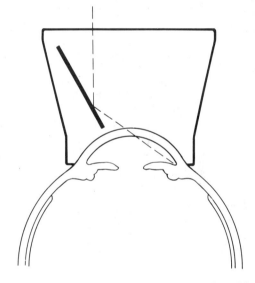

Fig. 9-31 Goniolens. A beam of light is deflected into the opposite angle of the anterior chamber.

lens type. The lens is placed on the anesthetized cornea, with a thin layer of fluid separating the lens from the cornea.

Contact goniolenses available are (1) the *children's goniolens*, which is small to conform to the small cornea; (2) the *single-sided goniolens*, which requires rotation to view the complete periphery of the angle of the anterior segment; (3) the *four-sided goniolens*, with all four mirrors inclined at the same angle, permitting the examiner to view the complete circumference of the angle without rotation of the goniolens; (4) the *Goldmann three-mirror contact lens,* with each mirror inclined at a different angle, permitting a view of the periphery of the retina and a view of the ciliary body, as well as the angle structures of the anterior chamber; (5) the *Koeppe contact goniolens,* which is applied to the cornea, with saline solution or methyl cellulose interposed, and which is used with the patient in a reclining position and the examiner viewing the angle structures through a hand-held gonioscope; and (6) the *operating goniolens,* which is similar to other contact goniolenses except that one side is partially removed to permit access of a goniotomy knife for surgery on the angle structures. (The first four lenses mentioned are used in conjunction with a slit-lamp microscope.)

The Posner diagnostic and surgical gonioprism

Although the principle of the Posner diagnostic and surgical gonioprism is certainly not new, the device is a good modification over existing instruments. This lens is used for viewing the anterior chamber, and it consists of a highly polished, truncated, silver-surfaced pyramid, with a plain anterior viewing surface over four mirrors—all inclined at 64 degrees—forming the sides of a pyramidal lens. The lens is used with a 45-degree angle so that the entire 360 degrees of the anterior chambers can be observed by locating the lens 11 degrees in either direction,

making a small adjustment in the slit-lamp beam. It is an ideal lens for use in children or in patients with a small palpebral fissure. A modification of this lens is the lighted surgical gonioprism, which was designed by Jerald L. Tennant. This lens is illuminated by a lighted halogen fiberoptics system that aids in the viewing of the alignment of feet of the anterior chamber that support an intraocular lens. It was designed primarily for viewing anterior chamber lens implants, particularly at the conclusion of the implantation procedure. The gonioprism is placed on the cornea at the position of the feet of the intraocular lens and is examined in relationship to the angle.

Gonioscope

The gonioscope is essentially a hand-held microscope and illuminating system used in conjunction with the goniolens for gonioscopy of the angle structures. The gonioscope may be balanced on counterweights over ceiling pulleys for ease of handling. In using the gonioscope, the examiner places a contact goniolens on the patient's cornea while the patient is in the recumbent position and then examines the complete angle structure through the magnification of the hand-held gonioscope (Fig. 9-32).

INSTRUMENTS USED TO ASSESS THE CORNEA
Keratometer

It is necessary to obtain the exact radius of curvature of the cornea. This can be accomplished with the ophthalmometer (keratometer), which is used in fit-

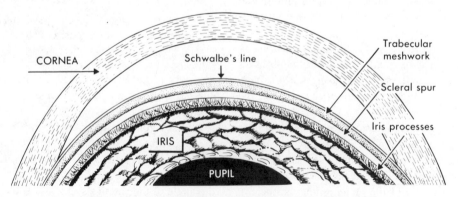

Fig. 9-32 Angle structure as viewed through the goniolens.

ting contact lenses. Keratometry is the measurement of the central anterior curvature of the cornea. It is valuable in eye examinations, particularly for detecting and measuring corneal astigmatism. The keratometer consists essentially of a target that is imaged by the cornea and telescoped to observe this image. The measurement of the target image reveals the corneal curvature in diopters with the variation in curvature (astigmatism). The keratometer is invaluable in cases of irregular astigmatism, asymmetric astigmatism, oblique astigmatism, conical cornea (keratoconus), and nystagmus. The Bausch & Lomb keratometer is the standard on which other keratometers are based (see Chapter 13).

A lightweight, hand-held autokeratometer recently was developed by Alcon Systems, Inc. (Fig. 9-33). A rechargeable battery located in the handle provides for several hours of use. Its accuracy appears comparable with that of traditional keratometers. It is of clinical value in hospitals, permitting early postoperative measurements after cataract and corneal transplantation. Because of its easy portability, its use in the clinical setting can minimize

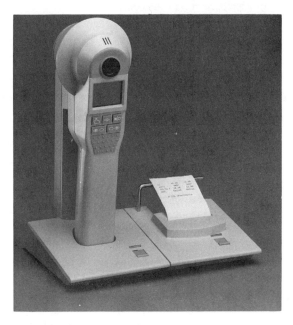

Fig. 9-33 Hand-held automated keratometer. (Courtesy Alcon Systems, Inc., Fort Worth, Texas.)

the number of keratometers required for a well-equipped office.

This keratometer, which is fully automatic and computerized, allows the operator to measure the vertical and horizontal base-curve values of the cornea, the angle of maximum difference between the two base curves; and to calculate astigmatism. These measurements, which can be taken while the patient stands, sits, or reclines, are stored automatically in terms of the right and left eyes and are displayed in either diopters or millimeters. An automated line-up system ensures that the keratometer is in line during measurements.

To take a measurement, one presses on either the right- or left-eye button. When a ring of green lights illuminates, the pupil is centered in the ring and a red blinking light is centered over the pupil. The patient is asked to fixate on the central blinking red light, and the keratometer is stabilized by the examiner's free hand on the patient's forehead. The keratometer lights are then aligned until eight green lights are located in an "x" formation around the red fixation light. The holding button is then released. The green lights turn off and there is a long chirp. This records the measurement of that eye. The procedure is then repeated on the fellow eye.

The Humphrey autokeratometer shows both the shape and the vault of the cornea. It uses infrared rays and measures an area 2.6 mm centrally. The Canon automatic keratometer K1 uses a xenon light and does the keratometer measurement in one tenth of a second.

Specular microscope

The specular microscope is used to examine the endothelium of the cornea, which is the layer of the cornea in contact with the aqueous humor. Without a good intact endothelium the cornea would swell, lose its transparency, and become a painful debilitating organ such as occurs in bullous keratopathy.

The specular microscope is an instrument in which light passes through a slit aperture into a system of mirrors with a direct light, moves out through an objective lens, and is attached to a "dipping cone." This cone lens is a flat surface extension of the $\times 20$

water immersion objective. It applanates the cornea just as in applanation tonometry. A focusing knob adjusts the movement of the cone lens to focus the image on a cornea for different thicknesses. This process is used for an objective measurement of the corneal thickness. The light that is reflected from the endothelium and back through the objected eyepiece at $\times 200$ magnification can be observed through an eyepiece or directed into a single-lens reflex camera. The xenon flash cube permits clear photographs despite continuous small eye movement. Endothelium counts are expressed as cells per millimeter squared. The average central endothelium cell count rate is from 1800 to 4000 cells/mm^2, with an average of 2800 cells/mm^2. A significant decrease in cell density occurs with age, indicating a continuous cell loss throughout life. The endothelial cell has no capacity for cell division and reproduction so that when loss occurs, there is no replacement. The endothelial cell population of the human cornea decreases from approximately 1 million cells from the first year of life to one third the number by the eighth decade of life.

The greatest impact of specular microscopy has been in the area of cataract extraction, particularly with regard to intraocular lens insertion. It has been shown that patients with routine cataract extraction have endothelial cell losses ranging up to 8%. With intraocular lens insertion, however, cell losses ranging from 24% to 62% have been reported. It has now been established that this endothelial cell loss is a result of the touch of endothelium by the intraocular lens. However, effective remedies to this endothelial cell loss have been achieved by maintaining the anterior chamber with air during the insertion of the lens, thus avoiding the touch of the corneal endothelium to the intraocular lens. The introduction of sodium hyaluronate (Healon) has significantly minimized the endothelial trauma during the surgery. The use of the specular microscope has made the practitioner aware of factors that encourage a concerted effort to minimize irreparable endothelial damage.

The clinical specular microscope has become an important clinical aid helping the surgeon operating on the anterior segment to plan a more rational presurgical approach. In those practices in which a great deal of surgery is being performed and a specular microscope is employed, it is important for the ophthalmic technician to learn how to employ this instrument, to understand its significance, and to know how to use it for taking pictures of endothelium for the surgeon to examine.

INSTRUMENTS USED TO MEASURE INTRAOCULAR PRESSURE (TONOMETER)

The tonometer, designed to measure the intraocular pressure, is used in the most important single test in the detection of glaucoma. There are two instruments in common use: the applanation tonometer and the indentation tonometer (for example, the Schiøtz tonometer). A comparison of these two types is presented, and a number of instruments employing these principles are discussed in Chapter 22.

Tonography

Tonography is a measuring and recording of intraocular pressure over a period of 4 minutes, during which time the weight of the Schiøtz indentation tonometer is held on the cornea.

Tonography can be done with an ordinary indentation tonometer and a stopwatch; readings are taken at regular intervals during the 4 minutes and the results are graphed after the test is complete. Many tonometers have been designed to draw the graph automatically. The movement of the plunger on the standard Schiøtz tonometer is amplified mechanically by the long pointer. The measurement of this movement is registered on the scale at the top of the instrument.

Electronic tonometers essentially use the same principle: the movement of the plunger through the footplate is transmitted to an electronic amplifier, and the resulting amplified signal activates the meter needle. The scale behind the needle is calibrated using the same figures as are on the standard Schiøtz instrument. The needle movements are transmitted to a writing pen, which draws a line on a roll chart passing under the nib; thus any movement of the plunger over the 4-minute period automatically appears on a chart.

SPECIAL INSTRUMENTS
Exophthalmometer

The exophthalmometer is an instrument designed to measure the forward protrusion of the eye. This instrument provides a method of evaluating and recording the progression and regression of the prominence of an eye caused by disorders such as thyroid disease and tumors of the orbit. Instruments commonly in use are the Luedde and the Hertel exophthalmometers.

Luedde exophthalmometer. The Luedde exophthalmometer is fundamentally a transparent ruler calibrated in millimeters. One end is notched to fit easily into the bony prominence of the lateral orbital margin. The observer, standing at the side of the patient whose gaze is directed forward, sights the apex of the cornea through the transparent plastic rule and then records the forward protrusion of one eye at a time in millimeters.

Hertel exophthalmometer. This instrument consists of a horizontal calibrated bar with movable carriers at each side. Each carrier consists of mirrors inclined at 45 degrees to reflect both the scale reading and the apex of the cornea of profile. Notches on the side carriers are placed on the bony lateral orbital margins of the patient. The patient is then asked to fixate on a point on the examiner's forehead. The apex of the cornea of each eye is superimposed on the millimeter scale reading by the inclined mirrors. The measurement of each eye is recorded by the examiner, alternately viewing with the right and left eye. The distance along the horizontal bar also is recorded as the base figure so that the carriers will be set at the same base for comparison at subsequent readings. This instrument provides a reliable comparison of the forward protrusion of each eye in relation to the bony orbit (Fig. 9-34).

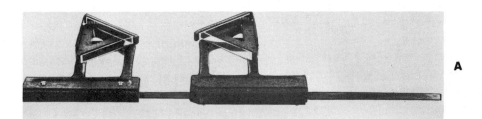

A

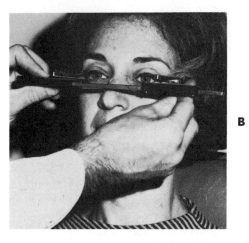

B

Fig. 9-34 A, Hertel exophthalmometer. **B,** Measurement of eye protrusion.

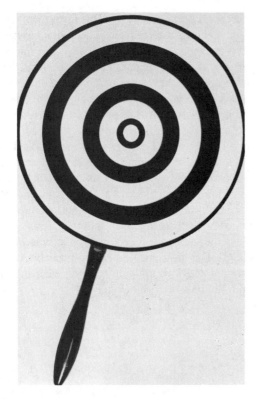

Fig. 9-35 Placido's disk used to identify corneal irregularities.

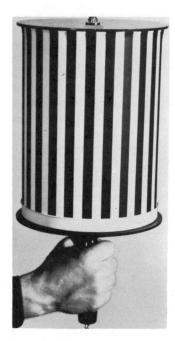

Fig. 9-36 Optokinetic drum.

Placido's disk

Placido's disk is a flat disk on which has been painted alternating black and white rings that encircle a small central round aperture (Fig. 9-35). Placido's disk is used in evaluating the regularity of the anterior curvature of the cornea. Its relative simplicity makes it a useful instrument in detecting early stages of keratoconus.

In an examination using Placido's disk the patient is placed with a strong light behind one shoulder; the examiner observes the cornea through the central hole of the disk. The reflections of the rings on the cornea are free of distortions if the cornea is normally curved. If the cornea has an irregular curvature, considerable distortion of the concentric rings will occur. An electric Placido's disk, or keratoscope, has been designed for controlled illumination and convenience.

Optokinetic drum

The optokinetic drum consists of a handle and a drum that can be readily rotated on the handle. The drum is covered with alternating vertical white and dark stripes or pictures (Fig. 9-36). The patient is seated and asked to observe the stripes as the drum is slowly rotated. The drum is held 1 foot away and rotated slowly from right to left, then from left to right, and finally upward and downward. The quick, jerky refixation movements the patient has to make in viewing the revolving stripes produce a jerk nystagmus of the patient's eyes. Normally this jerk nystagmus can be elicited with rotation of the drum in each of the directions tested. A failure to elicit a jerk-nystagmus type of response in one direction often indicates severe and serious neurologic disease.

A simplified optokinetic tape, designed by Dr. J. Lawton Smith, is a useful alternate to the larger drum. Its chief virtue is that it can be carried in the pocket. It consists of a series of 2-inch red squares sewed onto a 4-inch tape approximately 1 meter in length (Fig. 9-37). A further refinement is the black

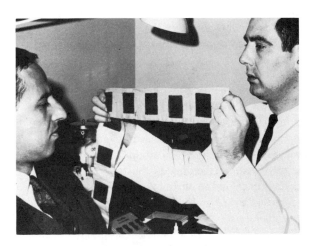

Fig. 9-37 Optokinetic tape.

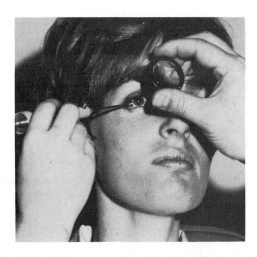

Fig. 9-39 Measurement of ophthalmic artery pressure by use of the ophthalmodynamometer.

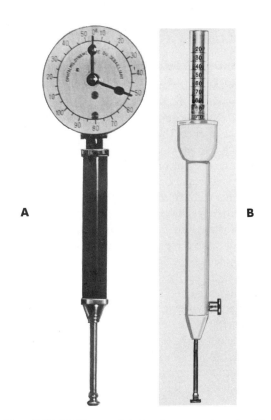

A

B

Fig. 9-38 Bailliart ophthalmodynamometer. **A,** Dial type. **B,** Plunger type.

and white optokinetic tape, which retracts into a carpenter's type of measuring tape cartridge.

Ophthalmodynamometer

The ophthalmodynamometer is an instrument designed to measure the pressure in the ophthalmic artery and its parent vessel, the internal carotid artery (Fig. 9-38). It is employed primarily to diagnose conditions resulting in a lower pressure in these main arteries. In particular, it is used in the diagnostic work-up of cases of carotid insufficiency, carotid thrombosis, and carotid stenosis.

For this test it is best if two examiners are present. One examiner applies the instrument to the globe, increasing the force applied in small increments, while the other visualizes the state of the retinal vessels (Fig. 9-39). Visualization can be achieved by use of either the direct or the indirect ophthalmoscope.

The patient should be seated comfortably and the pupils dilated with a mydriatic agent. Local anesthetic drops are instilled into the eye before application of the ophthalmodynamometer. The assistant places the instrument over the bulbar conjunctiva in the horizontal meridian of the eyeball, temporal to the limbus, and gradually increases the force to the eye as the examiner regards the retinal vessels on the surface of the disk. Once the intraocular pressure has been raised sufficiently to cause a pulsation of the central retinal artery, a reading is taken. This is the diastolic pressure recorded in grams. As the compression of the globe is continued, the central retinal artery finally ceases to pulsate, collapses, and appears completely blanched. At this point another reading is taken, and this reading represents the systolic pressure in grams.

For best results three readings of both the systolic and the diastolic pressure for each eye are made, with the patient in both the upright and the reclining positions. The recordings of pressure in grams can be converted to millimeters of mercury with tables.

Most ophthalmologists, before performing ophthalmodynamometry, also record the intraocular tension in each eye and the blood pressure in each arm.

A pressure difference of 20 between the two eyes is considered significant. Because one third of patients with a diagnosis of a stroke are found to have disease of the carotid arteries, this test has proved most valuable. It is a simple, nontraumatic method of detecting cerebrovascular disease. Because false positive and negative results do occur with this test, the results always must be correlated with other clinical investigations.

A new instrument by American Optical Company has been introduced to overcome some of the defects inherent in applying scleral pressure to the globe to cause collapse of the central retinal artery. The Dynopter is used with the slit lamp in a manner similar to that for the applanation tonometer. No ophthalmoscope is required. The eye must be anesthetized because the pressure is applied to the cornea rather than to the sclera, as is done with the older types of instruments. After the eye is anesthetized, the slit beam is used to view the optic disc through the microscope while a contact lens exerts increasing pressure on the cornea. The graded pressure dial is turned until the first pulsation of the central retinal artery is obtained. This is the diastolic pressure. The observer then turns the dial until sufficient pressure is exerted to stop all blood flow. This is the systolic pressure. Readings are then taken and recorded. This method provides a greater degree of accuracy and repeatability than others. It is not pos-

sible, however, to obtain measurements on the recumbent patient.

Doppler test

The Doppler test has virtually replaced the ophthalmodynamometer as a test of carotid flow. The test measures the flow of the internal and external carotid arteries directly. The Doppler is less subject than the ophthalmodynamometer to instrumental and operator errors. If the internal carotid artery of the neck is narrowed by atheromatous plaques, then the flow pattern distal to the obstruction site will be reduced and irregular. The turbulence of flow may be so great that the sound may be audible with a stethoscope placed directly over the internal carotid artery. This sound is called a *bruit*. With transducers in the instrument, however, the precise measurement of flow can provide more accurate information regarding carotid artery patency. This test is used for persons with central retinal artery occlusions, transient ischemia attacks, and cerebrovascular accidents.

Automatic refractors

Sophisticated automatic refractors that, in effect, do retinoscopy and in most cases are designed to be operated by the ophthalmic assistant have been coming on the market. These instruments do not produce a refraction from which a pair of glasses should be made. The present ones do no more than an automatic retinoscopic or objective refraction. It is essential that the results obtained with these machines be refined by a subjective refraction. In a busy office, however, they save a great deal of time.

Some of the errors that occur with automatic refractors include the following.
1. The individual patient can accommodate to the instrument.
2. Reflection over the patient's current glasses can occur.
3. Some autorefractors do not provide vision as an end point; consequently, if there is an error in the printout, the examiner does not know if the measurement is reliable.
4. Peripheral light from the room can affect the reading; thus a dark chamber is required.

In our experience, autorefractors act as an automatic retinoscope and do not provide good subjective refraction. The examiner must place the findings in a phoropter or trial lens case and test the patients subjectively. Autorefractors, however, do provide a reliable starting point in a refraction procedure and for an inexperienced practitioner may be even more reliable than a retinoscope. Many of the newer autorefractors allow subjective refinements on the machine.

See Chapter 11 for a more detailed description of these instruments.

Visual field equipment, tangent screens, and perimeters

See Chapters 16 and 17 on the subject of visual fields.

DIAGNOSTIC ULTRASOUND: A-SCAN AND B-SCAN*

Ultrasound was first used in World War II; the sound waves were employed to locate submarines under water. In a variety of ophthalmic disorders diagnostic ultrasound provides information that cannot be obtained in any other way. This is especially true in eyes with opaque media that preclude ophthalmoscopic examination. Intraocular use will be stressed because space does not permit a detailed description of the somewhat more difficult field of orbital diagnoses.

Ultrasound consists of high-frequency sound waves in the range of 8 to 10 MHz for most ophthalmic equipment. Electrical impulses are converted to sound by a vibrating quartz crystal (transducer). These sound waves are propagated through tissues at varying speeds and are reflected from interfaces between tissues of different acoustic density (a property related to the density of the tissue and the speed at which sound moves through it). After emitting a pulse, the transducer "waits" for the reflected waves to return, strikes the quartz crystal, and initiates the reverse process. The impulses are then electronically modified to produce the familiar A-scan and B-scan displays.

*Portions of this section from Pavlin CJ: *Diagnostic and therapeutic ultrasound, Ophthalmic Surgeon*, Feb 1986.

Two common types of ultrasound waves are used. The A-wave is a single-beam, linear wave that is directed in a probing manner to detect interference along its pathway. It travels like a beam of light in a straight direction. The B-wave is a radiating wave that gives a two-dimensional effect to the echoes that are returned. This not only minimizes possible missed areas but gives a clearer picture of the underlying pathologic condition. The B-waves are used to detect tumors of the orbit or eye that cannot be identified by any other means. The sound waves, like light waves, pass through certain tissues and are reflected by others. When the sound wave meets firm tissue such as would be found in a tumor mass, the waves are reflected off its surface. The rebounding waves are received by a microfilm, which turns the sound energy into electrical impulses that are amplified and displayed on an oscilloscope in a visible wave pattern called an *ultrasonogram* or *echogram* (Fig. 9-40). Homogeneous tissue, such as normal lens vitreous or aqueous humor, does not reflect ultrasound and produces no echoes. A cataractous lens produces intralenticular echoes. In some centers, ultrasound is used to aid the surgeon in locating a foreign body in the eye.

Ultrasonographic diagnosis with use of the B-scan also has been effective in the diagnosis of many ocular tumors, especially choroidal malignant melanomas. Drs. K. Ossoinig and Fred Blodi reported a 95% accuracy using a standard B-scan echogram in a large series of choroidal malignant melanomas.

B-scans differ from A-scans in that they are more complex. An A-scan is a linear echo, and the bounce of this linear ultrasound can indicate the position of the cornea, the lens, and the retina. The B-scan is similar, but it extends above and below the horizontal to sweep the contents of the globe.

A fine transducer probe, utilizing the A-scan, can be attached to slit-lamp or head fixating apparatus and employed to obtain the axial length of the eye. This measurement is used frequently today to determine the power requirement of an intraocular lens for cataract surgery (Fig. 9-41). The axial length measurements along with the keratometer may be directly converted to lens power requirement either

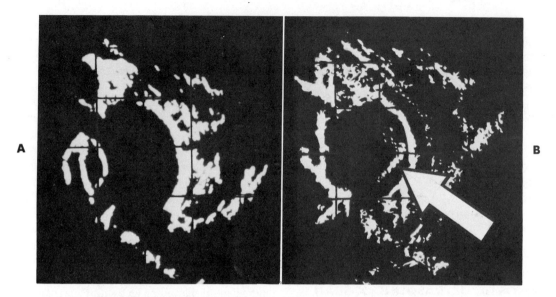

Fig. 9-40 B-Echogram. **A,** Normal. **B,** Showing retinal detachment *(arrow).*

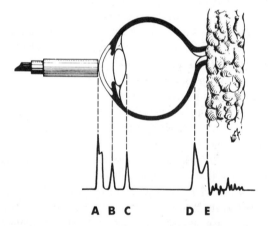

Fig. 9-41 Schematic representation of A-scan ultrasonogram made with transducer tip at left in direct fluid coupling to cornea. Opening deflection (opening bang) is shown at corneal surface, *A*. Reflection from anterior lens capsule is shown at *B* and posterior lens capsule is shown at *C*. The clear lens presents no echoes within its depths. Similarly, the clear vitreous presents no echoes. The posterior bulbar wall complex is represented by *D* and *E*. The retrobulbar fat at far right shows decreasing irregular spikes.

by the machine itself or by using a Texas Instruments calculator.

Ultrasonic echoes at various frequencies from the surfaces of the lesions in the eye and the orbit provide excellent information on the measurement of distance by the one-dimensional echoes of the A-scan or the two-dimensional cross-sectional view of the B-scan. The consistency of a lesion can be determined by the ultrasonographic findings; for example, solid tumors have a well-demarcated surface with much absorption of sound at an internal reflection as contrasted with cystic tumors or inflammatory lesions. C-scan techniques also are available and are used in the diagnosis of orbital disease. The C-scan employs a transducer to cover a small aperture. The C-scan image is soft tissue within the span of a corallar plane that is recorded on Polaroid positive-negative film. The corallar plane scans across the axis of the optic nerve. C-scan techniques are primarily used for optic nerve lesions, especially tumors.

Technique of B-scan

The use of a contact ophthalmic B-scan is best considered as analogous to the use of an ophthalmoscope. Ideally the practitioner has an ultrasound unit in the office and does a scan whenever ophthalmoscopy is difficult or impossible. The B-scan display represents a two-dimensional cross-section through the globe. In a manner much like ophthalmoscopy, the ultrasound beam can be swept through the eye, making correlations along the way and stopping the field on anything of particular interest. With most units an emphasized line on the B display indicates where the A display will be. Switching from one to the other is easily done with a foot pedal.

The most productive ultrasound examination is the one performed by the practitioner. There is a wealth of information obtained at the time of examination that cannot be duplicated by looking at photographs. The three-dimensional correlation of information as the probe is swept through the eye and the appreciation of movement of intraocular structures require the presence of a knowledgeable observer.

Machine settings

Ultrasound machines have a large number of switches and dials, most of which are rarely touched. It is best to determine the settings that produce the best results in the average patient, mark them, and then leave them alone. Most settings, including the magnification of the display, should be left constant to facilitate comparison on future examinations. The only change made during an average examination is to vary the sound intensity, and this is done only to bring out particular features such as the brightness of a foreign body. Leaving the settings constant allows one to turn on the machine and scan with the ease of picking up an ophthalmoscope.

Basic examination

The B-scan probe always has a mark near the end that indicates the top of the oscilloscope display. By convention, this mark is oriented superiorly for vertical scans and nasally for horizontal scans. It is best to hold the probe horizontally or vertically unless there is some reason for an oblique position.

The examination can be done on the open eye or through closed lids. The latter is more convenient for the patient and examiner and allows somewhat greater range of probe movement. The lens produces

considerable sound absorption and should be avoided. The limbal area is easily found through closed lids, with the examiner observing the anterior segment image while scanning.

The optic nerve image is located first. This provides a landmark that aids in determining the position of any pathologic condition. A routine examination of the posterior segment would involve placing the probe at the medial, temporal, superior, and inferior limbus and sweeping the probe through the eye at each of these positions. If any pathologic condition is detected, the probe is placed diametrically opposite. The form, location, and other B-scan features of the abnormality are then delineated. Having the patient move the eye while the examiner holds the probe steady produces valuable information on the mobility of intraocular structures. An A-scan can then be done through the area of greatest interest to further define internal tissue characteristics. Polaroid photos are taken to document these findings.

Water bath

Pathologic conditions in the anterior segment are not well-defined by the contact technique. A water bath allows one to hold the probe further from the eye and greatly improves resolution in this region. A standard operating room plastic drape is attached around the eye, with colloidin used to improve adhesion. The drape is then clipped to a large ring holder. A large chemistry retort holder attached to an intravenous (IV) pole works well for this purpose. A speculum is inserted and the bath filled with saline. The scanning probe is held in the water bath and examination done in the conventional manner.

Office biometry

It is possible to obtain useful information from the office biometry unit. This ability largely depends on the sophistication of the A-scan display. Machines with no display should be avoided; in addition to the lack of diagnostic capabilities, it is impossible to monitor the accuracy of axial length readings. A machine with a classic A-scan display would provide the most information. Between these two are electronic displays of varying merit.

The most common problem encountered in routine

cataract work is the patient with an opaque lens precluding a view of the fundus. While performing a biometry on these patients, one should watch for any indication of abnormal echoes between the lens echo and the echo from the posterior pole. Artifacts can occur, but the presence of any persistent echo in this region should alert the operator to the need for further assessment before surgery. It is a useful habit to sweep the probe through the globe to check for any pathologic condition outside of the axial position. This process is much easier if B-scan capabilities are available.

Ultrasound biomicroscopy

A new form of ultrasound imaging has been developed in Toronto by Drs. Charles J. Pavlin and F. Stuart Foster and colleagues. This technique, *ultrasound biomicroscopy,* is so-named because of similarities to slit-lamp biomicroscopy, that is, the ability to examine living tissue at microscopic resolution. The method uses very high-frequency ultrasound to produce images below the surface of the living eye that are similar to the images that could be obtained by a low-power optical microscope. For the first time, extremely detailed images of various eye structures in their normal living state can be viewed without violating the eye (Fig. 9-42). Resolution exceeds that of conventional eye ultrasound by a factor of approximately 10. Measurement of various ocular structures can be made with greatly increased accuracy. The examination is performed in a fluid bath in a small eyecup. Examination takes approximately 15 minutes and is of minimal discomfort to the patient.

This technique opens the door to a new way of studying eye diseases such as glaucoma and tumors. Many types of glaucoma have a structural abnormality as the cause. This is especially true of angle-closure and congenital glaucoma. For example, ultrasound biomicroscopy has already proved that the cause of plateau iris syndrome is anteriorly placed ciliary processes that prevent the iris from falling back, which results in continuing angle closure after treatment with laser iridectomy. Ultrasound biomicroscopy also has been shown to be helpful in dealing with anterior segment tumors. This method can im-

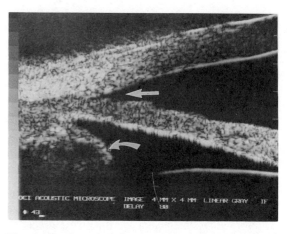

Fig. 9-42 Cross-section of normal anterior segment of eye as imaged by ultrasound biomicroscopy. Details of the angle between the cornea and iris can be seen *(straight arrow).* The ciliary processes *(curved arrow)* and their relationship to the iris are also shown. (From Pavlin CJ, Harasiewicz K, Foster FS: Ultrasound biomicroscopy of anterior segment structures in normal and glaucomatous eye, *Am J Ophthalmol* 113:381, 1992.)

age extremely small tumors, differentiate cysts from solid tumors, and define the depth to which these tumors have invaded. Many other types of eye diseases currently are being examined by this new imaging method.

RADIOACTIVE PHOSPHORUS

One test to detect whether an ocular or retroocular tumor is benign or malignant is determination of the radioactive uptake of the tissues. It is known that cancerous tissues proliferate rapidly. Certain highly malignant tumors (especially malignant melanomas) take up and retain certain radioactive elements, particularly ^{32}P (radioactive phosphorus), to a greater extent than do normal tissues. In this test the ^{32}P is injected intravenously, and the radioactivity is assessed on the surface of the eye by a Geiger counter 24 and 48 hours after the injection. The major difficulty in this test is that the counter has to be directly over the tumor. With tumors at the back of the eye it is difficult to accurately place the tip of the counter. In addition to this mechanical difficulty, some tumors simply do not give a high count. Other tumors such as retinoblastoma, the most common eye tumor in children, rarely show any alteration in the radio-active uptake of ^{32}P.

A positive ^{32}P test result, then, is of value in providing corroboration for the presence of an actively growing malignant tumor, but a negative result is of little value because it does not indicate the absence of a tumor.

ELECTRORETINOGRAPHY

Electroretinography (ERG) responses are described as photopic (light-adapted) or scotopic (dark-adapted). Although the rods outnumber the cones 13 to 1 in the normal human retina, the cones account for 20% to 25% of the ERG response amplitude. The response of the dark-adapted eye to white light breaks down to an early corneal negative A-wave, a corneal positive B-wave, a slower, usually positive C-wave, and in some mammals a small D-wave. The resting potential of the normal retinal axis is measured by a silver disc electrode mounted in a scleral contact lens.

An electrical potential exists between the cornea and the retina of the human eye. This potential can be altered by changes in the intensity of light entering the eye, the wavelength of that light, and the state of adaptation of the eye, that is, whether it is light-adapted or dark-adapted. In some disease states the resting potential is altered, and the ability of the electrical potential to be changed by these other factors is abnormal.

There are basically two types of retinal receptors: the rods that serve vision in dim light and the cones that mediate daylight vision and color vision. The electroretinogram will reveal disease of either the rod population or the cone population, or both.

For this test, electrodes incorporated into a contact glass are placed directly on the eye. Eye movements disrupt the values of the test, so the patient must be old enough to fixate on a target, which keeps the eyes still. Because they are unable to cooperate, very young children do not make good subjects for this test.

Total loss of electrical activity can be recorded in siderosis bulbi (caused by retained iron foreign bodies in the eye), in stages of retinitis pigmentosa, and in severe vitamin A deficiency. Selective de-generation of the rods, as manifested by night blindness, also can be detected by this method because the electrical reaction during dark adaptation would be faulty. Selective involvement of the cone, as seen in congenital total color blindness, also would be revealed by the inability of the eye to electrically respond during conditions of light adaptation.

The electroretinogram generally is performed in university centers. Expert technical knowledge is required to perform the test and to interpret its results.

LASERS

The laser, covered more completely in Chapter 29, is a device that amplifies light waves. The name itself is taken from the beginning letters of *l*ight *a*mplification by *s*timulated *e*mission of *r*adiation. Intense beams of light have many practical implications, but in the eye their virtue is that the laser beam may be directed through the pupil to the retinal structures for the repair of retinal holes and tears and for the destruction of blood vessels. The ruby laser emits a beam that creates a heat reaction in the pigment epithelium of the retina, binding the epithelium of the retina to the underlying choroid; it also aids the sealing of retinal holes in curing a retinal detachment when the retina is adjacent to the choroid. The blue-green light of the argon laser is superior to the red light of the ruby laser in treating certain eye blood vessel diseases because it is absorbed by the red blood pigment, which resists the red light of the ruby laser. The argon treatment is a feature in diabetic retinopathy and in such other retinal ills as Eales' disease, in which vessels grow abnormally and bleed easily; in sickle cell anemia, which produces sludging of blood in peripheral eye vessels; and in several congenital vascular conditions that cause blindness.

It has been well established that argon or neodymium YAG laser treatment is a good alternative to the surgery of a peripheral iridectomy in producing a hole in the iris. The former is painless and causes minimal inflammation, which normally is handled by application of steroid drops for about a week. It is most useful in treating angle-closure glaucoma or aphakic pupillary block glaucoma or in opening an incomplete surgical iridectomy. The Abraham iridectomy lens, a modified Goldmann type of fundus lens, may be valuable in the delivery of a more intense laser beam to the iris. Blue eyes are more difficult to penetrate than brown eyes because of the lack of the heat-absorbing pigment in blue irides. Trabeculoplasty involves using the laser for shrinkage of the trabeculum.

The excimer laser is being developed for two specific uses. One, it will enhance vision so that combined myopia and astigmatism, or hyperopia, can be eliminated or refractive errors can be significantly reduced. Second, it has significant use in removing corneal scars, clearing corneal infections, and smoothing out corneal surfaces after surgery for conditions such as pterygium. The influence on refractive errors is more thoroughly discussed in Chapter 31.

SUMMARY

The ophthalmic assistant should become knowledgeable about the workings of each instrument in the office. It is important to keep the instruments clean and all lenses free of dust and grease by using a lint-free cloth. The ophthalmic assistant should be able to change bulbs in every instrument inasmuch as the use of the instrument depends on a functioning bulb and an intact power supply. An active inventory of the replacement bulbs in the office should be kept so that bulbs always are available. Another area of expertise that should be developed is calibration of the tonometers. In addition, the ophthalmic assistant should know the purposes of each piece of equipment and what information can be derived from its use.

QUESTIONS FOR REVIEW AND THOUGHT

1. What is the purpose of the red-green test on the projection equipment? Explain the test.
2. Discuss the power and range of the various types of lenses and auxiliary lenses on the lens tray that you are familiar with.
3. How can you tell the power of a prism in the standard lens tray?
4. How can you differentiate a cylindric lens from a spherical lens in the lens tray?
5. What is the purpose of the pinhole disk?
6. What is meant by a retinoscopy lens in a standard refractor? What is its power? Why?
7. What is the difference between phoria and tropia? What instrument is used in detecting these conditions, and how?
8. Explain the principle of either the spot or the streak retinoscope.
9. What is meant by vertex distance? How is it measured in a trial frame? In spectacle? In a refractor?
10. What are the prisms used for?
11. What is the prism cover test?
12. Discuss the relative merits of direct and indirect ophthalmoscopy.
13. What is the purpose of a goniolens?
14. Draw the end points of the two half circles from the applanation tonometer as seen when a true reading of the intraocular pressure is to be obtained.
15. What is the value of the ophthalmodynamometer? What does it measure?
16. How can you determine whether a lens is concave or convex without using instruments?
17. What is the exophthalmometer? Describe how either the Luedde or the Hertel exophthalmometer is used.
18. How is ultrasound of value in ophthalmology?

SELF-EVALUATION QUESTIONS

True-false statements

Directions: Indicate whether the statement is true (T) or false (F).

T or F   1. In the duochrome test, a nearsighted person sees the letters more clearly on the red panel.

T or F   2. Trial frames and lenses are better than the Phoroptor in determining the refractive status of the aphakic person.

T or F   3. The Maddox rod is used to dissociate the eyes and prevent them from fusing.

Missing words

Directions: Write in the missing word in the following sentences.

4. The radius of curvature of any lens can simply be measured by using a _____.

5. Phenylephrine is an excellent mydriatic for dilating pupils. The best concentration of this drug is _____.

6. The optic disc is best examined with _____.

Choice-completion questions

Directions: Select the one best answer in each case.

7. If the media are opaque, which of the following tests can be employed to determine if an intraocular tumor is present?
   a. Transillumination
   b. Ultrasound—A- or B-scan
   c. ^{32}P
   d. All of the above
   e. None of the above

8. The Hruby lens is:
   a. A -55-diopter lens
   b. A jeweler's loupe
   c. A lens for detecting the intraocular pressure
   d. A lens for viewing Schlemm's canal
   e. None of the above

9. The corneal thickness can be best measured with:
   a. A specular microscope
   b. A slit lamp
   c. A pachymeter
   d. A goniolens
   e. None of the above

ANSWERS, NOTES, AND EXPLANATIONS

1. **True.** Green normally is focused in front of the retina because of its short wavelength. Therefore a nearsighted person whose entire image is focused in front of the retina would see letters on the red side of the chart more clearly. Red has a longer wavelength and would be seen more clearly by the larger eye of the myopic person. The person whose nearsightedness has been overcorrected, however, will see the green letters more clearly. The duochrome test is useful in determining the type and end point of the refractive error.

2. **True.** It is useful that the correcting lenses and spectacle lens the aphakic patient finally wears are similar with respect to the distance of the lens from the eye and its tilt. With four-drop lenses, trial aphakic spectacles are provided so that margin of error is minimized. Even without minimal effective diameter (MED) lenses or four-drop lenses, trial frames are still the best way of arriving at the aphakic person's final prescription inasmuch as the measurement for vertex distance is more reliable.

   The Halberg clip is an excellent method for determining the true spectacle correction.

3. **True.** This is done by changing the shape and color of the image of one eye. The rod converts a point of light to a linear rod by virtue of cylindric rods that run across it. The red line always runs perpendicular to the axes of the Maddox rod.

4. **Geneva lens measure.** The disadvantage of this instrument is that the gauges are calibrated for crown glass only. Moreover, the axis of the cylinder is not precisely determined.

5. **2.5%.** Recently, deaths have been reported with the use of 10% phenylephrine. It should not be used for routine dilation. The weaker solution should be used routinely. Phenylephrine should not be given to persons with hypertension or to those with active cardiovascular disease. When it is given, care should be taken to occlude the punctum so that minimal drainage into the nose and minimal systemic absorption occur.

6. **The direct ophthalmoscope.** The direct ophthalmoscope permits greater magnification so that the fine details of cupping of the disc are easily observed with this instrument.

   The indirect ophthalmoscope offers a wider field of vision, but it is not as good for examining disc detail such as mild cupping, slight pallor, pits or holes, and the growth of delicate new blood vessels off its surface.

7. **d. All of the above.** Probably the most widely used test for an intraocular mass when the media is too cloudy to permit direct examination is the B-scan ultrasound. It is precise, easy to perform, and painless. Permanent records can be obtained. The location and type of retrolental mass often can be detected with this method.

8. **a. A −55-diopter lens.** The Hruby lens is a −55-diopter lens for viewing the fundus. It is not as good as a fundus contact lens, but it has the advantage that the retina can be examined without placing an instrument on the eye.

9. **c. A pachymeter.** Many slit lamps have attachments to measure the thickness of the cornea and the anterior chamber depth. The pachometer has two models, each designed to measure either the depth of the anterior chamber or the thickness of the cornea.

   Corneal thickness is important to detect minimal corneal edema in surgical cases of cataracts, grafts, and corneal disease and in doing contact lens work. For instance, patients with keratoconus reveal a progressive thinning of the cornea.

   Anterior chamber thickness is used to decide the type of intraocular implant to be employed in cataract surgical cases, in research work, and in some postsurgical follow-ups such as after glaucoma surgery.

CHAPTER 10 Refractive errors and how to correct them

- Emmetropia
- Ametropia
- Refractometry and refraction
- Retinoscopy
- Subjective refining
- Anisometropia
- Aphakia
- When to refract after cataract surgery
- Presbyopia
- Complaints: how to anticipate them
- Glasses checks and how to handle them

Almost all patients who enter an ophthalmologist's office require a determination of the refractive status of their eyes, either for diagnosis or treatment. Only by correcting the patient's refractive error can the ophthalmologist distinguish between visual loss caused by organic disease and that caused by a refractive error. Visual loss not amenable to correction by lenses is regarded as a pathologic condition. Unexplained visual loss not corrected by glasses must always be investigated.

Many patients, regardless of their problem—be it fatigue with driving or headache—expect to receive a pair of glasses to remedy their complaints. Some patients are methodic about having their glasses changed every year or every 2 years; they believe that glasses, like tires, will wear out after a period of time. Others think that glasses have a therapeutic effect on the eyes, maintaining them in good performance and preserving their integrity. Vision, especially in younger persons and the presbyopic

patient, may deteriorate with time, necessitating a change in correction, but the health of the eye is not affected, for better or worse, regardless of changes made in the glasses. There is some evidence, however, that in the young, plus correction may prevent the normal loss of hyperopia, and minus correction may exacerbate the development of myopia.

Glasses function to improve visual performance, to relieve the symptoms of refractive errors and muscular imbalance of the eyes, and to prevent suppression of one eye in children younger than the age of 5 years, when the refractive difference between the two eyes is great. This chapter deals with the signs and symptoms of refractive errors and the therapy available for their treatment.

EMMETROPIA

The emmetropic eye is a normal eye in which the rays of light from a distantly fixated object are imaged sharply on the retina without the necessity of

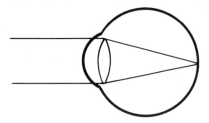

Fig. 10-1 Emmetropic eye. Parallel rays of light come to a focus on the retina.

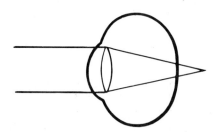

Fig. 10-2 Hyperopic eye. Parallel rays of light come to a focus behind the retina in the unaccommodative eye.

any accommodative effort. This is a relatively uncommon condition (Fig. 10-1).

AMETROPIA

There are three basic abnormalities in the refractive state of the eye: (1) hyperopia, or hypermetropia, (2) myopia, and (3) astigmatism.

Hyperopia

The hyperopic, or farsighted, eye is one that is deficient in refractive power so that rays of light from a distant object come to a focus at a point behind the retina with respect to the unaccommodated eye (Fig. 10-2). Consequently, the image that falls on the retina is blurred and can be brought into focus only by accommodation or by placing a plus, or convex, lens in front of the eye. The convex lens supplies the converging power that the eye is lacking.

Cause. In most cases of hyperopia, the chief cause is a shortening of the anteroposterior axis of the eye. Such an eye is smaller than the normal, or emmetropic, eye. At birth almost all human eyes are hy-

peropic to the extent of 2.00 or 3.00 diopters. With growth, the eye lengthens and approaches the normal length of an adult eye. Each millimeter of shortening of the eye is represented by 3.00 diopters of refractive change. This shortening of the globe results in *axial hyperopia*.

Another cause of hyperopia is found when the front surface of the eye (the cornea, or lens) has less curvature than normal so that the image formed is focused at a point behind the normally placed retina. This is called *curvature hyperopia*.

Types. From a practical standpoint, the cause of the hyperopia is not of great importance. What is significant is whether the accommodative system of the eye can supply an additional plus power to correct the hyperopic error. Young people are usually not handicapped by hyperopia because of their excellent range of accommodation.

Hyperopia may be latent, manifest, or absolute. A *latent hyperopia* is the portion of the hyperopic error that is completely corrected by the eye's own accommodation. The compensation is so complete that any attempt to place a plus lens in front of such an eye will merely blur the vision. *Manifest hyperopia* (facultative hyperopia) is the element of the refractive error that can be corrected either by convex lenses or by the patient's own accommodation. In both latent and manifest hyperopia the *patient has normal visual acuity* (Fig. 10-3). *Absolute hyperopia* is the portion of the refractive error that is not compensated for by accommodation (Fig. 10-4).

To understand the three types, consider the following case. A young man, 32 years of age, is found to have a visual acuity of 20/50. A +1.00 lens is given, which improves his vision to 20/20. This means that the patient has 1.00 diopter of absolute hyperopia. It is found, however, that the patient can still see 20/20 if an additional 1.50 diopters are placed before the absolute correction. Thus the patient is found to have 1.50 diopters of manifest hyperopia. A cycloplegic examination is performed, and it is found that the patient requires 3.50 diopters of plus lenses to enable him to see 20/20. Of the 3.50 diopters, 1.00 diopter we know has been accounted for in the form of *absolute hyperopia*, 1.50 diopters were present as *manifest hyperopia*, and 1.00 diopter remains in the form of *latent hyperopia*.

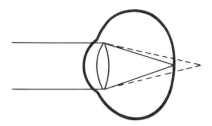

Fig. 10-3 Manifest hyperopia. Accommodation by the lens of the eye brings parallel rays of light to focus on the retina.

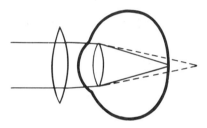

Fig. 10-4 Absolute hyperopia. A convex lens is required to bring rays of light to focus on the retina.

Such a patient requires 1.00 diopter, will accept up to 2.50 diopters, but cannot be given the full hyperopic correction of 3.50 diopters.

Role of cycloplegia. Cycloplegic drops paralyze accommodation and thereby prevent the accommodative effort required to compensate for hyperopia. Therefore, under cycloplegic examination all of the hyperopia is uncovered. Full correction of hyperopic errors, however, can never be based on cycloplegic findings, because correction of the latent factor will only blur distance vision. The findings may be unreliable, however, in the management of accommodating esotropics. Cycloplegic examination indicates the magnitude of the refractive error. Noncycloplegic examination reveals the acceptability of a particular correction.

Symptoms. In the young the condition may cause no symptoms, because a healthy youngster has an ample reserve of accommodation and if hyperopic, accommodates for distant and near objects without being conscious of the act. Thus a 5-year-old may have 4.00 diopters of hyperopia and not require any spectacle correction whatsoever. It is usually in older persons that the symptoms of hyperopia become apparent, as educational demands and the time allotted for close work increase (Fig. 10-5). The symptoms

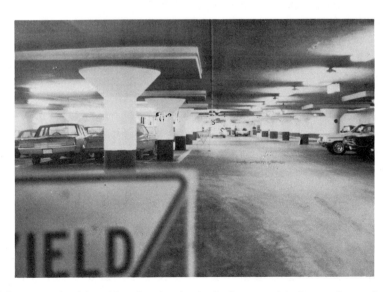

Fig. 10-5 Hyperopic vision. Note that the sign in the foreground is fuzzy, whereas the distance is clear.

of eyestrain are many and varied. They include headaches, burning of the eyes, and a pulling sensation of the eyes. These symptoms generally are related to the constant excessive accommodation that is required for close work. In older patients no symptoms may appear until the power of accommodation has diminished to the extent that the near point is beyond the range of comfortable reading distance so that close work has to be held farther away than usual to be seen clearly. The greater the degree of hyperopia, the sooner this symptom will arise; therefore, presbyopia commences at an earlier age than usual in the uncorrected hyperopic eye.

Treatment. The treatment of hyperopia is based on the patient's symptoms, occupation, and ability to compensate for close work. In the very young the treatment of hyperopia is usually unnecessary. The only exception to this rule occurs with accommodative strabismus. In this condition part or all of the strabismus may be corrected by the use of convex lenses, which decrease the need for accommodation and thus for the associated excessive convergence.

In older persons hyperopia always is corrected to improve near vision. Some believe the facultative component is never fully corrected unless the patient complains of fatigue and headaches. Whereas a 5-year-old child may be oblivious to 4.00 to 5.00 diopters of hyperopia, a young college student may be very distressed by the presence of even 1.00 diopter of hyperopia. Such a patient needs to wear glasses only when the demands on accommodation are the greatest, that is, for performing close work. Some ophthalmologists, however, believe that the facultative component should be fully corrected.

In the middle-aged person, reading glasses become a necessity. The decline in accommodative power becomes so great that the patient is totally unable to see at a comfortable reading distance without convex lenses. Moreover, the power of the lenses exceeds the absolute and facultative demands of the hyperopia, so that the patient can see comfortably with reading glasses for close work, but the vision is totally blurred when these lenses are used for distance vision.

Older persons, particularly those between 55 and

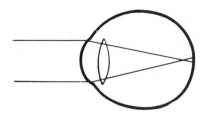

Fig. 10-6 Myopic eye. Parallel rays of light are brought to a focus in front of the retina.

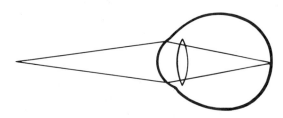

Fig. 10-7 The myope can see clearly out to his or her fixed far point in front of the eye.

65 years of age, find it difficult to accommodate even 1.00 diopter. This type of hyperopic patient usually needs convex lenses for both distance vision and close work.

Myopia

Myopia, or nearsightedness, is that condition in which parallel rays of light come to focus at a point just in front of the retina with respect to the unaccommodated eye (Fig. 10-6). The myopic eye has basically too much plus power for its size. The myope has a fixed far point in space. For example, a person with 1.00-diopter myopia can see an object clearly if it is 1 meter from the eye (Fig. 10-7).

Types. In *axial myopia* the eyeball is too long for the normal refractive power of the lens and the cornea. Parallel rays of light are brought to a converging point usually somewhere in the vitreous in front of the retina. This type of eye is larger than normal.

In *curvature myopia* the eye is of normal size, but the curvatures of the cornea and lens are increased.

Index myopia is a result of a change in the index of refraction of the lens. This is witnessed in two pathologic states, diabetes and cataract. In diabetes the lens loses water because of the high level of blood sugar in the anterior chamber, and therefore its index of refraction increases. In the cataract patient, the lens becomes increasingly hard because of the constant lamination of lens fibers being pushed to the center of the lens. The hard inner core increases the index of refraction of the entire lens structure, thereby increasing the converging power.

Cause. Almost everything has been blamed as a cause of myopia: diet, obesity, allergy, lighting conditions, vitamin deficiencies, and even wearing glasses too much or too little. Controversy and heated debate have raged about whether excessive close work or reading is a primary cause of myopia.

A great deal of research and clinical investigation have been carried out in trying to understand the development of myopia. The results, however, have been inconclusive.

In the great majority of cases the nearsighted eye is longer than the normal eye. Just as some people are tall and some are short, so some people are farsighted and some are nearsighted. The nearsighted eye has grown longer than normal.

Most authorities agree that some myopia is familial in nature and is passed from one generation to another as a dominant trait. In fact, it is uncommon to find a myope whose parents or siblings do not have a similar condition.

In the past the causes of myopia were a subject of heated debate, and its treatment often was based on speculative theories. One school of thought held that myopia was due to an excessive accommodative effort. In this regard children often were given bifocals to prevent them from using their own accommodation to see objects at near. Often there were limitations placed on them at school, and the child was allowed to use the eyes for homework only for a period not exceeding 1 hour. A variation of this line of thinking led to the undercorrection of myopia. Because these children could never see adequately at a distance, they would not use their accommodation. It was believed that not making an effort at accommodation would prevent the progress of the myopia. Another group believed that myopia was

caused not by excessive accommodation but by a lack of it. The contention was that a myope has to make less of an accommodative effort at near than an emmetrope or a hyperope. Therefore, to increase the circulation to the ciliary muscle and improve the health of the eye, this group advocated overcorrecting the myopia so that the individual would have to accommodate more than necessary. Another prevalent speculation was that myopia was a result of a vitamin deficiency, especially during the growing years. To cope with this deficiency calcium and vitamin D were prescribed during the active growth period, especially during adolescence, when myopia was thought to increase the most. One group believed that myopia was related to improper lighting conditions while children were reading. With this in mind many parents became alarmed if they discovered their children reading in bed during the twilight hours and using only the available light.

Recently, surgery has become popular as a way of treating myopia (See Chapter 31). With the higher degrees of myopia, removal of the lens has been advocated as a way of countering myopic effects. Some of these patients were treated by replacing the lenses of their eyes with artificial ones, a practice in vogue in the 1950s and no longer considered justifiable. Other operations for the relief of high myopia included shortening the eyeball or flattening a central portion of the cornea.

The overwork theory of accommodation excess in myopia has been recently resurrected. It has been shown that some groups of students seem to have a higher incidence of progression of their myopia than do individuals who leave school at an early age and who do not do any close work. Furthermore, some doctors are now treating myopia by placing some atropine or homatropine drops into myopic eyes to relax the ciliary muscle.

Progress. Myopia is rare at birth. It usually manifests after the fourth year of life. Its progression is relatively constant until the time of puberty. At that time the myopia may change alarmingly and progress rapidly, requiring changes of glasses every 6 months. Normally the myopia becomes arrested when full maturity is reached. Therefore the ages between 20

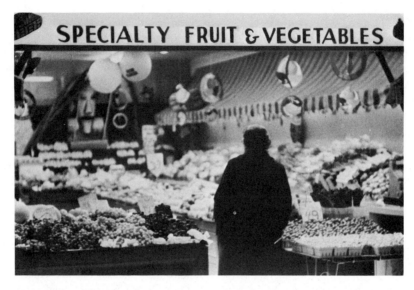

Fig. 10-8 Myopia. Note the clarity of the foreground and the haziness of the background.

and 40 years are relatively quiet, and the myope's correction may remain virtually unchanged during this period.

Symptoms. The most outstanding symptom of myopia is inability to see objects clearly at a distance. Near vision is always good (Fig. 10-8). Myopic children often regard this as the natural order of life—objects in the distance are fuzzy, whereas those at close range are clear. In many cases the myope is not detected until the school runs a visual screening program. Older children often learn of their condition when they discover that classmates sitting beside them can see the blackboard with ease, whereas they see it only with difficulty.

The antics of the nearsighted movie cartoon character Mr. Magoo are well-known. The humorous episodes in which Magoo mistakes a gorilla for his wife make us laugh, but they also make us aware of the danger and menace that a nearsighted person can be to society. Just imagine what a hazard Magoo would be on today's highways!

Many myopic children have a tendency to squeeze their lids around their eyes to create the effect of a pinhole camera. This is one expedient the myope uses to obtain better vision in the distance. The con-

stant squeezing of the lids, however, may lead to headaches and general eyestrain.

Progressive myopia. Occasionally myopia develops in early childhood and reaches alarming degrees. Children younger than the age of 10 years who have myopia of −6.00 diopters or more often develop secondary visual complications because of the elongation of the eyeball and a thinning of the sclera (Fig. 10-9). These complications, such as seeing spots before the eyes because of vitreous degeneration, may be relatively harmless. Others, such as retinal degeneration and detachment and macular hemorrhage, may be more serious. Invariably, all myopia over 10.00 diopters in magnitude is axial, that is, associated with an elongated eyeball. Because of these complications, the myope in particular should be examined yearly, not only for alteration of the spectacle correction but also for a thorough retinal examination.

Treatment. Myopia should be fully corrected at all times so that the person can enjoy comfortable and clear distance vision (Fig. 10-10). Some ophthalmologists, however, believe that myopia should be undercorrected and that the myope should read without glasses. They believe this prevents a

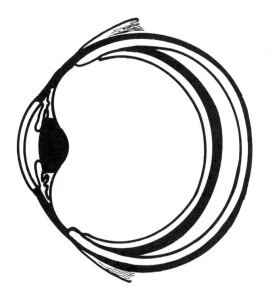

Fig. 10-9 Progressive myopia resulting in a longer eye with thinning of the sclera.

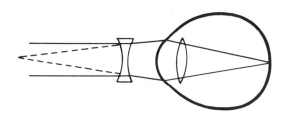

Fig. 10-10 Myopic eye. A concave lens brings parallel rays of light to a focus on the retina.

further increase in myopia. The full correction, however, enables the myope to establish a normal relationship between accommodation and convergence. Myopic children require no special inducements to wear their glasses. These children, on receiving their glasses, soon learn to enjoy the sharp, clean edges of clear vision and will reach for their glasses the first thing on arising in the morning.

Moreover, myopes are among the most conscientious regarding reappointments. Although they do not initially recognize their own visual defect, once they receive glasses, they become acutely aware of the progress of their myopia and changes in the clarity of things.

Persons with myopia of high magnitude, such as −4.00 diopters or greater, are slightly handicapped by the fact that their image size is smaller. A high myopic lens placed at a distance from the eye has a minifying effect. This effect may be offset by the use of contact lenses. Not only is the image size more normal with contact lenses but also the aberrations of the thick lens are eliminated and the field is enlarged. The use of contact lenses in high myopia—that is, −10.00 diopters or greater—is especially recommended, because in these ranges secondary disadvantages of spectacle correction are great.

Astigmatism

Astigmatism is the condition in which rays of light are not refracted equally in all directions, so that a point focus on the retina is not attained.

Types

Regular astigmatism. Regular astigmatism is that refractive condition which is amenable to correction by cylinders. The axes of the principal meridians of the astigmatism are at right angles to each other. If the axis of the astigmatism deviates from either horizontal or vertical meridians, generally the deviation is symmetric in the two eyes.

Regular astigmatism may be subdivided into the following groups.

In *simple astigmatism* one of the focal lines always falls on the retina; that is, one meridian is emmetropic. The other meridian may have its focus behind the retina or in front of the retina. The condition then is referred to either as *simple hyperopic* or as *simple myopic astigmatism,* respectively (Fig. 10-11, *A* and *B*).

In *compound astigmatism* the rays of light are refracted so that both focal points lie either in front of the retina or behind it. The former is referred to as *compound myopic astigmatism* and the latter as *compound hyperopic astigmatism* (Fig. 10-11, *C* and *D*).

In *mixed astigmatism* one focal point lies behind the retina, whereas the other focal point lies in front of it (Fig. 10-11, *E*).

Irregular astigmatism. If the cornea has been damaged by trauma, inflammation, scar tissue, or develop-

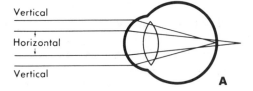

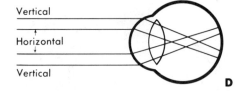

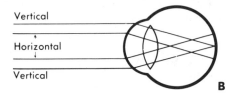

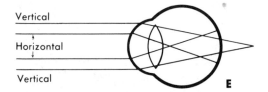

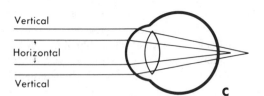

Fig. 10-11 A, Simple hyperopic astigmatism. The vertical bundle of rays is focused on the retina; the horizontal rays are focused behind the retina. **B,** Simple myopic astigmatism. The vertical bundle of rays is focused on the retina; the horizontal rays are focused in front of the retina. **C,** Compound hyperopic astigmatism. Both focal points fall behind the retina. **D,** Compound myopic astigmatism. Both focal points lie in front of the retina. **E,** Mixed astigmatism. The vertical rays come to a focus behind the retina; the horizontal rays focus in front of the retina.

mental anomalies so that a geometric form is not adhered to, the resultant condition is called *irregular astigmatism*. In view of the irregularity of the corneal surface and the lack of any geometric form, this condition usually cannot be completely corrected by cylinders.

Cause. In most instances astigmatism results because the radius of curvature of the cornea is not equal in all directions. Although at birth the cornea usually is a perfect sphere, by the age of 4 years it loses its spherical qualities. The horizontal axis (vertical radius) of the cornea becomes more steeply inclined so that rays of light are refracted more acutely than those rays being refracted along the vertical axis of the cornea. This type of astigmatism commonly is referred to as *with the rule* astigmatism. The astigmatism in which the vertical axis (horizontal radius) of the cornea is stronger than the horizontal one is referred to as *against the rule* astig-

matism. In the formative years astigmatism may alter in small increments, but its axis usually remains relatively unchanged.

Although astigmatism most commonly results from a cornea that is not spherical, in some instances the astigmatism may be the result of an unequal bending of light by the crystalline lens, the so-called *lenticular* astigmatism.

Problems of astigmatic persons. Because neither the horizontal nor the vertical axis forms a point focus, the person with an astigmatic condition usually chooses the more normal, or emmetropic, axis for seeing. If the two axes are equally in focus, then the vertical focal line is, as a rule, preferentially chosen. The object being viewed will appear somewhat indistinct.

Consider an individual with an astigmatic problem in which the vertical axis is focused on the retina and the object of regard is a cross. Each point of the

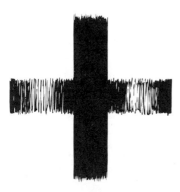

Fig. 10-12 Distortions of points of light are in a vertical direction. The horizontal band is fuzzy except at the end; the vertical band is sharp except at the end.

cross that is imaged on the retina will be elongated in a vertical direction. The horizontal line therefore appears as a series of short vertical lines, which elongate into a broad, blurred band; in the vertical line, the vertical strokes are superimposed and cover each other so that the whole line appears sharply defined and black, with only the uppermost and lowermost of the vertical lines having a vertical, brush-like appearance (Fig. 10-12).

Obviously the most common complaint of the patient with astigmatism is inability to see at both distance and near, whereas the hyperopic person normally can see efficiently at a distance, and the myope sees quite adequately at near.

As with other refractive errors, the astigmatic patient employs many compensatory movements to improve vision. There may be a tendency to half close the lids to make a horizontal slit between the lids and cut off the rays in one meridian. Reading matter may be held very close to the eyes to obtain a large, even though blurred, retinal image.

REFRACTOMETRY AND REFRACTION

Refractometry is defined as the measurement of refractive error, and it should not be confused with the term *refraction*. Refraction is defined as the sum of steps performed in arriving at a decision as to what lens or lenses (if any) will most benefit the patient. These steps include, in addition to refractometry, measurement of visual acuity, measurement of ac-

commodative ability, and the exercise of clinical judgment. Refraction, often referred to as an art, generally is considered to require a license for its practice and constitutes a major activity of ophthalmology and optometry.

Refractometry, on the other hand, is strictly limited to clinical application of optical principles. This measurement function can be performed at the highest level of precision by technicians and, in some cases, even by sophisticated instruments and computers.

The exercise of clinical judgment included in the foregoing definition of refraction refers to a consideration of such factors as the patient's occupational requirements, muscle balance, impairment of vision by other than refractive error (such as cataract, macular degeneration, or suppression amblyopia), the extent and type of refractive error present, and even the emotional "set" of the patient with respect to wearing glasses. (For some patients, even though there may be a significant error, the maximum benefit will be achieved by prescribing no lenses at all.) Refractometry may be classified several different ways: preliminary versus refining, objective versus subjective, and cylinder versus sphere. These classifications are integrated in Table 10-1.

Methods of refractometry

For convenience, refractometric methods will be considered here under two headings: objective and subjective. Objective methods provide the advantage of permitting measurements to be made without re-

Table 10-1 Classifications of refractometry

	Sphere	Cylinder
Preliminary		
Objective (retinoscope and objective separators)	Approximate	Approximate
Subjective (dials and cylinders)	—	Precise
Refining		
Subjective (cross cylinder)	—	Precise
Subjective (duochrome)	Precise	Precise

Table 10-2 Drops used in refraction

Drug	Onset of maximum cyclophegia	Duration of activity	Comment
Atropine sulfate 1%	6-24 hr	10-15 days especially in a blue-eyed child	Not used routinely except for the assessment of accommodative strabismus in children
Scopolamine hydrobromide ¼%	30-60 min	3-4 days	Used in patients allergic to atropine
Homatropine hydrobromide 1.25% to 5%	1 hr	1-2 days	Requires an hour to take effect and last 2 days; not used routinely
Cyclopentolate hydrochloride 1% (Cyclogyl)	10-45 min	12-24 hr	Is active in 20-45 min; two sets of drops given 5 minutes apart—a good rapid-acting cycloplegic for office use
Tropicamide (Mydriacyl) 0.5%	20-30 min	4-10 hr	A good drug for office use with an effect similar to Cyclogyl

quiring the patient to give answers; adequate measurements can be made in patients who are unable or unwilling to answer questions but who will cooperate to the extent of fixating a distant target. The disadvantages of objective methods are that they require a moderate-sized or dilated pupil, and they cannot be relied on to provide data sufficiently accurate to provide the basis of a prescription. The advantages of subjective methods are that they can be performed even when the pupil is very small, and they provide data that are much more precise and reliable; their use, however, is limited by the amount of patient judgment and participation required.

Steps for refractometry

At the beginning of any refraction, a decision must be made about whether to use drops and, if so, what drops to employ (Table 10-2).

Cycloplegic drops. Most refractionists would use cycloplegic drops on anyone up to the age of 20 years. The drops impair the power of accommodation by inhibiting the ciliary muscle. They also dilate the pupil. Thus the drops have two basic functions.

1. They arrest accommodation or focusing, which in a young person with a powerful accom-

modative ability may not be achieved any other way.
2. They dilate the pupil to make a retinal examination more complete by exposing a greater part of the peripheral retina.

The drawback to drops is that adult patients who drive to the examination have to return home with blurred vision, photophobia, and fear.

Systemic absorption of the drugs in Table 10-2 can cause a toxic reaction. For instance, atropine can cause a fast pulse, a fever, and a skin rash. To minimize the systemic absorption of these drops, pressure should be exerted with a cotton ball or tissue held over the tear sac for a minute after the drop is instilled into the eye.

The next step in the process of refraction is to check the old glasses for power and optical centration. Frequently the refractionist will use this information as a basis for refinement of the prescription or for the overrefraction.

Lensmeter. A lensmeter records the optical center of the lens, its power, and the axis of the correcting cylinder, including its power. The newer lensmeters are fully automated and digitalized. These basic mechanical lensmeters are accurate but require some technical expertise. Details are presented in Chapter 8.

Notation of the axis of the cylinder must be precise inasmuch as a patient will not tolerate a large deviation from his or her old prescription, especially in high degrees of astigmatism.

RETINOSCOPY

The retinoscope is the most useful instrumen[t] refractionist's armamentarium. Retinoscopy chief objective method of determining the ref error of an eye. (See Fig. 9-5). It is the on to assess the refractive error in children, illit people who speak a different language from t aminer's, and persons who are too confused, or ill to add a precise subjective component total refraction.

The retinoscope has a viewing system and luminating system. The viewing system consi a small aperture at the head of the retinoscop enables the examiner to see. The illuminating sy shines diverging rays of light into the patient's This light enters the patient's eye and is refl back again as a reflex in the patient's pupil. reflex appears as a red-orange glow with a s shadow around it. The vergence of the rays of that leave the patient's eye depends on the refra error of that patient. In a myope the rays leave verging, in a hyperope the rays leave diverging, in an emmetrope the rays leave parallel.

The degree of divergence of the rays that le the illuminating system of the retinoscope depe on the distance of the retinoscope from the patie eye. Most ophthalmologists use a working lens the phoropter or trial frame to account for distance. The working lens conventionally is h at 66 cm, being a +1.50-diopter lens, or at 50 c being a +2.00-diopter lens. If the patient is f sighted, the examiner will see, in the patient's ey a reflex that moves *with* the movement of the re noscope. In this instance plus lenses are added un there is no movement at all—in other words, un the refractive error has been neutralized. The wor ing lens is then removed or subtracted, and wh is left in the trial frame is a measure of the hype opia.

If the patient is a myope, the movement of th examiner's retinoscope will create a movement

the reflex that is opposite to the movement of the retinoscope. In this instance the examiner will place concave lenses or minus lenses in front of the patient's eye until the *against* motion is converted to a nonmoving ref the patient's pupil becomes ves much faster as the refrac duced. In other words, small e a bright and fast reflex, ve a dull and slow reflex. The upillary space when the re eliminated.

rovides aids to retinoscopy. e looking at a distant object feet away.

e should be examined with ye and vice versa.

be employed in astigmatic is easier to see "with" mo

astigmatism are difficult to atism is 1.00 diopter or less. rrecting cylinder should be ackward as a check for ac

asured should be fogged or should not be told to close scopy.

appear in the following

nses m poorly fitting hard con

of retinoscopes: the spot retinoscope. The Cope been the most popular. e the Nikon, the Welsh- Reichert. The last three g the bar on the handle

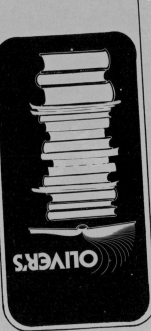

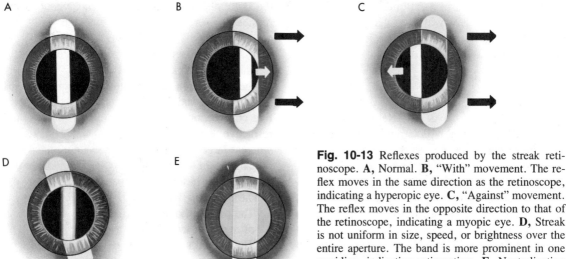

Fig. 10-13 Reflexes produced by the streak retinoscope. **A,** Normal. **B,** "With" movement. The reflex moves in the same direction as the retinoscope, indicating a hyperopic eye. **C,** "Against" movement. The reflex moves in the opposite direction to that of the retinoscope, indicating a myopic eye. **D,** Streak is not uniform in size, speed, or brightness over the entire aperture. The band is more prominent in one meridian, indicating astigmatism. **E,** Neutralization point. There is no movement of the reflex, and the pupil is filled with a red glow.

down, whereas the Copeland and the Nikon work by holding the bar up.

Many ophthalmologists today use the streak retinoscope (Fig. 10-13). The streak reflex illuminated in the pupil can be aligned easily with an astigmatic error. Moreover, it can be rotated to any desired meridian. With the streak retinoscope, the point of neutrality sometimes is evidenced by a cleavage in the streak (scissors reflex) so that half the streak moves in one direction and the other half moves in the opposite direction.

The light source for the streak retinoscope has a linear filament. From this source a divergent collection of light rays strikes the person's pupil. The alignment of the rays from the linear filament is made possible by the adjustable sleeve on the instrument, which provides rotation of the bulb.

Streak retinoscopy is largely plus cylinder retinoscopy, that is, corrected with plus cylinders.

A mirror in the instrument bends the path of light at right angles to the vertical orientation of the handle so that light can move across the space between examiner and patient. When the sleeve is up, a plano mirror effect is created. The sleeve-down position produces a concave mirror effect. Thus with sleeve

up, the most traditional position, diverging rays are emitted (planomirror effect), whereas in the sleeve-down position, converging rays are formed (concave mirror effect).

A retinal reflex is found in the pupil when light from the retinoscope is shined into the patient's eye. The movement of this fundus reflex will yield information as to the presence of myopia, hyperopia, or astigmatism. The instrument must be moved to elicit the reflex in the pupil. The movement is perpendicular to the axis of the streak. When the streak is vertical, the movement of the instrument is sideways.

It is important to remember that the light in the patient's pupil is reflected from the retina so that a total picture of the refraction is obtained.

The working distance must be taken into account in retinoscopy. Most refractions employ a 66-cm (22-inch) distance, which, translated into diopters, is an added plus lens of +1.50 diopters. If the person is emmetropic, with this lens no movement will be present in the light reflex of the patient's pupil. The neutralization point can be as much as 0.50 diopter of accuracy. If the patient is hyperopic or farsighted, the reflex will become a with movement. (The reflex

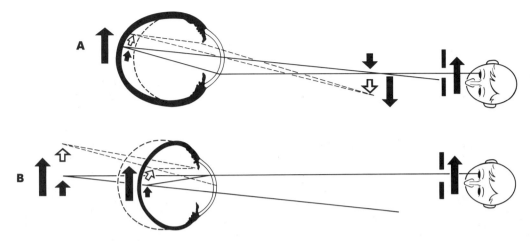

Fig. 10-14 Movement of images on retinoscopy. **A,** Myopia: real upside-down image creating against motion. **B,** Hyperopia: virtual upright image creating with motion.

moves in the same direction *with* the movement of the retinoscope.) If the eye is myopic, there will be an against motion from the neutral state (Fig. 10-14).

With a farsighted eye, plus lenses are added until neutralization occurs. The added plus spheres are then a measure of the total hyperopic refractive error. The same approach occurs with myopia, except that concave lenses are employed.

Many practitioners prefer to use the with motion, as it is easier to see as compared with an against motion. This can be done by overcorrecting myopic eyes or by reversing the position of the sleeve.

Neutrality of the objective refraction can be determined by the following:

1. The brightness of the reflex. The closer one comes to neutralizing the refractive error, the brighter is the reflex.
2. The speed of the light movement. When the light movement is dull and slow, it means the refractive error is still considerable.
3. The size of the reflex. The reflex fills the entire pupil when the neutrality is reached.

A large pupil makes it easier to recognize the motion of the reflex. For this reason, pupillary dilation is helpful in most cases.

With astigmatism, the speed, brilliance, and size of the reflex will be considerably different in one meridian as compared with the other principal meridian. Each band of light is neutralized separately, and the difference in diopters measures the degree of astigmatism. It should be remembered in all computations to deduct the value of the working lens by +1.50 or +2.00 diopters.

SUBJECTIVE REFINING

Once a preliminary estimate of the refractive error has been made by retinoscopy, the information is placed in a phoropter or trial frame. The patient's clinical responses to changes of spherical and astigmatic lenses are then noted while progressively smaller and smaller visual acuity letters are presented to the patient for evaluation. A number of special procedures often are employed in the refining of the final refractive error. These procedures include tests for astigmatism and the duochrome test.

Astigmatism tests

Two methods are primarily used for determining the axis and the power of the correct cylinder: the astigmatic dial or clock and the cross cylinder.

Astigmatic clock. The astigmatic clock has black lines intersecting at a common point, with the ends separated by 30-degree intervals or by 10-degree intervals (Fig. 10-15). The patient is seated at the normal refracting distance from the chart, that is, 20

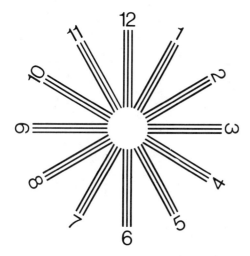

Fig. 10-15 Astigmatic clock.

feet, and asked to select the blackest line on the chart. The blackest line corresponds, of course, to the axis of the rays of light that are most in focus. Therefore the correcting cylinder is placed 90 degrees away from the blackest line; either positive or negative cylinders may be used. Positive cylinders will bring the most hyperopic focal point forward and collapse the astigmatic interval so that the focal point is either on the retina or in front of it. Minus correcting cylinders will reduce the astigmatic interval and push the point of focus either on the retina or behind it.

When the astigmatic dial is being used, it is usually wisest to use minus cylinders and reduce the astigmatic component by eliminating the myopic focal point.

The astigmatic component is resolved when the two principal axes on the clock are equally distinct and all lenses are equally in focus. Before asking the patient which line on the clock is the darkest, the examiner should blur the patient's vision to about 20/50 on the myopic side. This is done because a myopic state tends to inhibit accommodation. After the patient has selected the blackest line on the multiple dial chart, his or her attention is directed to a second chart that has only two lines that can be maneuvered to any position. The lines are set according to the most in-focus and out-of-focus axis.

Then minus cylinders are placed before the eyes, with the axis 90 degrees from the blackest line, increasing their strength at approximately 0.25 diopter at a time, until the blackness and distinctness of the two lines are the same. To ensure that the eyes are maintained on the myopic side or in a fogged state, it is advisable to add 0.25 diopter of plus sphere for each 0.50 diopter of minus cylinder that is employed. Once all the lines appear dark and equally distinct, then the myopic error can be reduced by use of minus spheres.

In employing the astigmatic clock with the spokes set 30 degrees apart, the examiner should ask the patient, in terms of hours on the clock, which line appears blackest. The smaller number of the clock hours is then multiplied by 30 degrees to determine the correcting axis. For example, if the 2 to 8 line is the blackest, then 2 times 30 is 60, and 60 degrees is the axis of the correcting cylinder.

If two lines appear equally black—that is, 1 to 7, and 2 to 8—then a mean between the two is taken and the axis of the correcting cylinder is determined that way. In the latter case it would be 1.5 times 30, and 45 degrees would be the axis of the correcting cylinder.

Cross cylinder. A cross cylinder is a lens consisting of two cylinders of equal power but of opposite designation, one being plus and the other being minus, their axes set 90 degrees apart. In most cross cylinders the red marks indicate the minus axis, and the white the plus axis. The entire lens is mounted in a ring, with a handle placed halfway between the plus and the minus axis (see Fig. 9-7).

A cross cylinder is employed to determine (1) the axis of the correcting cylinder and to check on this axis and (2) the power of the correcting cylinder.

The cross cylinder produces a mixed astigmatism of equal amount but opposite power in the two principal axes of the cylinder. To determine the *true axis of the correcting cylinder,* the patient wears full correction in the trial frame or the refractor, as determined by either a subjective astigmatic dial test or retinoscopy. The patient is then instructed to fixate on a line of letters that he or she can comfortably read. The handle of the cross cylinder is placed in alignment with the *axis* of the correcting cylinder already in the trial frame. The cross cylinder is then flipped from position 1 to position 2, and the patient is asked to comment on the clarity of the two positions of the cross cylinder. If the letters appear equally blurred at position 1 and at position 2, then the axis of the correcting cylinder in the patient's trial frame or phoropter is assumed to be correct. If one position is clearer than the other, the correcting cylinder is shifted in that direction. If the refractionist is using minus cylinders, the cylindric correction is shifted in the direction of the red dot that indicates the minus power of the cross cylinder. The opposite is true if the refractionist employs plus cylinders. A cross cylinder is most successfully used when it is held in a stationary frame, such as the refractor. This ensures proper alignment of the handle of the cross cylinders when the cross cylinder is changed.

Once the axis of the correcting cylinder has been determined, then the *power of the correcting cylinder* is investigated. This is accomplished by placing the handle 45 degrees away from the axis of the correcting cylinder in the trial frame or refractor. In this position the plus or minus cylinder of the cross cylinder are parallel with that of the correcting cylinder. Again the patient is asked to observe if there is any difference in the clarity between positions 1 and 2. If there is a difference in the clarity, cylinders are added or subtracted, depending on whether plus or minus cylinders are used, until the clarity of the letters becomes the same, regardless of which side of the cross cylinder is flipped.

There is an instrument in the cross-cylinder technique that is incorporated in the Topcon refractor and is available as an accessory for other refractors. This new device doubles the image so the patient is able to view two test charts simultaneously with one eye and to determine the clarity of the charts with the two positions of the cross cylinder. Additional cylinder or axis shift can be altered until the ultimate end point is reached when both lines are equally distinct.

It is immaterial whether one uses a cross cylinder or an astigmatic dial chart for the correction of astigmatism. The results are equally valid with both techniques. The efficiency by which one obtains a good refraction depends more on the skill of the refractionist than on the technique employed.

Irregular astigmatism. In irregular astigmatism the refraction in different meridians is irregular. Usually when irregular astigmatism is found, there is an associated pathologic condition of the cornea. Two of the most common causes of irregular astigmatism are corneal scarring from any cause and the developmental condition called *keratoconus.*

The diagnosis of irregular corneal astigmatism is best facilitated by employing Placido's disk. Placido's disk is a large, flat disk painted with concentric black and white circles (see Fig. 9-35). It is held in front of the eye, and the reflexes are observed through a hole in the center of the disk. The distortion of the circles on the cornea is usually readily visible.

The treatment of irregular astigmatism by conventional cylinders is virtually impossible. The best method of treating either corneal scarring or keratoconus usually is with a contact lens. If the treatment of irregular astigmatism by contact lenses is unsuccessful, often a corneal transplant becomes necessary.

Spherical equivalent. Occasionally in refraction, especially if the patient is an adult who has never worn glasses and requires a large astigmatic correction, the refractionist employs the spherical equivalent. Essentially what is done is that the cylinder is reduced, and half of that reduction is added algebraically to the sphere. For example, assume that the patient's correction is a $+3.00$ sphere combined with a $+6.00$-diopter cylinder, axis 180. Let us say in this instance that the refractionist decides that this cylindric correction would be too great for the patient to accept at once, and the decision is to reduce the cylinder by 1.50 diopters. Then the refractionist would add $+0.75$, or one-half the reduction, to the sphere. The resulting prescription would then read $+3.75$ sphere combined with $+4.50$ cylinder at axis 180.

Duochrome tests

Duochrome tests are based on the fact that light of longer wavelengths (red) is refracted by optical systems less than light of shorter wavelengths (blue or green). In the red-green duochrome test the projector screen is illuminated through a filter that is red on one side and green on the other. Another form of duochrome test requires the patient to look at a point source of light through a cobalt-blue glass filter. This type of glass is peculiar in that it transmits light in two "bands" of wavelengths, which are widely separated, one in the red and the other in the blue.

If the red-green test is used and the patient has insufficiently corrected myopia, then the letters on the red side will stand out blacker, clearer, and sharper. They will require more minus for the green to be as distinct as the red. On the other hand, if the same myopia is overcorrected and made artificially hyperopic, then the letters against the green background appear blacker, clearer, and sharper. The sphere is adjusted until letters on both sides are of equal quality. In the latter case, they will require plus levels for the red to be equally distinct. Similarly, with use of the cobalt-blue test, the person with undercorrected myopia will perceive a blue circle with a red center, whereas the person with overcorrected myopia will perceive a red circle with a blue center. The red-green test is in more common use than the cobalt-blue test.

Duochrome tests are useful only in refining spherical power, contributing nothing to the determination of cylinder power or axis. Therefore the most appropriate use of a duochrome test is as an end-point determination in refraction.

ANISOMETROPIA

Anisometropia is a condition in which there is a difference in the refractive error of the two eyes.

If the difference in the refractive error of the two eyes is slight, binocular vision is easily attained. Each 0.25-diopter difference between the refraction of the two eyes causes 0.5% difference in size between the two retinal images, and a difference of 5% is probably the limit that can be tolerated. Moreover, inasmuch as accommodation is a bilateral act in that it occurs equally in both eyes, there is no internal adjustment that one eye can make to compensate for this difference in refractive error. Because of difference in image size, fusion of images

of unequal size becomes impossible. Normally a 1.50-diopter difference in the refractive errors between the two eyes is quite easily managed with the retention of binocular vision. In large errors, in which the difference amounts to 1.50 to 3.00 diopters, fusion can take place for large and gross objects. With greater differences, some adjustment in binocular vision occurs. For example, the child may learn to alternate his or her vision, that is, to use one eye for distance and one eye for near. This is especially apt to occur when one eye is farsighted and the other nearsighted.

If the refractive error is negligible in one eye and great in the other eye, the individual tends to suppress the image in the eye with greater refractive error. This is especially true if the eye involved has a large astigmatic error, so that vision for both distance and near is foggy. The constant habit of suppression leads to loss of vision, or amblyopia from disuse. This condition is preventable because useful vision can be retained if the error in the defective eye is corrected early enough in life and the use of the eye is encouraged at the time by suitable patching or other exercises.

Another problem caused by unequal refractive errors is the development of *aniseikonia*. In this condition the differences in the size of the retinal image affect the patient's spatial judgments. This is not a common complaint, and it is most readily found in persons who use spatial judgments in their daily work at all times. Persons such as carpenters, interior designers, engineers, and artists are most prone to speak of disorders in spatial perception. These patients complain of visual discomfort, fatigue, headaches, distortion of objects, slanting of tables, dipping of surfaces, and so forth. Diagnosis of this condition is made with the patient's history and simple screening tests; for example, the patient reports a rectangular card as trapezoidal. Measurement of aniseikonia can be performed with a special instrument called a *space eikonometer*.

Treatment

When anisometropia occurs in children, especially those younger than 12 years old, every attempt should be made to induce them to wear the full correction. For adults, especially when the difference is only between 2.00 and 4.00 diopters, the full correction again should be given, and they should be encouraged to bear with this correction despite symptoms. Often after 3 to 4 weeks of wear, the symptoms of eyestrain disappear and adults becomes comfortable with their lenses. In older patients the visual discomfort often becomes intolerable, so that it is frequently advisable to undercorrect the eye with the higher refractive error.

Anisometropia and aniseikonia are being treated more successfully today by the use of contact lenses, particularly in the young child who has not yet developed amblyopia. Prisms to correct the secondary muscular imbalance and iseikonic glasses are other expedients used in treating this problem.

APHAKIA

Aphakia is that condition in which the crystalline lines is absent from the eye. This may be caused by removal of a cataractous lens or the displacement of the lens from the pupillary space by trauma.

Correction of aphakia is perhaps the most difficult task for the refractionist. Despite a perfect pair of glasses, the aphakic individual suffers from tremendous visual problems associated with this new refractive state. Dr. Oliver Dabezies, Jr., has made a significant contribution in clarifying some of the problems associated with aphakic spectacle vision. With aphakia, objects are magnified by at least one third. The magnification induced by this new refractive state poses considerable problems for the aphakic patient. Even the simplest of tasks can result in an embarrassing experience. In reaching for a cup of coffee, the aphakic person may underreach and spill its contents because the cup appears larger and therefore closer than it really is. Aphakic persons also must learn to move their heads rather than their eyes to avoid the distortions created by the prismatic effect of the lens periphery; they can see clearly only through the center of their glasses. The prismatic distortions of the thickened lens can affect them in other ways. Walking toward a door can be jarring to the aphakic person because the sides of the door appear to bulge inward as it is approached. The optical distortions lead to confusion, uncertainty, and

even fear. Walking down the stairs can be a calamity if persons with aphakia look down through their spectacles. The entire staircase seems to fall away, and affected persons feels themselves without support.

Perhaps one of the most disturbing aspects of aphakic vision is the jack-in-the-box phenomenon. In this situation the aphakic person finds an object through the corner of the eye and looks toward it, only to see that it is gone. *Aphakic vision, even though it results in 20/20 vision, requires a complete visual reorientation.* Spatial relationships, distances, and spatial judgments are all altered with this new type of vision.

An aphakic eye can never work together with a normal eye. This is because an aphakic eye essentially is a very farsighted eye, and the anisometropia induced is too great to overcome. Unless one uses a contact lens on the operated eye, it will not coordinate with the unoperated eye. Readiness for cataract surgery usually implies a diminution of visual acuity to at least 20/50 in the better eye, inasmuch as functional normal vision is a far better asset than the clear, distorted vision of aphakia.

When an aphakic correction is prescribed, the following must be kept in mind.

1. The optical centers must be exact because even a slight error causes a prismatic displacement with the thickened aphakic correction.
2. The distance of the trial lens from the eye and the eventual spectable glass also must correspond. The distance of the eye from the trial lens (vertex distance) can be measured with a distometer. If this notation is put down on the prescription card, the optician can make the suitable adjustment in power (see Fig. 9-9 and Appendix 9).
3. The periphery of the lens may be ground off. This type of lens is referred to as a *lenticular aphakic lens*. The lenticular lens serves to reduce the weight of the glass and abolish the extreme aberrations occurring from the periphery of a normal aphakic spectacle. Newer forms of aspheric spectacles are less curved in the periphery with use of an aspheric front surface instead of a lenticular design.

4. The frames must fit comfortably on the nose and be set straight.

The intraocular lens today represents the most suitable form of visual rehabilitation after cataract surgery. In situations in which it is indicated, a comfort lens may be used. With a contact lens the magnification is only 7%, as compared with 33% for an aphakic lens. The visual adjustments and distortions with a contact lens are considerably reduced compared with those with spectacles.

WHEN TO REFRACT AFTER CATARACT SURGERY

It used to be taught that at least 6 weeks were required after the cataract operation before aphakic lenses could be prescribed. The final prescription was then given when, after a recheck 1 week later, the prescription was still the same. Some surgeons use the keratometer as a guide and perform refraction when the K readings are stable between two visits.

There has been a marked change in cataract surgery. The phacoemulsification method has become more widespread and popular; this method requires a 3-mm incision. These patients are mobile almost as soon as the procedure is finished, and they can undergo refraction early. Extracapsular surgery has given the eye more protection from the forward movement of the vitreous. Extracapsular surgery, however, also may mean a discission by YAG laser of the posterior capsule weeks after surgery, which may delay refraction. Almost all patients today are receiving lens implants, and the refraction must be performed over the implant. Often glare of the implant can be a problem to the retinoscopist. The surgeon must make the decision as to the timing of a preliminary refraction.

Refractive points specific to the aphakic and pseudophakic person

The aphakic and pseudophakic person may not have a healthy eye, and the vision may not be refined to 20/20 or 6/6. The eye may have suffered surgical trauma, such as cystoid edema of the macula, or may have macular degeneration. Cataract patients generally are elderly and may have degenerative ocular manifestations such as glaucoma or optic atrophy.

A multiple pinhole may be used to start refraction to assess the potential of the eye.

The use of retinoscopy may be awkward in many ways. The patient who has no accommodation and has hazy vision cannot fixate accurately. The eye may move because of lack of fixation or lack of attention and concentration. If the patient does not hold the eyes steady, erratic and confusing scissor movements of the retinoscopy reflex may occur. Also, the axis and the amount of astigmatism will be difficult to gauge.

We have found keratometry an important reference starting point in pseudophakia, particularly when the retinoscopy shadows are poor.

In pseudophakia, with an entroocular lens, the problems are different. The pupil after an implant procedure may be small, and the retinoscopy shadows are more difficult to assess. If the pupil is small, frequently the surgeon will authorize the use of a mydriatic agent for the refraction. An ophthalmic assistant should not even consider dilating the eyes of a patient with an iris-supported intraocular lens without instructions from the surgeon. Fortunately, these are uncommon today. Dilation in iris-supported implants may be a pivotal step in dislocating the lens. In pseudophakia, retinoscopic examination in the direct visual axis frequently causes disturbing reflections from the intraocular lens surface. These annoying reflections can be avoided by moving side to side until a good reflex is obtained.

In aphakia with no implant, the trial frame should be placed close so that the lenses just clear the lashes. In the higher powers of aphakia, vertex distance should be taken into account.

The patient's old glasses may be suitable for an overrefraction or correction of an old prescription. The lenses are centered, and the vertex distance is correct. A regular refraction can then be done.

The refractionist always has to bear in mind the vertex distance. As much as 1.00 diopter may be off in the final prescription. The Halberg trial clip placed over spectacles eliminates the need for vertex adjustment for the aphakic patient.

Often a patient will be given a proper prescription only to find that the frame has been fitted incorrectly.

The heavy glasses in a heavy frame slide halfway down the nose, and the careful refraction measurements are worthless. The fit of aphakic spectacles should be checked because it is as vital as the prescription itself.

Procedure after cataract surgery

After cataract surgery, keratometric reading, which provide the starting point for refraction, can be obtained. Often the glare induced by the intraocular lens implant makes retinoscopic examination difficult. Once the keratometric readings are stable between visits, the final refraction can be considered. The autorefractor, used with dilated pupils, also may provide a good starting point for refraction. In extracapsular surgery astigmatism often is present; consequently the surgeon may elect to cut one or more of the sutures in the direction of the high plus cylinder to reduce the astigmatism.

The cataract lens

Aphakic lenses for the person who has had cataract surgery without benefit of an intraocular lens are fast-disappearing. Up until the early 1970s almost all patients underwent this procedure and required cataract glasses. Many cases today have been reversed by secondary implants or the benefits of contact lenses, thus eliminating the problems induced by aphakic glasses. Despite these advances, many individuals still are wearing these glasses.

The bull's-eye lenticular lens, a bulbous lens mounted on a plano carrier, has given way to the more cosmetically acceptable, highly aspheric lenses. These lenses are lighter and can be dispensed in a fashion frame. The optical effect is outstanding. The field of clear vision is enlarged, and the pincushion distortions are reduced to a minimum.

These lenses commonly have up to a 4.00-diopter drop in power at the periphery of the lens. This aspheric effect creates a marked improvement in the patient's cosmetic and functional rehabilitation.

The patient still has a 30% magnification of image size, but other features of lens scotoma, jack-in-the-box phenomenon, distortion, and field limitation, which are present in regular aphakic lenses, are greatly reduced with the highly aspheric lenses.

These lenses also are lighter and more comfortable, with less tendency to slide down the nose.

These lenses are prescribed a little differently. A trial set of spectacle lenses, fully mounted, is available to the practitioner. These lenses are used as a basis for refraction to eliminate vertex distance computations. The correct starter spectacle is easily derived from a rough retinoscopic examination. After the first trial lens is selected, an overrefraction is performed in the routine way.

Some refractionists advocate an overplus of 1.00 diopter for the elderly aphake who is not working or driving, so that indoor near vision is relatively clear at the expense of sharp distant vision. This approach depends strictly on the practitioner.

Despite these wonderful achievements in aphakic spectacles, it must be conceded that the best aphakic spectacle device is still inferior to a correcting contact lens or an intraocular lens.

PRESBYOPIA

Everyone becomes presbyopic with age. The accommodative ability decreases because of loss of the strength of the ciliary muscle and hardening of the lens. However, not everyone who is 45 or older needs reading glasses. Myopic persons do not because they can simply take off their glasses to read. Those who are nearsighted in one eye may not be aware of this anomaly and may carry on happily without a reading aid indefinitely. Also, the needs of people differ. An architect will require reading glasses long before a waiter will. Some people do not read or sew and have little use for a reading assist at any time. Thus the correction of presbyopia is not just optical. The needs of the individual must be kept in mind. What does the person do? What lighting is available? How much reading is done and at what distance? Does the person need to look up and down to see distance and near for occupational reasons? Are the person's symptoms genuine or is stress or anxiety making reading difficult?

Symptoms

The primary feature of presbyopia is an inability to do close work. Initially it manifests as difficulty in seeing the telephone book ("the print is grayer now") or a problem in seeing the menu in dimly lit restaurants. Presbyopic persons cannot see small print nor can they see without good illumination. They may increase lighting to see clearly. Light adds contrast and also constricts the pupil to a pinhole aperture. Some people complain that they have to hold the print farther away, and eventually they are reading with an uncomfortable reach, complaining that their arms have become too short. Other symptoms include fatigue with reading, grittiness of the eyes with prolonged close work, and trouble with threading a needle.

Treatment

Two types of spectacle lenses are available for the treatment of presbyopia: the reading glass and the bifocal. Psychologically, most new presbyopes are much more receptive to the idea of reading glasses. They are referred to as *working glasses, sewing glasses, library glasses*—in other words by any term that denotes their use rather than the patient's advancing age. Bifocals conjure up a picture of one's elderly grandmother and represent the first step toward declining vigor and old age.

If the patient's distance vision is adequate, reading glasses usually are prescribed first. The patient is, however, warned that the glasses will help only to read at near. They will blur things if they are used for distance work. The patient also is told that, with time, the reading glasses now prescribed will no longer suffice as accommodation declines. Many patients think that with time the glasses seem to get worse, rather than thinking that an intrinsic disorder of the eye is becoming more pronounced. Even if the patient requires glasses for distance, it often is best to give the patient a separate pair of reading glasses for close work. Most patients have several friends or relatives who have had difficult times in adjusting to bifocals, and the patients will relate these stories with great relish. For this reason and for psychologic considerations, the patient is best left to cope with trying to use two pairs of glasses. Once patients have become sufficiently harried trying to use two pairs of glasses, they will return, asking for bifocals, and will adjust to them quite comfortably. The optician can be of great service in helping patients choose the proper bifocal. For individuals who are conscious of their appearance, no-line bifocals are available (progressive "no line" lenses).

Most presbyopes complain that their glasses are too strong. When bifocals are prescribed, the near point of accommodation is measured in each eye with the patient's distance spectacles in place. It is customary to give the weakest possible lens that will enable the patient to see at a comfortable working or reading distance. The stronger the lens given for a bifocal addition, the shorter will be the patient's range of focus. This loss of range can be quite disabling for the executive who must see the corner of the desk or for the typist who has to look away at approximately 30 inches to see the typing. Therefore, when lenses are prescribed, it always is advisable to leave some accommodation in reserve. In fact, the rule in prescribing near corrections is to give that correction which will leave half the amplitude of accommodation in reserve.

When strong bifocal additions are required, such as $+2.00$ to $+2.50$, the range of focus is compromised by necessity. For those patients whose occupations demand an intermediate zone—that is, an ability to read at 1 meter—trifocals are used, the trifocal being one half the strength of the bifocal. Trifocals should not be prescribed with abandon because to most patients trifocals mean three times as much trouble as bifocals. It is important to realize that an individual with a $+2.50$ correction can see clearly only objects located at 40 cm, or about 16 inches away. Anything farther than this distance is fuzzy.

Tests for the correct power

The simplest way to test for the correct power is to allow the patient to hold a reading chart at his or her own reading distance and prescribe that lens which gives the needed clarity. A reading add of less than $+1.00$ diopter will not offer real assistance, and anything over $+2.50$ to $+3.00$ diopters makes the focal point too close and the reading distance too narrow to work in.

Why not give all patients a $+2.50$ add when they are 45 years of age and let them grow into that prescription at 65 years of age? A good idea cost-wise, but an ophthalmologist could lose his or her entire practice. The stronger the lens, the greater the weight factor, the aberrations, and the distortions and the closer the work distance. Ophthalmologists should always prescribe the weakest lens that a person can use.

At ages 42 to 45: a +1.00 to +1.25 is appropriate.
At ages 45 to 50: a +1.50 to +1.75 is a common strength.
At ages 50 to 65: a +2.00 to +2.50.

The strength of the add will vary with the refractive error—greater with hyperopic persons and the presence of pathologic conditions. Cataracts or macular degeneration may demand the higher magnification gained by closer reading distance, and the strength of the add also will vary with the needs of the individual.

Each eye should be tested individually and a record made as 20/20 or J1, and so on. The reading chart is a simple ready test and is desirable because the patient selects the reading distance. A variable light source helps simulate the patient's own illumination at work or home.

Another method is to test the amplitude of accommodation. This is merely the closest focal point at a given print size. For example, if a person's vision begins to blur at 25 cm, the amplitude of accommodation is 4.00 diopters. The patient is given a lens that leaves one half the amplitude of accommodation in reserve. If the patient has to work at 33 cm and requires 3.00 diopters of accommodation, then only a +1.00-diopter add is needed. One half the amplitude of accommodation is 2.00 diopters. To summarize, the need of accommodation is 3.00; thus the added plus strength of the reading aid is +1.00.

The dynamic cross-cylinder test also is useful. A +0.50 cyl/−0.50 cyl is the one most commonly employed. A grid made up of horizontal and vertical lines is the test target. The patient wears the distance correction. If the astigmatism has been properly corrected, the grid lines should be equally clear. The cross cylinder, with minus axis vertical, is added. Plus spheres are added, increasing the power until the vertical lines are clearer. At the same time spherical power is reduced until the lines are again equally clear. The add is the difference between the total spherical power for near and the distance correction.

This test has application for patients in whom the amplitude of accommodation is difficult to measure. It is not a preferred method.

The prescription

Patients should be given what they need. A man who works in a factory and walks around with safety glasses requires bifocals. He cannot walk with reading glasses. The same may be said for the musician who must look at the music and see the conductor. This person cannot see in the distance with reading glasses.

Reading glasses should be given in the following circumstances:

1. As a first lens when applicable
2. Whenever one is in doubt about which lens to prescribe
3. For persons who spend most of the day reading, writing, or working at a fixed distance

Bifocals should be considered for the following patients:

1. One who requires distance and near vision within moments, for example, a teacher
2. One who already wears distance glasses; two pairs of glasses, one for distance and one for near, are too cumbersome for efficiency
3. One who is disgruntled with reading glasses (no other options are available in a spectacle design, and the menu is limited to bifocals or readers)

Do's and don'ts

1. Do not prescribe bifocals for a −1.50-diopter myope. The simplest and cheapest device may be to take off the glasses, which is similar to opening a window; it always is much clearer to look through an open window.

2. Do not overcorrect the patient's vision. The greatest source of aggravation is with lenses that are too strong.

3. Never prescribe trifocals as an initial lens. A trifocal is used for intermediate range and is one half

the strength of the bifocal. Usually the bifocal must be a +2.00 diopter in power before a trifocal is valid. The trifocal is +1.00 diopter. This is too complicated and heavy a prescription for a first-time user.

4. Do warn patients of the difficulties and limitations of seamless or no-line bifocals. The no-line or invisible bifocal, although popular for cosmetic reasons, may induce marked astigmatism when the eyes wander to the sides of the bifocal segment. Some invisible or no-line bifocal lenses have larger clear fields than others, but all contain some limitation of clear, undistorted field in the reading portion. Newer adaptations of these lenses, which go under the trade names of Varilux II, Multilux, and Omnifocal, have addressed this problem and have improved the quality of vision, but the fault remains.

These lenses are expensive and promise a great deal. Optically they remove image jump and sharp transitions of focal power. Patients should be informed. This problem is covered in more detail on page 266.

5. Do not change the prescription of a bifocal until the fit has been appraised. The top of the segment on flattop segment bifocals (used to minimize image jump in looking from near to far) should be at the level of the lower lid. If the segment is too high, it will cut into the distant segment. If the segment is too low, it will add plus power to the prescription and the patient will in effect have a stronger spectacle. The fit of a bifocal affects the power, the field of vision, the image size, and the distortion factor. Always look at what the patient is wearing before reordering lenses, especially if the complaint regards a new set of spectacles.

The flattop bifocal is conspicuous. If the patient has strong feelings about the symbolic act of moving into bifocals, then respect this attitude. Some people's jobs depend on looking "young"—for example, entertainers, sales people, and media people—and these individuals frequently prefer a no-line bifocal.

6. Always check the reading segment monocularly. Sometimes a difference in the prescription between the two eyes will indicate a fault in the distance correction. Most people have equal accommodative reserve, and the bifocal addition should usually be the same. If unequal adds are required, an error in distance correction or some pathologic condition should be suspected.

7. Do not prescribe a bifocal if patients can read with their distance glasses. If patients can read through the distance segment, they will never get used to the bifocal segment. It is an intrusion in the field. Besides, they do not need a reading addition.

8. Look at the reading pattern when deciding between bifocals or reading glasses. Bifocals work well for persons who drop their eyes to read, because bifocals will not upset any ingrained visual habits, but for those who lower their heads and always look through the center of the lenses, reading glasses should be considered.

Myths to be dispelled

The following myths need to be dispelled.

Myth 1. Reading glasses ruin powers of accommodation and contribute to the aging of the eye. In reality, new bifocal wearers quickly become dependent on the reading additions, and further loss of accommodation would not have occurred anyway.

Myth 2. Bifocal wearers, in the main, have a difficult time adjusting to bifocals. In reality, the vast majority (a clinical "guestimate" would be over 90%) have no difficulty adapting to bifocals.

Myth 3. Bifocals are a hazard when a person walks down stairs. In reality, myopeic persons with vision of this power, without glasses, have no difficulty descending stairs.

Myth 4. Bifocals should be worn for racquet sports to see the ball close in. In reality, they should *not* be worn. Only distance spectacles are needed. Bifocals are not only unnecessary, they are a hazard to the game itself.

Myth 5. Presbyopia is a disease and the eyes become weaker with age. In reality, presbyopia is a normal change in the refractive error associated with the aging process. The crystalline lens of the eye loses its ability to accommodate because of changes in the lens fibers. Presbyopic persons see 20/20 for distance and near and merely require different lens to accommodate their needs. Presbyopic eyes are healthy.

COMPLAINTS: HOW TO ANTICIPATE THEM

Most frames are designed by fashion people in Paris or New York and are not particularly practical from an ophthalmic point of view. In the merchandising of lenses, style has become paramount and function downgraded.

A few key points will provide assistance to the patient and prevent much grief at a later date.

1. Jumbo frames are a very poor idea for someone with a large refractive error. Persons who have worn small frames before and want to move into a high-fashion style should not be encouraged. Large lenses induce large aberrations and increase the weight of the lenses. People will complain of ocular vertigo and blurred vision because of the sliding effect every time they look down.

2. Impact-resistant lenses should always be ordered. In many states and provinces this is law, but an ever present element of neglect or indifference exists and somehow the cheaper lenses occasionally find their way into the market. A lens should be a protection, not a liability.

3. Bifocals less than $+1.25$ diopters should not be prescribed. The disadvantages of a new bifocal do not warrant a new device with minimal advantages. Also, people tend to like high magnification when being tested and resent the same prescription in their ordinary lives. The ophthalmologist should not overplus a bifocal. When in doubt the rule is, do not change the glasses.

4. Tints should not be prescribed in lenses for indoor use. A tinted lens reduces contrast and makes reading more difficult. A tint, even though slight, makes driving in dim illumination hazardous. Besides, tints can distort colors. A blue tint can make the person more myopic. With driving at night, it enhances the normal night myopia.

5. When a high prescription has been given, it is important to check that the base curve has not been changed. A change of base curve or a change in the tilt of the lens may induce unwanted aberrations.

6. Glasses for elderly persons should not be changed unless significant visual gains can be made—at least two lines. Frequently, vision of elderly persons is undercorrected because of slight hardening or sclerosis of the lens of the eye. These patients often like being a little undercorrected for distance and overcorrected at near.

7. Plastic tends to be softer than glass and scratches more easily. This disadvantage is compensated by the lightness. Plastic lenses also do not shatter—a fact of importance when dealing with a high myope who has lenses that are very thin at the center.

Plastic frequently results in a thick lens and may not be desirable as a social lens. This consideration can be dealt with by making the lens one third thinner with flint glasses, which have a higher index of refraction. These lenses should not be used for children or adults working in industry inasmuch as these lenses are more brittle.

GLASSES CHECKS AND HOW TO HANDLE THEM

When a complaint is received from a patient who is unhappy, public relations are important. The ophthalmologic personnel may have made a mistake—it is best to check the total prescription. Arrogance, dismissal, and clichés like "You will get used to your prescription" will drive the patient to obtain a second opinion and jeopardize the ophthalmologist's reputation with that family. The following should be checked.

1. Poor centration. It is possible that the lenses are not centered properly. The optical centers of the lenses should be checked and aligned with the eyes.

2. Large frames. The frames may be too large compared with the patient's old glasses. If so, the patient will experience new distortions, particularly from the periphery of the lens. It may be necessary to go back to the old size of frames.

3. Incorrect prescription. The lenses should be checked on the lensmeter. They may not be correct. Not only can the ophthalmologic personnel make a mistake, but the optician and laboratory also are capable of the same sin.

4. Vertex problem. The distance the present lenses are set from the eyes should be compared with that of the old spectacles. If the vertex distance is not the same as the old lenses or has not been corrected in the prescription with refractive errors over

4.00 diopters, then the power will be wrong.

5. Frame problems. Do the frames slide up and down the nose with head movement in reading? Parallax may be a factor here.

6. Unwanted prism. Because of faulty centration, prisms may be introduced that cause induced phorias, either vertical or horizontal. This is more common in strong reading glasses.

7. Base curve. Have the new lenses been made up on the same base curve as the old ones? A change may cause difficulty. A Geneva measure may be useful.

8. Stress lines. Are there stress lines in the lenses? Have the lenses been crimped into the frames? A polarizing lens filter may be helpful.

9. Thick lenses. Are the lenses thicker than they need to be for the power involved, resulting in excessive glass to look through centrally?

10. Tilt. Are the lenses tilted adequately for reading, or is the patient reading obliquely through the lenses?

11. Correction of nondominant eye. Has the nondominant eye been corrected so that it has far better vision than the dominant eye? This may result in some difficulties.

12. Segment line of bifocal. Is the lens set too high or too low and interfering with some of the visual pathways, particularly during walking or working? Are the leg heights symmetrical?

The prescription should be reviewed. The ophthalmologist should re-refract and check the sphere cylinder and axis. An axis change of 10 degrees from previous glasses may not be tolerated even if correct.

In higher-cylinder corrections, an axis change of more than 5 degrees may not be tolerated.

If the prescription is wrong, the patient should be told. It is better to have an honest mistake than a subterfuge.

Cycloplegic drops should not be used for recheck. The prescription may be different with a smaller pupil. Also, the smaller the pupil, the greater the depth of focus, a factor that must be taken into consideration.

SUMMARY

Refraction is an art that requires patience, practice, and contact with many people before excellence is attained. It is important to remember that glasses must fill a particular need, and in the final analysis it is the need and not the refractive error that is paramount. The acme of visual efficiency—20/20 or 20/15 vision—is totally unnecessary in a 5-year-old child, but it may be vital to a young college student. Experience teaches us how to handle the presbyopic mechanic who must lie on his back and look directly at the undersurface of an automobile; the 65-year-old receptionist-typist who must be able to see across the room, type at 26 inches, and read at 16 inches; and the elderly, illiterate person who comes in for a checkup and neither reads, sews, nor does any close work whatsoever. In addition to knowledge of optics and the method of refraction, the refractionist must be congenial and a little talkative, at least enough to be able to assess the patient in terms of profession or work, hobbies, and special interests.

QUESTIONS FOR REVIEW AND THOUGHT

1. Illustrate the convergence of parallel rays in an emmetropic eye, a myopic eye, and a hyperopic eye.
2. With full cycloplegia, one measures +3.00 diopters of hyperopia. Will the patient accept this amount in a pair of glasses? Explain.
3. Why does a young person not require as much hyperopic correction as an older person?
4. What is meant by axial myopia?
5. What are some of the causes that have been advocated for myopia? Which are possible?
6. When does myopia usually stop changing?
7. What is with-the-rule astigmatism?

8. Where is the axis of a minus cylinder in with-the-rule astigmatism? Of a plus cylinder?
9. What is irregular astigmatism? How is it treated?
10. Explain how the cross cylinder is used.
11. What is Placido's disk? What is its purpose?
12. Outline some of the problems inherent in the correction of aphakia by spectacles.
13. In a strong plus prescription, such as after cataract surgery, of what importance is the distance of the spectacles form the eye? Explain.
14. What is the cause of presbyopia?
15. Discuss the shadows seen on retinoscopic examination of myope.
16. What is the most common problem in the correction of presbyopia?
17. What is the purpose of a cycloplegic refraction?
18. What is a manifest refraction?
19. What is the greatest difference between the refractive errors of two eyes that is compatible with good fusion?
20. What is meant by eyestrain?
21. Outline methods of dealing with a patient who complains of an inability to wear prescribed glasses.

SELF-EVALUATION QUESTIONS

True-false statements

Directions: Indicate whether the statement is true (T) or false (F).

T or F   1. The duochrome test is based on the fact that green is refracted behind the retina.
T or F   2. Myopia is largely a hereditary disorder.
T or F   3. Fogging involves discouraging accommodation by blurring the patient's eyes with plus spheres.

Missing words

Directions: Write in the missing word in the following sentences.

4. Retinoscopy and the correction of astigmatism are best done with a _____ cylinder.
5. Retinoscopy can yield information of an irregular cornea because of _____ reflexes in the pupil.
6. Vertex distance measurements can be avoided by _____.

Choice-completion questions

Directions: Select the one best answer in each case.

7. Aphakic spectacles cause which of the following problems?
   a. Magnification by 10%
   b. Barrel distortion
   c. Jack-in-the-box scotoma
   d. Variable vision
   e. Induced astigmatism
8. Presbyopia should first be corrected by:
   a. Reading glasses to prevent it from getting worse
   b. Taking off the glasses if the patient is myopic
   c. Vitamin A
   d. Bifocals if the patient does not need a distance correction
   e. A decrease in illumination

9. Aphakic spectacles may have:
   a. A drop in power in the periphery of the lens
   b. A plano carrier
   c. A mild gray tint
   d. A bifocal segment that aligns with the top of the lower lid
   e. All of the above

ANSWERS, NOTES, AND EXPLANATIONS

1. **False.** Green is refracted by the optical system of the eye so that a person with normal vision will have green focus in front of the retina and red focus behind the retina. A person who finds the letter on the green side more clearly in focus than that on the red requires plus correction.
2. **True.** Myopia is largely a hereditary disorder, but this is still debatable. Other causes have not been conclusively proved. Other claims of the causes of myopia that are without scientific validity are the following:
   a. Poor illumination
   b. Reading too much, with the eyes too close to the page, or without the proper reading posture
   c. Dietary problems, particularly insufficient vitamins
   d. Glasses that have been fully corrected instead of being undercorrected
   e. Wearing glasses (that is, proper correction) too early in life
   f. A disease that makes the eyes "weak"
   g. A lack of proper eye exercises
3. **True.** It is vitally important in the refraction of the eyes of children or young adults to control accommodation so that this element can be eliminated from the tabulation of a proper prescription. With children, short-acting cycloplegic drops are used. With many adults, and in some practices, cycloplegic drops are not routinely used because of practical problems such as a patient with fully dilated pupils trying to drive an automobile on a bright day. Instead of "dropping" the eyes, fogging may be used to eliminate the accommodative component of the refraction. The pupils are not artificially dilated, and a visual hazard is not created. The patient can drive home in safety or return to work or school. In addition, no deleterious side effects occur with fogging. It is a natural way to eliminate or reduce accommodation.
4. **Plus.** Plus cylinders are desirable because a with movement is easier to view in the pupil than an against movement. Because of this optical effect, the chance of making an error of retinoscopy is least when the reflex is neutralized from the plus side.
5. **Distorted or irregular.** The reflexes in the pupillary aperture should be regular and even. A distorted reflex means the corneal surface is irregular. This could be a result of surgery to the anterior segment, early keratoconus, "warping" of the corneal surface by an ill-fitting contact lens, or inflammation such as an old herpes scar.
   Whatever the cause, a proper refraction cannot be performed because there is no valid method of treating irregular astigmatism with regular lenses.
6. **Overrefraction.** There are two ways of handling vertex problems. One method is to make the calculation with a distometer and make the adjustment from distometer tables.
   A more accurate method is to overrefract over the patient's present spectacles and use the resultant power in a new prescription for the same frame.
7. **c. Jack-in-the-box scotoma.** Aphakic spectacles do cause an increase in magnification of the image size, but it is 30%, not 10%. They also cause distortion, but the effect of this distortion is a pincushion type, with the sides sloping inward. Variable vision does not really occur with proper lenses. However, many aphakic persons get a poor fit, and the lenses may slide down

the nose with reading. This slide is due strictly to the weight of the lens. The newer, lighter lenses control this variability caused by the slide of the frames. Chromatic aberration is a feature of many lenses, not just aphakic ones. Chromatic aberration is the breakup of white light into a spectrum of colors. The jack-in-the-box scotoma does occur with aphakic spectacles, and objects appear to suddenly dart into the peripheral field of the person wearing aphakic spectacles.

8. **b. Taking off the glasses if the patient is myopic.** Presbyopia should be corrected by the simplest device possible. A person who must work and walk around requires bifocals. A presbyope who is in industry requires safety glasses; thus there is no other option but bifocals.

If the patient is nearsighted, an easy solution is to have that person remove the glasses. It is fast and inexpensive, and the optical effect is the best if the vision is between -1.00 to -2.50 diopters.

Reading glasses do not make presbyopia better or worse. One practical way to postpone presbyopia is simply to direct more light on the page. An increase in illumination adds contrast, which is an excellent way to obtain greater clarity. It also makes the pupil smaller, thereby producing more of a pinhole effect.

9. **e. All of the above.** The newer aphakic lenses are aspheric. The peripheral curves are reduced so that the lenses are no longer spherical. The drop in the peripheral curves makes the lenses lighter and reduces peripheral aberrations and limitations of the visual field. It also reduces the effective power of the high plus lenses in the periphery and makes the lenses more in focus for distant objects.

A plano carrier is another way of reducing the mass of the lens. It does not take away from field of vision because the periphery of the regular lens contributes very little to clear vision.

A gray-tint No. 1 is helpful in reducing some of the photophobia some aphakic persons dislike. Gray is a color that distorts color appreciation the least.

CHAPTER 11

Automated refractors

DAVID L. GUYTON

- Historical development
- Modern Instruments
- Accuracy of measurement
- Future of automated refraction

Through modern technology, more than 20 automated refracting instruments have been introduced, including manual objective refractors, automatic infrared retinoscopes, and sophisticated subjective refractors. Some are fast and easy to use; some take longer and require more operator skill. All of the automated refractors are designed to be managed by the ophthalmic assistant without the need for extensive knowledge of refractometry techniques.

HISTORICAL DEVELOPMENT

Automated refractors date back more than 100 years, but only recently have some of them become successful. There have been three major problems in obtaining the necessary accuracy. First, many automated refractors have used only small portions of the patient's pupil to make the measurement. Because of the optical irregularity present in many eyes, the refraction obtained through small portions of the pupil may not be valid for the entire pupil. Such optical irregularities are easily visible during retinoscopy, and the automated refractors have no better

Dr. David L. Guyton is a professor of ophthalmology at Johns Hopkins University School of Medicine, The Wilmer Ophthalmological Institute, Baltimore, Md.

way to deal with these than does retinoscopic examination. Second, maintaining proper alignment of the automated refractor with the patient's eye was difficult with many of the early instruments. To lessen this problem, automatic tracking capability has been added to some of the newest automated refractors. Third, and most important, most automated refractors have been placed in box-shaped instruments that cause the awareness of near. Patients tend to accommodate when looking into these boxes, even though the visual targets within the boxes may be imaged optically at infinity. Accurate refraction is impossible in the presence of accommodation, and this so-called instrument myopia has been a continuing problem for automated refractors. Various fogging techniques or "free-space" techniques are now used to try to overcome the problem of instrument myopia.

MODERN INSTRUMENTS

Currently available instruments may be grouped into various categories according to the degree of automation and the objective or subjective nature of the instruments. Objective refractors require minimal cooperation on the part of the patient, usually requiring only that the patient hold still and look straight ahead. Subjective refractors, on the other hand, require responses from the patient, particularly in the final refinement steps of the refractive measurement.

Manual objective refractors

In the 1930s several instruments, known as *objective optometers,* appeared in Europe. The operator focused or aligned a target pattern on the patient's retina to determine the refraction. These manual objective refractors still are used in many parts of the world in preference to retinoscopy. They are less expensive than the other automated refractors but require more time and more operator skill. Patient cooperation is essential, and instrument accommodation is common when cycloplegia is not used. The objective optometers use only small portions of the eye's optics for the measurement, and alignment is critical, limiting the accuracy of the findings. One of these refractors, the Topcon uses infrared light for the alignment and measurement process so that the patient is not dazzled by the bright white-light target pattern used in other models. Currently available manual objective refractors include the following:

Rodenstock PR-50
Zeiss Objective Refractometer 140
Möller Reditron

Automatic objective refractors

Automatic objective refractors first became available in the 1970s, using infrared light to automatically refract the eye either by retinoscopy or by similar principles. The first instruments in this group were the Safir Ophthalmetron, the 6600 Auto-Refractor, and the Dioptron, now all discontinued. The infrared light refractors give good results in healthy eyes with medium to large pupils, but accuracy decreases in the presence of immature cataracts or pupils less than 3 mm in diameter. Operation is extremely simple, and the measurement time is rapid, requiring only one second or less for most of the instruments. The refractive results obtained, however, must be regarded as only preliminary. Accuracy is good enough to identify "no-change" refractions and to monitor postoperative refractions until stable, but the results are not reliable enough to serve as the basis for prescribing glasses or contact lenses. Refinement

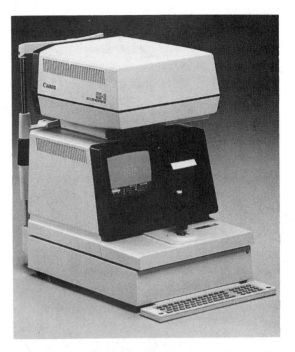

Fig. 11-1 Canon Auto Ref-Keratometer RK-2, an automatic objective refractor/keratometer. (Courtesy Canon U.S.A.)

by subjective techniques is recommended before prescribing. The automatic objective refractors currently on the market are the following:

Canon Autoref R-2
Marco/Nidek AR-800
Topcon RM-A2000
Nikon NR-5100
Shiu-Nippon QR-007N

An automatic keratometer has been added to some of these instruments, as in the Canon RK-2 (Fig. 11-1).

Combination objective/subjective refractors

Subjective capabilities have been added to several automatic objective refractors. For example, visual acuity can be measured through these instruments both before and after the refraction. Also, sphere, cylinder, and axis can be adjusted manually according to the patient's responses to various targets that are presented. Cross-cylinder testing is incorporated into most of these instruments, with successive

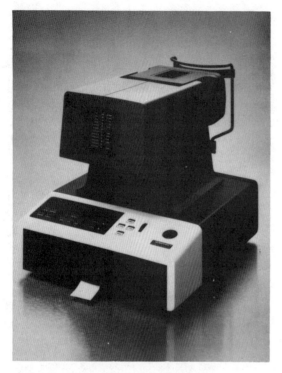

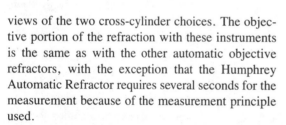

Fig. 11-2 Humphrey Automatic Refractor, Model 530, a combination objective/subjective refractor.

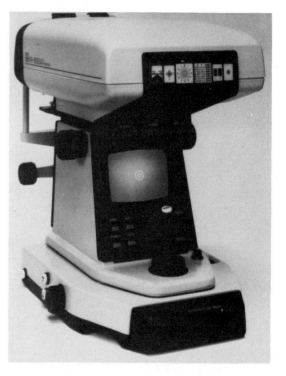

Fig. 11-3 Marco/Nidek AR-1600, a combination objective/subjective refractor.

views of the two cross-cylinder choices. The objective portion of the refraction with these instruments is the same as with the other automatic objective refractors, with the exception that the Humphrey Automatic Refractor requires several seconds for the measurement because of the measurement principle used.

The subjective capabilities of each of the combination refractors may be used, if desired, for refinement of the refraction. Considerable operator skill and knowledge of refracting techniques are necessary for optimal subjective refinement with these instruments, and there is still the problem of instrument myopia in patients up to the age of 40. The combination objective/subjective refractors now available are the following:

Humphrey Automatic Refractor (Fig. 11-2)
Marco/Nidek AR-1600 (Fig. 11-3)
Topcon RM-A2300G (Fig. 11-4)

The most recent addition to these instruments has been glare-testing capability.

Automated subjective refractors

Two automated refractors with purely subjective capabilities were on the market for about 10 years. The first to appear was the Humphrey Vision Analyzer in the mid-1970s. The Vision Analyzer used a novel optical system to refract the eyes in "free space," using a concave mirror three meters from the patient. Even the method of refraction was novel, using smeared-out astigmatic line targets in two independent meridians 45 degrees apart to arrive at the final cylinder and axis. The Vision Analyzer required an entire room, however, and was somewhat complicated to administer. It provided both binocular and near testing capabilities, unique among the automated refractors.

Because hyperopic patients often accommodated

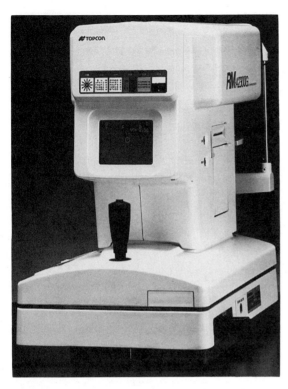

Fig. 11-4 Topcon RM-2300G, a combination objective/subjective refractor.

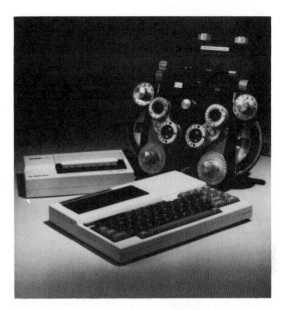

Fig. 11-5 Clinicon Refraction System, using a simplified technique for manual subjective refraction.

to the plane of the mirror of the Vision Analyzer, overrefraction capabilities were added, creating the Humphrey Overrefraction System. The eyes were refracted while the patient wore glasses, and the results were trigonometrically added to the power of the glasses.

The other automated subjective refractor was the Reichert (originally American Optical) SR-IV. Programmed Subjective Refractor, introduced in 1980. The sequence of refracting steps with this instrument was automated, so that the operator did not have to remember which step came next. A cross-cylinder system was used for the astigmatic portion of the refraction, with both of the cross-cylinder target choices seen simultaneously for ease of response and efficiency. As with some of the objective/subjective instruments, two different refractions could be compared quickly back-and-forth by the push of a button,

allowing comparison, for example, between the old glasses and the new results. As with the Vision Analyzer, the SR-IV allowed an experienced operator to obtain highly accurate refractive results, often usable as the basis for prescription. The operator had to be able to recognize, however, when the patient had difficulty with the measurement process and when instrument myopia was occurring. If instrument myopia was suspected, or for young patients in general, cycloplegia was administered, and the automated refraction was repeated. (I was the inventor of this instrument and hold patent right to some of the principles used.)

Another attempt to simplify subjective refraction is in the Clinicon Refraction System (Fig. 11-5). The cross cylinders on a Reichert Ultramatic RxMaster Phoroptor are replaced with variable power cross cylinders (Stokes lenses). The cylinder lenses inside the Phoroptor are replaced with cross cylinders, and a vernier axis scale is added. A manual refraction is performed, over the patient's old glasses if possible, using a "blur-to-clear" technique with the variable cross cylinders and axis dials.

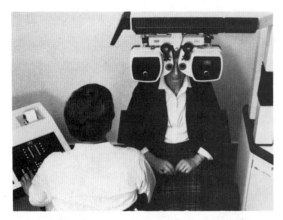

Fig. 11-6 Möller Visutron, a remote-controlled refractor.

Overrefraction results are added to the power of the glasses with the use of a special-purpose keyboard calculator.

Remote-controlled refractors

Several refractors or phoropters have been motorized in recent years and equipped with remote-control keyboards. These are designed to be operated by the skilled refractionist, because the techniques of refraction are not automated and still require full knowledge of refractive procedures. These remote-controlled refractors are somewhat expensive. Their major advantages are to impress the patient and to ease the practitioner's back strain. Retinoscopy can be performed in the usual manner through these instruments, and accuracy is comparable to that obtained with conventional manual refractors. Currently available remote-controlled refractors include the following:

Möller Visutron (Fig. 11-6)
Nikon Auto Optester OT-8A
Topcon CV-2000
Marco/Nidek TRS-1200
(TRS-1200)

Another remote-controlled refractor, which has been discontinued, was the Bausch & Lomb IVEX System (Fig. 11-7). This instrument was actually the combination of a vision tester with a remote-controlled refractor, intended to replace the conven-

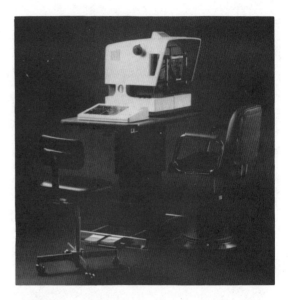

Fig. 11-7 Bausch & Lomb IVEX System, a self-contained vision tester and remote-controlled refractor. (Courtesy Bausch & Lomb, Rochester, New York.)

tional refracting lane. It had self-contained binocular distance and near targets and provision for retinoscopy through the rear of the instrument. The major problems with this refractor were instrument myopia and complexity of operation.

ACCURACY OF MEASUREMENT

The automatic objective refractors still create problems of irregular refraction in the patient's eye, maintenance of alignment of the instrument with the eye, and instrument myopia. Although accuracy is within a quarter diopter of the subjective refinement in over 80% of cases, it is not always obvious which measurements are incorrect, necessitating subjective refinement of most refractions. With a visual acuity check built into some of the objective instruments, valid information can be obtained at least to identify "no-change" refractions and to monitor the stability of the refraction after surgery.

The automated subjective refractors were highly accurate but required more operator skill. They also were not free from the problem of instrument myopia, and repeat measurement under cycloplegia was sometimes necessary in younger patients. The patients had to be 8 or 9 years old to respond reliably to the subjective refractors, whereas with the objective instruments, refraction sometimes can be affected in patients as young as 3 or 4 years old.

To this date, neither a purely objective instrument nor a purely subjective instrument has fully replaced conventional refracting techniques; that is, it is precisely the combination of an objective starting point and subjective refinement that yields the most reliable results throughout the widest range of patients. It is not surprising that automated refractors are now evolving into combination objective/subjective instruments, but the subjective portion still requires knowledge of refracting techniques and at least a moderate amount of experience for optimal results. It is likely that more sophisticated methods for subjective refinement will be developed within the next few years, decreasing the operator dependence of the present instruments.

FUTURE OF AUTOMATED REFRACTION

With the accuracy of some of the automated refractors now equaling that of conventional techniques, there is no question that the concept of automated refraction is here to stay. Combination objective/subjective instruments with full subjective refinement capability appear to be the final common development pathway for both the objective and subjective types.

In spite of the impressive capabilities of the newest instruments, their incorporation into an office practice must be carefully planned. Scheduling of patient appointments and proper sequencing of examinations must be arranged to prevent the automated refractor from obstructing the flow of patients. Operators must be trained properly, and substitute operators must be available. Service and maintenance for the instruments must be arranged and be available quickly when needed. Operators of the instrument must learn to recognize when either the patient or the instrument is having problems and to "flag" such cases for special consideration or repeat refraction by conventional techniques. Practitioners must learn when to trust the instruments, and when not to, and must provide feedback to the ophthalmic assistant if any learning is to occur. It is precisely the absence of such feedback that has limited the usefulness of automated refractors in many practices.

Patients generally are impressed with the automated instruments, and most do not seem annoyed that less time may be spent with the practitioner. Most practitioners initially expect too much from the automated refractors but eventually come to regard them as a valuable "second opinion" unbiased by knowledge of the patient's old prescription. The time will come, however, when the instruments are made less operator-dependent, simpler, and more reliable. Then the practitioner will need only to exercise the art of prescribing rather than to take time with the tedium of manual refraction.

QUESTIONS FOR REVIEW AND THOUGHT

1. Outline the value of automated refractors in clinical ophthalmology.
2. Compare the advantages of automated refractors versus retinoscopy and subjective refraction.
3. Outline the disadvantages of automated refractors versus retinoscopy and conventional subjection refraction.
4. If you are using an automated refractor, discuss inherent errors that can occur.
5. What is instrument myopia?
6. What are the drawbacks to introducing an automated refractor in practice?

SELF-EVALUATION QUESTIONS

True-false statements

Directions: Indicate whether the statement is true (T) or false (F).

T or F   1. Manual objective refractors require significant operator skill and time.

T or F   2. Automated objective refractors require significant operator skill and time.

T or F   3. Some automated refractors provide for subjective refinement.

Missing words

Directions: Write in the missing word in the following sentences.

4. Objective refractors may be used to replace _____.

5. Automated objective refractors still require _____ testing.

6. When an assistant using an automated refractor requires the patient to provide responses to questions, this is considered a _____ refraction step.

Choice-completion questions

Directions: Select the one best answer in each case.

7. The results of an automated refractor are least affected by:
   a. Large pupils
   b. Cataract
   c. Small pupils
   d. Irregular astigmatism
   e. Corneal scarring

8. To incorporate an automated refractor in a practice, one usually does not need to:
   a. Designate a staff person to be responsible for testing
   b. Provide more housing space
   c. Increase the capital cost
   d. Have a maintenance service agreement
   e. Have a large-volume practice

9. An accurate automated refraction result usually will be found in:
   a. A patient with moderate cataract
   b. Improper alignment of the patient's eyes
   c. High astigmatism (greater than 7 diopters)
   d. Macular degeneration
   e. Irregular corneal surface

ANSWERS, NOTES, AND EXPLANATIONS

1. **True.** To operate manual objective refractions, a person needs skill and time for the alignment and adjustment steps.

2. **False.** Automated objective refractors require little skill by the ophthalmic medical assistant. Skill is required when the patient is not aligned properly or moves during the testing procedure.

3. **True.** Some automated refractors have a subjective component in which the assistant will question the patient as to changes in vision. The instrument can add or subtract both sphere and cylinder to refine the prescription. This is considered a subjective refinement.

4. **Retinoscopy.** The automated refractors can give a beginning prescription for refinement on a

subjective basis. This simulates retinoscopy and becomes a starting point for refraction.

5. **Subjective.** Subjective testing is most important after using an automated objective refractor. The refractor provides only the starting point; one must still obtain individual responses to the given refractive finding.

6. **Subjective.** The word *subjective* means that the patient, who is the subject, has input into the final results.

7. **a. Large pupils.** Large pupils do not affect the result of the automated refractor. In fact, the opposite is true. Small pupils may yield no information, often because of misalignment.

8. **e. Have a large-volume practice.** Automated refractors can be valuable in any type of practice, whether it is small volume or large volume. They can provide a reference point similar to retinoscopy. The cost effectiveness may have to be questioned if the practice is relatively small.

9. **d. Macular degeneration.** Macular degeneration is a dysfunction of the cones present in the eye. The actual refractive error is not altered, although the vision is markedly reduced centrally. Consequently, the automated refractor usually provides reliable results as far as the refractive finding is concerned.

CHAPTER 12

Facts about glasses

- History
- Frames
- Dispensing spectacle frames
- Lenses
- Production of prescription lenses
- Care of glasses

Virtually every patient who enters an ophthalmologist's office receives a refraction, and most receive a prescription for spectacles. Thus the ophthalmic assistant should know something about the construction and types of spectacle frames and the types of lenses currently used. Despite an accurate prescription many patients are unhappy with their glasses because of the design, fit, or construction. Treatment of refractive errors of the eyes is finished only when patients have received glasses, can see 20/20 (6/6) with each eye, and find the design of the spectacles satisfactory in terms of their jobs, hobbies, and other needs. The purpose of this chapter is to provide a brief résumé of the types of optical appliances available to the patient, stressing the advantages and disadvantages of each.

HISTORY

The use of spectacles has its origin in ancient history. The first authentic record is a note written by Marco Polo when he visited the court of Kublai Khan in China in 1270. He noted that convex lenses were used by the aged to read fine print. In Europe the famous English Franciscan monk Roger Bacon was the first to recognize the value of convex lenses for those who were old or had weak sight.

The first primitive spectacles were balanced precariously on the nose, tied to the ears by means of thread or string, or held in the hand as one holds a present-day lorgnette. Their use was confined solely to monks and other learned men of the day. By the seventeenth century, spectacles were in common use and were elaborately fashioned of gold or silver for members of the aristocracy, whereas tortoiseshell frames were used by members of the upper middle class.

In 1784 Benjamin Franklin invented the bifocal by dividing his lenses for distance and near vision. The split parts were held together by the frame. Cemented bifocals were invented in 1884, then fused, and one-piece types followed in 1908.

In the early periods the optical glass was of poor quality and was made from scarce pebbles of quartz or semiprecious stones. The first high-quality glass was introduced for spectacle making in Europe, and the center of its manufacture was Venice. Not until the end of the nineteenth century, however, were spectacle lenses made of glass of high quality. Even as late as the early 1900s, spectacles were sold as merchandise, to be bought as one would buy a new coat or tie. A person would go to the spectacle maker's store and try a selection of spectacles already glazed with matching pairs of differently powered lenses, each of which was considered suitable for older persons.

Despite the improvements and refinements in the

manufacture and dispensing of frames, the final choice of the right set of spectacles is a personal one, derived not by any scientific formula but by the whims, fancies, and needs of the individual person.

FRAMES

Spectacles can be defined as an optical appliance comprised of lenses and a frame with sides, called *temples,* extending over the ears. The front, main part of the frame holds the actual lenses in front of the eyes, the pads give support on the nose, and the temples hold the front part in the correct position before the eyes. Frames may be either of metal or plastic, or a combination of metal and plastic.

Fig. 12-1 illustrates the anatomy of frames. Bridge size may be noted as distance between lenses (DBL), which should not be confused with the distance between the optical centers (DBC). Temples often are marked with the overall temple length expressed in either inches or millimeters. When two numbers are found on the temple, both overall length and length to the bend are given.

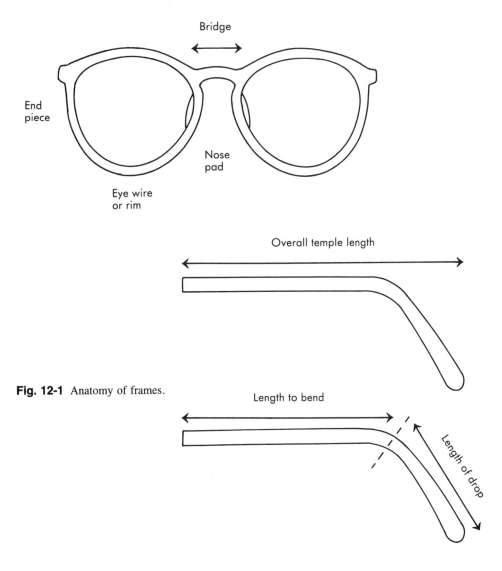

Fig. 12-1 Anatomy of frames.

Table 12-1   Metal frames: characteristics of the most common metal type of frames in current use

Material	Composition (%)	Features	Adjustment considerations
Nickel/silver	Nickel (18) Copper (64) Zinc (16)	Shock-resistant flexibility Suitable hardness for precision metal work Some anticorrosion	Cold bend tools Excess heat in solder- ing will weaken
Monel	Nickel (66) Copper (27) Various (7)	Harder than nickel/silver Very high heat resistance; no weakness from soldering Uses: bridge, temples, sometimes eye wire be- cause material is more rigid and stronger	Cold bend tools Monel and nickel/sil- ver solder well to- gether
High-nickel alloy	Nickel (85-90) Chrome (10-13)	10 times more expensive than nickel/silver Extremely hard; used in bridges and end pieces where pressure is high	Cold bend tools sol- derable
Stainless steel	Nickel (10) Iron (65) Chromium (19) plus carbon, manganese, phosphorus, sulfur (6)	Extremely flexible Extremely hard Can be made thinner, thus lighter Corrosion immunity	Cold bend tools Cannot be soldered by conventional means
Titanium	A silver-gray element alloyed with other elements	Maximum flexibility of materials used to date Extremely strong; can be made very thin High memory retention Lightest of all metals Immune to corrosion High heat resistance	Cold bend tools Cannot solder with existing techniques
Aluminum	Aluminum (96%) Alloyed with copper, sili- cone, iron, bronze, man- ganese, zinc, chromium	Lightest of all frame materials Must be made thicker to increase strength Poor corrosion resistance unless colored	Cold bend tools Excessive bending re- sults in weak spots and breakage
Bronze	Zinc (92) Tin (8)	Used only in temples High elasticity while retaining tensile strength Withstands bending	Cold bend tools Adjust at end piece

Metal frames

Originally, frames were designed and handmade of silver or solid gold for the aristocracy. These metals gradually have been replaced by other metals, such as gold-filled, nickel, and aluminum (Table 12-1).

Plastic frames

There are two types of plastic frames: (1) those molded to shape from *plastic materials* in an injection-molding machine and (2) higher-quality frames cut to shape from a flat piece of plastic, which is then machined and polished to form the finished frame.

The *higher-quality ophthalmic plastic frames* start as a flat sheet of plastic of the appropriate pattern or color. The frames are then cut to shape by machine and polished. All good ophthalmic plastic frames may be manipulated by applying heat to soften the material and shape it to conform to the face.

Ophthalmic frames are made of five types of plastic: (1) cellulose nitrate, (2) cellulose acetate, (3) Lucite, (4) nylon, and (5) a material called *Optyl*. Frames are made from precolored sheet stock, except those made of nylon and Optyl, which are created by injection-molding processes.

Cellulose nitrate (Celluloid, xylonite "XYZ") is now found only in a very few imported frames. This material will burn fiercely if a flame is brought into

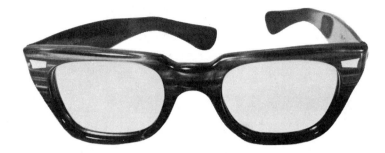

Fig. 12-2 Saddle-bridge frame.

contact with it. It is not used in modern plastic frames, and some states have passed laws forbidding the use of nitrate material for spectacle frames. Nitrate materials will become brittle, and clear nitrate tends to yellow with age.

Cellulose acetate is the most common plastic used today. Although it will burn if a flame is held in contact with the material, it is self-extinguishing; that is, if the flame is removed, the plastic will cease to burn. Cellulose acetate comes in various colors and patterns. Clear acetate will not change color or yellow with age, and acetate does not become brittle.

Lucite (Plexiglas, Perspex) is a much tougher plastic and is available in solid colors only (or two-tone or fade-away patterns, produced by laminating two colors). Once the frame is fitted, it retains its shape better than acetate or nitrate, and Lucite does not change color. Manipulation requires much more heat than do other materials.

Nylon frames are injection molded and thus of one solid color. Some types, however, also are dyed after completion to give the appearance of stock sheet materials also found in acetate. With age, the nylon frame becomes brittle.

With the development of *Optyl* in Austria in 1968, a whole new process of frame manufacturing emerged. The material is a thermosetting epoxy resin, which can soften when heated to 80° to 100° C. The frame is cast in vacuum molds, producing a neutral transparent product. The manufacturer then adds the required color to the finished frame by a secret dyeing process. The result is complete flexibility of color. The frames can be transparent, translucent, solid, in gradient shades, or even a wide variety of colors. The material is 30% lighter than acetate or nitrate and has a superior ability to stay in shape once fitted properly. Because of this memory, the plastic will return to its original position after some distortion by undue tension. The material is hypoallergenic because it is biologically inert, and it is excellent for those with contact allergies. It has better fire-resistant properties than acetate.

Advantages. The plastic frame is basically rigid, and it keeps its adjustment well, once fitted. The colors, patterns, and styles available in plastic are almost limitless. Most frames have fixed plastic pads that rest on the side of the nose.

Bridges. There are two basic types of bridge: the *saddle* (Fig. 12-2) and the *keyhole* (Fig. 12-3). The saddle bridge rests lower on the nose and creates the illusion of shortening a long nose. A keyhole bridge is more flattering to a round, short nose. Most plastic temples have a metal core for rigidity and strength. Some fronts are braced with metal, buried in the plastic, running across the top of the front from hinge to hinge. These frames are desirable for children and athletes.

Combination frames

A combination frame consists of a metal chassis with a decorative metal or plastic top and two fully adjustable pads (Fig. 12-4). The advantage of movable pads is that they can be moved in the up-and-down adjustment and backward and forward to fit the patient's face. Combination frames with movable pads are thus ideal for patients with cataracts and for high myopes, inasmuch as the distance of the lens from the eye can be accurately placed, as can the height

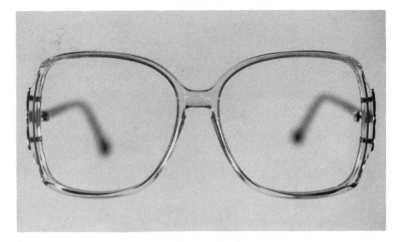

Fig. 12-3 Keyhole-bridge frame.

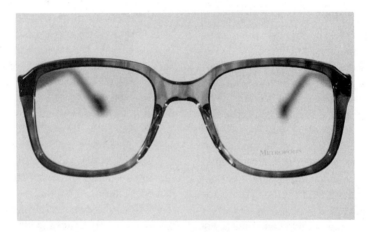

Fig. 12-4 Combination frame with adjustable pads.

of the bifocal or trifocal segment. In prescriptions for a heavy lens, such a frame should be ordered with jumbo pads—oversized plastic pads—which give a larger bearing surface on the nose and consequently have less tendency to leave marks.

Rimless frames

Rimless frames look much like combination frames in that there is a decorative top but no apparent metal holding the lens shape. Rimless frames may be of metal or plastic construction. In the case of plastic, there is actually a nylon cord fitted into a groove cut in the edge of the lens that holds the lens to the top. This nylon cord is almost invisible and gives the frame a rimless appearance.

In some metal rimless frames the lenses are held in position by hidden notches in the glass or optical plastic lenses. The notches are engaged by tabs protruding from the top but, when the frame is viewed from the front, out of sight behind the top.

Older-model rimless spectacles actually had holes drilled through the lenses and small nuts and bolts

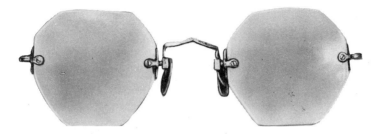

Fig. 12-5 Rimless frame.

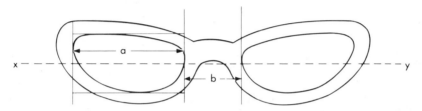

Fig. 12-6 Frame measurements. *a* represents the eye size; *b* represents the bridge size. The dotted line *xy* is the datum line.

placed through these holes to hold the lenses in position (Fig. 12-5). This type of rimless frame was easily shattered when dropped and therefore is now practical only when plastic lenses are used.

Frame measurements

Most frame measurements are based on the box system, whereby the lens is enclosed in a rectangle and the distances between opposite sides are taken as the eye size.

On the back of a frame are a few figures, such as 46 × 22, which represent the size of the bridge and the eyepiece (Fig. 12-6). The distance *a* is the *eye size,* that is, 46 mm; the distance *b* is the *bridge size* of 22. All measurements are in millimeters. The dotted line *xy* represents an imaginary line running through the center of the lenses and is called the *datum line*. This is a very important line, because all measurements are taken at this point.

The other measurements are for the temples; they vary according to the use for which the glasses are intended and the consequent shape of the temples.

Temples

The temple is the long strut that extends from the lateral aspect of the eyepiece and rests on the ear. The temple length (e.g., 140 mm) is expressed as the overall length from the hinge end to the end that rests behind the ears.

Several varieties of temples are available. The more commonly-used types are considered here.

Cable temples (Fig. 12-7, *A*). Cable temples sometimes are known as *riding bow* temples or *curl side* temples. The cable temple is either metal or plastic, with the ear portion made of a flexible metal that can be shaped to fit the contour behind the ear. Another type of riding bow temple has a much stiffer metal core covered with plastic. A comfortable fit is possible only when this temple is contoured to the back of the ear. This type of temple is ideal for children and active persons, and for those who are constantly looking down, or positions in which the spectacles might otherwise slide off the face.

Straight temples (Fig. 12-7, *B*). Straight temples sometimes are called *library* temples. They may be

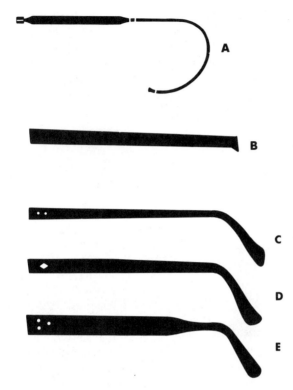

Fig. 12-7 A, Cable, riding bow, or curl side temples. **B,** Straight or library temples. **C** to **E,** Paddle, skull, or hockey-end temples.

plastic or metal and are bowed to fit around the sides of the head. These are ideal for persons who constantly take their glasses off and for those in religious orders whose ears are concealed under a habit, making it difficult to put on or take off glasses that have riding bow or other paddle temples.

Paddle temples (Fig. 12-7, *C* to *E*). Paddle temples are sometimes called *skull* temples or *hockey-end* temples. They may be made of plastic or metal, and the ends are angled. These temples are ideal for general use and are the most common type used today.

Specialty frames

Frame manufacturers produce a number of frames for most persons with standard eye sizes and bridge sizes. This leaves a small proportion of the population with unusual facial measurements unable to obtain a correct fit with the commercially produced frames. Fortunately some optical companies will hand make frames for this group and will produce frames for special vocational or medical requirements. A few of these are mentioned here.

Frames for infants and Orientals. Because Oriental persons and infants have practically no bridge to their noses, the ordinary plastic frame fits too low on the face and is so close to the eyes that the lenses interfere with the eyelashes. A handmade frame with special nose construction can be made to look like a standard frame yet have the necessary low-set and thickened portion to the bridge so that the spectacles can be properly adjusted in front of the patient's eyes. Before this development, such patients had to be fitted with frames that had adjustable pads to raise the frame and move it away from the face.

Hemianopic glasses. In homonymous hemianopia, one half the field of vision is lost on the same side (right or left) in both eyes, and the blind area becomes a danger to the patient so afflicted. There are two types of hemianopic glasses available. One incorporates a small side-view mirror mounted on the nose of the spectacle frame, reflecting objects from the blind area into that portion of the vision that still remains. The patient therefore is aware of some motion on the blind side and can turn his or her head to see it. A second type uses a beam-splitting filter lens (a semitransparent type of mirror), hinged at the bridge of the nose so that it can be adjusted by the patient. With a beam splitter, reflected images take on a pink hue, but objects looked at through the mirror are gray. Because this mirror is as large as the eyewire of the frame, it gives results superior to the small side-view mirror, which is the older of the two designs.

Side shields. There are conditions, such as an anesthetic cornea or a "dry eye," for which it is necessary to enclose the eye between the frame and the face. There are many ways of doing this, but most side-shield constructions are not attractive and usually are bulky, hard, and poor fitting. With the use of a soft, transparent plastic a shield can be produced and trimmed with a pair of scissors to exactly fit the individual patient. An added bonus is that it is almost invisible, and being soft and pliable it does not in-

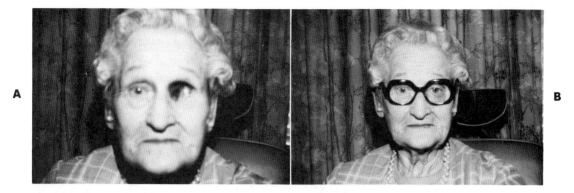

Fig. 12-8 A, Exenteration of orbit after a malignancy. **B,** Spectacle frames support a matching prosthesis.

terfere with the glasses being folded up in the standard manner.

Floating fronts. Some patients who require a refractive correction need a pair of glasses that does not touch the front of the face at all. Temple-grip glasses can be provided for this purpose. These are designed so that the transparent paddle that gently rests on the temples is at the point of balance of the frame, and consequently movement of the head does not cause the glasses to ride up or down.

Ptosis crutch. Although the ideal solution in the case of ptosis is an operation, there may be contraindications to surgery. Frames can be fitted with a ptosis crutch, which is a small piece of wire or plastic affixed to the inside of a spectacle frame. This wire can be adjusted to raise the eyelids of the patient so afflicted.

Frames to support prostheses. Frames may be used to support an artificial prosthesis combined with full upper and lower eyelids and socket. Fig. 12-8, *A,* shows a patient who had an orbital malignancy with complete extenteration of the orbit and eyelids. She was rehabilitated by using spectacles that supported a matching prosthesis (Fig. 12-8, *B*).

DISPENSING SPECTACLE FRAMES

It is important that spectacles are produced so that the patient, when viewing distance objects, looks through the *optical centers* of both lenses. Consequently it is essential to know the distance between the visual axis through the pupils of the patient, so that the lenses may be correctly mounted in the spectacle frame at the same interpupillary distance. The term *pupillary distance* is abbreviated *PD*.

Unfortunately the visual axis through the human eye does not pass, as one might expect, through the center of the pupil but varies from patient to patient and is on the nasal side of the pupil. Therefore any mechanical device that measures from the center of the pupil of one eye to the center of the pupil of the second eye will give a measurement greater than the actual distance between the visual axes of the two eyes.

This error is of little significance if the prescription is a weak one. For high myopes and cataract patients who have binocular aphakia, however, a few millimeters of error will produce a decidedly uncomfortable pair of glasses.

Because it is difficult to assess the visual axis, or the center of the pupil, the practice is to measure (if both pupils are the same size) from the nasal edge of the pupil on the patient's right eye to the temporal side of the pupil on the patient's left eye (Figs. 12-9 and 12-10).

Two PDs are taken, one for distance, where the visual axes are parallel, and one for near, which is the close working distance of the patient.

There is only one accurate method of measuring PD—the light reflex method—the result of which gives the distance between the visual axes of the two eyes, rather than the distance between the center of one pupil to the center of the other. The difference

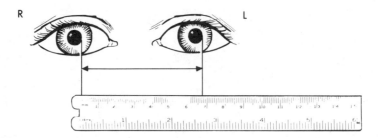

Fig. 12-9 Measurement of pupillary distance. Measurements are made from the nasal edge of one pupil to the temporal edge of the other pupil.

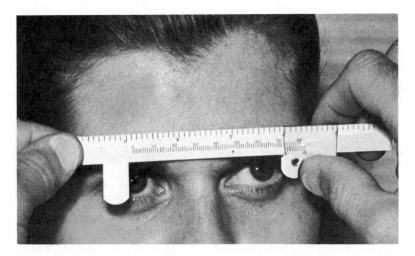

Fig. 12-10 Measuring pupillary distance.

between the two methods of measurement may be 2 to 5 mm. There are many optical interpupillary gauges that can give the measurement from pupil to pupil very accurately for distance vision; the PD can then be converted for near vision by means of tables. There is one gauge on the market today that uses the accurate reflex method (Fig. 12-11).

Special considerations in measuring PD include the following:

1. If the patient has pupils of different size and the standard method with a PD rule is to be used, the measurements should be made from the nasal side of the limbus of the patient's right eye to the temporal side of the limbus on the other, ignoring the measurements from the pupil.

2. If the patient can see from only one eye, the measurement can be taken for the good eye from the center of the bridge of the nose to the center of the pupil, because an inaccuracy of a few millimeters one way or the other has no significance.

3. If the patient has a squint, the measurement can be taken from the inner canthus of one eye to the outer canthus of the opposite eye, giving a reasonably accurate PD. A better way is to occlude the turning eye and measure from the center of the bridge of the nose to the center of the uncovered eye and then repeat with the other eye covered. The sum of the two measurements is the PD.

The PD is taken so that the optical centers of the lenses will be directly in front of the visual axes through the pupils (Fig. 12-12). If the optical centers are not so placed, an unwanted prism is incorporated in the glasses.

The *optical center* can be defined as the thinnest

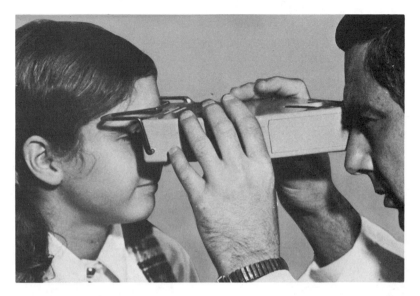

Fig. 12-11 Measuring pupillary distance by pupillary gauge.

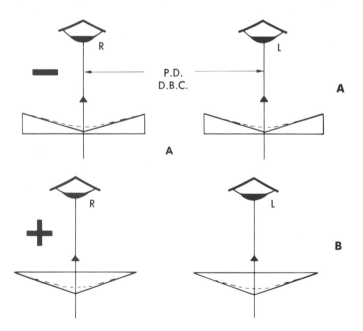

Fig. 12-12 A, Minus, or concave, lens. Optical center is at its thinnest part. **B,** Plus, or convex, lens. Optical center is at its thickest part. *P.D.,* Pupillary distance; *D.B.C.,* distance between centers of lenses.

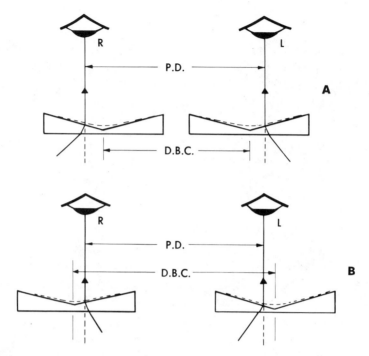

Fig. 12-13 A, Prism base-out effect is created by inward displacement of the optical centers of two concave lenses. **B,** Prism base-in effect is created by outward displacement of the optical centers of two concave lenses. *P.D.,* Pupillary distance; *D.B.C.,* distance between centers of lenses.

part in the center of any minus lens or the thickest part of the center of a plus lens. Only at the optical center do rays of light go through the lens without bending. To make this clearer, a minus lens can be represented by two prisms, bases out, and a plus lens, base in. When these lenses have their centers in line with the visual axes, they are correctly positioned in front of the patient's eyes (Fig. 12-13).

If the PD is wrong and the lenses are off center, the vision is bent by the lenses toward the base of the prism in each case, and the object would appear to be displaced laterally. The eyes would have to turn in or out to try to correct this, causing discomfort to the patient. If the lenses are high power, plus or minus, so much prism can be introduced that double vision will result. In the case of a cataract lens of + 10.00 diopters, if the PD is out 1 mm, 1.00 diopter of prism that has not been prescribed is introduced into the prescription.

Measuring PD with a ruler and the reflex method

The following equipment is required:

1. Small PD rule, graduated in millimeters
2. Pinpoint of light, such as a bare bulb of an ophthalmoscope battery handle or a penlight

To take a *distance PD,* the procedure is as follows.

1. Sit approximately 16 to 18 inches from the patient to be examined.
2. Hold the light source immediately under your left eye. Place the PD rule across the bridge of the patient's nose so that it will extend to cover the lower half of both pupils.
3. Make sure the patient looks directly at the light bulb.
4. Place the zero mark of the ruler on the pinpoint reflection of the light on the cornea. Use your left eye for this purpose.
5. Without disturbing the PD ruler, and without the

patient moving the head, move the light to a position underneath your right eye.

6. Make sure the patient is still looking at the light.
7. Note the measurement on the PD rule of the reflection of the light on the cornea of the patient's left eye. (In doing this you will observe that the pinpoint of light is not in the center of the pupil, but at some point nasally of center. The measurement is an accurate one of the distance between the visual axes of the two eyes [incorrectly termed the distance PD for want of a better term].)
8. Note the measurement at the center of the nose (this may be useful if the patient's face is grossly asymmetric).

Obtaining the *PD for near* is done in a similar manner, but the distance between the patient's eyes and the observer's eyes should be adjusted to the appropriate near distance. (It varies from person to person and from occupation to occupation.) The observer proceeds as before. Then the light is placed under one eye, and the patient looks at the light. A measurement is taken with the PD rule from the reflection on the cornea of one eye to the reflection on the cornea of the other eye, without moving the light. This will be the "near" PD.

Spectacle frames often have to be chosen for their physical advantages in supporting lenses that are required. The heavier the lenses, the greater the distribution of weight on the nose. The new technology that has made possible a larger selection of eye fashion may limit the choice of frames for the high myope and the aphake.

Spectacle frames should also provide cosmetic enhancement to the wearer. The design of the frame should take into consideration the contours of the face. In persons with unusually long faces, frames that are noticeably longer horizontally than vertically are very effective in reducing the long appearance of the face. An unusually long nose can optically be diminished by a low-fitting bridge bar. Dark colors accentuate this shortening effect. A small nose can be made to look longer by a slender bridge bar set high up or a keyhole bridge. Frames that are greater in depth at their outer ends than at their middle help to make eyes that are too closely set together appear

to be more widely separated; the opposite type of frame helps to mitigate the effect of eyes that are set unusually wide apart. Thus an illusion of wide-set eyes can be created by having the frame color fade away at the bridge.

Brightly colored frames complement the natural tones of a light-haired individual, whereas darkly colored frames blend better with a dark complexion. Dark-colored frames draw attention to nose width and should be avoided by persons with very narrow or very wide noses.

The actual choice of frames or style is highly personal. A variety of frames is available for both indoor and outdoor sports, for motoring, and for business and social occasions.

The frames should hold both lenses firmly in a direction perpendicular to the visual axes because tilting can introduce optical errors that may be considerable in lenses of high power. Glasses for distance should sit vertically, whereas glasses for reading should be slightly lowered and tilted downward. The frames should be comfortable at all times and cause no irritation of the skin on which they rest, and the lenses should be as close to the eyes as possible without touching the eyelashes.

LENSES

Spectacle lenses are made from either plastic or a high-quality glass. Most single-vision lenses are made up in a curved form rather than the flat form (Fig. 12-14).

Although many types of glass are used for optical purposes, the primary glass used for ophthalmic lenses is a *crown glass* of 1.523 refractive index. Exacting demands are required in its manufacture because the lens must be perfectly homogeneous—free of flaws, bubbles, and irregularities on its surface. *Flint glass* with a refractive index of 1.62 is used when a higher refractive index is desired, as in the making of bifocal or achromatic lenses. Flint glass contains lead, which is absent from crown glass.

The highest-index glass available today is *Hidex* (1.806). The lenses used for persons with high myopia or hyperopia are remarkably thin. High-index glass is very compatible with antireflection coating,

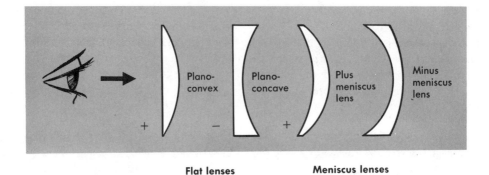

Flat lenses   **Meniscus lenses**

Fig. 12-14 Types of lenses. Meniscus lenses are designed with a base curve.

giving a superior effect to the appearance of crown glass. For obvious reasons, such glasses are not possible in fused bifocal form. The glass is a complete barrier to x-rays. It is heavier than crown glass, but because the lenses are thinner than crown glass for a given prescription, the net increase in weight of the lenses is slight.

Plastic lenses are about half the weight of glass and are highly impact-resistant. With a center thickness of 3.0 mm they can be considered as safety glasses without special hardening techniques. Plastic lenses have a thicker profile than does glass, scratch more easily, and do not protect the eye from ultraviolet light unless properly tinted. Glass lenses, unlike plastic, must be treated to resist breakage. They can be hardened by chemical processes or by heat.

Corrected lenses

Each manufacturer has an individualized series of base curves for toric meniscus lenses. In theory the inside curve, to give a "perfect" lens with no distortions, should have a radius that coincides with the radius of the rotating eyeball. Thus there would be the same vertex distance between the cornea and the spectacles no matter which way the eye turned behind the spectacles. This would give undistorted vision from edge to edge. However, if glasses were made in this way, the front surface of a high plus lens would be so bulbous and thick, and the lens would be of such a small diameter, that it would never fill the spectacle frame. It would be cosmetically unacceptable. Therefore all manufacturers'

"corrected" lenses are truly corrected only in the weaker powers. Beyond 5.00 diopters, plus or minus, no lens other than an aspheric lens is a "corrected" one.

A corrected lens is a compromise designed to avoid or minimize the distortions created through the edges of an ophthalmic lens. These distortions include the following:

1. *Chromatic aberration,* in which white light is broken up into its spectral components and observed as color fringes.
2. *Spherical aberration,* in which a lens fails to focus a broad beam to a single point.
3. *Distortion,* which is an aberration that causes objects to appear in other than their true shape. With strong concave lenses, the square is distorted to barrel shape; with plus or convex lenses, the square is distorted to a pincushion shape (Fig. 12-15). Distortion occurs when the eye looks toward the periphery of a lens. It is overcome chiefly by using deeply curved lenses, high *base curves,* or aspheric lenses.
4. *Astigmatism,* which occurs when an oblique ray of light strikes a spherical surface. This type of astigmatism also is reduced to a minimum by deeply curved lenses.

Corrected lenses have many designs. There are meniscus lenses, which generally are ground on a 6.00-diopter base curve. A toric lens is curved like a meniscus lens but also contains a cylinder that formerly was ground on a convex surface in single-vision glass lenses and on a concave surface in bi-

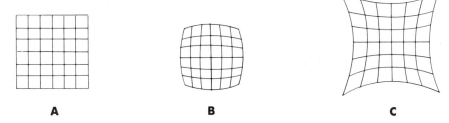

Fig. 12-15 A, Normal square pattern. **B,** Strong concave lenses distort a square to a barrel shape. **C,** Strong convex lenses distort a square to a pincushion shape.

focals. In plastic lenses the cylinder is on the concave surface. Most modern cylindric lenses have the cylinder on the concave side and are referred to as *minus cylinder lenses.*

Aphakic lenses

Today modern surgery involves inserting an intraocular lens so that the thick aphakic spectacle is no longer required. The new condition is called *pseudophakia,* in which a cataract is removed and an intraocular lens implanted. There are, however, still several thousand persons of an age at which a cataract was removed by the intracapsular route without an implant. These patients still wear either contact lenses or aphakic spectacles. The aphakic spectacles have a distortion inherent in their manufacture because of the strong correction. To avoid these distortions, special lens designs have been created to minimize both the distortions and the weight of these lenses. The types most commonly used are (1) lenticular lenses, (2) aspheric lenses, (3) hard-resin (plastic) lenses, and (4) combinations of 1, 2, and 3.

Lenticular lenses. The lenticular lens may be described as a small-diameter, circular or oval prescription lens (too small to fit a modern frame) mounted on a longer-diameter, thin planocarrier, which is edged to fit the frame (Fig. 12-16). The resulting lenticular lens weighs less and is thinner than a full-sized lens of the same power.

The main disadvantage of the lenticular lens is that it gives a bull's-eye effect, making it more conspicuous than the full-sized lens. Decentration of a

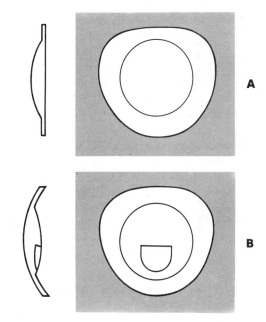

Fig. 12-16 A, Lenticular lens, single vision. **B,** Lenticular bifocal lens. Note that the periphery of the lens is ground off.

full-sized lens creates a heavy prismatic shape and heavy physical weight.

Aspheric lenses. A standard plus lens suitable for a patient who has had a cataract operation may be optically correct through its center, but it gives a progressively stronger effect as the patient's vision moves away from the center to the edge of the lens. This increase in plus power toward the edge, re-

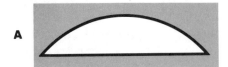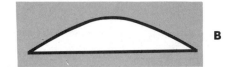

Fig. 12-17 A, Spherical lens, side view. **B,** Aspheric lens, side view. Note the flatter curve in the periphery of the lens. This eliminates many of the aberrations of the periphery of the lens and permits a greater field of vision.

sulting from an increase in vertex distance, causes the pincushion distortions previously mentioned, as well as blurred vision in these areas. Therefore, if a lens is ground with correct power at the center and a drop-off of power toward the edges, distortions and blurring of vision are eliminated or at least minimized. This is the aspheric lens, which is available in glass and in plastic (Fig. 12-17).

An aspheric lens is designed to eliminate the pincushion distortions of the aphakic patient who wears a strong plus lens.

Plastic lenses. Plastic lenses are made from a very high-quality synthetic resin and have the same qualities as glass but only half the weight. They are also highly impact-resistant and are rated as *safety lenses*. They have a cosmetic disadvantage, being thicker than equivalent glass lenses in the higher prescriptions. Plastic lenses are not quite as resistant to scratching as glass, but some manufacturers are now applying a coating on the plus (outside) surface to make them more scratch resistant. There are two types of plastic lenses: the original plastic lens, made of methylmethacrylate, and the modern hard-resin lens. The modern lens, made of allyl diglycol carbonate, is much harder and more resistant to scratches and can be ground the same way as glass lenses. Because of their lightness, plastic lenses are highly advantageous in prescriptions requiring high-powered lenses. Most of the cataract lenses today are of hard resin and not glass.

Safety lenses

No glass lens yet devised is shatterproof. However, glass can be treated to resist blows of tremendous force, and should glass safety lenses break, they would crumble into "hailstones" with no sharp splinters to lacerate the eye.

Plastic hard-resin lenses. These can be considered to be safety lenses with no additional treatment, because they will take abuse much greater than that required to shatter a standard glass lens. A shattered hard-resin lens does not have the sharp splinters typical of broken glass. Hard-resin lenses are superior to hardened glass for welding, where hot metal may splatter on the lens.

Polycarbonate lenses. First introduced in plano-safety goggles for industry, polycarbonate lenses are by far the most impact-resistant lenses now on the market. In this regard they outperform plastic and glass heat-treated or chemically-treated lenses. The material, however, is soft and flexible and thus prone to scratches. Polycarbonate is now being molded into ophthalmic prescription lenses that are coated to substantially reduce their tendency to scratch.

Heat-treated impact-resistant glass lenses. Today the emphasis is on discouraging glass and recommending plastic for patient safety. However, when these lenses are used in industry, they are made of the standard ophthalmic glass; the only prerequisite is that the lens must not be less than 3 mm thick at its thinnest point. For general wear (as in sports or for children) the minimum thickness is 2.2 mm. The lens must be ground, polished, and edged to fit the frame before hardening. The lens is not "case hardened"; that is, the surface is no tougher after treatment than before. It is therefore no more resistant to scratching after treatment than before. Industrial impact-resistant lenses will withstand a blow from a 1-inch steel ball dropped from a height of 50 inches (Fig. 12-18).

The finished lens is heated in an oven almost to its melting or softening point, removed, and then rapidly cooled by blasts of cold air on both surfaces simultaneously. The surfaces cool and contract faster

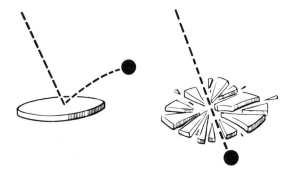

Fig. 12-18 Safety lens on the left does not shatter when a steel ball is dropped on its surface.

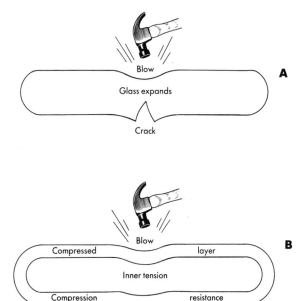

Fig. 12-19 Effect of tempering a glass lens to prevent breakage. **A,** Untreated lens. **B,** Treated lens. A firm outer compressed layer of glass is created by heat. This compressed layer prevents the lens from breaking at a point opposite that of the impact.

than the interior of the lens. Eventually the interior of the lens cools and contracts and pulls the surface of the glass lens into a compression condition (balanced by tension in the interior).

Glass is very strong in compression but pulls apart easily in tension. When one strikes a pane of glass, it does not shatter on the side that is struck. The bending force of the blow exerts itself as a tension (pulling apart) on the opposite side to that struck, and the glass breaks (Fig. 12-19).

A blow on the surface of the heat-treated lens (creating the bending force) must be great enough to overcome the compression of the opposite surface and must then put this surface under enough tension to tear the lens apart. Thickness plays a part, and in the criteria of the American National Standards Institute (ANSI) a minimum of 2 mm at the optical center and 1 mm on the edge is advised.

All heat-treated glass lenses may be identified by the fact that they unpolarize polarized light. The polariscope is an instrument used to identify an impact-resistant lens. This device consists of two sheets of polarizing filters set with their axes at right angles. Thus no light comes through the combination of the two filters. Inserting the treated lens between the filters upsets the polarized light so that a pattern is now seen through the combination of the filters and the spectacle lens. The shape (Maltese cross) of the pattern seen is no indication of the strength of the lens.

Some glasses on the market are labeled "toughened lenses." These are heat-treated, "hardened"

lenses that will withstand blows that would shatter ordinary glass. They are not treated to the point where they would be labeled safety glasses and should not be considered as such.

Another type of safety lens is the *laminated lens,* in which a sheet of plastic is sandwiched between the two pieces of glass. If the lens is shattered, the glass particles adhere to the plastic. These laminated lenses are seldom used today, except for polarized lenses.

Another type of impact-resistant lens is popular. A *chemical treatment* is employed that results in a lens with far superior impact-resistant qualities to those produced by the heat-treating method. The chemical hardening process consists of placing the finished glass lens in a hot solution of a potassium salt for about 14 hours. In that time the sodium ions in the glass are replaced by potassium ions (which are physically larger than the sodium). During cooling, the potassium ions place the surface into a state of compression, which gives an impact-resistant property to the lens.

Unlike the heat-treated lens, this process cannot be detected by polarized light. Failing other indications that the lens has been chemically treated, the drop-ball test is the only way to check such a lens!

Safety lenses are recommended for all children, persons engaged in sports, and industrial workers.

The role of protective lenses in sports

For individuals who do skeet shooting, there is the risk of being hit by ricochet pellets glancing from targets. Broken pieces from clay targets can careen from the flight path and strike the shooter. Game hunters may risk eye injury directly from tree branches or from pellets deflected off rocks or tree branches and even from the stray shots of other hunters when hunting in heavy grouse or woodcock cover. All shooters should be aware of the danger of blow-back that results from a defective shell or gun. Pieces of lead or copper jacketing can sail back to endanger shooters. For shooting range officials and spectators, eye protection is essential.

In the shooting sports, tints may be required. Polycarbonate today provides the best protection but lacks the optical clarity in the range of tintability required by shooters. The object of the lens coloration is to develop contrast between the target or game and the background. In trap and skeet shooting, there are four basic colors of clay targets—white, black, yellow, and fluorescent orange. To see these when thrown under different light conditions, colored lenses are needed to bring out the color of the target against the sky. Thus the serious shooter should own more than one pair of glasses to select interchangeable lenses in shooting frames. Shooting lenses should be in light to medium shades so that the pupils will contract more and give a greater depth of focus. Lenses may be coated but can still transmit 99.9% of the light to give the sharpest image possible. In overcast weather conditions, light scattered by water particles in the atmosphere produces a blue coloration. This blue dominance tends to compress the chromatic range and flatten color. The most negative effect on vision is that the blue light is not well focused on the retina but rather

in front of it. As the level of blue light increases, visual acuity decreases. Lenses with a light gold or amber color will neutralize the blue effect on overcast days. Skeet shooting or hunting ducks early in the morning or late in the evening requires the use of a high transmission lens that permits maximum light transfer.

Hockey is another high-risk sport in which there is a likelihood of sustaining eye injuries with permanent loss of vision. In 1974 there were 257 eye injuries in amateur sports in Canada, in which 17% caused legal blindness. Through efforts of safety committees, manufacturers began developing certified face protectors, which resulted in a marked decrease of injuries to the eye. All nonprofessional players are now required to wear these protective masks that meet the safety standards.

In racquet sports, more than 700 serious eye injuries have been reported in the past 10 years. Through efforts of Drs. Pashby and Easterbrook, eye guards have been developed that withstand the impact of a ball traveling up to 144 kilometers an hour. These guards must have full lenses and must not obstruct the player's peripheral view. Attention is now focusing on developing shields for badminton players because the badminton birds can travel at speeds up to 217 kilometers an hour.

By far the most popular protective lenses are polycarbonate lenses. As mentioned previously, these are impact-resistant and outperform plastic, glass-heated, and chemically treated lenses.

Antireflection (no-glare) coating

Artificial office light and computer video display terminals can cause reflections in untreated glass and create ghost images. This is particularly true with high-index glasses. When light passes through a spectacle lens, some is reflected by the front and the back surface of the lens. Street lights in the driver's field of view may be duplicated or triplicated. Coat the lens and only one image is seen.

Coating a lens with magnesium fluoride—one fourth of the wavelength of yellow-green light—is sometimes referred to as *blooming* a lens. The name comes from the distinctive purplish sheen, similar to the bloom on a ripe plum, that is seen on the surface of the lens. All camera lenses and optical instrument lenses are bloomed to cut out internal reflections and permit greater light transmission through the glass.

Coating is placed on a finished ophthalmic lens in a vacuum. Magnesium fluoride is heated in a crucible and "fumed" onto both surfaces of the lens. This material is very tough and usually lasts the life of the lens.

The coating, one quarter of a wavelength of yellow-green light, works by causing the reflection of light off the front and back surfaces of the *coating* to be out of step exactly one-half wavelength; thus the waves cancel each other out and the reflection is not there. The reflections that *are* seen are from the red and the purple ends of the spectrum, giving the bloomed color in reflection.

Almost all lens coatings are not multicoatings. These coatings, which are almost invisible, eliminate the red and the blue end of the spectrum. The multicoated lenses require special cleaners and antistatic and antifog solutions, as well as a very fine wiping cloth. Hard-resin lenses are commercially available, and they too can be coated.

Sunglasses and tinted lenses

By use of the appropriate chemicals, white glass lenses may be color coated almost any shade or color, or even mirrored. If a mask of appropriate shape is placed between the fuming crucible and the lens, a gradient color or gradient mirror coating can be produced. Popular colors available commercially are green, neutral gray, brown, rose, and transparent (one-way) mirror surfaces.

Color coating of ophthalmic lenses gives an even coloring across the whole surface of the lens, whether it is a strong plus or a strong minus lens. The coating, whether it is antireflection, mirror, or color, may be removed chemically in about 10 seconds, should this be necessary.

Almost all sunglasses are white lenses coated to the chosen color. However, colored-glass lenses are still available that are perfectly satisfactory for plano or weak prescriptions. If the prescription is a high plus, then the color of the glass is darker at the center than at the edges. Conversely, a high minus lens

would have a center light spot. Before the advent of the coating process, evenly spread color was obtained by laminating a colored plano lens to a clear prescription lens—an expensive process that is no longer necessary.

Plastic colored lenses are clear lenses dyed the appropriate color. Therefore they have an even color no matter how strong the prescription may be. Gradient tints, or even several colors on the same lens, can be produced.

Neutral gray tint has been the most popular color for sunglasses in North America for almost half a century. Because of its neutral absorption of all colors of the visible spectrum, light intensity is reduced without color distortion or imbalance—a very important factor when proper color perception is essential—for instance, a pilot having to read various colored dials, gauges, or maps; a telephone lineman distinguishing between color-coded telephone wires; a driver who might have difficulties differentiating colors of traffic signals; a participant or spectator at a sporting event where each team is denoted by the color of their uniforms; a naturalist watching birds, animals, or flowers. The list could go on. In short, gray lenses should be recommended whenever a patient wants protection from intensive light or glare without loss of color differentiation.

A green lens will absorb most of the ultraviolet and infrared light, and transmission peaks roughly at the same point as the luminous curve of the eye. Naturally, violet, blue, orange, or red colors are less distinguishable. Green lenses are recommended for situations with high amounts of reflected light (which will contain large amounts of ultraviolet), such as glaciers and open water. They should be recommended for vacations in the tropics and for use during hot weather to protect against (heat) rays. In industry, green lenses of various densities are used for welding and other high light and heat situations. They also have the psychologic effect of "coolness" during hot weather and thus provide comfort to the wearer.

For many years brown tints were very popular in Europe. Brown-tinted lenses are now being dispensed more commonly in North America. As can be seen by the graph of the spectrophotometer, brown lenses will absorb almost all of the ultraviolet and have a very even progressive curve throughout the visible spectrum. Brown lenses are most useful in moderate-to-cold climates to protect against ultraviolet radiation and excessive radiation with the added benefit of creating a "warm" visual environment. Three different tints of brown are available in either glass or plastic lenses.

Except for the cobalt blue lenses that are being used to judge the temperature in a blast furnace, blue-colored lenses are more a whim of fashion than eye protection.

Yellow-tinted lenses are good absorbers of ultraviolet, violet, and blue. Suppressing this area of the spectrum will enhance contrast in the rest of the visible spectrum. A yellow lens therefore is preferred to increase contrast in marginal light conditions, such as hunting at dawn or dusk or driving in foggy conditions, but should not be worn to protect against excessive light.

Other tints, such as pink, purple, and mauve, are deviants of the aforementioned tints and are used mainly as fashion accents.

Cheap sunglasses, usually in injection-molded plastic frames, are sold widely. These are not ground and polished lenses, although they may appear to be. Some lenses are plastic and can be identified as such by "bending" the lens in the frame.

Cheap sunglasses are produced from flat, colored-glass sheets of low quality. Circles are cut from the flat sheet, and each circle is placed in a metal concave dish having a curve of about 4.00 diopters. The dish is placed in an oven and left until the glass sags, or "drops," to the shape of the dish. The "lens" now has the shape of a ground lens. Lenses made in this manner are called "dropped lenses" and may be identified as such by (1) the shallow curve, (2) the distortions of objects *reflected* on the surface of the lens, and (3) usually some unwanted and unprescribed power. A properly ground and polished lens will show no distortions of reflected light and is usually on a base curve of about 6.00 diopters.

A popular type of sunglass on the market is the polarized sunglass. Such lenses usually are made of plastic but sometimes are found in a laminated form, in which the polarizing filter is sandwiched between two sheets of glass. Polarized sunglasses are available in prescription form.

Apart from the color of the lens, the axis of the polarizing material is placed in the frames so that glare coming off a flat horizontal surface is further darkened. The glasses are good for driving into the sun, because a white, glaring highway will appear dark. Persons who fish or go boating find that glare off water is reduced considerably. In rough-surfaced areas, such as grass, they are no improvement over tinted lenses.

The American Academy of Ophthalmology has suggested some guidelines for consumers to follow when purchasing sunglasses (see box, p. 265).

Densities. In dispensing tinted lenses, it is important to know the light conditions and environment the lenses are going to be used in. Lenses that are too dark will dilate the pupil, and visual acuity will be reduced. Should light intensity vary rapidly, such as driving in bright sunlight through shaded areas, driving could be impaired. Therefore very dark lenses may be recommended only for sailors, fishermen, and hikers. Naturally, for driving long distances through prairies and urban areas, a dark shade will be most comfortable.

Providing a medium tint with a gradient mirror will give the patient an opportunity to select the density according to the prevailing light conditions. Naturally, in this respect, the photochromic lenses fill a specific void in the eye protection field. Their ability to adapt to the varying light intensities has made them one of the most sought-after lens material. Unfortunately, they are not as yet available in higher-index glass or in a sunglass tint in plastic.

Photochromic (indoor-outdoor) glasses. Photochromic lenses have the chameleon-like ability to change from light to dark and back again. The silver halide microcrystals in the glass, which impart this changeability, never wear out. The halides darken when exposed to ultraviolet or the blue end of the spectrum. These lenses help the light-sensitive patient. The range of the darkening of photosensitive glass has been developed to the point where a pair

---

TIPS ON PURCHASING SUNGLASSES

1. Ultraviolet (UV) absorption. Check for the manufacturer's label indicating whether the sunglasses are UV absorbent and if they meet the American National Standards Institute's guideline for eyewear.
2. The color of the lens and the darkness of the tint are not good indicators of the glasses' ability to filter out UV light. Lens color should cause as little color distortion as possible. Dark gray or dark green tints permit the most normal color vision.
3. The price of a pair of sunglasses is absolutely no indicator of their ability to absorb UV light.
4. Polarized lenses tend to reduce reflection and glare and are especially effective around water and snow.
5. Photochromic lenses change color in response to sunlight, often preventing the need for two pairs of prescription glasses. These lenses, however, may not change quickly enough to accommodate comfortable transition between inside light and bright outdoor light. In addition, they may appear dark for a short while when one comes from outdoors to indoors.
6. Special coatings are available, which are UV absorbers, and can be applied to everyday glasses. These often are applied to glasses used for skiing, high-altitude flying, and outdoor sports.
7. The FDA requires that all eyeglass lenses, including sunglasses, be made of impact-resistant glass or plastic. The frames also must be nonflammable. This does not mean that the lenses are shatterproof but that they can withstand moderately sharp impacts.

---

of glasses can be a perfectly clear lens indoors and a satisfactory sunglass outdoors. The average sunglass is designed to permit 85% of the visible light to be filtered out by the lens, but the clear photosensitive indoor-outdoor glass darkens only to the point where 15% of the light is filtered out—not really dark enough when compared with standard sunglasses.

The cycling of the modern photochromic glass requires 60 seconds for the lenses to darken. They lighten less rapidly. The range of dark to light is greater in cold weather (winter skiing) than in hot (summer beach wear).

Ultraviolet and blue-blocking lenses

Through-and-through tinted lenses that filter out over 98% of blue and ultraviolet light were developed by Corning Glassworks and Younger Optics. The latter are made in C39 plastic. These lenses, which range in color from amber to red, are called plastic CPF by Corning and PLS by Younger. They are photochromic in that they darken outdoors and lighten indoors. For the normal individual these lenses provide comfort from glare, reduce haziness, and

sharpen vision. The light-colored CPF lenses (CPF 511, CPF 527, and PLS 530) may aid persons with developing cataracts, and the darker red lenses (CPF 550, PLS 540, and PLS 550) may improve functional visual acuity for such conditions as retinitis pigmentosa, albinism, aniridia, and intense photophobia.

The best method of evaluating these lenses is to place a plano-CPF lens over the existing lenses of the patient. Then the examiner turns up the lights of the room and rechecks vision. The patient is asked to go to a bright window and observe the change. If significant, the lenses should be prescribed.

Mirrored sunglasses. In glass a one-way mirror surface can be placed on a white or colored glass lens to convert it to a sunglass for special purposes.

There are situations in which patients do not wish anyone to see their eyes (perhaps because of permanent or temporary disfigurement). Mirrored sunglasses give this protection, and the patient has no trouble seeing through the mirrored lenses. In terms of the patient's vision, the tint can be neutral gray, pink, green, or any other color found in ordinary sunglasses.

Table 12-2   Bifocal types

Type	Advantages	Disadvantages
Cement	Inexpensive	Line of demarcation very visible and collects dirt
		Poor durability; segment tends to loosen and fall off
Kryptok	Inconspicuous segment	Distinct chromatic aberration when reading segment is over
	Inexpensive	+1.75
		Prism displacement at junction of distance and near segments very noticeable
		Increases thickness of lens
Ultex	Segment practically invisible	More costly
	No chromatic aberration	Prism displacement
	Light in weight	
	Reading segment on inside of lens and thus protected	
Flattop	No prism displacement	More costly than Kryptok
	Because of barium segment, chromatic aberration almost eliminated	

Multifocal lenses

Multifocal lenses include all types of bifocals, trifocals, and the so-called invisible bifocals, or continuous-vision lenses (such as Younger and Varilux II).

There are two basic types of multifocal lenses: the one-piece, or Ultex, and the fused.

The *one-piece* is so named because the material (glass or plastic) is the same throughout the lens, and the power is varied by changing the curvature of the surface on the convex or concave side of the lens. The following types of bifocals and trifocals are of the one-piece construction:

1. All-plastic lenses, with segments on the convex side in almost every case
2. Ultex (one-piece) lenses with segments on the convex side (These are used to be produced with the segment on the concave side.)
3. Younger (round-segment) invisible bifocals, with segments on the convex side
4. Varilux and Multilux lenses, with no segments, but with curvatures on the convex side
5. Executive, or president, type of bifocals or trifocals in glass or plastic, with segments on the convex side

The *fused* multifocal lens uses glass of two or more indexes of refraction. When the segment with the higher index is countersunk (fused) into the main lens, the surfaces of a fused lens have no change of curvature. The add (that is, the plus dioptric power of the bifocal or trifocal) is governed by two factors: (1) the difference in the indexes of refraction of the various types of glass and (2) the depth of the countersink into which the segment is fused. The following are fused-type glass lenses:

1. Kryptok or Achromat round-segment bifocals, with segments fused into the convex side
2. Flattop bifocals and trifocals, with segments fused into the convex side
3. Catraconoid bifocals, with a glass aspheric convex surface, and with a flattop segment buried in the lens (aspheric curvatures are before the reading segments as well as the distance portion; plastic aspheric bifocals have aspheric surfaces for the distance portion of the lens only)

Falling into a category between one-piece and fused lenses are *cement bifocals* (Table 12-2). Two lenses of the same type of glass having the same index of refraction are fastened together to form a lens with the characteristics of the one-piece lens. The original cement used was Canada balsam, chosen because it has an index of refraction close to that of glass. Lenses cemented with Canada balsam usually are temporary lenses. The cement can be expected to turn yellow after a period of time, and the

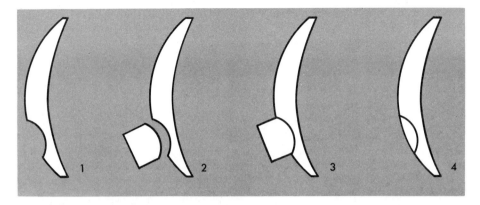

Fig. 12-20 Fused bifocal. *1,* A countersink is placed on the lens blank. *2,* Segment of a higher index of refraction is ground to fit into the countersink. *3,* Two lenses are fused together in an oven and cooled slowly. *4,* Excess lens is ground off and polished.

segment will drop off. With the use of a modern thermal cement, a lens can be made in which the segment will remain permanently affixed to the main lens and will not discolor. Cemented segments are useful because the segment can be made of any power and positioned anywhere in the main lens. These lenses are particularly useful for a patient with low visual acuity who might require an add of +20.00 diopters. A high-powered lenticular lens can be constructed using the thermally cemented segment process.

The following shows how a fused bifocal is made.

1. A countersink is placed in a lens blank of appropriate depth, and the countersink is finished by polishing (Fig. 12-20, *1*).

2. The segment that is merely a small lens of glass with a higher index of refraction than the main lens also is ground and polished to exactly fit the curvature of the countersink (Fig. 12-20, *2*).

3. The two are fused together in an oven and allowed to cool, slowly (annealing), so that no strain is set up inside the lens (Fig. 12-20, *3*).

4. The button is then ground off and the whole convex side finished to a polish. This is the Kryptok or Achromat bifocal with a round segment (Fig. 12-20, *4*).

For a flattop bifocal the process is much the same. The countersink in the main blank is made as previously mentioned. The button, however, is a different shape (Fig. 12-21).

A carrier is fused to the top of the flat segment after the contacting surfaces are fined to an optical flat. In fining (the manufacturer's term), a lens curvature is brought from a frosted-glass appearance to a satin finish.

The carrier is the same type of glass as the main lens, both in color and in index of refraction. The segment, however, is a glass of a higher index of refraction than the main lens. After the carrier is fused to the segment, the combined lens is finished and polished to fit the countersink in the main lens (see Fig. 12-21).

When the button is fused to the main lens and ground off, and the convex surface is polished, the carrier is invisible, but the segment, being a different type of glass, can be seen.

The purpose of the carrier is to maintain the flat top of the bifocal. If the carrier was not present and the button was ground off, the segment would return to a small circular one or a deep groove would be left in the surface.

A flattop trifocal is made in the same manner as a bifocal, but three types of glass form the button (Fig. 12-22). The carrier matches the main lens in color and index of refraction, as in the bifocal. The intermediate segment is made of a glass with more

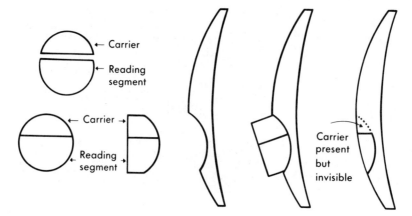

Fig. 12-21 Flattop bifocal. The reading segment is combined with a carrier of similar properties as the main lens. This button is then inserted into the countersink of the main lens, fused, and ground off to produce a flattop bifocal. The carrier is invisible, but the segment, being of a different type of glass, can be seen.

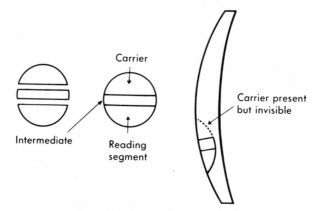

Fig. 12-22 Flattop trifocal. This lens is manufactured similarly to the bifocal, with an intermediate segment interposed between the carrier and the reading segment.

bending power (higher index of refraction) than the main lens or carrier but with less bending power than the reading segment. The intermediate segment is half the dioptric power, in the finished lens, of the reading segment. For example, trifocals with a +3.00 add would have an intermediate segment power of +1.50. Spectacle lenses are made of crown glass with an index of 1.523. Segments are made of barium glass or flint glass (index of refraction from 1.625 to 1.690).

Special flattop bifocals and trifocals. The Exec-

utive bifocal, in glass or in plastic, is a modern version of the original Benjamin Franklin bifocal, which has two lenses in one eyewire, the lower half for reading, the upper half for distance (Fig. 12-23, A).

The modern equivalent is of one-piece construction. The prescription is ground on the concave side, and there is a distinct ridge on the convex side where the two powers join. Trifocals are constructed the same way.

Invisible bifocals (progressive-add bifocals).

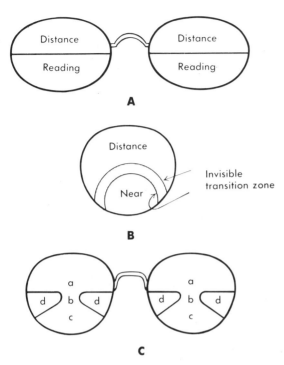

A

B

Distance

Invisible
transition zone

Near

C

a

d b d

c

a

d b d

c

Fig. 12-23 A, Benjamin Franklin bifocal. **B,** Invisible bifocal. **C,** Multilux or Varilux lens: *a,* clear distance vision; *b,* gradual increase in power on axis to coincide with convergence of eyes; *c,* clear reading area; *d,* distortion area.

There are several invisible bifocal lenses on the market. These lenses gradually increase in power as the line of sight travels downward through the lens. An early version of this lens was the Beach bifocal. Other names in this category are Flexsite, Omnifocal, Progressive R, Younger, Truevision, Varilux, and Multilux, the last two being one and the same. The latest to enter the market is the Varilux II, an improvement over the original.

The main difficulty in any lens that gradually increases in power is that vision on either side of a vertical line through the optical center produces unwanted, unprescribed cylindric power, causing great distortion. This is a fault of the Omnifocal and the Beach and, to a lesser degree, of the original Multilux or Varilux lens. The Varilux II is a great improvement over the first generation.

The Flexsite and Younger bifocals are an attempt

to create a one-piece round segment lens, with the segment on the convex side and the dividing line blended on the surface of the lens so that it is invisible. The result is a lens with a correct prescription for reading and for distance vision but with a blurred transition zone between the two. The Younger bifocal is useful in presbyopia when the prescription is not greater than a $+1.75$ add (Fig. 12-23, *B*).

The Multilux lens is constructed with a top portion that is a correct distance prescription, which gains in dioptic power toward the periphery; a bottom portion that is a correct near prescription, losing dioptic power toward the periphery of the reading area; and a transitional zone gradually increasing in power from distance to near.

The chief disadvantage is that there are distortions through this lens in the lower right and lower left quadrants with induced astigmatism (Fig. 12-23, *C*). They are successful (as are the Younger bifocals) with some patients who are not bothered by the areas of distorted vision.

Multivision lenses from patient's point of view (vocational lenses). Unfortunately, there is no one type of bifocal or trifocal that universally meets the visual requirements of all patients. The following are examples of some of the special needs of patients.

1. A presbyopic truck driver may need tinted bifocals, with segments set high enough so that the instrument panel is visible only through the bifocal, and an add of "intermediate" power to give clear vision at 24 inches. These glasses, because of the tint, would be unsuitable both for driving at night and for reading, because 24 inches is too far for this purpose.

2. A barber needs large segments set much higher than usual because he or she is working at near, with vision almost straight ahead.

3. A bookkeeper or an executive spends most of the working day at a desk, using bifocal segments, and a fraction of the day looking across the office. Thus this person should have "desk bifocals" of the Executive type, with segments set much higher than normal.

All these multivision lenses might be termed *vocational bifocals and trifocals*. With the flexibility of thermally cemented segments, almost any type of

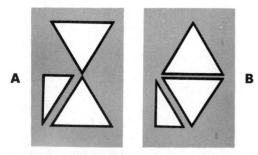

Fig. 12-24 A, Prism base-up effect of the flattop bifocal segment counterbalances the base-down effect of the adjoining distance concave lens. **B,** Prism base-down effect of the bifocal segment counterbalances the base-up effect of the adjoining distance convex lens.

segment, shape, size, or positioning—trifocal or bifocal—can be produced economically.

Most popular types of multifocal lenses. The essential factors in a bifocal lens should be that the line of demarcation is inconspicuous, involving no sudden break, that the additional strength of the add does not augment the weight of the lens, and that the segment is large enough to give an adequate field of vision for reading. The line of demarcation, even though inconspicuous, should not interfere with distant vision. Bifocals have an inherent disadvantage in that there is an image jump—an apparent displacement of objects—when one changes the direction of vision from distance to near. Efforts to minimize this image displacement are made by incorporating additional segments with optical centers designed to produce a compensating prismatic effect. There are basically two types of bifocal segments available.

Flattop segment. The flattop segment is fused with the optical center lying at the upper portion of the segment; this is of value in treating low hyperopes and all myopes. It eliminates image jump when looking from near to far. The base-down prism of the main lens is partially neutralized by the base-up prism of the flattop segment (Fig. 12-24, *A*).

Round top fused segments (Kryptok, Achromat). The Achromat looks like a Kryptok but is a superior lens because it has less chromatic aberation (color fringing around objects) than the Kryptok. This lens is

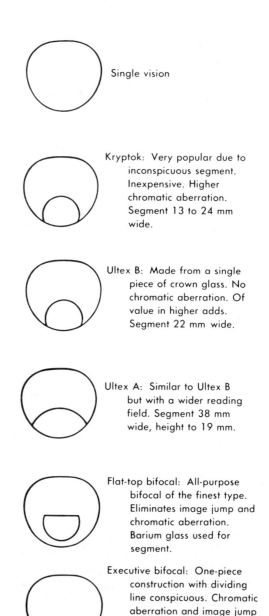

Single vision

Kryptok: Very popular due to inconspicuous segment. Inexpensive. Higher chromatic aberration. Segment 13 to 24 mm wide.

Ultex B: Made from a single piece of crown glass. No chromatic aberration. Of value in higher adds. Segment 22 mm wide.

Ultex A: Similar to Ultex B but with a wider reading field. Segment 38 mm wide, height to 19 mm.

Flat-top bifocal: All-purpose bifocal of the finest type. Eliminates image jump and chromatic aberration. Barium glass used for segment.

Executive bifocal: One-piece construction with dividing line conspicuous. Chromatic aberration and image jump virtually eliminated. Suitable where large reading field required.

Fig. 12-25

used for hyperopic patients. In stronger powers the base-up prism of the main lens is neutralized by the base-down prism of the round segment (Figs. 12-24, *B*, to 12-27).

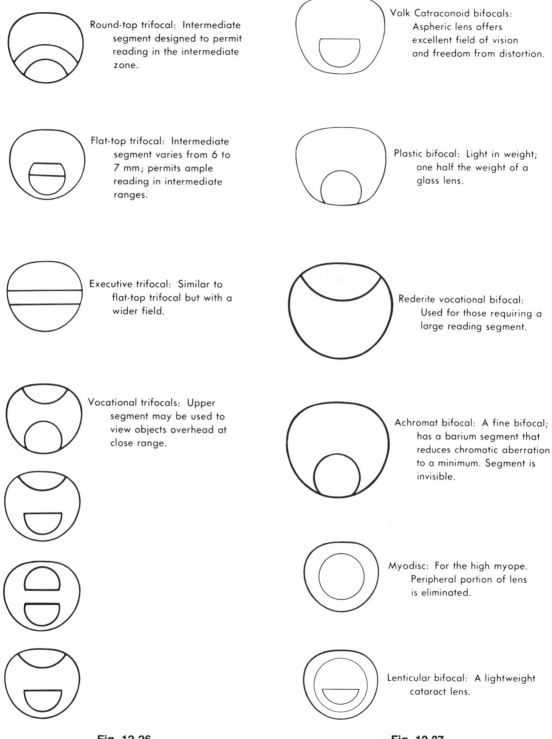

Round-top trifocal: Intermediate segment designed to permit reading in the intermediate zone.

Volk Catraconoid bifocals: Aspheric lens offers excellent field of vision and freedom from distortion.

Flat-top trifocal: Intermediate segment varies from 6 to 7 mm; permits ample reading in intermediate ranges.

Plastic bifocal: Light in weight; one half the weight of a glass lens.

Executive trifocal: Similar to flat-top trifocal but with a wider field.

Rederite vocational bifocal: Used for those requiring a large reading segment.

Vocational trifocals: Upper segment may be used to view objects overhead at close range.

Achromat bifocal: A fine bifocal; has a barium segment that reduces chromatic aberration to a minimum. Segment is invisible.

Myodisc: For the high myope. Peripheral portion of lens is eliminated.

Lenticular bifocal: A lightweight cataract lens.

Fig. 12-26

Fig. 12-27

Progressive lenses

Progressive-addition lenses such as the Varilux series, are capable of providing a more flexible presbyopic correction. The Varilux I was the first generation of these lenses, which are characterized by a distance and near spherical zone that are linked vertically by a progressive corridor and laterally by a continuous surface. Varilux II was designed to provide not only a progressive surface but visual comfort as well. Each point on the surface is matched as closely as possible to natural vision. It eliminates unwanted aberration, and there is a specific increase in power in the central and peripheral areas. The Varilux Infinity lens is a multidesigned progressive-addition lens, with specific changes based on the reading power. It upgrades the Varilux II insofar as it refines the surface characteristics of each level. A complete range of addition designs range from 0.75 to 3.5 diopters, which maximizes patient satisfaction at each stage of presbyopia. This lens takes into account not only central vision but also peripheral vision, which is important for patient adaptation and comfort; it also allows easier adaptation than did previous lenses.

The fitting of the Varilux Infinity is the same as for the Varilux II. The manufacturer suggests that while a patient looks at one point at eye level, the distance from the center of the pupil to the edge of the frame should be measured. The fitting height must be at least 22 mm. One chooses the smallest vertex distance possible between 12 and 14 mm and a panascopic tilt between 10 to 15 degrees. The examiner uses the pupillometer to measure PD for far vision; fitting heights are measured from the center of the pupil to the edge of the frame just below. The centering chart is used to check the accuracy of the mounting. The lens is marked for far-vision prism and near-vision power. The fitting cross always should be placed at the center of the pupil (Fig. 12-28).

Centering of lenses

Glasses should be centered so that the patient looks through the optical center of the lens; otherwise a prismatic effect will be introduced. The prismatic effect of 1.00 prism diopter is produced for every 1

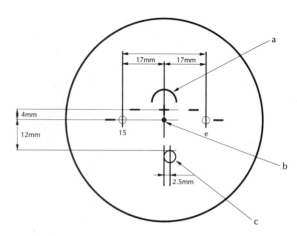

Fig. 12-28 Measurements for Varilux II and Varilux Infinity progressive addition lenses. *a*, Far-vision Power; *b*, prism power; *c*, near-reading power.

cm of decentering of a 1.00-diopter lens. Thus a 10.00-diopter lens will produce 1.00 prism diopter of deviation for every millimeter that its optical center is displaced. The amount of prismatic deviation can be shown by the formula

$$P = hd$$

where:

P = Prismatic deviation
h = Distance the lens is displaced in centimeters
d = Dioptric power of the lens

Decentering often is intentionally produced. Reading glasses normally are decentered 2.5 mm inward and 6.5 to 8 mm downward inasmuch as the eyes are converged and turned down for reading. Decentering of lenses has been employed to correct minor disturbances of ocular muscle imbalance.

Panascopic angle

The panascopic angle of the frame is the angle in which the frame front angles to the face when the glasses are worn. When viewed from the side, it is normal for the lower rims of the frame front to be closer to the cheeks than are the upper rims. Proper panascopic angle may range from 4 to 18 degrees. Often those with extremely protruding eyebrows may exceed this range. This angle permits the eye to focus downward from distant gaze to near gaze and maintain a constant vertex distance. It enables the patient to view reading print directly through the center of the reading addition. This is a very critical aspect of the fitting procedure.

Use of prisms in glasses. Vertical muscle imbalance of over 1.00 diopter cannot be tolerated by the patient. To compensate for a vertical muscle imbalance, the amount of prism correction needed is determined by the Maddox rod test. Suitable compensating base-up or base-down prisms are incorporated into the lenses. For example, an individual with + 2.00 diopters of right hypertropia would require 2.00 diopters of vertical prism to correct the imbalance. This may be given as 1.00 diopter, base down, in front of the right eye, and 1.00 diopter, base up, in front of the left eye. Prisms may be used for the treatment of large horizontal phorias and for convergence insufficiency.

If the difference in the refractive error between the two eyes is large, an undesired prismatic effect and a secondary ocular muscular imbalance may be induced when the patient is looking through the bifocal segment. In this situation, a "slab off" or a bicentric lens may be required to neutralize the induced prismatic effect. Slab off is the most common technique used to correct vertical imbalance at near. Slab offs often are used when the imbalance is greater than 1.5 prism diopters. They are, however, useful only for those with 5 prism diopters or less in vertical imbalance on looking downward.

Fresnel lens

The Fresnel lens has been used in various ways for many years and has found its way into ophthalmic lenses. It is used in ships' lanterns and in lighthouses as a light-condensing lens, but its most modern application is in condensing lenses in projectors and in many of the single-lens, reflex camera viewfinders, where it gives a brilliance to the image projected on the ground-glass focusing screen. It would make the ideal cataract lens, being paper thin and therefore almost weightless, but it exhibits a pattern of fine concentric circles, which is unattractive cosmetically. In the future, however, modern methods of manufacture may be able to produce lenses with these concentric circles almost invisible. In their present form they may be used by application to the back of the patient's spectacles, thus making excellent loaner "cataract glasses," with a spherical power near to that required when the patient's eye is "settling down" after the cataract operation and before the final stabilized prescription can be given (Fig. 12-29).

Fresnel prisms

A development in ophthalmic prisms is the Fresnel press-on prism (Fig. 12-30), which is as thin as a piece of paper but has powers up to 15.00 prism diopters. Like the Fresnel lens, it has visible lines. The thin plastic prism is cut to the shape of a spectacle lens and is pressed onto the lens surface without the use of a cement. The prism can be easily removed and changed in a few seconds. The advantage of the Fresnel prism is its light weight. It is ideal for a temporary prism over the patient's existing prescription.

PRODUCTION OF PRESCRIPTION LENSES

On receipt of the prescription from a patient, the dispensing optician notes whether multivision (bifocal or trifocal) or single-vision lenses are specified. If a single-vision lens is required, the optician or the optical laboratory can select from stock an uncut, finished, single-vision lens of the exact power of sphere and cylinder needed. This lens is *laid out* and *edged* (shaped to fit the frame) so that when it is mounted in the frame, the axis of the prescription is as specified. Most single-vision prescriptions do not require surfacing of the lens. Consequently, single-vision glasses can be produced to prescription in a matter of hours, if necessary.

The story of bifocals and trifocals is somewhat different. A stock of finished bifocal lenses that can be edged and put into a frame is just not possible (except a limited stock of sphere bifocals). The possible permutations and combinations of sphere powers, cylindric powers, axes, bifocal or trifocal addition powers, bifocal or trifocal segment shapes, and the position of the segment in the finished glasses mean a stock of finished bifocals or trifocals cannot be maintained by even the largest optical companies. These lenses must be custom made. However, lens

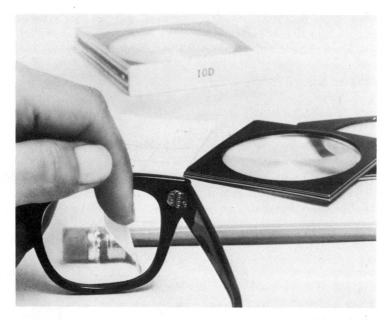

Fig. 12-29 Fresnel lens used for a temporary cataract lens. Note the magnification.

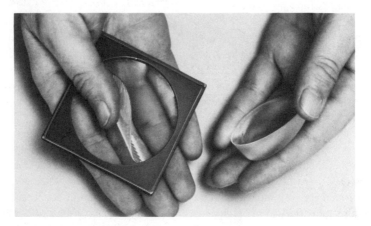

Fig. 12-30 Fresnel prism applied to glasses. Note the thinness as compared with a prism of comparable strength.

manufacturers do semifinish multifocal lenses to the point of providing an uncut lens finished on one side with the bifocal or trifocal segment of predetermined power. The patient's prescription as to spherical and cylindric power and axis must be produced on the other side.

In the case of hard-resin lenses and fused-segment bifocals and trifocals the prescription is placed on the concave surface by diamond-tooled *generators*. The result is a *frosted glass* appearance to the lens. The second step is termed *fining* (Fig. 12-31). A cast-iron lap that exactly fits the prescription generated on the lens is rubbed against the lens under a mixture of fine emery and water. The result of the

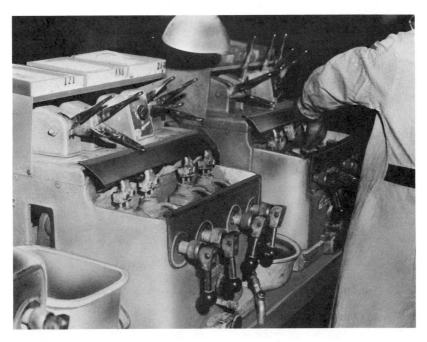

Fig. 12-31 Fining and polishing machine for glass lenses. (Courtesy Imperial Optical Co. Ltd., Toronto, Ontario.)

fining stage is a satin-finished surface. The third and last step again uses a lap, but this time a polishing pad is placed between the glass and the cast-iron lap. A polishing material (such as cerium oxide in water) produces the high polish of the finished lens.

From this point the procedure is similar to that for the single-vision lens; that is, the lens is laid out, edged to the shape of the frame, and inserted into the patient's frame.

Because of the necessity of surfacing one side of the bifocal and trifocal lenses and the additional time required for this, multifocal lenses cannot be produced as quickly as can single-vision lenses. They must go to a laboratory capable of doing more than just edging a single-vision stock lens to shape. Very few dispensing opticians have surfacing facilities on their premises. A few have edging machinery, but most send their work to optical laboratories.

CARE OF GLASSES

Patients should understand the need for care and cleaning of their glasses. Too often the patient comes

to the ophthalmologist wearing a dirty, scratched pair of glasses that has undoubtedly caused blurred vision. The following rules should be observed in the maintenance of spectacles.

1. The frames should be kept clean. The collection of grease and dirt on the frames and the lenses is best removed by washing in lukewarm water. Spectacle lenses should not be cleaned or polished when they are dry, because they may become scratched.

2. Spectacles, when not in use, should be kept in their case. If this is not possible, they should be laid so that they are supported by the folding sidepieces or left standing on their rims.

3. Spectacles should be removed by taking them off with both hands, holding them firmly and close to the hinges. Removing them with one hand causes the frame to bend out of shape or even break.

4. During the winter, lenses frequently mist over and blur vision. This can be avoided by smearing a piece of dried soap over them and polishing them. The thin film that results will stop misting for several

days. A number of defogging solutions also are available commercially.

5. In hardened lenses the surface compression layer is only three or four thousandths of an inch in depth, and a fairly deep scratch could exceed this and thus weaken the safety feature of the lens.

6. Screws in glasses may become loose. They may be fixed in position by applying clear nail polish.

QUESTIONS FOR REVIEW AND THOUGHT

1. Discuss the manufacture and types of ophthalmic frames.
2. What are the advantages and disadvantages of the different types of ophthalmic frames?
3. How is pupillary distance measured?
4. What is the temple length? What points are measured?
5. What type of glass is used commonly for ophthalmic lenses?
6. What are some of the distortions that are inherent in lenses?
7. Cataract lenses usually present a special problem because of their thickness and weight. What type of special lenses is available to overcome these problems?
8. Safety glasses are recommended for children, persons engaged in sports, and industrial workers. How are they constructed?
9. Sunglasses filter out certain of the color components of white light. Discuss some types of sunglasses that are available.
10. Bifocals are used to provide two focal distances in the same glass. They may be of one-piece or fused construction or even cemented bifocals. Draw diagrams to illustrate how fused bifocals are constructed.
11. Special occupations, such as garage mechanics, may require the worker to use a bifocal segment in an uncommon position. Name as many occupations as you can in which the bifocal segment may be required in an unusual position.
12. What are the advantages of the Fresnel prism?
13. Does a large stylish frame size improve or diminish visual acuity in a person with a large refractive error?
14. What lenses would you recommend for night driving?
15. Does a blue lens affect visual acuity?
16. How can thick glasses be made lighter?
17. What types of frames should be avoided because of their flammable potential?
18. What kind of glasses should a welder use?
19. What are the advantages and disadvantages of trifocals?

SELF-EVALUATION QUESTIONS

True-false statements

Directions: Indicate whether the statement is true (T) or false (F).

T or F   1. Cellulose nitrate is the most common plastic employed in the fabrication of spectacle frames.

T or F   2. The pupillary distance is the distance from the center of the pupil of one eye to the center of the pupil of the other eye.

T or F   3. The optical center of a lens is the thinnest part of the lens in a myopic correction, and the thickest part of a lens in a hyperopic correction.

Missing words

Directions: Write in the missing word in the following sentences.

4. The primary glass employed by opticians is _____ glass.
5. Aphakic lenses tend to distort to a _____ shape.
6. Coating a lens often is referred to as _____ a lens.

Choice-completion questions

Directions: Select the one best answer in each case.

7. Photogray lenses:
   a. Are sunglasses for outdoor use
   b. Are completely transparent indoors
   c. Work in an automobile
   d. Are recommended for reading
   e. None of the above
8. The invisible bifocal offers:
   a. Great vision over the whole lens
   b. Great vision just in a band on either side of the optical center
   c. Great vision nasally where the eyes turn in to read
   d. Best vision in powers above $+1.50$
   e. None of the above
9. A Fresnel lens is a press-on lens and:
   a. It can be cut to any shape
   b. It comes in prisms up to 15.00 diopters as well as in a range of positive and negative lens powers
   c. It gets dirty easily, peels off, and has to be replaced often
   d. It causes a drop of vision because the optics are not sharp
   e. All of the above

ANSWERS, NOTES, AND EXPLANATIONS

1. **False.** Cellulose nitrate burns fiercely if a flame is brought to it. Today the use of such flammable plastics is not allowed in the makeup of spectacles. One of the popular plastics employed presently is cellulose acetate, which is desirable because it comes in a variety of colors. It can burn if a flame is held to it, but it does not ignite and spread on its own. Lucite, a much tougher material, frequently is used. For children, nylon and Optyl frames are popular because they are flexible and virtually indestructible. Flexibility allows the frame to fit any face and prevents snapping, which can occur with the more rigid plastics. Nylon is made up in a limited number of colors, but Optyl can be dyed to any color combination.

2. **False.** This distance actually exceeds the true interpupillary distance, which is measured from the visual axis of one eye to the other. The visual axis is a little nasal to the center of the pupil in most instances. Because of the inherent difficulties in measuring visual axis, the PD is normally taken from the nasal edge of the pupil of the patient's right eye to the temporal side of the pupil of the left eye.

    Light reflexes off the pupil can indicate the visual axis of the eye, and they are more accurate. Two readings should be taken—one for the distance and one for near.

    The PD is an important measurement, as many complaints and glass checks stem from a failure of the optician to center the lens to the visual axis of the eye. When this happens, unwanted prism is introduced and the patient has symptoms.

3. **True.** The optical center of the lens should be marked inasmuch as it does not coincide with the midpoint between the nasal and temporal sides of the frame. Most lensometers have a marking device to indicate the true optical center of the lens. Some frames are so large and eccentric that the optical centers of the lenses never approximate visual axes of the eyes. Checking optical centers should be performed on every glass check because centering is the largest source of complaints.

4. **Crown.** Crown glass has been a favorite lens for opticians because it has a lower refractive index, and there is less tendency to color dispersion. These lenses are heavy and are particularly cumbersome in higher powers. The lens of tomorrow undoubtedly will be polycarbonate, which is a tough, hard plastic capable of resisting the impact of a bullet yet light to wear.

5. **Pincushion.** A lens that is thick causes distortion because the bending of light at the edge of the lens is not the same as in the middle of the lens. In an aphakic lens, the thickness is in the center of the lens, and the lens profile drops off sharply toward the edge. In high myopes, the thickness of the lens is toward the edges, and the distortion created by the thin center moving out to thicken at the periphery causes barrel distortion.

   In aphakic lenses remedies to distortion include (a) lenticular lenses because they get rid of the lens edge and (b) lenses that are flatter in the periphery because they eliminate the drastic change in power. The four-drop lens does this job well. Basically these lenses fall into the category of aspheric lenses.

6. **Blooming.** The lenses are coated with magnesium fluoride, one fourth of the wavelength of yellow-green light. The coating imparts a purplish sheen to these lenses, similar to bloom on a ripe plum; hence the name.

   The coating is tough and lasts the lifetime of the lens. The purpose of coating the lens is to eliminate annoying light reflections from lights and bulbs.

   A coated lens allows greater light transmission while depressing the amount of internal reflections.

7. **e. None of the above.** Indoors, photogray lenses never turn transparent but remain slightly tinted at all times. In an automobile they are shielded from the sun so that they never darken enough to offer minimal comfort and protection from sunlight. As a sunglass, one requires Photosun lenses, which turn a darker shade and are more suitable as a sunglass. The hazard comes while driving at night or in dim light. A tinted lens under reduced illumination makes driving more difficult. This is especially true in winter, when people wear dark clothes and the driver wearing tinted lenses has to find that dark figure in the darkness. Because the lens never drains its color, the tint also makes it harder to read; it provides a gray background to black type, thereby reducing contrast.

8. **b. Great vision just in a band on either side of the optical center.** This lens has become very popular because it eliminates the visible presence of bifocals, which to many people means aging. Optically it offers some advantages. It eliminates image jump as the transition between the distance and near portion is not abrupt. It also confers a continuous increase in power looking down so that a longer band of near focal points is available to the wearer. However, this lens does create lateral astigmatism on either side of the central band of the lens. Many people find the distortion disabling for reading. Some of the newer models of this seamless bifocal are better because the diameter of the clear central zone has been expanded.

9. **e. All of the above.** A Fresnel lens is basically a temporary lens. The advantages of this lens are that it is flexible and lightweight. However, the disadvantages of hazy vision and of lower durability and reliability preclude constant wear.

   It is a good temporary lens for postsurgical cataract cases and for those persons with temporary diplopia who require bridge prisms to carry them along until their condition improves.

CHAPTER 13

Rigid contact lenses: basics

- Development of contact lenses
- Optics of contact lenses
- How the corneal contact lens works
- Terminology
- Designs of corneal contact lenses
- Examination for contact lenses
- Fitting corneal contact lenses
- Evaluating contact lenses
- Instructions for insertion and removal of contact lenses
- Care of contact lenses
- Evaluating the fit of contact lenses
- Adjusting contact lenses
- Problems associated with overwearing contact lenses
- Uses of contact lenses

Contact lenses have become a routine part of our armamentarium for visual rehabilitation of the eye. Their use and demand are constantly increasing. Over 20% of the North American population are myopic, many of whom are dependent on visual correction. Coupled with the increasing use of contact lenses, many myths and fallacies have arisen regarding their indications and contraindications. At the very minimum, the ophthalmic assistant should be able to discuss with the patient the function of a contact lens, its purpose, and its limitations. The ophthalmic assistant can also be of value in some of the technical aspects of contact lens wear, such as method of insertion and removal, and particularly, proper care and storage of the lens itself. This chapter deals with the practical aspects of management of the patient who desires contact lenses.

DEVELOPMENT OF CONTACT LENSES

As early as the sixteenth century, Leonardo da Vinci conceived and sketched prototypes of modern contact lenses. He experimented by neutralizing his own refractive error by placing his face in a container of water. In the following century René Descartes described and illustrated a glass type of scleral contact lens (Fig. 13-1). However, the first practical type of contact lens was produced in 1887. This lens consisted of a glass capsule containing gelatin that was placed in contact with the cornea, with the glass being molded to correspond to the shape of the eye. In 1932 the first major advance in the design of the contact lens was made. Investigating impressions made from the human eye, Dr. Joseph Dallos found that no two were identical. From this he concluded that it was impossible to fit a contact lens manufactured to a preconceived formula. Dallos then devel-

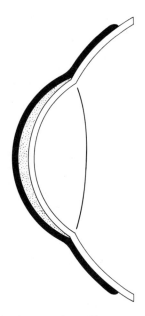

Fig. 13-1 Scleral contact lens. The contact lens fits over the cornea and sclera.

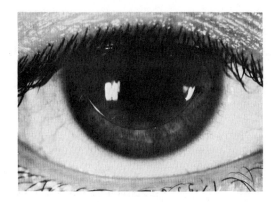

Fig. 13-2 The silicone-acrylate contact lens is gas permeable. It may be fitted larger than conventional PMMA rigid lenses. Note that the upper eyelid margin is covering the upper portion of the contact lens.

oped a technique of making negative casts of the anterior segment of the living eye. However, Dallos' lenses could be tolerated only for limited periods of time because of the excessive weight of the glass, and they were difficult to manufacture. In 1938 the first molded scleral contact lens that overlaid the sclera was made from a plastic material called polymethylmethacrylate (PMMA). This lens had many advantages over glass, because it was lighter, shatterproof, and easily moldable. It was not until 1948 that Kevin Tuohy introduced the first fluidless corneal lens, which was designed to rest on the corneal tear layer. These were large, but later smaller microcorneal lenses were introduced, which made possible a great step forward in the successful wearing of contact lenses.

Further developments in rigid lens manufacture came with the introduction of intermediate curves, the practice of refining the edges, and the development of toric lenses. Today rigid lens technology has made another leap forward by the introduction of silicone and fluorocarbon as materials. When combined with PMMA, these materials make the plastic material gas permeable (Fig. 13-2).

OPTICS OF CONTACT LENSES

The contact lens, for all practical purposes, eliminates the cornea as a major source of refractive power of the eye, because it is the same refractive index as the fluid in front of it. The fluid interface between the contact lens and the cornea fills out irregularities in the contours of the anterior corneal surface, converting the cornea to a sphere. Thus the fluid may be considered a forward extension of the cornea. If the radius of curvature of the back surface of the contact lens is the same as that of the front surface of the cornea, the refractive power of the PMMA contact lens will be the same as that of the cornea. The change in refractive power is produced by altering the curvature of the contact lens.

HOW THE CORNEAL CONTACT LENS WORKS

A contact lens rests on the cornea just as a small fragment of paper adheres to the wet fingertip by just touching it. The natural moisture on the surface of the cornea is sufficient to create a surface tension and permit the lens to adhere quite strongly.

The back surface of the lens is contoured so that it exactly fits the curvature of the cornea. This curvature can be measured by an instrument called an *ophthalmometer* or *keratometer*. It is vital that this measurement be exact because if there is any contact or touch between the cornea and the contact lens, a scratch, abrasion, or erosion can occur in the superficial layers of the cornea. The contact lens, therefore, rests on a liquid cushion (tear film) and never on the eye itself. Injury to the cornea is one of the most damaging complications that can result from a poorly-fitted contact lens. Not only does it produce a painful red eye that obscures vision, but it also provides a portal of entry for bacteria and other pathogenic organisms to form a corneal ulcer.

The front surface of a contact lens—that is, the surface exposed to the air—contains the prescription, which is the power of the lens. The profile of this surface, of course, varies with the individual's refractive error.

The edge of a contact lens is thin and polished so that it can gently slide underneath the lid without being dislodged and also prevent lid irritation when blinking.

TERMINOLOGY

To appreciate contact lens technology, the reader should have an understanding of lens jargon. The following terminology applies to both rigid and soft lenses.

The *ophthalmometer* is an instrument designed to measure the corneal curvature by using the cornea as a front surface mirror. The instrument is most commonly referred to as the *keratometer,* even though this is a trade name of Bausch & Lomb, Inc.

In *astigmatism with the rule* the vertical corneal meridian has the steepest curvature, whereas in *astigmatism against the rule* the horizontal meridian has the steepest curvature (Fig. 13-3).

In performing *keratometry* some authors record the flattest meridian first and the steepest meridian next so that a keratometer (K) value, for example, of 44.00 diopters × 46.00 diopters × 85, indicates that the horizontal meridian has a radius of 44.00 diopters and that the vertical meridian has a radius of 46.00 diopters with the axis at 85 degrees. Other authors prefer to always record the horizontal meridian first, regardless of which is the flattest. This value may be expressed in either diopters or millimeters of radius. Table 13-1 gives a comparative value of the *K reading* in diopters and millimeters.

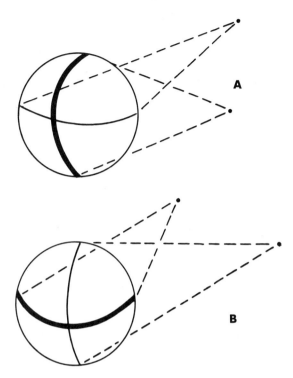

Fig. 13-3 A, Astigmatism with the rule. The vertical corneal meridian has the steepest curvature. **B,** Astigmatism against the rule. The horizontal meridian has the steepest curvature. (From Stein HA, Slatt BJ, Stein RM: *Fitting guide for rigid and soft contact lenses, a practical approach,* ed 3, St Louis, 1990, Mosby.)

Each 0.05 mm is equivalent to approximately 0.25 diopters, so that a 0.5 mm radius equals approximately 2.50 diopters. Expressed another way, each 1.00-diopter change in the K reading equals approximately a 0.2 mm radius change.

In lens work one usually first considers the flattest K reading. If the back surface of the lens is to be the same radius as K, this is referred to as *fitting on K.* One may fit *steeper than K* as in rigid lens design or *flatter than K* as in soft lens design. In the latter situation the lens will have a posterior radius flatter than the flattest K reading.

The *corneal cap* is the central zone of the cornea. This has a radius of approximately 4 to 6 mm and has a relatively constant spherical radius of curvature (Fig. 13-4) referred to as the *central posterior curve*

| **Table 13-1** | Diopter to millimeter conversion | | |

Keratometric reading (D)	Radius convex (mm)	Keratometric reading (D)	Radius convex (mm)
47.75	= 7.07	43.75	= 7.72
47.50	= 7.11	43.50	= 7.76
47.25	= 7.14	43.25	= 7.80
47.00	= 7.18	43.00	= 7.85
46.75	= 7.22	42.75	= 7.90
46.50	= 7.26	42.50	= 7.95
46.25	= 7.30	42.25	= 8.00
46.00	= 7.34	42.00	= 8.04
45.75	= 7.38	41.75	= 8.08
45.50	= 7.42	41.50	= 8.13
45.25	= 7.46	41.25	= 8.18
45.00	= 7.50	41.00	= 8.23
44.75	= 7.55	40.75	= 8.28
44.50	= 7.59	40.50	= 8.33
44.25	= 7.63	40.25	= 8.39
44.00	= 7.67	40.00	= 8.44

(CPC). The *peripheral* or *paracentral zone* of the cornea is the area surrounding the corneal cap and extending to the limbus. It has a much flatter curvature than does the central curve. The rate of flattening does not conform to a mathematic progression; that is, the cornea is not a true ellipse. It is generally described as being aspheric.

Most rigid corneal lenses used today are either bicurve or tricurve. A *bicurve lens* has one base curve and one secondary curve (Fig. 13-5). A small lens is usually bicurve. An *intrapalpebral lens,* a lens that fits within the palpebral fissure limits, is bicurve. This type of lens is small and steep, with narrow peripheral curves of 0.2 mm and small diameters of 7.5 to 8.8 mm.

A *multicurve lens* has a base curve and three or more peripheral curves. A *tricurve lens* usually has a large diameter (Fig 13-6). A contour lens is basically a tricurve lens with a narrow intermediate curve. The *blend* is the point of transition between the radii of curvature from one curve to another. The sharp junction is removed by making the zone of transition with a curved tool that has a radius value between the values of the two adjacent curves.

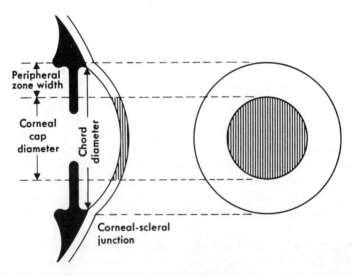

Fig. 13-4 Corneal cap, representing the theoretic spherical central zone of the cornea. (From Stein HA, Slatt BJ, Stein RM: *Fitting guide for rigid and soft contact lenses, a practical approach,* ed 3, St Louis, 1990, Mosby.)

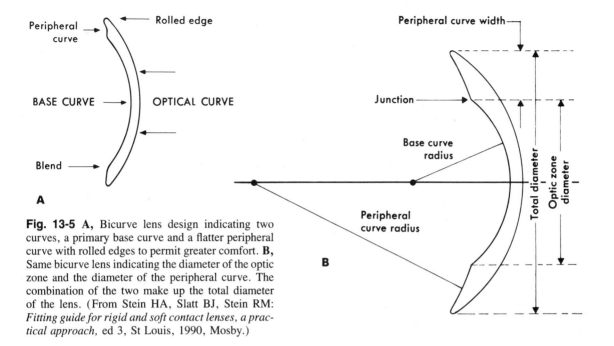

Fig. 13-5 A, Bicurve lens design indicating two curves, a primary base curve and a flatter peripheral curve with rolled edges to permit greater comfort. **B,** Same bicurve lens indicating the diameter of the optic zone and the diameter of the peripheral curve. The combination of the two make up the total diameter of the lens. (From Stein HA, Slatt BJ, Stein RM: *Fitting guide for rigid and soft contact lenses, a practical approach,* ed 3, St Louis, 1990, Mosby.)

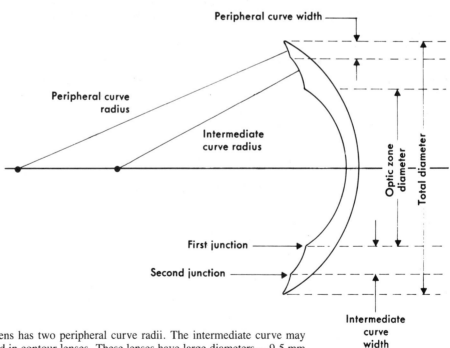

Fig. 13-6 A tricurve lens has two peripheral curve radii. The intermediate curve may be very narrow, as found in contour lenses. These lenses have large diameters—9.5 mm or greater—with an optic zone of 6.5 to 7.5 mm, which is just large enough to clear the maximum pupil diameter. The peripheral curves are slightly flatter than the base curves by 0.4 to 0.8 mm with a width of 1.3 mm. With a standard tricurve lens the intermediate curve is 1 mm flatter than the base curve. The peripheral curve is a standard 12.25 mm radius. (From Stein HA, Slatt BJ, Stein RM: *Fitting guide for rigid and soft contact lenses, a practical approach,* ed 3, St Louis, 1990, Mosby.)

An *intermediate curve* is a curve between the base curve and the peripheral curve.

The *total lens diameter* or the *chord diameter* is the measurement from one edge of the lens to the opposite side. This is a linear measurement and is not related to the circumference of the lens. Most rigid lenses used today have a chord diameter between 8 and 9 mm, whereas the cord diameter of a soft lens usually ranges from 12 to 15 mm. Depending on which end of the scale they fall into, lenses may be referred to as small or large.

The *peripheral curve width* is the diameter from one edge of a secondary curve to another.

The *central thickness* of a lens is the separation between the anterior and posterior surfaces at the geometric center of a lens. The higher the minus power, the thinner the center, whereas the higher the plus power, the thicker the center.

Tints refer to the coloring available in a lens and may be blue, brown, gray, or green for rigid lenses. They may be numbered 1 to 3, with number 1 the lightest and number 3 the darkest shade of each color.

A *ballasted lens*, often referred to as a *prism ballast lens,* is one that is weighted with a heavier base that will orient inferiorly when the lens is worn. A *truncated lens* is one that is cut off to form a horizontal base. The amputation of the base is usually at the inferior pole of the lens. Truncation is frequently used to add stability to a soft toric lens and to prevent rotation.

Back vertex power refers to the effective power of the lens from the posterior surface. The distance from the back surface of the lens to the focal point is the back focal length; its reciprocal is the back vertex power.

The *primary base curve,* as well as all other curvatures of a lens, may be expressed in terms of millimeters of radius of curvature. It can also be expressed in diopters—a primary base curve of 43.25 diopters is equal to 7.8 mm. The primary central posterior curve of a lens is designed to conform to the optic zone of the cornea.

The *optic zone* of a lens is the central zone that contains the refractive power and generally corresponds to the central corneal cap of the cornea.

Toroidal or toric lenses, derived from Latin *torus,* meaning "a bulge," are lenses with different radii of curvature in each meridian. The meridian of the shortest and longest radii are called the *principal meridians,* and they differ by 90 degrees. These lenses are used to correct astigmatism.

A *front surface toric lens* has an anterior surface that has two different radii of curvature but a central posterior surface that is spherical. Usually a prism ballast is required for orientation.

A *back surface toric lens* has a posterior surface that has two different radii of curvature and an anterior spherical surface.

In a *bitoric lens* both the anterior and posterior surfaces have two curvatures on the front and back surface. The axis of the anterior and posterior toroidal surface may coincide or be oblique to one another, but usually they coincide.

The *lenticular bowl* refers to the diameter of the optical portion of a lens and is used with higher power lenses.

The *posterior apical radius (PAR)* refers to the radius of curvature of the back surface of a lens at its apex. This is the area of curvature that will conform to the front surface of the apex of the cornea. This is particularly applicable to the Bausch & Lomb spin-cast Soflens, whose posterior curvature is not uniform. Lenses are labeled by the posterior radius at the apex of the lens.

When a base curve of a lens is said to be made steeper, this means that the posterior radius of curvature is decreased (e.g., from 8.4 to 8.1 mm), so that the curvature is now steeper. When the base curve is said to be made flatter, it means that the posterior radius of curvature of the lens is increased (e.g., from 8.1 to 8.4 mm), so that the curvature is now flatter.

The *sagittal depth* or *height* of a lens is the distance between a flat surface and the back surface of the central portion of the lens. Thus for two lenses of the same diameter but of different sagittal depths, the lens of the greater sagittal depth would produce a greater "vaulting" of the lens and in effect would be steeper. This is often referred to as the *sagittal vault*.

There are two important variables in understanding the mechanism of loosening or tightening a lens.

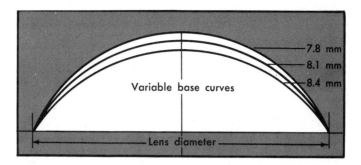

Fig. 13-7 If the diameter is held constant, by decreasing the radius of curvature from 8.4 to 7.8 mm the sagittal height or vault of the lens is increased. (From Stein HA, Slatt BJ, Stein RM: *Fitting guide for rigid and soft contact lenses, a practical approach,* ed 3, St Louis, 1990, Mosby.)

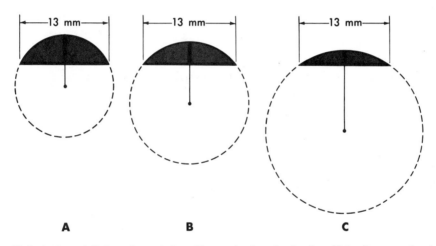

Fig. 13-8 A, B, and **C** show three circles of increasing length of radius. If the diameter of a given arc of the circle is kept constant, the sagittal height will decrease from **A** to **C.** (From Stein HA, Slatt BJ, Stein RM: *Fitting guide for rigid and soft contact lenses, a practical approach,* ed 3, St Louis, 1990, Mosby.)

These variables are the diameter and the radius of the lens. If the diameter is kept constant, by changing the radius to a longer radius (e.g., from a 7.8 to an 8.4 mm radius), the sagittal vault or sagittal height of the lens becomes shorter and the lens becomes flatter. The converse is also true (Figs. 13-7 and 13-8).

If the central posterior curve (radius) of the lens remains the same but the diameter is made larger (e.g., from 13 to 15 mm with soft lenses or 8 to 9 mm with rigid lenses), the sagittal vault or sagittal height of the lens is increased and the lens becomes steeper. The converse is also true (Fig. 13-9).

For example, if we consider the lens as being part of a similar circle (Fig. 13-10) and we take two parts of the circle with different diameters or chord lengths, the portion of the circle with the larger diameter will have a greater sagittal vault.

The wettability of a surface is measured in terms of its contact or *wetting angle.* In the case of a contact

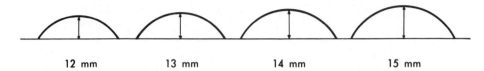

| 12 mm | 13 mm | 14 mm | 15 mm |

Fig. 13-9 When the radius is kept constant and the diameter increased, the sagittal height of the lens is increased and the lens becomes steeper. (From Stein HA, Slatt BJ, Stein RM: *Fitting guide for rigid and soft contact lenses, a practical approach,* ed 3, St Louis, 1990, Mosby.)

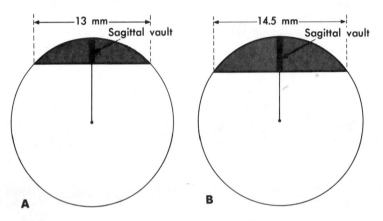

Fig. 13-10 If portions of two similar circles are cut off, each with a different diameter, portion **B** with the larger 14.5 mm diameter will have a greater sagittal depth or vault than portion **A** with the smaller 13.0 mm diameter. (From Stein HA, Slatt BJ, Stein RM: *Fitting guide for rigid and soft contact lenses, a practical approach,* ed 3, St Louis, 1990, Mosby.)

lens this is the angle that is formed between the tangent to the edge of a drop of water with the surface of a contact lens. The wetting angle, called *theta,* is expressed as zero if the material is completely wetted by the liquid (Fig. 13-11). As the wetting angle becomes greater than zero, the solid surface cannot be completely wetted. As an extreme, if a drop of mercury were to be placed on a glass slide, it would not spread out on the surface but would form a small blob whose angle would be greater than 90 degrees (see Fig. 13-11). Some plastics have smaller wetting angles than others; the lower the wetting angle of the plastic, the better the tears will spread evenly over the surface of the contact lens. "Wetting" solutions reduce this angle and permit better flow of tears and comfort. The lower the wetting angle, the greater the spread of tears.

Terminology pertaining to oxygen studies has taken on increasing importance in the contact lens literature because of the development of extended-wear lenses and gas-permeable contact lenses.*

The oxygen transmission through a given material is a laboratory measurement, often referred to as the DK value, where D is the diffusion coefficient for oxygen movement in lens material, and K is the solubility coefficient of oxygen in the material. It should be noted that a coefficient is a measure of a physical or chemical property that is constant for a system under specific conditions. The DK, or permeability, is characteristic of a material obtained in

*For a more extensive reference on terminology, consult Stein HS, Slatt BJ, Stein RM: *Ophthalmic terminology: speller and vocabulary builder,* ed 3, St Louis, 1992, Mosby.

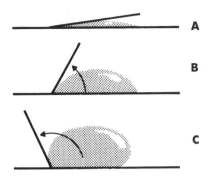

Fig. 13-11 Wetting angles. The smaller the angle of contact (0), the greater the spreading of a liquid over a solid. A hard lens is hydrophobic and has a 60-degree angle of contact with water. **A,** Low-wetting angle; **B,** wetting angle of methyl methacrylate hard lens; **C,** large wetting angle with droplet of mercury. (From Stein HA, Slatt BJ, Stein RM: *Fitting guide for rigid and soft contact lenses, a practical approach,* ed 3, St Louis, 1990, Mosby.)

a given condition at a given temperature in the laboratory only. The oxygen flux refers to the amount of oxygen that will pass through a given area of the material in a given amount of time driven by a given partial pressure difference of oxygen across the material. It is a function of the DK of the material, the lens thickness (L), and the pressure drop across the lens, ΔP.

Of more clinical importance is how much total oxygen passes through a lens and is permitted to reach the cornea. These are in vivo measurements, which involve the total lens and account for not only the material but also the design of the lens and its thickness in the center and the periphery. This measurement is called the equivalent oxygen performance, often referred to as the EOP.

DESIGNS OF CORNEAL CONTACT LENSES

Sophisticated corneal contact lens technology has made possible the manufacture of numerous widths, thicknesses, curvatures, and edge designs to aid the modern practitioner.

The contact lens can vary in diameter from 6 to 12 mm. The majority wear lenses with diameter of 8 to 10 mm, plus or minus 0.5 mm. The optic zone of the lens varies widely in diameter and may range

from 5 to 8 mm, depending on the overall diameter of the lens. Contact lenses are available in monocurve, bicurve, tricurve, multicurve, and aspheric designs.*

A secondary, or intermediate, curve is often put on a lens next to the base curve of the optic zone to accommodate the flatter periphery of the cornea. This intermediate curve may be 2.00 to 7.00 diopters flatter than the base curve. A tricurve lens is designed to have secondary curves. The width of these curves is relatively small, such as 0.2 mm. Occasionally, multicurve lenses are designed.

The resurgence of aspheric designs in rigid lenses has aimed to mimic the peripheral flattening of the cornea in a controlled and reproducible manner, thereby eliminating the need for progressively flattening peripheral curves.

The peripheral curve is the outermost curve and is much flatter than the other curves of the lens to conform to the flatter periphery of the cornea. The peripheral and intermediate curves permit a free flow of precorneal fluid under the lens.

To eliminate the sharp edges of the junction lines of these curves, the junctions are blended to give smoothness to the transition of the different curvatures. The blend may be light, whereby the zones are readily identified, or heavy, whereby the zones blend into each other.

Fenestration of hard lenses is valuable only from a historical perspective. Most rigid gas-permeable lens materials cannot be fenestrated because this increases the fragility of the lens. The ability of rigid gas-permeable lenses to transmit gases negates the functional need of fenestration.

Central thickness is an important factor in contact lens comfort. The thinner the lens, the more comfortable, but also the less stable the lens, the more likely it is to warp and break. When a gas-permeable lens is used, the thinner the lens the greater the oxygen transmission through the plastic.

Edge design of a contact lens is important and

---

*For additional lens design information, refer to Stein HA, Slatt BJ, Stein RM: *Fitting guide for rigid and soft contact lenses, a practical approach,* ed 3, St Louis, 1990, Mosby.

frequently the cause for patient rejection. The edge must be carefully designed, rounded, and polished. If the edge is too thick, it will irritate the eyelid margin. If it is too thin, it will be too sharp (knife edge) and also irritate.

Contact lenses can also have cylinder ground into the back surface *(back toric lenses)* into the front surface *(front toric lenses)* or into both the front and back surfaces *(bitoric lenses)*. Prism ballast can be incorporated in a contact lens to give weight to the lens and thus prevent rotation. Bifocals of varying design are also available (see Chapter 14).

EXAMINATION FOR CONTACT LENSES

Although a careful eye examination is mandatory for a practitioner to perform before evaluating whether a patient is a suitable candidate for contact lenses, certain areas must be delineated in more detail. Not only is a complete history of the eye relevant, but a history of systemic medications such as oral contraceptives or the possibility of pregnancy should also be recorded. During the inquiry, an assessment should be made not only of the person's reasons for desiring contact lenses but of personal hygienic habits and ability to look after the lenses and persevere with the required routines. For obvious reasons, the patient's manual dexterity should be evaluated. Also, the patient's temperament and emotional maturity should be evaluated so that introduction of contact lenses will ensure success rather than frustration and problems for both the practitioner and the patient. In those patients who were dissatisfied with previous contact lenses but wish to try again, one should establish the reason for the previous failure.

Over 95% or more of patients can wear contact lenses. The following instances preclude their use:

1. Blepharoconjunctivitis—chronic—from any cause such as seborrhea or acne rosacea
2. Pterygium formation—with small pterygiums, contact lenses can be fitted, but larger pterygiums may require removal first.
3. Seventh nerve palsy (Bell's palsy)
4. Poor hygiene—people who do not keep their hands clean will not keep their lenses clean. Clean fingernails trimmed short are mandatory.
5. Industrial hazards—welders' flash burns, people who deal with highly volatile acids or bases (alkalis)
6. Severe allergies—most allergic reactions can be suppressed by the use of local antihistamines. However, allergic reactions can reduce wearing time in soft lens wearers and cause papillary conjunctivitis.
7. Age—if the need is present, age is no barrier. One-day-old newborn children who have had cataract surgery have been fitted with contact lenses. The elderly, until intraocular lenses became popular, routinely wore aphakic contact lenses.

A careful slit lamp microscopic examination of the cornea before the patient begins contact lens wear will permit detection of small scars or opacities of the cornea that cannot later be blamed on the contact lens. The eyelids and in particular the undersurface of the upper eyelid should be examined for follicles, papules, and signs of inflammation. The lid margins must be free of blepharitis. Any ghost vessels or signs of new vessel formation on the cornea should be noted and their cause determined.

The patient's eyes should be refracted and the best possible visual acuity recorded. Any muscle imbalance should be measured by prisms, and particular attention should be paid to the phorias.

The corneal diameter can be measured with a ruler or by use of a pupillometer or a contact lens of known diameter. The most accurate method of measuring a cornea is by applying a contact lens. The size of the pupil may be measured by a ruler under room lighting conditions or estimated by a pupillary gauge. The height of the palpebral fissure and the area where the upper eyelid crosses the cornea should be recorded. These factors have an important bearing on the lens design. Lid tension can be estimated by grasping the lid between thumb and forefinger, pulling slightly down, and letting go. This will give a rough indication whether the eyelid is loose or tight. The practitioner should observe the patient to see if the blink rate is reasonably normal. Adequacy of tear production may be measured by the filter paper (Schirmer's) test. Keratometry (described later) is an important basis for the initial lens design required.

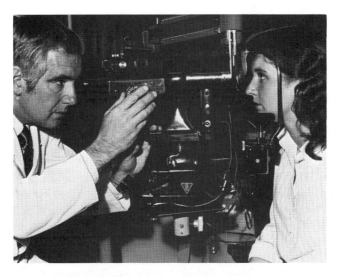

Fig. 13-12 Taking a keratometer reading.

FITTING CORNEAL CONTACT LENSES
Measurements

To fit a contact lens the following measurements are required: (1) the refractive error of the eye, (2) the dioptric power of the cornea, (3) the lens diameter, (4) the lens thickness, (5) the optic zone, and (6) the peripheral curve blending.

The *refractive error of the eye* is determined by conventional methods. Once the prescription for distance vision has been determined, the prescription is transposed to minus cylinders. The cylinder is disregarded by the fitter. The vertex distance of the spectacles should also be recorded, because the dioptric power of a plus lens will be increased and that of a minus lens decreased when the spectacle prescription is converted for contact lenses. These changes in the power of the lens are related to the distance from the original spectacle to the cornea and the power of the lens itself.

The *dioptric power of the cornea* is determined by keratometer readings (Fig. 13-12). For keratometer measurements, the patient is seated before the keratometer, with the chin placed on the chin rest. The room should have dim illumination. Two illuminated targets, called mires, are positioned to be reflected from the center of the cornea. The observer views the cornea through the telescopic system of the keratometer. This light is split by a prism into the images of the vertical and horizontal axis.

The keratometer should be calibrated on a steel ball of known radius at least once every two months. Before measurements are taken, the eyepiece should be adjusted to the observer's prescription. The patient should be comfortably seated and the keratometer placed so that the patient must lean slightly forward to rest his or her chin in the chin rest. The patient should then be instructed to press his or her head firmly against the forehead rest and to grasp the base of the instrument firmly with both hands in order to steady the head and to steadily fixate the eyes. The patient should be encouraged to open the eyes widely and to blink occasionally. The fitter should be seated with both feet flat on the floor, to operate the instrument without having to strain the neck or slump forward. Once the instrument has been aligned, the mires are positioned to be reflected from the center of the cornea. The fitter should constantly keep one hand on the knob that controls the clarity of the mire images and the other hand on the knob that controls the separation of the mire images; otherwise the instrument may be out of focus at the moment the final setting is made.

The Bausch & Lomb keratometer is typical of other keratometers in use (see the box on p. 289). The illuminated targets, or mires, consist of three illuminated circles, with one circle having a plus sign as an appendage. The central circle has both a plus and minus sign. At first the central circle will appear doubled (Fig. 13-13, *A*) until the focusing knob is used to produce a single central circle (Fig. 13-13, *B*). The black control cross should always be in the center of the right bottom circle. The next step is to rotate the axis of the keratometer so the plus and minus signs are aligned (Fig. 13-13, *C*). Then the horizontal measuring drum is turned so that the plus signs overlap and become single (Fig. 13-13, *D*). This is the first K reading. The vertical measuring drum is then turned so that the minus signs overlap (Fig. 13-13, *E*). This is the K reading of the second curvature. In exceptionally flat or steep corneas, readings cannot be taken without accessory lenses to extend the range of the keratometer.

It is common practice to record the horizontal reading first. The difference between the horizontal meridian and the vertical meridian constitutes the corneal astigmatism. As mentioned previously, when the horizontal meridian is flatter than the vertical meridian, the corneal astigmatism is referred to as *with the rule*. If the horizontal meridian is steeper than the vertical meridian, the corneal astigmatism is referred to as *against the rule*. When the corneal astigmatism of the eye differs from the refractive cylinder of the prescription, this difference is referred to as *residual astigmatism*.

Because the keratometer measures the central zone, or optic cap, of the cornea, which has a diameter of 5 to 7 mm and also includes the visual

---

BAUSCH & LOMB KERATOMETER

I. Adjusting the eyepiece:
  A. Position the occluder.
  B. Turn the eyepiece cap counterclockwise as far as possible; the user should see a blurred cross.
  C. Look through the eyepiece and turn the eye focus. Note the reading on the outer periphery of the eyepiece. Repeat the same set several times to verify the results.
II. Seat the patient comfortably before the instrument and fit the chin securely on the chin rest with the head against the headrest.
III. Level the keratometer to the patient's eye. Set the instrument at 90° and 180°. Put the instrument to one side to align it with the eye. Raise or lower the instrument until the silver pin on the side of the lamp house are lined with the patient's pupil. The patient's head must be positioned vertically and not tilted.
IV. Patient fixation—turn the instrument so that it points directly at the eye to be examined. One should see a tiny bright ring (the mire) in the center of the cornea. The mire should be aligned with the pupil, and the patient should see the reflection of his or her own eye.
V. Take the reading—to obtain the proper measurement the following steps should be followed:
  A. Focus the instrument carefully with the focusing knob. The double circle is seen with black crosshairs near the center when out of focus (Fig. 13-13, *A*). By turning the knob you should see a single clear circle with a clear cross in the center (Fig. 13-13, *B*).
  B. Rotate the instrument to locate the axis plus signs tip to tip. The axis of the cylinder is found when the tips of the two plus signs just touch. Turn the horizontal measuring drum until the plus signs are barely separated and the lines of the plus cylinders appear to be continuous (Fig. 13-13, *C*).
  C. Measure the horizontal meridians. Turn the left measuring drum until the plus signs are superimposed (Fig. 13-13, *D*).
  D. Measure the vertical meridians. Turn the right measuring drum until the minus signs are superimposed (Fig. 13-13, *E*). Actual diopter power of the corneal curvatures can be obtained.
  E. The difference between the two measurements is the amount of astigmatism. Read the axis on the scale and record.

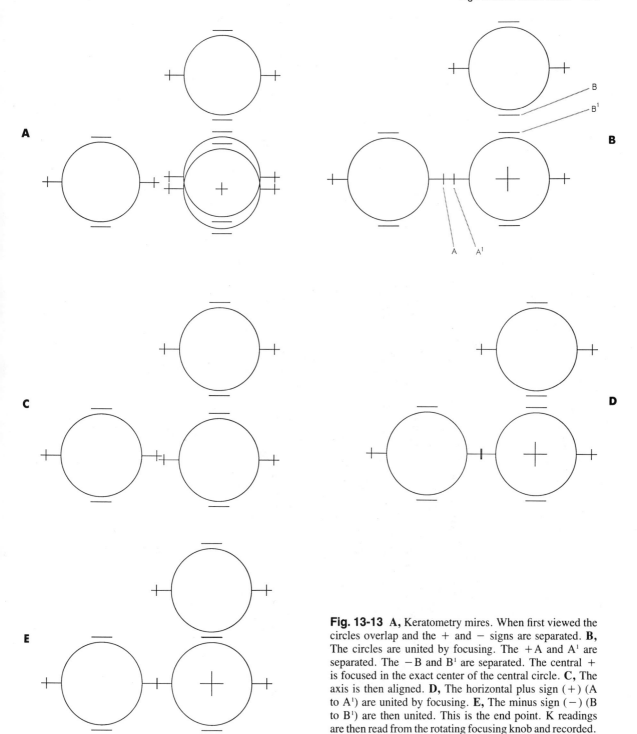

Fig. 13-13 A, Keratometry mires. When first viewed the circles overlap and the + and − signs are separated. **B,** The circles are united by focusing. The +A and A¹ are separated. The −B and B¹ are separated. The central + is focused in the exact center of the central circle. **C,** The axis is then aligned. **D,** The horizontal plus sign (+) (A to A¹) are united by focusing. **E,** The minus sign (−) (B to B¹) are then united. This is the end point. K readings are then read from the rotating focusing knob and recorded.

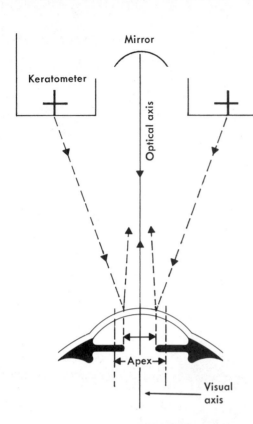

Fig. 13-14 The principle of the keratometer. The visual axis is aligned along the optical axis of the instrument so the central front surface of the cornea reflects the mires of the keratometer. (From Stein HA, Slatt BJ, Stein RM: *Fitting guide for rigid and soft contact lenses, a practical approach,* ed 3, St Louis, 1990, Mosby.)

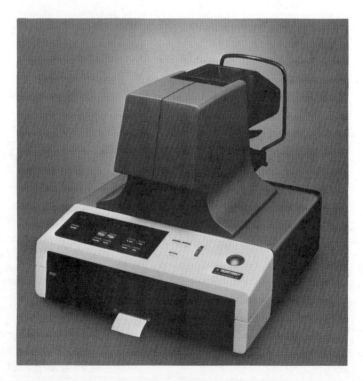

Fig. 13-15 The Humphrey automatic keratometer that provides a printout of the corneal curvature both centrally and peripherally to provide the shape factor of the cornea.

axis of the cornea, this reading should represent the base curve of choice (Fig. 13-14). However, the periphery of the contact lens actually rests on the intermediate zone of the cornea, which is somewhat flatter than the optic cap. Therefore the choice for the base curve for a contact lens is often steeper than the flattest ophthalmometer, or K, measurements.

Automated keratometers provide not only the dioptric K value of the central cornea but other data such as the shape of the cornea (Fig. 13-15). The corneoscope is another instrument that provides a photographic representation of the curvature of the portions of the cornea central to peripheral.

Topographic corneal analysis is today the most sophisticated way of analyzing the corneal dioptric values. By a sophisticated computerized readout with color analysis a person can determine 500 keratometry points on the cornea. This provides considerable new information and data on the cornea, which in turn can help determine how much flatter the periphery of the lens should be to the central radius of curvature. Details of this topographic analysis are addressed in Chapter 31.

The *size of the rigid contact lens* is important. Of historical importance is the *Topogometer*, which is an instrument designed to measure the optic cap, or apex of the cornea. In spherical corneas this optic cap is the same in all diameters, but in astigmatic corneas, there is a difference in curvature at different meridians. PMMA contact lenses are often ordered for each eye individually on the basis of the flattest radius of the optic cap plus 2 mm. Other factors that determine the size of the lens are the width of the palpebral fissure, the prominence of the globe, and the spasticity of the eyelids.

The *thickness of a lens* is an important factor in comfort. Again, thinner rigid lenses are more comfortable but are less stable and more likely to warp and break. Lenses should be ordered with minimal thickness and be verified by a thickness gauge. In powers greater than -6.00 diopters or $+2.50$, a lenticular design is frequently employed to reduce the thickness and consequently the weight of the lens. Some ultrathin lenses are available that will flex and provide less irritation.

The *optic zone* is generally referred to as the primary posterior curve (PPC). This is determined by the width of the *peripheral curves,* which are flatter than the base curve. The peripheral curves are designed in order to allow tear flow under the lens at the flatter corneal periphery.

Trial lenses

Trial lenses are simply a set of corneal contact lenses of known diameter, power, base curves, and peripheral curves. Most experienced practitioners use a fitting set of corneal contact lenses in conjunction with a keratometer. The use of a fitting set practically eliminates the need for exchanges of lenses. Most experienced fitters will agree that the best instrument to evaluate a fit is a contact lens on the eye.

Materials and manufacture

Corneal rigid contact lenses have for many years been constructed of PMMA. This material absorbs fluid minimally (less than 2%) as compared to the soft lenses which vary in hydration from 25% to 80%. PMMA has excellent optical qualities but requires some adaptation because of some discomfort associated with the use of this lens. These lenses are fitted smaller than the visible iris diameter but larger than the pupillary diameter and are known as corneal lenses.

The PMMA lens has for the most part been superceded by gas-permeable rigid contact lenses. To date, these lenses have been made of (1) cellulose acetate butyrate (CAB), (2) silicone acrylate, (3) styrene, (4) silicone resin, (5) fluoropolymer, and (6) fluoronated silicone-acrylate combinations. These lenses are often referred to as semisoft or flexible rigid contact lenses. These lenses are more flexible than standard PMMA lenses and have greater oxygen permeability, which is not found in the standard PMMA lenses. They have the advantage of being able to correct several diopters of corneal astigmatism and, because of their gas permeability, are able to maintain corneal detergescence and relieve some of the symptoms of corneal hypoxia.

Fitting gas-permeable lenses

The ideal fit for any gas-permeable lens is one in which the lens position is high, even when the lens

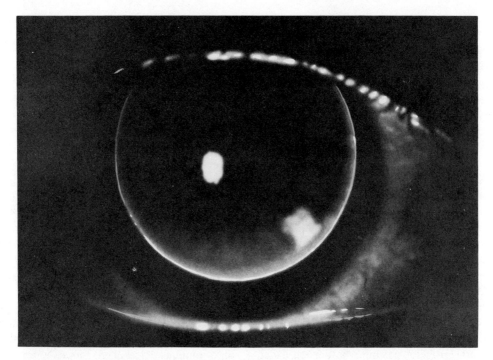

Fig. 13-16 Large gas-permeable rigid contact lens with upper edge under upper lid. Normal fit. (From Stein HA, Slatt BJ, Stein RM: *Fitting guide for rigid and soft contact lenses, a practical approach,* ed 3, St Louis, 1990, Mosby.)

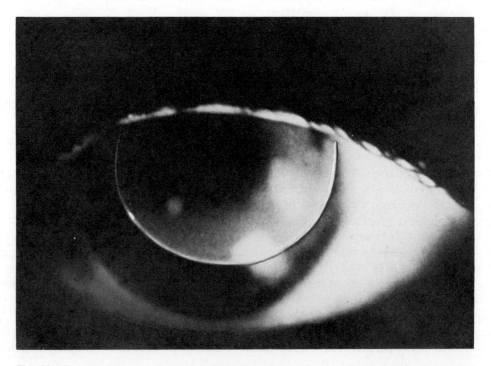

Fig. 13-17 A flat-fitting lens riding too high. (From Stein HA, Slatt BJ, Stein RM: *Fitting guide for rigid and soft contact lenses, a practical approach,* ed 3, St Louis, 1990, Mosby.)

overlaps the superior limbus (Fig. 13-16). The upper lid should cover a position of the lens during the full cycle of each blink. The purpose of the high-riding lens is to tuck the edge of the lens under the lid to avoid lid impact. This "full-sweep" blink also enhances lens surface wetting. The engagement of the upper lid margin with the edge of the lens is a major cause of discomfort. Even a soft hydrogel lens will be uncomfortable if it is made small and interpalpebral.

At times, the ideal may not be achieved (Fig. 13-17). The position of the upper lid may be too high to cover the upper position of the lens, or there may be excessive astigmatism, which because of the corneal topography resists the upper motion of the lens. In these cases, the central position may be accepted, provided that the patient accepts this type of fit, or modifications can be made. The lens diameter may be reduced to increase the lid lift, or a flatter base curve can be chosen. A central fit on the cornea is adequate, but a low-riding lens is unsatisfactory. When the lens is low, the blink rate is frequently suppressed to a minimum or the blink itself is incomplete. Also, a low lens is frequently a source of lid gap, which causes 3 and 9 o'clock-position staining of the cornea. The margin of the upper lid slides over the low lens, and it bridges the nasal and temporal cornea between the edge of the lens and limbus. Lid gap is especially common with highly myopic refractive corrective lenses because the edges of the lens are prone to be thicker than usual and the trough between the edge of the lens and the margin of the cornea is likely to be deep. Because these lenses are usually of large diameter, the proper edge treatment is essential. A plus edge or configuration for myopic lenses with power greater than −4.00 D and a minus edge for lenses +4.00 D or greater are usually designed.

Systems for fitting

Inventory fitting. There is a belief among some fitters that lens design and manufacturing is of primary importance and that soft lens systems may be applied to the gas-permeable lens. In effect, one manufacturer (Syntex Ophthalmics) believes that three diameters of lenses, 8.5, 9.0, and 9.5 mm, for

myopia will satisfy almost all requirements for patients, and they recommend 9.5 and 10.0 mm for aphakia. If adequate base curves are available, these lenses will simplify fitting.

For myopic patients, the larger 9.5 mm diameter is recommended for levels of high astigmatism and also for flatter corneas.

Inventory fitting by lenses with preselected diameter simplifies fitting because one has fewer variables to deal with. In addition, one can rely on the quality control in providing lenses and controlled edge designs by one manufacturer.

Lid sensation is directly dependent on the edge finishing. It must not be left thick, but thinned out to minimize lid sensation and the uncomfortable fitting of a lens that lies under the upper lid (Fig. 13-18). A good reliable laboratory is most important. A soft lens may be more comfortable, because of its relatively large diameter and its constant edge position underneath the upper eyelid.

Polycon, in an effort to maintain as high a per-

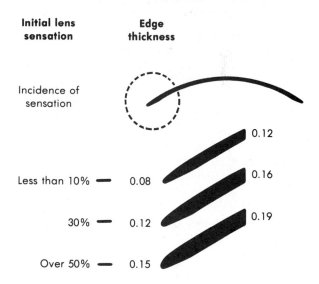

Fig. 13-18 Sensation of lens is directly related to edge thickness. Lens edges must be made thin to reduce lens sensation. Over 50% of patients with a lens edge 0.15 mm as noted in the lower lens will complain of sensation because of lens-lid impact. (Courtesy Syntex Ophthalmics, Inc., Phoenix, Ariz.) (From Stein HA, Slatt BJ, Stein RM: *A fitting guide for rigid and soft contact lenses, a practical approach*, ed 3, St Louis, 1990, Mosby.)

Table 13-2   Harrison-Stein nomogram: initial lens selection

If corneal cylinder <0.75:   select flattest K.
1.00 to 2.00 D: add ¼ of difference of 2 K's to flattest K.
>2 D: add ⅓ of the difference of 2 K's to flattest K.
(All plus prescriptions over +2.00 D should be in lenticular form.)

| Base curve (D) | Diameter (mm) | | Peripheral curves (mm/D) | | |
	Minus power	Plus power			
40.00 and 40.25	9.6	9.8	0.2/36.00	0.2/31.00	0.2/27.50
40.50 and 40.75	9.5	9.7			
41.00 and 41.25	9.4	9.6	0.2/36.00	0.2/31.00	0.2/27.50
41.50 and 41.75	9.3	9.5			
42.00 and 42.25	9.2	9.4	0.2/32.00	0.2/27.50	
42.50 and 42.75	9.1	9.3			
43.00 and 43.25	9.0	9.2	0.3/33.00	0.2/27.50	
43.50 and 43.75	8.9	9.1			
44.00 and 44.25	8.8	9.0	0.3/34.00	0.2/29.00	
44.50 and 44.75	8.7	8.9			
45.00 and 45.25	8.6	8.8	0.2/36.00	0.2/29.00	
45.50 and 45.75	8.5	8.7			
46.00 and 46.25	8.4	8.6	0.2/36.00	0.2/30.00	
46.50 and 46.75	8.3	8.5			

From Stein HA, Slatt BJ, Stein RM: *A fitting guide for rigid and soft contact lenses, a practical approach,* ed 3, St Louis, 1990, Mosby.

meability as possible, manufactures all minus lenses to a center thickness of 0.08 to 0.1 mm. This may not allow for lens flexure on high astigmatics. Custom lenses of greater center thickness may be better for these cases because the thicker lens marks the corneal toricity.

Inventory systems for rigid gas-permeable lenses may see a resurgence because a number of good aspheric and spherical stock lenses exist that fit a broad range of prescriptions and topographies with a relatively small number of lenses (250 or less). Many manufacturers are offering their particular design on a nationally available one, e.g. Boston Envision. This type of inventory system is good for the moderate to larger rigid gas-permeable practice. The important factor in making any of these systems work is the fitter's ability to select and diagnose the fittable lens.

Harrison-Stein nomogram method of fitting.*

*From Harrison R, Stein HA: *Nomogram for gas permeable silicone acrylate lenses, CLAO J* 9(4):324-326, 1983

The ideal method of fitting silicone-acrylate lenses is from a trial set where the lens is placed on the eye. There are a number of low-volume fitters and occasional fitters who do not wish to have and maintain a standard fitting trial set. We have developed, over the past few years, a nomogram that is designed to be a guide for the best possible starting point in lens selection (Table 13-2). With a nomogram, one may order the lens directly by referring to the nomogram for the initial lens factor.

The nomogram takes into account the progressive increase in diameter required for flatter corneas and the decrease in diameter for the steeper corneas. The second factor takes into account the increased thickness required for the soft silicone-acrylate lenses to avoid flexure on the cornea. The base curve is selected according to the corneal toricity. If the corneal cylinder is 0.75 D or less, we select the flattest K. If the corneal cylinder is between 1 and 2 D, we add one fourth of the difference of the two K's to the flattest K reading. If the corneal cylinder is over 2 D, we add one third of the difference to the flattest K.

Table 13-3   Harrison-Stein nomogram for fitting fluoronated silicone-acrylate lenses

Initial lens selection:
If corneal cylinder 0.75 D   Base curve 0.75 flatter than the flattest K
If corneal cylinder 1.00-1.75 D   Base curve 0.25 flatter than the flattest K
If corneal cylinder 1.75 D   Base curve 0.25 steeper than the flattest K

Base curve (D)	Diameter (mm) Plus and minus power	Peripheral curves (mm/D)		
8.44 and 8.39 mm	9.8	0.3/ 9.10 mm	0.2/10.50 mm	0.2/11.50 mm
40.00 and 40.25 D				
8.33 and 8.28 mm	9.7			
40.50 and 40.75 D		0.3/37.00 D	0.2/32.00 D	0.2/29.00 D
8.23 and 8.18 mm	9.6	0.3/ 9.10 mm	0.2/10.50 mm	0.2/11.50 mm
41.00 and 41.25 D				
8.13 and 8.18 mm	9.5			
41.50 and 41.75 D		0.3/37.00 D	0.2/32.00 D	0.2/29.00 D
8.04 and 7.99 mm	9.4	0.2/ 8.90 mm	0.2/10.00 mm	0.2/11.50 mm
42.00 and 42.25 D				
7.94 and 7.89 mm	9.3			
42.50 and 42.75 D		0.2/38.00 D	0.2/34.00 D	0.2/29.00 D
7.85 and 7.80 mm	9.2	0.2/ 8.90 mm	0.2/10.00 mm	0.2/11.50 mm
43.00 and 43.25 D				
7.76 and 7.71 mm	9.1			
43.50 and 43.75 D		0.2/38.00 D	0.2/34.00 D	0.2/29.00 D
7.67 and 7.63 mm	9.0	0.2/ 8.70 mm	0.2/ 9.50 mm	0.2/11.50 mm
44.00 and 44.25 D				
7.58 and 7.54 mm	8.9			
44.50 and 44.75 D		0.2/38.75 D	0.2/35.50 D	0.2/30.75 D
7.50 and 7.46 mm	8.8	0.2/ 8.70 mm	0.2/ 9.50 mm	0.2/11.50 mm
45.00 and 45.25 D				
7.42 and 7.38 mm	8.7			
46.00 and 46.25 D		0.2/38.75 D	0.2/35.50 D	0.2/30.75 D
7.34 and 7.30 mm	8.6	0.2/ 8.40 mm	0.2/ 9.20 mm	0.2/10.50 mm
46.00 and 46.25 D				
7.26 and 7.22 mm	8.5			
46.50 and 46.75 D		0.2/40.00 D	0.2/36.75 D	0.2/32.00 D

From Stein HA, Slatt BJ, Stein RM: *A fitting guide for rigid and soft contact lenses, a practical approach*, ed 3, St Louis, 1990, Mosby.

If the flattest curve of the cornea was 42.0 D and the cylinder axis was less than 0.75 diopters, we would select a lens 9.2 mm in diameter and provide the lab with the details of the peripheral curves.

In developing this nomogram, we have analyzed the fit of 987 eyes. We found that 75% could be fitted on a first-fit basis using this nomogram and most of the remainder fitted with less than two subsequent lenses.

We have developed a nomogram for the newer fluoronated silicone acrylate lenses, based on the fitting of 1,578 eyes (Table 13-3), which is similar to the silicone-acrylate nomogram. If one knows the K reading and the refractive findings, one can select the first lens which will fit 80% of the time.

Special solutions are required for silicone-acrylate lenses. The wetting and soaking solutions used at least 15 minues before insertion conditions the lens and improves its wetting angle. They also remove any accumulation of surface deposits.

Special problem solving with gas-permeable silicone acrylate and fluoronated silicone-acrylate lenses

Many of the major and disabling complications of PMMA lenses have been eliminated by the use of the new generation of gas-permeable lenses. There are still, however, a number of lens-regulated problems of the gas-permeable lenses that need to be addressed. By an understanding of these problems and solutions, practitioners are able to direct their attention to achieving happiness and success in a lens wearer.

Three o'clock and nine o'clock position staining. There are several causes of 3 o'clock and 9 o'clock position staining.

Lid gap. A lid gap occurs mostly with large-diameter rigid lenses. It is particularly prone to occur with gas-permeable lenses whose edges have not been properly thinned.

A gap occurs between the margin of the lens and the cornea. The meniscus of tears becomes very thin or absent at this border. It creates a lens-induced dry spot. The degree of staining is intense, often associated with episcleritis and formation of dellen. The staining of the cornea is attributable to desiccation of the corneal epithelium and not to corneal hypoxia. It is particularly prone to occur with lenses that ride low, that is, not brought up to a high position with a blink. Poor lid adherence is another cause of a low-riding lens.

The treatment is to make the lens flatter, thinner at the edges or smaller in diameter.

At times, the lens will rise with a blink and then suddenly drop to a low position. Such a lens requires a little alteration; flattening the blend and peripheral curves will frequently solve the problem and permit tear flow.

Poor blinking. The incomplete blinker dehydrates the exposed portion of the eye at the 3 and 9 o'clock positions. Lines of protein accumulation caused by dehydration across the lens indicates its presence.

Poor tear film. Some people have an insufficient tear film to support a large-diameter lens. With these people, supplementary tears during the day and a bland ointment at night may be enough to remedy the problem.

Comment. Three and 9 o'clock position staining is more common with large gas-permeable rigid lenses. Despite the intensity of the corneal erosions and episcleritis, patients do not seem to have much pain. Some fitters do not treat it because it may be an asymptomatic condition. This is an error. Breaks in the epithelial integrity should not be tolerated. More often than not, these patients primarily complain of the redness of their eyes.

Lens-flexure problems. The softer silicone component that is added to the silicone-acrylate mixture combined with the thin-designed lenses permits the lens to flex with each blink because of the pressure effect of the eyelid on the lens, which may rock on a toric cornea. This phenomenon results in blurring of vision, along with a residual astigmatism that is not corrected by the tear film.

Against-the-rule corneas create even more lens flexure as the lid sweeps over the lens. Steeper fitting of the lens also will create more opportunity for lens flexures. Smaller lenses may produce even more flexure than the larger-diameter lenses, which have a greater stabilizing force.

The newer fluorocarbon lenses combined with silicone acrylate are even more prone to produce flexure. They are also capable of wrapping on the cornea and creating a glued-on syndrome. The fluorocarbonated silicone-acrylate lens should be fitted at least 0.5 D flatter than one would fit the silicone-acrylate lens.

These problems of lens flexure are problems that are presenting themselves because the new generation of lenses is being used to correct astigmatism. These problems were apparent with soft HEMA lenses in the early years. Their use for corneal toricity was minimal because one soon learned that the soft HEMA lenses draped entirely over the cornea, since they did not have any hard component. These lenses did not significantly correct large measures of corneal astigmatism.

To remedy this problem, the practitioner needs to increase the thickness of the lens. This will vary with the degree of corneal cylinder present. As a general rule, the thickness should be increased by 20% to 30% for larger lenses, and 40% to 60% for the smaller lenses, which are more subject to flexure.

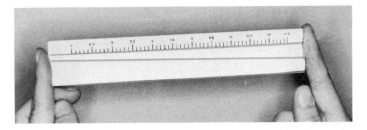

Fig. 13-19 V groove to measure hard lens diameter.

The lens should also be fitted high under the upper lid to minimize flexure, which may occur with an interpalpebral lens.

EVALUATING CONTACT LENSES

Contact lens practitioners should accept only high-quality lenses furnished by the manufacturing laboratory. Lenses arriving from the laboratory should be verified that they have been made to exact specifications. By doing so and by rejecting lenses that fall below standard, the practitioner will keep the laboratory on guard to furnish high-quality material. In addition, adequate evaluation of the lens dimensions will eliminate frustrations in fitting that might be attributed to faulty lens construction. Many unnecessary lens modifications may be prevented if proper lens inspection is performed.

Measuring diameter

The total diameter of a contact lens may be measured by a magnifier that basically consists of a plus lens with a scale. The contact lens is held between thumb and forefinger until one edge is aligned with the zero portion of the scale. The diameter can be read directly from the scale.

An alternate method is to place the contact lens, concave side down, into a ruler with a V-shaped groove (Fig. 13-19) until it slides into the lowest area in the groove in which it can no longer move. The measurement is then read directly from the adjacent scale on the plastic bar.

The contact lens may also be measured on the Shadowgraph and its diameter read off against the scale of the Shadowgraph (see Fig. 13-22).

Contacto Gauge and Radiuscope

Either the Contacto Gauge* or the Radiuscope[†] may be used to measure the base curve of a contact lens (Fig. 13-20). This measurement enables the examiner not only to check the accuracy of the lens received from the manufacturing laboratory but also to detect possible warpage of a lens that would be responsible for improper fitting. Some examiners feel that the peripheral curvature of a contact lens

---

*The Neitz Instrument Co Ltd, Tokyo, Japan.
[†]American Optical Co, Buffalo, NY.

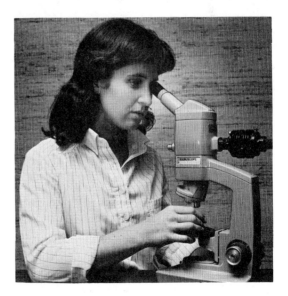

Fig. 13-20 Measuring curvature of a contact lens with the Radiuscope.

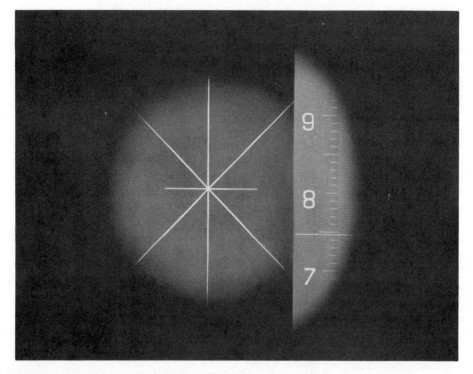

Fig. 13-21 Pattern and inside measuring scale in Radiuscope. (From Stein HA, Slatt BJ, Stein RM: *Fitting guide for rigid and soft contact lenses, a practical approach,* ed 3, St Louis, 1990, Mosby.)

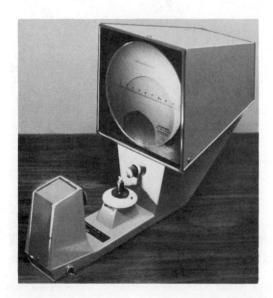

Fig. 13-22 Shadowgraph used to magnify and measure a contact lens.

may be measured with these instruments, but others feel that these latter measurements are unreliable.

Following are rules for measuring the concave curve of a contact lens with the Contacto Gauge:

1. Mount a concave lens mount horizontally on the mount holder. Put one drop of water in the hollow of the mount. Place the contact lens horizontally in the mount with its concave side upward.

2. Turn on the light. Move the microglide stage to center the contact lens in a position just beneath the objective.

3. While looking through the eyepiece, rotate the coarse adjustment knob clockwise until the spoke-pattern target comes into view. Center the target in the eyepiece by moving the microglide stage. Bring the target into sharpest focus by using the coarse and fine adjusting knobs.

4. Set the dial gauge on zero.

5. Continue to rotate the coarse adjustment knob until the target disappears and the filament comes into view. Continue through the filament until the target reappears (real image). Refine the sharpness of the target by using the coarse and fine adjustment knobs.

6. The radii of curvature reading is now taken from the dial gauge. The short hand in the inner dial is the whole number, for example, 5, 6, or 7 mm. The long hand in the outer dial is the fraction of the whole number expressed in decimal equivalents of hundredths of a millimeter, for example, 0.23, 0.59, or 0.101.

The Radiuscope operates in a similar way. If the convex radius of curvature measurement is desired, the examiner should proceed with either instrument exactly as for the concave measurement but should place the lens initially in a convex lens mount and float the contact lens with the convex side upward. (Fig. 13-21).

Shadowgraph and Contactoscope

The Shadowgraph* and Contactoscope† (Fig. 13-22) use light transmitted through the lens for inspecting contact lenses. The shadowgraph magnifies a contact lens in cross section or in front view. Magnification of the contact lens to 20 times its size is accomplished by internal projection on a ground-glass screen. On the screen is a reticule scale graduated in 0.1 mm, which can be used to measure (1) the diameter of the lens, (2) the width of the peripheral curve, (3) the width of any blending area, and (4) the width of the intermediate curve. The blending zone cannot be seen by the naked eye but can be evaluated only under the large magnification created by the Shadowscope. The Shadowscope is also useful in showing scratches on the optical surface of the contact lens, as well as any cracks or nicks in the edge.

The cross-section view of the contact lens shows up the contour of the edge so the edge thickness can be measured, which should be no thicker than 0.12 mm.

Use of Shadowgraph and Contactoscope. The contact lens is first placed on a vertically-mounted stage to provide a front view of the lens. The image is focused on the screen by a lever under the stage. The lens should be scrutinized for scratches, nicks, and cracks. The screen image can be raised or lowered by a knob on the stage so that the lens can be placed against the measuring scale. The diameter of the lens can then be measured on the scale. The peripheral curve width, the blend width, and the intermediate curve width can then be inspected and measured.

To view the lens on the edge either rotate the lens perpendicular to the screen or lay the lens on its convex surface on the stage. Refocus to get a sharp image of the edge. Move the stage laterally to project the image of the edge on the reticule scale for measuring edge thickness.

Measuring power

The power of a contact lens may be measured on the standard Lensometer. By holding the lens between thumb and forefinger, concave side down, the examiner can measure the back vertex power of the contact lens. A small error in the power will arise because of the impossibility of placing the concave surface firmly against the instrument. With low-power lenses this is of such small magnitude that it will not interfere with practical use of the information regarding the power of the lens. It will, however, introduce a significant error in high plus–power lenses.

Profile analyzer

Proper evaluation of the peripheral curves and the blend at the junction is probably the most important feature of evaluation of a contact lens. It is the blending and proper curvature in the periphery that will permit adequate tear exchange and a satisfactory wearing time without corneal trauma.

The profile analyzer (Fig. 13-23) is an instrument designed to show the profile of a contact lens and is invaluable in any office where contact lens work is performed. It will detect whether the zones between the central and peripheral curve are sharp or whether they have been blended and smoothed out, thereby adding to proper venting and comfort of the lens (Fig. 13-24).

---

*Urocon, Inc, Hollywood Calif.
†Wesley-Jessen, The Plastic Contact Lens Co, Chicago, Ill.

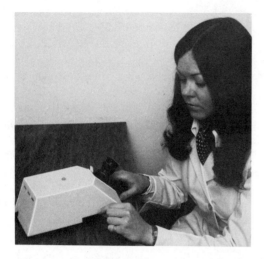

Fig. 13-23 Profile analyzer used to evaluate the blend of the peripheral curves of a lens.

Measuring thickness

For measuring thickness, a contact lens is inserted in the thickness gauge, convex side down.

The pin of the gauge is allowed to descend slowly until contact is made with the concave surface. The measure is read from the dial (Fig 13-25).

INSTRUCTIONS FOR INSERTION AND REMOVAL OF CONTACT LENSES

It is important that the patient be carefully instructed on how to insert, remove, and care for contact lenses.

Insertion

The hands should always be carefully washed and dried before insertion of the lens. The lens should be cleaned and wet before inserting; it should be balanced concave side up, on the tip of the index finger (Fig. 13-26). The lens should be moistened with contact lens solution or methyl cellulose. The right hand should be used for the right lens, and the left hand for the left lens, although this may vary with patient preference. The patient should look

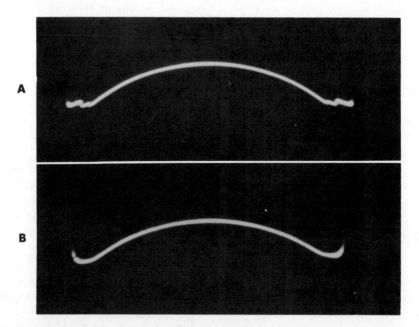

Fig. 13-24 A, Poorly finished transition zone as determined by the profile analyzer. **B,** Perfect transition zone with ski contour at its periphery. (From Stein HA, Slatt BJ, Stein RM: *Fitting guide for rigid and soft contact lenses, a practical approach,* ed 3, St Louis, 1990, Mosby.)

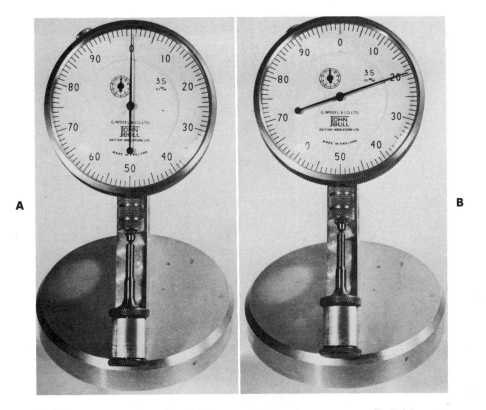

Fig. 13-25 A, Prior to measuring, thickness gauge must be set to zero. **B,** Thickness gauge. (From Stein HA, Slatt BJ, Stein RM: *Fitting guide for rigid and soft contact lenses, a practical approach,* ed 3, St Louis, 1990, Mosby.)

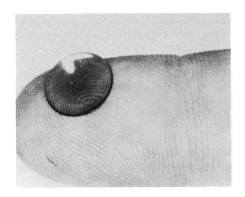

Fig. 13-26 Contact lens placed concave side up.

straight down, chin on chest, keeping both eyes open. The upper lid should then be held at the lashes with the fingers of the opposite hand pressing up and against the bony margin of the brow. The lower lid should be held at the lash margin with the fourth finger of the hand that is holding the lens, pressing down and against the cheek. The lens finger should then be brought straight up to the eye until the lens touches the eye (Fig. 13-27). An instant afterward, the lower lid should be released, and then slowly the upper lid. It is important to impress on the patient that he should not look away at the last moment. The head must always be kept straight and the temptation to turn must be avoided.

In the early stages of learning to insert the lenses, the use of a mirror will help. The patient should

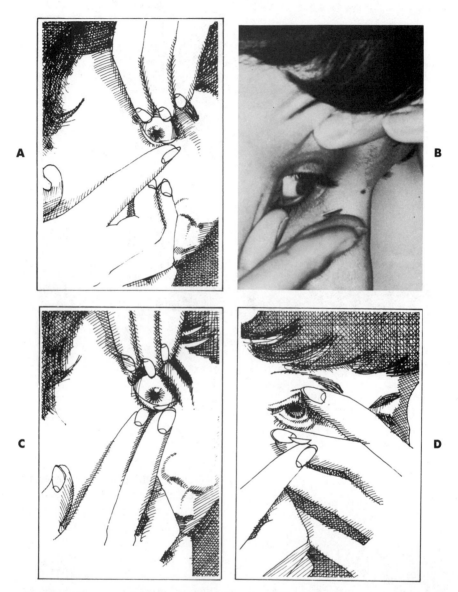

Fig. 13-27 Insertion by the patient. **A,** The upper lid is retracted by grasping the lid near the margin and retracting it. The left hand is used to elevate the right upper lid. The patient's gaze is directed downward, and the lens is carried to the eye by the index finger of the right hand. **B,** Incorrect method—the upper lid should be grasped near the lid margin, and the lens should rest on the tip of the finger. **C,** For the unsteady or tremulous patient, the middle finger carrying the lens rests on the index finger. **D,** The lids are separated by the index finger retracting the upper lid and the middle finger depressing the lower lid. The index finger of the free hand brings the lens to the eye.

Common fluorescein patterns

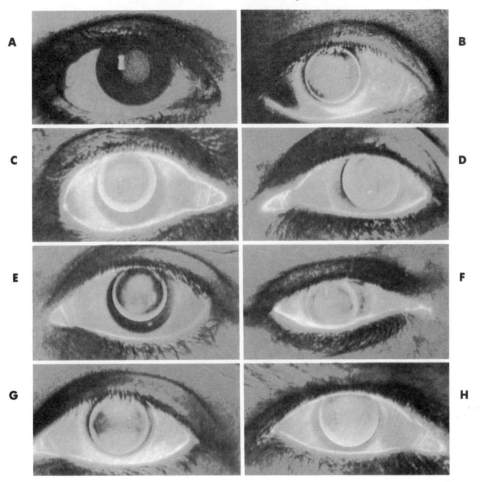

Plate 1 *Corneal lens.* **A,** Normal fluorescence of the crystalline lens without the instillation of fluorescein. This is a source of confusion to the novice in assessing the fit. **B,** Minimal apex-clear fitting in a corectopic patient with the pupil at the limbus at the 12 o'clock position. Note that a more apex-clear lens would show a broader dark band of contact adjacent to the peripheral curve. **C,** The apex-clear pattern in the normal eye. Note the fluorescence of the crystalline lens within the pupil. **D,** Flat-fitting lens. There is touch at the apex of the lens. **E,** Flat-fitting lens. A pool of fluorescein with a curved lower limit is seen above the central touch. **F,** Flat-fitting lens. A pool of fluorescein with a curved upper limit is seen below the central touch. **G,** Flat astigmatic picture. The other eye of the patient with corectopia is seen in **B. H,** Apex-clear astigmatic pattern in a normal eye. (Reproduced by permission from Duke-Elder S (editor): *System of ophthalmology,* vol V, Ophthalmic optics and refraction (by Duke-Elder S, Abrams D), St Louis, 1970, Mosby.)

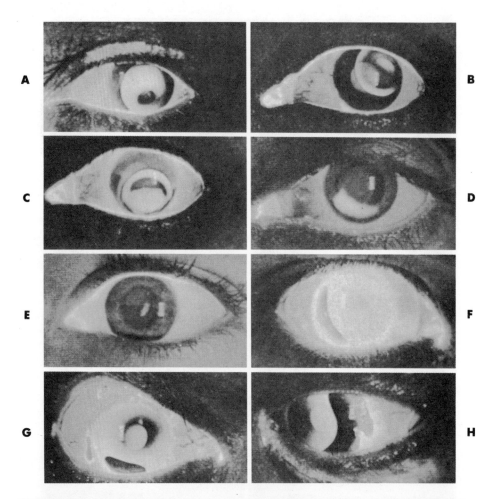

Plate 2 *Corneal lens*. **A,** Keratoconus. A hard touch in the area of the cone, lifting off the lens in other areas. **B,** Keratoconus. A thin, small lens fitted to the flattest keratometry reading. This lens proved satisfactory. **C,** Same case as in **B,** with the lens in a lower position, showing a completely different fluorescein pattern. **D,** Asymptomatic corneal stain of a superficial punctate type, 6 days after cessation of corneal lens wear. **E,** Transient crescentic staining of a granular or punctate type with a corneal lens, differing from that resulting from central corneal edema and not giving rise to any serious complications.

Scleral lens. **F,** Normal eye, scleral lens. There is a light corneal touch with adequate limbal clearance and a sausage-shaped bubble associated with the fenestration. **G,** Central corneal touch. Poor limbal clearance. **H,** Nasal corneal touch and enlargement of the bubble on adduction. (Reproduced by permission from Duke-Elder S (editor): *System of ophthalmology,* vol V, Ophthalmic optics and refraction (by Duke-Elder S, Abrams D), St Louis, 1970, Mosby.)

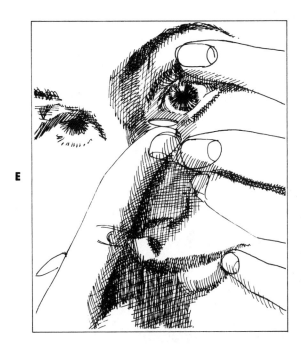
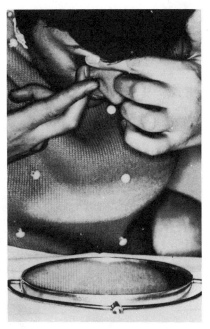

Fig. 13-27, cont'd E, The lids are separated laterally between the index and middle fingers while the hand opposite the eye carries the lens. **F,** Use of a mirror for insertion of a lens. (From Stein HA, Slatt BJ, Stein RM: *Fitting guide for rigid and soft contact lenses, a practical approach,* ed 3, St Louis, 1990, Mosby.)

learn to insert the lenses as soon as possible without a mirror, because one may not be handy at all times.

Some individuals are more successful in placing a lens on the eye when they do not have to look at the lens coming toward the eye. These individuals should look downward, with the upper lid lifted by the forefinger or middle finger. The lens is then placed on the sclera above the cornea, and the upper lid is released. The lens will usually center itself on the eye. As an alternative, one can look up and place the lens on the lower sclera, pushing the lens up with the lower eyelid margin.

Removal

Removal of the lens is much easier. The lens should always be centered before removal is attempted. The patient should be instructed to look down and to cup the opposite hand under the eye to catch the lens. The forefinger is placed on the outer corner of the eyelid and the lid is pulled aside at the same time

the patient blinks (Fig. 13-28). The lens will usually "pop" out.

Another method of removal is the scissor method. In this method the upper lid is held by the forefinger and the lower lid is held by the middle finger of the same hand. The lids are then separated at the lateral margin like a pair of scissors is opened. The patient is asked to blink at the same time that this maneuver is done.

The two-handed method actually pushes the lids under the lens. One finger of one hand grasps the upper lid, and the index finger of the other hand grasps the lower lid. The lids are then pushed toward the contact lens, squeezing it out of the eye.

Centering

Lenses may lodge off-center and thus may appear (1) under the upper lid, (2) under the lower lid, (3) in the outside corner of the eye, or (4) in the inside corner of the eye. The wearer should never panic

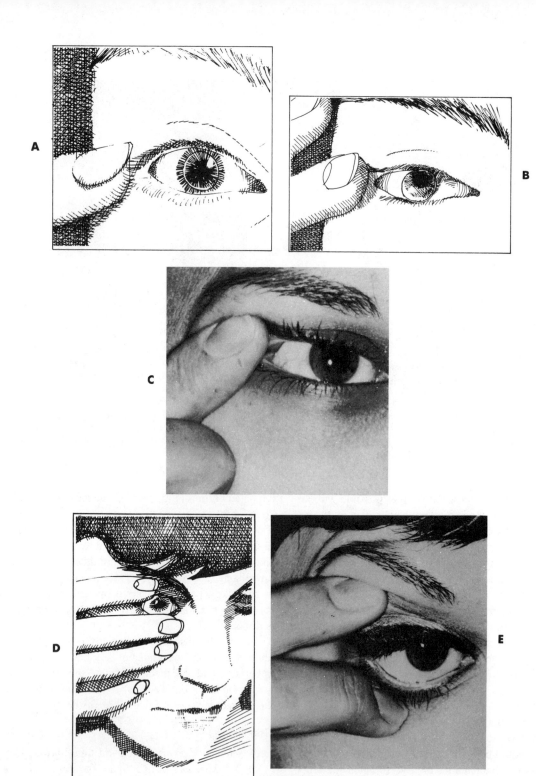

Fig. 13-28 Removal by the patient. **A** through **C,** The index finger tugs at the lateral canthus in an outward and upward direction. If the lids are held widely open, the edge of the lid margin should engage the lens and dislodge it. **D** and **E,** The open-handed scissors method. The lids are opened widely and the index and middle fingers are applied to the upper and lower lids to squeeze the lens off the eye.

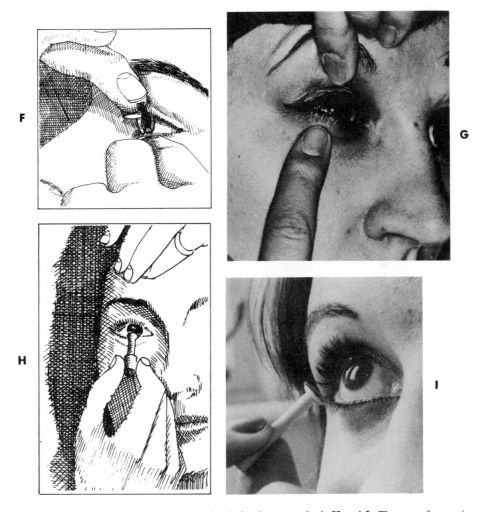

Fig. 13-28, cont'd F and **G,** The two-handed scissors method. **H** and **I,** The use of a suction cup is best delegated to an assistant to avoid inadvertent application of the cup to the cornea. (From Stein HA, Slatt BJ, Stein RM: *Fitting guide for rigid and soft contact lenses, a practical approach,* ed 3, St Louis, 1990, Mosby.)

under these circumstances, since a gentle push in the appropriate direction will be able to center the lens easily.

The lens can be centered by feeling for it through the closed eyelid. The patient is instructed to place his four fingers on the eyelid and to gaze straight ahead. The lens is then massaged toward the center of the eye (Fig. 13-29). This can also be done with one finger (Fig. 13-30).

Do's and don'ts with contact lenses

1. The hands should be washed before the handling and insertion of contact lenses.
2. It is helpful to wet the finger before balancing a lens on it.
3. The eye should not be rubbed with the lens in place.
4. After removal of the lenses, they should be rinsed in tap water to remove secretions.

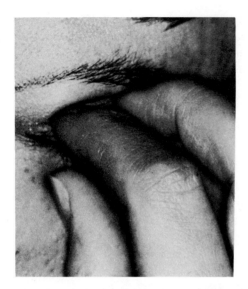

Fig. 13-29 Centering the lens by massage.

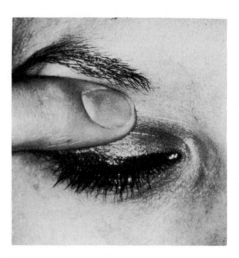

Fig. 13-30 Centering the lens with the index finger.

5. Storage of the lens is wet storage in contact lens solution. This permits the lens to be more comfortable on initial wearing.

6. Lenses should not be rinsed or placed in hot water, because the lenses may warp under extreme heat.

7. Beauty aids such as mascara should be used sparingly around the eyes. It is important to insert contact lenses before any cosmetic is applied to the lids. Any cosmetic with an oily base should not be used, since any oily agent will gather on the lenses and cause distortion of vision. Similarly, if a facial cleansing agent is employed to wipe away a cosmetic, a liquid, nongreasy material is preferable to cold cream or other products with an oily base. Mascara should be used sparingly on the lashes, and only the waterproofed brands are advisable. It should be placed on the very tips of the lashes only. Also, liquid eyeliner is preferred because it does not run or flake as does pencil eyeliner. False eyelashes should be used sparingly or not at all. They are made from human hair, animal hair, or synthetic fibers and are applied with adhesive to either the underside of the lid or the outside lid margin. In many cases the adhesive breaks off and enters the eye, interceding between the cornea and the contact lens and causing irritation and abrasions. Hair spray is also irritating to the corneas. Certainly, anybody wearing contact lenses should use hair spray with caution. The eyes should be closed when the hair spray is used and kept closed for several moments until the air clears. Similarly, the eyes should be kept closed when the head is placed under a hot hair dryer because the dryer causes evaporation of tears and a dry eye, which in turn can result in a corneal abrasion.

8. The lens wearer should avoid swimming while wearing rigid contact lenses; swimming is possible while wearing contact lenses but they are easily washed out.

9. Body-contact sports such as hockey and football should be avoided. These sports require large contact lenses that can be worn without fear of having them dislodged. These individuals may be best suited with soft lenses. For other types of activities such as golf, jogging, tennis, or badminton, regular contact lenses can be worn with confidence.

CARE OF CONTACT LENSES

Much has been written about the care of contact lenses. Of primary importance are the solutions that are used to minimize the possibility of bacterial contamination and permit relative safety for the eye. Also important is that the lens remain optically clear, free of debris and secretions, so that the lens will be comfortable when placed in the eye. The number of solutions available is legion, with many having combination features of wetting, cleaning, and soaking.

Superpermeable rigid contact lenses are slightly flexible. The lens wearer should not bend or flex the lenses, because they may warp or change shape so as to alter its fit. In addition, they are more fragile and may chip or crack.

The newer rigid lenses should be cleaned after each removal by placing them in the palm of the hand and cleaning the outer as well as the central portions with a suitable cleaner.

The lenses should be kept hydrated when not worn by soaking them in the recommended solution. This will not only disinfect the lenses but make them more wettable.

Care of gas-permeable lenses

Giant papillary conjunctivitis, which is an autoimmune papillitis of the upper tarsal conjunctiva, occurs with gas-permeable lenses but not with the same frequency as with hydrogel lenses. Allergic reactions occur in 1% to 5% of hard lens wearers and increases to 10% to 20% in soft lens wearers.

It is important to keep gas-permeable lenses clean. Daily nonsensitizing surface acting cleaners assist in reducing the incidence of papillary conjunctivitis. After cleaning, a saline solution, preferably without preservatives, should be used to rinse the lens. At times, reactions can occur to the saline solutions and the cleaners. Usually, it is the preservative thimerosal that is the sensitizing agent. In such cases, nonpreserved saline solution made fresh daily or dispensed from an airtight container should be used. Weekly or bimonthly cleaning may be necessary. Soft-lens weekly cleaners can be best employed for the more thorough cleaning. How does a patient know the lenses are dirty? After cleaning, the lenses should be clear and transparent. If the lens is exposed to a light source, the dirty deposits will become visible instantly.

Wetting solutions

The main function of a wetting solution is to convert the water-repelling surface of a rigid lens into a water-loving, or hydrophilic, surface. Ordinarily, the dry plastic, when dipped in water, will dry rapidly as the beads of water accumulate in little bubbles on the surface. Once a wetting agent has been used, the water forms a uniform film over the surfaces of the plastic. Thus when a wetting agent is used on a contact lens, the tear film spreads easily and evenly on both surfaces of the lens, not only making the lens comfortable by acting as a cushion but providing excellent refractive properties.

In addition to the wetting propery, the use of a wetting solution tends to maintain the cleanliness of the lens by preventing smudging by the fingers. Once the wetting solution bottle has been opened, sterility cannot be guaranteed, and hence most commercial solutions contain a preservative to maintain sterility of the solution.

The practice of using saliva as a wetting agent before insertion is to be condemned. Although it does have good wetting characteristics because of a polysaccharide present, the risk of bacterial contamination to the lens is so real as to make the procedure totally unjustified. In addition to other microbes, *Pseudomonas aeruginosa* is found in 6.6% of the population. Urine is much more sterile than saliva!

Soaking solutions

Soaking solutions are designed to clean the lens of oily and sebaceous secretions that accumulate from the eyelid and conjunctival glands. Soaking the lens overnight in properly designed solutions removes these secretions from the lens. If the lenses are stored dry without adequate cleaning, they will accumulate secretions, which harden on the lens surface to form a film that will be difficult to remove except by polishing.

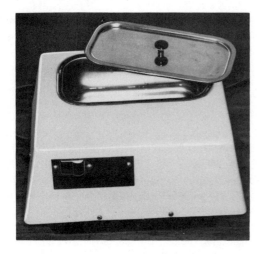

Fig. 13-31 Sonic cleaner for cleaning contact lenses.

In addition to the function of cleaning, soaking solutions contain germicidal agents that act to disinfect the contact lens. Although this action is by no means complete, certainly having little if any sterilizing effect on fungi and viruses, it does render some asepsis to the lens.

Another valuable benefit of overnight soaking of a lens is the ability of the plastic to absorb some water. This maintains the lens in a constant curvature, reduces irritation, and maintains good vision.

Cleaning solutions

When a lens is removed from the eye, it will be covered with oily secretions, mucus, or crystalline deposits. These materials must be removed before storage. Household detergents are not recommended, because they often leave a film on the lens. Patients should clean the lens before storage by applying a few drops of a lens cleaner on the lens and rubbing the lens between the thumb and forefinger and then rinsing the lens well in water. They must avoid such agents as alcohol, acetone, kerosene, or lighter fluid in cleaning plastic lenses. Mechanical (swirl clean) and electrical (sonic clean) cleaning instruments are available for cleaning contact lenses adequately (Fig. 13-31).

Eye drops with contacts

Some practitioners recommend eye drops with high viscosity to reduce lens sensation. Also available are drops that clean and rewet the lens while the patient is wearing them.

Lens cases

Lens cases are frequently the harbinger of germs that can contaminate contact lenses. It is important that lens cases be kept scrupulously clean. A good routine to follow is to scrub the lens case at least once weekly with a toothbrush and soap.

EVALUATING THE FIT OF CONTACT LENSES

An ideal fit is one in which wear is comfortable, vision is clear and comfortable with minimal spectacle blur, and there are no disturbances of the corneal integrity.

Subjective criteria

Adaptation symptoms. Initially the patient must adapt to the presence of the contact lens, which is basically a foreign body that rides on the surface of the cornea. The adaptive symptoms the patient has in early wear are normal and are distinguished from symptoms caused by poor fit in that they consistently decrease until they disappear as wearing time is increased. The following are some of the symptoms the patient may experience with early contact lens wear:

1. *Awareness of the lens.* Normally the patient is expected to be aware of the presence of corneal lenses. With time this awareness abates.
2. *Photophobia, or light sensitivity.* Photophobia that persists after the adaptation period is a symptom of corneal irritability. The patient has discomfort and even pain when exposed to normal thresholds of light.
3. *Spectacle blur.* Foggy vision occurs when the contact lens is removed and glasses are worn. The spectacle blur is caused by edema of the central portion of the cornea, which may be a result of inadequate oxygen transport to the cornea, either from inadequate tear transport

to the cornea or a material that has insufficient oxygen permeability characteristics.

4. *Reflections.* Internal reflections may occur from the contact lens itself or from a lens that decenters.

5. *Burning sensation.* This symptom of corneal irritability may represent corneal edema, corneal erosion, or excessive eyelid contact.

During the adaptation period, because the patient may have tearing, lid irritation, and excessive sensitivity to light, activities that require good visual acumen should be avoided. Until the adaptation period is complete, the patient should avoid driving a car, working on lathes, grinders, and other high-velocity moving equipment and doing prolonged close work.

Abnormal symptoms. Symptoms may be caused by poor technique on the part of the patient in the insertion or removal of the lenses. A poor insertion method is a common failing of the novice. Among the hazards of improper insertion are the tendencies of the patient to flinch, move the eye quickly, thrust the lens against the cornea, or squeeze the lids around the lens.

Symptoms caused by low oxygen (hypoxia) to the cornea tend to become more severe and more constant as the lenses are worn. Lenses that prevent adequate tear and oxygen exchange are referred to as "tight" lenses, but they are essentially caused by starvation of oxygen from the cornea. The symptom of corneal hypoxia is a burning sensation that appears after a comfortable induction period of 2 to 3 hours. Such a lens may not lag with eye movement, will not drop when the lids are pulled away, and shows little or no excursion with blinking. These are the signs of a "tight" lens. On the other hand, if the lens is too "loose," it may frequently slip off the cornea or fall out of the eye.

Poor vision may be a result of a variety of conditions. The power of the lens may be in error, the fit of the lens may be poor, the lens may be warped, or the lens may have been inserted in the wrong eye.

A distinction should be made between foggy vision that occurs upon insertion of the lens and that

which arises 2 to 3 hours after contact lens wear. The former is usually caused by improper cleansing or mucus under the lens. The latter is usually indicative of corneal edema or corneal hypoxia and is a pathologic finding.

Excessive awareness of a contact lens can be a psychologic problem, as it is only an extension of the normal conscious feeling of something foreign on the eye. However, the normal contact lens wearer usually has many periods during the day when he is free of this sensation. If the patient should *suddenly* become aware of his contact lens, this symptom may be indicative of roughened and scratched edges of the lens or the presence of dried secretions on its surface.

A burning sensation is generally attributed to a tight lens, to stagnation of tear fluid between the lens and cornea, corneal anoxia, or to damage of the corneal epithelium. In the first three causes the symptom abates on removal of the lens, while in the last it does not.

The patient with a foreign body sensation will either harbor a tiny foreign body between his lens and cornea, particularly in dusty areas, or have erosions of his cornea because of contact between the lens and the cornea.

Any patient who has pathologic symptoms should be told to remove the lenses and be reassessed before wear is resumed.

Abnormal symptoms and signs and the corrections required to eliminate them are discussed further in Chapter 14.

Objective criteria

The fit of a contact lens may be objectively evaluated according to its relationship to the lid margins and its position on the cornea. Ideally, the upper margin of the lens should fit under the upper lid and be free of the lower lid (Fig. 13-32). Blinking action of the lids should raise the lens slightly. The contact lens should be well centered on the cornea and not displaced to either side.

Other objective criteria used to evaluate the fit of a contact lens include (1) fluorescein patterns, (2) alteration of the blink rate, (3) scratches, chips, and

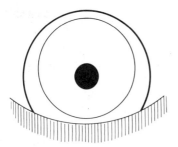

Fig. 13-32 Normal position of the contact lens lies 1 to 2 mm above the edge of the lower eyelid.

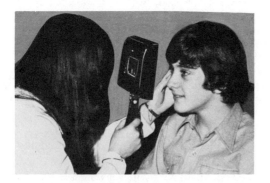

Fig. 13-33 Burton lamp to evaluate fit of contact lens.

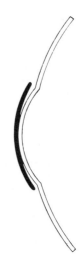

Fig. 13-34 Flat contact lens resting on apex of cornea.

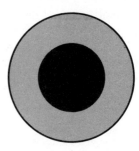

Fig. 13-35 Fluorescein pattern of a flat lens. Note absence of dye centrally.

roughened edges of the contact lens, and (4) changes in the cornea.

Fluorescein patterns (Plates 1 and 2). If the size and movement of the lens in the patient's eye appear satisfactory, the fluorescein test should follow. In this test, fluorescein is placed on the superior margin of the cornea, and the fluorescein patterns are best seen with an ultraviolet lamp source for illumination and a slit-lamp microscope or handheld magnifier for inspection (Fig. 13-33). The fluorescein dye forms a thin layer between the contact lens and the cornea. The distribution of the dye enables the observer to evaluate the adequacy of the precorneal fluid layer between the contact lens and the cornea.

The patient with a normal corneal contour will have an even and thin layer of dyed tear film centrally surrounded by a slightly deeper ring of fluid peripherally. At the area of marginal touch at the extreme periphery of the lens, the depth of the tear film is minimal. A flat lens, which is a lens with a flatter posterior curvature than the anterior central surface of the cornea, tends to rest on the optic cap of the cornea and touch it (Fig. 13-34). At the area of contact there is an absence of the green fluorescein dye (Fig. 13-35). A steep lens has a steeper posterior curvature than the cornea and bridges it, making contact at its margin with the peripheral portion of the cornea (Fig. 13-36). Peripheral contact tends to cause central pooling of the dye, with a ring of touch marginally (Fig. 13-37).

Alteration of the blink rate. Blinking properly is an important factor in the successful wearing of a contact lens. With blinking there occurs an inter-

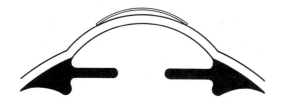

Fig. 13-36 Tight lens—base curve is too steep. (From Stein HA, Slatt BJ, Stein RM: *Fitting guide for rigid and soft contact lenses, a practical approach*, ed 3, St Louis, 1990, Mosby.)

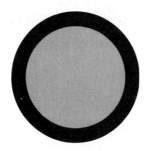

Fig. 13-37 Fluorescein pattern of a steep lens. Note absence of dye at the periphery due to marginal touch.

change of tears between the contact lens and cornea, thereby bringing fresh oxygen and nutrients to the cornea. As tears are produced, they form a small ring around the lid margins. When the lids close, as occurs in blinking, the lids act like a windshield wiper and sweep the tears over the cornea. When a contact lens is worn, the lids move the lens and a new precorneal tear film is interchanged to replace the existing tear film.

A patient whose lenses fit comfortably blinks normally, is free of squinting, and shifts gaze in a normal manner. If excessive blinking develops, it is usually in response to a lens that has excessive movement. Normally the lens makes a small, quick excursion upward with the blink, and then gently falls. A loose lens is generally indicative of a flat lens–cornea relationship. A loose lens slides more easily off center, and the patient begins to blink excessively to recenter the lens.

If the blink rate is reduced and the patient is given to staring, the contact lens may be irritating the eye-

lid. By opening the eyes wide and controlling the blink rate, the patient avoids the unpleasant contact of the superior margin of the contact lens and the upper lid. The nonblinker may show a reduction in the blink rate from the normal of twelve times a minute, or once every 3 or 4 seconds, to three or four times a minute.

Changes in the blink rate often occur because of awareness of the contact lens, and persist despite a perfect contact lens fit. To avoid this habit, many fitters advocate blinking exercises. The patient is asked to fixate on a distant object and perform voluntary closures of the lid until the lid awareness diminishes in intensity.

Scratches, chips, and roughened edges of the contact lens. Scratches may occur from improper handling of the contact lens. If the scratches are central and numerous, they can cause scattering of light and a diminution of visual acuity. Chips and roughened edges may cause erosion of the corneal epithelium by scratching it. Roughened edges may be caused by improper cleansing of the lens if the normal secretions and sediment are allowed to collect and dry at the margin of the lens. A contact lens should be examined under magnification to ensure that the lens is free of surface defects and adherent deposits.

Changes in the cornea. Alteration of the surface of the cornea occurs either in the form of diffuse or localized corneal edema or in the form of erosion of the epithelium. Corneal edema results if the contact lens fits so tightly against the cornea that the surface epithelium cannot breathe, or become oxygenated. Depriving the cornea of oxygen interferes with its metabolism, which in turn causes the formation of edema. The factors that cause corneal edema are (1) a flat lens, which causes compression of the apex of the cornea, (2) a steep lens, which causes stagnation of tears, (3) a poorly-centered lens that causes pressure in one area, (4) improper blinking, and (5) improper cleansing of the lens.

Patients complaining of spectacle blur or photophobia that persist beyond the first week or two should be examined for edema. By retroillumination the edema will appear as a smoky area in the center third of the cornea. Another method of detecting

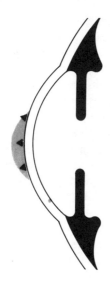

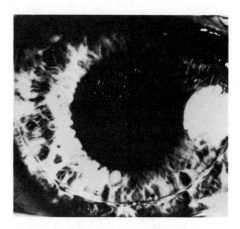

Fig. 13-39 Punctate staining of the cornea. (Courtesy Dr. J. Dixon.)

Fig. 13-38 The rigid lens produces a discreet type of corneal edema, confined to the corneal cap, which does cause spectacle blur because it produces a radical steepening of the corneal curvature. (From Stein HA, Slatt BJ, Stein RM: *Fitting guide for rigid and soft contact lenses, a practical approach,* ed 3, St Louis, 1990, Mosby.)

edema is by keratometry (follow-up K readings). Edema will often produce K readings higher than those originally found (Fig. 13-38).

During the adaptation period edema is almost inevitable. It should not, however, be present after 2 or 3 weeks. If edema persists it will be accompanied by subjective complaints of photophobia, burning smokiness, and spectacle blur. The usual cause of edema is a tight lens resulting from too steep a base curve. However, the peripheral curve may be too shallow or poorly blended, or the lens may be too large.

Erosions of the corneal epithelium may occur because of the incarceration of tiny foreign bodies between the cornea and lens. They are visible as slightly depressed spots that tend to take up the fluorescein stain (Fig. 13-39). Other causes of corneal erosions, or punctate staining, of the cornea are (1) a chipped or roughened edge, (2) flat peripheral curves, (3) a flat lens, (4) improper recentering of a lens, (5) poor insertion and removal techniques,

(6) dust or other particles under the lens, and (7) overwearing of lenses.

A patient with corneal edema will complain of blurred vision or veiled vision. In punctate staining the most common symptom is a foreign body sensation of the eyes either during contact lens wear or after the lens has been removed. If a patient continues to wear his contact lenses despite signs and symptoms of a punctate keratitis, he can easily develop a corneal scratch or abrasion or, eventually, a corneal ulcer. The occurrence of corneal erosions requires immediate removal of the contact lens and reevaluation of the fit.

ADJUSTING CONTACT LENSES

The most common problems with contact lenses are that they are either too loose or too tight. If the lens is too loose, it may be redesigned to provide greater adherence to the cornea by:

1. Increasing the optic zone diameter
2. Increasing the overall diameter of the lens
3. Decreasing the radius of the optic zone
4. Decreasing the radius of the intermediate or peripheral curve

All modifications that would produce a tighter-fitting lens require the manufacture of a new lens. A lens can always be adjusted to fit more loosely but never more tightly.

PROBLEMS ASSOCIATED WITH OVERWEARING CONTACT LENSES

Moderate to severe pain, lid edema, lacrimation, and marked photophobia can occur if contact lenses are worn too long. These symptoms usually occur if the patient has been too ambitious in the early adaptive period in trying to prolong the wearing time. They may occur as a result of carelessness, as typified by the person who falls asleep while wearing contact lenses. The pain usually occurs 2 to 3 hours after the lenses have been removed and is intense. The patient is usually very agitated and in such distress that examination of the cornea can be made only after local anesthetic drops have been instilled in the eye. The cornea shows diffuse erosions over its apex and stains intensely with fluorescein. This condition usually responds to patching of the eye. Within 24 hours the surface of the cornea is usually clear.

Acute hypoxia of the cornea was a common event with PMMA lenses, but is a rare occurrence with any of the gas-permeable lenses. Most of the hazards of insufficient oxygen to the cornea, whether acute or chronic, have been eliminated with gas-permeable lenses, and with the newer type of these lenses, extended wear for varying periods is a reality. The oxygenation of the cornea under the closed lid is sufficient to sustain metabolism despite the presence of a contact lens.

USES OF CONTACT LENSES

The popular thought regarding the use of contact lenses is that they are of value only for cosmetic purposes. It is true that many patients experience a tremendous psychologic emancipation when freed from the burden of heavy, thick, and unsightly glasses, but this is not their primary function. Contact lenses are a wonderful visual aid that can provide vision unobtainable by any other means. They are of particular value to a patient with high myopia. Myopes constitute the largest group of contact lens wearers, probably because of their high degree of motivation.

Contact lenses offer a more normal image size because they are closer to the eye. Just as high plus cataract spectacles magnify the image on the retina by virtue of lying in front of the eye with an air interspace, high minus spectacles tend to minify the retinal image. When contact lenses are used for myopia, the retinal image is more normal, enlarging about 10% for a -6.00-diopter lens and much greater for a higher minus lens. Therefore, contact lenses result in a retinal image of more normal size and better visual acuity. They allow an unrestricted field of view since the lenses move with the eyes, and the appearance is like that of unaided vision.

Contact lenses also treat irregular astigmatism caused by corneal scarring.

Hyperopic patients form a small portion of those desiring contact lenses, because a farsighted person needs a comparatively low-powered lens and can usually obtain satisfactory distance vision without glasses.

The patient who has had cataracts removed suffers the same visual disabilities as the high myope, and therefore enjoys the same advantages with contact lenses, such as freedom from the weight of heavy glasses, a wider range of field of vision, and a more natural-appearing image. For the aphakic or post-cataract patient, spectacles enlarge the image by 33%. With contact lenses, there is a restoration to more normal image size, since the contact lens reduces the magnification to only 7%. In addition, the aphakic individual suffers from many aberrations while looking through the periphery of the spectacle lens. With contact lenses distortion never ocurs, because the lens moves with the eye and vision is always obtained through the central portion of the lens.

Today, intraocular lenses are inserted after all cataract removal operations. For patients who have had the procedure performed before the advent of intraocular lenses, the contact lens offers restored normal vision. Contacts may make the image size approximately the same size as the image seen by the fellow eye or at the very least only slightly larger. For patients in whom this is not possible, contact lenses offer a solution to restore normal vision, because it makes the image seen approximately the same size as the image seen by the fellow eye.

Contact lenses have also been employed for chil-

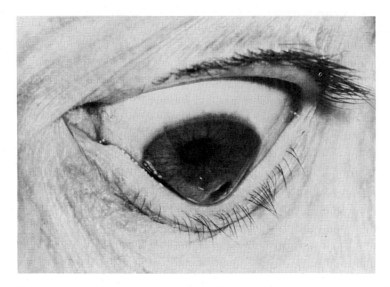

Fig. 13-40 An advanced case of keratoconus. (Courtesy Dr. Dean Butcher, Australia.)

dren who have undergone surgery for congenital or traumatic cataract.

Keratoconus is a development anomaly of the cornea, characterized by progressive thinning and an apical bulge of the central portion of the cornea (Fig. 13-40). This condition results in irregular myopic astigmatism that cannot be corrected by glasses. Contact lenses flatten the cornea, tend to stabilize the condition, and by virtue of the fluid interface between the contant lens and the cornea, eliminate irregular astigmatism and permit clear vision.

Besides correcting refractive errors, contact lenses may be used to cover *unsightly eyes*. In these cases the contact lens is colored to disguise disfiguring features of the eye.

Contact lenses have also been useful in the treatment of patients with nystagmus. In these cases vision is improved because the correcting lens moves with the eye. Another use for contact lenses is for the patient with congenital albinism. A small pupillary opening is provided and a collarette of darkly-tinted lens is produced to protect the patient from excessive glare.

Many professional persons, including actors, politicians, and public speakers, wear contact lenses to improve their appearance before the public. Professional athletes such as hockey players and football players can participate in competitive sports only by being free of the encumbrance and hazard of spectacles. However, soft contact lenses may be the wiser choice because they are less likely to be lost than are rigid lenses.

SUMMARY

One of the major problems with contact lenses is education of the contact lens patient. Each patient should be instructed about the symptoms that can be expected and tolerated, and those that are danger signals and indicate immediate consultation. Also, each patient should be shown the methods handling the lenses, their insertion and removal, and their storage and hygiene.

Each phase in the adaptation period should be clearly outlined to the patient. The patient must be given an orderly schedule to follow and a routine to perform.

The patient should also be told the function that the contact lens will perform. This function may be optical, therapeutic, or cosmetic. The wearing of contact lenses demands the payment of a price, in attention, care, and finances. The patient should know the benefits and be aware of the hazards.

QUESTIONS FOR REVIEW AND THOUGHT

1. Name factors that contraindicate the wearing of rigid contact lenses.
2. List the advantages and disadvantages of corneal rigid contact lenses.
3. What holds a contact lens in place?
4. What are the characteristics of the plastic used in rigid lens manufacture?
5. Outline a method of evaluating a patient before prescribing contact lenses.
6. The keratometer is an important instrument in evaluating the anterior corneal curvature. Outline a method of performing keratometry.
7. How can you verify the diameter of a contact lens? The radius?
8. Given a patient with -2.75, $+0.75$, $\times$ 90, and K readings of 43.50 $\times$ 44.50 $\times$ 90, with normal lid and pupillary opening, how would you compute a possible type of rigid lens for initial trial?
9. What effect would contact lenses have on the visual field of a patient with a -6.00-diopter lens?
10. Describe spectacle blur and its causes.
11. Describe how you would instruct a patient to clean and insert contact lenses.
12. Describe three methods of instructing the patient in lens removal.
13. What is the value of a wetting solution? Name several that are available.
14. What is the value of a lens cleaner? Name several that are available.
15. What are the advantages of using a trial set in contact lens fitting?
16. What is the importance of blinking?
17. What causes corneal edema after wearing of contact lenses?
18. How can a lens be adjusted that is too tight? Too loose?
19. Contact lenses are frequently used for cosmetic or refractive purposes. However, after cataract surgery they aid considerably in overall vision. Why?
20. What is your routine wearing schedule for rigid lenses?
21. What symptoms may be attributed to a loose lens and to a tight lens?
22. List the features of a contact lens that can be modified without making a new lens.

SELF-EVALUATION QUESTIONS

True-false statements

Directions: Indicate whether the statement is true (T) or false (F).

T or F
1. The keratometer is an instrument that is used to measure the radius of curvature of the front surface of the cornea.

T or F
2. If the keratometer measurements show a difference in dioptric power from one meridian to the opposite meridian, then irregular astigmatism exists.

T or F
3. With fluorescein staining, if a dark area appears centrally, then the corneal lens is considered too steep.

Missing words

Directions: Write in the missing word in the following sentences.

4. With the rule astigmatism is present when the horizontal meridian is _____ than the vertical meridian.

5. The optic cap is the _____ zone of the cornea.
6. The power of a rigid contact lens may be measured by an instrument called the _____

Choice-completion questions

Directions: Select the one best answer in each case.

7. Defects in lens material or edge design may be identified by which piece of equipment?
    a. Radiuscope
    b. Shadowgraph
    c. Lensmeter
    d. Keratometer
    e. Profile analyzer
8. A rigid lens that is too loose may result in
    a. Spectacle blur
    b. Burning sensation
    c. Blurring of vision after blinking
    d. Night blindness
    e. Pain after lens removal
9. Fluorescein patterns may be most helpful in identifying a poorly fitting lens. A lens that shows a large dark central area with an absence of fluorescein is indicative of:
    a. A normal fit
    b. A steep lens
    c. A flat lens
    d. Improper fenestration of the lens
    e. None of the above

ANSWERS, NOTES, AND EXPLANATIONS

1. **True.** The keratometer measures the front surface of the cornea, which acts as a convex mirror reflecting the mires or images of the keratometer. The keratometer measures only a very limited circular area of the cornea, approximately 2 to 4 mm apart depending on the manufacturer of the keratometer. The keratometer makes an assumption as to the index of refraction of the cornea.

2. **False.** If the dioptric power from one meridian to the opposite meridian is different, then regular astigmatism is said to exist and the difference in diopters between the two meridians indicates the amount of corneal astigmatism present. When irregular astigmatism exists, the mires are distorted and it is difficult to obtain satisfactory reflecting images from the cornea. Such conditions as keratoconus and scars of the cornea produce irregular astigmatism.

3. **False.** The dark area is indicative that there is no fluorescein pattern centrally, which signifies that the lens is touching the central portion of the cornea. This exists when the lens base curve is flatter than the curvature of the cornea so that the central portion of the lens rests on the central portion of the cornea and prevents the dye from entering into the center and pooling centrally.

4. **Flatter.** The eye is shaped in some ways like a football whose long axis is positioned horizontally in the palpebral fissures so that the steeper meridian is vertical and the flatter meridian is horizontal. This is known as with the rule astigmatism. When this occurs in the opposite direction, it is considered against the rule astigmatism.

5. **Central.** The optic cap lies in the central 5 to 7 mm of the cornea, which involves the visual axis of the cornea. This is the area that should be measured with the keratometer in determining the central corneal radius of curvature. This is the area that becomes involved when a rigid contact lens is overworn and edema results, causing fogginess of vision.

6. **Lensmeter.** By holding a rigid contact lens between the thumb and forefinger or letting it rest concave side down, the examiner may measure the back vertex power of a contact lens. The lens should always be placed so that the concavity of the lens lies toward the instrument so that the back power is measured. This is of minor significance in low powers, but in high minus or high plus powers, this may become significant.

7. **b. Shadowgraph.** The Shadowgraph is a type of magnifier and projector that permits the examiner to check the details of the lens material and edge design for chips, roughness, or sharpness. Important features such as sharpness or roughness of a rigid lens may be fundamental to the comfortable wearing of rigid contact lenses. It is the edge design, which must ride against and under the eyelid, that tends to produce the lid awareness of a contact lens. The surface quality of the lens as well as defects in material can be identified with the magnification of the Shadowgraph instrument.

8. **c. Blurring of vision after blinking.** A loose lens will often decenter after a person blinks and will ride either to the side or low, resulting in poor vision and fluctuating vision. Burning sensations are a result of hypoxia that develops from stagnation brought on by the accumulation of metabolites centrally from a steep lens that does not permit adequate venting and exchange of tear film. This is a tight lens symptom. Spectacle blur is a result of hypoxia with edema that develops in the central portion of the cornea and is usually a result of either overwear of a contact lens or a tight lens that does not permit adequate tear exchange. Pain following lens removal is also a symptom that there has been corneal hypoxia or complete anoxia brought on by improper venting or tear exchange and indicates a tight lens rather than a loose lens.

9. **c. A flat lens.** The absence of fluorescein is indicative that the lens is touching the apex of the cornea so that fluorescein does not intervene between the lens and cornea. This central touch may cause warpage of the cornea with compression changes on the surface of the cornea. If the lens is too flat, it may rock and usually decenters. Also, there may be a flattening of the cornea, and an undesirable type of reduction of myopia at the expense of possible permanent structural changes in the cornea. The principle of orthokeratology is to provide very slight changes by central touch so that small degrees of astigmatism can be reduced on a regular basis in this manner. This, however, may result in irregular flattening of the cornea by compression with resulting induced irregular astigmatism.

CHAPTER 14 Soft contact lenses

- History of hydrophilic lenses
- Advantages and disadvantages
- Patient evaluation
- Manufacture
- Inventory versus diagnostic lenses
- Lens inspection
- Evaluation of fit
- Disinfection
- Cleaning
- Insertion and removal techniques
- Taco test
- Precautions for wear
- Wearing schedules
- Thin and ultrathin lenses
- Correction of astigmatism
- Medical uses
- Extended-wear lenses
- Disposable lenses
- Innovations in design
- Contact lenses in industry
- Special occupations
- Common questions and answers
- Role of the ophthalmic assistant

The soft lenses currently available rival rigid lenses in the quality of vision and surpass them in the realm of comfort and ease of adaptation (Fig. 14-1). The two basic types of soft lenses used are

(1) the *hydrogel* (hydrophilic) lens, which owes its softness to its ability to absorb and bind water to its structure, and (2) the *silicone* lens, which owes its softness to the intrinsic property of the rubbery material.

HISTORY OF HYDROPHILIC LENSES

In 1960 two young New York lawyers established a company with a unique function of promoting patent

For a more extensive reference on contact lenses, the ophthalmic assistant is urged to consult Stein HA, Slatt BJ, Stein RM: *Fitting guide for rigid and soft contact lenses: a practical approach*, ed 3, St Louis, 1990, Mosby.

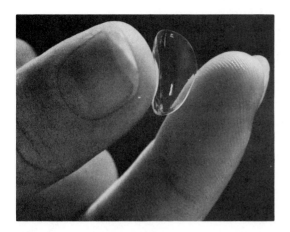

Fig. 14-1 A soft contact lens will fold completely

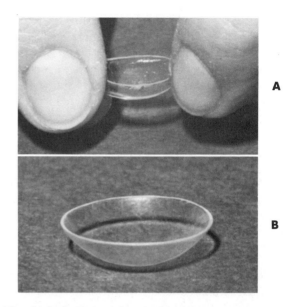

Fig. 14-2 A, The soft lens is sturdy despite its flexible quality. It can be stretched, dried, or crumpled and still retain its integrity. **B,** After stretching, the hydrogel lens retains its "memory" and returns to its original shape.

exchanges among corporations. Their specialty was combing through the dusty corporate files for idle patents and setting up licensing agreements with other companies interested in putting the dormant ideas to use.

In 1965 the men who had established the National Patent Development Corporation suddenly dissolved their patent law business. They had uncovered a patent with so many exciting possibilities that they decided to pick up a license themselves. In effect, they became their own client, eliminating their role as middlemen.

The new material was a plastic, which they called *hydron*. It was developed by Dr. Otto Wichterle, head of the Institute of Macromolecular Chemistry of the Czechoslovakian National Academy of Science and a leading expert on polymer chemistry, and by Dr. Drahoslav Lim. The new material appeared to be like other plastics in that it was a hard transparent substance that could be cut, ground, or molded into a variety of shapes. When placed in water or an aqueous solution, however, the tough, rigid plastic became soft and pliable. In the wet form it could be bent between the fingers until the edges met or could be turned easily inside out; yet it would snap back into its original shape quickly. When allowed to dry, the supple water-logged material became dry as a cornflake and crushed to a powdery dust if smashed. The substance was subjected to rigorous biologic tests and was found to be inert and

fully compatible with human tissue. One of its properties was that although highly elastic when wet, it remained strong and able to hold its shape (Fig. 14-2).

The plastic is hydroxyethyl methacrylate (HEMA), a plastic polymer with the remarkable ability to absorb water molecules. Chemically the polymer consists of a three-dimensional network of hydroxyethyl methacrylate chains cross-linked with ethylene glycol dimethacrylate molecules about once every 200 monomer units. As the water is introduced to the plastic, it swells into a soft mass with surprisingly good mechanical strength, complete transparency (97%), and the ability to retain its shape and dimensions.

Over the years, many modifications of the plastic have been introduced, new polymers added, and new lens designs created. Five vigorous years of improvements and clinical trials were conducted on the soft lens before the Federal Drug Administration (which considered the lens a drug) approved the lens as a safe prosthetic device of good optical quality.

The FDA's caution, after the thalidomide tragedies in which a drug produced severe deformities in the babies of pregnant women, was understandable. Both the public and the practitioner needed protection. In the first phase of research the soft lens was tested with laboratory animals to ensure that it was nontoxic; later it was given to selected practitioners and independent research workers for clinical trials on human beings.

It soon became apparent that the soft lens was an innovation of major importance, with widespread application not only as an instrument for treating diseased corneas but also as a superior contact lens. In the early stages, however, the therapeutic possibilities of soft lenses overshadowed any other consideration, because it appeared that these lenses would replace many conventional treatments of external diseases of the eye.

As the number of soft lens companies expanded throughout the world, a search for newer and better lens designs as well as lens plastics resulted in some companies emphasizing and developing research activities directed toward correcting astigmatism with soft lenses, developing bifocal soft lenses, and tinting soft lenses for cosmetic purposes. Ultrathin lenses and those with high water content have opened up new significant areas in contact lens development. In the manufacturing area, the emphasis has been on automated and semiautomated systems to produce a soft contact lens.

ADVANTAGES AND DISADVANTAGES

The advantages of hydrophilic contact lenses are as follows:

1. Comfort
2. Rapid adaptation
3. Lack of spectacle blur
4. Ability to be worn intermittently
5. Minimal lens loss
6. Minimal overwear reaction
7. Lack of glare and photophobia
8. Difficulty in dislodging
9. Protection of entire cornea
10. Attractive alternative for rigid lens dropouts
11. No serious corneal abrasion on insertion

Comfort. These lenses are exceptionally com-

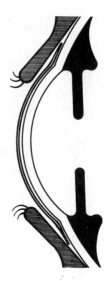

Fig. 14-3 Soft lens fits under eyelid margins, and the advancing lid edge just glides over its surface. This accounts for part of its comfort factor. (From Stein HA, Slatt BJ, Stein RM: *Fitting guide for rigid and soft contact lenses: a practical approach,* ed 3, St Louis, 1990, Mosby.)

fortable from the initial period. It is impressive to witness the rapid tolerance of the cornea to the presence of the contact lens. The lack of awareness of a soft lens is due partly to the flaccidity, water content, and the thin edges of the lens, which mold to the white of the eye (the sclera). Therefore there is almost no interference from the upper lids during normal blinking. The lens hugs the eye so closely that the advancing surface of the eyelid just glides over it (Fig. 14-3). Its supple quality when wet also contributes to the easy acceptance of the soft lens. Being hydrophilic, or water loving, it forms a cushioned fluid buffer between itself and the cornea. It also contours itself to the unique shape of the individual cornea. With no hard edges to irritate the eyelid edge and no rigid structure to compress delicate living tissue, the soft lens cannot abrade or crush the cornea. Because of its soft qualities, the lens flexes with each blink, permitting a normal tear exchange to take place by a pumping action.

A rigid lens has to be fitted according to the precise shape of the cornea. If the fit is poor or if the lab-

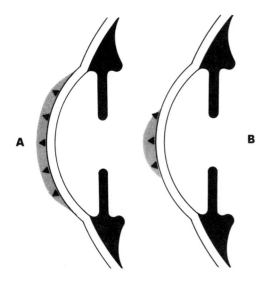

Fig. 14-4 The soft lens (**A**) produces a diffuse area of corneal edema that does not alter the radius of curvature of the cornea and does not cause spectacle blur. **B,** The hard lens produces a discreet type of corneal edema, confined to the corneal cap, which does cause spectacle blur because it produces a radical steepening of the corneal curvature. (From Stein HA, Slatt BJ, Stein RM: *Fitting guide for rigid and soft contact lenses: a practical approach*, ed 3, St Louis, 1990, Mosby.)

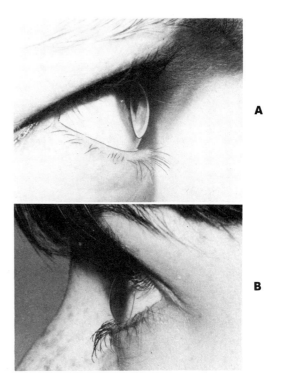

Fig. 14-5 Comparison of hard and soft lenses. **A,** The hard lens is smaller than the cornea and can be easily dislodged with the edge of the lid. **B,** The soft lens is larger than the cornea, hugs the eye tightly, and seldom is displaced even during body contact sports.

oratory does not make the lens according to exact specifications, a rigid lens will irritate the eye. This is not so with the soft ones. A wide latitude is possible without corneal injury, and less exacting measurements are required.

Rapid adaptation. Tolerance is extremely rapid as compared with that of the rigid lens. The lenses frequently are comfortable to a new patient within 30 minutes. Wearing schedules can be rapidly increased to full-time day wear.

Lack of spectacle blur. Removal of the lenses permits patients to switch directly to their glasses without the spectacle blur that occurs with rigid lenses. Spectacle blur is uncommon because of the diffuse nature of any edema, which spreads evenly over the cornea and does not alter its radius (Fig. 14-4).

Ability to be worn intermittently. Unlike rigid lenses, which require daily wearing to maintain corneal tolerance, soft lenses may be worn intermittently without a disciplined schedule. In this respect

the actor or athlete can wear the hydrophilic lenses only for the day or the time that is required. Any individual can wear them occasionally just for social activities.

Minimal lens loss. Most rigid lenses are lost in the first 3 months, when handling is still somewhat clumsy. Rigid lenses also will dislodge at inappropriate times. The technique for removal of a soft lens is such that loss is less frequent than that of a rigid lens. The larger size of the soft lens, coupled with the firm adherence of the lens to the cornea with minimal sliding effect, reduces the loss factor considerably. It is rare for a patient to report the loss of a soft lens (Fig. 14-5).

Minimal overwear reaction. Every ophthalmologist remembers cases of the overwear syndrome experienced by the rigid lens wearer, who appears

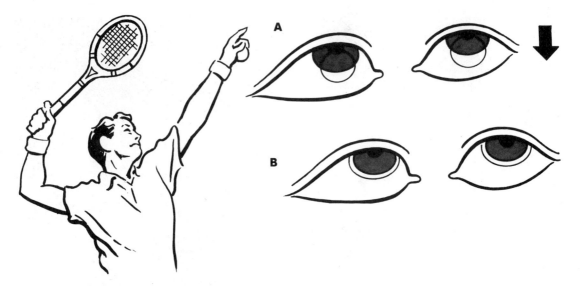

Fig. 14-6 A, With hard lenses the lenses drop when the tennis player moves his eye up to hit the ball. **B,** Soft lenses move with the eye and show only minimal lag; thus they are an ideal sports lens. (From Stein HA, Slatt BJ, Stein RM: *Fitting guide for rigid and soft contact lenses: a practical approach,* ed 3, St Louis, 1990, Mosby.)

at the hospital emergency room in the middle of the night with excruciating pain, having worn the rigid lenses longer than the normal time limit. This problem is virtually eliminated with the soft lens. Although 2% have been reported to show slight corneal edema with halos about lights and a burning sensation of their eyes, at the end of the day no serious disabling disorder has occurred. From this standpoint the soft lens is much safer than the rigid lens.

It is known that oxygen is carried to the cornea through the tear film and is replenished through the circulation of tears under it. This is the same method by which the cornea receives its oxygen supply under a rigid lens. The evidence of a good tear layer between the soft lens and the cornea has been demonstrated by a French ophthalmologist, Dr. Paul Cochet, who showed spherical particles 1 to 3 µg in diameter passing underneath the lens. When the tear layer has been stained, it has been shown to ripple with the blinking motions of the lids. The respiration of the cornea is provided by tear exchange during blinking.

Lack of glare and photophobia. Glare and light sensitivity are seen almost routinely in the early weeks of rigid lens wear. These symptoms are virtually absent with the soft lens, making it the ideal lens for outdoor athletes such as golfers and tennis players. Also, the generous size of the optic zone means that the pupil is always covered; this minimizes glare.

Difficulty in dislodging. The firm adherence of the soft lens to the eye permits the lens to be used in body contact sports and reduces embarrassment associated with dislodgement for the actor or politician (Fig. 14-6).

Protection of entire cornea. Hydrophilic lenses cover the entire cornea. They can be used to reduce corneal exposure for such conditions as facial paralysis and corneal insensitivity, and after ptosis operations (Fig. 14-7). In this sense these lenses are used as bandage lenses.

Attractive alternative for rigid lens dropouts. A significant percentage of rigid lens patients are unable to persist in wearing their lenses. This intolerance may be the result of pregnancy, birth control pills, or a change of environment. Most of these

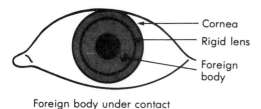

Foreign body under contact

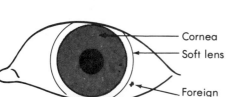

Fig. 14-7 The rigid lens permits foreign particles to enter under the lens, whereas the soft lens tends to prevent the tracking of foreign bodies under it by its scleral impingement and minimum movement. (From Stein HA, Slatt BJ, Stein RM: *Fitting guide for rigid and soft contact lenses: a practical approach,* ed 3, St Louis, 1990, Mosby.)

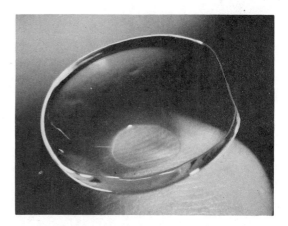

Fig. 14-8 Soft toric lens used to correct astigmatism. Note the truncated flat edge.

patients readily accept soft lenses and are able to wear them comfortably.

No serious corneal abrasion on insertion. Unlike the rigid lens, in which improper insertion can cause an abrasion of the cornea, this problem does not occur with the soft lens because of its soft nature.

The disadvantages of soft contact lenses are as follows:

1. Lack of ability to correct astigmatism
2. Variable vision
3. Lack of durability
4. Faulty duplication
5. Deposit formation
6. Modifications impossible
7. Sterilization problems

Lack of ability to correct astigmatism. Astigmatism is not readily corrected or covered by conventional soft lenses. The soft lens contours to the eye, and corneal astigmatism frequently remains uncorrected. There are, however, a number of special designs of toric soft lenses available to correct astigmatism of dioptric powers up to 4 diopters (Fig. 14-8).

Variable vision. Despite good fittings, a small per-

centage of patients become disenchanted because of either poor vision or variable vision. These problems may result from fitting failures, uncorrected astigmatism, or a dehydration effect from the water-laden lenses. They also may result from deposit formation and lens spoilage.

Lack of durability. Soft lenses are much more fragile than rigid lenses, and any rough handling will often scratch or tear the lenses. Even with careful handling, they may become sliced with the fingernails and may develop nicks at the edges because of the constant pinching and flexing of the lenses during insertion and removal. The higher the water content, or the thinner the lenses, the more fragile the soft lenses are.

Faulty duplication. Lenses will break or tear and require replacement. Often a duplicate set may be necessary, and sometimes the duplication is not exact if the laboratory does not have good quality control.

Deposit formation. With long-term wear, mineral precipitates occur on the lens, and protein, mineral, and lipoid deposits may accumulate on the surface (Fig. 14-9). Although special cleaning and protein-removing agents are available, strict adherence to their schedules for use is required to eliminate these build-ups and preserve the life of the lens. New lens developments may minimize the deposit adherence.

Modifications impossible. Although a soft lens can be dehydrated to the dry state, it does not form a

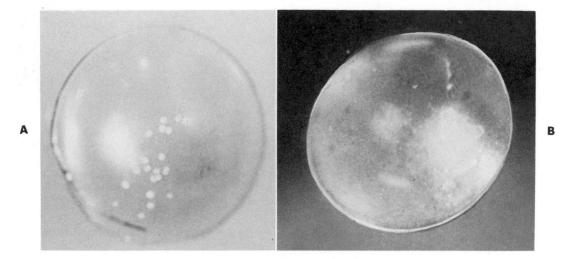

Fig. 14-9 A, Deposits on a soft lens. **B,** Protein build-up on a soft lens will vary with the duration of wear, the method of sterilization, and the tear composition and concentration of individual patients. (From Stein HA, Slatt BJ, Stein RM: *Fitting guide for rigid and soft contact lenses: a practical approach,* ed 3, St Louis, 1990, Mosby.)

regular shape in the dry state, and accurate modifications are impractical.

Sterilization problems. The routine of disinfecting must be rigidly adhered to, or infection may occur. This applies if the lenses sit in the drawer during illness or vacations or if there is a temporary "holiday" back to glasses.

Both the boiling method and chemical method of disinfection have their advantages and drawbacks. In any event, rigid adherence to disinfection procedures is most important both for the practitioner who keeps an inventory and for the patient who wears the lenses only occasionally. Fungus growth has been reported occasionally, as well as bacterial contamination of the lenses. Because soft lenses can be scratched and damaged more easily, the lens can be penetrated by infectious organisms. They are theoretically more dangerous than rigid lenses. In addition, the adherence of protein to the lens surface can harbor bacterial organisms. One source of soft lens contamination results from human neglect. Patients neglect to boil their lenses as instructed or neglect to use fresh solutions daily for disinfection. In some instances the distilled water has been shown to be contaminated. *Acanthamoeba* organisms

abound in warm water. Unlike rigid lenses, it is unwise to recommended a duplicate pair of soft lenses because the patient usually neglects the sterilization routine required of the unused soft lenses. As a result fungal contamination may occur.

PATIENT EVALUATION

Each patient who comes for a contact lens examination requires a complete history and physical eye examination. In addition to obtaining a pertinent history of previous eye diseases, such as recurrence of infections, corneal ulcerations, and history of herpes simplex, one must question persistently about the presence of any past neurologic disorders or any present medication that is being taken. Age factor and personality will be of significance in determining whether contacts should be prescribed. A history of allergies might sway the patient to the use of nonpreserved solutions for rinsing and boiling. Of utmost importance is the patient's motivation.

External examination consists of careful inspection of the cornea, the conjunctiva, and the fornices. The lids should be everted to detect any underlying pathologic condition, and in particular, notation should be made of papillary formation of the con-

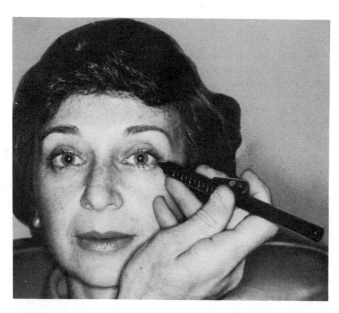

Fig. 14-10 Testing corneal sensitivity with fine hair of the Cochet-Bonnet esthesiometer.

junctiva. Routine slit-lamp biomicroscopic examination is performed to detect the presence of any corneal disease or scarring. Schirmer's test should be performed to evaluate the adequacy of tear formation. The corneal sensitivity test can be used to detect corneal oversensitivity (Fig. 14-10). The palpebral fissures should be measured; the findings may alter the fitter's judgment about the diameter of the soft lens to be employed. Lid tension can be evaluated by grasping the upper lid between thumb and forefinger and holding it upward. A careful refraction should be performed along with keratometer readings. The pupil and horizontal visible iris diameter should be measured either by a ruler, a pupillometer, or the slit-lamp biomicroscope. These measurements also may affect the diameter of the lens that is selected.

Patient selection

Soft lenses are ideal for the following persons:
1. Persons who have given up wearing rigid lenses because of the irritation, a bad experience with overwear, or the difficulties in maintaining a rigid daily wearing schedule

2. Intermittent wearers, such as public speakers, athletes, or actors, who want to wear their lenses only occasionally
3. Industrial workers, where the fear of losing a lens at work can be very disrupting (soft lenses rarely fall out)
4. Aphakic patients (Any residual astigmatism can be incorporated into the glasses)
5. Elderly persons who are impatient with the prolonged routine in following the rigid lens–wearing schedule

The decision to dispense contact lenses to any patient is, of course, a professional judgment and should be made by a professional contact lens fitter.

MANUFACTURE

There are various methods of manufacturing soft lenses:
1. Spin casting
2. Lathe cutting with manual or automated lathes
3. Molding methods

Most steps today are relatively automated, with quality control being performed by random sampling.

Spin-cast lenses

The spin-cast process, devised by Bausch & Lomb, produces a highly reproducible lens with a very smooth surface. This means that the lens is so standardized that all replacement lenses are duplicates of the original regardless of where in the world they are purchased. Although this is no mean feat for a Coca Cola bottle, it is a triumph for contact lens assembly.

Bausch & Lomb manufactures its Soflens by means of the spin-cast method. It is derived from a revolving mold that whirls the liquid plastic at high speed. The mold gives the lens its outside curvature. The inside curvature is formed as a result of the speed of rotation, the various surface tensions of the liquid, and the precalculated mathematic relationship between gravitation and rotation. The result is a parabola with inside curvature that can shorten or lengthen, depending on the speed of rotation. The procedure is basically a kind of pressureless molding.

Because the posterior surface of a spin-cast lens is aspheric, the traditional K readings and the posterior surface's relationship to the base curve do not apply with spin-cast lenses. The basic fitting system is based on measurement of the horizontal visible iris diameter and selection of a suitable diameter of lens with proper power. The numeric suffix on the label denotes the lens diameter. A label ending in 4 is a 14.5-mm diameter, a 3 is a 13.5-mm diameter, and the absence of a number is a 12.5-mm diameter.

A combination of the spin-cast and lathing processes has been developed by Bausch & Lomb. The Optima spherical lens, Medalist, and Sequence II employ the lathe-cut posterior and spin-cast anterior surface. This design permits more variables in fitting while combining the high quality of front surface for crisp optics.

Lathe-cut lenses

In the lathe-cut manufacturing process the lens, in the dehydrated state, behaves like a rigid lens. It is cut on a lathe to exact specifications similar to those of a rigid lens. Automated lathes currently are in fashion and reduce labor. Initially the back surface is ground with a diamond tool, and then the front surface is polished and edged. In this method, peripheral curves, blends, and even intermediate curves can be cut for better lens design. Lathed lenses are individually or custom made, and a wide variety of parameters can be ground for a better fit. The most important factor in the grinding of the soft lens is that one cannot use the usual polishing compounds that contain water; thus the whole process of grinding and polishing must be performed without any contamination by water.

Lathe-cut lenses are produced both for stock and custom orders, with most using high-tech computer-controlled systems for excellent quality and reproducibility. The most important consideration in cutting soft lenses from a dry button that is later to be hydrated into a hydrogel lens is that the entire process of lathing must be performed under a very strict climate control. Too much humidity in the laboratory can cause variations in the finished product because it is possible for the button to absorb moisture from the air. After completion of the grinding process in the hard inflexible state, the lens is placed in a water bath for several hours where it undergoes swelling and expands to its final state. This swell factor must be taken into account in the grinding of the lens in the hard state.

When the finished lens in a dry state is hydrated for final wet inspection or quality control, the difference or swell factor is 20% to 40%, depending on the polymer and water content. This factor makes it extremely important for the "dry state" lens to be made to exact specifications. In years past the criticism of lathe-cut lenses was inconsistency, and the reproducibility could be suspect. Today's lathe-cut lenses, however, compare favorably in quality and reproducibility with any other manufacturing process.

Molded lenses

The cast-molding process uses precision injection molding of engineered thermoplastic resins to produce lens replica molds. The lens replica molds are used in a monomer-casting process to convert cross-linkable lens monomers directly into a finished contact lens form. This process produces an optically finished surface from the mold, thus ensuring accurate reproduction of the lenses.

The FDA receives a constant parade of applications for approval of new lenses. With each lens comes an innovative approach to solving some of today's contact lens problems.

INVENTORY VERSUS DIAGNOSTIC LENSES

Soft lenses may be fitted in one of two ways: (1) from an inventory of lenses by selecting the lens that gives the best fit and the best visual acuity or (2) from a trial set of standard diameters and base curves to obtain the proper fit. The fitter can then overrefract to obtain the correct power of the lens and order directly. Alternately, lenses may be ordered after the fitter makes an educated guess according to K readings, horizontal corneal diameter, and refraction, realizing that a few changes of lenses may be required before the correct lens fit is achieved.

As a result of the large diameter of soft lenses and its effect on sagittal depth, their fit must be much flatter than that of rigid lenses. The average diameter of soft lenses used today is 13.8 to 14.5 mm, requiring that they be fitted 1.0 to 1.5 mm, or 5.00 to 7.00 D, flatter than K. Because of the large diameter of these soft lenses, they should be fitted

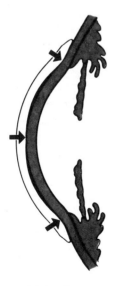

Fig. 14-11 Three-point touch—a normally fitting soft lens will rest lightly at the apex and at the periphery of the cornea. (From Stein HA, Slatt BJ, Stein RM: *Fitting guide for rigid and soft contact lenses: a practical approach,* ed 3, St Louis, 1990, Mosby.)

appreciably flatter than the flattest K reading of the cornea. Lens diameter and base curve are inversely related. To arrive at essentially the same fit, the base curve of the lens selected should be flattened as the lens diameter is increased; for example, a 12- to 13-mm diameter lens usually is fitted approximately 2.00 to 3.00 diopters flatter than K, whereas a 14- to 15-mm diameter lens will have to be fitted approximately 3.00 to 5.00 diopters flatter than K.

Lens selection may be based on one of three methods: (1) selection of soft lenses based on probable corneoscleral profiles, in which the fitter may select a lens diameter based on the horizontal iris diameter and observe how the lens performs on a given eye, (2) selection of soft lenses with a posterior curvature of radius based on K readings of the cornea, determined by actual measurement of the cornea, and (3) selection of soft lenses based on the sagittal value of the lenses, which requires the K reading of the cornea and takes into account not only the posterior radius of the lens curvature but also the diameter of the lens.

The fitting criteria are similar for all daily-wear soft lenses. Some basic guidelines apply.

1. The hydrophilic lenses are fitted as large as or larger than the diameter of the cornea and range in size from 12 to 15 mm.

2. Small eyes will require smaller diameters and consequently steeper base curves, whereas larger eyes are fitted with larger lenses and flatter base curves.

3. Soft standard-thickness lenses generally are fitted flatter than the flattest K reading, usually about 2.00 to 3.00 diopters for the smaller lenses and 3.00 to 5.00 diopters for the larger lenses. The thinner soft lenses (0.06 and less) are fitted 4.00 to 7.00 diopters flatter than K because they tend to drape themselves over the corneal surface (Fig. 14-11).

4. A normal-fitting lens should show 0.5 to 1 mm lag in the downward direction with each blink and provide good vision before and after blinking.

5. A soft lens that moves excessively (more than 1 mm with each blink) is too flat; a soft lens that moves less than 0.5 mm with each blink is too steep and will limit tear exchange.

6. A soft lens that decenters usually is too flat or too small (Fig. 14-12). To correct this problem, a

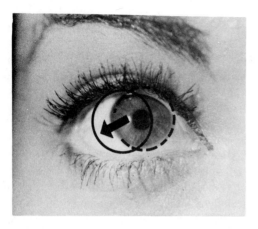

Fig. 14-12 Decentration. Soft lens does not center properly; it has decentered outward.

Table 14-1		Sagittal relationship of various base curves and diameters	
Diameter	**Radius**	**Diameter**	**Radius**
Flatter		14.0	8.1
12.0	8.7	13.0	7.2
12.0	8.1	14.5	8.4
12.5	8.7	13.5	7.5
12.0	8.4	15.0	8.7
12.5	8.4	14.0	7.8
12.5	8.1	14.5	8.1
12.5	7.8	15.0	8.4
12.0	7.8	15.5	8.7
13.0	8.7	13.5	7.2
13.0	8.4	14.0	7.5
13.5	8.7	14.5	7.8
13.0	8.1	15.0	8.1
13.5	8.4	15.5	8.4
14.0	8.7	14.0	7.2
13.0	7.8	14.5	7.5
13.5	8.1	15.0	7.8
14.0	8.4	15.5	8.1
13.0	7.5	15.0	7.5
14.5	8.7	15.5	7.8
13.5	7.8	*Steeper*	

larger-diameter lens or a steeper lens should be selected.

7. The fitter may determine increased steepness or flatness from a table showing the relationship of the diameter to the radius (sagittal values) (Table 14-1). To loosen a lathe-cut lens, smaller diameters in 0.5 mm steps may be fitted or the radius increased in 0.2 to 0.3 mm steps.

8. The lower the water content of the lens, the more durable the lens becomes. The higher the water content, the more fragile the lens.

9. The thinner the lens, the greater the oxygen permeability to the cornea. However, a thin lens will tear easily, and some optical quality may be lost by wrinkling.

10. Hazy vision caused by oxygen deprivation may occur from wearing too thick a lens.

11. Contact lens decentration can be caused by tight eyelids, large corneas, against-the-rule astigmatism, or asymmetric corneal topography.

12. Routine soft lenses do not mask large amounts of corneal astigmatism. In general, astigmatism over 1.0 diopters requires correction by toric soft lenses or rigid lenses.

13. With soft lenses, regular fluorescein cannot be used to study tear exchange because it permeates the lens. High-molecule fluorescein can be used, but it is no more effective than evaluating tear exchange by noting the movement of the lens. Fluorescein is helpful in highlighting and assessing corneal pathologic conditions.

14. Heavier lenses usually have to be fitted larger. The lens weight is influenced by its thickness and water content. Polymers of high water content usually are weaker than those of lower water content and require lenses of greater thickness. The increased gravitational pull on a heavier lens has to be offset by use of a larger diameter.

15. The rigidity of a lens is a function of its thickness, its water content, and the unique properties of the polymer from which it is made.

16. When fitting soft lenses, the fitter should aim at fitting the flattest possible lens that will provide good clear vision, will center well, and will have no effect on the corneal integrity.

LENS INSPECTION

The following routine is important for checking the quality of the lens received. For all soft lenses each factor should be assessed.

Edge and surface inspection. This should be per-

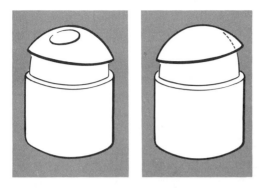

Fig. 14-13 Use of the template to measure base curve of soft lens. The lens on the left has a bubble under the center, indicating that the lens is too steep for the template. The lens on the right has edge standoff, indicating that the lens is too flat for the template.

formed with the lens under the microscope. The lens may be held in the hand or placed on a clear glass slide. It may be compared with white paper placed behind it to see if discoloration has occurred. The lens also can be examined under a hand magnifier.

Diameter. The lens is viewed through a magni-

fying gauge with a millimeter scale. No pressure must be exerted on the lens to distort the surface.

Base curve. A simple plastic template of varying graduated radii must be used. The lens is placed on the plastic spherical gauge. If there is an air bubble under the lens, the lens base curve is steeper than that of the ball (Fig. 14-13). If the edge does not align itself with the gauge but shows convolutions or if there is standoff at the edge of the lens, the lens is flatter than the gauge. One simply finds the gauge of which the lens fits perfectly and reads the base curve from the gauge.

One instrument, the Soft Lens Analyzer by Hydrovue, Inc., was developed to measure the base curve of hydrogel lenses. In addition, it measures diameter and center thickness and provides close surface and edge inspection on soft lenses as well as rigid lenses (Fig. 14-14). Because hydrogel lenses all contain some percentage of water, accurate measurement is best obtained in the hydrated state. The Soft Lens Analyzer provides a wet cell in which the lens is immersed in saline. The lens is then measured against a series of hemispheric standards with known

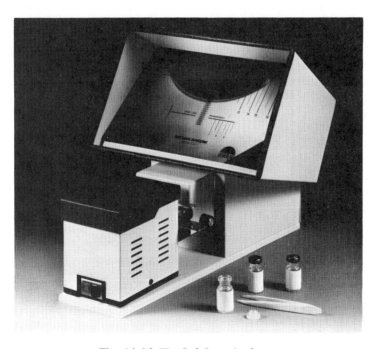

Fig. 14-14 The Soft Lens Analyzer.

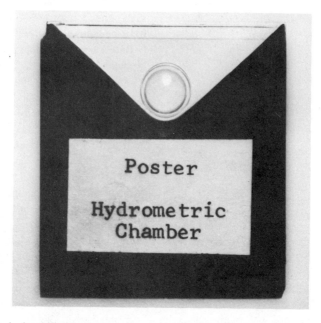

Fig. 14-15 The hydrophilic lens is floated in a normal saline-filled Poster chamber and measured in a regular lensmeter. Factor of 4 × is used to arrive at the true power. For thicker lenses additional factors may have to be calculated. (From Halberg GP: Contact lenses in aphakia. In *Transactions of the New Orleans Academy of Ophthalmology:* Symposium on contact lenses, St Louis, 1973, Mosby.)

radii from 7.6 to 9.8 mm in 0.20-mm increments. A beam of light is projected through and around the lens positioned on the standard. This image is projected onto a small built-in screen at × 15. The operator determines the base curve in terms of the lens-bearing relationship to the standard on which it is centered. This system for measuring the base curve of a lens is applicable to all lathed lenses. There is no reliable office system for measuring the base curve of a spin-cast lens.

Power. This can be performed with a fair degree of accuracy for spin-cast and lathed lenses. The lens is cleaned well and blotted dry with lint-free tissue. It is placed concave side up under a lensmeter. The measurement must be read quickly because it becomes impossible if the lens dries too much. As mentioned before, the hydrogel lens also can be measured in a small wet cell that contains saline solution (Fig. 14-15). An allowance factor must be made for the fluid surrounding the lens so that this factor is used to multiply the recorded power to obtain the correct power.

The value of in-office inspection of a soft lens before dispensing it is questionable. Sterility can be compromised, and the ability to check lens quality in the practice is poor at best when compared with the manufacturer's capability.

EVALUATION OF FIT

Because fluorescein cannot be used with soft lenses, the evaluation of a good fit depends on the positioning of the lens and its movement on the eye. The basic fitting philosophy is to fit the flattest, thinnest lens that will provide crisp vision before and after the blink, comfortable wear, stable positioning, and minimum metabolic interference.

A well-fitted lathe-cut lens will be about 1 to 2 mm larger than the cornea, will center well, and will result in a lag of 0.5 to 1 mm or slightly less on upward gaze. If the eye is moved sideways, the lens will lag slightly but will quickly center and will follow eye movements. The eye should be white and the patient able to wear the lenses comfortably all

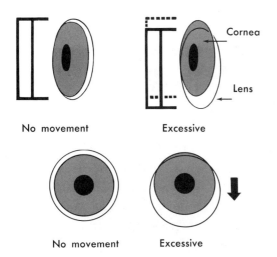

Fig. 14-16 Movement of a soft lens may vary from none (tight) to excessive (loose).

day. The lenses, however, may be too tight or too loose (Fig. 14-16).

Tight lens

A tight lens is really a large, or steep, lens and does not appear to have any movement after a blink (Fig. 14-17). It is uncomfortable to the wearer and may cause circumcorneal injection and indentation of the sclera adjacent to the limbus. The lens centers well, but vision frequently is blurred or fluctuating (Fig. 14-18); after a blink there may be a temporary clear-

ing that lasts a few seconds. Retinoscopy may reveal a dark shadow in the center, which may momentarily clear after a blink. Keratometry will show distortion of the mires, which clear after a blink. All these signs of a tight lens are caused by a lens that is steeper than the central cornea, which results in a gap that separates the lens from the cornea. During a blink the lid smooths the lens across the cornea, and there is a temporary central adherence of the lens to the cornea. Sometimes a lens that fits well initially will gradually tighten (Fig. 14-19).

Symptoms and signs of a tight lens are indicated in the box below.

**SYMPTOMS AND SIGNS OF
A TIGHT LENS**

---

1. Fluctuating vision that clears immediately after blinking
2. Initial comfort that changes to increasing discomfort as the day progresses
3. Corneal injection or redness around the circumference of the cornea (see Fig. 14-19, A and B)
4. Certain corneal indentation; compression of the conjunctiva at the limbus and a dishlike depression that obstructs the normal flow of vessels
5. Absent or minimal movement after blinking (Fig. 14-20)
6. Keratometry results in which distorted mires before a blink clear after a blink
7. Retinoscopic reflex, which is fuzzy at first and clears momentarily

---

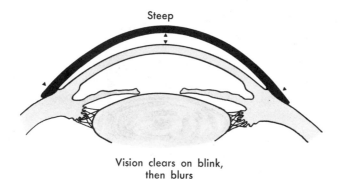

Fig. 14-17 Cross section showing steep lens. (From Uotila M, Gasset AR: Fitting manual for Bausch & Lomb and Griffin lenses. In Gasset AR, Kaufman HE, editors: *Soft contact lens,* St Louis, 1972, Mosby.)

Fluctuating visual acuity

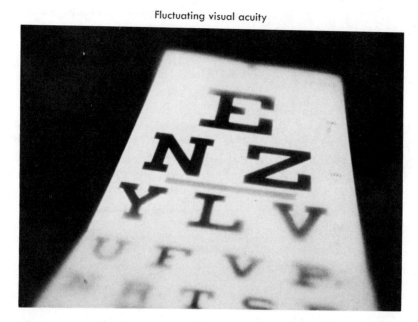

Fig. 14-18 A poor fit may produce fluctuating vision. (Courtesy Bausch & Lomb, Inc. Rochester, New York)

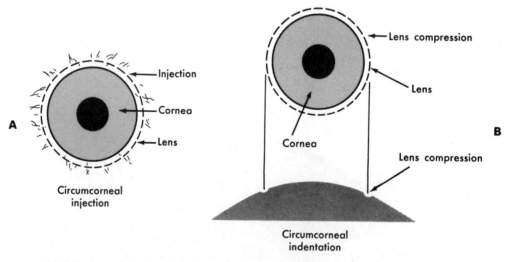

Fig. 14-19 A, Circumcorneal injection. Note the considerably vascularity at the limbus. **B,** Circumcorneal indentation. The tight lens compresses the peripheral limbal tissues. (From Stein HA, Slatt BJ, Stein RM: *Fitting guide for rigid and soft contact lenses: a practical approach,* ed 3, St Louis, 1990, Mosby.)

To correct a tight lens syndrome, the fitter must switch to a flatter lens by decreasing the base curve or by reducing the diameter of the lens.

Loose lens

A loose lens is a small, or flat, lens, has excessive movement, will lag 2 to 4 mm on downward excursion, and if extremely loose, may slide off the cornea entirely on lateral gaze (Fig. 14-21). A loose lens will center poorly and give poor, unstable vision. Vision may be good initially but may decrease two or three lines after each blink, although it may recover rapidly. Keratometer readings may show slight distortion of the mires, which is increased after each blink. With a loose lens, the edge may roll out and become dehydrated and may fall out of the eye on a blink.

The signs and symptoms of a loose lens are listed in the box on p. 336.

To correct a loose lens, one must switch to a lens that is steeper by decreasing the base curve or by increasing the diameter of the lens.

DISINFECTION

Disinfection of both spin-cast and lathe-cut soft lenses has been tested and found reliable. The major concern is that germs can enter the plastic of the lens and contaminate it. The molecular openings of the hydrogel plastic are so tiny that bacteria and fungus spores cannot invade it. The only way bacteria can contaminate an intact lens is by multiplying on its surface or if the surface of the lens is broken. This is more likely to occur if bacteria is present.

There are essentially two methods in practice today for disinfecting hydrophilic lenses: (1) by heat and (2) by chemicals.

The heat, or thermal, method consists of two steps.

1. The lenses are stored in normal saline solution in the patient's lens case.
2. The lenses are boiled daily in a specially designed automatic shut-off unit. Tests have shown that no actively growing pathogens will survive this treatment at a temperature of 180° F.

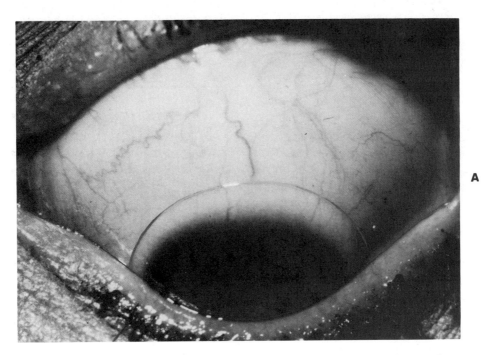

A

Fig. 14-20 A, Slightly tight lens as indicated by minimal movement up on downward gaze.

Continued.

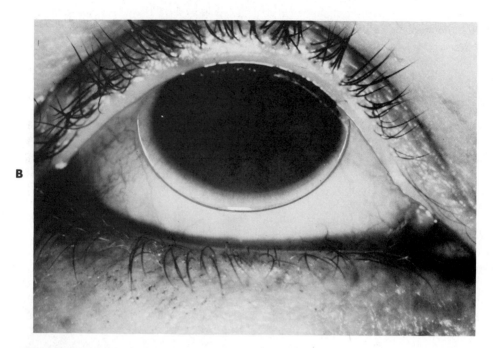

B

Fig. 14-20, cont'd B, Tight soft lens. Note the lack of lag on upward gaze and indentation in perilimbal area. (From Stein HA, Slatt BJ, Stein RM: *Fitting guide for rigid and soft contact lenses: a practical approach,* ed 3, St Louis, 1990, Mosby.)

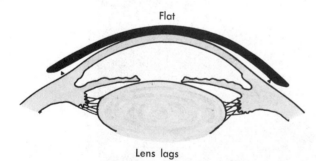

Flat

Lens lags

Fig. 14-21 Cross section showing flat lens. (From Uotila M, Gassett AR: Fitting manual for Bausch & Lomb and Griffin lenses. In Gassett AR, Kaufman HE, editors: *Soft contact lens,* St Louis, 1972, Mosby.)

SYMPTOMS AND SIGNS OF A LOOSE LENS

1. Variable vision; clear at first but poor after time
2. Excess awareness of lens
3. Poor centering
4. Excess movement (Figs. 14-22 and 14-23)
5. Edge standoff (Fig. 14-24, A)
6. Lens falling out (Fig. 14-24, B)
7. Bubble under a lens
8. Keratometry findings that show clear mires that blur after blinking
9. Retinoscopy results that are clear at first and blurs after blinking

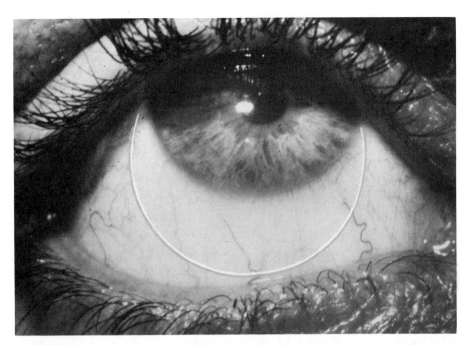

Fig. 14-22 Loose lens indicated by lag on upward gaze. (From Stein HA, Slatt BJ, Stein RM, *Fitting guide for rigid and soft contact lenses: a practical approach,* ed 3, St Louis, 1990, Mosby.)

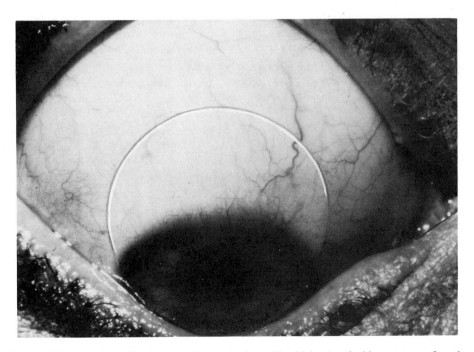

Fig. 14-23 Loose lens. On downward gaze the lens rides high. A valuable test to confirm the fitting of a soft lens. (From Stein HA, Slatt BJ, Stein RM, *Fitting guide for rigid and soft contact lenses: a practical approach,* ed 3, St Louis, 1990, Mosby.)

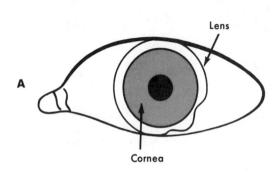 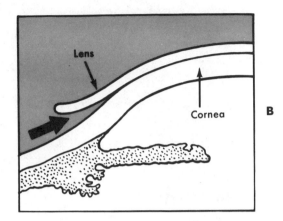

Fig. 14-24 Loose lens with edge stand-off. **A,** Shows the edge lifting of the scleral rim. **B,** Schematic side view interpretation of the edge lift-off of a loose lens. (From Stein HA, Slatt BJ, Stein RM: *Fitting guide for rigid and soft contact lenses: a practical approach,* ed 3, St Louis, 1990, Mosby.)

Several methods of chemical disinfection are available. These are based on chlorhexidine, thimerosal, quaternary ammonium compound, sorbate, and other disinfecting agents as preservatives. Thimerosal, which was found to be a common offender, has been removed from many solutions.

Boiling routines are a little cumbersome but effective. The only drawback to boiling is that the mucus and protein debris, if not cleaned from the lens beforehand, becomes coagulated and baked onto the surface of the soft lens. The replacement rate is higher with the thermal method than with the chemical method of disinfection. With chemical disinfection the germicide rapidly passes into the lens, cleans it, and disinfects it. The lens must be carefully rinsed. If not, it is irritating, and thus the forgetful are punished. Also, some individuals may be sensitive to the chemicals or preservatives in the solution. Thimerosal is a common offender.

Of recent concern has been the devastating parasite *Acanthamoeba*. It can cause severe keratitis, with pain and ring infiltrates into the cornea. The cyst form is killed primarily by heat and is resistant to chemical disinfection.

CLEANING

Protein is a natural component of human tears. In time, this protein or mucin secreted by the glands of the eyelid and found in the tears will have a tendency to stick to the surface of the soft lens and coat it. These deposits are often not normally seen until they become thick and vision becomes blurred or the lens becomes slightly irritating. These deposits develop rapidly in some persons, whereas others may never have a problem. They can interfere with the action of antibacterial agents in soaking solutions.

Lenses also may become dirty from dirty fingers, hair spray, or smoke. Cleaning is an important part of their care. Because cleaning can result in the removal of microorganisms, it aids in the disinfection of contact lenses. Theory dictates that the less concentration of microorganisms on a lens, the less challenge there will be to the disinfectant, therefore making the disinfection step as effective as possible.

Several prophylactic cleaners for hydrophilic contact lenses are on the market for daily care of the lenses. They contain various salts at physiologic concentration, preservatives to maintain control of microorganisms, and long-chain nonionic detergents. These surface-acting (surfactant) detergents provide the cleaning efficacy. Manufacturers claim that they remove mucoproteins, lipid deposits, and other forms of debris from the contact lens before the lenses are disinfected. These cleaners are not 100% effective, and eventually most soft lenses require replacement. The hands are carefully washed. Special soaps for contact lens wearers are preferred inasmuch as many commercial soaps contain moisturizers such as lanolin, which may be transferred to the lens surface. The hands are then dried with a clean, lint-free towel before removing the lens. The lens is rubbed on both sides on the palm of the hand with a clean finger, using the lens cleaner for at least 20 seconds.

Enzyme cleaners are intended for removal of protein deposits, which accumulate over a period of time and which are resistant to prophylactic cleaning regimens. The enzyme works differently from a detergent. The enzyme is capable of breaking down proteinaceous deposits, whereas the detergent can remove only loosely deposited matter on the surface. After the lens is rinsed with saline solution, it is soaked in the enzyme solution for a minimum of 15 minutes to overnight. Exceptions are the high-water lenses in which the soaking time may be considerable to prevent enzyme retention by the lens. Then the lens is rubbed and rinsed with freshly prepared saline solution and disinfected before wearing. This procedure should be undertaken at least twice monthly for the soft lenses, and even every week if the lenses easily become coated.

Surfactant cleaning both before and after lens wear increases the surface clarity and reduces the rate of solution reaction. Dirty lenses are more likely to bind high concentrations of preservative to their surface, thus creating a toxic keratitis or conjunctivitis that results in red eyes. Most patients' lenses will be somewhat dehydrated after a normal day of wear, and this makes it more difficult to properly clean the lenses in the evening. If surfactant is applied again in the following morning after the lens has been fully hydrated, the likelihood of adequate surface cleaning is much improved.

Hydrogen peroxide systems are almost too numerous to mention. It is advisable to refer to the manufacturer for details concerning each of the specific products. The standard of hydrogen peroxide systems is ophthalmic-grade hydrogen peroxide 3% to be used after surfactant cleaning. The recommended time for disinfection is a minimum of 20 minutes. Many suggest overnight storage before neutralization of the hydrogen peroxide. Neutralization usually is affected by means of a catalyst such as sodium pyrevate or catalase. The catalyst can be in the form of a saline storage step, that is, a saline-containing neutralizer into which the lenses are placed after hydrogen peroxide disinfection or a sodium-catalyst tablet placed directly in the hydrogen peroxide to convert it into saline.

The American Optical AO Sept system adopted by CIBA is unique in that it uses a saline that contains 3% hydrogen peroxide as a disinfecting solution, combined with a specially treated disk that is in the case at the same time to affect neutralization for a 6-hour period.

Cleaning routines, either daily or weekly, are part of a preventive maintenance program to ensure longer, more comfortable lens wear as well as longer lens life. The section on disposable lenses discusses at length how regular replacement of soft lenses can be more practical and effective.

INSERTION AND REMOVAL TECHNIQUES

The insertion and removal of soft contact lenses are different from the techniques used for conventional lenses. The soft lens is inserted on the lower part of the sclera and gently pushed onto the cornea with the lower eyelid. In the removal technique of soft contact lenses, it generally is recommended to first slide the lens down the index finger to the lower sclera and then to pinch off the lens.

Elderly patients may have difficulty in placing, removing, and handling the contact lenses. Normally, if this problem cannot be overcome by in-office training, the patient should not receive the lens. In some cases, however, another person might be taught to place, remove, and handle the lenses for the patient. The same is true with children who are being fitted with hydrophilic contact lenses. Insertion devices are available for the soft lens, but they should not be used unless manual attempts have failed.

Insertion by the fitter

The following technique is used for lens insertion by the fitter.

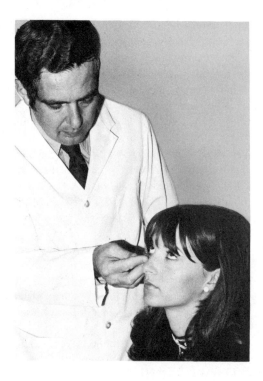

Fig. 14-25 Insertion of contact lens by the practitioner. The middle finger retracts with lower lid while the contact lens is gently offered with the index finger to the lower conjunctiva.

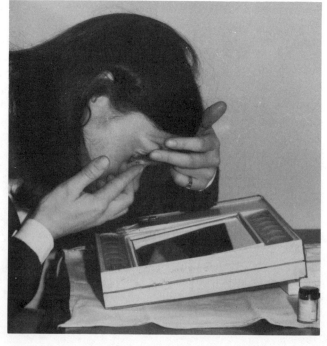

Fig. 14-26 A large mirror is a helpful adjunct in inserting a lens. (From Stein HA, Slatt BJ, Stein RM: *Fitting guide for rigid and soft contact lenses: a practical approach*, ed 3, St Louis, 1990, Mosby.)

1. Keep nails short at all times.
2. Wash hands and rinse thoroughly to remove all traces of soap. Dry with a lint-free towel. Avoid using oils and creams on your hands before handling the lens.
3. Remove the right lens from the vial or case. Lenses that have been soaked in germicide must be rinsed thoroughly with normal saline solution. Do not touch the inside lens surface after rinsing.
4. Place the lens on the tip of the index finger, concave side up. Have the patient look straight ahead. Retract the lower lid with your middle finger (see Fig. 14-25).
5. Have the patient look up and stare at a point on the ceiling. Roll the lens onto the lower white of the eye and express the air bubble. Swirling the lens on the sclera also helps to make the lens comfortable by introducing tears into the lens and making the lens isotonic with the tears.
6. Have the patient close the eyes, and lightly massage the lid to help center the lens.
7. Repeat the same procedure for the left lens.

Removal by the fitter

The following technique is used for lens removal by the fitter.

1. Hands must similarly be washed before removal as for insertion.
2. Be sure the lens is on the cornea before attempting removal.
3. Have the patient look up. Place the middle finger on the lower lid, and touch the edge of the lens with the forefinger.
4. While the patient is looking up, slide the lens down onto the white of the eye. Bring the thumb over, and compress the lens lightly between the thumb and index finger so that the lens folds and comes off easily.

Insertion by the patient

Careful patient instruction in the care and handling of soft contact lenses frequently is left to the ophthalmic assistant. It is important that the patient understand carefully the procedure and care system and comply. Failure to comply with instruction is the greatest single cause of difficulties with well-fitted soft contact lenses.

The following technique is used for lens insertion by the patient. For beginners, a large mirror is helpful (Fig. 14-26).

1. Keep the nails short, and carefully wash and dry the hands.
2. Take the right lens out of the vial either with forceps or by pouring the contents of the vial into the palm of the hand.
3. Rinse the lens with normal saline solution.
4. Place the lens on the tip of the index finger of the dominant hand. With thin lenses, permit the lens to dehydrate for 1 to 2 minutes in air and dry finger.
5. While looking up, retract the lower lid with the middle finger; while still gazing upward, apply the lens to the lower white of the eye (Fig. 14-27, A).
6. Express any air, remove the index finger, and then slowly release the lower lid.
7. Close the eyes and gently massage the lids to help center the lens (Fig. 14-27, B).

Removal by the patient

The following technique is used for lens removal by the patient.

1. Check vision in each eye separately to be sure the lens is in place on the cornea.
2. Wash hands and rinse thoroughly.
3. Look upward. Retract the lower lid with the middle finger, and place the index fingertip on the lower edge of the lens.
4. Slide the lens down to the white of the eye.
5. Compress the lens between the thumb and index finger so that air breaks the suction under the lens. Remove the lens from the eye (Fig. 14-28).
6. Prepare the lens for cleaning and sterilizing according to the recommendations of the manufacturer and the practitioner.
7. An alternative method of removal is to look nasally and slide the lens to the outermost portion of the eye before removal.

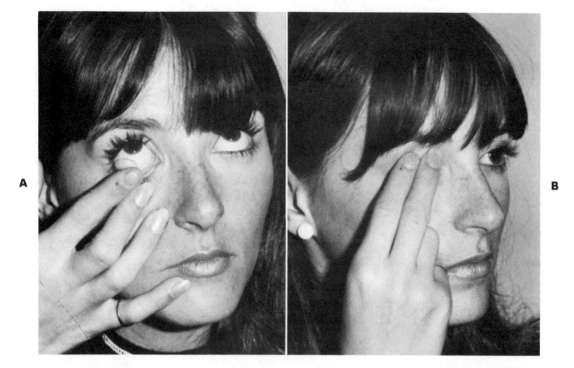

Fig. 14-27 A, Inserting the soft lens. **B,** Centering the lens through the closed eyelid.

TACO TEST

If there is any question of whether the lens is inside out, the "taco test" should be performed (Fig. 14-29). In this test the lens is flexed between the forefinger and thumb. If the edges are erect and point inward like a taco, the lens is in the correct position. If the edge appears to fold back in the fingers, the lens is everted and must be reversed. For new ultrathin lenses the taco test may not be valid. The inside-out shape is less regular than the correct position at the lens margin.

PRECAUTIONS FOR WEAR

1. Do not insert lenses if eyes are red or irritated.
2. Do not use tap water, distilled water, or spring water directly in the eye; always use saline solution.
3. Do not use any solutions with contact lenses other than those specifically recommended.

4. If the lens becomes uncomfortable when first inserted or while wearing or if vision becomes blurred, foreign material may be present on the inside surface of the lens. The lens should be immediately removed, cleaned, rinsed, and reinserted.
5. Lenses should not be worn in the presence of irritating fumes or vapors.
6. Lenses should not be worn overnight unless specifically advised.
7. If the lens is difficult to remove or difficult to slide down, rinse the eye with normal saline solution, and the lens should soon once again move freely and be easily removable.
8. If vision is blurred while wearing the lens, consider the possibility that the lens may be inside out, off center, not clean, or that the right and left lenses have been switched.
9. If the lens is left exposed to air, it will dry

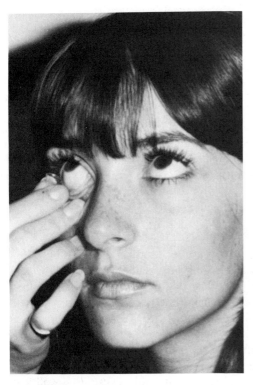

Fig. 14-28 Removing the lens. The lens is gently pinched between the thumb and forefinger.

out and become hard and brittle. Should this occur, handle it gently and place it in saline solution, and it will again become soft and flexible.

10. If hair spray is used, keep the eyes closed for at least 60 seconds to allow the spray to dissipate.

WEARING SCHEDULES

Because soft lenses are much more comfortable than rigid lenses, the wearer may be inclined to overwear the lenses the first few days beyond corneal tolerance. The manufacturers' routine wearing schedules usually are conservative in build-up but are designed to give maximum protection with minimum risk of corneal edema in the early stages while the eye builds up tolerance to the soft lens.

The difficulty in permitting overnight wear with standard lenses is that blinking does not occur, and consequently there is tear stagnation between the soft lens and cornea, with subsequent anoxia to the cornea. For many persons, this may result in serious corneal edema in the morning.

Lenses designed for extended wear are discussed in detail later in this chapter.

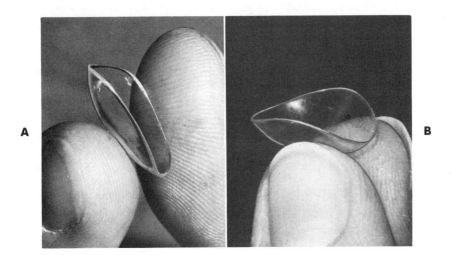

Fig. 14-29 Taco test to determine correct side of the lens. **A,** Edge is erect and points slightly inward. **B,** Edge appears to fold back on the fingers, indicating the lens is inside out and must be reversed.

ADVANTAGES AND DISADVANTAGES OF THIN SOFT LENSES

ADVANTAGES

Initial comfort and adaptation

Higher oxygen permeability

Decreased incidence of overwear

Can be fitted tighter for stable vision during sport activities

Alternative for highly sensitive individuals

Reduced risk of giant papillary conjunctivitis

Reduced risk of corneal warpage

DISADVANTAGES

Exaggerated dehydrating effect

More difficult to handle

More easily damaged

Less masking of corneal astigmatism, resulting in poorer quality of vision

More difficult to manufacture, and thus quality control may not be as precise

---

THIN AND ULTRATHIN LENSES

A major technologic change in soft lens manufacture has been the development of the thin and ultrathin soft lenses, with center thickness on both measuring less than 0.1 mm and even as thin as 0.02 mm.

The advantages and disadvantages of these thinner soft lenses are outlined in the box above.

The importance of thin and ultrathin lenses is that these lenses provide exceptional initial comfort. Being thin, these lenses provide some diffusion of oxygen and minimize corneal edema formation from hypoxia. Because of their oxygen permeability characteristics, these lenses may be fitted slightly tighter than regular soft lenses and consequently produce more stable vision; thus they are useful for sporting activities. They also appear to reduce the incidence of giant papillary conjunctivitis.

One of the disadvantages of thin and ultrathin lenses is the fact that they are harder to handle and require more patience by the fitter and patient in instruction. They also have an exaggerated dehydration effect in dry environments. These lenses may damage more easily. In addition, they may not mask as much astigmatism as regular soft lenses and thus may give a poor quality of vision in those with corneal astigmatism.

CORRECTION OF ASTIGMATISM

Most failures for soft lens wear occur because the lenses do not adequately correct astigmatism and, as a result, vision is poor. The soft lens conforms to the shape of the eye, and only about 1.00 to 1.50 diopters of astigmatism can be ignored. This low amount of astigmatism is what usually is found in most lens wearers. There are, however, a number of patients with astigmatism over 1.50 diopters who can be fitted with soft toric lenses.

Toric lens design

To correct astigmatism the lens must be stabilized so that it does not rotate on the eye. When this is accomplished, the cylinder is ground on either the front surface or the back surface. Current methods available to prevent rotation are (1) prism ballast lenses, (2) truncation, (3) a combination of prism ballast lenses and truncation, and (4) double slab-off or thin-zone lenses. Once lens rotation has been eliminated the lens can be constructed with the cylinder incorporated along a given axis.

Prism ballast. Just as in a rigid lens a prism can be incorporated into the lens so that the thicker, heavier edge will orientate to the inferior aspect of the eye (Fig. 14-30). A front or back surface toric lens can then be ground in the proper axis to compensate for the astigmatism. These lenses should be fitted accurately so that they will rotate to the final resting position and the cylinder will not be misaligned.

These lenses depend entirely on adequate movement and rotation. The eyelids influence the final position of the lens. Tight lids have a considerable influence on rotation of the soft lens and are difficult to fit with an astigmatic soft lens. The position of the lower lid will have an influence, and lenses must be fitted larger for those with wider palpebral fissures.

Truncation. By cutting off a small segment of the lens, the rotation of the lens will be stopped by the edge of the lower lid. Consequently the lens can have a toric or cylinder portion ground on its anterior

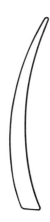

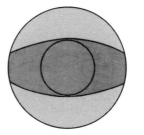 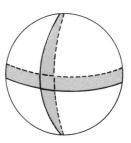

Fig. 14-31 Double slab-off soft lens used to correct astigmatism. The lens is made thinner superiorly and inferiorly so that the thinner portions tend to rotate and come to rest under the upper and lower eyelids. (From Stein HA, Slatt BJ, Stein RM: *Fitting guide for rigid and soft contact lenses: a practical approach,* ed 3, St Louis, 1990, Mosby.)

Fig. 14-30 Prism ballast to provide weight and stop rotation of a lens. (From Stein HA, Slatt BJ, Stein RM: *Fitting guide for rigid and soft contact lenses: a practical approach,* ed 3, St Louis, 1990, Mosby.)

surface. Truncation is useful when combined with prism ballast lenses because it eliminates the heavy, thick edge of the prism that lies below.

Truncation and prism ballast. Several forms take advantage of both truncation and prism ballast. The lower portion is truncated by 0.75 to 1.5 mm to eliminate the excess weight, the prism ballast. Lid configuration affects the final position of the inferior truncations. The truncated edge must be beveled; otherwise the lens could cause corneal abrasions.

Double slab off. In this method of correcting astigmatism, the superior and inferior portion of the lens is "slabbed off" from the anterior surface, resulting in a lens that is thinner at the top and bottom but thicker in the exposed portion of the lens (Fig. 14-31). The lens rotates so that the thinner portions lie under the upper and lower eyelids. The lids tend to hold the lens in the proper position, and a toric front surface can be ground on the lens to correct the astigmatic portion.

Configuration of the eyelid, blinking reflexes, and tension of the eyelids will have an affect on the final rotation of the lens. Thus each patient must have a trial fitting with a set of trial lenses, with markings that identify the position of the soft lens at all times. By using a soft lens as a diagnostic lens, the practitioner can incorporate correcting values to arrive

at the final lens for incorporation of the cylindric power and axis.

MEDICAL USES

A revolution has occurred in the treatment of corneal diseases by judicious use of soft contact lenses. A large number of patients who could not be helped before can now be helped by use of the soft contact lens, which can act as a bandage. It is not a panacea for all diseases, but if well fitted and wisely used with well-selected patients, contact lenses can be of inestimable value.

The soft lens acts by delicately covering the cornea and thereby protecting it. Its water-absorbing qualities keep the surface of the cornea moist and well-lubricated under the agreeable protective shell. The soft lenses that are best to use as a bandage are those that are extremely thin or those that are of high water content.

Blisters of the cornea (bullous keratopathy)

Bullous keratopathy in its late stages is characterized by blind and excruciatingly painful eyes. In this condition the cornea becomes swollen, and the superficial layer of the epithelium is raised into convex mounds. Some of these corneal blisters rupture and of course when they do so, there is a raw, burning feeling and often pain in the eyes, along with marked reduction is visual acuity. The attendant scarring and irregularity of the cornea that follow the rupture of these blisters can, on a cumulative basis, cause permanent loss of vision. This condition is brought on not by lack of oxygen to the epithelium but by damage to the inside layer of the cornea, the endothelium, so that aqueous humor from the anterior chamber can percolate through the cornea.

The introduction of the soft therapeutic contact lens and its popularization by Dr. Herbert E. Kaufman revolutionized the treatment of the disease. A bandage lens is a safe, simple, nonsurgical method of relieving both the pain and the profound visual loss. It can be performed in the office rather than the operating room. Its application does not require sophisticated surgical expertise and therefore can be applied by virtually every ophthalmologist or ophthalmic technician in any part of the world. Numerous reports in ophthalmologic literature confirm that these lenses are well-tolerated and can be worn continuously for prolonged periods on diseased corneas without adverse effects. In each case the patient is not only comfortable but may experience improvement in vision as long as the lenses remain in place. In some cases in which the cornea was terribly scarred, the only improvement is freedom from pain. Some patients have become so frightened of possible reactivation of discomfort that they have worn their soft contact lenses for 24 hours a day for months without removal for replacement purposes.

Fitting of the soft lens for bullous keratopathy is more challenging than fitting for refractive errors. Trial lens fitting is the method of choice. A properly fitted lens has both central and peripheral contact so that it does not flex in the center with each blink. In some cases it may be necessary to fit the lens with minimal or no movement. Because patients with bullous keratopathy wear soft lenses continuously for 24 hours per day, dehydration of the cornea and a change in corneal shape result. Thus a change or several changes of the lens often is required to achieve a good fit and improve vision. For aphakia one can use a planolens to achieve the corneal change; once the cornea improves, however, the refractive power needs to be considered. In some cases it is necessary to use medication, such as hypertonic saline 5%, along with the lens.

Corneal ulcers

An ulcer is a large defect in the tissues, and its appearance on the cornea is viewed with alarm. If a corneal ulcer increases in size and grows deep, it can cause perforation of the cornea and a loss of the structures inside the eye, which can herniate through this defect. This usually means loss of the eye. The likelihood of such a contingency is quite real. There is a certain pressure within the eye itself, which can burst through if there is a weakness of the coats of the eye, such as a thinning of the cornea or sclera. Furthermore, because the cornea is devoid of any blood vessels (a factor that aids in its transparency but prevents the successful mobilization of the body's resources to a damaged site), it is an extremely vulnerable organ. The cases in which soft lenses have been tried have been those in which antibiotics and pressure dressings have failed, and the surgeon has had to perform corneal transplantation. The largest cause of infection and corneal ulcers is poor hygiene. Dirty hands, nails, and contact lens cases are the most responsible sources. Contaminated distilled water also is a common cause (Fig. 14-32).

Recurrent corneal erosion

Many people at one time or another have had a piece of grit fly into the eye and have required professional help to remove it. Once the eye is patched for 24 hours, the cornea repairs itself and the mishap is forgotten, relegated to the domain of unpleasant minor memories. If, however, the eye is injured by anything organic, such as a fingernail, the cornea may heal but break down again weeks or months later.

The entire sequence of the initial accident is relived, and the person suffers pain, sensitivity to light, watering eyes, redness of the eye, and marked blurring of vision. The event may seem unreal because there is no antecedent injury the second or third time. Soft lenses may prevent this recurrent breakdown.

Keratitis sicca (dry eyes)

The primary disturbance in keratitis sicca is a result of a gross deficiency of tears, which parches the cornea and causes dryness of its surface so that it

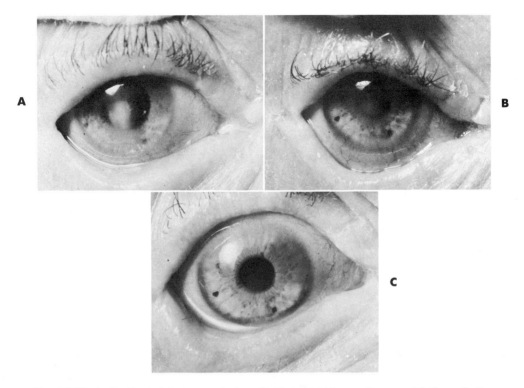

Fig. 14-32 A, Sterile, indolent corneal ulcer. **B,** Forty-eight hours after use of Soflens. **C,** Two weeks after wearing Soflens. (From Buxton JN, Locke CR: A therapeutic evaluation of hydrophilic contact lenses. In Bitonte JL, Keates RH, editors: *Symposium on the flexible lens; the future of flexible lenses vs. rigid lenses,* St Louis, 1972, Mosby.)

develops pits and erosions. Patients with dry eyes complain of a terrible burning sensation that is much worse when indoors. They are constant visitors to the drugstores and will buy anything that comes out of a dropper, provided it is wet.

In mild cases artificial tears (which are really a type of wetting agent) are effective, and people can be comfortable as long as they keep placing drops in their eyes every few hours. In severe cases when the tear production is virtually nil, wetting agents, regardless of how frequently they are applied, fail to work and the cornea and conjunctiva become dry. The use of the soft lens has been the salvation of some of these patients who are faced with a condition that was incurable.

Again, the mechanism by which soft lenses achieve these clinical results is not clear. They do act as a protective bandage, and their tendency to retain water probably accounts for their successful lubricant value. In patients affected with this condition, improvement in their general corneal status has not only given them symptomatic relief but has invariably improved their vision and in some instances in a spectacular fashion. These lenses are often effective if used in conjuction with artificial tears and local antibiotics that do not contain preservatives. In some cases, however, soft lenses will fail to be of help.

Conclusion

Soft lenses have added a new dimension to the treatment of severe external ocular diseases. They act basically as a protective cover for the cornea, shielding it from irritants and allowing it to rest much in the same way as a cast permits a broken leg to mend. With the introduction of extremely thin lenses and lenses of high water content, their potential use been expanded.

EXTENDED-WEAR LENSES

Extended-wear lenses are lenses that are worn for 24 hours or more on a continual basis. The manufacturing technology has advanced to produce thinner and thinner soft lenses that provide more comfort and more oxygen under the lens. In addition, lenses can now be made with high water content, which also provides more oxygen to the underlying cornea. It has been clearly shown that if a person halves the thickness of a soft lens, its oxygen transmission will be doubled.

A second factor that has resulted in the availability of extended-wear lenses has been the ability to polymerize soft lens materials and manufacture lenses that will absorb more water in their substance. For every 10% increase in water absortion of these materials there is a corresponding 50% increase in oxygen transmission, so that if water content increases 20%, the oxygen transmission doubles. Hydrophilic lenses that retain up to 79% water have been developed. Polymer chemists working in this specialized area developed materials that have satisfactory tensile strength and that are durable.

A third thrust has been the development of silicone-PMMA and fluorocarbonated silicon—PMMA rigid lenses. At present, however, two types of hydrophilic lenses that provide satisfactory extended wear are those that are either (1) manufactured very thin or (2) of high water content, over 55%.

The direction and emphasis in ophthalmology have been to provide a better method of visual rehabilitation with contact lenses for the myope. The myope who wants spectacle-free vision 24 hours a day and the competitive advantages in social, recreational, and occupational environments can now benefit from the extended-wear lens.

Myopic versus aphakic extended wear

Extended wear for myopia is a completely different problem from extended wear for aphakia. The myopic person usually is younger, with healthier corneas and better tear production, and usually is more capable of learning the insertion, removal, and care

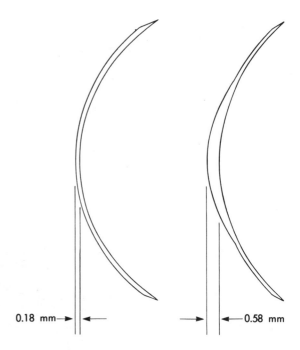

0.18 mm→ ←   → ←0.58 mm

Fig. 14-33 Comparison of a regular soft lens *(left)* with an aphakic lenticular lens *(right)* Note the considerably thicker central portion of the aphakic lens that may contribute to corneal edema by impairing oxygen transmission. (From Stein HA, Slatt BJ, Stein RM: *Fitting guide for rigid and soft contact lenses: a practical approach,* ed 3, St Louis, 1990, Mosby.)

techniques for the lenses. In addition, having myopia aids an individual in seeing lenses for insertion, as well as in following care routines. The aphakic person, on the other hand, usually is elderly; has poor hand coordination, poor tear production, and a tendency to form increased lens deposits; and usually is less mobile for return visits to the office or clinic. In addition, the aphakic lens is considerably thicker to achieve suitable power in the lens (Fig. 14-33), and this impairs some of the oxygen transmission qualities of the lens. The inability of aphakic individuals to accommodate or visualize the lens on their finger makes insertion and removal very difficult.

Problems with extended-wear lenses

The patient is under some risk unless the fitter is prepared to provide careful monitoring. In addition, there are medicolegal implications for improper monitoring if serious problems arise. The most troublesome problem has been deposit formation and coating of the lenses. This results in a lens that not only interferes with vision but also increases the mass of the lens, alters the parameter of the lens, and reduces the oxygen transmission of the lens, with attendant risks of corneal hypoxia. Deposits also add an immunoglobulin factor that may result in giant papillary conjunctivitis and a red eye. Careful cleaning on a regular basis is an important factor in the satisfactory wearing of extended-war lenses. With the current anxiety concerning AIDS in tears, hydrogen peroxide is an effective cleansing and disinfecting system. Apparently there also have been outbreaks of acanthamoebic infections. In this situation, thermal disinfection is the best form to destroy this organism.

Corneal hypoxia is a reality in aphakia, with the attendant hazards of neovascularization, diffuse corneal edema, and corneal alteration. A lens that is quite permeable for a myopic eye and that is 0.1-mm thick may show no permeability at an aphakic-level thickness of 0.35 to 0.50 mm.

Extended-wear lenses should be fitted with the flattest lens that will remain centered on the eye and that will provide good vision. A lens that may appear a little loose the first day may become tighter the next day because of dehydration. Thus a 24-hour examination is very important.

Recently, *Acanthamoeba,* a parasitic organism found in hot tubs, swimming pools, and contaminated distilled water, has been shown to cause serious eye infections in contact lens wearers.

Extended-wear lenses have come under greater attack because of reported cases of corneal ulcers directly related to extended-wear lens use. Some clinicians even advocate banning extended-wear soft lenses. Although the preponderance of medical opinion does not go that far, precautions should be taken.

1. Patients should be screened, and those with corneal disease, dry eyes, allergies, and chronic blepharitis should not be fit.
2. All new candidates should be day-adapted.
3. Patients should be educated about the need for hygiene procedures with respect to wearing of lenses.
4. Lenses should be removed, cleaned, and disinfected at least once weekly.
5. The lenses should not be worn longer than 1 week, with 1 night's rest.
6. Follow-up examinations are essential. Patients should be seen at least twice a year by the ophthalmologist.
7. Any complications, such as a red eye or pain in the eye, should be reported immediately.
8. We advocate a hydrogen peroxide disinfecting and cleaning system for most extended-wear patients. This has been shown to kill the AIDS virus. Hydrogen peroxide does not adequately kill *Acanthamoeba* organisms, although some studies are beginning to show that the organism will be killed if the contact time is long. This parasite requires heat to kill.
9. It is recommended that any patient wearing extended-wear lenses be offered a form of disposable lenses or planned replacement lenses.

With long-term wear of extended-wear lenses, or daily-wear soft lenses, vacuoles and microcysts may occur in the epithelium of at least 40% of patients. This condition probably occurs because of prolonged low levels of cell death by hypoxia. It usually clears up after lens use is discontinued.

The sucked-on lens syndrome, reported by Wilson and others, involves a tight, nonmovable lens that is associated with red eye. Its cause is still controversial, but it may result from chemical changes that alter the steepness of the lens. It may be relieved by the use of alkaline drops such as balanced salts on solution.

Conclusion

The search for a lens that can be worn for prolonged periods of time was risky and adventurous. Today new plastics and better manufacturing techniques are available, although risk factors still are present with extended-wear lenses.

The fitting of the young myopic person with extended-wear lenses is much easier and more successful than that of the aphakic person because of the thinner lens centers, the healthier corneas, and the better tear film often found in the myopic individual.

Lens technology has continued to advance so that disposable lenses are now available. These disposable lenses may be thrown away on a weekly basis. For our own patients, about 20% wear these lenses on an extended-wear overnight basis, whereas 80% wear them on a daily-wear basis.

DISPOSABLE LENSES

The development of disposable contact lenses has ushered in a new era in contact lens safety. Lenses such as the Vistakon Acuvue and SureVue, Bausch & Lomb SeQuence, and Ciba Vision New Vues are lenses that can be worn on an extended-wear basis for 1 week or on a daily-wear basis for 2 weeks and then discarded. The SureVue is a slightly thicker lens that is easier to handle. All these lenses have extended-wear capability on the basis of a high DK or oxygen permeability.

Disposable lenses are not available in every power. When they are introduced, however, a new safety factor occurred that has changed the entire concept in the way we think of soft contact lenses. Planned replacement of lenses is now a practical choice. A person can purchase two to four pair of lenses per year and discard them frequently.

Disposable lenses have the following advantages.
1. Clearer vision is obtained because clean lenses are introduced on a regular basis.
2. The cost of lens-care solutions is greatly reduced.
3. Because lenses are discarded before significant deposits form, there is minimal deposit formation.
4. Better compliance occurs because daily-wear disposable lenses require minimal care compared with the cleaning routines necessary for regular soft lenses.
5. Loss or tearing of a lens is not as much of a problem as the wearer has a purse-size extra lens to carry and insert in emergencies.
6. Disposable lenses offer convenience for travel in that a small package is available, which ends the need to pack a great number of care-system bottles.
7. The incidence and degree of giant papillary conjunctivitis are reduced.
8. The incidence of corneal infection is reduced.

It should be noted that any disposable lens that is removed from the eye with the intent of reinserting it again must be disinfected. It is our recommendation that all disposable lenses should be worn on a daily-wear basis unless some occupation or special reasons require extended wear.

On the negative side the disposable system is more expensive than traditional lenses. Patients may skimp and save and try to wear lenses long beyond their recommended time factor.

With frequent replacement the lenses are dispensed on an annual or semiannual basis, and the patient picks up new lenses periodically. Planned replacement, sometimes called *programmed replacement,* often is less expensive than disposable lenses. The intervals of anywhere between 2 weeks and 6 months may be used.

With all disposable and frequent replacement lenses, patient compliance in discarding the lenses on a timed arrangement and in adhering to care systems are mandatory. Patient compliance generally is regarded as high because of less confusion concerning the proper solutions and their application. The system is safe and simple and provides the best in long-term ocular health for patients. Most of these lenses at the present time do not mask very effectively any astigmatism over 1.25 diopters. Because of the minimal base-curve availability for these lenses, the "one size fits all" concept is not applicable. However, about 80% of this group can be fitted with the currently available disposable lenses. The others may be put into a planned-replacement program.

Daily-wear disposable lenses and frequent-replacement lenses are problem solvers for many patients with lens deposits, short lens life, and frequent damage to conventional lenses. The current disposable lenses stand up well to normal insertion and short-term removal.

There is now a significant pool of dropouts from contact lens wear who can be reintroduced to a safe and more convenient system of soft lens wear.

INNOVATIONS IN DESIGN

As soon as a person puts pen to paper, innovations appear in the soft lens field, making old lenses and

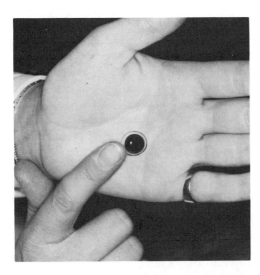

Fig. 14-34 Colored soft lens to cover cosmetically disfigured eyes.

methods of cleaning and disinfecting obsolete. Soft lenses have become thinner and more durable. Their manufacturing techniques have become more automated and more reproducible.

Soft lenses are available in a variety of colors to cover cosmetically disfigured eyes (Fig. 14-34). They may be used to occlude pupils for amblyopia and may be tinted red to correct color blindness. Slight handling tints are available for better identification of the lenses. Laser mark impregnation of size and power can be made directly on the soft lenses. Bifocal soft lenses are available for the presbyope. Lenses with dark irides and a clear central portion are available for albino or light-sensitive persons. The rapidly expanding technology in daily and extended-wear lenses continues to enhance the practitioner's therapeutic armamentarium. UV-blocking lenses are becoming more common, and disposable, toric, color-changing lenses are available.

CONTACT LENSES IN INDUSTRY

The following statement by the Contact Lens Association of Ophthalmologists (CLAO) addresses the use of contact lenses in industry.

1. Contact lenses may be worn in industrial environments, in combination with appropriate industrial safety eyewear, except where there is likelihood of injury from intense heat, massive chemical splash, highly particulate atmosphere, or where specific federal regulations prohibit such use.
2. Employees wearing contact lenses must be identified and known to their immediate supervisors, and to the plant safety and medical personnel.
3. First aid personnel should be trained in the proper removal of contact lenses.
4. Employees whose central and peripheral vision can be increased by the wearing of contact lenses, as contrasted to spectacle lenses, should be encouraged to wear contact lenses in industry. Examples of such employees are those who have had a cataract removed from one or both eyes, those with irregular astigmatism from corneal scars or keratoconus, and those who are extremely nearsighted.
5. Employees must keep a spare pair of contacts and/or prescription spectacles in their possession on the job to avoid an inability to function if they should damage or lose a contact lens while working.
6. Safety and/or medical personnel should not discriminate against an employee who can achieve visual rehabilitation by contact lenses, either in job placement or on return to a job category.
7. Safety and/or medical personnel should determine on an individual basis the wearing of spectacle or contact lenses in jobs which require unique visual performance. The Occupational Safety and Health Administration and the National Institute for Occupational Safety and Health recommendations must be considered.

SPECIAL OCCUPATIONS

Persons such as flight attendants, aircraft pilots, police, firefighters, and military personnel have special occupational requirements. For them, contact lenses may be a hazard because clear vision is necessary at all times. Flight attendants need to read warning labels, circuit-breaker labels, and controls; at the same time they must be able to see a small child at the rear of the airplane in case of an emergency.

Similar good vision is required of police and fire-fighters. Contact lenses may be hazardous for these workers because of downtime, discontinuance of wear, loss or removal of the lenses, or other problems.

Downtime

Downtime can amount to as much as 10% to 15% of the wearing time. Contact lenses may have to be temporarily discontinued at critical moments.

1. Some individuals have difficulty with contact lenses because of allergies and sensitivity to smoke and other pollutants. Women who take birth control pills have diminished tear secretion and subtle changes in the cornea that make contact lenses difficult to wear.
2. Some individuals have recurrent conjunctival infections. Corneal ulceration can occur in 20/10,000 extended-wear contact lens users and 4/10,000 daily-wear lens users.
3. Proper care and maintenance of contact lenses are important. Failure to follow directions and reliance on shortcuts, particularly during busy times, affect 75% of wearers. This can result in more contamination of the lenses.
4. Inflammation may be caused by cosmetic lotions in and around the eyes.
5. The carrying cases of contact lenses may harbor microorganisms.
6. A lens can alter its shape and consequently its fit so that it may become too tight or too loose.
7. Some contact lenses may chip or crack and may cause a corneal abrasion that requires removal and downtime. Breakage occurs in 4 to 5% of rigid contact lenses, and soft lenses may tear at a similar rate.
8. Warping of a rigid contact lens is fairly common. This warping causes a change in the curvature and an imperfect fit, resulting in downtime.
9. Fatigue plays an important role in the wearing of contact lenses. When fatigued, the wearer tends to stare, with reduced blinking time. This results in dehydration of the soft lens, and irritation begins, often resulting in removal.

Discontinuance of wear

Situations occur, such as eye injury, during which the patient may have to discontinue contact lens wear for several months until the eye is healed. In this case the patient may have to rely on spectacles. Other reasons for discontinuance of wear follow.

1. Warped rigid lenses may require discontinuance for several months to allow the cornea to restore its normal curvature.
2. Some persons are more prone to infection with contact lens wear. This infection may cause severe ulceration and keratitis, resulting in several weeks of downtime.
3. Care systems may be time-consuming and cause an individual to discontinue using the lenses and revert to spectacles.
4. Many persons are sensitive or become hypersensitive to the disinfectant solutions that are required for contact lens care and may be required to discontinue contact lens wear.
5. Allergic conjunctivitis can occur in 1 to 5% of persons who wear hard lens and in at least 20% of those who use extended-wear soft contact lenses.

Loss or removal of the lenses

Loss of a lens is a common occurrence, particularly with rigid lenses.

1. Lenses can become lost during activity in certain occupations or sports.
2. Cigarette and pipe smoke can force the wearer to remove contact lenses.
3. In case of fire, both smoke and toxic gases may become trapped behind the contact lens and irritate the eye, making removal necessary.
4. Foreign particles underneath a contact lens may scratch and irritate the eye, requiring removal of the lens.
5. Soft lenses dehydrate relatively quickly in low-humidity environments such as aircraft, which may cause their removal because of discomfort.

Problems of contact lenses

1. Contrast sensitivity in the everyday world often is reduced with contact lenses. In critical areas of visual function, this may become a hazard.

2. Scratches may occur on hard and soft contact lenses and require replacement of the lens for improved vision.

3. Debris may accumulate on the surface of the contact lenses as a result of mixtures of lipids and proteins. Not only can this make the eye uncomfortable; it also can impair the vision.

4. Poor fitting can result in tightness of the lens.

COMMON QUESTIONS AND ANSWERS

1. Is a contact lens to be removed before evaluation with use of the air tonometer?

   Yes. The practitioner does not obtain reliable results of pressure unless the contact lens is removed before this measurement.

2. Are lenses required to be removed before a field test?

   No. The best visual acuity is required to perform a field test. If the lenses provide this, then the lenses may remain in the eyes.

3. How long should a contact lens be removed before an eye examination?

   If the examination does not involve a refraction, the contact lens need not necessarily be removed. All major examinations can be done during this procedure. It will, however, require removal during the tonometric examination.

4. How long should a contact lens be removed before refraction?

   To obtain a suitable refraction, a contact lens should be removed at least 24 to 48 hours before examination. This permits the corneal epithelium to regain its full corneal curvature and thus provide a suitable refraction. Sometimes epithelial edema is present, which clouds the refraction and produces an error in the refractive surface.

5. Can patients who wear contact lenses be considered for implant surgery?

   Yes. The correct lenses provide no impairment to implant surgery. The use of biometry provides a new measurement for an intraocular lens that often will eliminate contact lenses.

6. Can contact lenses be used after refractive surgery?

   Yes. The keratometer readings often are misleading. These patients should be fitted according to their original K readings. Soft lenses, if worn for any extended basis, will provide some vascularization at the knee of the depression. Consequently, the patient should receive instructions for daily wear and minimal wearing times. Hard lenses probably are more suitable and will reduce any corneal toricity that may be present.

7. Can soft or rigid lenses be worn after implant surgery?

   Yes. Usually, however, these are not required. On the other hand, in cases of higher astigmatism or residual refractive error they may provide a very useful form of visual rehabilitation.

8. What are the major problems in care of contact lenses?

   The most common problems are those caused by lack of compliance; that is, the patient does not follow the regimen given by the instructor. Because patients often become haphazard about lens care, care must be emphasized at almost every repeat visit. Reduced vision, discomfort, red eye, infections, and allergic responses are the problems that occur most frequently.

ROLE OF THE OPHTHALMIC ASSISTANT

A high percentage of the tasks in an efficient contact lens practice may be delegated to the ophthalmic assistant. Supplies and inventory of lenses add a dimension of expense to a practice that must be supervised and continually looked after. Unlike rigid lenses, soft lenses will spoil and deteriorate once the vial has been opened unless cleaning and sterilizing routines are applied to trial sets and unopened vials. The ophthalmic assistant in a clinical contact lens practice often will be primarily responsible for maintaining inventory and helping in cost efficiency.

The following list indicates some of the duties of the ophthalmic assistant in a busy contact lens practice:

1. Maintain inventory and cost efficiency
2. Handle insurance programs
3. Provide instruction on lens care and handling

4. Schedule appointments
5. Make follow-up calls for dropouts, particularly those prescribed extended-wear lenses
6. Handle telephone
7. Understand adaptive and abnormal symptoms
8. Perform office cleaning of lenses
9. Perform collections
10. Order replacement lenses

The assistant must become familiar with telephone communication with patients and in particular must be able to distinguish purely adaptive symptoms for both rigid and soft lenses from the abnormal symptoms. Abnormal symptoms such as persistent red eyes, blurring of vision, excessive glare, and unusual discomfort require an emergency appointment with the ophthalmologist. When in doubt, assistants should exercise caution, turn the call over to someone more experienced, or schedule the patient for an examination. They should not assume responsibility for diagnosis on the telephone.

QUESTIONS FOR REVIEW AND THOUGHT

1. Why is a soft lens so comfortable?
2. Describe a method of teaching a patient insertion and removal of a soft lens.
3. What are the advantages of soft hydrogel lenses compared with rigid lenses?
4. Review the fitting method of one type of soft lens.
5. How are soft lenses sterilized?
6. How are soft lenses cleaned?
7. How can you inspect and evaluate a soft lens returned by the patient?
8. Name some medical uses for the soft contact lens.
9. If the diameter of a lens is increased, is the lens made flatter or steeper?
10. How can you determine whether a soft lens is inside out?
11. Can fluorescein be used with a soft lens? Explain.
12. Which candidates are not suitable for soft lenses?
13. If the water content of a soft lens is increased, is its durability increased or decreased?

SELF-EVALUATION QUESTIONS

True-false statements

Directions: Indicate whether the statement is true (T) or false (F).

T or F   1. Soft lenses are better than rigid lenses in reducing glare and photophobia.
T or F   2. Measurement of a soft lens is labeled in the fully hydrated state.
T or F   3. Thin soft lenses are better for occasional wear such as sporting activities.

Missing words

Directions: Write in the missing word in the following sentences.

4. Circumlimbal compression and injection are characteristic of a soft lens that has been fitted too _____ .

5. Ultrathin lenses have _____ oxygen transmission as compared with lenses of standard thickness.

6. Soft lenses worn in a dry environment should not be thin but be of _____ thickness to reduce dehydration.

Choice-completion questions

Directions: Select the one best answer in each case.

7. Soft lenses can be of great therapeutic value as a bandage lens. Which of the following conditions would possibly indicate the need for a bandage soft lens?
   a. Bullous keratopathy
   b. Recurrent corneal erosion
   c. Keratitis sicca
   d. All of the above
   e. None of the above

8. Which of the following are true for present-day extended wear lenses for myopia?
   a. Difficult to handle lenses
   b. Loss factor common
   c. Deposit formation common
   d. Infection common
   e. Neovascularization

9. To maintain corneal integrity and proper cornea-lens relationship, the fit should exhibit:
   a. Central touch
   b. No movement
   c. Apical vaulting
   d. Three-point touch
   e. Slight edge lifting

ANSWERS, NOTES, AND EXPLANATIONS

1. **True.** Soft lenses reduce foreign body sensation and thus reduce the incidence of lens-induced photophobia. Also, the large optic zone eliminates the flare that can be experienced when light passes through the peripheral curves of a rigid lens or when the pupil dilates.

2. **True.** All soft lenses contain some percentage of water content. The expressed parameters are measurements when the lens is fully hydrated. A lens will tend to shrink and steepen as it dehydrates. In the manufacturing process of a soft lens, the measurements usually are made initially for the manufacture of the soft lens while it is still in the hard state. An allowance factor for the constant swelling of the material in the hydrated state is taken into consideration to arrive at the final dimensions of the required hydrated lens. The soft lenses are then measured in the fully hydrated state.

3. **True.** Thin and ultrathin lenses show better oxygen transmission and may be fitted larger and tighter and thus track with rapid movements of the eye. This reduces loss and prevents particles from getting under the lenses. This can be a most useful feature in the stability of vision required for most sports.

4. **Tightly or steeply.** A lens that is too tight will show minimal or no movement and cause inadequate tear exchange under the lens, along with compression of the vessels at the limbus.

5. **Higher.** Oxygen permeability is a function of the material, whereas oxygen transmission takes into account the thickness of the material as well. When any material thickness is reduced by 50%, the transmission of oxygen is doubled. Thus the thinner the lenses, the better oxygen transmission through to the cornea.

6. **Standard.** In a dry environment the standard-thickness lenses perform better because they carry more water and permit greater evaporation before they become depleted of their water reservoir.

7. **d. All of the above.** These are but a few of a long list of indicators for the soft lens as a medical device in the therapeutic armamentarium against corneal disease processes.

8. **c. Deposit formation common.** Build-up of minerals, protein, and lipids is still the single main feature of contact lenses that are not cleaned on a daily basis. Although weekly or semimonthly cleaning routines are recommended for most patients with extended-wear lenses, those who fail to follow this regimen often will allow deposits to build up and cause spoilage of their soft lenses.

9. **d. Three-point touch.** The proper cornea-lens relationship for a soft lens involves slight central touch with touch of the lens at the periphery. For the smaller-diameter soft lenses, this peripheral touch may be at the limbus, whereas for the larger lenses this may be on the sclera. With each blink there is some movement of the lens and a small amount of tear exchange under the lens.

CHAPTER 15

Advanced techniques in soft and rigid contact lens fitting

- Abnormal symptoms and signs
- Follow-up keratometry
- Special lenses
- Manufacturing and modification
- Gas-permeable lenses
- Tinted contact lenses
- Recommendations for selection of rigid or soft contact lenses

Many ophthalmic assistants play an expanded role in contact lens delivery and thus require detailed knowledge of contact lenses. Although the changing and ordering of lenses may be beyond the scope of the ophthalmic assistant, an understanding of how to order and modify lenses and a review of abnormal symptoms and signs are not. This chapter only highlights some of the problems encountered; further information may be obtained from our textbook, *Fitting Guide for Rigid and Soft Contact Lenses: A Practical Approach* (ed 3, St. Louis, 1990, Mosby).

ABNORMAL SYMPTOMS AND SIGNS

It is important to recognize purely adaptive symptoms and differentiate them from pathologic symptoms that could result in corneal damage. The ophthalmic assistant may be the first to hear of these symptoms and should alert the ophthalmologist to patients' complaints that might lead to serious corneal damage.

Flare or streaming of lights or glare from oncoming headlights is a symptom that may occur when the lens or the optical portion of the lens (optic zone) is too small. This symptom occurs because the pupil of the eye dilates at night or in a darkened room,

and the patient begins to have interference in his vision from the edge of the optic zone or the edge of the lens. It can be corrected by making the lens larger or increasing the size of the optic zone.

Blurring of vision in daytime through the normal pupil may be a result of the lens riding too high or gravitating too low after each blink. This can be observed directly by watching the patient view a vision chart or distant object. The patient may respond by producing streaming opposite to the displacement of the lens (Fig. 15-1). Lenses that ride high may be because of a high minus power and edge thickness that cause the lens to be lifted up by the upper lid. A small lens under a tight lid will also ride high. A lens that rides low may be too heavy because of thickness or because of high plus power, or there may be insufficient edge thickness that will not permit the upper lid to grasp the lens and lift it. Redesigning the edge to provide proper compensation will permit the lens to center better. If this fails, smaller lenses may be required. Occasionally the lens will slide nasally or temporally because of an abnormally-centered cornea. These lenses should be replaced with lenses of larger diameter or a larger optic zone.

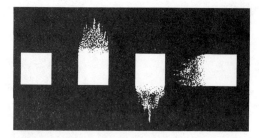

Fig. 15-1 Flare: The zone of streaming is always opposite to the displacement of the lens. Such a lens requires re-centering. Uniform flare indicates that the optic zone of the lens is too small. (From Stein HA, Slatt BJ, Stein RM: *Fitting guide for rigid and soft contact lenses, a practical approach,* ed 3, St Louis, 1990, Mosby.)

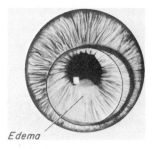

Edema

Fig. 15-2 Corneal edema created by a contact lens. (From Rosenthal, P: *Int. Ophthalmol. Clin.* **8**:611, 1968, Little, Brown and Co.)

Central corneal edema (Fig. 15-2) with consequent blurring of vision occurs when there is insufficient oxygenation of the cornea brought about by poor tear exchange. The edematous area appears hazy on the slit lamp microscope, particularly if the light is shone off to the side of the area to be viewed so the area is illuminated from behind rather than directly. When the epithelial edema advances, some cells may die, causing central stippling, which will stain with fluorescein dye. The stippling may represent only a few small, discreet spots at the beginning, but the spots may increase in number as the condition progresses. If the condition progresses, *punctate staining* is said to occur. Patients who develop these objective signs will often complain of spectacle blur for some time after the lenses are removed. To correct this situation, the tear exchange

must be improved. This can be done in the original lens by (1) blending the junctions of the curve better, (2) flattening the peripheral curve, (3) reducing the total diameter, (4) reducing the diameter of the optic zone by increasing the width of the peripheral curve, or (5) fenestrating the lens.

Corneal abrasion (Fig. 15-3) may follow corneal edema caused by lack of oxygen but may also result from too flat a lens rubbing on a portion of the cornea. Evaluation of the fit of the lens to indicate that the abraded area lies just under the touch area of the contact lens will determine that the lens is rubbing the cornea and is too flat, too loose, or both. The excessive movement adds to the friction of the cornea and can be corrected with a new lens by (1) increasing the lens diameter, (2) increasing the optic zone diameter, (3) reducing the edge thickness, (4) steepening the optic zone, (5) steepening the peripheral curve, and (6) increasing the base curve.

Three o'clock and nine o'clock staining (see Fig. 15-3) of the cornea with fluorescein refers to erosions at the 3 and 9 o'clock positions in the exposed portion of the palpebral fissure. It is usually believed to be a result of dryness because of inadequate blinking while wearing the contact lens, so that the small exposed portion of the cornea on each side of the lens becomes dry. This symptom is not usually seen with the smaller and thinner lenses. Various methods, such as a smaller, thinner lens, blinking exercises, or artificial tears, may help eliminate this problem.

Insertion abrasions may result from improper or clumsy insertion. Abrasion causes either immediate pain or pain after removal of the lens. Further practice in insertion under observation of the instructor should be undertaken.

Foreign bodies trapped under the lens will show varying types of zigzag scratch marks on the cornea, which will stain with fluorescein. Common substances such as mascara and cosmetics may be the offending agents and should be used with caution.

Arc staining may occur either from poor insertion technique or most commonly from a sharp junction line between the central posterior curve and the intermediate or peripheral posterior curve. A proper blend is required.

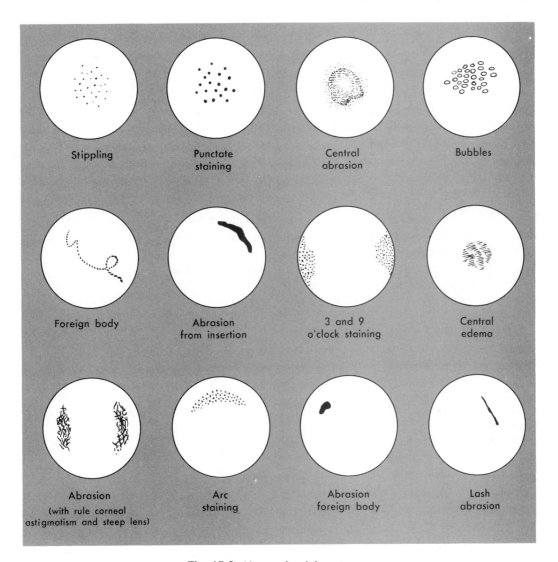

Fig. 15-3 Abnormal staining patterns.

Bubbles with staining occur when the lens is steep and there is too much sagittal depth to the lens so that air is trapped under the central curve. A flatter lens is required.

Blurring after reading may occur in the myope nearing the age of 40. The introduction of contact lenses requires a further accommodative effort and convergence that the patient cannot compensate for. Reading glasses may be required.

If the blur in the nonpresbyope occurs soon after insertion, it may be due to the lower lid pushing the lens upward, thus causing poor centering of the lens in the reading position. This may be corrected by making the lens smaller.

If blurring occurs after prolonged reading, it may be because of inadequate tear exchange and corneal anoxia. Concentrated reading reduces the blink reflex, induces staring, and consequently permits less tear exchange. A smaller lens, a flatter peripheral curve, or a material with a higher DK may alleviate this problem. Blinking exercises with prolonged reading is also helpful.

Corneal warpage or induced astigmatism, both regular and irregular, can occur, resulting either from poorly fitting lenses that alter the corneal curvature or from chronic hypoxia of the cornea by over-wearing the contact lenses. A complete reassessment of the fit is called for, and even a change to a gas-permeable material may be necessary.

FOLLOW-UP KERATOMETRY

By performing keratometry on repeat visits, one can detect any molding or distortion of the cornea or induced astigmatism. One should record the difference in the K readings at subsequent visits. Such a notation as K + 1.25 + 0.50 indicates that the cornea has steepened by this amount in each meridian. Any changes over 1.00 diopter indicate that the wearing time should be reduced or the lens adjusted. Distortion of the mires also indicates a change is needed.

SPECIAL LENSES

The methods of contact lens fitting for correction of the commonest defects of the eye have been described in Chapter 13. The techniques and devices available have proved highly successful for the majority of cases. However, as with other natural systems, variations in the anatomy and physiology of the eye are quite broad. Thus for those defects associated with more extreme variations, corrective devices and methods must be custom built to a highly sophisticated level. For example, patients with extremely high myopia (− 6.00 diopters or greater) or aphakic patients (+ 8.00 diopters or greater) require modifications of the normal lens design because of the extra thick (myopic) or extra thin (hyperopic) peripheral edge of the corneal contact lens. Similarly, extreme cases of keratoconus require bicurvature lenses for effective apposition to the eye, whereas highly astigmatic cases require an asymmetric (nonspherical), nonrotating lens design. Many eye patients older than 40 years require bifocal lenses, and special lens systems with bifocal lens characteristics can be prepared for their accommo-

dation. Certain pathologic cases requiring telescopic lenses also present a need for specially designed lenses.

Contact lenses for high myopia

Myopia is the most common reason that a patient seeks contact lenses. Contact lenses for high myopia have not only the added feature of cosmetic enhancement by discarding glasses, but also that of increased optical benefit because the contact lens rests on the eye and thus the retinal image is larger and more normal than it would be with spectacles. In addition, the high myope no longer has a visual field restricted by the edges of glasses and frames.

However, as the minus power of a contact lens increases, so does the edge thickness. This increase in edge thickness creates a base-up wedge effect, which causes the lens to be pulled up by the upper lid and consequently to ride high so that the patient fails to look through the center of the lens. To reduce the thickness of the edge, it must be shaved off to prevent the upper lid from tugging upward on the lens. This in effect results in a lenticular-designed lens for high minus powers. The higher the minus power, the more the anterior edge has to be reduced (Fig. 15-4).

Aphakic lenses

With the more common use of intraocular lenses, aphakic lenses have declined in use. Aphakic contact lenses are primarily used when an intraocular lens is not appropriate. It is obvious why intraocular lenses are preferred; they generally offer better vision and freedom from the daily handling of contact lenses. For an elderly person who may have a tremor of the hand, lax eyelids, or a tear deficiency, this freedom from the hazards of contact lens wear is important. Yet not all cataract extractions are treated with intraocular lenses. They may not be inserted if the following occurs:
1. Angle-closure glaucoma
2. Recurrent iridocyclitis
3. Any surgical contingency that makes the insertion of an intraocular lens hazardous

In addition, there are many aphakic patients wearing spectacles who were operated on when indications

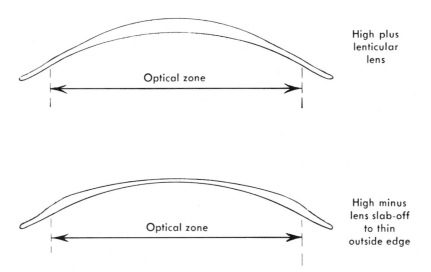

Fig. 15-4 Lenticular lenses. (From Soper JW, Girard LJ: Special designs and fitting techniques. In Girard LJ, editor: *Corneal contact lenses,* ed 2, St Louis, 1970, Mosby.)

for implants were not quite as liberal. Thus a knowledge of aphakic contact lenses should be acquired despite a definite downgrading of their importance in the management of a cataract patient.

Aphakic individuals require strong plus lenses. As the power of a plus lens increases, so does the central thickness of the contact lens. This increase in central thickness creates a base-down wedge effect at the upper edge of the lens, and thus the upper lid forces the lens downward. The high plus lens is also heavy, which causes it to gravitate downward. One way of reducing the thickness and thus the weight of a high plus lens is to keep the overall diameter of the lens very small. Unfortunately, this does not solve the problem if the patient has large pupils or keyhole iridectomies, in which case the patient may be looking through the lens edge. A more practical way of fitting a high plus lens with a reduction in the thickness and weight is to add a lenticular design on the lens (Fig. 15-5). It is important that the lenticular optic portion of the lens completely cover the pupil; otherwise the patient will complain of blurry vision and glare. Another solution is to put a myopic edge finish on any high plus lens, which will help the upper eyelid elevate the lens.

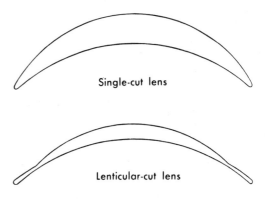

Fig. 15-5 Single-cut and lenticular-cut lenses.

Nonrotating lenses

Patients with a moderate or high degree of astigmatism will experience difficulties in wearing spherical contact lenses. Symptoms of blurred vision, excessive awareness of lens edge, and slipping of the lens off the cornea or even out of the eye will be encountered because of the rocking effect of the lens over the flatter meridian. Residual astigmatism, where the cornea is spherical but the patient has a cylindric spectacle prescription, is another indication for nonrotating lenses. In these cases the astigmatism comes from the lens of the eye and it is necesssary to add prism to the lens in order to add weight to one section of the lens and thus to stop lens rotation and to properly orient the cylinder over the correct optical axis. Several types of bifocals indicate another use for nonrotating lenses.

Several types of nonrotating lenses have been designed.

Noncircular shapes. A *truncated* lens is really a circular lens in which the bottom or top portion or both (double-truncated lens) have been cut off. The corners at the edge of the truncation are smoothed off. A double-truncated lens, while infrequently used, will tend to stabilize so that the flat portion lies adjacent to the upper and lower lid edges. If the edges are rounded off more, the lens assumes an oval shape; but this type of lens rotates frequently and thus negates the use it was intended for. Rectangular and triangular lenses have been designed, but they have shown little practical value.

Toric curve lens. A lens may be cut so that it is not spherical on its back surface. It is called a *toric back curve lens* when it has two meridians of curvature on its back surface. They are designed to conform somewhat to the two meridians of curvature of the front surface of the cornea. It is used to correct a high degree of astigmatism. When the lens is placed in the eye, it tends to align its curvature with that of the cornea. However, an optical problem of astigmatism may exist that may require the grinding of a toric surface on the front of the lens, the so-called *front surface toric lens*. These are used primarily to treat residual astigmatism in patients with spherical corneas. In some instances toric surfaces may be ground on both the front and back surfaces, the so-called *bitoric contact lens.*

Prism ballast lenses. When prism is ground into a contact lens, the heavier base of the prism will swing the lens around so that the heavier base will ride low, attracted by gravity, and thus further rotation of the lens will be eliminated (Fig. 15-6). One can incorporate up to 3.00 diopters of prism in a lens to provide sufficient weight. In addition to preventing rotation, a prism may be used to create weight in a lens that tends to ride high or may be

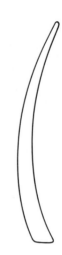

Fig. 15-6 Prism ballast to provide weight and stop rotation of a lens.

used to reduce excessive lens movements. The weight of prism ballast lenses and the thinner superior edge of the lens, which fits under the upper lid, provides stability and prevents rotation of the lens.

Contact lenses for astigmatism

Residual astigmatism occurs when a contact lens is placed on an eye and an astigmatic refractive error still results. Several conditions may contribute to this residual astigmatism, but it is most commonly induced by the crystalline lens of the eye (so-called lenticular astigmatism). If the amount is small, it will not significantly interfere with vision. If the amount of astigmatism is large, vision will be substandard unless one can compensate for this in the contact lens. Although this requires a complex type of lens, essentially a toric surface is ground on the front of the lens to prevent the lens from rotating, so that the toric surface is lined up with the axis of astigmatism. One must stop rotation of the lens by introducing a weight such as a prism ballast to the lens at the correct position.

Correction of high astigmatism

Astigmatism may result from corneal surfaces of different radii or from changes in the lens of the eye.

The latter is less common but nevertheless does occur and accounts for residual astigmatism when corneal astigmatism has been fully corrected.

Keratometer readings provide a good index of the amount of corneal astigmatism that is present. Most spherical-based lenses will be the first choice for fitting eyes with corneal astigmatism. Tear fluid readily fills in the interface and provides a good optical result in most cases. However, in some cases these lenses will not provide adequate tear interchange, rocking occurs, or poor staining is found. A back surface toric lens will be required that will conform to the corneal toricity. Diagnostic trial lenses may be a valuable adjunct. Frequently, changing the back surface to a toric surface causes residual astigmatism; this must be corrected by grinding a toric surface on the front of the lens. This constitutes the so-called bitoric lens.

Toric soft contact lenses. There are a wide variety of toric soft contact lenses on the market, and fitters must familiarize themselves with what is available on a lens-by-lens basis. Specific lenses are not discussed here since there are excellent fitting guides available from the manufacturers. Before choosing a specific lens, the fitter must make sure that the lens is available in parameters that match the patient's refractive error.

Some "off-the-shelf" toric lenses are available in a limited range of cylinders and axes. Manufacturers make and stock lenses in the most commonly requested power ranges, and these are available immediately. "Off-the-shelf" lenses are available in powers from -6.00 to $+4.00$ diopters (D), with cylinder powers of -0.75, -1.00, -1.75, and -2.00 D. (-3.00 D of cylinder is available in a more limited axis range, generally 20 degrees on either side of the 90 or 180 degree meridians.) Limited fitting sets are available. A diagnostic lens of the selected toric design must be evaluated on the patient's eye for fit and position of axis.

For "custom" work a fitting set must also be used. The fitting lenses are spherical designs with the diameters and orientation systems of the toric lenses that the patient will eventually wear. Toric lenses that can be fit in this manner are available in powers from -20.00 to $+20.00$ D, with axes of rotation available in 5 degree increments. A few manufacturers provide toric lenses made to order with even greater power and cylinder and with axes of rotation in 1 degree increments.

Several design alternatives are used to maintain the orientation of toric lenses. *Double slab off,* the creation of thin zones on the inferior and superior parts of the lens, allows lids to hold the lens in position (Fig. 15-7). As with bifocal soft contact lenses, prism ballasting (Fig. 15-8), peri-ballasting, and truncation are also used to maintain orientation.

Toric lenses have *orientation* (or scrib) *marks* near the edge, some at the 3 o'clock and 9 o'clock positions, others at the 6 o'clock position. The manufacturer can sometimes be verified by the marks or by the laser identification marks on the lens.

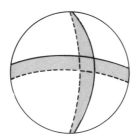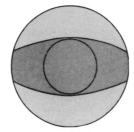

Fig. 15-7 Double slab-off soft lens used to correct astigmatism. The lens is made thinner superiorly and inferiorly so that thinner portions tend to rotate and come to rest under the upper and lower eyelids. (From Stein HA, Slatt BJ, Stein RM: *Fitting guide for rigid and soft contact lenses, a practical approach,* ed 3, St Louis, 1990, Mosby.)

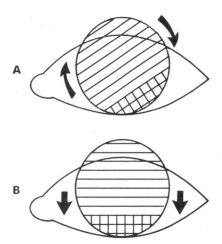

Fig. 15-8 A, Lens on immediate insertion. **B,** The weighted lens combined with the torsional effect of the eyelid muscles, rotates the lens to a stable position. (From Stein HA, Slatt BJ, Stein RM: *Fitting guide for rigid and soft contact lenses, a practical approach,* ed 3, St Louis, 1990, Mosby.)

Contact lenses for keratoconus

Keratoconus is a forward bulging of the central cornea with irregular astigmatism (Fig. 15-9). It usually begins in adolescence and progresses over the next several years. It is often bilateral, although one eye advances more than the other. Its cause is still unknown, but there is a strong hereditary feature.

This irregular astigmatism cannot be corrected by normal spectacles, but vision can be satisfactorily corrected in the majority of cases by contact lenses. In addition to vision correction, contact lenses tend to flatten and stabilize the cornea, although it does not change the progress of the disease. The apex of the cornea is very sensitive in early stages, giving rise to photophobia and lens-fitting problems; but in later stages the cornea becomes relatively insensitive.

The thinness of the cornea, ruptures in Descemet's membrane, and small apical tears may be detected in advanced cases by slit-lamp biomicroscopy, the hand keratoscope, or Placido's disk (Fig. 15-10). Keratoconus is often associated with patients who have hay fever, atopic dermatitis, eczema, or asthma.

A slit-lamp diagnosis is difficult to make in the early phase, whereas in the late stages the diagnosis becomes obvious with apical thinning. Fleisher's keratoconus ring, increased endothelial reflex, increased visibility of the nerve fibers, and scarring of Bowman's membrane. Keratometry is very helpful in the early phase of this disease, since the mire images appear distorted and irregular. The two principal meridians are not at right angles to each other, and the dioptric value of the readings is quite high—48.00 diopters or higher. The range of the keratometer may have to be extended to accurately record the full corneal curvature. The addition of a +1.25-diopter lens over the front of the keratometer either by hand or the INNS retention ring is most useful (conversion by means of a table is required for true K readings; see Table 15-1) (Fig. 15-11).

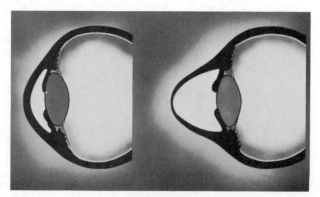

Fig. 15-9 A, Normal eye. **B,** Keratoconus. Note thinning of the cornea as well as the forward protrusion.

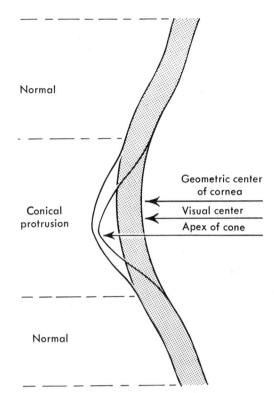

Normal

Conical
protrusion

Normal

Geometric center
of cornea

Visual center

Apex of cone

Fig. 15-10 Keratoconus. Note the forward protrusion and thinning of the cornea. (From Soper JW, Girard LJ: Special designs and fitting techniques. In Girard LJ, editor: *Corneal contact lenses,* ed 2, St Louis, 1970, Mosby.)

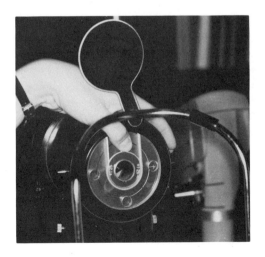

Fig. 15-11 INNS extension disk to extend range of the keratometer.

Table 15-1 Dioptric curves for extended range of keratometer

High power (with +1.25 lens over aperture)				Low power (with −1.00 lens over aperture)			
Drum reading	True dioptric curvature	Drum reading	True dioptric curvature	Drum reading	True dioptric curvature	Drum reading	True dioptric curvature
52.00	61.00	46.87	55.87	42.00	36.00	36.87	30.87
51.87	60.87	46.75	55.75	41.87	35.87	36.75	30.75
51.75	60.75	46.62	55.62	41.75	35.75	36.62	30.62
51.62	60.62	46.50	55.50	41.62	35.62	36.50	30.50
51.50	60.50	46.37	55.37	41.50	35.50	36.37	30.37
51.37	60.37	46.25	55.25	41.37	35.37	36.25	30.25
51.25	60.25	46.12	55.12	41.25	35.25	36.12	30.12
51.12	60.12	46.00	55.00	41.12	35.12	36.00	30.00
51.00	60.00			41.00	35.00		
		45.87	54.87				
50.87	59.87	45.75	54.75	40.87	34.87		
50.75	59.75	45.62	54.62	40.75	34.75		
50.62	59.62	45.50	54.50	40.62	34.62		
50.50	59.50	45.37	54.37	40.50	34.50		
50.37	59.37	45.25	54.25	40.37	34.37		
50.25	59.25	45.12	54.12	40.25	34.25		
50.12	59.12	45.00	54.00	40.12	34.12		
50.00	59.00			40.00	34.00		
		44.87	53.87				
49.87	58.87	44.75	53.75	39.87	33.87		
49.75	58.75	44.62	53.62	39.75	33.75		
49.62	58.62	44.50	53.50	39.62	33.62		
49.50	58.50	44.37	53.37	39.50	33.50		
49.37	58.37	44.25	53.25	39.37	33.37		
49.25	58.25	44.12	53.12	39.25	33.25		
49.12	58.12	44.00	53.00	39.12	33.12		
49.00	58.00			39.00	33.00		
		43.87	52.87				
48.75	57.75	43.75	52.75	38.87	32.87		
48.62	57.62	43.62	52.62	38.75	32.75		
48.50	57.50	43.50	52.50	38.62	32.62		
48.37	57.37	43.37	52.37	38.50	32.50		
48.25	57.25	43.25	52.25	38.37	32.37		
48.12	57.12	43.12	52.12	38.25	32.25		
48.00	57.00	43.00	52.00	38.12	32.12		
				38.00	32.00		
47.87	56.87						
47.75	56.75			37.87	31.87		
47.62	56.62			37.75	31.75		
47.50	56.50			37.62	31.62		
47.37	58.37			37.50	31.50		
47.25	56.25			37.37	31.37		
47.12	56.12			37.25	31.25		
47.00	56.00			37.12	31.12		
				37.00	31.00		

Courtesy Bausch & Lomb.

Perhaps the best instrument for diagnosis of keratoconus in the early stages is the retinoscope, which reflects irregular light reflexes from the surface of the cornea with scissorlike movements. Dr. Joseph Baldone has described and popularized remote ophthalmoscopy as another valuable diagnostic tool. In this method an ophthalmoscope qualitates the red reflex.

Corneal topographical analysis with the new computer-assisted keratovideoscopes offers a maplike correction of several thousand points of K readings on the cornea. This advancement has given us much more information than simple keratometry or corneoscopy. A more detailed explanation of topographical analysis of the cornea will be presented later in the text. One of the main values of corneal topographical analysis by computer-assisted keratoscopy is the detection of early keratoconus.

The purpose of the contact lens is to cover the irregular astigmatism and the disordered anterior surface optics of an ectatic cornea by providing a regular, spherical, optic surface before the eye. The lens does not retard the progression of the disease, which by itself may have long periods of natural remission. Both scleral and rigid lenses have been used in the treatment of keratoconus.

Scleral lenses

Scleral lenses have been employed in the past but have given way to rigid and soft lenses, which are simpler for both fitter and patient to handle.

Rigid lenses

It is controversial whether corrective rigid lenses should touch the apical cone lightly and rest on the peripheral cornea where there is little or no thinning, or whether they should just clear the apex of the cone. Lenses fitted excessively flat eventually cause corneal abrasions. Minimal apical clearance of the cone has been advocated, but this point of view does not represent the majority. Gas-permeable materials are the materials of choice for better maintenance of the corneal integrity.

The majority of early to moderate cones exhibit a manifestation of the irregularity at or below the midline of the cornea. Because keratometric readings can be misleading, it is important to remember that the superior portion of the cornea may be relatively normal or much flatter than the K readings suggest. These early to moderate and some more advanced oval cones can be effectively fit using spherical and aspherical designs that will align with the superior cornea. Diagnostic fitting and fluorescein evaluation are most valuable. The fitter should not be alarmed at the slight to moderate inferior edge lift of the lens if it aligns well superiorly. The upper lid especially aids in holding the lens in position. It is not uncommon to fit an oval cone with irregular K readings in the 50.00 diopter range with a lens such as the Boston, Envision, or Quantum with a base curve of 7.5 to 7.3 (45 to 46.25 diopters).

For more classic nipple-type cones, the Soper keratoconus lens can be of value. In our experience the Soper keratoconus trial lenses (Fig. 15-12), combined with fluorescein assessment of their fit, have been valuable in aiding the fit of lenses. These trial lenses have a steep central base curve to permit the bulging of the cone, and a much flatter peripheral

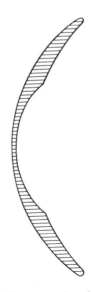

Fig. 15-12 Soper cone lens for keratoconus.

Table 15-2 Soper cone diagnostic lens set

Sagittal depth (mm)	CPC	Power	Lens diameter (mm)	Thickness (mm)	Diameter of OPC (mm)
0.68	48/45	−4.50	7.5	0.10	6.0
0.73	52/45	−8.50	7.5	0.10	6.0
0.80	56/45	−12.50	7.5	0.10	6.0
0.87	60/45	−16.50	7.5	0.10	6.0
1.00	52/45	−8.50	8.5	0.10	7.0
1.12	56/45	−12.50	8.5	0.10	7.0
1.22	60/45	−16.50	8.5	0.10	7.0
1.37	52/45	−8.50	9.5	0.10	8.0
1.52	56/45	−12.50	9.5	0.10	8.0
1.67	60/45	−16.50	9.5	0.10	8.0
(Optional)	52/43	−8.50	8.5	0.10	7.0
	64/45	−20.00	8.5	0.10	7.0

curve. Ten lenses make up the trial set, extending from a central curve of 48.00 to 60.00 diopters, with increasing sagittal depth to accommodate an increasingly projecting cone (Table 15-2). There is a range of dioptric powers in the set to approximate normalcy for the average keratoconus patient. From the trial set, a lens is selected that has either a slight central touch or slight vaulting at the apex.

Trial lens fitting

In the early phase of keratoconus, K readings are a guide to selecting a lens. As the condition develops, the mire image becomes irregular and the cone becomes steeper than 50.00 diopters so that the radius of curvature cannot be determined by ordinary keratometry. The only alternative is to fit the patient by trial and error.

The range of the keratometer can be extended to 61.00 diopters with an auxiliary +1.25-diopter lens. However, because of the disordered mires, problems in fixation, and optic defects in the system, the results merely serve as a guide to trial lens selection. Fixation can be improved by employing the viewing light of the Topogometer.

A good fit should have a central touch of 2 to 3 mm centrally with a thin band of touch at the lens periphery, as determined by the fluorescein test. The three-point touch adds to the stability of the lens on the cornea and distributes the weight of the lens not only over the apex but over other bearing areas as well. The peripheral touch area corresponds to the zone of the intermediate curve. The initial lens selected, using the K readings as a guide, should have a base curve flatter than K. Then employing the fluorescein test, the lens is exchanged until one is found that results in slight apical touch of 2 to 3 mm or from 1 to 4 mm flatter than K. A light, apical touch is desirable so that the lens can function as a pressure bandage on the thin, central, corneal apex (Fig. 15-13). Overrefraction is then performed to arrive at the correct power.

Piggyback lenses

Piggyback lenses were introduced by Dr. Joseph Baldone for patients with irregular corneal astigmatism or keratoconus who could not tolerate a rigid lens. These lenses consist of a soft lens carrier for comfort, with a rigid lens riding in the soft lens to add usual definition. The soft lenses have been modified to provide a donut groove. The diameter and wall height of the groove can be varied according to the

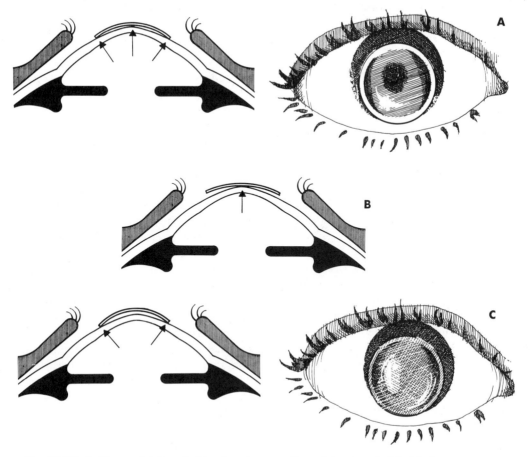

Fig. 15-13 A, Three-point fit—apical touch to the cone plus peripheral touch. Ideal for keratoconus because of the distribution of weight of the lens. **B,** Flat fit—apical touch but poor centration because of rocking on the corneal cap and edge stand-off. **C,** Steep fit—two-point touch with an air bubble between the lens and the cone. The apical cone is cleared. (From Stein HA, Slatt BJ, Stein RM: *Fitting guide for rigid and soft contact lenses, a practical approach,* ed 3, St Louis, 1990, Mosby.)

needs of the patient. The rules for fitting are simple.

1. Always evaluate the piggyback lens with the rigid lens in place.
2. Use the same disinfectant and storage solutions for both lenses.
3. The groove diameter when available should be 0.2 mm larger than the diameter of the rigid lens being used.

Softperm lens is a successor to the Saturn II lens. It has a base curve of 7.1 to 8.1 mm. The lens is 14.3 mm in diameter and ranges from +6 to −13. This is used in contact lens management of keratoconus. The Softperm lens consists of a hard styrene lens core or central button supported by a soft hydrogel lens skirt. The rigid lens button provides a clear, regular optical surface to yield good vision while the soft lens flange gives the patient stability and comfort. With a keratoconus patient, in whom the shape and position of the cone button is unpredictable, stability of the fit of the lens is vital.

METHODS OF FITTING A PRESBYOPIC PATIENT

1. Reading glasses over contact lenses
2. Monovision
3. Bifocal contact lenses
   a. Segmented bifocal
   b. Annular bifocal
   c. Aspheric bifocal
   d. Central add bifocal

Bifocal contact lenses

Before fitting a patient with bifocal lenses, the practitioner would be wise to explore alternate solutions to the problem of presbyopia (see the box above). In early presbyopia the patient, particularly the hyperope, may be sufficiently able to accommodate with single-vision contact lenses.

However, some practitioners will put more plus in one or both lenses so that although distance vision is slightly blurred, the patient is still able to read at near. In addition to these methods, many patients are content to wear auxillary spectacles for reading over their contact lenses. This is by far the simplest solution to the problem if the patient is not concerned with the cosmetic disadvantage of glasses.

Bifocal contact lenses are designed in two different ways: (1) those that provide alternating vision so the lens moves and permits the individual to see at times through the distance and at other times through the reading portion and (2) those that provide simultaneous vision so the individual selects either distant or near vision. In principle, when a patient looks down to read, the lower lid edge pushes up the near vision area of the contact so that it overlies the pupil (Figs. 15-14 and 15-15).

Bifocal lenses have been designed in a large variety of ways. Most popular are those lenses in which the central optic zone of the lens contains the distance prescription and an outer peripheral ring contains the near prescription. This is called an *annular bifocal*. The lenses are fit loosely so the lower lid pushes the lens up to the reading portion when the eye looks down (Fig. 15-16).

An alternate method is to construct the lens with the reading prescription in the center and the distance prescription in the outer ring. This is the central add type of bifocal made by University Optics (Fig. 15-17).

Other bifocals have been designed similar to the standard spectacle bifocal, with a stonger dioptric power segment below. These lenses must have a

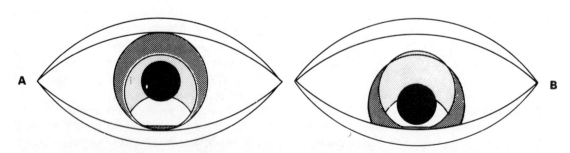

Fig. 15-14 Action of a contact bifocal lens. **A,** Vision through the distant portion. **B,** The bifocal segment is pushed up for reading. (From Stein HA, Slatt BJ, Stein RM: *Fitting guide for rigid and soft contact lenses, a practical approach,* ed 3, St Louis, 1990, Mosby.)

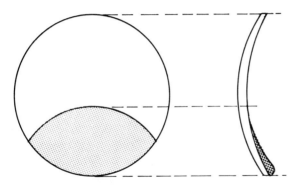

Fig. 15-15 Fused bifocal lens. (From Stein HA, Slatt BJ, Stein RM: *Fitting guide for rigid and soft contact lenses, a practical approach,* ed 3, St Louis, 1990, Mosby.)

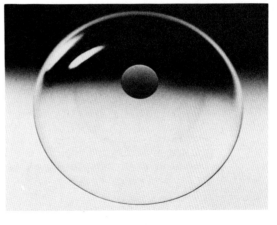

Fig. 15-17 Central add bifocal contact lens.

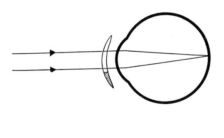

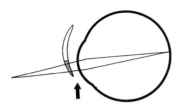

Fig. 15-16 Bifocal contact lens. When the eye looks down, the lower eyelid moves the lens up to reading position.

prism ballast or truncation to weight the lenses and prevent rotation. The segments on these bifocal contact lenses may be either fused or one piece (Fig. 15-18).

Of recent origin is a type of aspheric one-piece contact lens that provides a distance correction at the center, a reading correction off center, and an intermediate correction at midway points. This is available in both a soft lens and a rigid lens (VFL) design (Fig. 15-19).

The latest soft lenses of multifocal designs are the reverse type of aspheric lenses such as the PS 45 and Unilens. These designs combine the maximum prescription in the center of the lens with progressively more minus as you move away from the center. This helps to eliminate peripheral distortion at a distance, especially under low illumination.

All bifocal lenses are affected by ambient light. The most affected are those with either a central distance optical zone surrounded by a collarette of reading prescription or the opposite type in which the reading portion is central (Fig. 15-20). Success in fitting a presbyope depends on the following conditions:

1. Suitable patient screening
2. Understanding the strengths of each type of lens

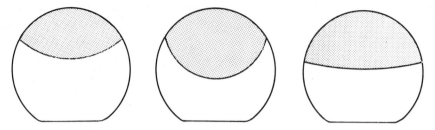

Fig. 15-18 Variations in design of one-piece bifocal lens. *1,* Standard lens design; *2,* concave lens design–this lens affords greater side-to-side viewing for a near object; *3,* flat lens design–this lens affords a wider sweep for distance vision. (From Stein HA, Slatt BJ, Stein RM: *Fitting guide for rigid and soft contact lenses, a practical approach,* ed 3, St Louis, 1990, Mosby.)

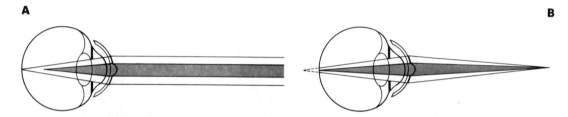

Fig. 15-19 A, Central add bifocal contact lens. Light from distant objects focuses on the retina. Light from near objects is ignored. **B,** Light from near objects focuses on the retina. Light from distant objects is ignored.

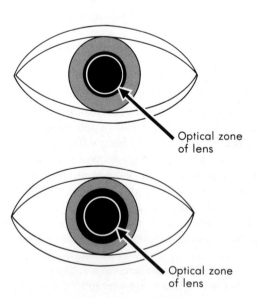

Fig. 15-20 Ambient lighting affects the size of the pupil. A large dilated pupil may result in ghosting.

3. Using the strengths of each lens to the best advantage for a particular patient
4. Good patient education and motivation
5. Enthusiasm of the fitter
6. An increased success with the experience of the fitter

With well-motivated patients and knowledgeable, experienced, and enthusiastic fitters, success can be as high as 60% to 70%. If any of the conditions are missing, the results can be devastatingly poor and disappointing.

Magnification with contact lenses

Patients with low visual acuity may benefit from contact lenses for two reasons. First, many visual defects may be a result of small corneal scars, which produce areas of irregular astigmatism. Rigid contact lenses overcome these surface irregularities of the cornea by providing a smooth tear film interface, which eliminates irregularities and can significantly improve vision. Second, visual improvement may be achieved by a telescopic system devised by a combination of a minus contact lens with high plus glasses, which produces a magnified retinal image. This is the same system found in standard opera glasses, which magnify four, five, six, and even seven times. The greater the magnification, however, the narrower the field of vision, as can be appreciated when one looks through strong field glasses.

Contact lens combination with spectacles, such as a − 30.00-diopter contact lens and a + 20.00-diopter spectacle lens, provides a magnification of 1.5 times when there is 17-mm separation between the contact lens and spectacles. Often this magnification is a great help to the patient with markedly reduced vision. It certainly is a more pleasant and cosmetically better method than wearing only thick telescopic lenses.

One problem in addition to the limited field of vision is that each time the patient turns his head there is a rapid movement of the visual field in the opposite direction. Also, all the disadvantages of magnification appear making objects appear closer than they really are.

NRK lenses

Nick Siviglia has developed a lens called NRK lens. This lens design is based on corneal topography and uses the new modeling systems. The NRK lens may be used as a retainer lens, or it may have the power to reduce refractive error. The lens, which is extremely comfortable, has good centering and optical alignment. The lens moves well and fits both the central and peripheral steepened portion. The lens can be put on any hydrophilic material. The peripheral curve is anaspheric design. The lenses are almost always over 10.5 mm, with an optical zone of at least 7.5 to 8 mm.

The NRK lens is designed to be fitted after radial keratotomy. This unique design in a refractive surgery lens retains the stability of the cornea and may incorporate power.

Bandage lenses

Bandage lenses are contact lenses used for therapeutic purposes to enhance epithelial regeneration and corneal healing. They should provide sufficient oxygenation to the cornea in order to minimally disturb corneal physiology. In addition, bandage lenses provide ocular comfort and act to protect the cornea from eyelids, eyelashes, and environmental conditions.

Therapeutic (bandage) lenses help to:
1. Promote healing
2. Provide splinting over lacerations, perforations, and wound leaks
3. Provide comfort
4. Protect the eye
5. Improve corneal architecture and vision
6. Act as a drug reservoir

Bandage lenses may be made of the following materials:
1. Thin or high-water HEMA lenses
2. Silicone
3. Collagen 12-, 24-, or 6-week lenses
4. CSI lenses

The thickness of the lens affects the oxygen permeability. The thinner the lens, the greater its oxygen permeability. Bausch & Lomb pioneered the Plano T series, which has a water content of 38%. Since then numerous other lenses have become available that provide greater oxygen permeability. Disposable lenses are often used because they allow extended wear with good oxygen permeability. Collagen lenses that biodisintegrate in 24 to 48 hours or in 6 weeks provide good oxygen permeability.

MANUFACTURING AND MODIFICATION

Contact lens practitioners fall into three categories: (1) those who make their own contact lenses from blanks, (2) those who order a finished lens or fit from an inventory system and then modify existing lenses depending on the fit and the requirements, and (3) those who order finished lenses and return them to the laboratory for modification. An understanding of what can and cannot be done to contact lenses is mandatory for a full understanding of contact lens technology. The ophthalmic assistant is well advised to spend some time in a contact lens laboratory, grinding and modifying at least a few lenses (Fig. 15-21).

Today the majority of rigid contact lenses are lathe

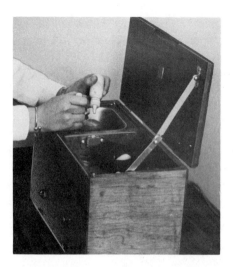

Fig. 15-21 Modification unit for rigid contact lenses.

cut, rather than molded, in the following manner:

1. Buttons are cut from a rod of plastic that looks like a curtain rod.
2. The inside curve is then cut and polished. In this stage the lens is referred to as a *semifinished blank*.
3. The front surface is then cut and polished. This is now referred to as an *uncut lens*.
4. Intermediate and peripheral curves are applied.
5. The edge is then finished. This is now a completed lens.

Modifications of finished lenses

Diameter reduction. The diameter of a rigid lens can be reduced by means of a razor blade, knife, file, emery, or sandpaper. The lens is mounted, concave side up, on a rotating spindle, and the blade of the razor or knife is rocked back and forth on the edge. Care must be taken not to allow the lens to overheat or to scratch the front of the lens. The file and emery are used mainly for small reductions in lens diameter. When a lens has been reduced, the intermediate peripheral curves and the edges must be applied and blended.

Blending (Fig. 15-22). Blending is done to smooth out the junction between the optic zone and the intermediate peripheral curve and between the intermediate and peripheral curves. When the transition zones are blended, a tool having a radius of curvature halfway between one curve and the next is used. The lens is held by a suction cup and rotated on the tool in the opposite direction of the tool rotation.

Edge shaping. If a lens has a secondary curve but no bevel, some edge shaping is usually necessary. The edge should be smoothly rounded by means of a file or razor blade. If the edge is relatively thick, it may be made thinner by means of a front surface bevel. Once the edge has been shaped, it is polished by means of a rag wheel, a felt disk, or a sponge.

Power change. Velveteen and a drum tool are used. The velveteen is first thoroughly soaked in

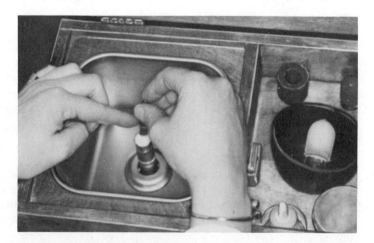

Fig. 15-22 Blending the junctional zones of a contact lens.

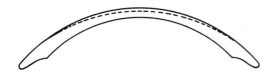

Fig. 15-23 Adding minus power. (From Stein HA, Slatt BJ, Stein RM: *Fitting guide for rigid and soft contact lenses, a practical approach,* ed 3, St Louis, 1990, Mosby.)

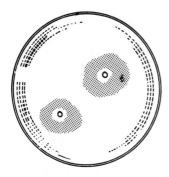

Fig. 15-24 Fenestrations reduce corneal edema in a 1 or 2 mm zone around the aperture. (From Stein HA, Slatt BJ, Stein RM: *Fitting guide for rigid and soft contact lenses, a practical approach,* ed 3, St Louis, 1990, Mosby.)

water and then pulled over the sides of a drum tool and fastened tightly with rubber bands. A depression is formed in the tool. The lens is held by means of a brass lens holder or suction cup. To add plus power, the lens is held in such a manner that its convex surface is held against the velveteen and is exactly centered on the tool. To add minus power, the lens is held in such a manner that the convex surface is held against the velveteen at the outer edge of the tool. In either case the lens is rotated once or twice a full 360 degrees against the rotation of the tool (Fig. 15-23).

Peripheral curve. A peripheral curve can be applied by the use of a tool having a radius of curvature of 12.25, 11.5, 10.5, or 9.5 mm. The lens is carefully mounted on the lens block so that it is not on an angle, or it is fixed by means of double-sided tape. The block is held perpendicular to the tool, concave side down, by a sharp-pointed pencil acting as a spindle. The polishing agent (such as Silvo) is then applied to the surface of the radius tool. The lens is held so that the concave surface rests lightly against the tool, revolving at about 1500 rpm; the entire edge of the lens must touch the tool at the same time. Equal pressure should be exerted on all meridians of the lens.

Fenestration of rigid lenses. Small holes drilled through a contact lens permit better tear exchange and consequently better oxygenation of the cornea. This is also a remedy for moderately tight contact lenses. Practitioners vary as to whether one or several holes should be employed or whether the lens should be completely redesigned. In any event, these holes should be no larger than 0.5 mm, and the interior walls must be highly polished to prevent clogging with secretions and irritation to the cornea. The fenestrations, while they do not interfere optically, do have a tendency to allow warpage of a lens and to weaken its structure. The fenestrations should lie over the area of corneal edema, since they provide only a small amount of increased respiration to a very limited underlying area of the cornea (Fig. 15-24).

Removing scratches. Care must be exercised in removing scratches from a rigid contact lens so as not to ruin the optics of the lens. In many cases a new lens is preferred to trying to remove scratches. When scratches are removed from the front surface of a lens, the lens is held with a suction cup or spindle against the velveteen-covered drum while the drum is rotated (Fig. 15-25). As in other modifications of contact lenses, Silvo is the polishing compound used.

Removing scratches from the inside (base curve) of a lens can be done by use of a convex-shaped tool and Silvo as the polishing compound. Although this procedure can remove scratches to some extent, it is not recommended, because it can damage the optics and fit of the lens.

GAS-PERMEABLE LENSES

The gas-permeable polymer is a huge step forward in lens technology. The contact industry has not witnessed such a contact upheaval since the soft hydrogel lens was introduced over two decades ago.

Gas-permeable lenses are made from materials

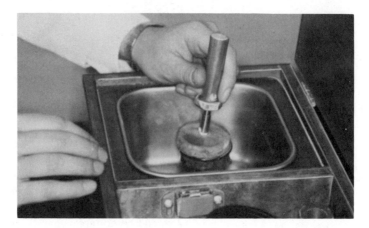

Fig. 15-25 Polishing the lens on velveteen with Silvo to remove scratches.

that have the ability to permit oxygen and carbon dioxide to diffuse through the plastic. These materials also wet more easily than the ordinary rigid lens and thus permit the tears to flow better under them.

Gas-permeable lenses have become well established in clinical practice. They have replaced the conventional PMMA lenses because they offer all the advantages of a rigid lens but add fewer complications. Gas-permeable lenses are also safer and more comfortable than rigid lenses.

The scope of gas-permeable materials is widening. The materials available to date include the following:
1. Cellulose acetate butyrate (CAB)
2. Silicone
3. Combinations of various materials, which include:
   a. Silicone-PMMA (silicone acrylates)
   b. PMMA-silicone-CAB
   c. Combinations of fluorocarbon-PMMA-silicone
4. Pure fluorocarbon material

The attractive feature of these lenses is their oxygen permeability. The permeability of these lenses is expressed as DK, where D is the diffusion coefficient for oxygen movement in lens material and K is the solubility of oxygen at room temperature.

$$\text{Oxygen transmissibility} = \frac{DK}{T}$$

where
D = the diffusion coefficient for oxygen movement in any substance,
K = the solubility constant for oxygen in that substance, and
T = the thickness of the center of the lens. (Sometimes the letter L is used for thickness, $\frac{DK}{L}$.)

The oxygen permeability varies from lens to lens and according to the method used for measuring this factor. The silicone combinations, mixed with PMMA, have a high rating. The lenses with the highest oxygen permeability are those made of pure fluorocarbon or those made of combinations of fluorocarbon and other proven contact lens materials.

The lens thickness of any given material must also be considered. The thicker the lens, the less its permeability. Thus a lens that is made 0.1 mm thick has much greater permeability than one that is made for aphakia and is 0.50 mm thick.

Rigid lenses have now been developed with a DK value of 50 and greater (the so-called super DK lenses). This means greater freedom from the complications of corneal hypoxia. This permits the application of such high DK lenses for extended wear.

Extended wear rigid lenses

With higher DK values, the oxygen permeability of these lenses is sufficient to maintain corneal physiologic needs so that overnight wear is possible.

These lenses can be worn for extended periods of up to 1 to 2 weeks. Ptosis, variable vision, and lack of tolerance have been reported with rigid gas-permeable lenses but not in alarming proportions.

Silicone-PMMA material

With the introduction of blends of material, the most popular has been the silicone-PMMA material often referred to as silicone acrylates. PMMA provides wetting, stability, and thinness; silicone provides oxygen permeability.

The better physiologic tolerance shown by these new plastics is not only a function of greater permeability but also of thermal conductivity. This is the ability of the plastic to allow heat to be dissipated through the lens so that the cornea has reduced oxygen demands. Clinically, the role of heat in lens comfort is seen with skiers. Most skiers find their rigid lenses work best on the hill when temperatures are low and the oxygen demands of the cornea are reduced. Hot, arid office buildings are the worst for lens tolerance because they increase corneal oxygen demand.

Silicone-PMMA lenses are fitted 0.1 to 0.3 mm flatter than the flattest corneal meridian. This allows the lens to ride high under the upper lid. The decrease or elimination of lid impact between the edge of the lid and the edge of the lens accounts for the excellent comfort that these lenses offer. These lenses have a diameter from 8.5 to 9.5 mm, with occasionally large 11-mm lenses prescribed.

It is important to note that the higher the silicone content, the higher the permeability of these combination lenses. However, a higher silicone content in the lenses also means a higher susceptibility to lipoid and waxy deposits forming on their surface and a greater fragility of the lenses.

In general the advantages of silicone-based combinations include (see box below):

1. Easier and faster adaptation.
2. Greater comfort.
3. Safety. Oxygen deprivation of the cornea is a prime cause of PMMA complications, which include spectacle blur, change in the shape of the cornea, and lack of full-day tolerance. The acute oxygen deprivation resulting from hypoxia (the so-called over-wearing syndrome) is extremely rare with gas-permeable lenses.
4. Greater application. Because of their large size they are centered more easily than PMMA lenses. They are used to advantage in keratoconus, irregular corneal astigmatism, aphakia, and large degrees of corneal astigmatism from 3.00 to 5.00 diopters.
5. Better vision. The larger lens diameter results in a larger optic zone diameter lens (8.4 to 9.5 mm). This reduces glare from lights at night despite the healthy movement of the lens with blinking.

Silicone-based combinations are a solution for

ADVANTAGES AND DISADVANTAGES OF SILICONE-ACRYLATE LENSES

ADVANTAGES

Greater oxygen transmission.

Surface tension 40% higher than PMMA.

Increased comfort and wearing time. Larger diameters mean a larger optic zone, which reduces annoying flare.

Reduced spectacle blur.

Design flexibility allows for a large or small diameter in spherical or aspherical profiles.

DISADVANTAGES

Softer than PMMA and scratches and chips easily.

Poor shape memory. The lens does not spring back when flexed or distorted. A change of shape of the lens is more likely to occur with fabrication or usage.

Deposit formation occurs.

chronic corneal edema in former rigid lens wearers. These lenses become a practical solution to refitting warped corneas from previously poorly-fitting rigid lenses. They increase the wearing time of rigid lens wearers who can wear conventional lenses for short periods. They eliminate spectacle blur in rigid lens wearers. They are excellent for corneas with marginal function, such as with recurrent viral keratitis.

The drawbacks to these lenses include the following:

1. There is greater fragility, which results in a tendency to chip or scratch. This is due largely to softness of the plastic.
2. The lenses require cleaning regularly, which adds to the maintenance.
3. There is a need for special lens solutions that are specific for these lenses in order to reduce the wetting angle and provide comfort.
4. Special compounds are required for modifying these lenses. For instance, these lenses must not be polished with compounds containing ammonia. Also these lenses cannot be exposed to alcohols, esters, ketones, and chlorinated hydrocarbons.
5. There is an increase in the frequency and severity of 3 and 9 o'clock staining. This is usually due to thick edges and resolves itself when the edge profile is reduced to 0.06 mm or the lens is made larger.
6. Larger diameter lenses seem to be more susceptible to protein deposits.

Cellulose acetate butyrate

Cellulose acetate butyrate (CAB) is not a new innovation. It was developed for photography by Eastman Kodak because it was less flammable than other materials. Although this plastic was discovered in 1938, it was not used for lenses until 1974.

The CAB lenses are fitted more steeply than conventional lenses, as the material tends to flatten because of softness or even molding by the surface of the cornea. This material is being challenged by newer materials that have greater stability.

ADVANTAGES AND DISADVANTAGES OF FLUORONATED SILICONE ACRYLATES

ADVANTAGES	DISADVANTAGES
High oxygen permability	More flexible than S/A
High deposit resistance	More brittle than S/A
In office adjustments possible	Glued on syndrome may occur (lens adhesion)
Low wetting angle	
Lighter in weight than S/A or PMMA	

Fluoronated silicone acrylates

The newest generation of rigid gas-permeable lenses are those that contain some form of fluorocarbon similar to the Teflon used in frying pans. The fluorocarbon component greatly increases the oxygen transmissibility of silicone-acrylate material. The lenses are lighter in weight and an ultraviolet blocker may be added. Even the earliest FSA type lenses have about double the DK/L of most silicone acrylates. Virtually all signs of clinical hypoxia are eliminated, thus increasing the extended-wear potential of rigid lenses. Deposit resistance is greater than any other soft or rigid lenses as a result of the Teflon or non-stick effect of the fluorocarbon (see box above). The FSA lens design has flexibility that permits larger or smaller diameters in both spherical and aspherical profiles.

Fitting fluorocarbon silicone-acrylate lenses usually requires a flatter base curve selection than when fitting S/A materials. This compensates for corneal cylinder correction better and reduces risk of "glueing on" or adhesion of the lens.

Pure fluorocarbon lenses

A pure fluorocarbon lens that contains no silicone or PMMA has been developed and manufactured by 3M. The material has an extremely high DK in the realm of 90. It is not brittle and is highly scratch resistant.

TINTED CONTACT LENSES

Tinted contact lenses have their role in many eye conditions. Their use over scarred corneas has been helpful in rehabilitating the individual and making the eye look cosmetically perfect. Tinted contact lenses have also had some use in patients with heterochromia. One lens is tinted to match up with the fellow eye. Tints may be used for cosmetic purposes or to make them easier to locate. Therapeutic applications of tinted lenses include scarred or opaque corneas, iris irregularities, iris coloboma, iridectomies, aniridia (absence or iris), fixed dilated pupil, photosensitivity resulting from albinism, and amblyopia.

We have treated two National League hockey players who had eye injuries with widely dilated pupils and photophobia, and required tinted lenses. In one case, a star forward with the Chicago Black Hawks had an eye injury with a dilated fixed pupil that finally responded to a diluted 1/64th% Pilocarpine. This caused an induced myopia of -6.00 D and he was unable to play hockey—a major disability. Because of the extreme glare reflecting from the ice, a very dark contact lens was provided and he is now able to play hockey.

Color enhancement lenses have been very popular. They make blue eyes bluer and green eyes greener. A retrospective study in patients we have fitted, showed that aqua was preferred by 60%, green by 20%, blue by 15%, and the other colors by 5%. Also, handling tints were often used in the lenses of many of our patients for ease of identification.

Another use for cosmetic lenses is to alter the color of the eye in which a brown-eyed patient can be made blue-eyed. Wesley Jessen, CooperVision, Ciba Vision and the Narcissus Medical Foundation have good lenses in this area. Pupil size is very important because ambient light can have a major influence on the "tunnel vision" effect created by these lenses.

Another use of these color-altering lenses, includes colobomas of the iris, where an opaque lens with a clear center can often give a very visually pleasing appearance.

The iris print method consists of placing an iris image on a dome of clear hema producing an opaque tint. A dot matrix is placed on the front surface of the contact lens to alter the iris color of the wearer. The Narcissus Medical Foundation, the Toya Lens Company, and CIBA Vision make a custom-designed tinted lens that is a combination of known and custom tinting. A sandwich process is involved that requires hand-painted or iris-printed images on hema plus lamination.

What affects a tint? Tints are often affected by noxious vapors and chemical agents, and they may also be affected by aging. Some cleaning agents will bleach some lenses. Leaching of the lens dye out of the lens may be a problem with continual wear. Some companies have minimized this effect by burying the material deep into the lens or directly into the buttons before cutting.

RECOMMENDATIONS FOR SELECTION OF RIGID OR SOFT CONTACT LENSES

In some patients the presence of astigmatism or other conditions makes it difficult to choose between rigid contact lenses and soft contact lenses. In others, this decision is made based on interaction with the patient. We currently recommend disposable soft contact lenses when the patient is suitable and powers are available. Throw-away soft lenses used on a daily or occasional-wear basis are also now available in limited powers. Below are some guidelines for recommendation for rigid and soft contact lens wearers.

PATIENTS RECOMMENDED FOR RIGID CONTACT LENS WEAR

1. Previous rigid contact lens wearers
2. Patients requiring sharp visual acuity
3. Patients with significant corneal cylinders over one diopter
4. Patients concerned with the cost of lens maintenance, replacement, and care
5. Patients requiring easy insertion and removal techniques

PATIENTS RECOMMENDED FOR SOFT CONTACT LENS WEAR

1. Failed hard contact lens wearers
2. Intermittent or part-time wearers for social functions
3. Patients with small corneal cylinders desiring more comfort
4. Patients working in high-particle environments
5. Patients participating in sports, particularly body contact sports
6. Patients requiring therapeutic use
7. Specialized areas such as colored soft lenses, iris-changing lenses and lenses for cosmesis

---

QUESTIONS FOR REVIEW AND THOUGHT

1. When a patient complains of blurring with his rigid contact lenses while in a movie theater, one physiologic mechanism occurs. How can this symptom be corrected?
2. What causes central corneal edema in a rigid contact lens wearer?
3. A patient has been wearing rigid lenses successfully for several years, but recently she has been unable to wear them longer than 4 hours. What might be some sources of trouble?
4. What causes 3 and 9 o'clock position staining? How can it be corrected?
5. What is the value of repeat keratometry of contact lens wearers?
6. What is the value of fenestration of rigid contact lenses?
7. Why are keratoconus cases a special fitting problem?
8. If the keratometer cannot read a steep corneal radius, as occurs in keratoconus, how can the range of the keratometer be extended?
9. What types of lenses are available to correct presbyopia?
10. Bifocal lenses present a particular problem in obtaining a small additional reading power in a small lens. How are lenses designed so that the lower eyelids push them up when one looks down to read?
11. What is the principle behind using contact lenses for magnification as an aid for patients with limited vision?
12. What are the advantages and disadvantages of rigid gas-permeable lenses of the fluorocarbonated silicone-acrylate material?

SELF-EVALUATION QUESTIONS

True-false statements

Directions: Indicate whether the statement is true (T) or false (F).

T or F   1. A thick, heavy plus lens will tend to ride high under the upper lid.

T or F   2. Corneal molding or distortion can be detected by taking keratometric readings at the repeat visits.

T or F

3. Keratoconus fitting is the same as any other rigid lens fitting and may be approached in exactly the same manner.

Missing words

Directions: Write in the missing word in the following sentences.

4. A front curve toric lens is held at its proper axis by means of a _____.
5. Spherical rigid lenses are usually the first choice for high degrees of _____ astigmatism.
6. Some bifocal lenses are fitted _____ so that the lower lid will push the lens up to the line of sight for near vision.

Choice-completion questions

Directions: Select the one best answer in each case.

7. If the keratometer cannot read a steep cornea, as in keratoconus, its range may be increased by which device?
   a. Placido's disk
   b. Soper cone lens
   c. INNS extension disk
   d. Fleisher's ring
   e. Prism ballast
8. In order to achieve better fitting characteristics with high refractive errors, what is the best design to incorporate into the lens?
   a. Lathe cut
   b. Wide flat peripheral curves
   c. Single cut
   d. Fenestrations
   e. Lenticular
9. What is the basic principle behind fitting high minus contact lenses and wearing high plus spectacle lenses over them?
   a. They overcome corneal surface irregularities
   b. They create a telescopic system
   c. They narrow the visual field
   d. They magnify by ×1.5
   e. Cosmetically they are better than telescopic lenses

ANSWERS, NOTES, AND EXPLANATIONS

1. **False.** A thick heavy lens such as a high plus lens will tend to ride low because of its weight and the force of the lid on its thinnest portion, the edge. The use of lenticulation reduces the weight and thickness of the lens thus enhancing its centering characteristics.
2. **True.** K readings taken at repeat visits are an excellent method of monitoring any corneal changes. If the K readings change it may be important to modify or change the lens.
3. **False.** The keratoconus cornea usually has a high degree of irregular astigmatism, and the keratometer may be of very little value. Moderate to extreme cases may require fitting purely by trial lens evaluation.
4. **Prism ballast.** A front curve toric lens is held at its proper axis by means of a prism ballast. This thicker portion is ground into the lens at the time of manufacture. Gravity will hold the heaviest portion of the lens along the lower lid stabilizing the cylindric correction.

5. **Corneal.** In general the corneal astigmatism is eliminated by the lens. However, certain fitting problems may indicate the need for a back surface toric lens.

6. **Loosely.** The peripheral ring that holds the near corrections raises slightly while the eye rotates downward thus giving the proper alignment for the near vision.

7. **c. INNS extension disk.** The INNS extension disk enables the use of a $+1.25$ lens to be placed over the keratometer face plate, thus extending its range of measurement by 9.00 diopters.

8. **e. Lenticular.** The lenticular design reduces thickness and weight of high-power lenses, thus giving better centering, comfort, and vision.

9. **b. They create a telescopic system.** The creation of a telescopic system that produces a magnified retinal image can be of great benefit to the low visual acuity patient. The lens can overcome the corneal irregularities and thus cause the magnifying effect of the plus spectacles to give better acuity.

Visual fields

In the determination of the visual field the perimetrist attempts to make a two-dimensional map of a patient's entire area of vision. Normally in everyday living we do not place much importance on the width of our vision, the emphasis being directed on seeing clearly straight ahead. However, those persons who have lost much of their peripheral field are just as incapacitated functionally as those who have lost much of their central field. Try rolling up two sheets of paper and placing them before your eyes so that you are basically looking through two large-diameter straws. Although you can see directly ahead clearly, it is very difficult to walk through a room without bumping into the furniture.

The circumference of the visual field depends on many factors. Obviously, the field of vision for seeing a mosquito flying about would be far less than for seeing a new jumbo jet. Thus the size of an object is important in referring to the dimensions of the seeing area. Also, the ability to perceive at the sides is not as great when the visibility is poor, as opposed to when it is clear; therefore illumination is an important factor in mapping the field of vision. The state of adaptation of the eye, whether light-adapted or dark-adapted, although not a critical factor, will influence the measurable size of the visual field area. These factors are objective and can in all instances be controlled by the perimetrist. The difficulty in qualitative or quantitative perimetry is not in assessing the factors of size, illumination, and adaptation but in assessing the patient. Perimetry depends entirely on obtaining an accurate and rapid subjective response. How does one compare the replies of a 72-year-old, belligerent, slightly senile patient who has recently had a stroke to those of an intelligent 25-year-old woman with no cerebral disease? Because it is difficult to evaluate such factors as reaction time, fatigue, and general health, what is done and noted in every case is a simple evaluation (good, fair, or poor) of the patient's cooperation and reliability.

Although perimetry is not an exact science because it is entirely dependent on subjective replies of the patient, the visual field for a given patient should be reproducible. Many methods have been devised for estimating visual fields. We discuss only those methods that have survived the tests of time, and their applications and limitations.

PRELIMINARY PROCEDURES

1. A general statement should not be made about the patient's visual behavior. If it is noted that the patient tends to bump into objects located on either the right or left, a right- or left-sided total loss of visual field (homonymous hemianopia) may be present.

2. The visual acuity, with and without glasses, should be noted before taking a visual field. As a general rule it can be stated that the poorer the patient's visual acuity, the larger the test object that must be employed to plot an accurate visual field. The manner in which the patient responds to visual acuity testing should be recorded. If the patient appears to see only the last three letters of all the lines on the chart, a loss of one half of the visual field may be present.

3. Color-vision testing should be used, especially if colored test objects are going to be used.

4. The purpose of the visual field always should be noted so that emphasis can be given to specific areas. Such instruction must come from the ophthalmologist who has made a complete ocular examination and a tentative diagnosis. For instance, for a patient with papilledema, the tangent screen might be thoroughly explored, with particular attention paid to the state of the blind spots, as opposed to the patient with retinitis pigmentosa, in whom a ring scotoma might be anticipated.

FACILITIES FOR FIELD TESTING

Ideally every office or clinic should have a visual field room that is quiet and out of the way of the normal traffic of the office or clinic. This room should be of simple design so that distraction is kept to a minimum. Approximately 7 foot-candles of illumination are necessary for adequate visual-field tests.

Realistically, most offices do not contain special field quarters because of the cost and lack of available space. Similarly, the equipment used varies from place to place. Although it is helpful to have the best ophthalmic equipment, the room and equipment always take a subordinate position to the skill and ingenuity of a competent perimetrist. If the patient understands what is expected and has rapport with the examiner, adequate perimetry can be performed.

CONFRONTATION TEST

Of all methods of perimetry, the confrontation test is the most widely used because it requires no special facilities or equipment and can be performed in the home, on bedridden patients, and in hospitals. This is essentially a screening test. Any pathologic condition discovered requires a more sophisticated test where possible to determine the exact nature of the visual defect.

In this test the examiner tests the range of the patient's field by that of his or her own, which may be considered normal. The examiner stands facing the patient at a distance of approximately 2 feet. Opposite eyes are occluded; that is, the patient's left eye is covered while the examiner closes his or her right eye. Each of them then fixes the exposed eye of the other. The examiner moves a finger or a white test object, such as a small hatpin mounted on a handle, from the extreme periphery and notes when it comes into the field of view; the patient and examiner should see it simultaneously (Fig. 16-1). The test is best performed while the patient's back is to the light and the background behind the examiner is uniform and dark. All four quadrants of the visual field should be tested, and two different approaches should be used in each quadrant. If any defect is indicated or suspected from this method, the field should be accurately mapped out and recorded with the perimeter and tangent screen. When vision is extremely poor, a small penlight may be used for a rough test. A modification of this test is to have the

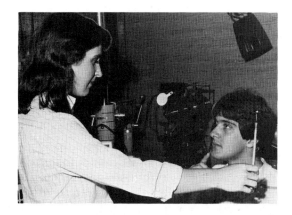

Fig. 16-1 Confrontation test. A test object is brought in from the periphery to the seeing area.

patient count fingers. While one eye is occluded, the examiner brings in from the periphery one, two, or three fingers and asks the patient to count the number of fingers brought in from each quadrant.

The confrontation test is an excellent method of screening patients and, if used skillfully, can be surprisingly accurate. It may be the only method of examining children, illiterates, and the mentally deficient. With children, a small article of interest such as a brightly colored plastic toy usually is used as a test object. The preservation of a field in a particular area is indicated when the child makes a quick glance at the object of interest detected in the peripheral field. Finally, when fixation is lost or essential vision is grossly impaired, this method may be more valuable than a more refined technique. For example, in a patient with a cataract, the accurate perception and projection of light or a hand in all four quadrants may be the only method of determining retinal function.

This test, however, should be regarded only as a rough test, and failure to demonstrate a field defect does not imply a normal field. Defects of large size may easily be missed by this method.

PERIMETERS

Perimeters are constructed in such a manner that the eye is at the center of rotation of a hemisphere that has a radius of curvature of 33 cm. Some perimeters consist of an arc of a circle that is rotated, and the

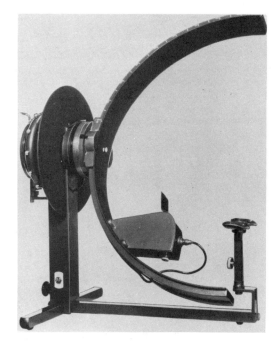

Fig. 16-2 Arc perimeter used for measuring the peripheral visual field.

test object is moved either manually or mechanically along this arc from the periphery toward the center (Fig. 16-2). The more elaborate perimeters, such as the Goldmann perimeter, are constructed from a half shell, in which the test object is projected (Fig. 16-3). In this type of perimeter, not only can the intensity of the illumination of the test object be controlled but the patient's fixation can be continually checked by a viewing device behind the perimeter.

Before use, the Goldmann perimeter should be aligned and calibrated.

1. Level the instrument so that the projector arm will swing back automatically into the protected position on the sphere when the instrument is not being used. Insert the chart paper, and position the vertical and horizontal lines with the V-notch on the frame. If a fixation light projector is used, the chart is positioned 5 degrees from the center line.

2. Use the 15-degree position to the right and left

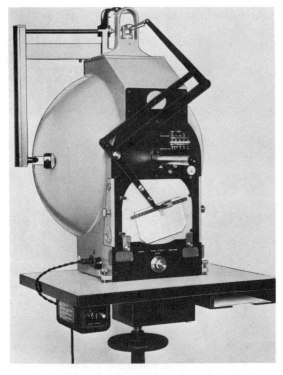

Fig. 16-3 Goldmann spherical projection perimeter, an excellent apparatus for both peripheral and central fields.

for examination when the central scotoma device is indicated.

3. Adjust the telescope so that the reticule and the patient's eye are clear and in plain focus. Proper adjustment of the light within the sphere and of the projected target is most important. The recording arm is positioned at the 70-degree mark on the chart. This will allow you to lock the projector arm in the proper position by pushing the centering pin on the operator's side into the socket on the upper left side of the instrument. When the arm is locked in, light from the projector will fall on the light meter.

4. Position the size and brightness control levers to the far right. Turn the instrument on and the room lights off. Turn the appropriate control knob, and adjust to a reading of 1,000 apostilbs on the light meter.

5. Set the gray filter level to the 0.0315 position.

This will produce an illumination of 31.5 apostilbs.

6. Interpose the white photometer shade between the projected light and the light meter.

7. At this point look at the photometer screen through the cutout on the opposite side of the sphere. Match the sphere's brightness to the brightness on the photometer shade or screen by moving the diaphragm up or down. To achieve reliable and accurate fields, calibration of the instrument should be performed before each examination. You are now ready to proceed with the visual field test.

When the visual field has been mapped out on a perimeter, the following notations should be made: (1) the size of the test object, which can vary from 1 to 25 mm, (2) the test distance, which is always 330 mm in a perimeter, (3) the color of the test object, and (4) the cooperation and reliability of the patient.

MEASURING A FIELD ON THE PERIMETER

Just before the actual perimetric examination, the patient should be told in detail what is expected during this test. It is essential that the patient be comfortable, relaxed, and alert. Glasses are not required. The patient is brought to the perimeter, and the chin is set on the chin rest. The chin should be placed comfortably on the rest so that the face is held vertically and not tilted to one side. One eye is covered. The other eye, situated in the center of the arc, fixes on the white fixation target at the center of the perimeter around which the arc revolves.

The size of the test object chosen for use depends on the accuracy of the patient's fixation and on reaction time. If the patient is young and alert and has 20/20 vision, then the examination is begun with a 1 or 2 mm white target. However, if the patient is confused and somewhat senile and has vision no better than 20/200, it would probably be best to employ a 10 mm, 20 mm, or even larger test object as the initial stimulus. The test object is always brought in from the periphery toward the center (from the nonseeing to the seeing area). The test object should be brought in slowly so that the time lag from the patient's response to the mark of the examiner will not be great. In many instances the ophthalmologist will request a perimetric examination to be performed with certain test targets. These different targets will show characteristically larger fields with the larger target. In follow-up visits it is important to reuse the same targets to show any regression or progression of the field changes. The different targets will show a different-sized field at a common illumination and distance; each of these completed mappings is called an *isopter*. The ophthalmologist will inform the ophthalmic assistant which isopters are desired.

The patient should be taught a series of signals to indicate (1) when the test object becomes visible, (2) when it disappears, and (3) when it flickers or grays out. The signal system is important because it reduces the length of time required for the completion of the test by eliminating needless conversation. Conversation during the test should be kept to a minimum inasmuch as it only serves to distract the patient. Approximately 12 meridians should be tested, and in each meridian the object should be carried up to the fixation point. The normal physiologic response to an object in the peripheral field is to turn the eyes toward it. When the field of vision is charted, this normal response has to be suppressed because fixation by the patient must be rigidly maintained on the central target. Therefore it is imperative to observe the patient's fixation at all times. In some of the more elaborate perimeters a viewing system at the back of the shell enables the examiner to constantly watch the patient's eyes during the entire examination.

It should always be remembered that field testing is taxing. Accuracy depends on the subject's accurate and quick response. It should not be laborious because prolonged visual field testing will tire a patient and cause erroneous results. Drooping eyelids or eyeglass frames interfering with a clear view of the test object can cause these erroneous results.

Errors in field testing can occur on the part of either the patient or the examiner. Errors attributable to the patient may include (1) following the test object rather than maintaining proper fixation, (2) tilting the head or moving the chin off the chin rest,

(3) not understanding the test or being generally uncooperative, (4) responding slowly, most often done by senile patients with low visual acuity or obvious field defects, and (5) physical, mental, or psychologic handicaps. Errors attributable to the examiner may include (1) poor patient instruction, (2) too-rapid movement of the test object, (3) improper monitoring of the patient's fixation, (4) poor or inaccurate marking of the chart, and (5) poor or improper adjustment of the perimeter.

TANGENT SCREEN

Determination of the central 30 degrees of the visual field is best performed by the use of a tangent screen (Fig. 16-4). A tangent screen usually is made of black felt material, and the test is conventionally conducted at 1 or 2 meters from the eye. The tangent screen should be kept clean by a gentle whisking from time to time. Test objects, whether flat or spherical, can be washed gently with mild soap and water.

Testing with a tangent screen is the most common visual field test. The test is simple, easy to perform, and offers the most information to the examiner. If the patient requires glasses for distance vision, the test should be performed while the patient is wearing his or her glasses.

Because a high percentage of the visual field defects detected on the perimeter in the peripheral field extend inward to within the 30-degree radius, as delineated on the tangent screen, many perimetrists advocate performing the tangent screen examination first and then following it with a perimeter examination.

The targets available are in the form of circular disks or balls varying in size from 1 to 50 mm in diameter (Fig. 16-5). These test objects are inserted into the end of a long wand. The holder, or wand, should be covered with a black cloth of the same material as the screen. Painted black wands cast a considerable amount of reflection and should be avoided because they are a distraction for the patient.

A spider-web pattern is stitched around the central fixation point into the tangent screen. The concentric circles represent the angle in degrees from the center. The radiating lines represent degrees of the circle around the fixation point. This pattern is stitched

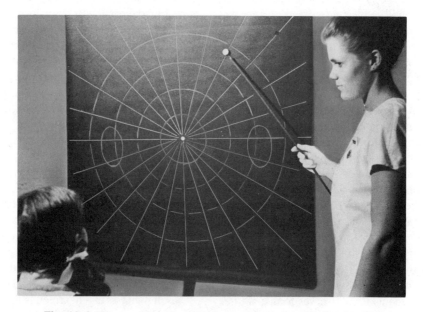

Fig. 16-4 Tangent screen examination measures the central field only.

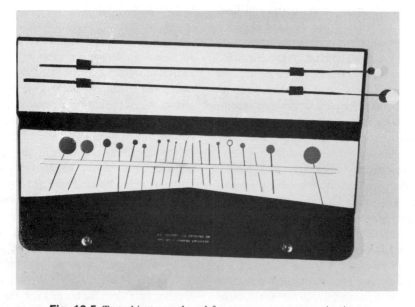

Fig. 16-5 Test objects employed for tangent screen examination.

into the screen to be as invisible as possible to the patient and is designed to assist in the mapping of the patient's central field on the appropriate recording chart. The position of the blind spot for both the right and left eye usually is stitched into the tangent screen.

PERFORMING A TANGENT SCREEN FIELD EXAMINATION

In a tangent screen examination it is essential that the patient who has a refractive error wear glasses. This is not essential in perimetric examinations. It is helpful to stabilize the head by means of a chin rest, but this is not necessary. The patient is seated on a chair or stool with the eyes exactly opposite the fixation point on the screen (usually a white disk) and 1 meter (or 2 meters) from the fixation point. One eye is occluded. The examiner usually stands to one side and watches the patient's eye to ensure that fixation is absolutely maintained. Again, the test object, the size of which is correlated with the patient's visual acuity, is brought in at 30-degree intervals from the periphery toward the center of the tangent screen. The patient indicates seeing the test object, either verbally—such as saying "yes"—or by tapping a coin or raising a hand. At all times the reliability of the patient's responses should be checked. The easiest check is to map out the patient's blind spot. At a distance of 1 meter the blind spot usually is 5.5 degrees wide and 7.5 degrees high and is placed approximately 15 degrees temporal to the point of fixation. In the aphakic person it is smaller and closer to the fixation point. The blind spot can and should be accurately measured on every patient with a tangent screen. Another way to check the patient's responses is to rotate the test object out of view so that it cannot be visible to the patient.

An old method of recording results is to insert black pins into the screen at the points indicated, transferring them to a chart after the examination has been completed.

If at any point during the test a defect appears, it should be explored for its *size, shape,* and *density.* This is accomplished by moving the test object from a blind area to a seeing area at right angles to the border of the defect. The size and shape of this defect should be outlined at least twice to check the patient's reliability. The density of the field defect is determined by the use of a number of test objects of various sizes. If a small test object was employed when the defect was initially discovered, then a larger test object should be used, and vice versa if the larger test object was employed initially. If the patient's responses are confusing and equivocal, it is probable that the test object was too small to be easily seen. In such an instance a larger test object should be chosen.

It is extremely important that the examiner have the patient's undivided attention at all times during a visual field test. In some instances the patient may have to be reminded to maintain undivided attention.

For younger children in whom the attention span is short and to whom the fixation spot and target are uninteresting, the examiner can use small figures for the target and the fixation spot. However, the dimensions of the target must be measured and a note of these made on the record. A target should never be oscillated to elicit an expected response, because this in effect increases the size of the target; thus the isopter is changed and an erroneous result is obtained.

For patients with poor vision who cannot see the fixation spot, it is permissible to enlarge the fixation spot until they can obtain some central fixation. This can be accomplished by cutting out a large star-shaped fixation spot or drawing a large cross and placing it over the original fixation spot. Vertical and horizontal strips of ½-inch white adhesive tape may be placed to intersect at the fixation center.

CHARTS

The visual field chart is merely a permanent record of the patient's responses at tangent screen and perimeter examinations. The best type of chart is that in which both fields are represented on a small pad that can be fastened to the patient's record of the rest of the eye examination, so that the whole picture of the patient's visual status can be seen at a glance. The right and left eye should be indicated, and the chart should be printed as the patient sees the visual field, and not according to the anatomy of the visual pathway; that is, the field for the right eye is on the

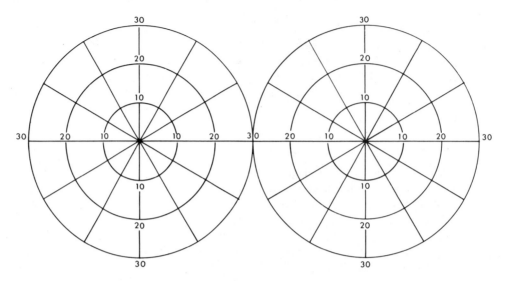

Fig. 16-6 Tangent screen chart.

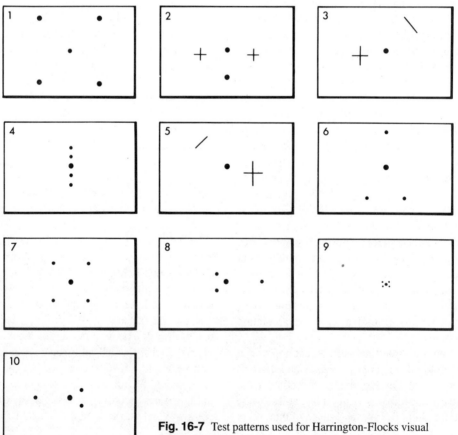

Fig. 16-7 Test patterns used for Harrington-Flocks visual field screener.

right side of the chart. A notation should be made of the *patient's name,* the *date,* and the *examiner's name.* In addition, the *size* and *color of target* used, the *corrected visual acuity,* the *pupillary size,* and also the patient's *cooperation* and *reliability* should be noted (Fig. 16-6).

An *isopter* is the map of the circumference of a visual field determined by a test object of a certain size, with the patient at a certain distance from the tangent screen or perimeter. The isopter, as indicated on the visual field chart, should be noted as a fraction, the numerator indicating the size of the test object employed in millimeters, and the denominator indicating the distance of the patient in millimeters from the field chart. Thus the fraction 5/1,000 indicates to anyone what test object was used and at what distance.

SPECIAL PERIMETRIC TECHNIQUES
Visual field screening

Visual field screening is a good method for rapidly determining the presence or absence of a field defect. It is useful as a preliminary procedure in offices or in testing large groups, such as military personnel or students.

Harrington-Flocks screener. This apparatus consists of a portable box; the open lid is used as a background for the screen. It has a series of 10 cards, each exhibiting a distinctive pattern printed in fluorescent material. An ultraviolet light source is switched on 0.25 second while the patient fixates the central point of each card. Each time the patient is asked to describe what he or she has seen. If the patient sees only three dots when four have been flashed, then the defect is explored further and analyzed by conventional perimetry and tangent screen examination (Fig. 16-7).

Automated visual fields. The automated perimeter or visual field plotter is a quick, randomized test to determine field defects. A complete discussion of the automated visual field equipment will be found in Chapter 17.

Reliable indications of a field defect include the following:

1. Two or more adjacent test spots that were missed at a single test intensity

2. A single spot missed at two or more stimulus intensities

3. Marked contraction of the visual field

Tests with the automated screener and the Goldmann tester may be comparable (Figs. 16-8 and 16-9). A device such as the Fieldmaster is not a replacement for the Goldmann perimeter and is not intended as such. Automated screeners are designed to distinguish between patients with normal visual fields and those requiring more detailed evaluation. In principle, the fieldmaster test screener is similar to the glaucoma screening technique developed by D.M. Armaly and modified by Stephen Drance.

The automated screener is extremely useful for preliminary visual field testing because it does not take up the amount of time required with the Goldmann perimeter. Those patients examined in the office whose responses to the Amsler grid are questionable or who reveal constriction during finger confrontation tests should be examined by the automated screener. If results are normal, generally no further testing is required. If defects are found during the automated screener test, however, then more detailed visual field examination must be done, with particular attention paid to the areas having defects as noted on the automated screener.

There are other models of visual field screeners, all employing these principles.

Fully-automated perimeter. Fully-automated perimeters include the Octopus, the Tübinger automated perimeter, the Heijl-Krakau perimeter, and the Pashley perimeter. All of these perimeters operate on the principle of nonmoving stimuli, and the automatic perimeter determines the thresholds of the points tested.

Amsler's chart

The Amsler chart was devised to detect abnormalities in the central 20 degrees in the field of vision. This chart consists essentially of grid lines with a central white fixation dot. The squares on the grid are 5 mm in size and subtend an angle of 1 degree at 30 cm. The Amsler chart is of greatest value in detecting microscopic areas of macular or perimacular edema in which visual distortion is a prominent sign (Fig. 16-10).

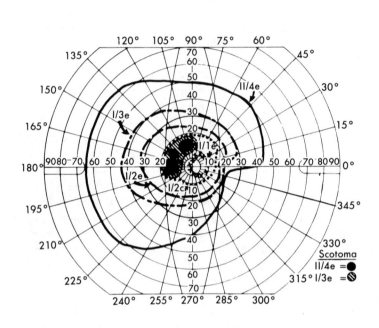

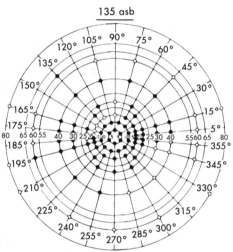

Fig. 16-8 Goldmann *(left)* and Fieldmaster *(right)* field plots in a patient with glaucoma.

A series of questions should be asked while the patient is viewing the central white spot:

1. *Is the center spot visible?* If not, a central scotoma may be present.
2. *While viewing the center, can you see all four sides?* If not, an arcuate scotoma or a cecocentral scotoma may be present.
3. *Do you see the entire grid? Are there any defects?* If any areas are absent, then a paracentral scotoma may be present.
4. *Are the horizontal and vertical lines straight and parallel?* If not, then metamorphopsia is

present. The parallel lines may bend inward, indicating micropsia, or bend outward, indicating macropsia.

Static perimetry

A detailed method of examining the visual field has been available since the manufacture of the newer perimeters. The sensitivity of the retina at any point can be determined by presenting the patient with test points of increasing brightness until the patient says he or she sees the light. In this way the retinal threshold can be determined at any point on the retina.

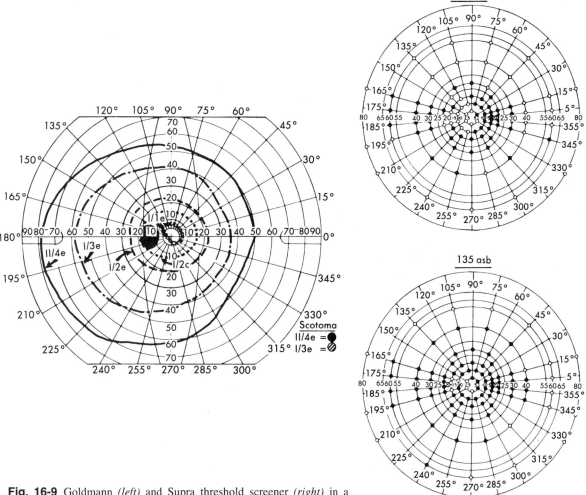

Fig. 16-9 Goldmann *(left)* and Supra threshold screener *(right)* in a patient with nutritional amblyopia and a central scotoma.

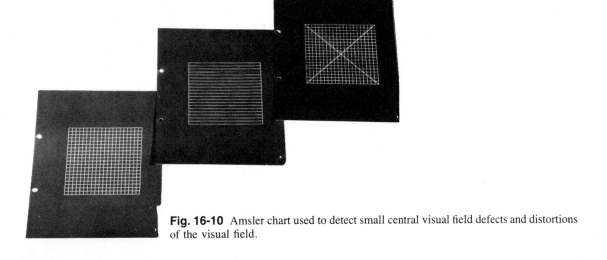

Fig. 16-10 Amsler chart used to detect small central visual field defects and distortions of the visual field.

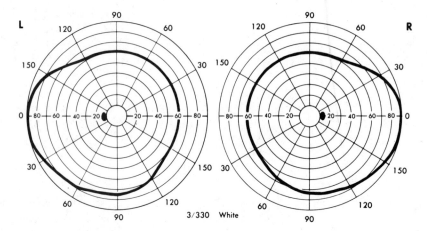

Fig. 16-11 Normal perimetric visual field.

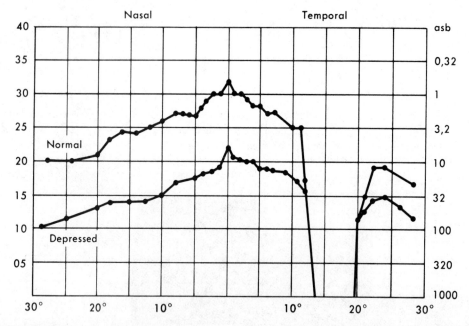

Fig. 16-12 Recording of section of sensitivity or static perimetry profile of normal and depressed visual field. (From Harrington DO: *The visual fields: a textbook and atlas of clinical perimetry;* ed 5, St Louis, 1981, Mosby.)

In static perimetry the field charts show a profile section of retinal sensitivity. In that profile the blind spot looks like a vertical tube. Areas of partial loss of vision are mapped as shallow to deep depressions extending below the normal range. The peak on the profile corresponds to an area of foveal fixation.

Static perimetry is considered more accurate than kinetic perimetry because of the lack of delay in the projected moving target and the patient's response. Regardless of which method is best, inasmuch as there are defenders of both, static perimetry is here to stay and probably is the best method for the detection of early glaucomatous field defects.

NORMAL VISUAL FIELD

The normal visual field, within limits, is determined by the size of the test object employed and the distance at which the test was made. With a 3-mm white target on a perimeter of a 330-degree radius, the average peripheral limit is about 95 degrees outward, 75 degrees downward, 60 degrees inward, and 60 degrees upward (Figs. 16-11 and 16-12). If the size of the target is increased, the temporal limit can be pushed outward to about 110 degrees. In many cases allowances have to be made for the contours of the face. Especially to be considered during field testing is the loss of field caused by the projection of the brow and the nose. If the visual field is taken without making allowances for these contours, the field is called a *relative* visual field. The *absolute* field is obtained by rotating the eye and the head to escape these limitations.

The *blind spot* marks a physiologic blind area of the retina. It corresponds with the entrance of the optic nerve to the posterior pole of the eye. This blind spot is located about 12 to 15 degrees to the outside of the fixation point, and about 1.5 degrees below the horizontal meridian. It measures approximately 7.5 degrees in height and 5.5 degrees in width.

PATHOLOGIC DEFECTS IN THE VISUAL FIELD

Pathologic field defects resulting from derangement within the optic nerve or its extensions to the occipital lobe of the brain cause a loss of vision but not a sensation of blackness. Only those field defects that arise from disturbances in front of the retina, such as those caused by a vitreous or macular hemorrhage, result in awareness of something black before the eyes. The distinction between the two is subtle. In disorders of the brain the patient complains of the effects of the field loss but not of any particular sensation associated with this loss. With retinal disease the patient will complain of both types.

Field defects are classified according to those that emanate from the periphery of the field and those that originate from within the confines of the field itself.

Scotoma

The scotoma is an area of partial or complete blindness within the confines of a normal or relatively normal visual field. Within a scotoma the vision is more depressed than in the area of visual field surrounding it. When the depressed area of a scotoma expands into the periphery of the field, it is said to have "broken through."

Scotomas may be divided into the following types:
1. *Central,* which involves the fixation area and is always associated with a loss of visual acuity (Fig. 16-13).
2. *Pericentral,* in which the fixation area is relatively clear and the field immediately surrounding it is deficient.
3. *Paracentral,* in which the area of depressed visual field is to one side of fixation (Fig. 16-14, *A*). These scotomas also may be denoted as to their position—whether they are nasal or temporal to the fixation point.
4. *Cecal,* which involves the area of the normal blind spot (Fig. 16-14, *B*).
5. The nerve fiber bundle scotoma. This is also referred to as an *arcuate, Bjerrum,* or *comet* type of scotoma (Fig. 16-14, *C*). This type of lesion extends around the fixation point from the blind spot in an arc and ends typically on the nasal field with a sharply demarcated border. It can occur either above or below the blind spot. In some instances it is not even attached to the blind spot but seems to issue from it (Fig. 16-15).

The intensity of a scotoma varies from absolute

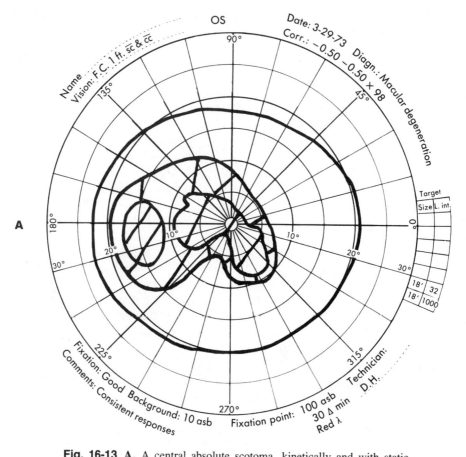

Fig. 16-13 A, A central absolute scotoma, kinetically and with static.

CONTRACTION OF VISUAL FIELD

blindness to a minimum detectable loss of visual acuity. If there is complete blindness to test objects of all sizes, the scotoma is absolute. If the area involves loss of only the smaller test objects, it is referred to as a *relative scotoma*.

Contraction usually occurs as an area of blindness emanating from the periphery of the field toward the center. If the contraction affects only one part of the field, it often is referred to as a *sector defect*. Sector defects bounded by vertical or horizontal diameters of the field are hemianopic defects. The term *hemianopic* is used to indicate a defect occupying half of the visual field; invariably it is a bilateral defect. A hemianopic defect is *homonymous* right or left

when the corresponding half of both eyes is affected (Fig. 16-16). In this instance there is total blindness in the temporal field of one eye and the nasal field of the other eye. The vertical dividing line between the seeing and the nonseeing portion of the field is midline. When a quadrant of each field is affected, a *quadrant hemianopia* is present (Fig. 16-17). A defect or loss of the upper or lower half of the visual field is termed an *altitudinal hemianopia;* it can be superior or inferior. A *bitemporal hemianopia* is a visual field defect in which part or all of each temporal field is depressed (Fig. 16-18). The defect may vary from the slightest depression of the upper temporal portion of the field to complete blindness in each temporal field.

A *congruous homonymous hemianopic defect* is

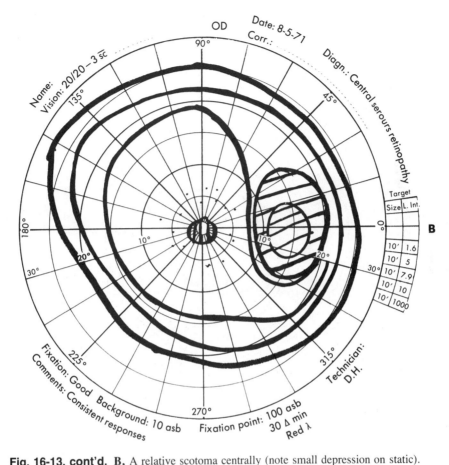

Fig. 16-13, cont'd. B, A relative scotoma centrally (note small depression on static).

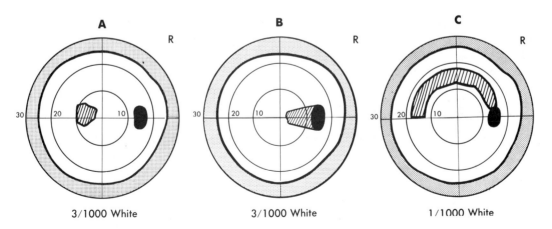

Fig. 16-14 Kinetic perimetry. **A,** Paracentral scotoma. **B,** Cecal scotoma. **C,** Arcuate, or Bjerrum, scotoma.

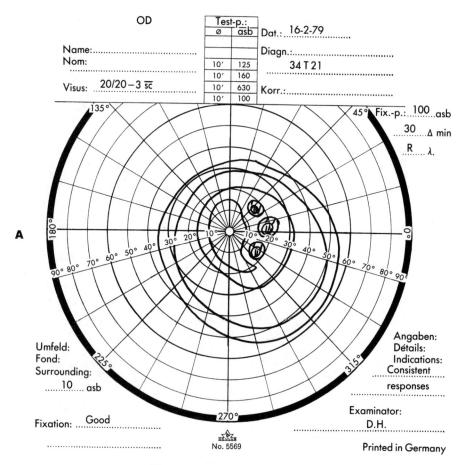

Fig. 16-15 A, Glaucoma field, early.

one in which the defect in the two fields is superimposable, that is, completely identical. In this instance, when the examiner maps the visual field of one eye, its margin will be identical to the visual field of the other (Fig. 16-19).

HYSTERICAL VISUAL FIELD

In some instances defects of the visual field will be functional rather than organic; that is, they will be due to disturbance of the patient's emotional status rather than to disease of the retina or its visual pathways. In this instance the most common field of vision seems to be narrowed down to only 10 to 20 degrees in diameter. If the patient is free of any organic disease, a tubular defect should indicate, or

at least give rise to suspicion, that the patient has hysterical fields (Fig. 16-20).

The presence of such a functional defect can easily be checked by moving the patient back another meter from the tangent screen and doubling the size of the test object. By doing this the visual angle of the field remains the same, but the diameter of the field on the tangent screen should double in size. If the diameter remains the same at 1 and 2 meters, the presence of hysteria should be strongly suspected.

If the diameter of the visual field increases as it should, organic visual loss must be considered. In this case the differential diagnosis of tubular fields would include (1) vitamin deficiency, (2) retinitis pigmentosa, and (3) glaucoma.

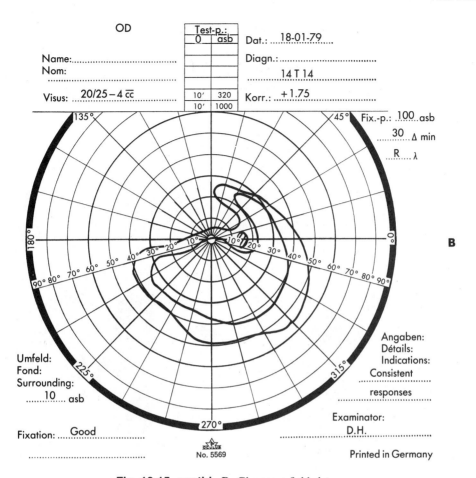

Fig. 16-15, cont'd. B, Glaucoma field, late.

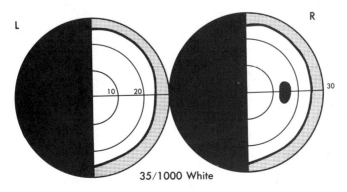

35/1000 White

Fig. 16-16 Left homonymous hemianopia.

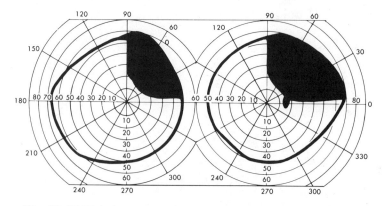

Fig. 16-17 Right incongruous homonymous superior quadranopia.

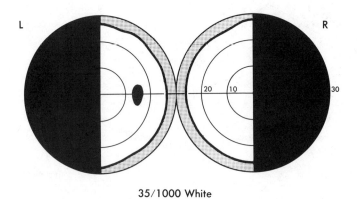

35/1000 White

Fig. 16-18 Bitemporal hemianopia.

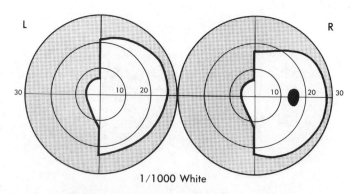

1/1000 White

Fig. 16-19 Left congruous homonymous hemianopia.

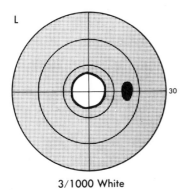

3/1000 White

Fig. 16-20 Tubular, or hysterical, field. The size of the field remains unchanged when testing at 1 or 2 meters.

With hysterical patients the size and shape of the field defect can virtually be suggested by the examiner. Other field defects that have been frequently noted with this type of situation are the spiraling field and the star-shaped field. With retinitis pigmentosa, the patient has true "tunnel vision." Driving a car with this type of field restriction would be hazardous (Fig. 16-21).

AUXILIARY AIDS IN KINETIC VISUAL FIELD TESTING

1. The examiner should always stand to the side of the patient and keep an eye on the patient's fixation. Test objects should never extend across the visual field chart, because this is a distraction.

2. The test object generally should be moved from a nonseeing area to a seeing area.

3. The patient should always be comfortable and well-rested for field examination. The examiner should not tire the patient with prolonged testing.

4. The eye with the best vision should always be tested first to obtain an idea of the patient's reliability and the extent of the normal visual field.

5. The test object to be used should be the smallest that will give a reliable and reproducible field. If this is unsuccessful, larger test objects should be employed. For example, if the patient's visual acuity is 20/20, a 1-mm test object can be used. If the visual acuity is 20/40 or 20/50, a 5-mm test object should be the smallest employed.

6. It is important that the test objects be kept clean, especially the white ones, as a change in the intensity of the color of the test object will affect the size of the field. Projection test objects are best.

7. The visual field examination should be demonstrated to the patient before the actual test. In the demonstration a large test object should be used so that the patient gets the idea of what is expected.

8. If the patient is lethargic or responds poorly, the confrontation test may be the test of choice.

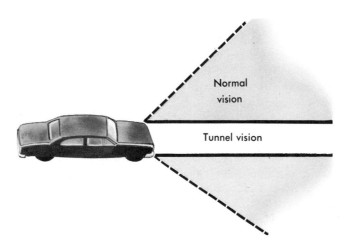

Fig. 16-21 Tunnel vision, with gross construction of the visual field as is found in retinitis pigmentosa. Driving would be hazardous.

9. Glasses, if required for distance, should be worn for the tangent screen examination.

10. In tangent screen examinations the test object should be hidden at various intervals to test the patient's reliability. Suspicious answers should always be double-checked.

11. The use of colored test objects presently remains a source of debate among neuroophthalmologists and perimetrists. The opponents of color-vision testing point out that colored test objects are difficult to standardize and to identify crisply on visual field testing. They also point out that the substitution of a colored test object for a white one is merely a convenient method of reducing its area. Because testing with colored objects is closely related to testing with reduced illumination, they believe that the disadvantages outweigh the advantages. The proponents of the colored test objects believe that they provide a meticulous test that can yield valuable information. All authorities agree that if color is to be used, the red test object is the most useful in detecting neurologic disease, especially for lesions of the optic chiasm. The end point in color-vision testing should not be a mere detection of the test object but the detection of the color red itself. Blue test objects sometimes are employed for disorders of the retina.

SUMMARY

The assessment of the visual field is vital to any complete ocular examination. It is of paramount importance in diagnosing lesions of the visual pathway, retinal lesions, and glaucoma. It is the mainstay of deciding whether glaucoma therapy has been adequate for an individual patient, because the entire principle of glaucoma therapy is to prevent loss of visual field. Its importance cannot be emphasized strongly enough. Many professionals believe that visual field testing is so important that it should be performed only by a trained visual field technician. We are in total agreement with this principle. We do believe, however, that the ophthalmic assistant, if properly trained to do a meticulous examination, can perform a valuable service in visual field testing as a preliminary examination. The final interpretation of the visual field must always be done by an ophthalmologist because only the physician can correlate the results of the visual field test with the patient's problem and the signs obtained on physical examination.

Instruction in visual field examination is best done by demonstration. Competence in visual field testing requires experience. The ophthalmic assistant should take every opportunity to perform routine normal visual field examinations to become familiar with the best techniques of visual field testing.

QUESTIONS FOR REVIEW AND THOUGHT

1. What is an isopter?
2. If a tangent screen examination is recorded as 3/1,000, what do the numerator and denominator stand for?
3. What are the pitfalls to avoid in obtaining a good visual field?
4. In a field examination when should the patient's spectacles be removed? When should they be left on?
5. Outline a method of performing the confrontation test.
6. Screening devices are rough guides to detecting possible defects. If a defect is found, what further examination is required?
7. If you find a defect during the tangent screen examination, how do you outline the size, shape, and density of the area?
8. What is the value of the Amsler grid?
9. How can you detect a hysterical field?
10. Lesion in the right side of the brain may show a defect on which side of the visual field?

11. Defects such as a retinal detachment in the lower half of the retina will show a defect in which part of the visual field?

12. In detecting a defect in the peripheral field, would you be more likely to use the tangent screen or the perimeter?

13. What effect does illumination have on the size of the visual field?

14. A patient who has nystagmus frequently sees better when turning the head in one direction. Is head turning permissible during a field test?

15. What is the field defect that may arise from pressure on the optic chiasm?

16. Contraction usually occurs in one or both eyes as an area of blindness emanating from the periphery. How can you determine if the field is contracted?

17. The eye with the best vision should always be tested first to obtain an idea of the reliability of the patient. Why?

18. Is the blind spot located nasally or temporally in the visual field? Is it more prominent in the lower or upper field?

19. Patients with macular disease complain of inability to see clearly straight ahead but retain good peripheral vision. What type of field would be found?

SELF-EVALUATION QUESTIONS

True-false statements

Directions: Indicate whether the statement is true (T) or false (F).

T or F 1. Static perimetry is performed by presenting test points of increasing brightness.

T or F 2. Static perimetry is accomplished with stationary targets with variable brightness in the test targets.

T or F 3. The fixation area of the field is the first to be affected in glaucoma.

Missing words

Directions: Write in the missing word in the following sentences.

4. A bitemporal defect always suggests a defect in the _____.

5. Static or profile perimetry utilizes projected light spots in which the luminance is increased by measured increments of light until the patient signals that the stimulus is _____.

6. The visual field defect most commonly found in hysteria is the _____.

Choice-completion questions

Directions: Select the one best answer in each case.

7. The following conditions cause a ring scotoma:
   a. Retinitis pigmentosa
   b. Glaucoma
   c. Ischemia of the optic nerve
   d. Vitamin A deficiency
   e. All of the above

8. Tobacco amblyopia usually is caused from:
   a. Smoking pipes and cigars
   b. Smoking cigarettes
   c. Common use of chewing tobacco and snuff
   d. Smoking marijuana
   e. None of the above

9. The most frequent visual field defect in patients with optic nerve disease is:
   a. An enlarged blind spot
   b. Peripheral contraction of the field
   c. A sector defect
   d. A central scotoma
   e. A centrocecal scotoma

ANSWERS, NOTES, AND EXPLANATIONS

1. **True.** The light is held stationary (static) and the illumination is increased until it is seen by the patient.

2. **True.** Most perimeters have an attachment that enables the perimetrist to chose a meridian on the visual field to discover the retinal sensitivity along a particular meridian. It is used to best advantage to plot out a field defect picked up by a screening device or with conventional kinetic (moving targets) perimetry. Initially, 1-second flashes of subthreshold intensity are employed, and these are increased until a profile of the field defect is uncovered. Any defect in the field of vision is delineated as an area of reduced light sensitivity (see Fig. 15-25).

3. **False.** The nerve fiber bundles first affected usually are 5 to 15 degrees away from fixation. The first defect appears as small isolated scotomas that become larger and denser, eventually fusing to form the sweeping arcuate scotoma. Typically these field defects follow the pattern of the nerve fiber bundle and end abruptly at the horizontal raphe. The raphe corresponds to the 180-degree axis on the field chart.

   The other early field defect is the nasal step. In fact, the very last areas to be afflicted by glaucoma in the visual field are fixation and a small temporal island of vision.

4. **Chiasm.** The only area in the visual system that can produce bitemporal defects is the chiasm. The chiasm is largely composed of crossed nasal fibers, which accounts for the loss of temporal fields of vision. The most common sources of compression of the chiasm are the pituitary gland and its congenital remnants and the hypothalamus. In adults, a tumor called *chromophobe adenoma of the pituitary* is the most likely cause of chiasmal compression, whereas in children the craniopharyngioma, derived from the congenital remnant of the pituitary, frequently is the major source of chiasmal distress. Other lesions that can affect the chiasm include meningiomas, aneurysms, and compression from a swollen third ventricle of the brain. Bitemporal hemianopias are pathognomonic for chiasmal interference, but the causes of such disturbances are myriad.

5. **Visible.** With static perimetry, the stimulus is not moved but rather increased from zero to visibility. This is repeated at 1-degree intervals within the central 15 degrees of the field and at 5-degree intervals in the peripheral field. Approximately 50 stimulus exposures are available along a single meridian. The stimulus size can be varied according to the diagnosis and visual acuity of each person tested. Adequate coverage of the field is provided by scanning along four meridians: 90, 180, 45, and 135 degrees. Static perimetry is regarded as being somewhat more accurate than the kinetic method but is less flexible. It should be noted that the Goldmann perimeter can be equipped to do both static and kinetic perimetry. A major advantage of kinetic perimetry is that it is less time-consuming.

6. **Tubular or contracted field.** The key to a hysterical field is that the field loss is the same size regardless of the distance of the test object from the patient's eye, be it 1 or 2 meters. The tubular field is remarkably constant in size, shape, and steepness or margin. It is commonly found in military personnel attempting to escape duty or in children where it is a device to avoid stress at home or at school.

Hysteria should be separated from malingering, which is a conscious simulation of visual loss and in which the field defect is used for monetary gain. The malingerer overstates the case, and the hysterical person seems indifferent to the disability. The malingerer often is a person involved in litigation, a motor vehicle accident, or an industrial mishap.

The hysterical patient is cooperative and reliable. The malingerer is snarly, hostile, and afraid to be uncovered. This individual often will not complete a test, complaining of lights, headaches, and watering of the eyes.

The discovery of a hysterical patient requires wit, shrewdness, and ingenuity. With the malingerer, the patient views the examiner with hostility and suspicion. The examiner must not only be creative in field testing but also careful lest the patient turn against the perimetrist.

7. **e. All of the above.** Retinitis pigmentosa is a bilateral condition, passed from one generation to another, that causes night blindness and patchy visual loss in a ring pattern in the midperipheral areas of the visual field (around 15 to 45 degrees from fixation). Eventually the rings expand and grow more dense until the patient is looking through tunnels of vision.

The clinical progress of vitamin A deficiency often is indistinguishable from retinitis pigmentosa.

With glaucoma, it is quite common to encounter a double arcuate scotoma that arises from the blind spot and arches above and below the fixation to meet in the nasal field as a ring scotoma. The fact that the blind spot always is involved in the ring serves to distinguish it from retinitis pigmentosa. Also, the two halves of the ring are rarely symmetric, so there is an overlap at the horizontal meridian.

Dr. Stephen Drance suggests that the basic disorder of low-tension glaucoma really is due to an ischemic process of the optic nerve head. Certainly the field defects are quite similar.

8. **a. Smoking pipes and cigars.** The most common cause of bilateral cecocentral scotomas from tobacco is created by pipe and cigar smoking. Most cases develop in elderly men who smoke frequently and use a dark strong leaf. Scotomas are rare in cigarette smokers but have been reported in snuff inhalers and those who chew tobacco. They appear to be a more common condition in northern England and Scotland and are not encountered with great frequency in North America because of different patterns of smoking habits.

9. **d. Central scotoma.** The central scotoma is the most common defect of optic nerve disease because of the predilection of these lesions for the pipillomacular bundle of nerve fibers. Perhaps the most common cause of such optic nerve lesions is multiple sclerosis. Retrobulbar neuritis that creates central scotomas occurs in at least 50% of all cases. It usually is unilateral, although bilateral involvement does occur. The scotoma is most commonly central, but other forms can occur, such as paracentral, pericentral, annular, or cecocentral. The scotomas are quite variable and may be present one day and absent on another.

CHAPTER 17 Automated visual field testing

HOWARD S. BARNEBEY and RICHARD P. MILLS

- Differences between manual and automated perimeters
- Understanding threshold
- Threshold testing
- Units of measure
- Automated perimetry: basic rules of testing
- Test selection

A dramatic revolution is occurring in perimetry. The way visual fields are tested and mapped is significantly different now than it was a few years ago.

In the past the standard of excellence revolved around the Goldmann perimeter and the perimetrist (Fig. 17-1). The visual field was plotted after a lengthy examination during which both kinetic (moving) targets and static (stationary) targets were presented in random fashion. Technicians required extensive training and, perhaps more important, considerable patience to perform this task accurately. They became skilled in testing a glaucomatous patient and knew how to spend the time searching for an abnormality. This approach was different, for example, from that of a neurologic patient suspected of having an occipital lobe tumor. If prior tests were available in this case, they were carefully studied before testing to minimize testing time and also to make sure that the results "made sense." Results became subject to bias of the previous test findings.

The opportunity for biased results quickly became apparent regardless of who performed the test—experienced technician or physician. Testing strategies also contributed to the problem of bias because of the selection and omission of areas of the visual field to be tested.

Other factors contributed to the problems with manual perimetry. Training an ophthalmic assistant or technician in the art of perimetry required months of work. Once technicians became experienced, there still remained variabilities in testing. This was substantiated in several studies in which up to 80% of paracentral scotomas were missed by experienced technicians using manual techniques. It was further detected that the patient's attention for the entire length of the test varied, and this affected the dependability of the results.

The problems with test results changed with the use of the microprocessor and the computer. At first glance, it seemed too easy. The computer was capable of performing the tedious task of testing by presenting targets in a random fashion, analyzing the results, and printing a map of the visual field.

Unfortunately, all the problems were not solved immediately. Automated perimeters were expensive, test strategies were slow to evolve, and data were difficult to understand and interpret. Problems were encountered when an attempt was made to program the perimeter computer to execute the complex ki-

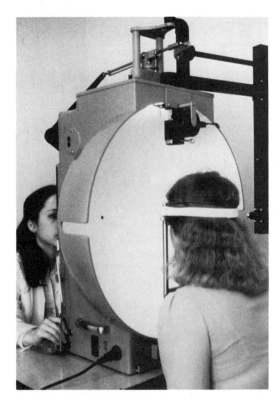

Fig. 17-1 Goldmann perimeter and perimetrist.

netic testing pattern performed by the technician. It was not unusual for the computer to spend 15 to 20 minutes "lost" inside a scotoma attempting to define its borders. When this happened, the computer was unable to complete the test.

Many of the software and hardware problems have since been solved and the automated testing process has been standardized. Kinetic testing has been almost exclusively replaced by static techniques. Infrared and mosaic video cameras now monitor fixation. Patient consistency is constantly evaluated during the test by catch trials designed to elicit false positive and false negative responses.

In spite of these advances, perimetry remains a subjective test. The entire process depends on the patient's ability to understand and respond to the test stimulus. The key person interfacing between the patient and the computer is the technician. It is his

or her responsibility to ensure that the patient understands the test and that the testing process runs smoothly. It is also the responsibility of the technician to ensure that fixation remains aligned, that the patient is given a break, and that the patient is reinstructed if fatigue is observed. No automated perimeter available today has eliminated the need for a technician to administer the test and monitor its quality.

With the advent of automated perimetry, the responsibilities of the technician have changed. Once a test begins, the technician no longer chooses where to project the test target. The task is implemented by the computer. In this chapter the technician's duties will be outlined and, where appropriate, suggestions will be given to make the task easier and more relevant to the patient's needs.

DIFFERENCES BETWEEN MANUAL AND AUTOMATED PERIMETERS

Both manual and automated perimetry ultimately perform the same function: they test the field of vision, but they do so in different ways. Manual devices highlight moving (kinetic) targets to map out the visual field (Fig. 17-2, *A*) and spend less time exploring the field with stationary or static techniques, whereas automated devices depend on static techniques almost exclusively (Fig. 17-2, *B*).

The best way to describe static perimetry is to contrast it with the more familiar kinetic perimetry. The analogy of the visual field to an island of vision sitting amidst a sea of blindness is a useful one (Fig. 17-3). The highest point near the center of the island corresponds to the area of greatest visual sensitivity (for the fovea of the retina). As a person moves toward the water's edge, the sensitivity falls to zero. In other words, the farther away from the area of greatest visual sensitivity a person is, the brighter a light target needs to be to be seen. At water's edge, in the analogy, not even the brightest target can be seen.

The task of perimetry is to map the island of vision. The problem is that the island is enshrouded in a fog bank (Fig. 17-4), and indirect methods of mapping it are required.

Kinetic testing can be likened to airplanes flying toward the visual island at different altitudes (Fig.

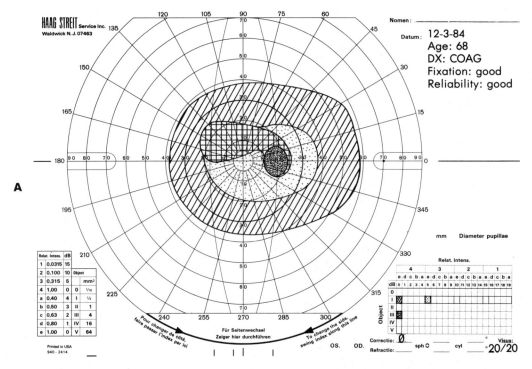

Fig. 17-2 A, Goldmann kinetic visual field. (Courtesy Humphrey Instruments.)

17-5). If we know the altitude at which the planes fly and if we record the coordinates of each "crash site" of many planes flying at the same altitude, then we can draw an "isopter" line connecting the points. With several isopters, the shape of the island unfolds.

There are disadvantages with kinetic techniques. Flat sections of the island are hard to map unless we use many closely spaced isopters. In a similar fashion, hollowed-out valleys in the interior portion of the island are hard to identify, often dependent on our luck in choosing the proper airplane altitude, or isopter, to detect its presence (Fig. 17-6).

Static perimetry uses an entirely different method of visual field exploration. Continuing the analogy, instead of flying airplanes at a known altitude into the island, parachutes are dropped onto the island from above and the altitude where each parachute lands is recorded. Once enough parachutes have landed, a topographic map of the island can be created because the coordinates of each parachute are known (Fig. 17-7). This circumvents the disadvantages associated with kinetic testing techniques, but this method is extremely time-consuming and imposes a practical limitation on the number of points to be tested.

To save testing time, variations on the static theme have been created. The helicopters flying near the island (Fig. 17-8) either land or remain in the air at any specified location. These methods use one of two testing strategies: (1) suprathreshold or (2) threshold-related.

Suprathreshold strategy tests the island of vision starting at a level where the person with normal vision is already expected to see. This may be done at two or three increments of illumination brighter than the patient's expected threshold. Patients report whether they can see the stimulus. Although this

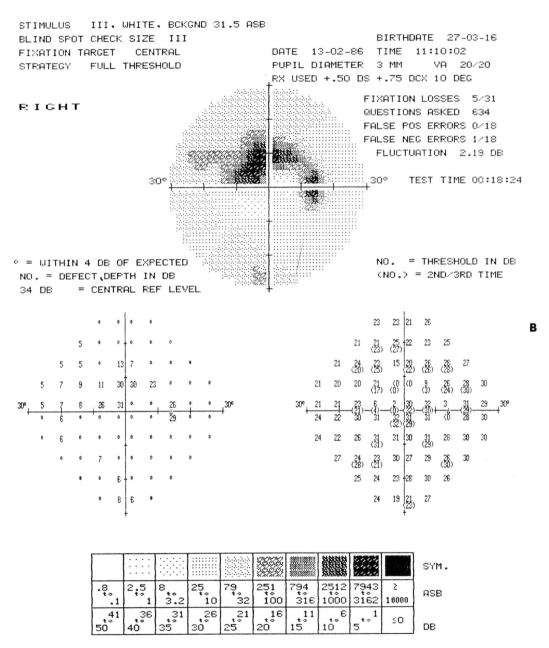

STIMULUS   III, WHITE, BCKGND 31.5 ASB
BLIND SPOT CHECK SIZE   III
FIXATION TARGET   CENTRAL
STRATEGY   FULL THRESHOLD

BIRTHDATE   27-03-16
DATE 13-02-86 TIME 11:10:02
PUPIL DIAMETER 3 MM   VA 20/20
RX USED +.50 DS +.75 DCX 10 DEG

RIGHT

FIXATION LOSSES 5/31
QUESTIONS ASKED 634
FALSE POS ERRORS 0/18
FALSE NEG ERRORS 1/18
FLUCTUATION 2.19 DB

30°   30°   TEST TIME 00:18:24

° = WITHIN 4 DB OF EXPECTED   NO. = THRESHOLD IN DB
NO. = DEFECT,DEPTH IN DB   (NO.) = 2ND/3RD TIME
34 DB   = CENTRAL REF LEVEL

Fig. 17-2, cont'd. B, Same patient examined with use of Humphrey visual field (static technique). (Courtesy Humphrey Instruments.)

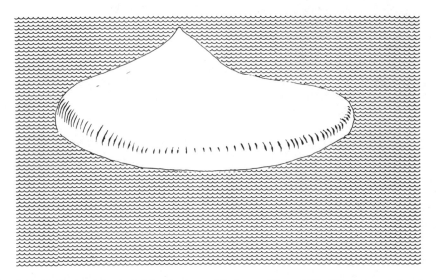

Fig. 17-3 Traquair's island of vision in a sea of darkness. (From Mills RP: Automated perimetry, Part I, *Am Intra-ocular Implant Soc J* 10:347, 1984.)

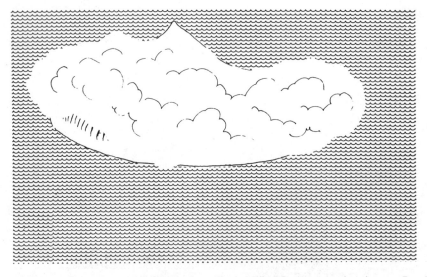

Fig. 17-4 Island of vision enshrouded in fog. (From Mills RP: Automated perimetry, Part I, *Am Intra-ocular Implant Soc J* 10:347, 1984.)

technique is useful in screening large numbers of points rapidly, many levels of illumination are needed to obtain a good idea of the shape of the island. It is easy to waste time if points are not selected wisely.

Threshold-related strategy circumvents this problem. With this technique, threshold static methods (parachutes) are used to obtain a general idea of the height of the island at a few points. Stored in the memory of the computer is a normalized contour of

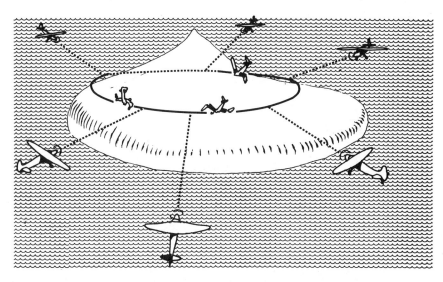

Fig. 17-5 Kinetic mapping of the visual field. (From Mills RP: Automated perimetry, Part I, *Am Intra-ocular Implant Soc J* 10:347, 1984.)

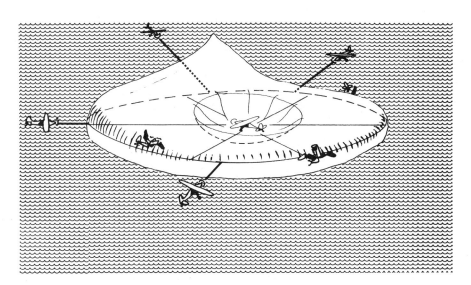

Fig. 17-6 Limitations to kinetic perimetry. (From Mills RP: Automated perimetry, Part I, *Am Intra-ocular Implant Soc J* 10:347, 1984.)

the visual island. Once the general height of the island is estimated from a few initial threshold determinations, the computer can interpolate the normal contour of the island and can project a stimulus slightly brighter than the expected threshold level at each point (Fig. 17-9). On this basis in our analogy, if we know that a helicopter lands or remains in the air, or if the patient responds to or misses the target that is near expected threshold, the information has more meaning and relevance. The test remains brief,

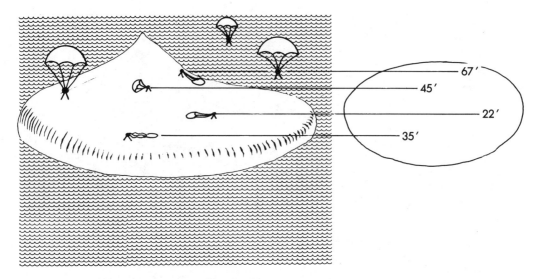

Fig. 17-7 Static mapping of the visual island with parachutes. (From Mills RP: Automated perimetry, Part I, *Am Intra-ocular Implant Soc J* 10:347, 1984.)

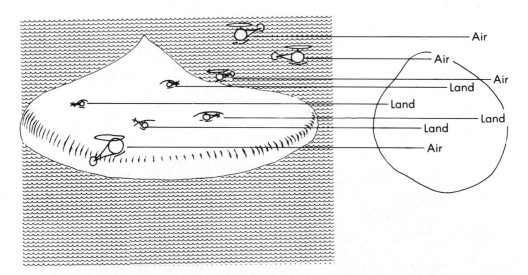

Fig. 17-8 Helicopter method of detecting the visual island's contour. (From Mills RP: Automated perimetry, Part I, *Am Intra-ocular Implant Soc J* 10:347, 1984.)

and fewer tested levels of brightness are required to produce a reasonable view of the island.

UNDERSTANDING THRESHOLD

Threshold is a relative term and represents the level where a stimulus can be seen 50% of the time. This means that the same stimulus also will be missed 50% of the time. Threshold is not an absolute number; rather it is a mathematical approximation described by the sigmoidal curve (Fig. 17-10). As the brightness of the stimulus increases, the likelihood of detecting it becomes higher and higher. This per-

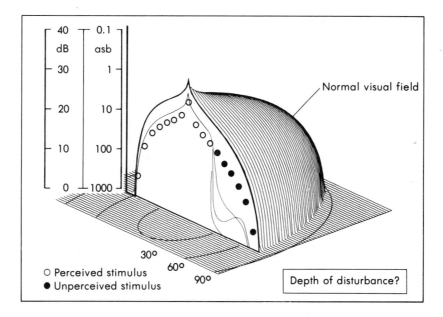

Fig. 17-9 Computer-calculated hill of vision. (From Choplin NT: *Octopus perimetry: a meaningful approach to interpretation, Interzeag AG,* 1985.)

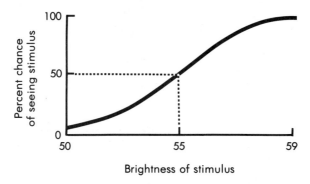

Fig. 17-10 Determination of threshold. (From Mills RP: Automated perimetry, Part I, *Am Intraocular Implant Soc J* 10:347, 1984.)

centage of seeing the stimulus does not approach 100% until it is brighter than threshold. In the example illustrated, a stimulus of 55 brightness is seen half of the time. When the stimulus is increased to 59 brightness, the likelihood of seeing it is 95%—yet it is still missed 5% of the time.

Accurate approximation of threshold requires multiple tests of the same points. Single-test determinations may inaccurately reflect the true threshold based on multiple determinations. For similar reasons, stimuli that are clearly suprathreshold still may be missed on chance alone.

The same variability affects kinetic testing when the patient responds to the same moving target at different eccentricities on multiple presentations. Not only is target illumination a consideration, but so is the actual target motion. The threshold level of seeing a moving test object reflects the patient's

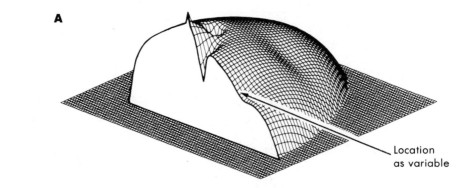

A

Location
as variable

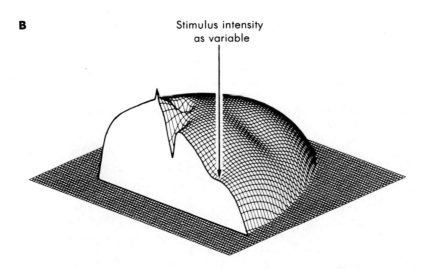

B

Stimulus intensity
as variable

Fig. 17-11 A, Kinetic perimetry: the test variable of stimulus movement. **B,** Static testing: the test variable of stimulus intensity. (From Choplin NT: Octopus perimetry: a meaningful approach to interpretation, *Interzeag AG,* 1985.)

ability to detect movement (Fig. 17-11, *A*). Therefore it may be stated that kinetic testing is affected by threshold considerations but in different ways than static testing (Fig. 17-11, *B*), and visual fields from kinetic and static perimeters cannot be directly and consistently compared.

THRESHOLD TESTING

In threshold testing the actual threshold level for each point tested is measured. Starting with a stimulus brighter than calculated normal threshold, the automated perimeter gradually reduces illumination in

4-decibel (dB) steps until no longer seen. At that point the computer brightens the stimulus in smaller 2-dB steps until the stimulus is seen again (Fig. 17-12). Using the 4-2 staircase technique, the threshold level is crossed at least two times, and the true threshold level is estimated efficiently.

To save time the threshold level start points may be calculated either from prior threshold tests or stored age-corrected normal information. If neither is available, four primary points, one in each quadrant of the field, are tested twice, and the overall level of the hill of vision and then the threshold start

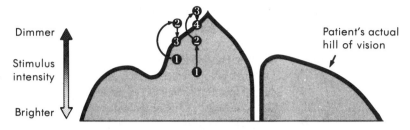

Fig. 17-12 Full threshold strategy determination. (From Haley MJ: *The field analyzer primer,* San Leandro, Calif., 1986, Allergan Humphrey.)

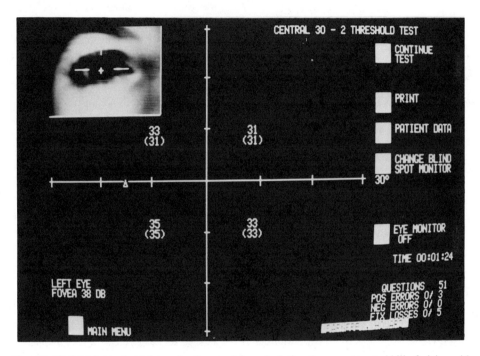

Fig. 17-13 Initial threshold determination used for calculating the age-corrected hill of vision with the Humphrey field analyzer.

point level are extrapolated from these four threshold points (Fig. 17-13).

UNITS OF MEASURE

Goldmann perimetry uses an alphanumeric code to denote target illumination. Each letter step from *a* to *e* represents 0.1 log unit (1 dB) brighter in illumination, and each number step from 1 to 4 is a 0.5 log unit (5 dB) change in intensity. Roman numerals from I to V indicate stimulus size changes and not variation in brightness. Because most automated threshold perimetry uses only intensity and not size changes, the automated devices use a different unit of measure, that is, decibels. The advantages of the Goldmann code are enhanced in decibel nomenclature with its direct logarithmic scale. For example, a 20-dB light source is 10 times brighter than a 10-dB stimulus.

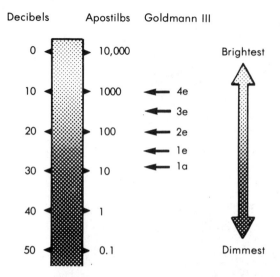

Fig. 17-14 Stimulus intensity scales compared (Humphrey and Goldmann equivalent). (From Haley MJ: *The field analyzer primer,* San Leandro, Calif., 1986, Allergan Humphrey.)

Unfortunately, not all manufacturers have adopted the decibel scale. Some have continued to use the apostilb notation, whereas others have adopted the decibel notation, which is nonlogarithmic. When compared with log units, the two scales are inversely related (Fig. 17-14). Note that 0 dB on the automated devices corresponds to the maximal stimulus intensity, and 0 apostilbs (asb) on the Goldmann refers to absolutely no illumination. Not all automated perimeters produce the same absolute levels of target brightness or use the same level of background illumination. The Octopus perimeters use a dimmer background level of illumination (4 asb) and do not need to produce a target stimulus brighter than 1000 asb. The Humphrey perimeters adopted the traditional Goldmann level of background illumination (31.5 asb); thus they produce a maximum stimulus of 10,000 asb. Other perimeters, such as the Dicon, have several different options for background illumination and use light-emitting diodes (LEDs) for targets instead of a projected target source.

Some perimeters have a maximum stimulus brightness of 1000 asb, and others have the capability to produce 10,000 asb stimuli. Because each machine is different, it is important for both the technician and physician to understand what units of measure are used and the breadth of the scale. In one automated perimeter the brightest possible stimulus, which is 0 dB, corresponds to 10,000 asb, whereas in another one, 0 dB corresponds to 1000 asb.

AUTOMATED PERIMETRY: BASIC RULES OF TESTING
Before the test

Preparing the patient. One of the greatest sources of error is the patient's not knowing what to expect. Even the most experienced kinetic perimetry patient will produce erratic results on static testing unless some education is provided. Therefore the patient must be provided with a rulebook to the game. Many perimeter manufacturers make this job easier by providing a script to read (Fig. 17-15). By using the "patient instruction" command on the monitor, an information outline can be read. Testing seems to be less traumatic if the patient can anticipate what will occur. For example, we know that threshold testing strategy projects stimuli that are visible only half the time. This means that the informed patient should expect to miss about half the presented stimuli.

The operator should share the importance of good fixation by letting the patients know about the telescope or video monitor. Often, simply telling the patient about the TV monitor that the operator watches during the test will minimize fixation losses (Fig. 17-16). If the patient complains of burning or watering of the eye, an artificial tear can be quite comforting.

Remember, do not neglect to patch the other eye!

Finally, the operator must determine whether the patient is fresh and alert. If not, consider rescheduling the test to minimize any patient wait in the office and ask if the patient has a preference for a morning or afternoon appointment. It is surprising how well people know themselves and prefer to schedule a visual field test at their best times.

Using best corrected vision. Another source of frustration and error is not incorporating the proper refractive correction. The visual acuity in each eye should be checked separately before testing, and the

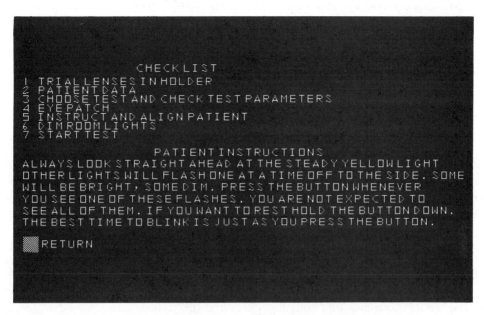

Fig. 17-15 Guide for patient instruction (Humphrey field analyzer).

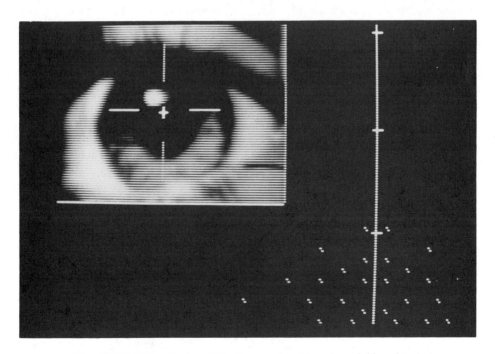

Fig. 17-16 Video display of fixation monitor (Humphrey field analyzer).

patient's medical record should be consulted for the most recent refraction. If one is not available, the technician performs refractometry (if allowed) unless the vision is 20/20. A good rule of thumb is to repeat the refraction if the visual acuity has dropped two lines or more since the last visual field.

Determining the proper trial lens to use

1. Ignore any cylinder less than 1 diopter and instead use the spheroequivalent. (Add +0.25 sphere for each +0.50 cylinder ignored.)

2. Calculate lens power for *near!* This depends on the patient's age and degree of cycloplegia. Not all perimeter bowls have a 33-cm depth; thus consult the manual provided by the manufacturer (Table 17-1).

3. Adjust the lensholder to barely clear the eyelashes (Fig. 17-17).

4. Use narrow-rimmed trial lenses (Fig. 17-18).

5. Remove the lens correction for testing the periphery outside the central 30 degrees.

Having carefully recorded the patient's best visual acuity and incorporated this refraction with the proper trial lenses for near, it is important to check pupil diameter to ensure that it is adequately dilated. Small pupils artificially induce a constricted or narrow visual field, which will return to normal proportions once dilated. It is important to remember that cataracts or corneal scars dramatically affect the field if the pupil is small. Optimal pupil diameter is 2.5 mm or larger.

It is important to check for droopy or ptotic eyelids capable of impinging on the superior portion of the field. Taping the eyelid up with adhesive or paper tape is permissible.

Preparing perimeter. Compared with the manual Goldmann perimeter, for which calibration of the light source and background illuminating light is required daily, the newer automated devices are easy. Most are programmed to automatically self-test and check calibration once the power switch is turned on.

A thorough database must be completed before starting the test on a patient. Each machine differs slightly, but most require the patient's name, including middle initial, birth date, visual acuity, lenses used for the test, and pupil size. The technician must avoid the temptation to skip over this step. It is crucial to properly record the information for interpretation and analysis of test results.

The machine is placed in a dimly lit room away from distracting noise. An adjustable, motorized table seems like a luxury at first, but soon the benefits are obvious. Comfortable and proper alignment for the entire procedure is important (Fig. 17-19). Comfortable chairs for both the patient and technician are needed.

During the test

The patient should not be left alone. Automation has not and never will eliminate the need to have a technician present during the entire test. A 12- to 20-minute field test can seem like an eternity, and fatigue is a common complaint. If you do not believe this, try a field test on yourself. What you will discover firsthand is that the technician feedback is important and encouragement very helpful.

Monitoring fixation. This is a tedious task, but very important. Different fixation devices are integrated into different field machines—some use the manual method with a telescope (Fig. 17-20), others use miniaturized infrared video monitors. Neither method is perfect and not without its problems. It is important that the technician viewing the monitors have patience and skill.

The technician's role changes dramatically once the person is behind the controls of an automated

Table 17-1	Guide for calculating proper near add using a perimeter with a bowl depth of 33 cm
Age	**Add for perimetry**
30-40	+1.00
40-45	+1.50
45-50	+2.00
50-55	+2.50
Over 55	+3.00

Courtesy Humphrey Instruments.

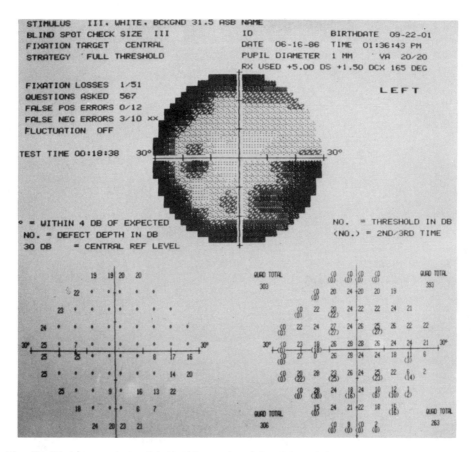

Fig. 17-17 Automated visual field with pseudoperipheral field defect created by lens holder and lens positioned too far from eye.

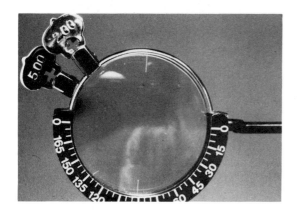

Fig. 17-18 Narrow-rimmed trial lenses.

perimeter. It is tempting for the technician to turn on, tune out, and completely disengage from the test. No one will know. As long as the perimeter keeps marching along and the patient keeps on pressing the buzzer, no one can really determine how attentive the technician really was. The computer does not know if really the technician is monitoring fixation. Yet, much like a pilot, the perimetrist needs to constantly scan the control panel, interpret information, and make adjustments. For example, pleasant 91-year-old Mrs. Johnson looks as if she is dozing off for a nap. This is understandable inasmuch as the test has taken nearly 18 minutes and is almost complete. It is important to stop the test, arouse Mrs.

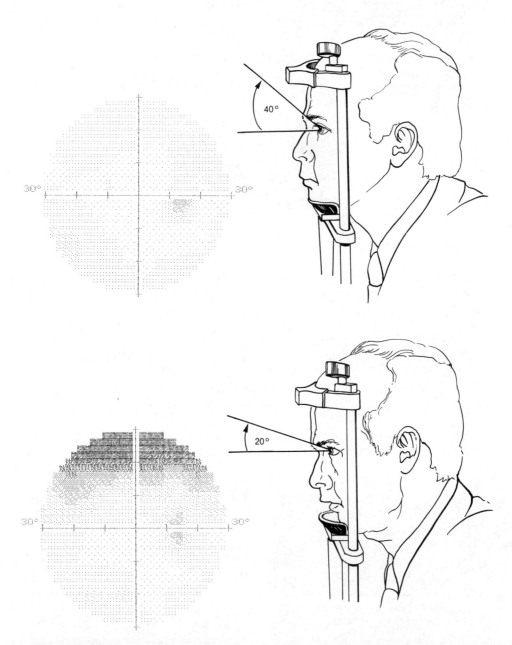

Fig. 17-19 Proper positioning of the patient minimizes artifacts such as illustrated here, where depression of the superior visual field is exaggerated because of incorrect patient alignment. (From Anderson DR: *Perimetry: with and without automation,* St Louis, 1987, Mosby.)

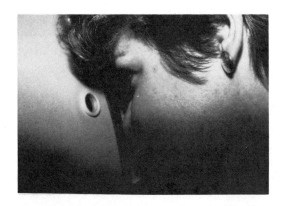

Fig. 17-20 Watching fixation via telescope (Dicon 2000).

Johnson, encourage her that the test is nearly completed, and perhaps even give her a brief break before finishing. Once done, it is equally important to note on the hard copy printout that Mrs. Johnson fatigued easily.

Choosing the best strategy. Initially the task of choosing the proper and best testing strategy is puzzling to both physician and technician. Many options are available—screening or threshold and short or long.

Two important precepts are important to recognize. One is that experience has dictated that only a handful of test strategies will be used on a regular basis. Glaucoma patients almost uniformly require a threshold 30-degree central field. If the Dicon is being used, then the selection is the central 25-degree threshold strategy. For the Humphrey Field Analyzer it is the 30-2 program, and for the Octopus 500E, it is the 38 or G1 program.

The second precept is to determine what question the field test is expected to answer. The test could be part of a large population screening study, or it could be looking for a specific problem—chloroquine maculopathy, for example. In most cases the physician will need to answer this question to direct the test and choice of strategy.

In the box at right is a guide that we have felt comfortable using. This can be a starting place to establish a set of criteria for a visual field protocol. The technician whose particular instrument is not listed

can review the possible testing programs and select the most similar ones available to fulfill individual needs.

Monitoring the test

Fixation. Different machines monitor fixation differently, but generally, fixation is recorded in a similar fashion—the number of fixation losses are relative to the number of fixation checks. Some perimeters will retest those spots evaluated just before the fixation loss, whereas others will simply note the loss and beep, and then continue with the test.

False positive. This is a measure of the patient's understanding of the test. Often, a click of the shutter opening is heard just before the light stimulus is flashed on. Patients may respond to the click and not the light. To evaluate this potential source of error, the computer will randomly click open the shutter but will not turn on the light. If the patient responds to the noise, then a false positive response is indicated. The more frequent number of false positive errors encountered, the less valid the visual field results.

False negative. This parameter attempts to quantify the patient's alertness during the test. During the test program, the computer will retest spots where the stimulus was previously seen. The retesting uses the brightest possible illumination. Thus, if the patient does not respond to the brighter light, then the assumption is made that the patient was not alert at that particular point to respond. Again, a high ratio of false negative responses to a number of false

---

GUIDE TO PROGRAM SELECTION

GENERAL SCREENING: FULL FIELD SUPRA-THRESHOLD
Humphrey/Dicon: 120 point full field
Octopus 500E: Program 07
GLAUCOMA, GLAUCOMA SUSPECT: CENTRAL THRESHOLD
Dicon 2500: Central 25-degree threshold
Humphrey: 30-2
Octopus 500E: Program 38 or G1

negative tests indicates a potentially serious problem with test reliability.

Fluctuation. Patient consistency is checked if a threshold test is done. Threshold is determined twice at multiple points during the examination. It is anticipated that there will be some variation of results at different times during the test because of the inherent variability of threshold measurement. This is calculated mathematically, and a number is generated to indicate the patient's short-term fluctuation. Low short-term fluctuation numbers suggest that the patient is highly consistent during the entire test period, whereas larger numbers imply less consistence and more variable responses. Please note that some disease processes may adversely affect fluctuation and produce a higher number. Thus, increased short-term fluctuation is not necessarily a reflection of a patient's inability to perform a reliable test but may also be an indicator of disease.

TEST SELECTION

As previously mentioned, it is important for each office to develop an office protocol dealing with test selection. This enables the office assistant to select and to perform the proper visual field examination.

New testing strategies evolve and provide advantages worthy of consideration. For example, one new test available for use with the Humphrey Field Analyzer significantly reduces the test time required to perform a threshold central examination. This test is called "FastPac" and clearly provides the inexperienced patient, or the patient with limited attention span, an opportunity to complete a threshold examination in a much shorter time period. The assistant and physician, however, need to recognize that using the faster test limits the computer's ability to interpret multiple sequential visual fields performed on a glaucoma patient. Powerful statistical packages, such as Statpac 2, are programmed only to analyze the traditional threshold central tests.

The point for all assistants to recognize is that along with the benefits of new tests, some limitations can be expected. The dynamics of these new test strategies are evolving rapidly as manufacturers address the problems of current visual field testing.

SUMMARY

It should be apparent that automated perimetry is here to stay. The power of the computer to perform redundant and complex tasks frees the perimetrist to perform better visual field tests than before. The key component is not the computer or sophisticated software programs; rather the key component continues to be the technician. Initial fears that computers would eliminate the need for a qualified ophthalmic assistant or technician are unfounded. There is no computerized perimeter currently available with enough artificial intelligence to replace the well-trained and knowledgeable perimetrist. The role of the perimetrist is continuing to evolve as the automated perimeter eases many aspects of testing. As this occurs, the attention of the technician is now directed toward other areas. In particular, the perimetrist has more time for guiding and encouraging the patient through the testing procedure.

Automated refractors can be as useful and reliable as manual refractors used by skilled technicians. Many clinicians feel that automated fields may be even more reliable than manual field examinations in that an important variable is eliminated, that is, the visual field technician. For patients whose attention span or understanding is weak, however, manual perimetry may be required. Such patients as the aged, children, and patients with decreased levels of consciousness, ptosis, or posture abnormalities may be suitable candidates for manual perimetry.

In the past decade, many new automated refractors have appeared in the marketplace and have been valuable in suprathreshold and threshold static perimetry, with detection rates as high as 90% to 98% and false positive findings of only 5% to 10%. Interpretation of field test results requires careful analysis for proper diagnostic interpretation.

CHAPTER 18 Ocular injuries

- Diagnosis of ocular injury
- Conjunctival and corneal foreign bodies
- Intraocular foreign bodies
- Contusion of the eyelids: black eye
- Contusions of the globe
- Penetrating eye injuries
- Lacerations of the lids
- Fractures of the orbit
- Chemical injuries
- Injuries caused by sports
- Injuries caused by radiant energy
- Prevention of traumatic injuries to the eye
- First-aid care by the ophthalmic assistant

The ophthalmic assistant should have knowledge in the prevention of eye accidents and the first-aid therapy of trauma both in industry and at home. Reports from the National Society for the Prevention of Blindness reveal that ocular injury is responsible for 5% of all blindness in children of both school and preschool age. Many athletic activities, including racquet sports, boxing, and hockey, carry the risk of visual casualties. Industrial eye injuries are virtually a daily occurrence in every ophthalmologist's office and in every emergency center of a hospital. The escalation of traumatic eye injuries is partly attributable to the progress achieved in the field of transportation, to the development of potentially dangerous consumer home products and children's toys, and to advancements in industrial mechanization, without corresponding advances in personal safety devices. Only in large industrial plants have safety programs been inaugurated to detect visual disabilities and to prevent eye accidents. From the

industrial safety organizations have sprouted the Wise Owl clubs in the United States, now numbering 26,000. Members are employees who have had one or both eyes saved from a serious injury by the use of protective lenses.

Despite rigid precautionary safety measures, however, eye accidents will continue to occur because of carelessness, chance, and the tendency of people to ignore the safety measures provided for them.

This chapter deals with first-aid therapy of eye injuries and preventive measures to help reduce the loss of vision from trauma.

DIAGNOSIS OF OCULAR INJURY

The diagnosis of an eye injury can be determined by a careful history of the injury in relation to the time and type of injury. A history of discomfort and the reduction in vision may indicate the severity of injury. Objective signs require careful external examination that includes comparison with the unaffected eye. Pressure in separating the eyelids should never be exerted, but the upper lid should be pushed up against the bone under the eyebrow and the lower lid depressed with pressure only on the bone of the cheek below. All injuries to the globe, until proved otherwise, should be examined as if the globe has been ruptured. If magnification is required, a ×2 loupe or slit lamp microscope can detect areas of damage not otherwise discovered.

CONJUNCTIVAL AND CORNEAL FOREIGN BODIES

Despite the many anatomic and physiologic protective factors around the eye, nearly everyone at one time or another has had a foreign body in the eye. In most instances the ensuing tearing and blinking of the lids have been sufficient to dislodge the irritant. It is when these natural mechanisms fail to remove a foreign body that one has to have it located and removed (Figs. 18-1 and 18-2).

When a foreign body has lodged in the cornea, examination should always begin by determining the patient's best corrected visual acuity of the injured eye with glasses on or with the addition of a pinhole disk if the vision is reduced. In this way any preexisting visual impairment will not be attributed to the trauma and removal of the foreign body. In taking the history, the examiner should attempt to ascertain the source of the fragment, because the type of foreign body will influence the amount of tissue destruction and rate of repair. Particles of copper and brass are notoriously more irritating to the eye than iron and steel. High-velocity foreign bodies—that is, those catapulted by hammering, chiseling, or lathing—are prone to penetrate the cornea deeply or even to perforate it, as opposed to the windblown particle that embeds itself in the superficial corneal epithelium.

It usually is expedient to place two or three drops of a local anesthetic, such as proparacaine hydrochloride (Ophthaine, Ophthetic) or tetracaine hydrochloride (Pontocaine), into the lower conjunctival sac to facilitate surface anesthesia. This makes the patient more comfortable and allows the examiner to scrutinize the injured eye with ease. The best instrument for examining the cornea is the slit lamp

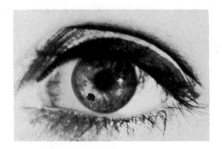

Fig. 18-1 Embedded corneal foreign body.

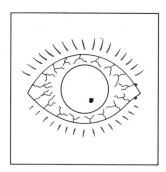

Fig. 18-2 Redness, foreign-body sensation, and photophobia occur in the presence of a corneal foreign body. (From Stein HA, Slatt BJ, Stein RM: *A primer in ophthalmology: a textbook for students,* St Louis, 1992, Mosby.)

microscope because it offers simultaneously high magnification and strong focal illumination. A useful alternative is an ordinary electric light or flashlight placed about 30 inches from the patient and slightly below the level of the eyes. The light can then be brought into focus on the eye by means of a condensing lens. Magnification is obtained with the use of jewelers' loupes or other types of binocular magnifying glasses. If a foreign body cannot be seen, a strip of fluorescein paper can be placed in the eye to stain the surface of the cornea inasmuch as foreign bodies become visible when surrounded by the stain. If the foreign body has become dislodged by the patient's blinking and tearing, the fluorescein will settle in the resultant corneal defect. In many cases the cornea will show many surface scratches, and the foreign body will be located on the undersurface of the upper or lower lid. Routinely, an examination

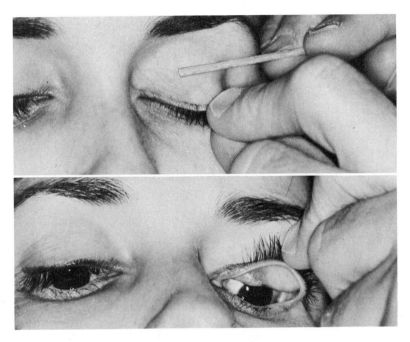

Fig. 18-3 Eversion of the upper eyelid over an applicator.

of the palpebral conjunctiva lining both the upper and lower lids should be performed. Inspection of the conjunctiva lining the lower lid is carried out simply by depressing the lower lid. The undersurface of the upper lid is examined by everting it. The patient is asked to look down while the eyelashes are grasped and pulled over a glass rod, toothpick, or tightly wound cotton swab (Fig. 18-3). Alternatively, this examination can be accomplished by everting the upper lid over a transilluminator or muscle light. The foreign body usually is revealed as an opaque speck in the red glow of the lid tissue.

The treatment of corneal foreign bodies is total removal. A superficial foreign body often can be dislodged by a gentle stream of saline solution delivered from an irrigator, or it can be wiped off by a tightly bound cotton toothpick swab. If these measures fail, the foreign body must be lifted from its base by the use of a corneal spud (Fig. 18-4) or burr (Fig. 18-5), preferably under magnification by a slit lamp microscope.

After a period of 6 to 8 hours a metallic foreign body may result in the formation of a rust ring in the corneal tissue (Fig. 18-6). This rust spot is much more difficult to remove because it becomes adherent to the surrounding corneal stroma. The tenacity of the rust is so great that often the corneal spud will only fragment the rusted spot. In such cases it is wise to have a corneal burr on hand to remove the rust ring completely (Fig. 18-7). Small dental drills make excellent corneal burrs. Some ophthalmologists advocate patching an eye that has a rust ring for approximately 24 hours because the slight necrosis of the tissue that results enables easier extraction.

Once the foreign body has been removed, a patch is placed over the affected eye. Adhesive tape applied firmly is used to keep the patch tight against the eyelid. The purpose of the patch is to immobilize the eyelid, thus allowing the corneal epithelium to regenerate without irritation from a moving eyelid. It is important that the patch remain firm to keep the eyelid from blinking. The patient should be advised to avoid excessive eye movements. If the tape securing the patch becomes loose, the patient should be told to refasten it. Most corneal defects that are

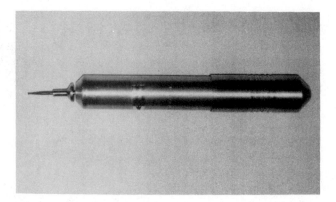

Fig. 18-4 Foreign-body burr for removing a corneal foreign body.

treated in this manner will be adequately repaired within 24 hours. If the foreign body is organic (for example, a fingernail, a piece of wood, or a piece of paper), corneal repair may take as long as 3 or 4 days. Most ophthalmologists tend to use antibiotic drops or ointment before applying an eye patch.

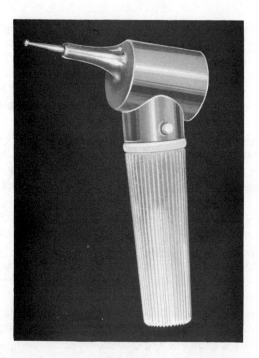

Fig. 18-5 Rotating burr for removal of deeply embedded corneal foreign bodies and rust rings.

A corneal foreign body should be treated as an ocular emergency. It is desirable but not mandatory that the foreign body be removed as soon after the mishap as possible. If there are extenuating circumstances, however, such as the ophthalmologist's being involved in surgery, the injured eye should receive some antibiotic drops and be firmly patched until it is seen. It is imperative, however, to relieve the patient's symptoms. The discomfort of a corneal foreign body can be intense. Satisfactory relief of pain can be obtained with compounds that contain codeine. The patient should never be given a local anesthetic ointment or drops to take home, because local anesthetics only interfere with wound healing and mask complications.

If the foreign body becomes dislodged by the forceful and frequent blinking activity of the lids and the profusion of tears, the patient may still feel that something is in the eye. This is because injury to the cornea, whether it is caused by inflammation, a foreign body, or an abrasion, yields the same symptom—a foreign body sensation.

Conjunctival foreign bodies do not, as a rule, give rise to pain or discomfort in the eye. If they lodge in the bulbar conjunctiva, they usually are easily visible because of the white background of the underlying sclera. Superficial conjunctival foreign bodies are removed either by the application of a moistened cotton-tipped applicator or by gentle irrigation with saline solution. If there is some blood around the foreign body, the ophthalmic assistant

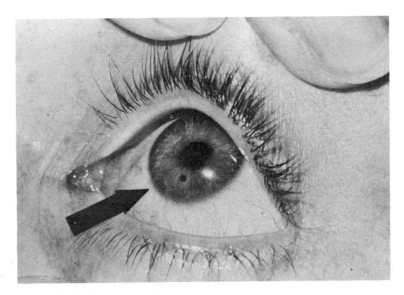

Fig. 18-6 Rust ring of the cornea.

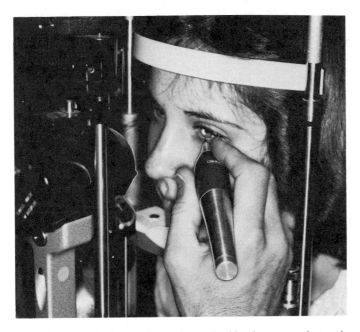

Fig. 18-7 Removal of corneal rust ring under biomicroscope observation.

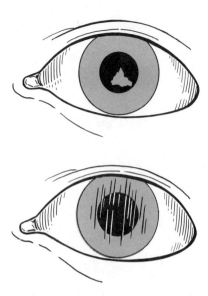

Fig. 18-8 Corneal abrasions.

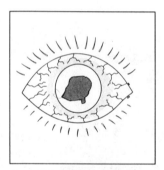

Fig. 18-9 Corneal abrasion is characterized by ciliary injection and an epithelial defect (which stains with fluorescein). (From Stein HA, Slatt BJ, Stein RM: *A primer in ophthalmology: a textbook for students,* St Louis, 1992, Mosby.)

should be aware that penetration of the eye may have occurred.

Corneal abrasions

Corneal abrasions are superficial scratches and erosions of the cornea (Fig. 18-8). They are found after corneal foreign bodies have been removed, either spontaneously or with treatment. They are most commonly found after injuries caused by paper, fingernails, wires, and so forth. A corneal abrasion,

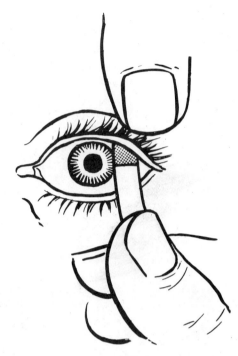

Fig. 18-10 Application of moistened fluorescein paper strip. Some practitioners find the lower cul-de-sac easier to use.

unless it is large, cannot be seen with the naked eye. Patients with a corneal abrasion complain of a foreign body sensation of the eye. Often these patients are seen by a nurse or a friend and told that there is nothing in their eye, and as a result they suffer until they are finally seen by the ophthalmologist. Any patient who complains of a foreign body sensation of the eye should be seen. Fluorescein strips should be placed in the eye (Figs. 18-9 and 18-10) to stain the area of the corneal defect, and the eye should be examined with magnifying glasses. Corneal abrasions are treated by firm patching for 24 hours.

Aftercare of patients with superficial injuries

The following points summarize the aftercare of a patient with a superficial corneal and conjunctival injury:

1. Arrangements should be made to have the patient driven home.

2. The patient should be warned that discomfort

in the eye may occur an hour or two after office treatment. This is the length of time that the local anesthetic given in the office usually remains effective. If a feeling of irritation continues, the patient should be instructed to take some pain-relieving drug.

3. The patient should be instructed not to remove the patch until he or she is seen again. Medication other than some general analgesics should not be given. The patient also should be told that it is best to return home and rest. Movements of the cheeks, such as in talking, only serve to loosen the patch and free the eyelid. A blinking lid causes pain and removes the regenerated epithelium.

4. The patient should be seen the following day and daily when necessary. Corneal abrasions caused by organic agents may take longer to heal and may require further attention. The rate of healing depends on the area of the tissue injured, the amount of tissue devitalized, the presence or absence of infection, and the nature of the injuring agent.

INTRAOCULAR FOREIGN BODIES

Intraocular foreign bodies constitute a surgical emergency. Often the site of penetration is not visible externally (Fig. 18-11). The ophthalmic assistant should not make a judgment on the gravity of a foreign body injury on the basis of the external appearance of the eye.

Because the severity of the intraocular damage depends on the size, shape, and composition of the foreign body, the assistant should attempt to obtain an accurate description of the nature of the type of metal embedded. Often it is possible to obtain the source of the fragment. This is very important because the success of the operative procedure depends to a large extent on whether or not the fragment is magnetic. The patient should be reassured that everything possible will be done but should not be promised a full recovery of the eye, because vision inasmuch as eyes that are injured by foreign bodies, particularly those lodged in the posterior pole (that is, in the retina or vitreous), often do poorly.

The ophthalmic assistant can serve the patient best by making sure that this type of injury is seen by the attending ophthalmologist immediately. Dispatch

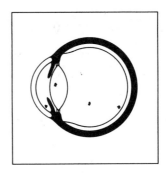

Fig. 18-11 Intraocular foreign bodies can be found in a variety of sites: in the anterior chamber, lens, vitreous, or retina. (From Stein HA, Slatt BJ, Stein RM: *A primer in ophthalmology: a textbook for students,* St Louis, 1992, Mosby.)

of the patient to the hospital should be smooth and comfortable. Relatives should be notified, and the hospital, particularly the operating room personnel, should be informed of the emergency. Transportation to the hospital should be arranged so that the patient is not kept waiting in the office. The patient's eye should be patched, primarily to prevent the patient from causing further damage to the eye by rubbing it or by cleaning it with a dirty handkerchief.

The ophthalmic assistant should always be aware of the possibility of the presence of an intraocular foreign body. Intraocular foreign bodies usually are high-velocity small missiles and should be suspected in accidents in which striking, grinding, or cutting force is applied to metal. Fast-moving particles may penetrate the eye without producing any pain, discomfort or gross visible signs and yet still may cause severe damage to the eye. Fig. 18-12 shows an air pellet in the eye that passed through the upper eyelid.

CONTUSION OF THE EYELIDS: BLACK EYE

A black eye is the result of an injury to the orbital margin or eyelids from a blunt object, such as a fist (Fig. 18-13). The appearance of a black eye is quite alarming to the patient because of the large extravasation of the blood underneath the skin. A patient with this type of injury should be seen immediately because examination of the globe is easiest in the

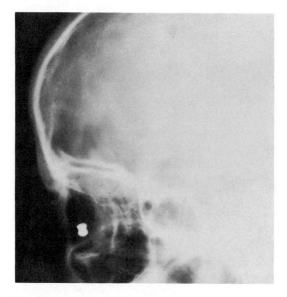

Fig. 18-12 Intraocular foreign body. Air pellet entry into the globe.

immediate period following the injury. After a period of 1 or 2 hours the lids become so swollen and taut that examination of the underlying eye becomes very difficult. Treatment of a black eye is the application of cold compresses in the immediate phase to reduce the swelling and the use of local analgesics to relieve the pain. Usually within a period of 5 to 7 days the swelling subsides, and the hematoma changes in color, gradually fading away as the blood decomposes underneath the skin. Although a black eye is quite innocuous, the secondary contusion to the globe can cause considerable disruption within the eye. The effects of contusion to the globe include traumatic hyphema, dislocated lens, vitreous hemorrhage, and tears in the choroid and retina. A black

eye also may be associated with a broken nose because the bones between the orbit and the nose are extremely thin. Consequently, an abnormal communication may arise between the nose and the soft tissues of the lids. When the nose is blown, air may be forced under the pressure into the lids, causing swelling and the development of a curious crackling feeling that is felt under the skin. Because there is a risk of spreading infection from the nose into the orbit and eyelids, the patient should be instructed not to blow the nose forcefully. Frequently a blow to the lids and globe is sufficiently strong to cause a blow-out fracture of the orbit. The muscles on the inferior surface of the globe, the inferior rectus, and the inferior oblique muscles may become incarcerated in the defect in the floor of the orbit, and the eye cannot be elevated. The patient complains of diplopia, especially when looking up. These cases are treated surgically by freeing the wedged muscles and placing an implant of bone or plastic over the fracture site. The results of surgical repair are best when the patient is treated early.

CONTUSIONS OF THE GLOBE

Contusions of the globe may be caused by an explosive force such as an air blast, a blow to the bony orbit, or direct injury to the eye itself. Initially the effects of a blow to the eye can be disastrous because perforation of the globe—with prolapse of the intraocular contents, vitreous hemorrhage, retinal detachment, and rupture of the choroid—may occur as an immediate complication. If the hemorrhage is confined to the anterior chamber, it is called a *hyphema*. If the hemorrhage involves the posterior chamber as well, it is referred to as a *black-ball hemorrhage*. In the event that the initial injury

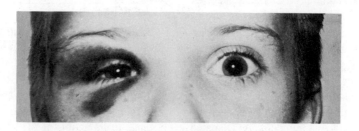

Fig. 18-13 Contusions of the eyelids with ecchymosis.

to the eye appears to be minimal, loss of vision can result from complications occurring later, for example, glaucoma, cataract, and sympathetic ophthalmia.

Early complications

Early complications of contusion injuries include (1) subconjunctival hemorrhage, (2) hyphema (hemorrhage into the anterior chamber) (Fig. 18-14), (3) iris involvement (iridodialysis, or separation of the iris at its base), tears of the sphincter muscle and iritis, (4) glaucoma, secondary to iritis or hyphema,

(5) dislocation of the lens, (6) vitreous hemorrhage, (7) retinal tears, detachment, and hemorrhage, (8) choroidal rupture, (9) scleral rupture, and (10) avulsion of the optic nerve.

Of the early complications, injury to the anterior segment of the eye is the most frequent because it receives the greater proportion of the force of injury. Frequently the injuries to the eye are multiple, the most common of which are tears either at the root or at the pupillary margin of the iris, combined with a hyphema (Fig. 18-15).

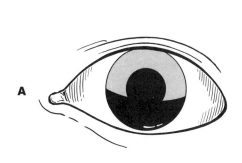
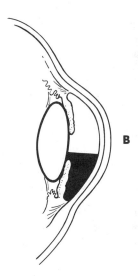

Fig. 18-14 Hyphema, or hemorrhage in the anterior chamber. **A,** Front view. **B,** Side view.

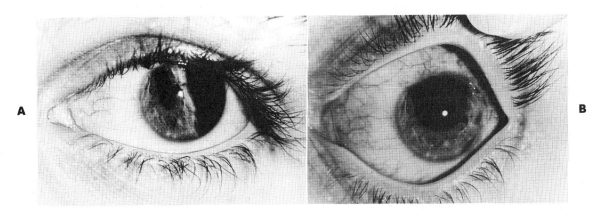

Fig. 18-15 A, Iris sector loss with iridodialysis from globe injury. Double vision and cosmetically poor. **B,** After iris repair.

Late complications

Late complications of contusions of the globe include (1) glaucoma, which may appear many years after the original injury, (2) sympathetic ophthalmia, (3) cataract, (4) band keratitis, and (5) phthisis bulbi (shrunken and disorganized eyeball).

Of the late complications, *sympathetic ophthalmia* is most feared. It occurs in the *noninjured eye* when the injured eye has had extensive damage to the iris and ciliary body. Sympathetic ophthalmia takes at least 2 weeks to appear, being most common 2 months after injury. It may even take 6 months to a year before it manifests. The early symptoms of this condition are slight pain, photophobia, lacrimation, disturbances in accommodation, and diminution in vision in the unaffected eye. This condition often leads to extensive loss of vision and even blindness despite treatment with steroids. For this reason many surgeons will enucleate a blind, disorganized injured eye within 2 weeks of the injury to avoid this dreaded complication of sympathetic ophthalmia. Enucleation after 2 weeks has no prophylactic value once the condition has commenced.

PENETRATING EYE INJURIES

Recognition of penetrating injuries is most important because prompt treatment may result in complete or partial recovery of vision. However, the examiner must be very careful not to press on the globe in trying to separate the eyelids. If blepharospasm exists and the eye does not open readily, it is best to leave the problem alone until the ophthalmologist arrives. Any medication instilled in the eye to relieve pain and blepharospasm should be administered only on the instruction of the attending physician, and the medication should have proper dating and be sterile.

Identification of a penetrating eye injury may be made by the following:

1. Black or brown uveal tissue showing through the white sclera
2. Iris protruding from the lips of a laceration of the cornea
3. Flat anterior chamber with collapse of the front portion of the eye
4. Irregularly shaped pupil
5. Any localized tears or holes in the iris

6. Purulent or cloudy material within the eye

The "management" of a penetrating eye injury is beyond the scope of an ophthalmic assistant. It will depend on the nature and severity of the injury, as well as the site of the injury. The ultimate concerns are the restoration of the functional capability of the injured eye to see again and the protection of the normal fellow eye from sympathetic ophthalmia.

LACERATIONS OF THE LIDS

Lacerations of the lids should be seen immediately. A delay of 6 to 8 hours in repairing a lid laceration may result in serious infection. A wound is considered contaminated if it is not closed within 6 to 8 hours after injury. Early surgery enables the surgeon to restore the tissues to their original position with greater accuracy than can be done if retraction and swelling of the tissues have been allowed to develop. Normally the ophthalmologist will prepare the patient by administering an injection of a broad-spectrum antibiotic and some tetanus toxoid or tetanus antiserum. The ophthalmic assistant should keep these materials on hand for such a contingency.

Lacerations of the eyelid are caused by explosive injuries, deflected high-velocity metal or wood, blunt objects such as the dashboard or steering wheel of a car, and careless play with knives, especially in children. Lid lacerations can involve any site on the upper or lower eyelid. In the upper eyelid the major structure that is disrupted by a large, through-and-through laceration is the levator palpebrae superioris muscle. Damage to this muscle and its subsequent retraction (Fig. 18-16) may result in post-

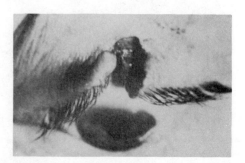

Fig. 18-16 Vertical lacerations of the upper eyelid.

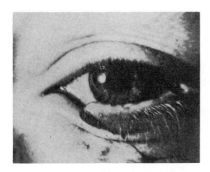

Fig. 18-17 Laceration of the lower canaliculus.

traumatic ptosis. In the lower eyelid the delicate canaliculus on the medial aspect of the lower eyelid may be severed (Fig. 18-17). Permanent tearing will result unless accurate apposition of the cut ends is immediately performed. Other complications of lid lacerations include notched lid margins, entropion, and ectropion.

In all major wounds to the lids or globe the ophthalmic assistant can best serve the patient by patching the eye with a clean patch and notifying the attending ophthalmologist immediately of the mishap.

FRACTURES OF THE ORBIT

Direct injury to the eye, as by a blow, a golf ball, or a piece of equipment, may result in a fracture of the orbital rim or wall (Fig. 18-18). Two types of fractures may occur. One type involves the bony rim of the orbit, along with part of the wall of the orbit, and usually is readily detected by x-ray film. A less commonly detected fracture is that of a blow-out fracture of the orbital floor. Any direct blow to the eye may drive the globe back into the orbit, where a sudden transfer of pressure to the thin orbital wall occurs. The weakest part of the orbital wall fractures relatively easily because the walls are adjacent to air-containing sinuses and are not supported by heavy fluids or tissue. Whenever a black eye is seen, a blow-out fracture of the floor of the orbit should be suspected, particularly if diplopia occurs in any direction of gaze. The diplopia is a result of entrapment of the inferior muscles that support the globe. Muscle-balance testing, along with x-ray tomograms of the floor of the orbit, will bring this defect to light. Surgical repair of an orbital fracture depends on the computed tomography (CT) scan findings or the clinical signs during the subsequent few days, or both. Surgery is indicated if there is soft tissue entrapment.

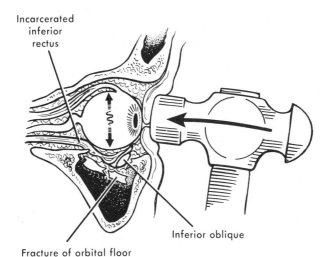

Incarcerated inferior rectus

Inferior oblique

Fracture of orbital floor

Fig. 18-18 Mechanism of blow-out fracture of the orbit. A blow on the eye causes internal pressure on the delicate floor of the orbit, resulting in a fracture. The inferior oblique and inferior rectus muscles may herniate into the maxillary sinus below.

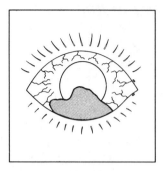

Fig. 18-19 Depending on the type and severity, signs of chemical injury may include conjunctivitis, superficial punctate keratitis, epithelial defects of the cornea and conjunctiva, blanching of blood vessels, and necrosis of tissues. (From Stein HA, Slatt BJ, Stein RM: *A primer in ophthalmology: a textbook for students*, St Louis, 1992, Mosby.)

CHEMICAL INJURIES

Alkali injuries often are more severe than acid injuries, because acids tend to coagulate tissue and inhibit further penetration into the cornea. Clinical findings of chemical injury vary with severity of the injury: a mild injury is characterized by conjunctivitis, superficial punctate keratitis, and an epithelial defect of the cornea and conjunctiva; a severe injury exhibits blanching of limbal blood vessels and opacification of the cornea (Fig. 18-19).

Acids

The acids used extensively in industry are sulfuric, hydrochloric, nitric, and acetic. In small quantity, either as fumes or as a fine spray, these acids can cause injury to the eye. The injury is minimal, with redness, watering, and irritation of the lids and conjunctiva occurring. With repeated or prolonged exposure, small erosions on the surface of the cornea may result. A copious splash of an acid can produce an extensive burn of the face and eyelids, in addition to serious local damage to the eye itself. Acid burns frequently are complicated by glass injuries as a result of flasks and bottles bursting. These injuries arise particularly in laboratories associated with industries, schools, research establishments, and universities.

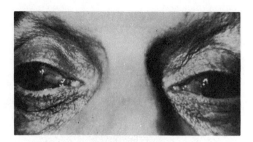

Fig. 18-20 Alkali burn of the eyes.

Alkalis

Sodium, potassium, ammonium, and calcium hydroxide are the common alkalis involved in burns in industry. In general, alkali burns are more serious and penetrate the eye more deeply than do acid burns (Fig. 18-20). In the home, ammonia is a common cause of corneal burns because it is used extensively as a cleaning material. It also is used in domestic refrigerating apparatus. Calcium hydroxide, or lime, burns are perhaps the most common alkali burns to the eye. Lime burn may occur whenever cements, mortars, whitewash, and plaster are used. The severity of lime burns is related to the fact that the alkali becomes adherent to the corneal and conjunctival tissues and produces chemical reactions between its products and the tissue proteins.

First-aid care

Because the degree of damage done to the cornea or conjunctiva is directly proportional to the concentration of the chemical at the time of injury and to the duration in which the chemical is in contact with the eye, it is vitally important to dilute the chemical and to start therapy as soon as possible. Water is the most nearly universal solvent; it also is the most universally available cleansing liquid in industrial establishments. It should be used abundantly and quickly. If there are no special irrigating facilities available in the plant, the patient's eye should be irrigated with water in a pail, glass, or any other available container. The personnel in charge of first aid should separate the lids to overcome the lid spasm and to allow the water to irrigate the conjunctiva and cornea. Separation of the lid is

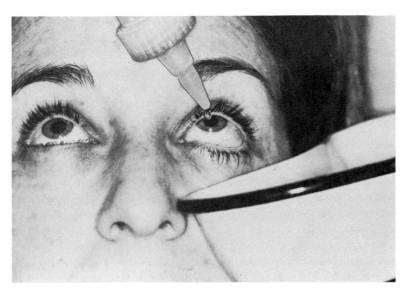

Fig. 18-21 Irrigation for chemical burn of the eye.

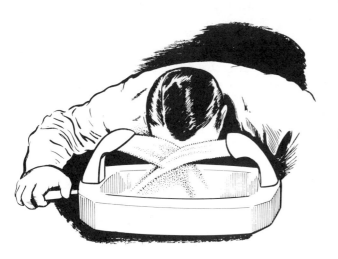

Fig. 18-22 Irrigation of the eye by a jet fountain.

difficult to maintain and is best accomplished by using a paper towel and pressing the lids on the bony prominences above and below the eye. For alkali burns this irrigation should be continued for at least 20 to 30 minutes until arrangements have been made to transport the patient to an ophthalmologist (Fig. 18-21).

If the industrial plant has many chemical injuries, thus constituting an occupational hazard of this par-ticular plant, a sterile wash fluid should be kept on hand. This can be distilled water, physiologic saline solution, or Ringer's solution. In other situations the sterility of the water is of secondary importance to the effectiveness of water as a diluent and an irri-gator. Irrigators that may be found in an industrial plant include jet stream drinking fountains and safety showers (Fig. 18-22).

The use of neutralizing or buffered solutions to

counteract the specific effects of the injurious chemicals has virtually been abandoned today. The reason for this is that the delay in discovering the proper buffer has been regarded as a greater disadvantage than the advantage obtained by having a direct counteracting chemical. Further, if the irrigation is sufficient, neutralization usually is unnecessary.

Second-stage emergency care

Once the patient has been seen by the industrial nurse or the ophthalmic assistant, the patient's vision should be tested to assess the degree of damage. In many cases the amount of lid swelling, pain, and redness is of such magnitude that a visual acuity assessment is not possible. The industrial nurse or ophthalmic assistant should place two or three drops of a suitable topical anesthetic in the eye to relieve the pain and lid spasm. Irrigation with sterile saline solution is continued if the previous attempts have been unsatisfactory. While this is being done, information should be obtained as to the nature of the chemical involved in the accident, its concentration, the method of the injury, and the duration of probable exposure. The upper and lower fornices should be thoroughly examined with a bright focal illumination for solid particles. These particles, if present, should be removed with a wet cotton-tipped applicator. Because of the copious tearing and lid spasm, it may be difficult to visualize the palpebral conjunctiva for embedded particles. To obtain better exposure, the lids should be pinioned against the orbital margin with a dry cotton cloth rather than with the fingers, which tend to slip. An alternate method would be to evert the upper lid over a retractor. Particles of calcium hydroxide, mortar, or plaster often adhere tenuously to the conjunctival or corneal tissue despite irrigation with water. In such instances the offending particles have to be manually removed or irrigated with a solution of 0.01 molar solution of ethylenediaminetetraacetic acid (EDTA).

It is imperative that any patient with an injury caused by alkalis, strong acids, or any other chemicals known to produce severe ocular injury be seen by an ophthalmologist after the emergency eye care has been given. It is helpful if the ophthalmic assistant or industrial nurse can give the ophthalmol-ogist a summary of the events that transpired, including the patient's visual acuity, the nature of the injury, the concentration of the offending agent, the chemical involved, the duration of chemical exposure, and the emergency therapy initiated. The patient should not be sent back to work without the consent of the ophthalmologist. Small particles of alkali that can be visualized only by using the slit-lamp microscope may still be embedded in the cornea. Also, damage to the cornea and conjunctiva may continue for some time after the accident has occurred. If the ophthalmologist is delayed and the patient cannot be seen immediately, the ophthalmic assistant should bandage the injured eye firmly after placing a few topical anesthetic drops on the conjunctival sac. The ophthalmic assistant should attempt to calm the patient during the period of stress but should not attempt to make any prognosis regarding recovery. This is the prerogative of the ophthalmologist.

Personal protection against chemical eye hazards

Many plants have rigid safety controls for the handling and transporting of dangerous chemicals. There are safety engineering systems for designing clear-air ventilation, segregating hazardous material from the rest of the plant, and designing automatic equipment for the handling of toxic materials in closed or semiclosed systems. The employee is best protected by some type of eye safety glass if the plant uses chemicals in abundance.

INJURIES CAUSED BY SPORTS

Eye protection in sports is an issue that affects everyone. A number of sports contribute to injuries that involve the eye and the adjacent tissues. In 1970 and 1971, there were 543 injuries in two seasons of Canadian hockey, in which 63 eyes were blinded. Most of these were caused by hockey sticks raised above the shoulder during the game. Since that time, certified face protectors attached to a certified helmet have become mandatory for most minor hockey players in Canada and are voluntary for professional hockey players.

In racquetball, tennis, and squash, a high inci-

| Table 18-1 | Incidence of eye injuries and blind eyes in major sports in Canada over a 12-year period |

Sport	Number of eye injuries	Number of blinded eyes
Hockey	1465	214
Racquet sports	705	31
Baseball	288	18
Ball hockey	199	19
Football	105	4
Golf	31	12
Skiing	16	7
War games	40	15
Other sports	151	20

dence of eye injuries is reported annually (Table 18-1). Even badminton has become a concern in eye safety programs. Approved eye protectors have been designed with polycarbonate lenses that replace unsafe open eyeguards in many sports.

INJURIES CAUSED BY RADIANT ENERGY
Ultraviolet radiation

The most common radiation injury encountered results from the absorption of ultraviolet by the cornea. The ultraviolet of the sun is absorbed mainly by the atmosphere. Except in high altitudes or on exceptionally clear days, the ultraviolet content of the sun seldom exceeds 1% or 2%. Sunlight reflected from the sea, snow, or bright sand, however, may contain 4% to 6% ultraviolet light, and such reflections constitute a greater ultraviolet light hazard than the sun itself. Industrial sources of ultraviolet include the carbon arc lamp, the arc used in welding, and sunlamps used for tanning the skin. The ultraviolet rays from these sources may be reflected, and that reflection, as well as direct viewing, may be a source of injury.

With ultraviolet burns to the cornea there are no immediate symptoms, but a few hours later the recipient's eyes begin to water and feel gritty. Later, as the symptoms progress, the foreign body sensation becomes extreme and the patient is in a great deal of pain. In addition to pain, tearing, congestion of the globe, and marked photophobia (inability to tolerate light) occur. Staining of the cornea with fluorescein reveals slight pitting of its surface that is caused by erosion of the superficial epithelium.

Before commencement of therapy the ophthalmic assistant should attempt to record the patient's visual acuity. The ocular examination is facilitated by placing in the patient's eyes an anesthetic agent, which relieves the distress and enables patient to cooperate for the ensuing eye examination. Patching of the eyes for 24 hours usually is sufficient to allow the cornea to heal completely. However, during that time the patient may experience a great deal of discomfort. One hour or so after leaving the ophthalmologist's office, the patient may have a recurrence of symptoms because the local anesthetic wears off. The patient should be warned that a scratching sensation and pain at home may occur. Most ophthalmologists will provide the patient with some pain-relieving medication. The patient is best advised to rest as much as possible with both eyes closed under the patches for 24 hours.

Once the patches are removed the next day, the condition usually is cleared. The patient should be told, however, that some blurring of vision and sensitivity to light may remain for a week or so after the accident. The patient also should be advised to wear protective lenses against ultraviolet radiation in the future.

Infrared rays

The most common infrared calamity to the eye is an "eclipse burn" to the retina. This follows direct observation of a total eclipse of the sun. The effect of this injury to the retina is a marked reduction in visual acuity that is permanent. Ordinary protective devices such as tinted glass, Polaroid lenses, and usual filters are of no value in protecting against this hazard. Direct viewing of eclipses should be avoided.

X-rays

X-rays are of very short wavelength, shorter than ultraviolet radiation, and considerably shorter than the visible violet end of the spectrum (see Fig. 3-4). Exposure to x-rays can produce many ocular complications, including glaucoma, cataracts, necrosis of the skin, loss of lashes, and iritis. Consequently great care has been taken in the clinical use of x-ray exposure about the eye—both to protect the patient from excessive dosage and the hospital staff from unnecessary exposure to dangerous radiation. As a result, the incident rate of eye complication among x-ray and radium workers is extremely low.

PREVENTION OF TRAUMATIC INJURIES TO THE EYE
Prevention in industry

At present the only effective area where safety measures have significantly reduced the number of ocular injuries is in industry. Most industrial safety programs revolve around four categories: (1) the detection of ocular disabilities before placement of workers in specific jobs, (2) the wearing of protective goggles, visors, or masks, (3) education of workers in eye safety, and (4) correct diagnosis and early treatment of eye injuries.

The use of safety glasses has been of greatest importance inasmuch as the glass itself becomes a protective shield for the eye. Although ordinary glasses for street wear and industrial glasses may look alike, the similarity ends there. The difference between the two types of lenses and frames is vast.

Regular street glasses, for example, can shatter easily into the eye. In contrast, industrial safety lenses are thicker and hardened so that they resist, without shattering, the impact of a standard steel ball dropped onto its surface (see Fig. 12-18). The best safety glasses are made of polycarbonate plastic. The frames of safety glasses also are of different construction. In addition to being flame-resistant, they are designed to retain safety lenses under heavy impact.

Contact lens wear may be hazardous in the fume- and chemical-laden environments of some industries. Contact lens wear, however, should not be considered a deterrent to employment in most industries. In some industries contact lens wearers must wear protective goggles as well, as a protection against flying missiles.

Prevention at home

Industrial safety lenses should be employed when work or hobbies are pursued that involve lathing, chiseling, grinding, or hammering. The hazard to the eye is even greater than in industry, because home lighting conditions are not always optimal and built-in safety guards are not always found in home machinery.

Children in particular should not be allowed to wear glasses that will shatter. Every pair of glasses given to a child should serve as a shield for the eyes. The safety glasses available include case-hardened lenses, tempered glass, and plastic lenses. Industrial glasses with industrial frames also serve as an excellent protective shield for the child. A sturdy frame, although not a requirement for safety, is an appreciated asset to the family who must repair frames frequently.

FIRST-AID CARE BY THE OPHTHALMIC ASSISTANT

1. Never place a miotic or mydriatic agent in an eye that has been injured.

2. Never put pressure on the globe when trying to separate the eyelids.

3. Never place any ointment in the eye before it has been seen by the ophthalmologist. It only makes the subsequent examination more difficult.

4. Never send a patient back to work who has pain in the eye, loss of vision, or congestion of the globe. Such a patient should be seen by the ophthalmologist first.

5. Never attempt to reassure the patient with a cheery prognosis. It may be wrong.

6. Do not attempt to use any ophthalmic instruments on an eye, especially corneal spuds, burrs, or curets.

7. When you are in doubt, patch the eye and call for help. The only exception to this rule would occur with a chemical burn of the eye. This must be irrigated immediately.

8. Keep accurate accounts and records of all injuries occurring in the office or clinic. The first step in the prevention of ocular trauma is to obtain statistics of their frequency, their mode of occurrence,

and the type of activity being pursued at the time of the accident.

9. Never evaluate the severity of an ocular injury by its external appearance. Superficial injuries are often more painful than deep, penetrating ones.

10. Be prepared. All emergency drugs, trays, and instruments should be available, sterile, and ready to use for any contingency. It also is important to have a blood pressure cuff, oxygen, epinephrine (Adrenalin) and meperidine (Demerol) in the office if a severe accident occurs and general systemic complications occur.

QUESTIONS FOR REVIEW AND THOUGHT

1. Sympathetic ophthalmia occurs in the fellow eye after a serious injury to one eye. For how many weeks should one be on guard for this dreaded complication?
2. In a through-and-through vertical laceration of the upper eyelid, name the anatomic structures that may be cut.
3. How can rust rings of the cornea best be handled?
4. What is the term used for blood in the anterior chamber? How does it occur after injuries?
5. What is the term used for tears of the iris from its root?
6. A patient is hit directly in the eye by a golf ball. Name the possible damage that can result.
7. What is the first-aid treatment by the ophthalmic assistant when the eye is perforated by a knife and before the patient can be seen by the ophthalmologist?
8. After grinding or chiseling accidents, the examiner must always be alert for the possibility of intraocular foreign bodies. How may they be detected?
9. After an emergency, it is important to check the patient's vision. Occasionally other procedures, such as irrigation, take precedence, but in general it is wise to assess visual acuity. Why?
10. The most common type of cut results from a twig, fingernail or piece of paper scratching the cornea. The immediate symptoms may be severe. What is the purpose of fluorescein, and how does it help determine the extent of the damage?
11. Injuries to the eye frequently result in a form of traumatic iritis. What are the symptoms of such as injury?
12. After lime burns to the eye, plaques of lime may adhere to the undersurface of the upper eyelid. How can the upper eyelid be averted?
13. Distortions of the iris and softness of the eye are signs that the eye has been perforated. The ophthalmic assistant must be careful to avoid any manipulations. What is the first-aid treatment?
14. A mother calls on the telephone and informs you that her young son was injured in the right eye by a tennis ball. When she looked at the eye, the pupil was red instead of black and the child could not see with the eye. What would you suspect?
15. Which foreign substance is apt to be more injurious to the eye—iron, steel, or copper?
16. The industrial nurse telephones saying that an employee has spilled a strong chemical in his eyes. What is your instruction to the nurse?

SELF-EVALUATION QUESTIONS

True-false statements

Directions: Indicate whether the statement is true (T) or false (F).

T or F 1. Alkali burns are more serious than acid burns of the cornea.

T or F 2. Sympathetic ophthalmia usually causes blindness in the fellow eye after an injury to one eye.

T or F 3. Corneal abrasions are often painful.

Missing words

Directions: Write in the missing word in the following sentences.

4. Blunt injuries may result in an intraocular hemorrhage. This hemorrhage, when confined to the anterior chamber of the eye, is called a _____.

5. Hemorrhage in the eye is called a *black-ball* hemorrhage when it is present in both the anterior and _____ chambers.

6. A patient has had an intraocular lens inserted and receives a blow to the eye. The lens is knocked into the vitreous. The intraocular lens is said to be _____.

Choice-completion questions

Directions: Select the one best answer in each case.

7. Which of the following is not an ocular injury?
   a. Corneal abrasion resulting from fingernail injury to cornea
   b. Painless loss of vision in one eye over a period of 3 months
   c. Loss of vision after hammering a nail
   d. Splashing caustic soda in the eye
   e. Double vision following a blow to the eye

8. A squash ball injury to the eye may result in damage to:
   a. The lids
   b. The lens
   c. The retina
   d. The bony wall
   e. All of the above

9. Penetrating injuries to the eye do not usually result in damage to:
   a. The cornea
   b. The lens
   c. The iris
   d. The retina
   e. Bone

ANSWERS, NOTES, AND EXPLANATIONS

1. **True.** Alkali burns can be devastating to the cornea because they continue to penetrate through the corneal thickness. Chemicals will persist even after copious washing for 10 minutes; thus irrigation should be continued for at least 20 to 30 minutes. Because alkalis continue to penetrate and destroy the cornea, a vascular response is created in which vessels grow into the cornea and preclude any possibilities for a successful corneal transplant later.

   Acids, on the other hand, precipitate the underlying layer and inhibit the progression of the acid into the cornea and the eye. Whereas acids may turn the outer corneal layer immediately white, the epithelium will fall off and a new coat of epithelium will regrow and leave the cornea transparent. Thus alkali burns are much more severe and require prolonged attention by copious irrigation.

2. **False.** Sympathetic ophthalmia is a rare occurrence that does follow an ocular injury to one eye, resulting with involvement of the uveal tissue of the fellow eye. It is not common, however, and its onset may be prevented or delayed by the systemic use of cortisone. However, eyes that are damaged beyond any hope of repair or restoration of visual function often are considered for enucleation to minimize this risk factor.

3. **True.** Corneal abrasions often are painful because of exposure of the corneal nerves. The epithelium has been denuded from an area of the cornea, leaving the corneal nerve endings exposed. A firm pressure bandage will minimize the exposure of these nerve endings and will provide a smooth contour for new epithelium to rapidly heal over a corneal abrasion. Topical anesthetics and ointments inhibit the growth of epithelium over a corneal abrasion, and consequently their use should be minimal in the treatment of corneal abrasions.

4. **Hyphema.** Hyphema is an intraocular hemorrhage confined to the anterior chamber. When small, it pools inferiorly, but if the hemorrhage continues, it may fill the anterior chamber and cause blood staining of the cornea. This is often irreparable and leads to loss of vision. It is most important for persons with hemophilia to be aware of this tendency and to prevent further bleeding. Hyphema frequently follows a blunt injury, and there may be recurrent bleeding 3 or 4 days after the initial injury. Consequently, the patient often is hospitalized and bed rest is prescribed, with one or both eyes bandaged.

5. **Vitreous or posterior.** When a black-ball hemorrhage, with blood both in anterior and posterior chambers of the eye, occurs, there is a grave prognosis in that the reabsorption of the hemorrhage from the posterior chamber or vitreous often is slow when hemorrhage becomes mixed with vitreous. If this is unresolved, a vitrectomy may be required for surgical removal of the vitreous hemorrhage in order to restore vision.

6. **Dislocated.** Intraocular lenses always carry the danger that trauma can dislocate them both posteriorly and anteriorly. Consequently, their use in children is still somewhat hazardous. This is particularly so in children who are involved in competitive sports. These lenses are loosely attached and do not have the firm fixation of a normal lens, which is retained by the natural zonular ligaments.

7. **b. Painless loss of vision in one eye over a period of 3 months.** This usually is a medical problem caused by a number of medical conditions that result is visual decrease. The other areas are all injuries that result from trauma.

8. **e. All of the above.** A squash ball injury may cause ecchymoses of the lid or a dislocation of the lens of the eye. The injury may result in contracoup injury involving the posterior globe and resulting in a tear of the choroid or a retinal detachment. The small ball may strike the eye directly and result in a blow-out fracture of the orbit.

   Racquetball injuries, particularly those incurred while playing squash, may be prevented by the use of special squash glasses. With their proper use, the incidence of eyeball damage has decreased considerably.

9. **e. Bone.** Any injury that penetrates the globe may perforate and injure all the structures within the globe and may cause damage to them. No particular tissue is spared. The corneal injury is often the least destructive and can be repaired with either suturing or, in small lacerations, a soft bandage lens. Lens injuries, however, may result in cataracts or may cause dislocation backward into the vitreous. In these cases the lens may have to be removed. Iris injury may result in tearing of the iris from its root or in a portion of the iris being exposed outside the globe and requiring a surgical removal. The retina may be damaged by tears and may result in retinal detachments. Bone, however, usually is damaged by blunt injuries, and sharp instruments tend to caroom off the bone into the soft tissues and particularly into the globe.

CHAPTER 19

The urgent case

- Ocular emergencies
- Urgent case: to be seen within the hour
- Urgent case: to be seen the same day
- Priority case: to be seen within days

The decision as to whether a patient requires an immediate examination is important, and it rests heavily on the shoulders of the ophthalmic assistant. Without previous medical training and amid the noisy clatter of the outer office or clinic, the assistant must be prepared to screen the incoming calls and decide in a period of 30 seconds or less which patient has a complaint that could be symptomatic of an ocular emergency. With industrial or traumatic injuries, this decision can be discharged rapidly and with authority. Obviously a patient who has suffered a flash burn of the cornea or a laceration of the eyelid cannot be kept waiting until there is an open appointment. On the other hand, each patient who calls to make an appointment has some ocular problem that is causing some real or functional derangement of vision. The high myope with lost glasses is just as incapacitated as the individual who has suffered an episode of acute chorioretinitis. Both patients cannot see and are incapacitated by the handicap. The only difference between the two situations is that the myope has a static problem that can be solved the moment spectacles are received, whereas chorioretinitis is a progressive problem that must be stopped before serious damage has occurred.

When patients are screened, a system of priority must be established that can be exercised rapidly and efficiently. In this section, instead of merely cataloging the diseases that constitute an immediate threat to an eye, we discuss their symptoms and signs and attempt to assemble them into a meaningful classification. As with all classifications, the purpose is to provide an orderly way of thinking about a particular symptom or disease, and it is impossible to cover all situations. Professionals cannot blame patients for not presenting their problems as the books and authorities lead them to expect, but with some flexibility they can realize that exceptions will occur. We favor, in cases of doubt, erring on the side of caution and providing an appointment rather than letting the single "functional patient," with a flashing-lights symptom, silently extend a retinal hole to a full retinal detachment while patiently awaiting that cherished appointment with the ophthalmologist three months hence.

OCULAR EMERGENCIES

A. True emergencies (therapy should be instituted within minutes)
1. Chemical burns of the eye
2. Central retinal artery occlusion
3. Penetrating injuries of the eye
4. Sudden loss of vision
B. Urgent situations (patients should be seen the same day)
1. Acute narrow-angle glaucoma (Fig. 19-1)
2. Corneal ulcer (Fig. 19-2)
3. Corneal foreign body
4. Corneal abrasion
5. Acute iritis (Fig. 19-3)

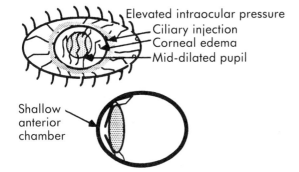

Fig. 19-1 Acute angle closure glaucoma. (From Stein RM, Stein HA, Slatt BJ: *Ocular emergencies: a practical approach to management,* Montreal, 1990, Medicopea.)

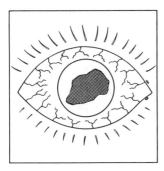

Fig. 19-2 In patients with corneal ulcers, the cornea will have a whitish infiltrate with an overlying epithelial defect that will stain with fluorescein. (From Stein HA, Slatt BJ, Stein RM: *A primer in ophthalmology: a textbook for students,* St Louis, 1992, Mosby.)

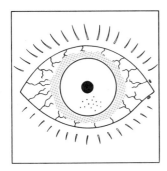

Fig. 19-3 In iritis, ciliary flush is prominent, the pupil is constricted, and slit-lamp examination reveals keratic precipitates. (From Stein HA, Slatt BJ, Stein RM: *A primer in ophthalmology: a textbook for students,* St Louis, 1992, Mosby.)

6. Retinal detachment
7. Hyphema (hemorrhage in the eye)
8. Lid laceration
9. Blow-out fracture of the orbit

C. Semiurgent situations (patients should be seen within days)
1. Optic neuritis
2. Ocular tumors
3. Protrusion of an eye
4. Previously undiagnosed glaucoma
5. Old retinal detachment

URGENT CASE: TO BE SEEN WITHIN THE HOUR
Sudden loss of vision in one eye without pain

This symptom in an adult usually means a *central retinal artery occlusion,* a *central retinal vein occlusion,* a *vitreous hemorrhage,* or a *massive retinal detachment.* A *retrobulbar neuritis* will cause a loss of central vision, but side vision (peripheral vision) usually remains intact. All these conditions require immediate examination and early therapy and therefore belong to the category of the urgent situation. The central retinal artery occlusion is the most urgent in terms of time.

If this artery remains occluded for one hour or more, the involved eye will go totally blind. If sight is to be salvaged, the ophthalmologist must attempt to dislodge the occlusion in the central retinal artery to a more peripheral branch. Only 15 minutes should be allowed to elapse between the initial event and the onset of therapy. However, some visual return has been noted if therapy is implanted before 90 minutes have elapsed. Not only must the patient be on hand but the emergency drug and instruments must be ready, prepared, and sterilized for immediate use.

The other conditions mentioned also require early treatment, but treatment in these cases can be measured in hours rather than minutes. On the basis of symptoms, the patient with a central retinal artery occlusion cannot be differentiated from the patient with a vitreous hemorrhage or retinal vein thrombosis. Therefore *any patient who complains of sudden loss of vision in one eye is an emergency case*

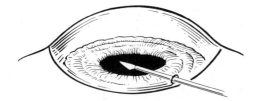

Fig. 19-4 Anterior chamber tap to promote lowering of intraocular pressure in central retinal artery occlusion.

and requires fire-alarm respect.

It is true that the ophthalmic assistant may experience many false positive cases and believe that he or she is gaining a reputation as an alarmist. A patient may state that vision in one eye is lost, whereas examination reveals that vision was merely blurred. However, one good result in a potentially serious case is worth the feeling of chagrin in finding 10 false positive cases. Some patients may lose sight in one eye insidiously and make this appalling discovery quite suddenly. This can occur in glaucoma patients who quietly lose sight in one eye and then inadvertently and casually rub their good eye, only to discover that they are momentarily blind. Therefore the discovery of blindness in one eye may be sudden, but the inciting sequence of events leading to this state can be chronic. This type of case must be added to the list of false positive ocular emergencies.

The ophthalmic assistant always should be prepared in any of the previously mentioned daily contingencies for a central retinal artery occlusion. Eye instruments in the office or clinic must be sterilized in case the attending ophthalmologist has to perform a sterile anterior chamber tap (Fig. 19-4). The following drugs should be available: tolazoline hydrochloride (Priscoline), acetazolamide (Diamox), lidocaine hydrochloride (Xylocaine), and amyl nitrate (Vaporole). Carbachol inhalant gas often can significantly relieve a central retinal artery closure. Small tanks of carbachol, which frequently are available in hospitals, should be used for immediate therapy. The purpose of all the various maneuvers used by the ophthalmologist is to lower the intraocular tension suddenly and promote rapid dilation of the retinal arterioles, thereby enabling any obstructing embolus to pass on to a more peripheral branch.

Chemical injuries to the eye require prompt attention. As soon as the patient arrives at the office, the ophthalmic assistant should institute initial therapy consisting of irrigating the eyes with water or saline for approximately 30 minutes. This is done to wash away any chemicals that still have the potential to cause ocular damage. The visual prognosis as a result of chemical injuries must initially be guarded inasmuch as the full effects of the injury may not be appreciated for several weeks.

Sudden loss of vision in both eyes is a rare event and does not require any degree of sophistication to realize that it also constitutes an ocular emergency.

Vein occlusion

A significant and acute loss of vision can result from the presence of a central vein occlusion (CRVO) or a branch vein occlusion (BRVO). In CRVO the hemorrhages are located primarily at the posterior pole but may be seen throughout the fundus. In BRVO the hemorrhages are located in the distribution of the occluded vein.

The intraocular pressure may be elevated, inasmuch as patients with vein occlusions often have a higher incidence of glaucoma. Fluorescein angiography may be performed to determine the extent of retinal ischemia or macular edema. Panretinal laser photocoagulation is indicated if the retina shows significant ischemic changes. This prevents the neovascularization of the anterior chamber angle, which can lead to glaucoma. In BRVO, focal laser photocoagulation may improve visual acuity and may be indicated for chronic macular edema. If neovascularization does occur, then focal laser photocoagulation may resolve the neovascular tufts and prevent vitreous hemorrhage.

URGENT CASE: TO BE SEEN THE SAME DAY
Painful red eye

Painful red eye, with or without a concomitant decrease in visual acuity, is a symptom complex that deserves immediate attention. Four conditions usually are responsible for a painful red eye: (1) acute glaucoma (a congested, tense eyeball caused by sudden blockage of the aqueous outflow), (2) acute con-

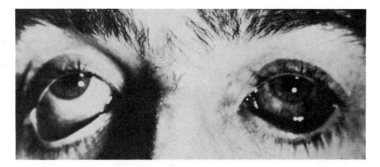

Fig. 19-5 Acute conjunctivitis.

junctivitis (inflammation of the outer eye) (Fig. 19-5), (3) acute iritis (inflammation of the inner eye), and (4) acute keratitis (which generally is caused by a corneal infiltrate or ulcer).

Diagnostic investigation may be required in cases of acute iritis, because this condition may be an incident in the course of a general body disorder. In particular, the ophthalmologist may want to investigate for tuberculosis, syphilis, sarcoidosis, arthritis, and other diseases.

After an attack of angle-closure glaucoma, the patient is treated with a number of pressure-lowering drugs before either a laser or surgical iridectomy. The following drugs should be kept on hand for emergency treatment: (1) acetazolamide, 250 ml in oral and injectable form, (2) glycerin or isosorbide, (3) pilocarpine, 2%, (4) timolol, 0.5%, and (5) meperidine hydrochloride (Demerol) or equivalent pain-relieving drug.

Keratitis, or corneal inflammation, is not commonly present as an isolated entity. It may result from a preexisting conjunctivitis or may be the initiating cause of a secondary iritis. Among the causes of a painful eye, *herpes simplex keratitis* warrants special mention (Fig. 19-6). It is commonly diagnosed as a simple conjunctivitis because the eye is red, is sensitive to light, and has a watery discharge. The patient experiences a gritty sensation of the eye that actually decreases in severity as the condition becomes worse. If the eye is left untreated, many complications can develop, including corneal scarring, secondary iritis, and glaucoma. In the more severe cases, the late corneal scarring can be so

extensive as to warrant a corneal transplant to restore vision. Early treatment in the form of antiviral drops (for example, trifluridine or idoxuridine [IDU]) or débridement of the involved corneal epithelium may reduce the frequency of these late complications. The ophthalmic assistant must always keep this condition in mind when presented with a seemingly innocent and common case of simple conjunctivitis.

Swollen eyelid

The most alarming aspect of an acutely swollen eyelid is the cosmetic disfigurement of the face, which causes the patient to believe that some terrible malady of the eye is present. In fact, the most common cause of acute lid swellings is an infection of the tiny sweat and oil glands emptying into the margin of the lids. The patient with an infection of a sweat gland, commonly known as a *stye,* usually exhibits

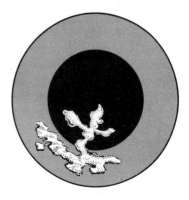

Fig. 19-6 Dendritic pattern of herpes simplex keratitis on the cornea.

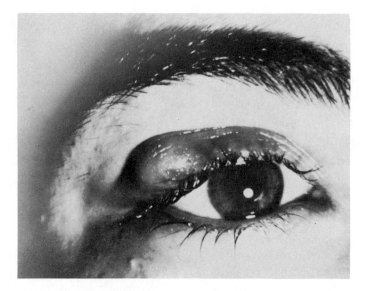

Fig. 19-7 Acute chalazion.

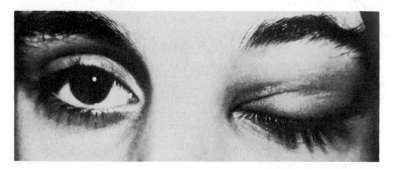

Fig. 19-8 Insect bite with edema of the upper eyelid.

diffuse swelling of the lid, with a tiny raised nodule on the lid margin that denotes the actual site of involvement. Inflammation of the meibomian or oil glands will result in an internal hordeolum that also can result in diffuse lid swelling. On eversion of the lid, however, the site of infection is denoted by a linear red area of congestion extending from the lid margin vertically across the tarsus along the full extent of the meibomian gland. With time an internal hordeolum may resolve, and the infection may become walled off by the formation of a capsule in the tissues of the lid. The patient then has a firm lump that can be felt through the skin surface of the eyelid. This is called a *chalazion*. If the initial infection is minimal, a chalazion may develop without any history of a swollen lid (Fig. 19-7).

Another cause of acute swelling of the eyelid is an *insect bite*. With insect bites the swelling of the eyelid tends to be so severe that the eyelid cannot be opened. Occasionally the site of the bite is visible as a tiny raised red mark on the surface of the eyelid (Fig. 19-8).

Allergic reactions also may give rise to the diffuse, painless swelling of the eyelids. The allergy may be a result of eye drops, skin creams, perfumes, mascara, or environmental causes (for example, dust, molds, and pollen). Most allergic reactions tend to be bilateral and often are accompanied by uncomfortable itchiness.

Flashes of light

Flashes of light coming across the field of vision often are a forerunner of a *retinal detachment;* therefore the patient with this symptom should be seen promptly. In this condition, however, time is not quite as critical a factor; that is, often days or a week can pass between the formulation of such a diagnosis and the initiation of therapy. Although flashes of light are a dangerous symptom, it should be noted that they occur in other conditions besides retinal detachment. Patients with *migraine* often experience a "lightning flash" of light that flickers on and off before onset of the headache. Also, vitreous detachment, an innocuous and common event in middle-aged or elderly persons, may also appear in a similar fashion. Although it is important, the symptom of flashes of light does not possess the urgency of an emergency condition, which usually is associated with pain or loss of function. Its association with an impending retinal detachment, however, is so constant that it does merit recognition as a symptom of paramount importance. Patients with this symptom in one eye should undergo wide dilation to permit a complete examination of the retina.

Double vision or lid droop

Any person older than 5 years of age will see double if a single extraocular muscle becomes weak or paralyzed. The eye may be turned in *(esotropia)* (Fig. 19-9) if a lateral rectus muscle is paralyzed, or turned out *(exotropia)* (Fig. 19-10) if a medial rectus muscle is paralyzed. Hypertropia occurs if there is paralysis or weakness of any of the muscles that move the eye up or down (Fig. 19-11). The symptom of double vision is of grave importance because it occurs as a result of disease within the brain itself, the nerves going to the extraocular muscles, or the muscles themselves. Among the more serious conditions that produce double vision are brain tumors, aneurysms, myasthenia gravis, and strokes.

The lid is primarily held open by the action of the levator palpebrae superioris, which is innervated by the same nerve that supplies many of the extraocular muscles of the eye. Weakness of the levator muscle results in lid droop, or *ptosis*. The significance of an acquired lid droop has the same gravity as the onset of double vision.

PRIORITY CASE: TO BE SEEN WITHIN DAYS

In the priority group the patients concerned are not involved in an ophthalmic emergency, but symptoms may herald an acute emergency, cause immediate functional loss, or indicate a chronic and serious derangement within the eye or brain. Again, our approach will be on the basis of the patient's symptoms.

Halos around lights

The symptom of seeing halos around lights is caused by the formation of droplets, somewhere in the optic media, that break up white light into its spectral components. The rainbow after a storm has a similar explanation, being formed by suspended droplets of rainwater, which spectrally divide light. In the eye the most common cause of seeing halos around lights is related to the formation of mucous deposits on the surface of the conjunctiva, occurring in association with chronic conjunctivitis, allergies, and ocular irritations. Early cataracts, if cystic spaces form in the lens, also can produce this symptom. The phenomenon of seeing colored halos around lights, however, has its major import as an impending sign of acute angle-closure glaucoma. In an eye predisposed to this condition, elevations in ocular tension occur that are insufficient to cause an acute attack but high enough to stretch the cornea and allow edema fluid to form in its substance. The episodes of seeing colored rings around lights usually are transient. They commonly are associated with some blurring of vision and some ocular discomfort. Often, these "small attacks" of intermittent elevations of ocular pressure are so mild that the patient does not seek advice on their account. The symptom of seeing colored rings around lights is a small one as far as the patient is concerned. The

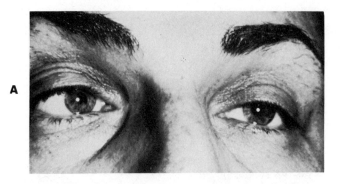

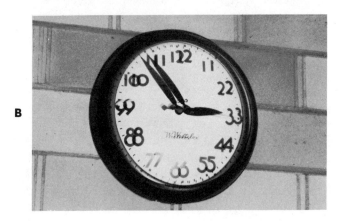

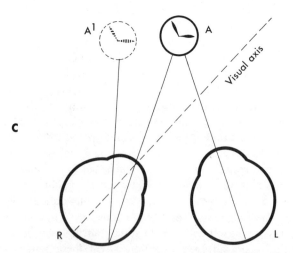

Fig. 19-9 A, Esotropia. Right eye is turned in because of paralysis of the right lateral rectus muscle. **B,** Horizontal diplopia. The patient sees two clocks side by side. **C,** Image of the clock falls on the macula of the left eye and a point on the retina nasal to the macula of the right eye. The projection of the image of the clock is displaced horizontally to A^1 and is on the same side as the turned eye.

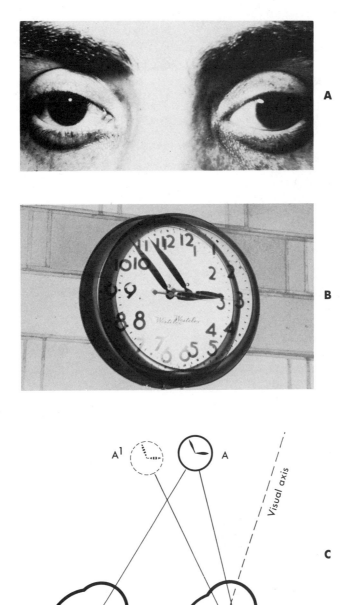

Fig. 19-10 A, Exotropia. Left eye is turned out because of paralysis of the left medial rectus muscle. **B,** Horizontal diplopia. The patient sees two clocks side by side. **C,** Image of the clock falls on the macula of the right eye and a point on the retina temporal to the macula of the left eye. The projection of the image of the clock is displaced horizontally to A^1 and is on the same side as the turned eye.

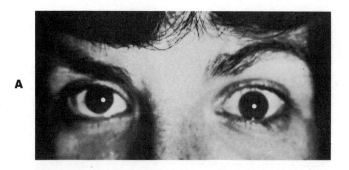

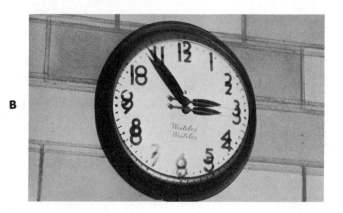

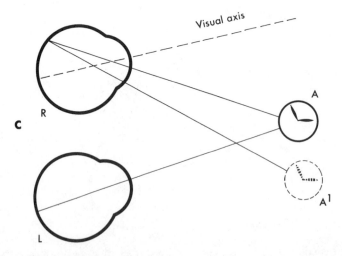

Fig. 19-11 A, Right hypertropia. The right eye is turned up because of paralysis of the right inferior rectus muscle. **B,** Vertical diplopia. The patient sees two clocks, one above the other. **C,** Image of the clocks falls on the macula of the left eye and a point above the macula on the right eye. The projection of the image of the clock is displaced inferiorly to A^1.

ophthalmic assistant should not regard it quite so casually.

Headaches

Headaches usually are prominent among the reasons for which patients are referred. The causes of headaches in or about the eye are numerous. They can include such varied conditions as sinusitis, tooth abscess, migraine, hypertension, and brain tumor. They also appear as a symptom of chronic anxiety and tension and of oculomotor disturbances. Of all of the causes of headaches, ocular dysfunction is quite low on the list.

Ocular headaches usually appear after prolonged periods of close work or after performing other tasks that require visual concentration, such as driving or watching movies or television. The pain is mild and is not associated with such symptoms as nausea, vomiting, or muscular weakness. It usually is relieved by rest, weekends, vacations, and so on. The site of the headache can be virtually anywhere in the cranium, but most often the headaches appear in or behind the eyes, around the eyes, or in the temporal regions. Commonly the patient with an ocular headache has recently changed activities, thereby becoming bothered by uncorrected refractive errors or disturbances in oculomotor balance. Such a patient often has, for example, decided to finish a university degree at night, been promoted to a desk job, or if a homemaker or widow, decided to return to work. Part of the discomfort may be visual, but the factors of anxiety in doing unfamiliar activities, in forced concentration, and in learning can be of significance as well.

The types of headache that should be included in the category of the priority case are nonocular because they may be indicative of serious neurologic or systemic disorder. Nonocular headaches may (1) occur at any time and be so severe as to awaken the patient during the night, (2) be associated with other systemic symptoms, such as nausea, vomiting, fainting spells, drowsiness, or stiffness of the neck, (3) be preceded by an aura of flickering lights and jagged lightning flashes lasting 15 to 20 minutes (an aura often precedes a migraine headache), (4) be throbbing in nature and occur in clusters, and (5) be ag-

gravated by the position of the head or movements of the body.

In practice, the ophthalmic assistant should be aware that a headache may be a serious symptom and give the patient with consequential associated findings priority treatment. (Many brain tumors are first noticed in ocular assessment.)

Lost or broken spectacles

Although lost or broken spectacles appears to be a minor problem, it can be a disabling event to the patient. A myope of -3.00 to -4.00 diopters without correction may not be able to see better than 20/200 and legally may be considered blind. The patient with a considerable refractive error who has lost his or her spectacles can be totally incapacitated. The high myope cannot drive a car, the presbyope cannot read, and the patient with high astigmatism cannot do either activity. For these patients, improving vision with glasses can be as dramatic, satisfying, and rehabilitating as any other form of therapy involving drops or surgery.

Gradual loss of sight in quiet eyes

Gradual loss of vision occurs in conditions in which a progressive deterioration develops without obvious external signs of ocular disease. In children this symptom generally is caused by uncorrected refractive errors. Once the child receives spectacles, the difficulty with vision is improved for a time. As the child grows, the refractive status constantly changes, until physical maturity is reached. These changes are particularly prone to occur in myopia. Once the age of 19 or 20 years is reached, the growth of the eye is complete, and changes in vision are less likely to be caused by errors of refraction. A quiescent period supervenes for about 20 to 25 years, and then most people find that focusing at near becomes difficult, and the era of the presbyope is ushered in. Again a reduction in the ability to see, this time at near, occurs, and the presbyopic patient's reading glasses must be strengthened from time to time.

Apart from uncorrected refractive errors, the most common pathologic causes of painless progressive loss of vision are cataracts and macular degeneration. They occur most commonly in elderly persons but are by no means restricted to this group. The patient with a cataract sees as though looking through a frosted window or gazing at something through a piece of paper. Objects appear hazy because of irregular refraction of light and are dim because some of the light is reflected by the opacities in the lens and does not reach the interior of the eye. Often the cataract patient complains of photophobia, or sensitivity to light, because the retina cannot adequately adapt to the vagaries of illumination coming through a semiopaque lens. Most cataracts are bilateral, but their development may be asymmetric, so that a patient may have a moderate reduction of vision in one eye and a severe visual loss in the other. It is only when the cataract becomes mature or totally opaque that vision drops to the point of mere light perception and projection. Most persons who have access to a medical center have their cataracts removed before the cataracts become mature. In areas where medical facilities are not available, cataracts are a leading cause of blindness.

The patient with macular disease has difficulty seeing clearly straight ahead because of destruction of this most vital region of the retina. Macular disease may be slow or acute in onset. Often it is bilateral, but rarely do both eyes become involved simultaneously. Central vision is lost, and the patient usually cannot see looking straight ahead. Side vision, or peripheral vision, however, is intact so that patients afflicted with this problem can still navigate

through a room without bumping into things even though their visual acuity is 20/200 or less. To envision what a patient with macular disease sees, close one eye, place your thumb close to your open eye in your line of vision, and look at a framed picture hanging on the wall. You will find that all you can see is the frame on the surrounding wall; the picture is blotted out.

SUMMARY

The task of screening or triaging patients on the telephone is difficult and a heavy responsibility for the ophthalmic assistant. It would be impossible even for a well-trained ophthalmologist to adequately screen large numbers of patients through a short conversation that lasts only minutes. The only method of solving this problem is to make errors of inclusion rather than exclusion. Far better to reward the functional patient with a bit of eye time than to turn away the patient with a serious remedial organic problem.

Every patient who calls an ophthalmologist's office believes he or she has a problem that is important, serious, and requires immediate attention. Even though all complaints do not fall under the category of urgency or priority, they should not be minimized and dismissed as trivial. Patience and understanding are required in the handling of all patients. Discretion must be used to ferret out the urgent patient.

QUESTIONS FOR REVIEW AND THOUGHT

1. A patient telephones, complaining of sudden loss of vision in one eye. What are the possible causes? When should the patient be seen?
2. Severe pain in an eye, accompanied by nausea and vomiting, is often an indication of what condition? How should the telephone receptionist handle such a call?
3. When a patient calls complaining of redness of one or both eyes, what is the common differential diagnosis? What are the common characteristics that differentiate types of red eyes?
4. What is the significance of flashes of light?
5. What is the significance of sudden onset of double vision?
6. Compose a list of possible causes of headaches.
7. A patient calls in and says that her baby scratched her eye. What advice would you give her?
8. What advice would you give an ophthalmic assistant who gives medical advice over the telephone?

9. A patient has been hit by a fist and has a simple black eye. Should that patient be seen the same day? Why?
10. A high myope loses his glasses. Is the problem urgent?

SELF-EVALUATION QUESTIONS

True-false statements

Directions: Indicate whether the statement is true (T) or false (F).

T or F   1. A central retinal artery occlusion can be salvaged if seen within 2 hours.
T or F   2. Pain in the eye represents a severe corneal malady.
T or F   3. A chalazion of the upper lid can cause a loss of vision.

Missing words

Directions: Write in the missing word(s) in the following sentences.
4. A person who has an esotropia will have the displaced image on the _____ side.
5. A headache that is preceded by flashing of lights for 15 minutes is invariably a _____ headache.
6. The most common cause of halos around lights is _____.

Choice-completion questions

Directions: Select the one best answer in each case.
7. Patients with cataracts:
   a. Have better distance vision than near vision
   b. Develop better near vision than distance vision
   c. Have variable vision depending on the time of day
   d. See better at night
   e. See better with miotics
8. The most common cause of headaches is:
   a. Eye strain
   b. Sinusitis
   c. Migraine
   d. Stress-anxiety-depression (SAD)
   e. Hypertension
9. Flashes of light can indicate:
   a. Syneresis of vitreous
   b. Migraine
   c. Retinal detachment
   d. A blow to the back of the head
   e. All of the above

ANSWERS, NOTES, AND EXPLANATIONS

1. **False.** A true central retinal artery occlusion rarely can be salvaged. Usually 20 minutes is all that the retina can take without oxygen before permanent damage sets in. It is unusual for the diagnosis and treatment to be done that fast once the incident occurs. Sometimes the occlusive

plug fragments and lodges in a branch so that the entire retina is not destroyed. The typical fundus picture is that of a retina drained of blood; thus the retinal arteries are narrow and the macula appears red because of the choroidal blush. The glowing epithet, cherry-red spot, applied to the condition of the macula does not really do justice to this blinding event.

2. **False.** Pain in the eye is commonly corneal and can be caused by anything from a foreign body in the cornea to herpes simplex keratitis. The pain of iritis and especially of acute glaucoma, however, is far more severe than corneal pain.

  Naturally everyone with pain in the eye should be seen right away. If the eye is fiercely red and the vision is hazy, the worst should be suspected. If the patient states that the pain occurred suddenly and reveals that the pupil is dilated, the assistant can almost start booking the hospital for an acute glaucoma admission.

3. **True.** Any mass, nodule, or lump on the upper lid can cause a slight ptosis of the lid and a flexure of the cornea by compression. It is like pressing on a balloon: the top goes in and the sides go out. The eye is not as flexible as a balloon, but alteration in the corneal curvature does occur. The radius of curvature becomes steeper and more toric in shape. Visual loss of one to three lines on the Snellen chart is common.

4. **Same.** Because the eye is turned in, the nasal side of the retina is exposed to the object of regard. The projection is straight ahead, and the false second image will be beside the real one and located on the same side as the paralyzed muscle.

5. **Migraine.** Migraine is characterized by the following:
   1. A family history of headaches
   2. An aura lasting 15 to 20 minutes of light flashes, off-and-on signals, and loss of visual field
   3. Precipitation of the headache by stress, drugs, birth control or diet pills, or trauma
   4. A tense, commonly compulsive personality
   5. Onset in young adults, although it can occur in childhood

6. **Mucous deposits on the cornea.** A halo is caused by the presence of water droplets breaking up white light into its colored components. Its most sinister importance is acute glaucoma, where episodes of corneal edema occur. Other causes of corneal edema, however, can produce halos.

  The most common causes are mucous droplets on the cornea is association with chronic conjunctivitis, atopic conjunctival allergies, and ocular irritations. Cigarette smoke, pollution, and dry office buildings are a common source of ocular irritation, mucous production, and halo formation. Thus the assistant should not panic over halos.

7. **b. Develop better near vision than distance vision.** Patients with cataracts often will see poorly in the distance but still manage to read. This occurs because the hardening of the lens of the eye increases the index of refraction of the eye. It is the reason that Granny gets "second sight."

8. **d. Stress-anxiety-depression (SAD).** Problems of living are the most common cause of headaches. It is the so-called tension headache that is so endemic. Eye strain rarely causes a headache. Further, the eye is a sensory organ, which cannot be overlooked. Anybody with persistent headaches should have a physical examination to rule out hypertension, sinusitis, or a neurologic disorder.

9. **e. All of the above.** Flashes of light is a dangerous symptom for the patient to report. The most urgent condition that it might indicate is a retinal detachment, which requires immediate surgery. Other symptoms to be worried about in association with light flashes include:
   1. A veil over the affected eye
   2. A shower of spots before one eye
   3. Loss of vision or distortion of vision in the same eye

  Migraine sometimes is a puzzle. On occasion patients have the flashes of light for 15 minutes and no headache.

Syneresis of vitreous is a result of the liquefaction of a part of the vitreous. The remaining gel-like vitreous bumps into the retina whenever the eyes move. The impact of the vitreous against the retina causes flashes of light.

CHAPTER 20

Common eye disorders

- The conjunctiva
- The cornea
- The lids
- Lacrimal apparatus

Perhaps the most interesting part of an ophthalmologist's professional life is the challenge presented in the diagnosis of diseases of the eye. It is toward this end that his or her training has been directed, first as a medical doctor, then as a specialist. Although refraction seems to occupy much of an ophthalmologist's time, it is merely a step in the process of defining disease.

For the ophthalmic assistant the study of disease processes can only aid in making the examination of the eye more rewarding. Despite the assistant's limitations in training and instrumentation, there are many common eye disorders seen daily that should be appreciated. The function of this chapter is not to make diagnosticians of ophthalmic assistants but to enrich their career through the study of the various disorders that are commonly seen.

THE CONJUNCTIVA (Plate 3, A to D)

The conjunctiva commences at the lid margin, lines the inner surface of the lids, forms a cul-de-sac, and then lines the surface of the eye itself, becoming circumferentially attached to the cornea at the limbus. It is translucent, moist, and membranous, has a rich vasculature, and is kept supple by the tear film.

Hyperemia

Hyperemia, or redness, of the conjunctiva is perhaps the most common condition seen. Everyone gets red

eyes at one time or another. The offensive redness is caused merely by dilation of the normal vascular channels in the conjunctiva. It can result from such transitory and innocuous events as exposure to dust, wind, or air pollutants, fatigue, excessive reading, exposure to strong light or heat, poor ventilation, excessive dryness, and even the moderate consumption of alcoholic beverages. Many people equate red eyes with infection or inflammation and become alarmed. It is for this reason that proprietary medications "to get the red out" are so successful with their in-depth media advertising. Many people think that by getting the red out they are nipping a diseased process in the bud, as well as removing a socially unacceptable disorder.

Transitory redness of the eyes requires no treatment because it is not a disease. People who find some relief with the use of eyewashes or astringent drops get only a temporary abatement of their symptoms and become addicted to drops for the rest of their lives. When the medication wears off, the conjunctival vessels have a tendency to dilate again, so that the redness becomes more prominent than before.

Subconjunctival hemorrhage

Subconjunctival hemorrhage is caused by a ruptured conjunctival blood vessel. It usually produces an irregular red patch because of pooling of blood under the conjunctiva (Fig. 20-1). Its appearance is par-

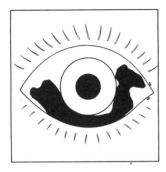

Fig. 20-1 A ruptured vessel with blood accumulation in the subjunctival space is diagnosed as a subconjunctival hemorrhage. (From Stein HA, Slatt BJ, Stein RM: *A primer in ophthalmology: a textbook for students,* St Louis, 1992, Mosby.)

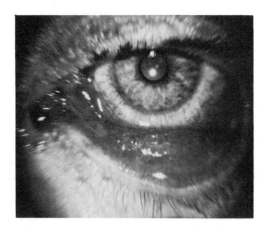

Fig. 20-3 Conjunctivitis.

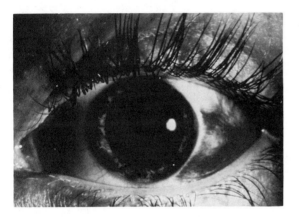

Fig. 20-2 Subconjunctival hemorrhage.

ticularly gruesome and alarming because it is accentuated by the white of the sclera (Fig. 20-2). Invariably, collection of blood, like any other bruise under the skin, spreads and seems to enlarge as the blood is disseminated. Eventually the blood pigment breaks down to its component parts until it is absorbed. This process can take anywhere from 7 days to 3 weeks, depending on the size of the hemorrhage. Subconjunctival hemorrhage occurs most often in elderly patients with diabetes or hypertension, but commonly no cause can be found. A predisposing cause appears to be events that produce a sudden rise in venous pressure, such as coughing, straining,

lifting, sneezing, or vomiting. There is no treatment for this condition, which is entirely innocuous, other than reassurance. Occasionally a subconjunctival hemorrhage is part of a general bleeding disorder, but it must be emphasized that such an event is rare.

Conjunctivitis (Plate 3, B)

Conjunctivitis is an inflammation of the conjunctiva characterized by redness of the conjunctiva, swelling, a discharge that can be watery or purulent, and congestion of the tissues (Fig. 20-3). The patient commonly complains of a burning or grittiness of the eyes. Characteristically, the discharge accumulates during sleep, and its resultant drying on the lashes makes the lids difficult to open in the morning. Usually the lids have to be bathed to open the eyes.

Conjunctivitis may have an infectious, allergic, or toxic cause. The most common infectious agents are viruses, bacteria, and chlamydial organisms. A virus is the most common cause of conjunctivitis. Unlike bacterial or chlamydial conjunctivitis, the discharge is characteristically watery. Adenovirus is the most common viral conjunctivitis. Certain serotypes of this infectious agent may be responsible for causing epidemic keratoconjunctivitis (EKC) or pharyngoconjunctival fever (PCF). EKC is highly contagious and often is associated with epidemic outbreaks in a localized area. This disease is characterized by conjunctival and corneal involvement.

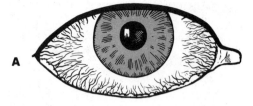

Acute conjunctivitis

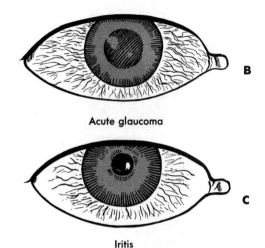

Acute glaucoma

Iritis

Fig. 20-4 A, Acute conjunctivitis, characterized by discharge, injection greater in the fornix, clear cornea, and pupil normal in size. **B,** Acute glaucoma, characterized by tearing, extreme injection of entire eye, hazy cornea, and pupil that is dilated, oval, and fixed to light. **C,** Iritis, characterized by absent discharge, circumcorneal injection, clear to slightly hazy cornea, and small pupil.

PCF differs from EKC in that patients usually exhibit symptoms of a sore throat, just preceding or at the time as their ocular symptoms.

Staphylococcus aureus is the most common cause of bacterial conjunctivitis. The organism also is responsible for such common conditions as boils or impetigo of the skin. Gonococcal conjunctivitis can be a severe infection resulting in blindness if appropriate treatment is delayed. The disease can be seen in newborns who contact the organism while traveling through the birth canal. The sequelae of neonatal conjunctivitis can be so devastating that it is mandatory in most countries for either antibacterial drops or 1% silver nitrate to be placed into the lower conjunctival sac of all newborns immediately after birth. Gonococcal conjunctivitis also can be seen in adults and is characterized by a significant purulent discharge. These patients and their sexual contacts need to be evaluated for a venereal disease that was probably the source for the conjunctivitis. *Haemophilus influenzae,* another bacterial organism, can cause pink eye, especially in children.

Chlamydial conjunctivitis can be caused by inclusion conjunctivitis of trachoma. The disease is characterized by a red eye and often a mucoid discharge. Inclusion conjunctivitis is the more prevalent of the two in North America and occurs in newborns and young adults. Trachoma is a more severe disease that can give rise to extensive scarring of the lids,

conjunctiva, and cornea. It is epidemic in some parts of the world, such as North Africa, the Middle East, and South Asia, where poor hygiene, poor sanitation, deficient diets, and crowding are the norm. It is a major cause of blindness in the world.

The features that distinguish acute conjunctivitis, acute iritis, and acute glaucoma are shown in Fig. 20-4 and Table 20-1. In cases of acute conjunctivitis, antibiotic drops should never be administered before the patient is seen by the ophthalmologist. Smears and cultures may be required in selected cases, especially in patients with ophthalmia neonatorum (conjunctivitis of the newborn), membranous conjunctivitis (diphtheria), and purulent conjunctivitis (gonococcal).

Allergic conjunctivitis is basically a hypersensitivity reaction. It may occur as a component of hay fever or as an independent ocular allergy. There may be large formations of papules or cobblestones under the eyelid (Fig. 20-5). At times the conjunctivitis may be an allergic response to an invading organism, such as the tuberculosis, protein, or staphylococcal bacillus. Contact allergies to drugs are a common occurrence and one of the main reasons why an inflammation can progress despite the copious applications of medication. Neomycin and sulfur preparations are particularly sensitizing.

Chemical conjunctivitis often is seen in the summer and is caused by irritation from chlorine in

Table 20-1   Differential diagnosis

Factor	Acute conjunctivitis	Acute iritis	Acute glaucoma
Pain	None to grittiness or foreign body sensation	Moderate to severe	Severe and radiating
Discharge	Watery or purulent	None	Tearing only
Sensitivity to light (photophobia)	Mild	Severe	Moderate
Cornea	Bright and clear	Clear or hazy	Hazy
Pupil	Normal	Constricted or small	Dilated, oval, fixed to light
Intraocular pressure	Normal	Usually normal	Elevated

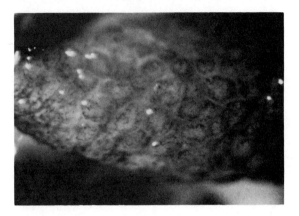

Fig. 20-5 Vernal conjunctivitis. Note cobblestone formation of upper tarsus when lid is everted.

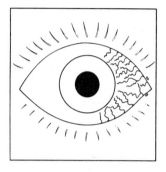

Fig. 20-6 Sectorial episcleritis is characterized by a salmon-pink color of the conjunctival and episcleral tissues. (From Stein HA, Slatt BJ, Stein RM: *A primer in ophthalmology: a textbook for students,* St Louis, 1992, Mosby.)

swimming pools. It also may occur in industrial workers after exposure to irritating fumes.

Obviously, the treatment of conjunctivitis depends on identifying its cause and applying the appropriate therapy. Local antibiotic drops that are effective for a bacterial conjunctivitis would obviously be of no value for a viral infection.

In most offices the diagnosis of conjunctivitis is made largely on clinical grounds and, if serious enough, enhanced with laboratory studies. For example, in a membranous conjunctivitis caused by diphtheria, swabs are taken from the discharge for a smear preparation, and samples also are cultured for growth identification and drug sensitivity. Routine cultures and sensitivity tests rarely are done because the time lag in obtaining the results of such investigation does not warrant the delay in treatment.

Where conjunctivitis is potentially serious, the ophthalmologist will do appropriate laboratory investigations but will institute therapy first. If the trial of therapy does not work, it can later be altered when the precise etiologic agent has been identified and the exact drug to which it is sensitive has been determined.

Episcleritis

Episcleritis is characterized by a salmon-pink hue of the superficial layer of the eye, with involvement of the conjunctiva and episclera (Fig. 20-6). At least one third of the lesions are tender to touch. Simple episcleritis may be sectorial in 70% or generalized in 30% of the patients. In nodular episcleritis, unlike nodular scleritis, the nodules that form are movable with a cotton swab (Q-tip).

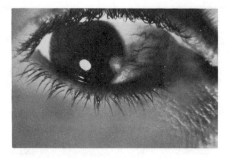

Fig. 20-7 Pterygium actively invading the cornea.

Pinguecula/pterygium

A pinguecula is a triangular, wedge-shaped thickening of the conjunctiva, usually found encroaching on the nasal limbus. If it invades the cornea, it is then referred to as a *pterygium* (Fig. 20-7). These lesions appear as yellowish or white vascularized masses. They are common in tropical climates where people spend a great deal of time outdoors and are exposed to sunlight and the harmful effects of ultraviolet light. Pingueculae usually do not cause symptoms. Occasionally they may cause some irritation or may be a cosmetic blemish. Treatment with artificial tears, vasoconstrictors, or rarely, surgical excision may be indicated. Pterygia occasion-

ally can extend across the cornea and eventually encroach on the visual axis and cause loss of vision. If there is documented evidence of growth, or if the lesion is close to the visual axis, then surgical excision is indicated. Unfortunately, there is a high incidence of recurrence; thus surgical removal is combined commonly with beta-radiation to minimize recurrences.

Conjunctival nevus

A nevus is a benign neoplasm that appears on the conjunctiva at birth or in early childhood. The most common appearance is that of a flat, slightly elevated brown spot (Fig. 20-8). It usually becomes pigmented late in childhood or in adolescence. It is uncommon for a nevus to become malignant. This condition should be differentiated from the acquired pigmented lesion that can occur by the age of 40 to 50 and that can, with growth, turn into a malignant melanoma.

THE CORNEA (Plates 3, *E* and *F*; 4, *A* to *F*)

The cornea, which forms the anterior one sixth of the globe and functionally is the main refracting surface of the eye, is the most vulnerable structure to injury or inflammation. It is almost completely exposed so that it receives the brunt of chemical

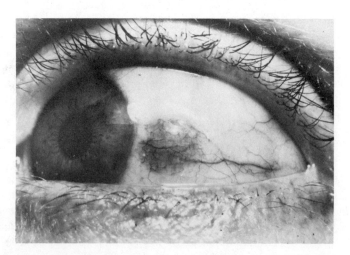

Fig. 20-8 Pigmented nevus of the conjunctiva. (From Liebman SD, Gellis SS, editors: *The pediatrician's ophthalmology,* St Louis, 1966, Mosby.)

injuries to the eye, foreign bodies, particulate matter, and organisms that can invade it from such contiguous sources as the conjunctiva and the lacrimal sac. It is avascular tissue, which means that it is robbed of the defense mechanisms that normally are marshalled against any inflammatory insult elsewhere in the body. The corneal epithelium provides a strong barrier against bacterial invasion. The integrity of this surface is best appreciated by applying fluorescein to its surface and noting any defects in the integrity of this layer by the accumulation of fluorescein pools.

Keratoconus

Keratoconus is a developmental abnormality in which the cornea progressively becomes thinned centrally and bulges forward in a conical fashion (Fig. 20-9). It is usually bilateral and occurs more often in females than in males. Keratoconus is often associated with patients who have hay fever, atopic dermatitis, eczema, or asthma.

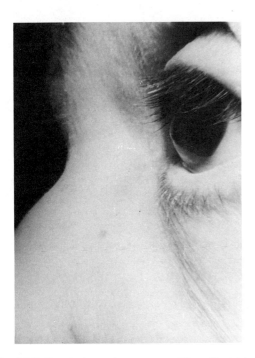

Fig. 20-9 Fourth-degree keratoconus. (From Hartstein J: *Questions and answers on contact lens practice*, ed 2, St Louis, 1973, Mosby.)

It creates irregular corneal astigmatism that defies correction by ordinary spectacles. Rigid contact lenses have been used to correct the visual defect. If the patient is unable to be fitted properly with contact lenses because of high irregular astigmatism, keratoplasty is necessary to restore vision.

Keratoconus can be detected by Munson's sign. This is observed when the examiner has the patient look down and notes from above the indentation of the lower lid by the cone of the cornea. The diagnosis may be made by slit-lamp examination; by the keratometer or retinoscope, which shows the presence of irregular corneal astigmatism; or by use of a keratoscope or Placido's disk, which reflects the images of disordered and irregular concentric circles on the surface of the cornea.

Herpes simplex keratitis

Herpes simplex keratitis is a common corneal inflammatory disorder created by the herpes simplex virus, which is the offending agent of the common cold sore. The first exposure to herpes simplex virus in 90% of cases results in subclinical, usually mild, disease. Characteristically, the young child is infected by salivary contamination from an adult who has labial herpes. The incubation period is three to nine days. The clinical features of herpes simplex are both ocular and non-ocular. The symptoms are relatively mild and consist of an irritating foreign body sensation, mild tearing with no frank pus or purulent discharge, and some haziness of vision accompanied by sensitivity to light. The classic herpes lesion is the dendritic figure, which when stained with fluorescein reveals a branchlike erosion of the cornea, sometimes as a single lesion or as multiple disturbances (Fig. 20-10).

The virus will remain dormant in the sensory nerves to the face, where it can be aroused by a variety of precipitating factors. These factors include the presence of emotional stress, trauma, menstruation, sunlight, or the use of steroid drugs either locally or systemically. The virus, when aroused, will travel down the sensory nerves to the face, lids, conjunctiva, and cornea to produce a recurrence of the disease. These recurrences may be frequent, adding insult to each previous episode, so that reduction

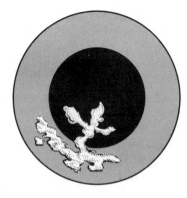

Fig. 20-10 Dendritic figure. Typical of herpes simplex keratitis.

of vision over the years is a common complication. If only the epithelium were involved, no scarring would occur. However, the inflammatory process commonly extends deep down toward the stroma, which heals with vascular proliferation from the limbus and results in corneal scarring.

This condition can be a diagnostic danger because it appears to be a simple conjunctivitis. Many patients treat themselves or are treated by their family physicians with antibiotics for a period of several days before the patient arrives in the ophthalmologist's office. Local antibiotics are of no value in this condition because it is caused by a virus. In many instances, self-medication severely aggravates the condition, because many antibiotic preparations are coupled with steroids, which cause the virus to proliferate even more, thus ensuring the spread of the ulcer and further necrosis of tissue.

The treatment of herpes keratitis is instillation of trifluridine (Viroptic) drops or application of idoxuridine (IDU) or vidarabine (Vira-A) ointment. The cornea usually heals in 7 to 14 days in approximately 85% of cases. Some ophthalmologists prefer to remove the offending virus by scraping off the diseased epithelium. This can be done at the slit-lamp with a dull blade.

Other forms of the disease include the following:
1. Gingivostomatitis. Symptoms are fever, malaise, and lymphadenopathy, along with sore throat.
2. Pharyngitis. Often pharyngitis occurs with vesicles on the tonsils.
3. Cutaneous disease. This usually manifests as type I that occurs above the waist and type II below the waist. The disease is seen in wrestlers and rugby players.
4. General infection. Type II infection, which is more common than type I, is characterized by fever, myalgia, extensive vesicular lesions, and inguinal and pelvic lymphadenopathy.

Recurrent herpes simplex

The virus develops a "symbiosis" with human beings. Interior mechanisms such as trauma, fever, sunlight, emotional stress, steroids, and menses, which provoke viral shedding and the immunologic functions, may be overcome. The trigeminal ganglion is a reservoir for the type I disease. The virus has a 50% recurrence rate over 5 years and may be highly localized in the lymph nodes, chin, eyes, and genitals. Cultures usually are unnecessary because this is chiefly a clinical diagnosis.

Superficial punctate keratitis

Superficial punctate keratitis consists of fine erosions in the corneal epithelium that can be diagnosed by means of the slit lamp and fluorescein staining. These lesions are common and can be seen in dry-eye conditions, infections such as adenovirus and herpes simplex, and chemical injuries. Treatment varies, depending on the cause of the superficial punctate keratitis.

Herpes zoster ophthalmicus

Herpes zoster ophthalmicus is caused by the varicella virus, which causes chickenpox in children. In the adult it is ushered in by a severe neuralgia type of pain, which usually includes the upper lid and extends upward beyond the brow to envelop the forehead through the scalp almost to the vertex of the head. After the pain a vesicular eruption of the skin usually occurs and the skin surface becomes swollen, red, and heavily blistered (Fig. 20-11). The severe pain and vesicular phase lasts approximately 2 weeks. With healing, the skin often is pockmarked with deep, pitted scars, and sensitivity to normal sensation is depressed.

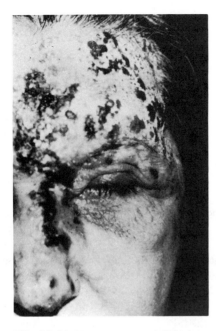

Fig. 20-11 Herpes zoster ophthalmicus.

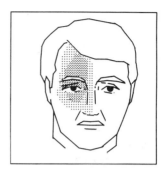

Fig. 20-12 Herpes zoster ophthalmicus is characterized by vesicular skin eruptions in the distribution of any of the branches of the trigeminal nerve. (From Stein HA, Slatt BJ, Stein RM: *A primer in ophthalmology: a textbook for students,* St Louis, 1992, Mosby.)

The virus has a predilection for dermatomes T3-L3, but the most common site is the trigeminal nerve. Cutaneous lesions of herpes zoster are histopathologically identical to varicella but have a greater inflammatory reaction, which can cause scarring. The dermatome pattern of herpes zoster may occur in three sites supplied by branches of the trigeminal nerve:

- The ophthalmic nerve distribution (V1) where it occurs 20 times more frequently than at the V2 or V3 sites. Frontal involvement is the most common, including the upper lid, forehead, and superior conjunctiva, which are supplied by supraorbital and supratrochlear branches (Fig. 20-12). Alternatively, it may spread to the lacrimal and nasociliary area, which supplies the cornea, iris, ciliary body, and the tip of the nose.
- The maxillary nerve distribution (V2).
- The mandibular nerve distribution (V3).

The virus may affect none, any, or all of these branches.

If the tip of the nose has a vesicular eruption, it usually means that the nasocilliary nerve has been affected and that the underlying eye also will be affected by the herpes zoster virus. This occurs in about 50% of the patients. Ocular disturbances include superficial and deep corneal ulcers, iritis, secondary glaucoma, and even paralysis of an extraocular muscle in the minority of instances.

Treatment may include the use of systemic steroids to decrease the scarring and pain that is so common after the inflammation has subsided. Ocular treatment may include topical steroids to decrease the inflammation and a cycloplegic agent to make the patient more comfortable. Acyclovir is a new antiviral agent, administered in an oral form, that has been shown to be effective in shortening the course of disease in herpes zoster.

Marginal corneal ulcers

Marginal corneal ulcers usually are secondary to inflammation caused by the toxin of *Staphylococcus aureus* combined with cells and other mediators involved in the body's immunologic response. It is an extremely painful condition, and most patients believe that they have a large foreign body in their eye. There is marked redness around the eye, and usually a white infiltrate extends from the limbus into the substance of the cornea for 2 to 4 mm. At times the cornea is ulcerated over the surface, but the epithelium also may be intact. The discharge is scant and usually watery.

Because this condition has an immunologic basis, it responds well to antibiotic-steroid medication. Other less common causes of marginal ulcers include nonimmunologic bacterial infections, herpes simplex, and inflammation secondary to a variety of systemic diseases, such as rheumatoid arthritis.

Recurrent corneal erosion

The typical history of recurrent corneal erosion is that the cornea is abraded by a fingernail, a branch of a tree, the edge of a piece of paper or cardboard, or any other organic agent. The actual injury heals temporarily, but a few days, weeks, or even months later the person experiences a complete recurrence of signs and symptoms of the original injury but does not have any recollection of having reinjured the eye. Invariably the symptoms occur in the morning and are thought to be caused by opening the eyes or by the trauma of rubbing the eyes, which removes the area of freshly healed epithelium on the cornea. The disorder is disabling because of the recurrent pain and is somewhat baffling because the features of the disorder are not evident in between attacks. The symptoms may last anywhere from 30 minutes to several hours or several days.

The use of hypertonic drops during the day and ointment at night is helpful in dehydrating the corneal epithelium, which makes it less likely to slough off. If this is unsuccessful, a therapeutic soft contact lens can be tried. A new treatment modality is the technique of anterior stromal puncture, in which a fine needle is used to make multiple puncture marks in the anterior third of the cornea. This technique decreases the recurrence rate by forming stronger bonds between the epithelium and the underlying tissue.

THE LIDS (Plates 5, E and F; and 6, A to G)

Certain anatomic features of the lids affect the manner of lid response. For instance, the skin of the lid, unlike that in the rest of the face, is extremely thin, loosely attached, and devoid of thick connective tissue and a fatty layer. Therefore any inflammatory swelling may cause the skin of the lid to balloon out and look puffy, whereas the weight of the collection of fluid is commonly sufficient to cause ptosis. The lid margins contain the openings of the meibomian glands (oil-secreting glands), as well as small sweat glands (Moll's glands). It is easy to understand why people who put eyeliner on their lid margins, get

recurrent cysts. They do so by obstructing the orifices of these tiny glands with their cosmetic pigments. The cilia or eyelashes are strong, short, curved hairs arranged in two or more closely set rows. They are longer and more numerous on the upper lid than the lower. They have a protective effect, eliminating debris from the eye except when they themselves are caked by debris of a heavy mascara brush.

Chronic inflammation of the lid margins results in thickened, heavily vascularized lids. At times lashes will fall out, and even worse, grow aberrantly. Instead of curving out, they turn in to rub against the sensitive cornea, creating erosions and even ulcerations.

Normally the upper lid just covers the upper millimeter or so of the cornea, whereas the lower lid skirts at its lower level. If the sclera is visible either above or below the cornea, it suggests either retraction of the lids or protrusion of the eye, which might be seen in hyperthyroidism, or orbital inflammation or a tumor.

If the lid droops more than 1 to 2 mm over the cornea, the eye seems smaller by virtue of narrowing the palpebral fissue. This condition, called *ptosis,* is caused by the weakness of the muscles that elevate the upper lid (Müller's smooth muscle or the levator palpebrae superioris muscle).

Epicanthus

Epicanthus is a common congenital variation in young white children. A vertical sign fold from the upper lid is present over the medial angle of the eye and the caruncle (Fig. 20-13). It makes the eyes seem closely set together, and many parents and general practitioners mistake this condition for strabismus. Invariably the condition is self-correcting with the growth of the root of the nose and the face. In Asians this variation persists throughout adult life. Surgical procedures that eliminate this fold to make the eyes look rounder or more like those of Westerners are quite popular in Japan.

Entropion

An entropion is an in-turning of the lids; usually one of the lower lids is affected (Fig. 20-14). The spastic type is more common in old age than in youth. Its

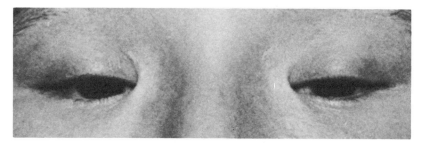

Fig. 20-13 Epicanthal folds.

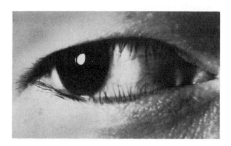

Fig. 20-14 Entropion with lashes involving the cornea.

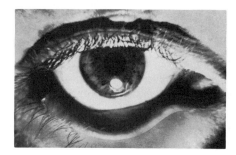

Fig. 20-15 Ectropion. The lower lid falls away from the globe so that the punctum can no longer function as the exit portal for tears.

major disability is created by irritation to the cornea by the in-turned lashes. The inversion of the lid margin is a spasm of the orbicularis oculi, the washerlike muscle under the skin of the lid, and the spasm closes the eye. This muscle spasm often is induced by ocular inflammation or irritation. In an elderly person it is an easy feat for a spastic muscle to turn in on an atonic lid. A more severe form of entropion is caused by sparring, which can follow inflammation of the conjunctiva such as in ocular pemphigus, trachoma, lacerations of the lid, and chemical burns of the eye with attendant scarring. Again, surgery is required to remedy the condition.

The treatment of entropion generally is surgical, although temporary relief can be obtained by drawing the skin of the lower lid down toward the cheeks by means of adhesive tape. The surgery is safe, simple, and effective and usually is performed with the patient under local anesthesia.

Ectropion

In this disorder the lid suffers a loss of tone and flops away from the eye so that the conjunctiva lining

the inner surface of the lid becomes exposed, irritated, and thickened (Fig. 20-15). It occurs primarily in elderly people and is aggravated by attendant tearing as a result of aversion or stenosis of the punctum. The wiping away of tears from the lower lid makes the lower lid drop further, setting up a vicious cycle of tearing and progressive ectropion. Exposure of the conjunctiva causes burning and irritation and predisposes the eye to secondary inflammation. Again, the most common type is a result of senile atrophy of the lid structures, which causes the lids to stay outward. Scarring also can produce the same defect and is caused by the same conditions that create cicatricial entropion. An ectropion is a mechanical defect of the lids that can be remedied only by surgery.

Ptosis

In ptosis there is a conspicuous droop of the upper lid, and the opening of one eye seems smaller than the other (Fig. 20-16). Commonly the lid fold will

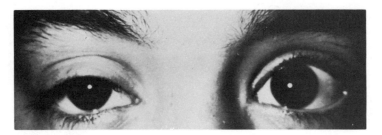

Fig. 20-16 Congenital ptosis, unilateral.

be absent or smooth on the affected side. It is evident when the individual has to look up, because the lid on the affected side does not move upward with the globe as compared with the opposite normal side. If both lids are involved, a child will develop a characteristic head posture with the head thrown back and the upper lids elevated as a compensatory mechanism to raise the drooped eyelids. Treatment of the condition is invariably surgical. It is directed toward shortening the levator palpebrae superioris muscle, the primary elevator of the lid. Resection of a section of this muscle and advancement of its insertion strengthen it and increase its leverage.

Exaggerated blink activity

Exaggerated blink activity is a common condition seen especially in children. The sole feature is the presence of conspicuous repetitive blinking motions of the lids. Invariably the ocular examination reveals the presence of normal eyes. The rapid reflex blinking is thought to be the mechanism by which anxiety and restless motor activity are released in a young child. It clears by itself, and parents are best advised to ignore this self-limiting condition, which disappears more rapidly if it is ignored. Constant attention to these repetitive blinking motions only increases the child's anxiety.

A corollary to reflex blinking in the adult is tremor of the orbicularis oculi muscle. Many adults will complain of a fine lid flutter that is like a current going through the lower lid. Other than the annoying spontaneous twitch, it dos not cause any other symptoms. The condition usually is caused by a mixture of tension and fatigue and disappears on its own.

Rarely, it can be caused by serious conditions, such as Parkinson's disease, multiple sclerosis, and hyperthyroidism.

Blepharochalasis/dermatochalasis

Blepharochalasis is a condition that often drives middle-aged persons to the plastic surgeon. It is caused by recurrent swelling of the upper lids and appears most prominently in the morning. The continuous stretching of the skin of the upper lids and the accumulation of edema cause the skin to lose its tone and hang lifelessly as a redundant fold or curtain over the upper lids. One disability is that it interferes with the application of eye make-up to the lids. In extreme cases it can even weigh on the lashs, creating a sensation of heaviness and ocular fatigue. It may cause restriction of the upper field of vision. At times this condition is accompanied by the protrusion of fat from behind the eye through the orbital septum just under the skin. These fat pads most prominently appear on the medial side of the upper lids and on the lower lids as rather large, unattractive mounds.

This condition is mainly, but not entirely, cosmetic and can be remedied surgically by removing the excess skin, removing the fat, and repairing the septum so that further protrusion of the retroorbital fat cannot occur.

Although blepharochalasis is largely innocuous, occasionally it is a manifestation of thyroid disease, kidney disorders, severe allergic reactions, or angioneurotic edema. This condition should be differentiated from dermatochalasis, which is predominantly an involutional aging change. Dermatochalasis is a result not of recurrent edema but of loss of elastic tissue and relaxation of the fascial bands that connect the skin and underlying orbicularis muscle.

Trichiasis

In trichiasis, instead of being directed outward, the lashes turn in toward the eye, causing irritation and sometimes erosion and ulceration of the cornea. Trichiasis may be a result of scarring of the lid, which can be caused from previous injury, chemical burns to the lids, and severe lid inflammations. Simple epilation of the offending cilia is really a palliative measure, because the lashes tend to regrow aberrantly. If only a few lashes are irritating, their base can be cauterized by electrolysis. In more severe cases a freezing technique applied to the base of the cilia, referred to as *cryosurgery,* or surgical reconstruction of the lid margin may be necessary to remove the aberrant lashes that rub against the conjunctiva or cornea and cause the irritation.

Blepharitis

Blepharitis is a common chronic inflammation of the lid margin. Patients usually complain of a sandy or itchy feeling of their eyes, especially in the morning. There usually is redness, as well as a thickening and irregularity of the lid margins. The disease may occur at any age. The two most common types of chronic inflammation of the lids are staphylococcal blepharitis and seborrheic blepharitis. Seborrhea is a common cause of dandruff. Telltale diagnostic patches of seborrheic involvement in such patients are commonly seen in the medial aspect of the brows, the forehead, and sometimes behind the skin of the ear or on the nose. The base of the eyelash usually is caked with a greasy type of scale that comes off easily, leaving an intact lid margin.

At times the blepharitis can be infective in origin; when this is the case, it invariably is a result of *Staphylococcus aureus.* The lid margins become ulcerated and congested, and adhesive exudate forms on the base of the follicles and on the lid margin. When the ulcerative scale is removed, it always reveals an ulcerative defect on the lid margin. The ulcerative type of blepharitis is more serious because if the inflammation reaches down to the base of the follicles, it can cause permanent scarring, with either loss of lashes or misdirection of lash and regrowth with accompanying trichiasis. Also, the cosmetic consequences are undesirable because the lids become thickened, heavily vascularized, and unattractive.

External hordeolum (stye)/internal hordeolum

A stye is an acute suppurative inflammation of small sebaceous glands on the lid margin that empty their secretion into the hair follicles of the cilia. These glands are known as the *glands of Zeis.* An internal hordeolum is an acute inflammation of the sebaceous glands that reside in the tarsal plates—the meibomian glands. In the early stages of the inflammation, the affected gland becomes swollen and the lid becomes red and edematous. An abscess forms with a small collection of pus, which usually points at the apex of one of these glands. Unless the suppuration is opened, the discomfort can be considerable. The inflammation generally results from invasion by bacterial *Staphylococcus aureus.* It is a common affliction of young adults, but it can occur at all ages, especially in patients with blepharitis.

Treatment consists primarily of hot compresses to rupture the gland in the early stage. If this is unsuccessful, the ophthalmologist can incise and drain the hordeolum or inject local steroids into the lesion in the hope of bringing about its resolution.

Chalazion

A chalazion is a chronic inflammatory granuloma of the large meibomian glands embedded in the tarsus of the lid. Multiple chalazia can occur in the upper or lower lids. Unlike the infectious causes of the internal and external hordeolum, chalazia are a result of a sterile process. Initially the orifice of the meibomian gland becomes occluded by a small inflammatory swelling, and the accumulative sebum ruptures the gland, creating a granulomatous type of inflammatory reaction in the lid itself. The lid becomes swollen, painful, and inflamed until eventually the inflammatory reaction is walled off and a cyst forms (Fig. 20-17). If the cyst is large and

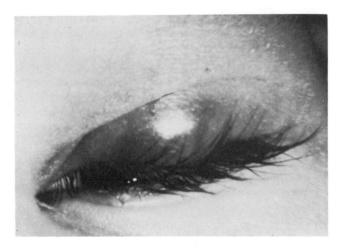

Fig. 20-17 Chalazion.

thickly walled, it must be opened surgically and evacuated with a curet and blunt dissection.

Occasionally the injection of localized steroids into the lesion may obviate the need for surgical drainage. Sometimes in the early stages, hot compresses will rupture it and can effect resolution of the inflammation. Many times the patient will come to the ophthalmologist with a nonpainful, localized swelling of the lid after the inflammation has subsided. The lesion may be surgically excised.

Tumors of the lid

Milia. Milia are small, white, slightly elevated cysts of the skin with a pedunuclated apex. They can create a cosmetic blemish when they appear in crops.

Xanthelasma. Yellowish fatty deposits, or plaque, occur in the upper and lower lids on the medial side. The condition is largely cosmetic, but it may indicate a more serious lipoid disorder, because it represents a deposit of circulating cholesterol or other lipids. The deposits can be destroyed or removed by trichloracetic acid, carbon dioxide snow, or surgery. The purpose of removing xanthelasma is strictly cosmetic.

Carcinoma. The most common malignant growth of the lid is the *basal cell carcinoma* (Fig. 20-18). It usually appears on the lower lid near the inner canthus, next on the lateral side of the lower lid,

and finally and least commonly on the upper lids. The tumor typically has a raised ulcerated surface. Its margin is pearly white, and despite the appearance of tissue destruction, it rarely causes any symptoms. If the tumor is treated early with either radiotherapy or surgery, a complete cure can be effected. The tumor is invasive if it is not treated and tends to spread directly to the tissues surrounding it.

A much less common form of carcinoma is the squamous cell carcinoma. It has greater malignant potential and can spread to distant sites.

Seborrheic keratosis (senile verruca). This is one of the most common lesions involving the eyelid skin. It appears as a well-defined, small, elevated, brown to brownish-black lesion on the eyelid, much like a button flush on the skin surface. It is benign.

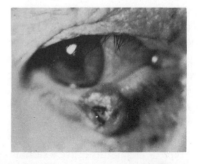

Fig. 20-18 Basal cell carcinoma of eyelid.

It may be surgically removed for cosmetic reasons.

Keratoacanthoma. This is a benign lesion, but because of its rapid growth, it often is mistaken for a malignancy. It grows rapidly but reaches maximum size in 6 to 8 weeks. There may be spontaneous regression, but it is usually excised.

Molluscum contagiosum. These are waxy, raised nodules, often with an umbilicated center. The lesions are caused by a member of the pox virus group. Toxic debris released from the lesion into the tears may give rise to a chronic conjunctivitis. The lesion usually has to be surgically excised.

LACRIMAL APPARATUS
Acute dacryoadenitis

Acute dacryoadenitis is an inflammation of the lacrimal gland that causes pain and discomfort in the upper outer portion of the orbit and swelling of the lid laterally. Eversion of the upper lid indicates a swollen, reddened gland on its lateral surface. Mumps and infectious mononucleosis are the usual systemic causes of this condition.

Lacrimal gland enlargement. Mass lesions of the lacrimal gland may manifest in a variety of ways. They may be painful or painless, they may be palpable, and they may be associated with swelling of the lid and ptosis. Enlargement of the lacrimal gland can be caused by tumor formation, such as the mixed tumor, adenoid cystic tumor, or lymphoma, or a granulomatous inflammation.

Tearing

Tearing may be the result of lacrimation, which is excessive tear formation of the lacrimal gland, or it may be caused by epiphora, which is defective drainage of tears. Lacrimation may result from psychologic stimuli as an expression of grief or depression, from irritation of the eye by wind or dust, or from irritative inflammatory disorders of the conjunctiva, cornea, or lids. These causes of lacrimation usually are self-evident and desist once the stimulus has stopped.

Persistent tearing, with overflow onto the cheek, usually is caused by obstruction somewhere in the lacrimal draining system from the punctum situated on the medial aspect of the lower lid to the naso-

lacrimal duct. The patency of tear elimination can be tested in several ways. Fluorescein solution, 2%, instilled in the conjunctival sac normally disappears within 1 minute. A cotton swab placed in the nasal passages usually can prove the patency of the system as it becomes stained with fluorescein. Irrigation of the lacrimal system with saline solution is less physiologic but at least can demonstrate that tears will flow from the punctum to the nasolacrimal duct and empty into the nasal passages. If there is obstruction of the nasolacrimal canal, the tears forced through the lower canaliculus will reflux out through the upper punctum. This reflux of tears through the upper punctum is plainly visible. An additional point is that the person being tested will not taste the saline solution, which should be coming through the nose. Another test of tear function employs the use of saccharin solutions that are placed in the conjunctival sac. If tears are being eliminated, 1 or 2 minutes later the patency is proved by the patient indicating the taste of something in the throat.

It is also important to note the presence of apposition of the lower lid against the globe. Tearing can occur if the lower lid is not in contact with the globe, as can be seen with medial ectropions.

Regardless of the cause, the treatment of tearing caused by defective drainage is largely surgical. No one has ever died from a bit of tearing; thus the decision to operate depends on the distress of the patient created by the mechanical reflux of tears and the association of secondary infections.

Dacryocystitis (Plate 6, *H*)

Dacryocystitis, an inflammation of the lacrimal sac, is indicated by an inflammatory swelling at the site of the sac. This inflamed swelling is seen as a visible red lump just below the caruncle overriding the inframedial aspect of the orbital bone (Fig. 20-19). Sometimes pressure over the sac will cause pus or mucoid material to regurgitate through the punctum. This condition usually results from the effects of stricture of a nasolacrimal duct arising from chronic inflammation, usually of nasal origin. Obstruction to the lower end of this duct can be caused by the presence of a nasal polyp and extreme deviation of the septum or a marked congestion of the inferior

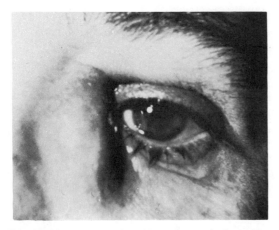

Fig. 20-19 Dacryocystitis. Note the marked swelling over the lacrimal sac.

turbinate. Surgery, called *dacryocystorhinostomy* (DCR), is required to establish a new canal for the tears to flow, thus preventing stagnation.

Dry eyes

Tear formation generally is measured by Schirmer's test, in which a 35 × 5 mm strip of No. 41 Whatman filter paper or standardized paper (Fig. 20-20) is folded over the midportion of the lower lid. Generally, if 10 mm or more of the paper from the point of the fold becomes wet in a 5-minute period, tear formation is considered normal. This test measures both reflex and basic secretion.

The basic secretion test is similarly performed but only after a local anesthetic has been placed into the eye. This eliminates the reflex production of tears from the test and measures basal secretion.

A dry eye, referred to as *keratoconjunctivitis sicca,* is one deficient of tears and is a far more serious problem than an eye bothered by an excess of tears. A deficiency of lacrimal secretion gives rise to chronic conjunctival irritation, which may be associated with erosions of the cornea and eventually corneal scarring.

If keratoconjunctivitis sicca is part of a general systemic disorder, which includes a variety of joint and skin diseases, then the term *Sjögren's syndrome* is used. Treatment of dry eyes consists primarily of the liberal use of artificial tears during the day and ointment at bedtime. Other modalities for more severe cases include occlusion of the puncta with cautery or laser. Vitamin A may offer some hope in patients with severe dry eyes.

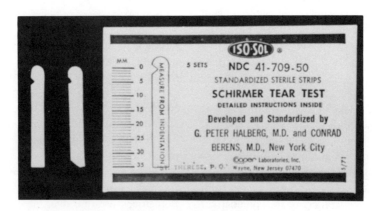

Fig. 20-20 Standardized filter paper for Schirmer's test.

QUESTIONS FOR REVIEW AND THOUGHT

1. Describe the typical contact conjunctival allergic response to neomycin.
2. What is a nevus? What type should cause concern?
3. What is a xanthelasma plaque? Does it have any significance?
4. What influence do cortisone drops have on the herpes simplex virus?
5. Keratoconus affects the cornea and is revealed by a forward protrusion of the globe. Why does it impair vision?
6. What are the external signs and symptoms that distinguish herpes zoster ophthalmicus?
7. What would you see if you stained with fluorescein the eye of a patient who has two marginal corneal ulcers? What is the usual cause of such ulcers?
8. What glands lie in the eyelid, and what are the conditions called when they become inflamed?
9. What causes repeated blinking in childhood?
10. Describe the typical picture of chronic blepharitis.
11. What is the treatment for a stye?
12. What causes persistent tearing?
13. What virus that produces cold sores on the lips also can cause a severe keratitis? What is the typical pattern of infection that it produces on the cornea?
14. Name three causes of purulent conjunctivitis of the newborn.
15. What is a basal cell carcinoma? Where is it usually located with respect to the lids? How is it treated? What is the prognosis after treatment?

SELF-EVALUATION QUESTIONS

True-false statements

Directions: Indicate whether the statement is true (T) or false (F).

T or F   1. Large cobblestones under the eyelid often are seen in vernal conjunctivitis.
T or F   2. A pterygium is a vascular invasive area on the cornea.
T or F   3. Keratoconus results in scarring and irregular curvature of the cornea.

Missing words

Directions: Write in the missing word in the following sentences.

4. The virus that causes a dendritic pattern of the cornea is called _____.
5. When herpes zoster ophthalmicus involves the eye, the tip of the _____ usually is involved and blistered.
6. A fingernail injury to the cornea may result in recurrent _____ of the cornea a few months later.

Choice-completion questions

Directions: Select the one best answer in each case.

7. Ptosis or blepharoptosis is a drooping of the upper lid caused by a paralysis of:
   a. The levator palpabrae superioris muscle
   b. Müller's muscle
   c. a or b
   d. The orbicularis oculi
   e. None of the above

8. A subconjunctival hemorrhage may occur in which of the following conditions?
   a. Trauma
   b. Blood disorders
   c. After sneezing
   d. Perforating injury of the globe
   e. All of the above
9. Abrasions of the cornea is not caused by:
   a. Entropion resulting from scarring of the conjunctiva
   b. Entropion resulting from spasm of the orbicularis
   c. Trichiasis
   d. Dacryocystitis
   e. Contact lenses

ANSWERS, NOTES, AND EXPLANATIONS

1. **True.** Although cobblestones or large papules on the undersurface of the eyelid are typically seen in vernal conjunctivitis, they also may occur in a number of allergic conditions. In addition, giant papillary conjunctivitis is seen in contact lens wearers with both rigid and soft contact lenses. It is believed in these cases to be caused by an allergic response to some protein constituent that builds up on the contact lens.
2. **True.** A pterygium is a locally invasive area that extends across the cornea and eventually may interfere significantly with vision. Once removed there is a significant incidence of recurrence, and each removal increases the risk of further recurrence. A number of surgical procedures have been advocated to try to overcome the recurrence rate of pterygia.
3. **True.** Keratoconus is marked by a cone-shaped protrusion of the cornea, resulting in irregularity of the spherical surface of the cornea. The cornea develops an irregularity that can no longer be corrected by spectacle lenses and requires correction by contact lenses. There are many microbreaks in the extremely thin cornea, resulting in scar formation and even hydrops of the cornea. Each small break in the cornea becomes devastating to the homogeneous regularity of the cornea and results in further scarring and reduction in vision.
4. **Herpes simplex.** The herpes simplex virus most commonly forms a dendritic pattern, usually in the central or paracentral area of the cornea. However, there is no set manner by which it manifests in the eye. It may manifest as a conjunctivitis or may extend deeply into the stroma of the cornea and become a necrotic central ulcer that fails to heal. However, the dendritic pattern, which represents an involvement of the corneal epithelium, is the most typical manifestation of the herpes simplex virus.
5. **Nose.** When the tip of the nose is involved, the ciliary ganglion is involved, through which the nasociliary branch of the fifth or ophthalmic nerve courses. Serious ocular damage often can be prognosticated if the tip of the nose is involved.
6. **Erosion.** Often any abrasion of the cornea by objects such as paper or a fingernail, which involves the corneal epithelium, also will interfere with the basement membrane sufficiently to result in inadequate attachment of the epithelium to the basement membrane. During the night the epithelium become relatively edematous. In the morning, on awakening, there is a tendency to dislodge the epithelium that is not firmly attached to the underlying basement membrane. This results in the typical symptoms of recurrent corneal erosion, with all the irritation and foreign body reaction that was present during the original injury.
7. **c. a or b.** The levator palpebrae superioris muscle may be affected in this condition, as occurs in most congenital ptoses and in many of the acquired paralytic ptoses. If Müller's muscle is

paralyzed, such as occurs in Horner's syndrome with paralysis of the sympathetic nerve, a slight ptosis will be present.

8. **e. All of the above.** Whereas a subconjunctival hemorrhage often is harmless, it is important to be aware that a subconjunctival hemorrhage may be an ominous sign of a small perforating wound of the globe from a sharp flying missile. Thus x-ray films and further detailed examination of the interior of the eye with a well-dilated pupil become important. In addition, the examiner should rule out medical conditions, such as blood disorders, hypertension, diabetes, and so on, that may be responsible for a subconjunctival hemorrhage.

9. **d. Dacryocystitis.** Dacryocystitis does not cause abrasions of the cornea. Contact lenses result in the most serious type of abrasions of the cornea, either by improper insertion or by overwear syndrome. Trichiasis, or an abnormal row of eyelashes, may result in a constant irritation and abrasion of the corneal epithelium. Entropion also may result in irritation of the cornea by eyelashes.

CHAPTER 21 Common retinal disorders

- Retinal artery occlusion
- Retinal vein occlusion
- Diabetic retinopathy
- Retinitis pigmentosa
- Retinopathy of prematurity
- Retinoschisis
- Retinal breaks
- Retinal detachments
- Central serous chorioretinopathy
- Changes in the retina from concussion
- Foreign body in the eye
- Eclipse burns of the retina
- Senile macular degeneration
- Ocular manifestations of common systemic diseases
- Infectious diseases of the retina and choroid
- Malignant melanoma

It is important that the ophthalmic assistant have hard facts about common disorders in clinical practice that are not seen on external examination. That is, retinal disorders require some type of ophthalmoscopic examination. Although this assessment is not within the regular domain of the ophthalmic assistant, patients with retinal disorders may ask questions of any member of the ophthalmic team to which they entrust the safety and security of their eyes. It is valid, then, to upgrade the assistant's knowledge both in breadth and in intensity. We identify in this chapter some of the common disorders.

The clinical evaluation of the retina includes refraction, ophthalmoscopy (both direct and indirect), visual fields for peripheral and central vision, color-vision assessment, dark-adaptation studies, electro-retinography, ultrasound tests to determine space-occupying lesions of the retina and the choroid, and fluorescein angiography.

RETINAL ARTERY OCCLUSION (Plate 6, C)

Retinal artery occlusion is a true ocular catastrophe. If the central retinal artery is blocked by an embolus, the anterior nine layers of the retina undergo necrosis, resulting in total loss of light perception of that eye.

If the condition is seen within 30 minutes, there is a possibility of salvaging the eye by dilating the retinal arterioles to allow the embolus to move into the peripheral circulation.

The diagnosis is simple. There is a sudden and total loss of vision, the retina is gray (cloudy swelling of the retinal layers), and the blood vessels are attenuated and segmented. Ischemic changes make the entire nerve fiber layer of the retina gray. However, the macula does not have this layer. Consequently it stands out, revealing the red blush from its choroidal vascular supply—thus, the quaint term for this sinister condition, the *cherry-red spot*. The usual prognosis is total and permanent loss of light perception for the involved eye.

RETINAL VEIN OCCLUSION
(Plate 6, *D* and *F*)

Central retinal vein occlusion generally is caused by a thrombus in a central retinal vein. Conditions that are associated with an increased risk of retinal vein occlusion include diabetes, hypertension, polycythemia, glaucoma, and any other condition that causes stasis of blood flow.

Because there is no pain, the patient may not be immediately aware of the onset of the condition. The profound loss of vision may not be detected until the patient "discovers" it by rubbing or closing the good eye.

On ophthalmoscopic examination, the entire retina may be covered with superficial hemorrhages that appear flame-shaped. There may be scattered cotton-wool spots, which are microinfarcts of the retina. The retinal veins appear dilated and tortuous distal to the site of occlusion. The macula usually is edematous, and this leads to cystoid macular degeneration with a permanent loss of vision. If a branch of the vein is involved, only that sector through which it passes will be involved. Therefore, in a branch vein occlusion the vision may not be affected. However, it is almost always the patients with visual loss that are seen in the ophthalmologist's office. The prognosis is for visual recovery is significantly better with a branch vein occlusion than with a central vein occlusion.

The chances for visual recovery in a central retinal vein occlusion generally are poor. There is no effective treatment modality for restoring vision. The most dreaded complication is neovascular glaucoma, which can result in severe pain that may eventually be managed by enucleation. With ischemia there is proliferation of new vessels that can occur on the iris and extend over the trabecular meshwork. This can lead to obstruction of aqueous outflow and neovascular glaucoma.

Once the diagnosis of a central retinal vein occlusion is made, a fluorescein angiogram usually is performed to determine the degree of retinal ischemia. If there is significant ischemia, laser photocoagulation to all areas of the retina, that is, panretinal, can be performed. This is thought to destroy areas of ischemic retina that probably are responsible for producing a factor that leads to new blood vessel formation. The use of laser photocoagulation in selected cases has markedly decreased the incidence of neovascular glaucoma.

In branch vein occlusions, if there is macular involvement, vision will be decreased. Studies involving branch vein occlusions have shown that if vision has been decreased for more than 3 months and the fluorescein angiogram shows leakage of fluid in the macula, laser photocoagulation in a sector distribution can improve the visual prognosis. The risk of neovascular glaucoma is not generally a concern with branch vein occlusions.

Patients with venous occlusive disease should have a general medical evaluation to rule out diabetes, hypertension, or blood dyscrasias. The ophthalmologist must evaluate the nonaffected eye to rule out glaucoma, which commonly is associated with vein occlusions.

DIABETIC RETINOPATHY (Plate 6, *G*)

Diabetes may have a juvenile or adult onset. Generally the incidence of diabetic complications increases with the duration of the disease. Complications may include systemic and ocular problems. Systemic complications include peripheral nerve disease, kidney disease, and vascular problems that can result in extremity pain and poor healing. Ocular problems tend to develop from no abnormalities to nonproliferative or background retinopathy and subsequently to proliferative retinopathy.

Background diabetic retinopathy includes the presence of microaneurysms (small vascular buds), dot and blot hemorrhages, and lipoid exudates from a serous leakage of the retinal vessels. Preproliferative retinopathy includes cotton-wool spots (microinfarcts of the retina) and intraretinal microvascular abnormalities (IRMA), which are capillaries within the retina that help supply ischemic areas. Proliferative retinopathy includes the presence of new vessel formation, that is, neovascularization on the disc, the surface of the retina, or the iris. These fragile aberrant blood vessels are easily ruptured, causing recurrent retinal and vitreous hemorrhages. The neovascularization can contract to form a fibrovascular mass that can pull on the retina and lead to a retinal detachment. New vessel formation on the iris, with extension over the trabecular meshwork, can lead to neovascular glaucoma, which is difficult to treat.

Ocular treatment modalities for diabetes depend on the stage of the disease and the absence or presence of a variety of complications. If neovascularization is present, then panretinal photocoagulation is the treatment of choice. Approximately 2000 to 3000 burns are made with the argon laser. This destruction of ischemic retina is thought to decrease the secretion of the vasoproliferative factory by the retina. This in turn usually causes shrinkage and often resolution of the neovascularization. If the vision is decreased by macular edema, photocoagulation of leaking microaneurysms in the macular area has been shown to improve the visual prognosis. If the patient has a vitreous hemorrhage that does not appear to be clearing after 1 to 3 months, or if there are fibrovascular bands producing a tractional retinal detachment, a vitrectomy is the surgical procedure of choice. The vitrectomy infusion suction and cutting instruments are introduced over the pars plana. The vitreous is removed and replaced with saline, and tractional bands are cut in the hope that the retina will fall back into its normal position.

The treatment of diabetes requires the entire coordinated effort of the ophthalmologist and the internist. Although technologic advances have been beneficial, diabetic retinopathy remains one of the leading causes of blindness in North America.

RETINITIS PIGMENTOSA (Plate 6, *H*)

Retinitis pigmentosa is a hereditary disorder that has a variable pattern of transmission. It can be passed on as a sex-linked trait or as an autosomal dominant or recessive trait.

It is a disease of the rods, so that the primary symptoms relate to a failure to see properly in dim illumination. The disease may be mild or may progress to cause total blindness, depending on the nature of the condition and its duration.

It is not inevitable that each case will develop and cause field loss that is constricting. Some cases of retinitis pigmentosa occur and then remain stable for a lifetime.

The diagnosis is made by a visible inspection of the retina with the ophthalmoscope. The following findings are characteristic:

1. Bone spicule-like pigment debris in the midperiphery of the retina
2. Retinal vessel attenuation
3. Tubular visual fields
4. A waxy pallor of the disc

Occasionally a case will be found with typical symptoms but no retinal pigment dispersion. The electroretinogram (ERG) will show the depressed rod function, despite the absence of characteristic retinal changes.

Night blindness also may be caused by vitamin A deficiency, syphilis, and glaucoma.

At times, retinitis pigmentosa may occur with other disorders, including deafness, mental retardation, and, in the eye, cataracts, myopia, and glaucoma.

At this time there is no specific treatment for this disease. It is important to elicit a genetic tree from the patient so that genetic counseling may be done. It also is imperative to follow the patient's progress. This is done to treat any complications that may occur and to ensure that the patient does not feel that the situation is hopeless. The handicap is great enough without gloomy predictions, which, in truth, may not be accurate. Many causes of retinitis pigmentosa are mild and either do not appear to progress or do so quite slowly. Naturally, persons who develop the disease in their first decade are worse off than those who seem to develop retinitis pigmentosa in their forties or fifties.

In many states and provinces, there are retinitis pigmentosa foundations. Patients should be directed to these groups for counseling, assurance, and a line to new therapies.

RETINOPATHY OF PREMATURITY

Retinopathy of prematurity is a proliferative vascular disease occurring in premature infants exposed to high concentrations of oxygen soon after birth. The fibrovascular proliferation can lead to retinal detachment or a white retrolental membrane (behind the lens of the eye). The disease usually is bilateral and, in severe cases, will cause blindness.

Prevention of this disease is of utmost importance. The pediatrician should try to use the lowest oxygen level that is compatible with good neonatal care. An eye examination should be done at the time of discharge from the hospital on all premature infants who received significant oxygen therapy. Careful follow-up examinations should be performed to rule out any fibrovascular proliferation. Treatment of retinopathy of prematurity may include observation for spontaneous regression, cryosurgery, vitrectomy, or retinal detachment surgery.

RETINOSCHISIS

Retinoschisis is a splitting of the retina that results in occasional partial-thickness hole formation. The condition usually occurs in the peripheral retina and therefore rarely affects central vision. This is a condition that occurs in 3% of the population and rarely leads to a retinal detachment.

RETINAL BREAKS

Retinal breaks may take the form of holes or tears. A retinal hole often is the result of an atrophic process that leads to a through-and-through defect of the retina. If it occurs in the macula, it causes a permanent loss of vision to 20/200 or less. A different type of hole and a tear can be produced when a detaching vitreous pulls off a small piece of retina. If the operculum, or everting lip of retinal tissue, is still attached to the retina, a retinal tear is produced. If the operculum is free from the retina, a hole is produced.

Most retinal tears and holes occur in the periphery of the retina, and detection requires a fully dilated pupil and visualization with an indirect ophthal-moscope. All retinal tears in which the retina is not detached should be sealed by the laser beam to prevent the possible entry of liquefied vitreous through the tear and between the pigment epithelium and the retina. The use of the laser in this manner usually will prevent the retina from detaching. All retinal holes in which the patient has recently exhibited symptoms of flashing lights or floaters should be treated with laser photocoagulation.

RETINAL DETACHMENTS (Plate 7, A)

Retinal detachments usually are rhegmatogenous (tear induced). The ingredients for a detachment are the presence of retinal hole or tear, liquid vitreous (which can get under the sensory layers and provide a fluid wedge), and a force to drive the liquefied vitreous as such. That force can be provided by minor trauma or even eye movement.

In aphakia, tears occur because of senile degeneration of the vitreous, which separates out to fluid and gel compartments, and because of disruption of the vitreous by the surgery itself. (This is more likely to occur with intracapsular cataract surgery as opposed to extracapsular cataract surgery.)

In myopia, characterized by an increase in axial length, there is a greater tendency for retinal and vitreous peripheral degenerative changes—and thus for a higher incidence of retinal detachments. Axial myopia is characterized by a posterior staphyloma, a tilted disc with a temporal conus, and a high refractive error—6.00 diopters or greater.

Holes or tears usually are sealed if detected early, which is likely if there is a family history of retinal detachment or a detachment in the opposite eye. Also treated are large holes, multiple holes, or those in the extreme periphery of the retina.

The detection of a retinal tear may be made at the time of routine assessment. The patient may, on the other hand, have no symptoms whatsoever. A common symptom is the shower of spots, which may be caused by small broken blood vessels that liberate free red blood cells which, in turn, cast shadows on the retina.

Vitreous traction is the major cause of retinal tears, and it almost always occurs spontaneously. Although trauma to the eye does cause vitreous traction, it is not the most common cause.

At times the retina can be detached and no holes found. This could be the result of trauma or inflammation. The most sinister cause of a nonrhegmatogenous retinal detachment is a malignant melanoma.

The symptoms may be absent for any detachment. Some patients have light flashes, some lose vision if the macula is involved, and others complain of a veil or curtain before the eyes.

A retinal detachment requires immediate repair. The object of therapy is to identify the holes or tears and close them with a freezing technique known as *cryotherapy*. After this is done, the retina is pushed inward, often with a Silastic band, toward the detached vitreous. The liquefied vitreous that has accumulated beneath the retina often is drained so that the retina will lie flat.

Most procedures are successful (over 90% of routine cases). If the macula is involved, a reduction in acuity may occur, but recovery can take place 6 months after surgery.

The best cases are fresh cases without heavy vitreous traction bands, vascular membranes, or macular detachment.

CENTRAL SEROUS CHORIORETINOPATHY

Central serous chorioretinopathy is a type of retinal detachment that involves the macula but is unassociated with a retinal tear or hole. Serous detachment of the macula is more common in males than in females, and typically occurs in patients 25 to 50 years of age. There appears to be strong association between stress and the development of this disorder.

The symptoms are often highly characteristic. The patient not only complains of blurred vision but will commonly describe distortion of vision with loss of color perception. Objects often appear curved, darker in color, and smaller.

Fluorescein angiography typically shows a leakage point in which fluid passes from the choroid, through a defect in the pigment epithelium, to a location beneath the retina. Most cases clear spontaneously and therefore require no specific therapy. Treatment may be indicated in cases that have prolonged visual loss or show degenerative changes in

the retina. Treatment is with laser photocoagulation to seal the defect in the pigment epithelium.

CHANGES IN THE RETINA FROM CONCUSSION
Commotio retinae (Berlin's "edema")

A blow to the front of the eye can cause a disalignment of the outer segments of the photoreceptors. The involved retina is not edematous. It has a whitish appearance resulting from structural changes of the photoreceptors. With time the whitish appearance resolves and some mild pigmentary changes of the retina can be seen ophthalmoscopicallly. If the macula is affected, a permanent reduction in vision can occur.

Retinal hemorrhages

Retinal hemorrhages may be in front of the retina (preretinal), under the retina (subretinal), or within the retina (intraretinal).

Birth injury is a common cause of traumatic retinal hemorrhage of the newborn.

Retinal detachment

Although retinal detachment is uncommon, patients with retinal injury must be watched because the detachment can occur months or even years after the injury.

FOREIGN BODY IN THE EYE

The degree of damage depends on the mechanical disruption of tissue, as well as the chemical injury specific to a type of metal within the eye.

A foreign body composed of relatively pure copper (greater than 90%) can cause a massive purulent inflammation. Copper in a concentration of 70% to 90% will cause chalcosis, with the deposition of copper in intraocular structures possibly leading to cataracts and glaucoma. If the foreign body is an alloy of copper in a concentration of less than 70%, it rarely will cause any intraocular problems.

Gold, silver, platinum, aluminum, and glass are chemically inert and do damage only by disruption of the tissues.

A retained iron foreign body can cause siderosis bulbi. In the retina it destroys the sensory elements and can cause a profound loss of vision indicated by a flat or extinguished ERG. The entire retina eventually becomes saturated with iron. The trabecular meshwork also can be affected, which can result in glaucoma. These changes can be observed for months to years after the accident. If the foreign body is removed at an early stage, the entire process of siderosis bulbi may be prevented.

Iron injuries are common. Fortunately, metallic foreign bodies are magnetic. This makes removal easier because the magnetic particle can be drawn out of the eye with relative ease.

Most retained ocular foreign bodies are a result of industrial accidents. The best treatment is prevention, which means advocating safety glasses. The most impregnable lens is made of polycarbonate, which will withstand the force of a bullet.

ECLIPSE BURNS OF THE RETINA

After an exposure of minutes, or even seconds, to an eclipse, the macular area may be burned by the infrared rays of the sun. Once a hole is made in the macula from an eclipse burn, the results are permanent.

There is no absolutely safe way to protect children against such mishaps. The best treatment is prevention. Even when proper dense filters are recommended for observing an eclipse, there is no guarantee of patient compliance, especially with young children.

SENILE MACULAR DEGENERATION
(Plate 7, *C*)

There are a great variety of clinical conditions that are labeled *senile macular degeneration*. The clinical findings that may be present include the following:

1. *Absent foveal reflex*. This is the most subtle of changes. The architecture of the fovea is slightly altered so that the reflex of the foveal pit is not seen.
2. *Pigment mottling*. These macular changes are caused by scattered areas of clumping and atrophy of the pigment epithelium.
3. *Drusen* (Plate 7, *B* and *E*). These are small, yellowish white lesions located between the retinal pigment epithelium and Bruch's membrane. They are a common aging change and

a predisposing factor of splitting of Bruch's membrane, which can lead to neovascularization from the choroid.

4. *Subretinal neovascularization*. These new vessels can leak serum or blood and cause a serous or hemorrhagic detachment of the pigment epithelium, resulting in a dramatic decrease in vision. When the blood has not broken through the retina, it may appear as a black mass and simulate a malignant melanoma. If these new vessels are detected early and confirmed with a fluorescein angiogram, laser treatment can be employed in an attempt to destroy the abnormal vessels and prevent subsequent leakage.
5. *Disciform degeneration of the macula*. If serum or blood leaks into the macula, the healing process can lead to gliosis, which leaves a flat grayish white scar. This scar results in permanent loss of central vision, whereas the peripheral field of vision is left intact. Degenerative changes also can occur if the pigment epithelium undergoes atrophy, which leads to death of the photoreceptors and a decrease in vision.

Senile macular degeneration is one of the most common causes of loss of vision in elderly persons. Generally, for most patients, no specific remedy can be offered. For a small percentage of patients, however, the laser can be used to coagulate subretinal neovascularization. This can prevent or slow down the degenerative process. Vitamin and/or zinc therapy may be of help. Because most elderly persons with bilateral disciform degeneration have a visual acuity often reduced to 20/200 or less, visual aids are necessary to enable them to read.

OCULAR MANIFESTATIONS OF COMMON SYSTEMIC DISEASES (Plate 7, *F*)
Hypertension

Patients with high blood pressure, or hypertension, commonly are diagnosed by the ophthalmologist.

In the early phase of the disease the only manifestation may be an attenuation of the retinal arterioles. This narrowing may be uniform, as found in older people, or focal, which may occur in a younger person.

In elderly persons, the changes may be mild as the retinal vessels become thicker, with a dulling of the light reflexes on the retinal arteriole surface. At the area of crossings, the retinal arterioles may compress the underlying veins and cause banking or arteriovenous nicking of the underlying blood column.

Younger patients with severe hypertension may display a florid type of retinopathy with flame-shaped hemorrhages, exudates, cotton-wool spots, and marked narrowing of the retinal arterioles.

The most ominous sign is edema, or swelling, of the optic disc. Patients with this symptom have an extremely poor survival rate.

Sickle cell disease (Plate 7, D)

Sickle cell hemoglobinopathies are most common in black people. The disorder is hereditary. The normal hemoglobin is replaced by the sickle hemoglobin in the red cell.

Retinal changes are common in the severe form of the disease. These include retinal arteriole occlusions and neovascular budding of vessels on the surface of the retina—leading to retinal and vitreous hemorrhages—and preretinal membranes. Comma-shaped capillaries in the conjunctiva are part of the general vascular pattern.

Thyroid disorders (Plate 8, B)

Ocular disease can be seen in patients with hyperthyroidism (excessive thyroid activity), hypothyroidism (depressed thyroid activity), and even euthyroidism (normal thyroid function after successful treatment for hyperthyroidism).

Persons with hyperthyroidism tend to have a rapid pulse, shortness of breath, and a loss of weight. Those with hypothyroidism show a deceleration of activity and may be dull mentally, with a low voice, reduced pulse rate, dry skin, and a gain in weight.

Patients with a thyroid disorder and specific eye findings have a condition referred to as Graves' disease. The etiologic factors of this condition are thought to be immunologic. A variety of tests can be employed for diagnosis of the thyroid condition: serum thyroxine, triiodothyronine (T_3) resin uptake, thyroid autoantibodies, thyrotropin-releasing hormone (TRH), and T_3 assay.

The ocular manifestations of Graves' disease include the following:
1. *Lid lag*. This is one of the earliest findings. When the patient looks down, the lid tends to lag behind the downward moving eye.
2. *Lid retraction*. The lids may leave a clear white space between the lid margins, both upper and lower, and the limbus.
3. *Exophthalmos, or protrusion of the eye*. Using either the Hertel or Krahn exophthalmometer, the degree of protrusion can be measured. It is usually between 20 and 28 mm of exophthalmos. The forward displacement of the globe is caused by an increase in the bulk of ocular muscles and orbital fat swelling. A computed tomography scan will document the swollen extraocular muscles.
4. *Exposure keratitis*. Lid retraction and proptosis lead to exposure of the cornea and its consequent drying effect.
5. *Motility disturbance*. Limitation of eye movements can ensue because of direct involvement of the extraocular muscles. The cellular infiltration of these muscles can lead to fibrosis, with a resultant tethering effect on their function. The most common muscles affected, in descending order of frequency, are the inferior rectus, medial rectus, superior rectus, and lateral rectus.
6. *Disc edema*. Flow through the optic nerve can be slowed by orbital compression. This can lead to disc edema. The swollen nerve is commonly a prelude to optic atrophy with a permanent visual loss.

Management of Graves' disease involves both the internist, to treat and manage the thyroid condition, and the ophthalmologist, to deal with the ocular complications. Guanethidine eyedrops, 10%, often are helpful in reducing the lid retraction, which is cosmetically disfiguring. The lid retraction also can be aided surgically by cutting Müller's muscle and a section of the levator palpebrae superioris.

Exposure keratitis can be managed by the liberal use of lubrication in the form of artificial tears and ointment. Therapy is indicated if the orbital congestion causes a decrease in either color vision or central vision, or a defect on visual field testing. Therapy may consist of systemic steroids, orbital radiation, or an orbital decompression (removing a wall of the orbit) to reduce the severe orbital pressure. If double vision results, muscle surgery can be used to relax the muscles and align the eyes.

INFECTIOUS DISEASES OF THE RETINA AND CHOROID
Toxoplasmosis (Plate 8, A)

Toxoplasma gondii is a protozoan parasite that can cause a chorioretinitis of the eye, especially in the congenital form. The congenital disease is a result of intrauterine infection. This disease is more severe because it is bilateral, and inflammatory deposits also may appear in the brain. The macular region is affected most commonly so that this infection results in considerable visual loss.

In the active stage the affected retina looks gray and edematous with overlying vitreous haze. In the healed phase there is chorioretinal atrophy so that a white punched-out area is visible, surrounded by a fringe of pigment.

The diagnosis of toxoplasmosis is basically a clinical one inasmuch as ocular cultures cannot be taken. A variety of blood tests, however, can be done to document whether the patient has ever been exposed to toxoplasmosis. The problem inherent in the results is that 50% of the population has been exposed to this organism; hence the only valuable result is a negative blood test. Active infection with involvement of, or close to, the optic disc or macula should be aggressively treated with systemic antibiotics. These may include sulfadiazine, pyrimethamine, or clindamycin.

Histoplasmosis (Plate 8, C)

Histoplasma capsulatum is a fungus that is commonly responsible for significant ocular morbity. The infection is most prevalent in certain river valleys in the zone from 45 degrees north latitude to 45 degrees south latitude. In the United States, people living in the Mississippi and Ohio River Valley areas are most commonly affected. The clinical features may include "punched out" chorioretinal scars, peripapillary scarring, and subretinal neovascular membranes. This last condition can lead to exudates and hemorrhages in a subretinal macular location, which can result in a permanent decrease in vision.

If the new vessels are detected early, laser photocoagulation may be employed to improve the visual prognosis.

MALIGNANT MELANOMA (Plate 8, D and E)

Melanoma, although rare, is the most common malignant neoplasm found in the eye. This tumor is 15 times more prevalent in white than in black persons, is more common in males than in females, and often is detected in the fifth and sixth decades of life.

Clinical symptoms may be absent unless the macula is involved, with a resultant decrease in vision, or if there is an overlying retinal detachment with a field loss. The tumor appears as a greenish-brown choroidal mass that in an advanced state may assume a mushroom shape if the tumor breaks through Bruch's membrane.

A variety of treatment modalities can be offered. The technique used depends on the size of the lesion. For small tumors, usually less than 1 cm in size, observation with sequential fundus photographs to detect growth may be the practice of choice. For larger tumors, management usually is a choice between the use of radioactive plaques (attached to the globe over the tumor site) and enucleation. This is an area of great controversy, because studies have shown an increase in mortality after enucleation and suggest that tumor shedding may occur during removal of the eye. Long-term results of radiation therapy are not well-known. Because of these uncertainties, the patient and the clinician often are faced with a difficult decision regarding the most appropriate management. A new technique of resecting only the tumor and leaving the remainder of the eye has proven to be therapeutically efficacious.

The prognosis with and without treatment cannot be given with certainty. Even after enucleations, spread of the tumor has been reported 20 years after the diagnosis has been made. The tumor has a predilection to metastasize to the liver, the skin, and bone. When the tumor has spread outside of the eye, the survival rate is usually less than 1 year. New developments in the field of immunology, in which cells are created to attack specific tumor cells, eventually may lead to an improvement in survival.

QUESTIONS FOR THOUGHT AND REVIEW

1. Discuss possible eye involvement of diabetes mellitus.
2. What is the use of the laser in ophthalmology?
3. What is the clinical picture of someone who has had a central retinal artery occlusion?
4. What symptoms suggest a retinal detachment?
5. What are the retinal findings that suggest retinitis pigmentosa?
6. What is retinopathy of prematurity? What is its cause?
7. An individual has a metallic foreign body that perforates the eye and enters the posterior chamber. What possible eye involvements may there be?
8. What are the clinical manifestations of hyperthyroidism?

SELF-EVALUATION QUESTIONS

True-false statements

Directions: Indicate whether the statement is true (T) or false (F).

T or **F** 1. Retinopathy of prematurity occurs in one eye of premature infants exposed to high concentrations of oxygen.

T or **F** 2. Every retinal hole should be sealed with either laser beam or cryosurgery.

T or **F** 3. Drusen of the retina rarely causes any loss of vision.

Missing words

Directions: Write in the missing word in the following sentences.

4. Central retinal vein occlusion can cause _____ glaucoma 3 months after the event.
5. Diabetic retinopathy is more prevalent with diabetics whose disease is poorly controlled and who have had their disease at least _____ years.
6. Retinitis pigmentosa causes _____ field defect in the early stages.

Choice-completion questions

Directions: Select the the one best answer in each case.

7. Retinal detachments are common:
   a. In high myopes
   b. After contusion
   c. With malignant melanomas
   d. With retinal tears with an operculum
   e. All of the above
8. Central serous retinopathy is a disease of:
   a. Elderly persons over 65
   b. Persons between 25 and 50
   c. Females
   d. Blacks
   e. Absent symptoms
9. Central retinal artery occlusion usually is caused by:
   a. A tumor of the optic nerve
   b. A thrombus

    c. An embolus

    d. Glaucoma

    e. Carotid artery stenosis

ANSWERS, NOTES, AND EXPLANATIONS

1. **False.** Retinopathy of prematurity is a bilateral disease occurring in infants born before 36 weeks of gestation or weighing less than 4.2 pounds at birth and having a history of significant oxygen therapy. These infants develop three signs, peripheral neovascularization (especially on the temporal periphery) vitreous bleeding, and retinal detachment.

   Infants exposed to high doses of oxygen should be examined with the indirect ophthalmoscope before discharge from the hospital and every 2 months until the condition is considered stable.

   The treatment of this condition is still not satisfactory despite the use of lasers, cryotherapy, vitamins C and E (tocopherol), and encircling retinal buckles.

   The most serious complication of retinopathy of prematurity is retinal detachment, which may not be evident until the age of 10 to 20 years.

   The difficulty in evaluating treatment of this condition results from the fact that many infants have a spontaneous regression.

2. **False.** Every break or retinal hole should not be sealed with laser beam or cryosurgery. Many retinal holes are not through and through or do not have an operculum or lip developed through traction. It is true, however, that in many retinal detachments a retinal break develops. A hole in the retina permits the accumulation of fluid between the pigment layer of the retina and the anterior nine sensory layers of the retina. The subretinal fluid that accumulates acts as a wedge between the retinal layers, and further detachment results.

   Most retinal holes occur in the extreme periphery of the retina. They are quite common, and most do not lead to detachment. If a retinal hole is found with a break in the retina, with evidence of a lip traction or a serous wedge, these breaks are treated. Although most retinal holes do not cause a retinal detachment, most detachments (over 85%) reveal multiple holes.

3. **True.** Drusen of the choroid are basically excrescences of Bruch's membrane of the choroid. They appear as yellow deposits in the posterior pole of the retina, sometimes surrounded by a collarette of retinal pigment. Unless associated with macular degenerative phenomena, these drusen usually are harmless. They may, however, involve the optic nerve and cause compression.

   Drusen of the optic nerve are quite another matter. They consist of hyalin or calcium, and these deposits take up and compress tissue in the optic nerve. Field defects are common and may be quite varied depending on the size of the drusen, their location, and their development.

   In addition to causing visual field defects, drusen may simulate the appearance of papilledema or swelling of the optic nerve head.

   Typically drusen are glistening pearl-like bodies, which when visible are seen in the surface of the optic disc. When they are buried, the disc is heaped up and its margins are quite blurred.

4. **Hemorrhagic.** Central retinal vein occlusion can cause a severe, intractable glaucoma within 3 months after the venous occlusion.

   The vascular ischemia of the venous occlusion causes neovascularization at the level of the retina and iris. In the retina macroaneurysms and vascular buds appear. These can create retinal hemorrhage and lead to retinal detachment. In the iris the vascular proliferation can sew up the angle structures with fibrovascular tissue. This leads to a permanent angle-closure type of glaucoma that cannot be satisfactorily treated medically or surgically. The term *hemorrhagic* actually is a misnomer because it is not the presence of the blood in the anterior chamber that causes the glaucoma. It is caused by the growth of active fibrovascular bands that invade and occlude the angle structures.

5. **15.** Diabetic retinopathy is a major cause of blindness in North America. Initially the retinopathy was thought to be a straight function of duration. Diabetics of 15 years or longer were the most susceptible to the disease. The duration factor is still valid inasmuch as it is uncommon to see diabetics of 25 years without some form of retinopathy. That is not to say that long-term diabetics invariably go blind, but they show a few microaneurysms, perhaps some neovascularization of the retina, or turgid retinal veins. In addition to duration, most researchers believe that hyperglycemia by itself is toxic, and proper control is important to minimize the disease. For years this point was contentious and appears now to be settled. Another area of dispute is the relationship of age to retinopathy. It was believed that maturity-onset (40 years or over) diabetics were free of the complications of retinopathy. This is definitely not true. Approximately 20% of maturity-onset diabetics develop retinopathy. When this occurs, it usually is more severe than in the juvenile diabetics. Some physicians believe that the division of juvenile diabetes and maturity-onset diabetes should be abolished and replaced by insulin-dependent and non–insulin-dependent disease. It is the group of diabetics who are insulin dependent that is more prone to retinal complications of this disease.

6. **Tubular or signet ring.** Retinitis pigmentosa can cause tubular field defects. Such defects in the visual field also can be caused by syphilis, glaucoma, quinine poisoning, eclampsia, and on occasion, hysteria.

   The diagnosis of this disease can be made by observing the bone spicule pigment deposits in the retina at the level of the midperiphery. Also, an ERG can reveal the flat electrical response of the rods, which is abolished under dim light. There usually is a family history of the disease. This may not be obvious because the disease can be transmitted as a dominant, recessive, or sex-linked type of heredity pattern.

   Occasionally, vitamin A deficiency can be uncovered, and this plus nutritional disorders, although rare in industrialized countries, may mimic retinitis pigmentosa. At present there is no cure for this disease. In many patients the evolution of this disease may be quite slow; thus so blindness may not be prognosticated for all afflicted patients.

7. **a. In high myopes.** The typical high myope has a tilted disc with an oblique entry of the optic nerve though the sclera, an elongated eye sometimes with a large posterior staphyloma, and a stretched vascular system for both the retinal and the choroidal circulations. As a result, through vascular ischemia, retinal holes (some leading to retinal tears and subsequent detachment) are common. A retinal tear with an operculum is merely a large retinal tear with a lip or edge that is everting. Such tears cannot be sealed by laser therapy and represent a further stage in the development or evolution of a retinal detachment. A malignant melanoma can cause a detachment by virtue of this solid mass derived from the choroid pressing forward from behind and pushing the retina anteriorly. Diagnostically the melanoma is one of the few instances in which a retinal detachment may be present without a retinal hole or tear. Injury also may cause retinal detachment as a result of the underlying presence of blood, edema fluid, and inflammatory debris. Injury is not the major cause, however, of most retinal detachments.

8. **b. Persons between 25 and 50.** Central serous retinopathy is a disease of young people. At times it may be related to stress or a prolonged period of anxiety or to an allergic reaction to drugs, vapors, or chemicals, but commonly it has no antecedent of any kind. The person invariably is made aware of the problem because of blurred and distorted vision. Lines appear curved, at times with missing pieces in the center, and color vision is depressed or darker in hue. The patient's symptoms are pathognomic of this condition. However, support for the diagnosis can be made by the Amsler grid or by looking for the telltale macular blister, which usually is clinically evident. The treatment, depending on the severity of the condition, is systemic steroids, laser beam obliteration of the leaking vessel if possible, and a tincture of time. Often

the condition improves without any drug or device. Angiography of the retinal and choriodal circulation should be done because simulating conditions include a small macular melanoma, histoplasmosis, hematoma, and an effusion of a hemangioma.

9. **c. An embolus.** Central retinal artery occlusion is invariably a result of an embolus from an atheromatous plaque of the carotid artery. It is commonly a mixture of fatty debris, platelets, and fibrin and appear as a glistening yellow plaque at the head of the optic nerve in the central retinal artery. At times, nothing is found at this location, but fragments of the embolus may be visible in the retinal circulation. Such an event invariably causes blindness unless heroic measures such as ocular paracentesis or heavy massage of the globe are undertaken within 5 minutes of the event. Such patients should receive the benefit of a neurologic investigation to direct attention to the carotid artery on that side, which too may be stenosed or compromised by the presence of an atheromatous ulcer in the wall of the vessel.

Patients with this disease often worry about a similar event occurring in the other eye. Of course it is possible, because atheroma in a person usually is not limited to a single vessel but is present more or less in all large blood vessels. Statistically the chances of such a catastrophe being bilateral are extremely remote and highly improbable.

CHAPTER 22 Glaucoma

- Primary angle-closure glaucoma
- Primary open-angle glaucoma
- Secondary and congenital glaucoma

It is estimated that more than 2 million persons in North America suffer from glaucoma. Over half of these are unaware of their condition. Open-angle glaucoma increases dramatically with advancing age. The prevalence rises from 2% in persons younger than 40 years of age to 9% in those aged 70 and older who have raised intraocular pressure.* Although not everyone with raised intraocular pressure has glaucoma, it is estimated that among those who do, 0.1% have glaucoma between the ages of 40 and 49 years and 2% to 3% among those older than 70 years. Apart from age there is significant individual variation in the apparent susceptibility of optic nerves to glaucomatous damage. Some persons have optic nerve damage at relatively low pressures whereas others withstand considerable pressure elevation for many years without damage.

Glaucoma is a localized ocular disease characterized by (1) elevated intraocular pressure, (2) optic nerve cupping, and (3) visual field loss. The hallmark of glaucoma is an elevated intraocular pressure, which leads to pressure and atrophy of the optic nerve and subsequent loss of visual field. Glaucoma falls roughly into four classifications (Table 22-1):

1. *Primary angle-closure glaucoma.* In this condition there is a sudden marked rise in the intraocular pressure caused by mechanical obstruction of angle structures of the eye at the root of the iris (see Fig. 2-14). The vision is lost rapidly, the eye becomes red, and the patient complains of excruciating pain.

2. *Open-angle, or chronic, glaucoma.* This condition is thought to arise from a progressive narrowing of the openings in the trabecular meshwork of the anterior chamber angle structures. The accompanying obstruction to outflow induces a slight rise in intraocular pressure. It is insidious and symptomless, initially causing erosion of the peripheral visual field. Most glaucoma falls into this group.

3. *Secondary glaucoma.* Secondary glaucoma can be of either the open-angle or the narrow-angle type. The elevated intraocular pressure results from some specific disease within the eye, such as iritis or tumor, which interferes with aqueous flowing out of the eye. It may occur after trauma or may follow neovascularization in the anterior chamber, as occurs after diabetes.

4. *Congenital, or infantile, glaucoma.* This condition is often referred to as *buphthalmos,* because the infantile eyeball distends as a result of the elevated intraocular pressure and comes to resemble the eye of an ox (Fig. 22-1).

---

*American Academy of Ophthalmology, Quality of Care Committee on Glaucoma.

Table 22-1   Types of glaucoma

Type	Cause	Symptoms	Comments
Chronic open angle	Gradual blockage of drainage channel; pressure builds slowly	Gradual loss of side vision; affects side vision first	Progresses very slowly and is a lifelong condition; considered the "thief in the night"
Primary angle closure	Total blockage of drainage channel; sudden increase in pressure	Nausea, blurred vision, severe pain, halos around lights	A medical emergency inasmuch as permanent blindness occurs rapidly without immediate treatment
Secondary	Injury, infection, tumors, drugs, or inflammation, which causes scar tissue growth, blocking the drainage channel	Gradual loss of side vision; affects side vision first	May progress slowly; similar to chronic open-angle glaucoma
Congenital	Fluid drainage system abnormal at birth	Light sensitivity, excessive tearing, enlarged eyes, cloudy cornea	Must be treated soon after birth if vision is to be saved

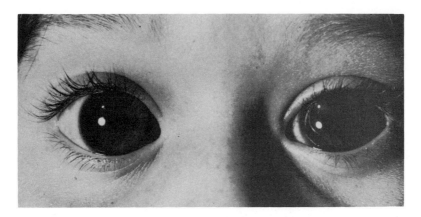

Fig. 22-1 Congenital glaucoma. Note the enlargement of the eyes. (Courtesy M. Shusterman.)

PRIMARY ANGLE-CLOSURE GLAUCOMA

Primary angle-closure glaucoma constitutes approximately 30% of all glaucoma. In the general population a higher incidence of angle-closure glaucoma occurs in women because of their shallower anterior chambers. Angle-closure glaucoma is less common among black persons and shows increased incidence among Eskimos.

Patients with this disorder have essentially normal eyes with the exception of a shallow anterior chamber and a narrow entrance into the angle. Crowding of the angle structure tends to occur more in hyper-

opia and increases as the patient becomes older (Fig. 22-2). The narrowing is mainly caused by the increased growth of the crystalline lens, which tends to push the entire iris diaphragm forward when the endocorneal angle of the anterior chamber is less than 20 degrees in width. Then a state of narrow-angle glaucoma is said to exist. The trigger mechanism that brings about closure of a critically narrowed angle is dilation of the pupil. Dilation of the pupil relaxes the iris and causes its tissue to bunch up toward the base of the iris, thereby effectively blocking off all the angle structures. Also, dilation

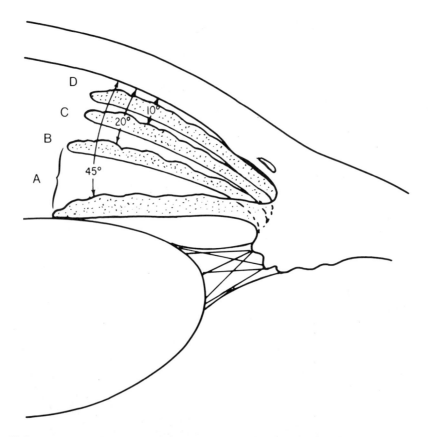

Fig. 22-2 Shaffer classification of anterior chamber angle, based on angular width of angle recess.

Angular width	Clinical interpretation
(A) Wide open (20 to 45 degrees)	Closure improbable
(B) Slightly narrow (10 to 20 degrees)	Closure possible
(C) Extremely narrow (<10 degrees)	Closure probable
(D) Partially or totally closed	Closure present

(From Shields, MB, editor: *Textbook of glaucoma,* ed 2, Baltimore, 1987, Williams & Wilkins.)

of the pupil may relax the periphery of the iris sufficiently so that the pressure in the posterior chamber exceeds that in the anterior chamber, resulting in further forward displacement of the iris and further crowding of the angle structures. If the pupillary border of the iris is bound down (as a result of inflammation) to the anterior lens capsule or if the pupil is blocked by a prolapsed vitreous body, pupillary block mechanism exists. This may lead to bowing of the iris, so-called iris bombé (Fig. 22-3). In this situation, the pupil is blocked so that the aqueous pressure from the posterior chamber bows the iris forward, and this blocks the angle of the anterior chamber and prevents the outflow of fluid.

An attack of acute angle-closure glaucoma can become fully developed within 30 to 60 minutes. The abruptness of the onset is so characteristic that a presumptive diagnosis of acute angle-closure glaucoma can virtually be made over the telephone. Commonly the attack begins under conditions that lead to pupillary dilation—for example, fear, emotional arousal, or conditions of dark adaptation (movie theaters). Many an attack may be precipitated by dilation during an eye examination. The pain can

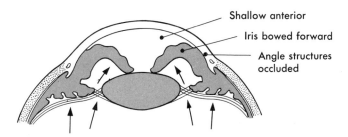

Fig. 22-3 Pupillary block glaucoma. The pressure in the posterior chamber exceeds that of the anterior chamber. The iris is bowed forward (iris bombé) and occludes the angle structures. Without treatment the iris becomes permanently adherent to the angle structures, and intractable secondary glaucoma ensues.

vary from a feeling of discomfort and fullness around the eyes to a severe, prostrating pain that can radiate to the back of the head or down toward the teeth. With severe pain the patient may be prostrated and nauseated and may even vomit. The vision usually is reduced to mere perception of light.

Drugs can precipitate an attack. The most common drugs are cyclopentolate and tropicamide. Other commonly used medications that can precipitate an attack are epinephrine derivatives. These drugs frequently are agents in common hayfever remedies, and the package insert indicates their contraindication in glaucoma; however, the phenylephrine derivative drugs are perfectly safe in open-angle glaucoma.

Examination reveals that the eyelids and conjunctiva are edematous and congested, especially around the limbus. The cornea appears steamy and hazy because of epithelial edema, which results from aggregations of tiny water droplets in the superficial layers of the cornea. The iris itself appears dull, gray, and patternless because of the edema. The pupil is typically dilated and may be oval, and it does not respond to light. The tension is extremely high, in the range of 50 to 60 mm Hg or higher.

This type of ocular catastrophe is preceded in nearly half the cases by premonitory self-limiting episodes of aching and blur, lasting a few hours each time and occurring with increasing frequency before an acute attack. Also, the patient may report seeing halos or rainbows around lights; they are caused by the slight edema of the cornea in these premonitory periods. These halos, although not pathognomonic

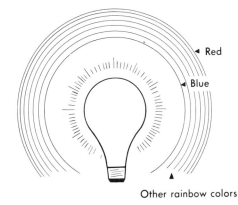

Fig. 22-4 Halos around lights. This is a prominent symptom in angle-closure glaucoma. These colors are related to the spectral colors of light through water droplets.

of glaucoma, are most significantly related to this disease, and they are caused by dispersion of light by the epithelial droplets. They are typically composed of two colored rings, an inner blue-violet ring and an outer yellow-red ring (Fig. 22-4). Between the attacks little abnormality may be noted.

The halos caused by subacute attacks can be distinguished from the permanent halos caused by lens opacities by placing a stenopeic slit across the line of vision. A glaucoma halo remains intact, but with diminished intensity, behind the slit, whereas a lenticular halo is broken up into segments that revolve as the slit is moved. The halos that are sometimes caused by conjunctival debris can be swept away by movements of the lid.

Diagnosis

The shallow-chambered, narrow-angled eye should be identified by a routine eye examination. The observer can easily see the convex iris diaphragm by illuminating the limbal area with a flashlight and noting the proximity of the iris periphery to the cornea. If there is any doubt as to whether the angle is narrowed, mydriatic drops such as cyclopentolate (Cyclogyl) or homatropine should not be used because they can, in such an eye, induce an attack of acute angle-closure glaucoma. It must also be emphasized that the finding of a normal pressure by tonometry before dilation is no guarantee that this type of glaucoma will not ensue. The only method of assessing such an eye is by examination of the angles themselves with the use of the gonioscope.

There are many tests that provoke an angle-closure attack and therefore confirm the diagnosis of angle-closure glaucoma. The *dark room provocative test* is the time-honored method of revealing this condition. In this test the patient is kept in a dark room for 60 to 90 minutes, following which the ocular tension is measured. A rise of 8.5 mm Hg or more is considered a positive reaction. Unfortunately, this test is not specific for predicting future angle-closure attacks and, although useful, is not relied on as much as the mydriatic test.

The *mydriatic test* for angle-closure glaucoma consists of instilling one or two drops of a weak-acting mydriatic agent, such as hydroxyamphetamine (Paredrine), into the conjunctival sac. Again, an 8-mm rise in pressure by the end of 1 hour is considered a positive reaction if gonioscopy confirms that the angle has been closed during the period of tension elevation.

Pupillary dilation plus gonioscopy provide the most thorough basis for confirmation of angle-closure glaucoma. After the pupil of one eye is dilated with a weak mydriatic agent, tonographic examination is performed in dim light. A decrease of 25% to 30% in the facility of outflow, if coupled with gonioscopic evidence of angle closure, is considered a position reaction.

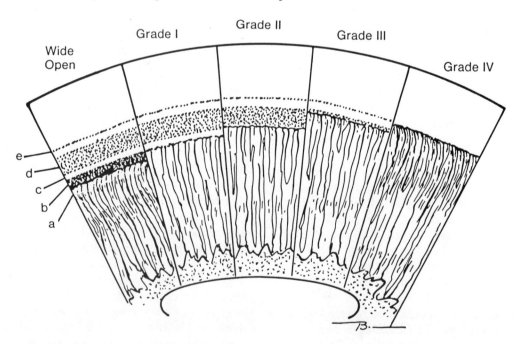

Fig. 22-5 Scheie's gonioscopic classification of the anterior chamber angle, based on the extent of visible angle structures: **A**, root of the iris; **B**, ciliary body band; **C**, scleral spur; **D**, trabecular meshwork; **E**, Schwalbe's line. (From Shields MB, editor: *Textbook of glaucoma*, ed 3, Baltimore, 1991, Williams & Wilkins.)

Table 22-2	Classification of angles based on gonioscopic appearance (Scheie's classification)

Classification	Appearance
Wide open	All angle structures seen
Grade I narrow	Difficult to see over the iris root
Grade II narrow	Ciliary band obscured
Grade III narrow	Posterior trabeculum hazy
Grade IV narrow	Only Schwalbe's line visible

Modified from Shields MB, editor: *Textbook of glaucoma,* ed 3, Baltimore, 1991, Williams & Wilkins.

A negative provocative test reaction certainly does not rule out the possibility of the patient's ever having an attack of angle-closure glaucoma. The most important diagnostic investigation into this condition is the use of gonioscopy (Fig. 22-5 and Table 22-2). If the angles are unduly narrowed despite negative provocative test reactions, the patient should be observed closely.

Gonioscopy

Gonioscopy is a clinical technique that is used to examine the structures of the anterior chamber angle. With this technique one can differentiate between the two major types of glaucoma; open-angle and angle-closure glaucoma.

Normally, light rays coming from the anterior chamber angle are reflected back into the anterior chamber, preventing the visualization of the angle. The answer to this interesting reflection is to eliminate the cornea optically. This is performed with a contact lens so that light rays flow onto the contact lens and the angle structures can be visualized.

Two major types of lenses are used in gonioscopy: the goniolens and the Zeiss four-mirror lens. The goniolens, which is used primarily for infants, is applied with the patient in the supine position; a viscous preparation such as methylcellulose is placed between the lens and the cornea. The gonioscope is held in one hand and the light source in the other (Fig. 22-6).

In indirect gonioscopy the light rays are reflected by a mirror in the contact lens (the gonioprism). The

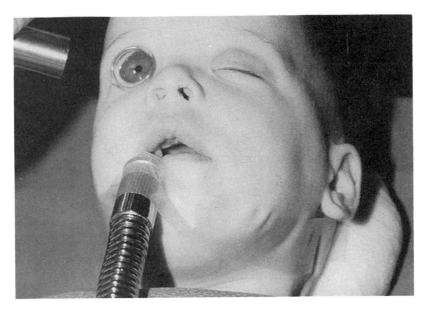

Fig. 22-6 A major use of direct Koeppe gonioscopy is examination of the angle in the operating room. In a child, it provides a direct view that is identical to the view during actual gonioscopy. (From Hoskins HD Jr, Kass M: *Becker-Shaffer's Diagnosis & Therapy of the Glaucomas,* ed 6, St Louis, 1989, Mosby.)

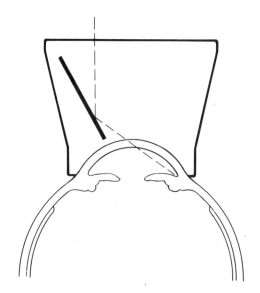

Fig. 22-7 Goniolens. A beam of light is deflected into the opposite angle of the anterior chamber.

mirror is usually inclined at an angle of 62 degrees. Frequently, two of the mirrors may be tilted at a steeper angle to permit examination of the surface of the peripheral retina (Fig. 22-7).

In the Zeiss four-mirrored lens, each of the mirrors is tilted at 64 degrees to permit examination of the angle without rotating the lens (Fig. 22-8).

The technique of using the goniolens is as follows. A local anesthetic is applied to the eye, and goniolens gel is applied to the lens. The lens is applied directly with the lids held apart, usually by an assistant. Examination of the angle is performed with the slit-lamp biomicroscope. The goniolens is more popular for examining the angle because it can be done with normal office instrumentation and techniques. Also, the slit lamp offers better optics and lighting.

The normal anterior chamber angle as seen through the gonioscope reveals the following structures (see Fig. 22-5):

1. *The ciliary body band*. The band is usually gray or dark and depends on the level above the iris insertion. It is a little wider in persons who are myopic.

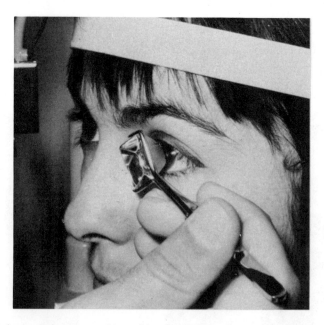

Fig. 22-8 Slit-lamp gonioscopy position of hand-held Zeiss lens, with hand resting against the cheek for maximum control. (From Hoskins HD Jr, Kass M: *Becker-Shaffer's Diagnosis and Therapy of the Glaucomas,* ed 6, St Louis, 1989, Mosby.)

2. *The scleral spur.* This is seen as a prominent white line between the ciliary body band and the trabecular meshwork. Frequently, fine pigmented strands may be visible crossing the scleral spur. These are the iris processes.

3. *Trabecular meshwork.* This is a pigmented band just anterior to the scleral spur. The appearance of the trabecular meshwork is variable. Usually it gathers pigment as an age-related change. The color is anywhere from tan to dark brown that may be irregular and more mottled in appearance.

4. *Schwalbe's line.* This is viewed as a fine ridge just anterior to the trabecular meshwork.

Oblique flashlight illumination, with the light coming from the temporal side of the eye, gives a fairly accurate evaluation of the depth. With a deep chamber the entire iris is illuminated. If the iris is bowed forward, its distal portions are in the shadows.

Gonioscopy is still the most valued technique used to determine the adequacy of the anterior chamber angle. Most of these evaluations are concerned with the angular width of the angular recess. This is largely based on the extent of the angle structures that can be visualized.

Treatment

The procedure of choice today is laser iridotomy (Fig. 22-9). It is simple, noninvasive, and can be performed with virtually no complications. It should be done bilaterally inasmuch as it has been shown that 50% to 70% of the patients with angle-closure glaucoma in one eye will have an attack in the fellow eye within 5 to 10 years despite miotic treatment.

A peripheral iridotomy is accomplished to relieve the pupillary block and to allow the anterior chamber to deepen. If the attack has not formed adhesions between the iris and the angle structure, the procedure is curative.

Medical therapy for angle-closure glaucoma is used only as a prelude to laser iridotomy. The pur-

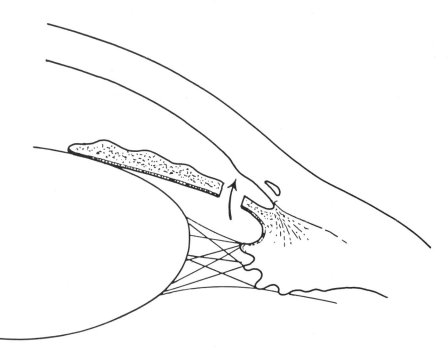

Fig. 22-9 Peripheral iridotomy eliminates pupillary block. (From Shields MB, editor: *Textbook of glaucoma,* ed 3, Baltimore, 1991, Williams & Wilkins.)

pose is to reduce the pressure and eliminate the corneal edema so that the subsequent procedure can be accomplished with greater safety and ease.

If the attack is not aborted early, permanent scar tissue can result in secondary glaucoma, and the vision can be permanently affected by damage to the optic nerve.

When one eye has been subjected to an attack of angle-closure glaucoma, the other eye has a strong chance of experiencing a similar attack. For this reason, most surgeons prefer to do a prophylactic iridectomy on the healthy eye to avoid the hazards of acute-closure glaucoma. The risks of an iridectomy are far less than the risks of a second attack.

Medical therapy for angle-closure glaucoma is useful only as a prelude to surgery. Its object is to lower the intraocular pressure and open the blocked angle so that the subsequent surgery can be performed more safely and with greater ease. Acetazolamide (Diamox) or methazolamide (Neptazane), carbonic anhydrase inhibitors, are used to temporarily lower the intraocular pressure. Acetazolamide may be given intramuscularly, intravenously, or orally. β-Blockers such as timolol, levobunolol, and betaxotol work in concert with carbonic anhydrase inhibitors (CAI) to lower intraocular pressure. Miotic agents are used to pull the iris away from the peripheral angle. Pilocarpine, 2%, or carbachol, 1.5%, is instilled in the affected eye two to three times, 5 minutes apart. The use of demecarium bromide (Humorsol) or echothiophate iodide (Phospholine Iodide) is to be avoided in angle-closure glaucoma because these medications only exaggerate the pupillary block and the congestive reaction of the eye.

In addition to acetazolamide, various hypertonic solutions have been used to gain a more prompt and rapid reduction of intraocular pressure. The agents most commonly used today are (1) mannitol, given in a dose of 1 to 2 g/kg of body weight (intravenously) and (2) glycerin, given in a dose of 1.5 g/kg of body weight (orally). Usually 1½ to 2 ounces of glycerin is mixed with orange juice or lemon juice to avoid the sickening effects of the sweet taste of the glycerin. For the relief of pain, morphine sulfate, 50 mg subcutaneously, is quite helpful. Meperidine (Demerol), 50 to 100 mg, is a good alternative.

The ophthalmic assistant should be familiar with this condition because it constitutes an ocular emergency. Over the telephone the abruptness of its onset is its most pressing clue. On examination, the dilation of the pupil fixed to light, combined with a steamy cornea, is its most imposing sign. Because treatment should begin as soon as the diagnosis is made, the ophthalmic assistant should keep all the medications used in the treatment of this condition available for immediate use.

PRIMARY OPEN-ANGLE GLAUCOMA

Primary open-angle glaucoma is a relentless bilateral chronic disease. There are no external signs of the disease at any time. In most cases the glaucoma develops in middle life or later, and the onset is gradual and symptomless.

The cause of this disorder is obstruction of the outflow of aqueous humor in the trabecular meshwork. Most cases of primary open-angle glaucoma are caused by an inability of aqueous fluid to leave the eye, and not by an overproduction of aqueous fluid (Fig. 22-10).

No symptoms may be found until the disease is far progressed or until the ophthalmologist has seen an excavated disc or elevated tension on a routine eye examination. The diagnosis of this condition depends on three objective signs: (1) raised tension, (2) cupping of the disc (Fig. 22-11), and (3) field defects.

Ocular hypertension

Some persons exhibit high intraocular pressures but do not show any changes in their visual field or in their optic discs. These may be individuals who can sustain higher than normal intraocular pressures without damage. Some ophthalmologists believe they may be preglaucomatous or "glaucoma suspects." However, ophthalmic personnel should label this condition *ocular hypertensive* to avoid using these other terms so patients do not look up in the dictionary the omnious meaning of glaucoma and become upset. The term *ocular hypertensive* creates a convenient category, without a gloomy label, for

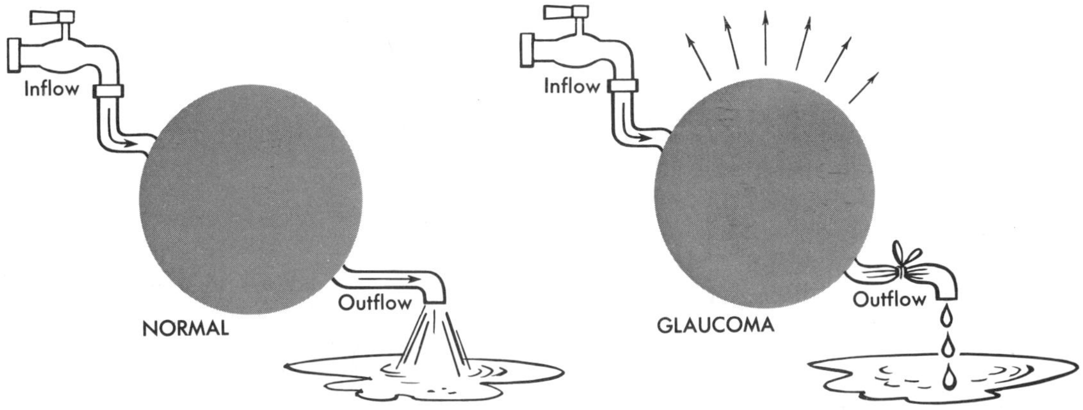

Fig. 22-10 Obstruction of aqueous outflow causes an elevation of intraocular tension.

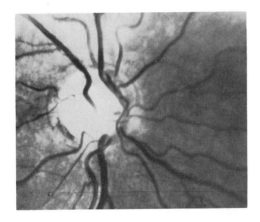

Fig. 22-11 Cupping of the optic disc. Note the dip of the vessels as they traverse the temporal margin of the disc.

keeping patients under observation. Actually, most of these persons will live most of their lives without therapy. However, they must remain under observation because some individuals in this group are at greater risk of developing true glaucomatous changes in their field and disc.

At one time persons older than 40 years of age with pressures greater than 21 mm Hg were considered to have glaucoma and were treated on the basis that field loss would inevitably follow. However, clinical evidence has shown that whereas 5% to 15% of the population over the age of 40 have pressures greater than 21 mm Hg, only 0.3% of the same population have detectable visual impairment. Of those with ocular hypertension, 10% have field loss, and another 4% will develop field loss during 5- to 10-year follow-up.

Therapy for those with ocular hypertension is not without risk. Therapy may limit the patient's ability to manage daily activities. It may affect pupil size. It may interfere with systemic medication or systemic conditions. It may cause periorbital pain and headache. Therapy may restrict a healthy person to the schedule of a disabled individual requiring medication two or three times daily. For these reasons the decision to treat this group of patients with high intraocular pressure is a judgment decision dependent on the perceived threat to vision. Thus observation and continued monitoring of ocular hypertension are commonly the choice today.

Tonometry

Measuring intraocular pressure, called *tonometry,* is an essential part of all eye examinations for adults and children. The reason is simple: routine tonometry can detect undiagnosed glaucoma. Glaucoma affects an estimated 2% of adults older than the age of 40; in fact, some investigations have found elevated intraocular pressure (greater than 21 mm Hg) among as many as 4.7% to 6.5% of normal individuals and 80% of untreated glaucoma patients.

Because eye pressure measurement is such an important parameter to record, more and more ophthalmologists are instructing their personnel to perform tonometry. It therefore behooves the ophthalmic assistant to understand the basic techniques and underlying physiologic principles of tonometry and to become comfortable, facile, and knowledgeable in this role.

Eye pressure is not measured directly. It simply is not practical or safe to place a small needle in the eye and record the actual intraocular pressure. Instead, the measurement can be accurately determined noninvasively. Noninvasive devices work with use of either an indentation or an applanation principle. Both work well. Each method has advantages, as well as limitations, which will be outlined in the next few paragraphs.

The accuracy of either technique is limited by the physical properties of the cornea. During the actual measuring process, the indenting apparatus deforms the cornea more than the applanating one. Therefore more aqueous fluid, normally in the anterior chamber of the eye between the cornea and iris, is displaced. The displaced aqueous ultimately distends the other structures inside the eye. These intraocular structures have an inherent elastic property that resists distention—that is, the eye does not expand like a balloon; rather, its natural elastic qualities maintain a constant volume. Because the volume does not change, the pressure inside the eye must change. Thus the intraocular pressure is "falsely" elevated. This phenomenon is well known, and calibration charts formulated to adjust for this abnormal "false" elevation of pressure are readily available.

The applanation technique differs from the indenting technique by displacing a minimal amount of fluid. Therefore any applanation tonometer–induced intraocular pressure elevation is not a real concern. This is the major reason that many ophthalmologists believe the applanation technique is more sensitive and accurate than the indentation technique.

Schiøtz tonometer. The Schiøtz tonometer is an instrument used throughout the world for the detection and determination of intraocular pressure, because it is convenient to use, portable, fairly reliable,

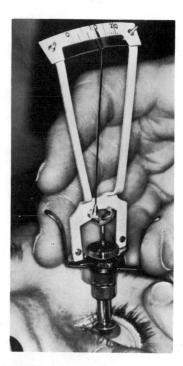

Fig. 22-12 Measurement of intraocular pressure with the Schiøtz tonometer. Note that the lids are pinioned against the bony orbit by the examiner's fingers.

and low in cost. When the Schiøtz tonometer is used, the patient usually is placed in a recumbent position and asked to look up at a fixation point directed vertically above (Fig. 22-12). The corneas are anesthetized with a topical anesthetic such as proparacaine. If the blinking motion is excessive, the examiner may pinion the lids against the margin of the orbit with his or her fingers, taking care not to press on the globe itself. The tonometer is allowed to rest on the patient's cornea, and the extent to which the plunger of the tonometer indents the cornea is, in effect, a measure of its intraocular pressure. The greater the distance the plunger indents the cornea, the softer the eye or the lower the intraocular pressure. This is recorded on a scale on which the scale reading reflects the excursion distance of the plunger. If the eye is soft, as the Schiøtz tonometer plunger moves, the recording needle moves further along the scale located at the top of the tonometer. The higher

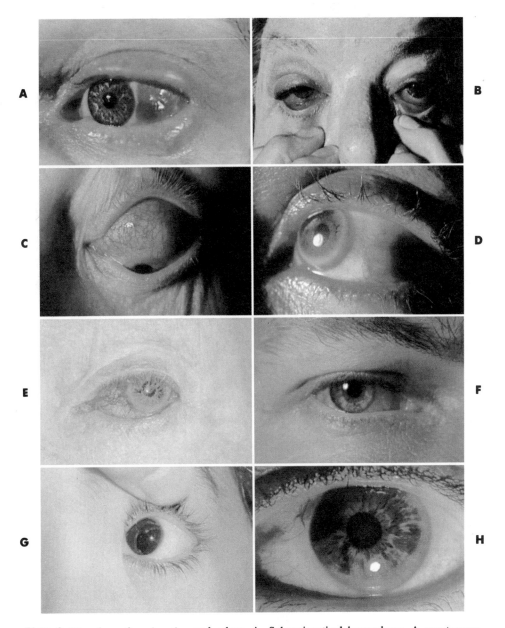

Plate 3 *Disorders of conjunctiva and sclera.* **A,** Subconjunctival hemorrhage. A spontaneous hemorrhage occurring under the conjunctiva and spreading over the globe. **B,** Acute bacterial conjunctivitis. Inflammation of the conjunctival lining caused by *Streptococcus.* **C,** Scleritis, Nonbacterial inflammation of the sclera. **D,** Nodular episcleritis. (Courtesy Dr. Ira Abrahamson Jr., Cincinnati, Oh.)

Disorders of the iris. **E,** Acute iritis. An acute inflammatory reaction of the iris resulting in pain, redness, and a constricted pupil. **F,** Subacute iritis. A less violent reaction of the iris with redness and blurring of vision. **G,** Congenital coloboma of the iris. A congenital defect in the iris inferonasally. **H,** Melanoma of the iris. A pigmented lesion of the iris. (Color plates made possible through a publication grant from Allergan Pharmaceuticals and Syntex Ophthalmics, Inc.)

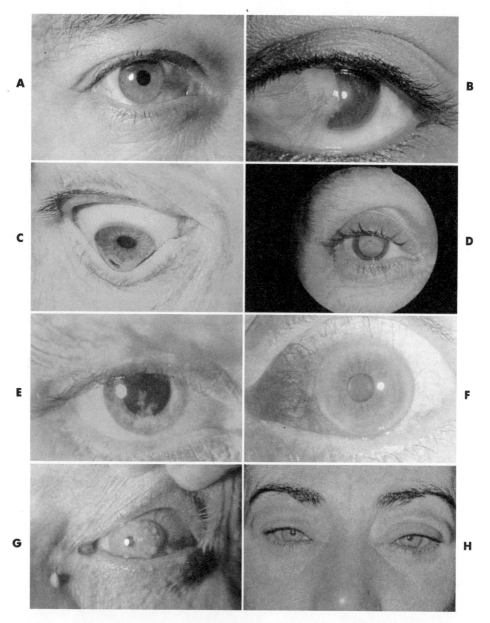

Plate 4 *Disorders of the cornea.* **A,** Pterygium. A triangular membrane extending from the conjunctiva over the cornea. **B,** Extensive recurrent pterygium. A history of two previous removals of the pterygium with a recurrence involving the visual axis. **C,** Advanced keratoconus. A cone-shaped deformity of the cornea with thinning of the cornea. (Courtesy Dr. Dean Butcher, Australia.) **D,** Keratoconus reflex. Retinal reflex as seen through a thin protruding cornea. (Courtesy Dr. Dean Butcher, Australia.) **E,** Herpes simplex—dendritic ulcer. Fernlike projection on the epithelial surface of the cornea from herpes simplex of the cornea. (Courtesy Dr. Ira Abrahamson Jr., Cincinnati, Oh.) **F,** Marginal corneal ulcer. Ulceration of the margin of the cornea resulting from *Staphylococcus* exotoxin. **G,** Squamous cell carcinoma of cornea. A cancer growth occurring at the limbus and invading the cornea. **H,** Ultraviolet keratitis. Inflammation of the cornea resulting from arc welding. (Color plates made possible through a publication grant from Allergan Pharmaceuticals and Syntex Ophthalmics, Inc.)

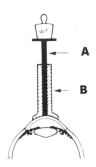

Fig. 22-13 Principle of the indentation tonometer. *A,* Plunger to indent cornea. *B,* Frame resting on cornea. (From Reinecke R., Stein H., Slatt, B: *Introductory manual for the ophthalmic assistant,* St Louis, 1972, Mosby.)

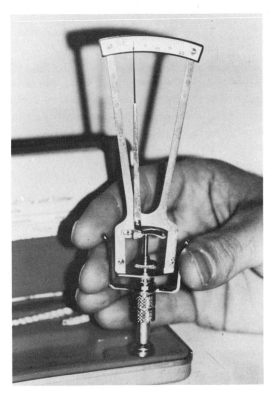

Fig. 22-15 Metallic test plate for Schiøtz tonometer.

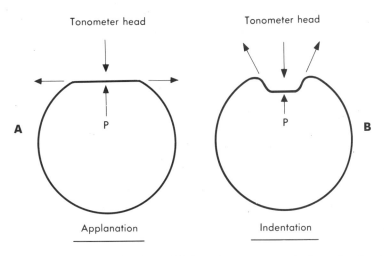

Fig. 22-14 Comparison of applanation and indentation tonometry. **A,** In applanation tonometry the cornea is flattened and the pressure is distributed evenly on each side; the pressure measurement is very close to that of the undisturbed eye. **B,** Indentation of the cornea causes buckling of the ocular coats because of the oblique distribution of pressure.

using a pipe cleaner or a brush moistened with alcohol or ether. The other parts, such as the plunger itself, are cleaned with a cotton cloth and alcohol.

Most ophthalmologists do not sterilize their tonometer. If desired, however, the base of the instrument can be sterilized by using a flame or burner, gaseous sterilization chamber, or small disposable rubber caps (Tonofilms) that are applied over the base of the instrument. Some ophthalmologists house the tonometer in an ultraviolet sterilizer. If possible, tonometry should be avoided on infected eyes as a prevention against spread of the infectious organisms.

Concern has been raised regarding tonometry and the potential transmissibility of infectious diseases, especially the AIDS virus (HIV) and the hepatitis virus. Whereas the AIDS virus has been isolated in the tears of patients with known AIDS, the infectivity of the virus through tears appears low, because there are no known instances where the virus has been transmitted in this manner. The concern about transmissibility, however, has led to recommendations for the sterilization of contact tonometer tips. It is recommended that gloves be used when high-risk patients are examined, especially if the examiner has scratches or skin lesions on the hands.

Instruments contacting the external eye surfaces should be wiped clean and disinfected with either hydrogen peroxide, 3%, for 10 minutes or a 1:10 dilution of liquid bleach (5000 parts per million). Please note that the bleach may remove the printed markings on the plastic tonometer tip. Ethanol or isopropanol, 70%, is an effective disinfectant, but both agents will discolor the plastic and create a haze on its surface.

The patient should be comfortable, well anesthetized with drops (proparacaine), and relaxed. Fixation should be maintained on one spot. Coughing, breath holding, and wandering eye movements will make pressure recordings inaccurate. The most common error in Schiøtz tonometry results from the patient's squeezing the lids together, thus either preventing the easy application of the tonometer to the cornea or gripping it like a vise. In such situations, the lids should be manually opened by the examiner without any pressure on the globe. At the same time,

the patient is asked to open the mouth and take a deep breath. This last maneuver serves to distract the patient and also takes advantage of a primitive reflex that prevents forceful closure of the lids with the mouth held wide open.

The examiner must be aware of two points in Schiøtz tonometry. *The fingers must never press on the globe at any time.* In addition to being uncomfortable to the patient and dangerous to the eye, such extraneous pressure will cause absurd elevations in the intraocular pressure. *The tonometer must be applied directly over the apex of the cornea and not allowed to slide over the surface of the cornea.* Sliding the tonometer is a certain way of producing corneal abrasions. Observing fine movements on the needle confirms good alignment, because the oscillations are from variations in blood pressure.

For inexperienced examiners, practice with the instrument may be performed on someone with an artificial eye. This will eliminate the worry of danger to the patient's or a colleague's eye.

Applanation tonometry. In applanation tonometry the ocular wall (cornea) is flattened, and the flattened area is measured. (The word *applanation* originates from the Latin *planare* or *ad planare,* meaning "to flatten.") The higher the intraocular pressure (the harder the eye), the smaller will be the flattened area, assuming that the same weight is used for flattening each time tonometry is performed.

Applanation tonometry eliminates some of the errors inherent in indentation tonometry. Indentation tonometry creates tension forces in the indented ocular wall, and these forces act against the plunger of the tonometer. In addition, during indentation tonometry the considerable weight of the tonometer itself artificially raises the intraocular pressure. However, in applanation tonometry the tension forces that are created in the applanated ocular wall are lying in the plane of applanation and are opposing each other; thus they cancel each other for all practical purposes. Also, in applanation tonometry the artificial increase of the intraocular pressure during tonometry caused by the weight of the tonometer is minimal.

A common source of error of indentation tonometry is underestimation of the intraocular pressure in

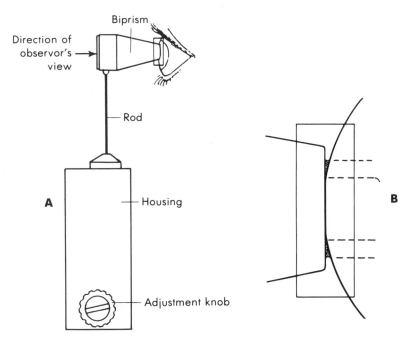

Fig. 22-16 Goldmann type of applanation tonometry. **A,** Basic features of tonometer, shown in contact with patient's cornea. **B,** Enlargement of **A** shows tear film meniscus created by contact of biprism and cornea. (From Shields MB, editor: *Textbook of glaucoma,* ed 3, 1991, Baltimore, Williams & Wilkins.)

eyes that have low ocular rigidity, such as the eyes of myopes. Applanation minimizes this error.

Goldmann applanation tonometer. The Goldmann applanation tonometer gives a reliable measurement of intraocular pressure to within ± 0.5 mm Hg. This tonometer, because it flattens the cornea and does not indent it, gives accurate information about the tension in the undisturbed eye. Scleral rigidity can be disregarded because it displaces less than 0.5 mm of volume. It also causes little increase in tension, so that no massage effect is produced by repeated measurements that might lower the pressure. A plastic tip is attached to a sensitive balance mounted on the slit lamp (Fig. 22-16). This small tip is designed to minimize both the "inward" pull from the liquid tear film on the cornea and the "outward" push from the elastic cornea. The volume of displaced fluid inside of the eye is so small that any variation in ocular rigidity can be ignored. When the circular tip

with only a 3.06 mm diameter is used to applanate the cornea, no significant elevation of eye pressure is created.

One disadvantage of the Goldmann applanation tonometer is its lack of portability. However, hand-held applanation tonometers have been devised to eliminate the difficulty. Other disadvantages are that the technique requires training for successful use. In addition, corneal distortion such as seen with scarring or high astigmatism creates difficulty in obtaining reliable end-point measurements. Corneal abrasions are always a potential hazard if the assistant is too aggressive during the pressure reading or if any underlying corneal problem is present. Infection is a potential risk as well.

The method of applanation tonometry is as follows. One or two drops of a local anesthetic solution are placed into the lower conjunctival sac. Then a drop of fluorescein from a fluorescein strip (small

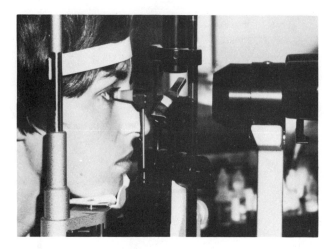

Fig. 22-17 Measurement of intraocular pressure with the applanation tonometer.

strips of filter paper impregnated with fluorescein) is instilled in the eye. After the drop is instilled, the patient's head is placed at the slit-lamp microscope with the chin on the chin rest and the forehead pressed firmly against the head rest (Fig. 22-17). Once the cornea is in focus, the appropriate blue filter is attached, and the slit diaphragm is opened completely. In the beam the whole surface of the patient's eye should glow in a bright greenish yellow. The blue light should be approximately 45 to 60 degrees to the side of the tonometer and should illuminate the front end of the prism head. The low power is used on the slip-lamp microscope. The patient's lids must be open and unblinking. It is necessary to avoid any contact between the tonometer and the lid margin or lashes because this contact only induces further blinking. The patient is instructed to look straight ahead or at some target device attached to the slit lamp to ensure fixation. Once the patient is ready, the tonometer, with the measuring drum set at 1 g, is brought forward by the joystick of the slit lamp until it comes in contact with the center of the cornea.

Looking through one eyepiece of the microscope, the patient sees, at the moment of contact, a bright yellow-green spot that quickly breaks into two bright yellow-green semicircular arcs as the tonometer is moved slightly farther forward. These arcs should be in sharp focus and of equal circumference both above and below the horizontal dividing line. Any necessary correction should be made by the control lever or the height adjustment control on the slit lamp. The calibrated drum on the side is conventionally set at 1. The drum is then turned toward the higher numbers corresponding to increasing force of applanation. As this occurs, the two semicircular arcs move until they overlap, the inner edge of the upper semicircle becoming aligned with the inner edge of the lower (Fig. 22-18). This is the desired end point at which the reading is taken from the drum. The scale is such that the reading obtained is multiplied by 10 to convert the number to an equivalent millimeters of mercury of intraocular pressure. Therefore, 1 on the drum would be equal to 10 mm Hg. It is best to take at least two readings on each eye to obtain an average set of values. If the values obtained on two successive readings are approximately the same, the technique is probably adequate.

Checking the calibration of the Goldmann applanation tonometer. Applanation tonometers may be checked for accuracy by the use of a central weight. For the Goldmann tonometer, a short rod of measured weight is attached to the balancing arm of the tonometer and the rod set at 0, 2, and 6, respectively. At each measure, the measuring drum should be placed at the corresponding stop. At each stop, the

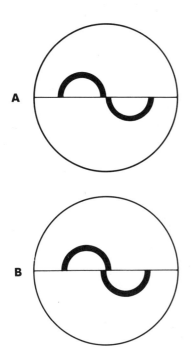

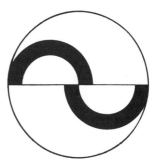

Fig. 22-20 Too much fluorescein has been instilled.

Fig. 22-18 A, Split half circles at beginning of applanation. Intraocular pressure is read when the inner half circles touch one another (end point), as shown in **B**.

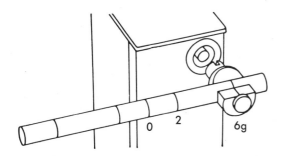

Fig. 22-19 Calibration bar for calibrating the Goldmann applanation tonometer.

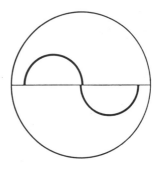

Fig. 22-21 Too narrow a fluorescein band because of too little fluorescein or evaporation of fluorescein.

3.06 mm—is flattened. The inner border of the ring represents the line of demarcation between the cornea flattened by applanation and the cornea not flattened. The measuring drum can regulate the tension to produce a force that is between 0 and 8 g.

Errors in Goldmann tonometry

1. If the fluorescein ring is too wide (Fig. 22-20), too much fluorescein may have been instilled. In this case a small cotton wad can be used to absorb excess fluorescein and the procedure repeated. Alternately, the measuring prism may not have been cleaned of previous fluorescein. A wide band will result in a high and erroneous reading.

2. If the fluorescein band is too narrow (Fig. 22-21), this results from evaporation of the stained tear layer during protracted measurement. The reading on the drum will be lower than normal. The patient should be told to blink several times and the measurement repeated.

tonometer head should move only plus or minus 0.05 g (0.5 mm Hg) of these settings (Fig. 22-19).

The applanation tonometer consists of a plastic prism with the anterior surface flat and having a diameter of 7 mm. This prism is brought into contact with a fluorescein-stained tear film of the cornea, which it displaces to the periphery of the contact zone until a surface of known and constant size—

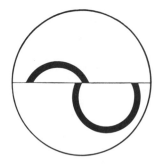

Fig. 22-22 Unequal semicircles because of improper centering of the tonometer head.

3. The two semicircles may not be on the middle field (Fig. 22-22). The patient may have moved slightly or the chin rest may not be properly adjusted; thus the fluorescein rings are not two exact semicircles because of improper centering of the tonometer head. This will produce a considerably elevated intraocular pressure. The slit lamp should be adjusted up or down to obtain two exact semicircles.

4. If the patient's head is not pressed firmly against the forehead bar, there may be intermittent contact of the prism with the cornea, resulting in apparent pulsations of the fluorescein rings.

5. With a spherical or near-spherical cornea, measurement can be made in any meridian. If, however, astigmatism greater than 3 diopters exists, the flattened area becomes elliptical rather than circular. In this instance, the tonometer prism head should be set with the axis corresponding to the axis of the minus cylinder.

6. Standard applanation tonometry with fluorescein cannot be used with a soft contact lens. Alternately the MacKay-Marg tonometer, a pneumatic tonometer, or the electronic tonometer may be used in this situation.

7. Breath holding or a tight collar will give a false high reading.

8. If it is necessary to hold the lids apart with the fingers and thumb, care must be taken to avoid pressing on the globe or this will falsely raise the intraocular pressure.

Evaluating the pressures. If the pressure was found to be 22 mm Hg or more with the Goldmann applanation tonometer recordings, the eye would be considered abnormal. A tension of 21 should be regarded as borderline. Tensions between 18 and 21 are generally normal, but the patient should be seen for repeated examinations.

The tension normally varies in an eye during the time of day. It is highest in most people at 6 o'clock in the morning and lowest during the waking hours, the time when ophthalmologists conduct their office hours or clinics. It is because of this diurnal variation that the tension may be borderline, or less than borderline, and the patient may still have glaucoma. In addition to the diurnal variation, there are other low-tension glaucomatous states in which the pressure recordings may be normal, or even below normal, and the patient may still have clinical evidence of the disease. Although applanation tonometry is the best method of discovering the most characteristic sign of glaucoma, it is not an infallible test for the reasons mentioned.

As mentioned previously, elevated intraocular pressure without demonstrable damage to the optic nerve and without visual field changes in sometimes called *ocular hypertension*. These cases require relentless and meticulous observation.

The diagnosis of glaucoma requires an evaluation of all three parameters: tension, optic disc, and visual field change.

Hints for use

1. *Educate the patient*. Less anxiety is created if the examiner tells the patient that the tonometer tip will touch the tear film instead of saying the tip will actually touch the eye.

2. *Instill topical anesthetic*. Again, tell the patient what to expect: "This drop may feel cold or may even sting for a few seconds." After the anesthetic is given, touch the conjunctiva with a strip of fluorescein-impregnated paper. Alternatively, a drop of a combination topical anesthetic-fluorescein mixture such as Fluress (a combination of fluorescein and a topical anesthetic) can easily be used.

3. *Alignment*. Rest the patient's chin on the rest, and press the forehead against the headband. The patient's eyes but not mouth should be open. Ask the patient to stare straight ahead and not at the blue slit light.

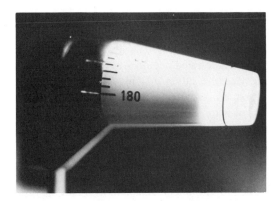

Fig. 22-23 Markings on the tonometer head for alignment with high cylinders.

4. *Slit lamp and tonometer alignment.* Set the magnification on low (this is much easier to use). Position the tonometer and light so that the tonometer tip is as brightly illuminated as possible—usually a 45-degree angle between the light and tip. Do not forget to use the blue filter! Remember, if corneal astigmatism is greater than 3 diopters, set the tip axis 43 degrees from the minus cylinder axis of the astigmatism (Fig. 22-23).

Move the slit lamp toward the patient with the joystick held back. Once 3 to 5 mm away from the cornea, slowly advance the slit lamp forward with the joystick. At this point the examiner can look through the left eyepiece and begin to see a faint purple semicircle created by the reflected corneal image of the prism tip. These arcs will touch one another just before the tip actually touches the cornea.

5. *Align tonometer mires.* Just as the tip touches the cornea, two bright-green semicircles appear. If this does not happen, pull the joystick back, recheck both the patient and tonometer alignment, wipe the tip, and start again. If the semicircles are slightly out of line, alignment can be adjusted without repositioning the slit lamp.

Proper measurement depends on the two arcs being sharply focused, symmetric, and bright. Rotate the dial on the tonometer scale until the inner edges of the two arcs exactly align (Fig. 22-24). To calculate the intraocular pressure, multiply the scale

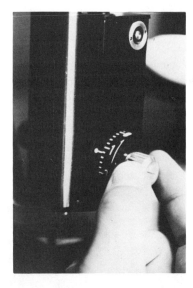

Fig. 22-24 Tonometer scale is adjusted to align the inner edges of the two fluorescein arcs on the cornea.

reading times 10. Pulsatile movements of the mires can be frustrating as the examiner tries to carefully touch the two inner edges together. A setting halfway between the two extreme pulse pressures will provide the truest pressure measurements.

The Goldmann tonometer has been miniaturized into a hand-held model that does not require a slit lamp for proper use. The two models presently available, Kowa and Perkins, are nearly identical in construction and use. The same plastic applanation tip used with the slit lamp mounted model is incorporated in the portable units and is counterbalanced with a small weight in the handle. Eye pressure is measured by applanating the tonometer tip to the central cornea until the familiar mires are identified and properly positioned. The tip is illuminated by a penlight also contained in the handle. By rotating a knurled knob on the handle, not only is the light turned on but also increased pressure is applied to the tonometer tip. Once the correct applanating force is applied, the intraocular pressure can be easily determined by viewing a scale and multiplying times a factor of 10. This technique is quite accurate, yet requires some perseverance to master because the patient's head is not firmly supported in a chin and forehead rest.

Tonomat. The Tonomat, another type of applanation tonometer, was developed from the Maklakov, the original applanation tonometer. The Tonomat consists of a standard weight with a variable flattened or applanated area—exactly the reverse principle of the Goldmann tonometer. This tonometer has a small, flat, disposable plastic footplate, which is lightly stained with a coating material supplied with the instrument. The usual problem in obtaining accurate results is use of too much stain on the footplate. The correct amount is a very light brown, dry coating.

The patient, recumbent and with anesthetized corneas, looks toward the ceiling, as in the case of Schiøtz tonometry, and the footplate is momentarily lowered onto the cornea and removed immediately. Inspection of the footplate will reveal that the cornea has printed a clear, lighter circle on the brown-stained footplate.

The footplate is then printed onto dampened filter paper (supplied with the instrument), resulting in a true imprint, which now can be measured with a magnifying loupe, also supplied with the tonometer. The diameter of the applanated area can then be measured and converted to pressure in millimeters of mercury. (A conversion table is provided with the instrument.)

Perkin's hand-held applanation tonometer. (Fig. 22-25) The principle of this instrument is the same as that of the Goldmann applanation tonometer, in that an applanating surface is placed in contact with the cornea, and the force applied is varied until a fixed diameter of applanation is achieved. In the hand-held instrument, the Goldmann doubling prism is mounted on a counterbalanced arm, and the change in force is obtained by rotation of a spiral spring.

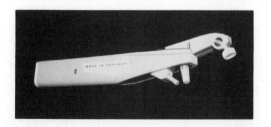

Fig. 22-25 Perkin's hand-held applanation tonometer.

The instrument operates on two AA batteries, and a tiny lightbulb underneath the doubling prism gives off a cobalt blue glow. The instrument can be used in any position and need not be held vertically. The patient can be sitting or lying flat.

The method of use is as follows. The eye is anesthetized with 1 drop Fluress, a fluorescein solution. The tonometer should be held so that the thumb rests on the thumb wheel, controlling the spring. The light is switched on by turning the thumb wheel until the scale reading is above 0, and the filter holder is adjusted to illuminate the end of the doubling prism, when the latter is at approximately its midpoint of travel, which is the position used for measurement.

The instrument has a forehead rest that can be used when the tonometer is positioned on the patient's cornea.

It is easier to hold the tonometer obliquely, with the handle slanted away from the patient's nose. Care should be taken that the prism is not touching the lids. Otherwise the readings obtained would be invalid.

The doubling prism is applied to the center of the patient's cornea, with the scale to read 1. Semicircles of fluorescein should now be visible through the viewing lens; force is adjusted by turning the thumb wheel until the inner margins of the semicircles coincide. The tonometer is then removed from the eye and the reading noted. The reading is multiplied by 10 to give the tensions in millimeters of mercury. The usual method is to repeat the reading for each eye twice and, if elevated, to take three readings.

If the semicircles appear large and are not reduced by altering the force of the spring, the tonometer has been pushed too close to the eye. Withdrawing it slightly will bring the prism within the range of free movement.

Airpuff tonometer. The American Optical Company has placed on the market a tonometer that measures intraocular pressure without any part of it coming in contact with the globe (Fig. 22-26). Basically it is an air pump that blows a jet or "puff" of air onto the cornea, flattening and applanating it.

This tonometer works on the principle of an interval timer, measuring the time it takes from the

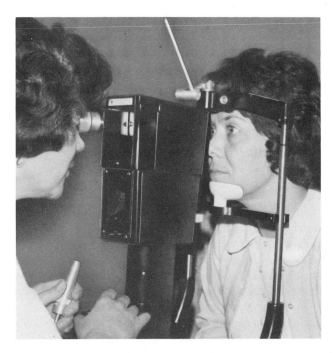

Fig. 22-26 American Optical noncontact applanation tonometer. A jet of air flattens the cornea, and the pressure is recorded electronically.

generation of the puff of air to the point at which the cornea is exactly flat; this time (usually about 3 msec) can be related directly to the intraocular pressure. Infrared light and photoelectric cells determine the point at which the cornea is flat, at which time the timing device stops. It takes less time for the puff of air to flatten a soft eye than it does a hard one, and hence an accurate relationship between time and intraocular pressure can be established. Digital readout numbers indicate the pressure in millimeters of mercury. We have found this to be an excellent screening device by the ophthalmic assistant. Its regular use will ensure a fair degree of accuracy in screening, but positive results should be rechecked with the Goldmann tonometer. We have found that the air puff tonometer tends to err slightly on the high side. High pressures should be rechecked with another tonometer.

Electronic applanation tonometer. Electronics represents the final adaptation of the applanation principle and is best represented by the MacKay-Marg tonom-eter or the Electro Medical Technology tonometer. With this technique, as the tip is applied to the eye, the pressure flexes an ultrathin membrane. This pressure is indirectly transmitted to a force transducer. The pressure waveform is converted into electrical impulses proportional to the applied pressure and recorded on a graph with a thermal stylus. This device is no longer available, but several miniaturized versions that function on similar principles have been developed and appear accurate and reliable.

Other applanation tonometers. Hand-held noncontact tonometers that are lightweight and portable are currently available. Also on the market are tonopens, which are penlike and which permit repeated accurate reading by applanation.

Also available is an applanation tonometer that can grade the intraocular pressures through use of an operating room microscope. This operating room device allows the surgeon to estimate whether the intraocular pressure is high, medium, or low at the end of intraocular surgery.

Comparison of the Schiøtz tonometer and the applanation tonometer

1. The Schiøtz tonometer indents the cornea, whereas the applanation tonometer flattens it.

2. The Schiøtz tonometer is portable; the conventional applanation tonometer is not.

3. The Schiøtz tonometer measures the amount of corneal indentation produced by a given weight. The applanation tonometer measures the amount of force required to produce a constant corneal flattening.

4. The Schiøtz tonometer raises the intraocular pressure because of indentation and the weight of the instrument itself. The applanation tonometer exerts only a small force on the cornea.

5. The Schiøtz tonometer may give an inaccurate measure because of the distortion of ocular coats. The footplate of the instrument is shaped to the average corneal curvature, but most patients' corneas are not exact fits. This poor fit introduces errors. Readings with the applanation tonometer are relatively independent of the rigidity of the ocular coats and are unaffected by corneal curvature variations.

6. Because of the buckling of the cornea and the resultant displacement of aqueous humor by the Schiøtz tonometer, second and third readings may be slightly lower as a result of massage of aqueous humor out of the eye. This does not occur with the applanation tonometer.

7. The Schiøtz tonometer measures tension with the patient in the recumbent position, whereas the conventional applanation tonometer measures tension with the patient in the sitting position. The new hand-held applanation tonometer can be used with the patient in any position.

8. The Schiøtz tonometer can be used for tonography; the applanation tonometer cannot.

Tonography

It is an old observation that massage of an eye lowers the intraocular pressure. The effect is marked in normal eyes but occurs at a slower rate in glaucomatous eyes. Tonography attempts to quantitate the massage effect by the use of an indentation tonometer applied to the globe to express fluid from the eye.

The value of tonography in helping to make the diagnosis or in follow-up of patients with glaucoma is controversial among ophthalmologists. However, because of its past widespread interest and its present interest in some centers, it is discussed.

The proponents of tonography point to its virtues, notably its effectiveness in diagnosing patients suspected of having glaucoma as a result of outflow trabecular damage, determining the adequacy of medical and surgical therapy, and assessing the patient with a complicated form of glaucoma. The opponents of the test decry many of its theoretic limitations, as well as the practical and abundant sources of error that limit its usefulness.

Certainly tonography should never be employed by the occasional operator who does not understand the fundamentals or the purpose of this test. If errors are compounded to whatever theoretic limitations are inherent in the test, the entire procedure becomes worthless.

Tonography is gradually becoming obsolete because of many features that are no longer applicable in evaluating glaucoma. Generally glaucoma can be evaluated by other means. Originally it was designed to map out the amount of aqueous that leaves the eye at a given time. Historically it had value in detecting glaucoma and in evaluating the outflow facility of the eye.

Theoretic considerations. Tonography measures the change in pressure that occurs when a constant weight (the tonometer) is applied to the eye for a period of 4 minutes. The application of some types of tonometers on the surface of the cornea indents the cornea and, by doing so, displaces aqueous out of the eye. The longer this pressure or weight is applied to the cornea, the greater will be the displacement of fluid from the eye and the lower will be the resultant pressure within the eye. In effect, the application of the tonometer on the eye for a period of 4 minutes decreases the volume of contents within the eye and therefore reduces the pressure of the eye. The time of 4 minutes is arbitrarily selected. If the tonometer were applied indefinitely, eventually a new relationship would exist between the amount of aqueous produced and the amount of aqueous leaving the eye, and further drops in intraocular pressure would not occur. With a normal eye the outflow

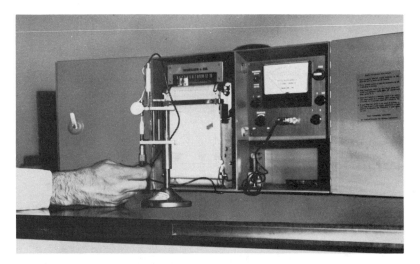

Fig. 22-27 Calibration of the Mueller electronic tonometer.

channels are open so that the application of the tonometer for 4 minutes will cause a marked drop in intraocular pressure. In a glaucomatous or hard eye the ability of aqueous humor to leave the eye is impaired, so that despite the application of a constant weight on the surface of the cornea, very little volume of the fluid contents of the eye is expelled, and as a result the decline in pressure is minimal.

Technique. Tonography is best carried out in a quiet, closed room that is free from the normal traffic of the office or clinic. The patient should be relaxed and reclining comfortably, either on a stretcher-type table or on a suitable reclining chair. The transistorized tonometer and recorders should be warmed up for at least 1 minute before actual use. The older tonometers required at least 10 minutes of warming up before calibration. Calibration should be employed routinely before the tonometer is used, just to ensure that the instrument is working normally. The 0 mark and the No. 7 mark of the tonometer are checked and recorded. If the calibration is inaccurate, adjustments should be made on the tonography machine to bring the needle into alignment at the 0 and 7 positions. Periodically the tonometer itself should be checked against a calibration gauge (Fig. 22-27).

A drop of topical anesthetic is placed into each eye. It is best that the upper lid be retracted and the patient asked to look down, because the contact of the drop on the sclera is not as jarring to the patient as the contact of the drop on the cornea. After topical anesthesia has been completed, the patient is asked to fixate on a target on the ceiling. The right eye is conventionally tested first. The examiner should be seated and comfortable because the test takes 4 minutes and can be fatiguing. The lids of the patient are grasped between the thumb and index finger of the left hand and then pinioned against the bony orbital margins (Fig. 22-28). It is important that the fingers of the examiner never touch the globe, because this would increase the ocular pressure. The tonometer is allowed to rest on the eye for a period of 4 to 4½ minutes. During this time the operator should observe the patient's eye to ensure that the patient's fixation is adequately maintained and that the tonometer is resting comfortably and centrally on the cornea.

The tonogram obtained should show an even and regular decline in pressure recordings between the initial and final pressure reading. The tracing should be sawtooth in nature, revealing good pulsations (Fig. 22-29).

Examination of the optic disc

Inspection of the optic disc is vital to a diagnosis of glaucoma. Because of the raised intraocular pres-

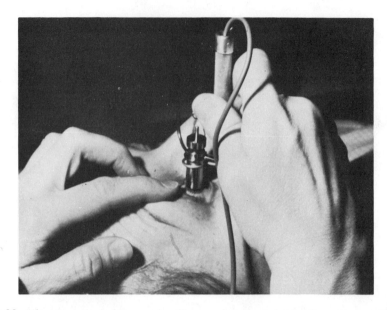

Fig. 22-28 Alternate method of tonography. The examiner stands behind the patient, and the index finger of one hand retracts the upper lid while the fourth finger of the hand applying the tonometer depresses the lower lid.

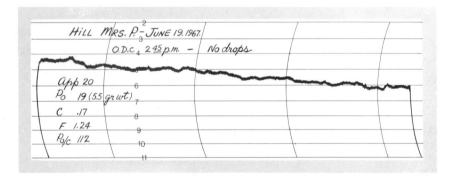

Fig. 22-29 Tonogram showing normal pulsations.

sure, the cumulative effect of this sustained pressure rise results in atrophy of the optic nerve at its entrance into the eye, the optic disc (Figs. 22-30 and 22-31). These changes consist of pallor and cupping of the optic disc. *Cupping,* usually manifested on the temporal aspect of the optic disc, results in the retinal vessels' dipping down over a saucerized edge at the margin of the disc, instead of running across it smoothly (Fig. 22-32). The disc also appears pale with glaucomatous atrophy.

Many ophthalmologists follow the course of glaucoma either by photographing the disc and noticing the changes or by making diagrams of it at regular intervals.

The fibers going to the optic nerve are called the *neural rim.* The central position of the disc head of the optic nerve contains a depression termed the *optic cup.* The ratio of the disc to the cup (cup:disc) is used by many ophthalmologists to follow the progress of changes in the optic nerve head. There is a

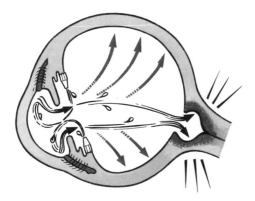

Fig. 22-30 Increased pressure causes excavation of the optic disc.

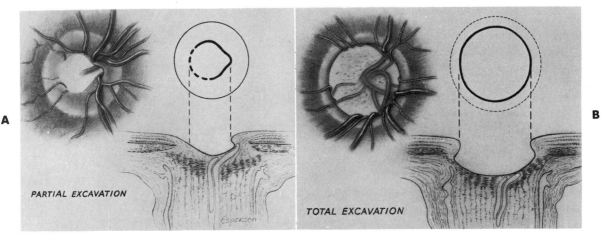

A

B

PARTIAL EXCAVATION

TOTAL EXCAVATION

Fig. 22-31 A, Diagram of moderately cupped disc. *Dotted line* indicates a sloping edge; *solid line,* undetermined edge of the cup. **B,** Diagram of markedly cupped disc. (From Kolker AE, Hetherington J: *Becker-Shaffer's diagnosis and therapy of the glaucomas,* ed 5, St Louis, 1983, Mosby.)

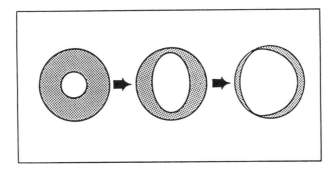

Fig. 22-32 Progressive cupping or increasing cup-to-disc ratio in the right eye in glaucoma.

very large variation of the cup-to-disc ratio in the normal population; however, the documentation of progressive cupping is one of the most important clinical findings in glaucoma. The optic cup normally has a horizontal oval shape. Thus the detection of a vertical cup suggests glaucoma. Notching and pallor are other important indicators of damage to the neural rim. Normally the cups are symmetric; thus significant asymmetry can indicate glaucoma. When the neural rim becomes severely atrophied, the retinal vessels crossing the sharpened rim will be acutely angulated at the edge of the disc, producing a picture of cupping. The ultimate course in this process leads to advanced glaucomatous cupping in which all the neural rim tissue is eventually lost. This is seen as a white disc that appears pale, with thinning of all the vessels at the margin of the disc.

Evaluation of the optic cups is a difficult procedure. Colobomas of the optic nerve, which are hereditary, with loss of optic neural tissue, can mimic variations of the normal appearance of the optic cup and may confuse the examiner. The disc may appear cupped and yet be perfectly normal. Photography offers a more objective assessment of the appearance of the cup. One can compare the appearance at one visit with the appearance at another without relying on memory. A reliable technique is the use of stereo photographs. This can be done by taking two photos in sequence on the same film with the use of a sliding carriage adapter or by applying two prisms that separate the pictures. The Donaldson camera is particularly good for stereoscopic fundus viewing. Glaucomascopes that provide optic disc imaging now can provide reliable pictures of the depth of the cupping. By repeating the imaging, one can detect subtle changes in the disc, and the computer of the machine will provide a change analysis for a printout.

Visual fields

Glaucomatous field defects arise as a consequence of damage to the optic disc. Field defects do not occur in glaucoma if the disc is normal. In most instances the ophthalmologist can predict the location of the field defect by noting the portion of the disc that is excavated. For example, if the pathologic cupping and atrophy are found on the lower outer

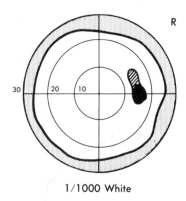

1/1000 White

Fig. 22-33 Enlargement of the normal blind spot.

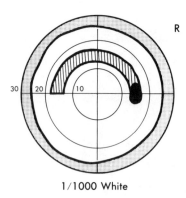

1/1000 White

Fig. 22-34 Nerve fiber bundle defect.

pole of the disc, as occurs in most early cases of glaucoma, the field defect will be found in the upper nasal regions.

The type of field defects to be expected in glaucoma are as follows:

1. *Enlargement of the normal blind spot* (Fig. 22-33).
2. *Nerve fiber bundle defect* (Fig. 22-34). This type of defect is scimitar-shaped and arches from the blind spot around the macula in the area between 10 and 20 degrees on the tangent screen. It usually ends in a very sharply demarcated border on the horizontal line. The nerve fiber bundle defect is a prototype of all glaucomatous field defects.
3. *Baring of the blind spot.* Baring of the blind spot is merely an arcuate or nerve fiber bundle defect

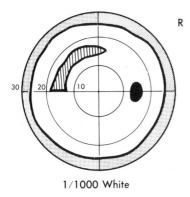

1/1000 White

Fig. 22-35 Arcuate defect, or Bjerrum's scotoma, not attached to blind spot.

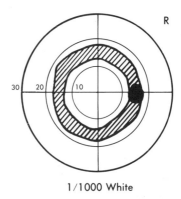

1/1000 White

Fig. 22-37 Double arcuate scotoma, producing a ring field defect.

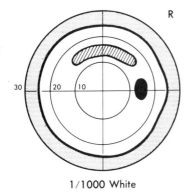

1/1000 White

Fig. 22-36 Arcuate defect, superiorly.

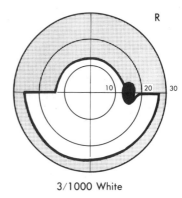

3/1000 White

Fig. 22-38 Advanced glaucomatous field defect.

emerging from the blind spot.

4. *Bjerrum's scotoma.* This defect is a complete type of nerve fiber bundle defect emanating from the blind spot, arching over the macula, and ending on the horizontal line. In its early stages this defect may not be attached to the blind spot and may extend only part way around the macular region (Figs. 22-35 and 22-36).

5. *Nasal depression of the field.* This type of defect may appear quite early in glaucoma and later merges with a nerve fiber bundle defect to create an area of considerable visual loss.

The presence of a typical glaucomatous field defect is virtually diagnostic of glaucoma, irrespective of the results of tonometric examination. The treat-

ment of glaucoma is directed principally toward avoiding further field loss, not merely toward reducing intraocular tension. If a patient is under treatment and the tension has been maintained at a satisfactory level, visual fields should be examined approximately two or three times a year. It is important in field testing to use an adequate-sized test object; many of these patients cannot see well because they have cataracts and small pupils, the latter caused by the miotic agents they are using. The examiner should use the smallest detectable stimulus that can be seen temporal to the blind spot.

The last area of involvement of the visual fields in glaucoma is the central fixation area. Thus the wave of darkness that comes from the blind spot first

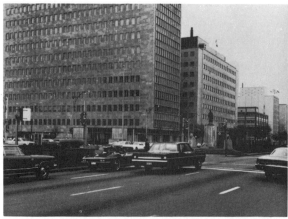 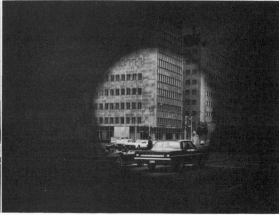

Fig. 22-39 Gradual constriction of field of vision caused by glaucoma. **A,** Normal field of view. **B,** Constricted visual field caused by glaucoma.

surrounds the central area (Fig. 22-37), extends to the periphery (Fig. 22-38), and leaves the individual at the end stage of the disease looking clearly straight ahead through a long tunnel of darkness—the so-called tunnel vision (Fig. 22-39).

Changes of the head of the optic nerve often precede detectable visual field loss. It has been estimated that almost half of the near fibers of the disc have to be lost before reproducible early field defects can be found. The correlation between optic nerve changes as noted by alterations of the disc and changes in visual function as detected by visual field assessment is usually parallel. If the correlation is not there, then one has to look for other sources of visual field changes such as defects or disturbances of the optic nerve or even further back in the eye.

Techniques of perimetry

Because perimetry is discussed in another chapter, the following points highlight its significance to glaucoma.

Kinetic perimetry involves moving the test object from a nonseeing area to a seeing area, whereas *static perimetry* involves the use of stationary test objects that are presented at random. The points at which the patient fails to recognize the spot of light are recorded.

Threshold static perimetry measures the intensity thresholds of visual acuity of the individual points

within the field of vision. This is accomplished by gradually increasing the target light on the subthreshold intensity and recording the level at which the patient first recognizes the target. The process also can be approached from the other direction— that is, decreasing from the suprathreshold level and recording the lowest value found.

Static perimetry has been shown to be more sensitive than kinetic perimetry at detecting early glaucomatous field defects. The use of colored targets has no advantage over white, which remains the most reliable and stable indicator as a test target.

Cataracts can cause visual field defects. In one study of 90 eyes with open-angle glaucoma and cataracts, 41% had a partial or complete scotoma after the cataract was removed. Reduced ocular clarity from other causes such as corneal scarring also may affect and reduce the visual field study. A small miotic pupil may depress central and peripheral threshold retinal sensitivity and exaggerate the field defect.

The treatment of myopia with glasses is not required with the use of a 300-mm perimeter unless the refractive error exceeds 3.00 diopters. With high myopia, refractive scotomas may appear that can be confused with glaucomatous field defects. Usually they are eliminated with appropriate correction of the refractive error. Astigmatic errors should first be corrected before visual field studies unless the condition indicates less than 1.00 diopter. Increasing age also causes a reduction in retinal threshold sensitivity.

Psychologic factors may depress the visual field and create false pockets of visual field loss. The field test is definitely influenced by the state of the patient's alertness, anxiety, calm, and degree of cooperation. A lack of familiarity with the test and heightened tension about performing well often lead to a poor first-test result, which invariably improves on the second or third visual field test. This improvement is not a reflection of a change in optic nerve status; rather it is due to familiarity with the test and better response to the visual stimuli.

The tangent screen is almost a historic relic of visual field testing. It suffers from the drawbacks of monitoring fixation and is limited by variations in background lighting. No visible record is automatically elicited, the area is strictly limited to the central 30 degrees, and the screen does not reveal the peripheral field where early glaucomatous defects may appear.

Approaches to glaucoma field testing

There are two approaches to glaucoma field testing. The first is a screening technique to detect the presence of a glaucoma field defect. The second is to measure accurately the breadth, depth, and density of the field defect so that it can be appropriately charted on subsequent dates to ascertain any progress in the loss of field.

The Armaly-Drance technique is used for visual field screening. A Goldmann perimeter tests for central field defects with use of suprathreshold static or kinetic perimetry. This test has the highest probability of showing a glaucomatous defect. The Goldmann type of perimeter maps out the size and shape of all scotomas by means of both central threshold targets and peripheral targets.

Early detection of glaucoma is an ideal goal. Many mass screening programs are faulty because they usually involve a single tonometer reading. The overreferral rate is enormous, ranging from 10% to 30%, which means that large groups of patients undergo costly follow-up examinations. On the other hand, some glaucoma cases are missed: low-tension glaucoma, diurnal variations in which higher pressures are not found during office visits, and angle-closure glaucoma in which the pressure may be normal between attacks.

Screening with a Schiøtz tonometer is ideal except that it produces lower intraocular pressures than the Goldmann applanation tonometer. It disturbs the coats of the eye (the scleral rigidity factor). The applanation tonometer (Perkins) is useful for its accuracy and portability, but this testing requires a skilled operator.

The noncontact tonometer, which uses air, is probably ideal because it eliminates contact with the cornea and therefore any threat of abrasion, infection, or topical anesthetic reactions. The major drawback is the cost of the instrument. Usually the criterion for referral is 21 mm Hg, a number that is influenced by the diurnal variation of pressure and any large amount of fluid taken before the test.

Screening test results are vastly improved if one includes an inspection of the optic disc. This usually requires the services of an ophthalmologist, who may not always be available. There are those who advocate screening only persons at high risk, such as those with a family history of glaucoma, high myopia, or vascular disease, especially diabetes. Although a comprehensive screening program is a desirable goal, unfortunately a good comprehensive screening program that is cost efficient and accurate is not currently available.

Treatment

Open-angle glaucoma cannot be cured, but it can be adequately controlled so that loss of visual function does not occur. Every patient with cupping of the optic disc and visual field changes should be treated. However, in every clinic or office there is usually a large group of patients who have ocular hypertension. These are patients with ocular tension greater than 22 mm Hg; yet their discs are normal, and there is no visual field loss. The decision as to whether this type of patient should be actively treated requires individual consideration. These cases of suspected or borderline glaucoma frequently can be followed without treatment for many years. If follow-up examinations are difficult to obtain or if the ophthalmologist has poor rapport with the patient, the patient often is treated with conventional glaucoma drugs.

Medical therapy. Glaucoma usually can be adequately controlled with drops. The most commonly used miotic agent is pilocarpine hydrochloride. Initially it is given in percentages of 1% to 2%. If stronger concentrations are required, pilocarpine, 4% to 6%, may be used. This miotic agent generally is given every 6 hours during the day. A good alternate to pilocarpine is carbachol chloride, 0.75% and 1.5%. The stronger, longer-acting miotic agents are demecarium bromide (Humorsol), 0.125% and 0.25%; isoflurophate (Floropryl), 0.025% and 0.1%; and echothiophate iodide (Phospholine), 0.06%, 0.12%, and 0.25%.

These powerful miotic agents, although they offer decreased frequency of application, have numerous side effects that make them undesirable unless absolutely necessary. They are contraindicated in persons who have a predisposition to a retinal detachment, high myopia, or angle-closure glaucoma. They also may lead to cataract formation. The systemic side effects include such symptoms as nausea, vomiting, intestinal cramps, and bladder cramps.

A medication that can be manufactured in a gel form and can be inserted as a wafer into the conjunctival sac has been shown to have some value in the long-term control of chronic wide-angle glaucoma. This medication tends to be more cumbersome to use and is more expensive than drops.

An excellent alternate to the use of miotic agents is one of the epinephrine derivatives. These drops, which come in concentrations of 1% and 2%, have a duration of activity of approximately 12 hours and therefore need be used only twice a day. Furthermore, epinephrine drops do not constrict the pupil or interfere with vision. Miotic agents, on the other hand, can severely reduce the vision if the patient has a small posterior incipient cataract. Many ophthalmologists find epinephrine the drug of choice to initiate glaucoma therapy because of the infrequency of application, lack of systemic side effects, and the absence of any visual disturbances caused by their use.

A newer form of epinephrine is called Propine. This compound is relatively inactive until it is enzymatically converted into active epinephrine. Fewer side effects occur with this preparation.

Timolol maleate (Timoptic), first described by Hall in 1970, has been the first of the β-adrenergic blocking agents that have been employed successfully for open-angle glaucoma. Solutions of 0.25% and 0.5% concentration are used once or twice daily, depending on the severity of the glaucoma. Timolol maleate and Betagen have minimal side effects and can be used for most patients except those with asthma, cardiopulmonary disease, heart failure, or 2% to 3% heart block. Betaxolol (Betoptic) is a newer, more selective β-blocker with apparently fewer side effects and similar potency and topical application.

Carbonic anhydrase inhibitors such as acetazolamide are employed in glaucoma therapy if drops are unsuccessful in controlling intraocular pressure. Although acetazolamide (Diamox) is effective in lowering intraocular pressure, it is used only as a last resort because of the extensive complications resulting from prolonged use. Many patients develop tingling in their fingers and toes, diarrhea, nausea, loss of appetite, and general debility. A few patients have even developed kidney stones. Other carbonic anhydrase inhibitors in use are methazolamide (Neptazane), 50-mg tablets; and dichlorphenamide (Daranide, Oratrol), 50-mg tablets.

Compliance with medication. A medication regimen should be as simple as possible. It has been estimated that anywhere from 20% to 40% of patients prescribed medication for open-angle glaucoma miss some or all of their drop dosages. Those who were asked to instill three times a day were more apt not to use the drops than those told twice a day. Other disturbing factors that lead to relative noncompliance or poor compliance are side effects of the medication, such as miosis and loss of focusing accuracy with pilocarpine, as well as failure to understand that the treatment preserves the visual field and the acuity already present. In many instances these patients do not believe they are sick, especially if no other disease is present, and are reluctant to undertake a treatment of medication when they have only the physician's pronouncement that they need it.

Laser trabeculoplasty. Laser treatment to the diseased trabecular meshwork has been proved quite effective in controlling open-angle glaucoma and obviating the need for surgery in many patients. The actual procedure involves lasing the middle to anterior portion of the trabecular meshwork. Approximately 80 to 100 burns are equally spaced over half of the angle's circumference. Often the remainder of the angle will need to be treated.

The argon laser reopens the blocked drainage channels and reduces the fluid pressure in the eye. The gonioprism is used to reangle the light toward the outflow channels. Whereas the success rates vary for different types of open-angle glaucoma, there does appear to be a relationship between laser success and a patient's age and degree of trabecular meshwork pigmentation. It is important to realize that laser therapy is an adjunct to medical therapy and does not ensure that medications may be stopped. More than 90% of patients experience successful results with argon laser trabeculoplasty. A second procedure may be required in the remaining semicircular angle of the eye.

When to treat. Most authorities believe that medical therapy should be initiated before laser therapy is attempted. Recently there has been a small shift in thinking toward the use of laser therapy as an initial treatment. Laser therapy does not require any compliance, does not cause any side effects from medication, and is virtually free of any complications from the procedure itself. It is performed on an outpatient basis in the hospital or during an office visit and requires no hospital stay whatsoever. The only real problem with this treatment is a possible rise in intraocular pressure occurring the first 2 weeks after laser therapy. Most ophthalmologists still use medical therapy first and reserve laser treatment for poor responders.

Surgery. Surgery is performed only if the patient continues to lose visual field despite the attempts by the ophthalmologist to provide maximum medical therapy. This usually means that the ophthalmologist has been unable to effectively lower the intraocular tension with the most potent drugs available, either singly or in combination with others. Although many types of surgical procedures are performed for open-angle glaucoma, they are all basically fistulizing operations; that is, they attempt to create an opening

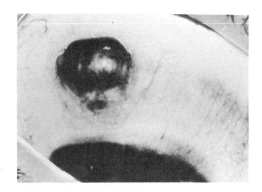

Fig. 22-40 Staphyloma in absolute glaucoma.

between the anterior chamber and the subconjunctival spaces or between the surgically prepared layers of the sclera (subscleral filtering procedures). These procedures are being performed less and less today because of the adequacy in most instances of medical management. However, *absolute glaucoma* with complete blindness and intolerable pressure in an eye is still a tragic entity (Fig. 22-40).

As glaucoma surgery becomes more sophisticated, attendant risks are decreasing. A major consequence of filtering surgery appears to be the development of a cataract. It is for this reason that early surgery is being advocated, especially in the presence of factors that place the patient at high risk.

Management of the patient by the ophthalmic assistant

The ophthalmic assistant should assist the patient through the regimen of glaucoma therapy. First, it is imperative that the patient be seen at regular intervals to maintain control of the disease. Usually the ophthalmologist will designate when the next appointment should take place. However, the ophthalmic assistant must call to remind the patient of this appointment. If a particular patient with glaucoma has been remiss in keeping appointments, the patient should be called and told about the dangers of lack of supervision.

Instructions should be given to each patient about the exact time of administration of the drops and the methods of placing them in the eye. Compliance with instructions is the most important feature in preventing loss of vision from glaucoma. Glaucoma medication is best instilled by depressing the lower lid and placing the drops in the lower fornix. If this procedure is difficult, the patient should be instructed to lie down, place the drops directly over the cornea, and close the eyes for a minute or two. Pressure should be applied to the inner canthus to avoid having the drops flow down through the nose and be absorbed systemically. Systemic absorption of the stronger miotic agents can cause unpleasant side effects in the rest of the body. Certain drops, such as echothiophate iodide, must be kept in a cool place. Others, such as epinephrine derivatives, should be kept out of the sunlight. The latter are no longer effective when they turn brown. The patient should be instructed in the management and care of the medications.

It is helpful if patients are given a card stating that they have glaucoma and indicating the nature of their medication. Each patient should know the name of the drug, the dosage, and the frequency of application. The card is invaluable for patients who lose their medication, especially during travel. Also, if the patient becomes involved in an accident, the attending physician will be in a better position to evaluate the consequences of the injury if the practitioner is aware of the cause of the pinpoint pupils.

In many instances patients have sinister ideas regarding the nature of this disease. Often they believe they have an incurable disease leading to blindness or that they will be invalided because of glaucoma. The glaucoma patient should be reassured that with good control there is no reason why vision or visual field should ever be lost. The patient also should be told that there is little or no evidence that limitations of activities, diet, tobacco, alcohol, movies, television, reading, driving, and so forth alter the control of the glaucoma.

Aids in diagnosis

In suspected cases of open-angle glaucoma in which the tension is borderline and the disc is equivocal in appearance, the ophthalmologist may resort to provocative tests to determine the presence or absence of glaucoma.

Diurnal variations. Normally the intraocular pressure is greatest at 6 AM and lowest during the day. This diurnal variation in the intraocular pressure seldom exceeds 3 or 4 mm Hg. However, in a glaucomatous patient this pressure difference often exceeds 7 to 8 mm Hg. In this test ocular tensions are taken throughout the day and during the night, especially at those times when the intraocular pressure is found to be the highest. Many authorities find that this test is the best method for the detection of glaucoma. The only drawback to its gaining widespread popularity is that the patient must be hospitalized for the test to be performed, which is costly.

Water-drinking and tonography tests. These used to be popular but have fallen out of favor because of a lack of specificity. Briefly, with the water-drinking test, a rise in ocular tension of 8 to 10 mm Hg after the rapid ingestion of 1 quart of water suggests glaucoma. A negative reaction does not rule out this condition. This test often was coupled with tonography because the number of positive reactions are very high in the combined test. This test is used with decreasing frequency.

Tonography. Tonography offers the ophthalmologist three important pieces of information: the P_o, or the intraocular pressure in the undisturbed eye, the flow of aqueous into the eye, and the C value, or facility of outflow. The P_o/C ratio has been found to be extremely helpful. A P_o/C ratio greater than 140 usually means a diagnosis of glaucoma in 90% of cases. (See p. 510.)

Time. Observation over a period of time is the most widely used method of proving glaucoma. In suspected cases patients usually are told that they have borderline glaucoma or that glaucoma is suspected, and they are asked to return to the office on three or four occasions during the year. On these occasions the tensions are tested, the discs are examined, and the fields are tested. The ophthalmologist basically looks for an alteration in any one of these three parameters before beginning therapy. The patient may show a pattern of gradually increasing pressures, slight cupping of the disc, or an early glaucomatous field defect. This method is quite justifiable in the treatment of open-angle glaucoma in view of the chronicity of the disease and slow loss of the visual field.

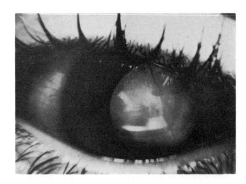

Fig. 22-41 Dislocated cataractous lens, causing secondary glaucoma.

SECONDARY GLAUCOMA

Secondary glaucoma occurs as a result of other disease within the eye. Because in essence there are two diseases in the eye—the precipitating cause of the glaucoma—the condition is often more difficult to treat.

The conditions that can lead to *secondary angle-closure glaucoma* are (1) dislocation of the lens (Fig. 22-41), (2) swollen lens, (3) scar tissue or peripheral anterior synechiae between the iris and the trabecular meshwork, and (4) posterior synechiae to the lens.

The most common cause of anterior synechiae is chronic angle-closure glaucoma, and the most common cause of posterior synechiae is chronic and severe iritis.

Some of the causes of *secondary open-angle glaucoma* are (1) invasion of the trabecular meshwork by tumors of the iris, ciliary body, and choroid, (2) iritis and cyclitis, and (3) trauma.

CONGENITAL GLAUCOMA

Congenital glaucoma is an extremely rare disease. It is estimated that an average ophthalmologist is unlikely to see more than one new case of congenital glaucoma in 5 years of practice. Despite its rarity, the signs and symptoms of the disease are so characteristic that a diagnosis should not be missed.

Often the parents are aware that the baby has something wrong with the eye in the first few weeks or months of life. The child appears extremely sensitive to light and tears profusely. Many infants even keep their eyelids tightly closed most of the day to avoid the light. However, it is the corneal haziness caused by the corneal edema that makes most parents suspect that something is wrong with the child's eyes. Because the coats of the eye are distensible in early infancy, the increased intraocular pressure causes progressive enlargement of the infant eye and cornea. Most infant corneas measure less than 10.5 mm in horizontal diameter. A measurement over 12 mm is considered diagnostic of congenital glaucoma. These eyes, hazy and enlarged, appear so grotesque that the term *buphthalmos,* or ox eye, has been commonly applied to designate this condition.

It is important that any child with a symptom of tearing be seen immediately because the earlier glaucoma is diagnosed and brought under control, the better is the prognosis. In most cases the tearing will be caused by a blocked tear duct, but the ophthalmic assistant should always be aware of the possibility of congenital glaucoma.

SUMMARY

The ophthalmic assistant should remember that the best management of glaucoma is early detection. Once vision is lost because of the disease, it can never be retrieved. Chronic glaucoma cannot be cured but its progress can be arrested. The patient with this disease, like the person with diabetes, must control the condition on a daily basis. For acute angle-closure glaucoma, it is important to be aware of the signs and symptoms. The ophthalmic assistant should help the patient understand the nature of the disease and help in the management of the patient's drops. The importance of early detection should be stressed. Public awareness is an important feature of glaucoma.

QUESTIONS FOR REVIEW AND THOUGHT

1. What causes angle-closure glaucoma?
2. List the characteristic symptoms that might suggest angle-closure glaucoma in a patient telephoning the office for an appointment.
3. What are the characteristic signs of angle-closure glaucoma?
4. Outline the medical treatment for an acute attack of angle-closure glaucoma.
5. What causes open-angle glaucoma?
6. What are the classic signs of damage from open-angle glaucoma?
7. What is the principle of applanation tonometry? How is applanation tonometry performed?
8. Discuss the usefulness of hand-held applanation tonometers.
9. How does one clean and care for the Schiøtz tonometer to maintain its accuracy?
10. Outline visual field changes that may occur in open-angle glaucoma.
11. Outline a plan for the medical therapy of open-angle glaucoma.
12. Discuss the value of tonography and of the water-drinking test.
13. Why does the eye enlarge in congenital glaucoma?
14. What causes pupillary block glaucoma, and how does this mechanism come about?
15. List ways to eliminate squeezing by the patient during indentation and applanation tonometry.

SELF-EVALUATION QUESTIONS

True-false statements

Directions: Indicate whether the statement is true (T) or false (F).

T or F 1. Patients with acute angle-closure glaucoma complain of halos or rainbows around lights.

T or F 2. Primary angle-closure glaucoma occurs more commonly in males than in females.

T or F 3. All patients with a high intraocular pressure (greater than 21 mm Hg) have glaucoma.

Missing words

Directions: Write in the missing word in the following sentences.

4. In children with congenital or infantile glaucoma, distention of the eyeball is referred to as _____.

5. _____ is the most common cause of posterior synechiae.

6. _____ is a convenient method of estimating the outflow facility or the flow of aqueous out of the eye.

Choice-completion questions

Directions: Select the one best answer in each case.

7. Chronic open-angle glaucoma is *not* characterized by:
   a. Raised intraocular pressure
   b. Sudden loss of vision associated with excruciating pain
   c. Slow erosion of the visual field
   d. Slow progressive loss of visual acuity
   e. Cupping of the temporal aspect of the optic disc

8. Which of the following are provocative tests available for the diagnosis of primary angle-closure glaucoma?

   a. Miotic test using pilocarpine
   b. Mydriatic test using hydroxyamphetamine
   c. Dark room provocative test
   d. Pupillary dilation plus gonioscopy
   e. All of the above
9. Which of the following field defects is *not* commonly seen in patients with chronic open-angle glaucoma?
   a. Nerve fiber bundle defect
   b. Loss of central vision (central scotoma)
   c. Paracentral scotoma
   d. Nasal depression
   e. Peripheral constriction

ANSWERS, NOTES, AND EXPLANATIONS

1. **True.** The halos around lights are caused by corneal edema. Light is dispersed by the droplets of fluid in the corneal epithelium, and the halos are typically composed of two colored rings, an inner blue-violet ring and an outer yellow-red ring. Halos are not pathognomonic of glaucoma. They also may occur in patients with cataracts (nuclear sclerosis) and excess conjunctival debris.

2. **False.** Primary angle-closure glaucoma occurs more commonly in females, particularly those over 50 years of age. Patients with this disorder have essentially normal eyes with the exception of a shallow anterior chamber and a narrow entrance into the angle. In addition, these patients are usually hyperopic and have a "smaller eye" than normal. Crowding of the angle structures tends to increase as patients become older because of an increase in size of the lens, which pushes the iris diaphragm forward.

3. **False.** *Glaucoma* is a term applied to a diverse group of ocular disorders characterized by an elevation of intraocular pressure to a level capable of producing damage to the ocular structures, the most important being the optic nerve head.

   About 2% of people over the age of 40 years have an increased intraocular pressure, but only 0.5% have raised intraocular pressure and field loss.

   Patients with an increased intraocular pressure and no field loss are referred to as having ocular hypertension. About 5% to 10% of these patients may develop field loss with time, and they should be carefully observed. Some physicians may treat these patients if the pressure reaches levels greater than 25 to 30 mm Hg.

   There is a group of patients who develop field loss with an intraocular pressure less than 21 mm Hg. These patients may have a compromised blood supply to the optic nerve head. In this group an intraocular pressure of 18 mm Hg may produce damage, and these patients are said to suffer from low-tension glaucoma.

4. **Buphthalmos.** If an increased intraocular pressure is present in an infant's eye, there is a progressive enlargement of both the eye and the cornea. This can result in a huge eye, which is referred to as *buphthalmos*, or ox eye. If pressure does not become elevated until after the age of 3 years, the eye usually resists distention. In infants, an increasing corneal diameter is a very significant sign of uncontrolled glaucoma. The enlarged cornea usually is associated with tears in Descemet's membrane. The stretching results in myopia and irregular corneal astigmatism.

5. **Iritis.** Iritis is inflammation of the iris and behaves like inflammation anywhere else in the body. Posterior synechiae form as a result of the iris becoming adherent to the lens or vitreous in an

aphakic eye. As a result, the aqueous cannot enter the anterior chamber and is forced to accumulate behind the iris, which is pushed forward, resulting in blockage of the outflow. At the same time there is an increase in intraocular pressure, and secondary angle-closure glaucoma results. This cycle of events may be prevented by treating patients with iritis with antiinflammatory agents and mydriatics. If secondary angle-closure glaucoma occurs, a surgical or laser peripheral iridectomy should be performed so that the aqueous can bypass the pupillary pathway and enter the anterior chamber from the posterior chamber.

6. **Tonography.** Tonography is used to measure the outflow facility of an eye. It is based on the principle that massage of an eye lowers the intraocular pressure. This effect is rapid in a normal eye but occurs much more slowly in a glaucomatous eye. Tonography measures the massaging effect of a tonometer to express fluid from the eye.

7. **b. Sudden loss of vision associated with excruciating pain.** The main purpose of this question is to emphasize the fact that chronic open-angle glaucoma is insidious in onset, and routine intraocular pressure should be performed on patients to detect this condition. Acute angle-closure glaucoma is characterized by a sudden marked rise in intraocular pressure. The vision is lost rapidly, the eye becomes red, and the patient complains of excruciating pain.

8. **e. All of the above.** An eye with a narrow angle should be investigated to determine its acutal capacity to occlude. There are many provocative tests available for diagnosis of primary angle-closure glaucoma. Answers *b, c,* and *d* are often used. The pilocarpine provocative test may be used in narrow-angle glaucoma patients with closure and elevated pressure to rule out the possibility of an open-angle glaucoma component. In addition, pilocarpine constricts the pupil and may cause an increase in pupil block and hence precipitate an attack of acute angle closure.

9. **b. Loss of central vision (central scotoma).** Central vision is classically spared in patients with chronic open-angle glaucoma. These patients may have a markedly constricted visual field (so-called tunnel vision) with good central visual acuity. The visual acuity may even be 20/20 with extensive loss of visual field. The last area of involvement of visual field in glaucoma is central vision.

Loss of central vision, so-called central scotoma, would cause profound loss of visual acuity with a relatively full peripheral field. Central scotomas are seen classically with disorders of the optic nerve, for example, optic neuritis secondary to demyelinating disorders.

CHAPTER 23 Examination of the newborn, infant, and small child

ALEX LEVIN

- Approach to the Parent and Child
- Vision Assessment
- External Examination
- Installation of Eye Drops
- Refraction
- Retina and Optic Nerve Examination

The ocular examination of a newborn, infant, or small child presents unique challenges that require special techniques and particular knowledge of the unique normal variations in eyeball anatomy and function of this age-group. Infants and small children may be unable or unwilling to participate in the examination in a way that would provide information regarding their visual function. The ophthalmic assistant also must remember that the child's caretaker is an integral part of the "patient team": attention to the needs of both parent and child is essential for optimum examination.

APPROACH TO THE PARENT AND CHILD

Children are unique patients in that they always are accompanied by a caretaker who is their advocate, communicator, and guardian. The parent must be enlisted as a positive participant in the child's eye examination. In taking the ocular history, it also is important to distinguish between the parental concerns and the child's symptoms that led to examination. Sometimes the parent may have observed a visual behavior that is of concern. In other situations the parent may not have observed a problem that was noted by the referring pediatrician or family physician. Parents usually are excellent historians because they are very observant of their children. One must never underestimate the value of parental observations, which should be noted on the patient's chart even if they refute the problem that initiated the referral. This is particularly important in assessing a baby who is thought to have poor vision or blindness. The first question should be, "Do you think your baby sees" Although some parents may deny that their baby's sight is poor, most will make an accurate assessment of the baby's ability to see objects and people. This assessment provides perhaps the single most valuable piece of information acquired in the initial stage of the visit.

Although it is important for ophthalmic assistants to introduce themselves to the parents, a self-introduction directly to the small child also is necessary. The child's individuality must be recognized and honored. Young children need to know that they have some control over the situation. They often are scared, unsure, or even tearful and combative. The initial introduction and conversation with the child can "make or break" the success or failure of the remainder of the examination. Before conversing with the parents, the assistant can chat with the child about issues unrelated to the visit, inquiring about the youngster's age, siblings, pets, or a toy the child is clutching. Seemingly inane comments often provide valuable reassurance to the child that the examiner has true interest and concern for the child's well-being.

Once this initial liaison is made with the child, one can then turn to the parent to establish the reason for the visit. If possible, it often is helpful to let the child roam about the examination room and touch objects and equipment that are safe. This also gives children some control over their environment, and their exploration leads to a decrease in their fearfulness. It is almost essential for the ophthalmic assistant to have several toys available to distract the child both before and during the examination.

Once the history has been completed and it is time for the eye examination to begin, young children, particularly those younger than 4 years of age, should be encouraged to sit on the parent's lap in the examination chair. The assistant can make the examination a game by constantly carrying on a playful banter while presenting the child with tasks and toys. It is important to glean as much information as possible without touching the child. Often one can assess eye movements, pupillary reactions, the external ocular anatomy, and even visual acuity with only the most minimal physical contact with the child. When the child is asked to answer questions or perform visual tasks, such as visual acuity testing or binocular vision testing, one should always be positive when responding to the child's answer even if that answer is incorrect. If the child makes a mistake, one can simply say "good job" and move on to the next letter. Undermining a child's confidence by indicating a poor performance on a visual test may decrease compliance with the examination. It also is helpful if the examination is conducted without external interruptions such as the answering of telephone calls or the movement of people walking in and out of the room. Because children in the younger age-groups have very short attention spans, the examination must be conducted swiftly in good humor with minimal extraneous distractions.

If the child becomes tearful or uncooperative, it often is best to "back off" and either undertake an unrelated conversation or ask the child how he or she would like to proceed. For example, some children will prefer to hold the penlight or direct ophthalmoscope themselves. They can hold the instrument along with the assistant who is conducting the examination. It may be helpful to perform part of the examination on the parents in a mock fashion to demonstrate that it is painless before carrying that step of the examination on to the child.

Children have certain biologic needs that must be satisfied if an optimum examination is to be completed. If a child appears cranky, one might inquire if the parent feels that the infant needs to bottle- or breast-feed. Quite a bit of information can be obtained while the child is being examined during a feeding. A pacifier or favorite toy also should be allowed because it may increase the child's level of comfort and security. Interruptions for diaper changes and visits to the bathroom must be permitted. If a sibling's behavior is distracting, the examiner can turn attention to that child and issue an invitation to participate in the delivery of care to the sibling. For example, a sibling can be asked to flip the switch when the lights are being turned on and off or can hand the examiner toys and tools that are being used.

VISION ASSESSMENT

Assessment of the visual acuity in neonates and infants often is limited to ascertaining whether vision is absent, present, or within normal limits for their age and equal in both eyes. Visual fixation is present at birth. Perhaps the best visual target for the neonate is the human face. All infants should smile responsively and briefly follow a stimulus by 2 months of age. In the second and third months of life, infants develop the ability to follow a target beyond the midline, although it may not be until the fourth month that they can follow completely from their

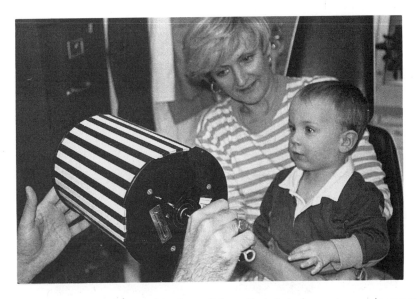

Fig. 23-1 The OKN drum is rotated in front of the patient, inducing nystagmus in any patient that is neurologically normal and sighted.

left side over to their right side (180 degrees). When the examiner presents an infant with a target, it is important to use a silent target to ensure that any following or responsive behavior that is observed results from visual rather than auditory stimuli. High-contrast (black and white) targets are particularly helpful.

Children who are blind or have very poor sight often manifest wandering, purposeless, dysconjugate eye movements or nystagmus. The presence of nystagmus at birth, however, does not necessarily imply poor vision. If the child has very poor sight, it is important to note response to light (light perception, LP). One can look for the "eye-popping reflex" by abruptly turning off all illumination in the room. A sighted baby or infant will demonstrate a reflex opening of the eyes. When the lights are then turned on abruptly, both eyes should squeeze shut. Even premature babies should respond to a bright light. If the child's eyes are closed, the bright light can be shone through the closed eyelid, and a reflex contraction of the eyelid and surrounding muscles should be seen. Although intermittent misalignment of the eyes, particularly intermittent exotropia, is common and within normal limits up to 3 to 4 months

of age, the presentation of a large target or human face should elicit fixation even if one eye is temporarily misaligned. The wandering eye movements of the poorly sighted or blind child will not stop in response to these stimuli.

More formal technical means are available to better quantify an infant's visual acuity. These techniques include visual evoked potential (VEP), preferential-looking tests, and graded optokinetic nystagmus (OKN). The VEP is a test designed to measure the ability of the occipital cortex in the brain to register a response to visual targets of increasingly difficult resolution by placing electrodes on the scalp that sense the passage of visual information from the eyeballs to the brain. The OKN drum (Fig. 23-1) will elicit nystagmus in anyone capable of seeing the stripes on the rotating drum. Preferential-looking techniques (Fig. 23-2) rely on the ability of an infant to distinguish between and favor a target that is variably different in terms of resolution of black and white stripes as compared with a bland gray target. The electroretinogram (ERG) is used to assess whether the retina is functioning in a child who is apparently blind or has poor sight. This test, however, does not measure visual acuity.

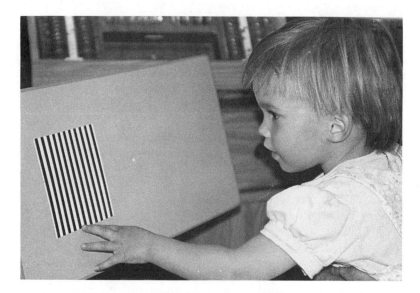

Fig. 23-2 Preferrential-looking technique. Given the ability to distinguish between the stripes and the other side of the board, the child indicates the striped target, which is a homogeneous gray. As the stripes get closer together, they become more difficult to distinguish and the target becomes less preferred.

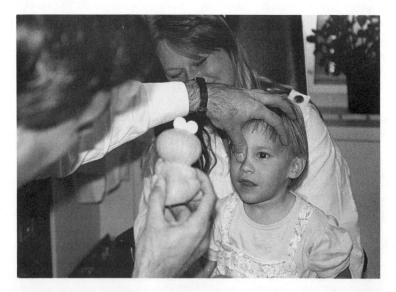

Fig. 23-3 Examiner covers the child's right eye while showing a toy for fixation. If the child has better vision in her right eye, she may become visibly upset or attempt to remove the examiner's thumb, indicating that the preferred eye is being covered. When the unpreferred eye is covered, the child may show no reaction at all.

If a significant difference exists in the visual acuity between the two eyes, the small child will object to the examiner covering the better eye. The eye can be covered by a piece of tape, the examiner's hand, or a commercially available occluder paddle. In response, the child may become visibly uncomfortable or may attempt to remove the obstruction only when a particular eye is covered. This test is best performed while presenting the child with a target of interest such as a bright toy (Fig. 23-3). When the good eye is covered, the child will object.

The visual acuity in infants and preverbal children is recorded as central-steady-maintained (CSM) or good-central-maintained (GCM). This indicates that visual acuity appears to be normal for the child's age, that the eyeball does not stray from fixation while viewing a target, and that nystagmus does not occur in the straight-ahead position. If an eye is clearly unpreferred but otherwise straight and steady when it is fixating a target, the examiner may record the child's vision as CSNM: central, steady, but not maintained. In other words, the child always will prefer to maintain fixation with the better eye even when both eyes are straight and open at the same time. If nystagmus or wandering eye movements are present, the vision may be recorded as CNSNM: central, not steady, and not maintained. Vision is not central when the patient appears to be fixating

COMMONLY USED QUANTITATIVE VISUAL-ACUITY TESTS FOR CHILDREN
Sheridan Gardiner test
HOTV matching game
Allen picture chart
Snellen's letter chart
Tumbling E's chart
Number chart
Preferential looking test
Visual evoked potential (VEP)

on a target although the eyeball is not pointing directly at what is being presented (eccentric fixation).

As children approach the third, fourth, and fifth years of life, they begin to be able to participate more voluntarily in the assessment of their visual acuity. Several types of charts that can be projected or posted for use in more formal visual-acuity testing are listed in the box, p. 527. It is absolutely essential that the method chosen be consistent with the child's developmental level and skills. Initially, projected pictures (Allen pictures) are the first test a child is able to perform. One might show the pictures to the child up close (Fig. 23-4) and ask that the figures

Fig. 23-4 Section of the near Allen picture card.

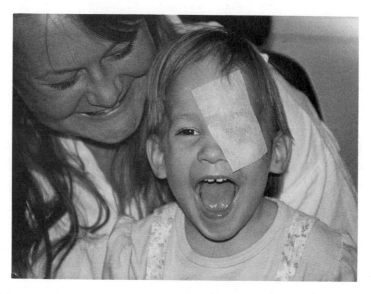

Fig. 23-5 Paper tape occlusion properly applied to left eye for testing of visual acuity in right eye.

be identified so that the examiner is aware of what interpretation the child gives to these somewhat abstract diagrams. For example, the birthday cake may be called a bag of French fries and the telephone a butterfly. As long as the examiner knows what the child calls that picture, testing can proceed. The use of letter charts (Snellen's letters) should be reserved only for those children whose ability to identify every letter is verified by the parent. For children in that intermediate stage in which they recognize "some of their letters," the Sheridan Gardiner test may be helpful because it allows the child to match projected letters or letter cards held by the examiner with a "cue card" the child holds. This approach gives children more confidence and allows them to guess letters they might otherwise not feel secure enough to try. Children in these young age-groups often are afraid of being wrong and even with the greatest encouragement will not read letters that they really are able to see. This underscores the constant need for building the child's confidence by indicating that the answer given is correct even when it is not. The "tumbling E" chart also can be used for children who do not recognize their letters. This test, however, can be difficult for small

children to interpret because they may not know left from right and they may have trouble indicating with their hands which direction the tumbling E is pointing to.

When the visual acuity of small children is tested, one eye must of course be covered. Children unconsciously will make every effort to use their better eye if there is a difference between the vision in their two eyes. Therefore the occlusion of one eye must be absolute. Children should never be allowed to hold their hand over their eye or to hand-hold a plastic occluder paddle. They will look through tiny holes between their fingers that actually create a pinhole effect and improve the vision in the covered eye or look around the occluder. It is recommended that paper tape be applied over the eye to effect complete occlusion (Fig. 23-5), although children must be observed constantly throughout the visual-acuity examination to be sure that they are not peaking between the tape and their skin (Fig. 23-6). This can be accomplished either by the use of a "cheater's mirror" placed behind the child, which allows the examiner to view the projected target behind them while still facing the child, or by having the examiner stand next to the chart at the end of the examination

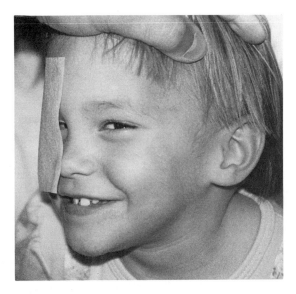

Fig. 23-6 Incorrectly applied paper tape occluder allows child to visualize the chart with the better right eye by peeking between the tape and the bridge of the nose at the fixation target.

lane while viewing the child and indicating which letters are to be read.

To accommodate the child's short attention span, it is helpful to have the child identify only a few letters from each line. Most children have normal vision so that it may be advisable to start at the 6/9 or even 6/6 line rather then start at the top of a chart and work the child down through many lines of letters/pictures. This may lead to a loss of the child's attention and artificially poor results. It may be helpful to ask the parent to remain silent during this examination, because distracting comments such as "you can do better" may serve to undermine a child's honest effort at good performance.

If a child objects to the covering of one eye by tape, the examiner can hold a +5.00 or greater spherical lens in front of the eye not being tested. This sufficiently blurs that eye in most children so that they actually are viewing with the eye that does not have a lens in front of it. Having the parent use a hand to cover the child's eye invites the same problems as having the eye covered by the child's hand.

Remember, some children just are not ready to perform formal visual acuity testing. It is more important to forgo this part of the examination when one senses that the child's cooperation is being lost than to persist and develop a negative relationship with the child that would make the remainder of the examination difficult. When the child is cooperative and the examination is successful, however, every child who is able to read a chart should have 6/6 vision by that age (with the use of Allen pictures, the distance chart allows only measurements up to 6/9). If not, an explanation must be sought. That explanation may be poor compliance with testing if nothing else is found on examination. A repeat visual acuity test performed 1 or 2 weeks later with a more confident and comfortable child may be successful. This conclusion, however, should be drawn only after a complete ophthalmic examination has ruled out the presence of refractive error or anatomic problems.

In most clinical situations it is not necessary to test the near vision of children because it can be assumed that the remarkable accommodative abilities of young children will allow for normal near vision in almost every case. Assessment of near vision is necessary only when there is poor distance vision. In these situations, near vision should be tested with both eyes open simultaneously. If the vision is normal at near but highly abnormal at distance, one might suspect that the child is either nearsighted or simply noncompliant with distance vision testing. In children who clearly have poor vision at distance, however, the knowledge of the maximum near vision allows for proper educational intervention at school.

In children with nystagmus, the vision also should be tested with both eyes open, as well as with one eye "occluded" with a +5.00 sphere. Covering the eye may make the nystagmus worse (latent nystagmus). Sometime the visual acuity with both eyes open is better. Some children with nystagmus may choose to hold their head in an abnormal position while viewing straight ahead. This abnormal position should be allowed because it is used unconsciously to help dampen the nystagmus (null point).

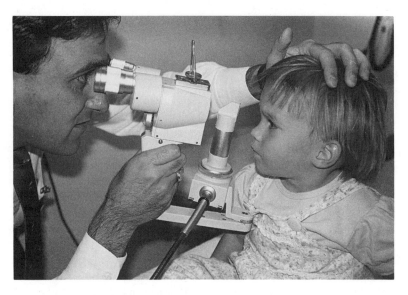

Fig. 23-7 Examiner using hand-held slit lamp.

EXTERNAL EXAMINATION

The anatomy of the eyelids, lashes, conjunctiva, cornea, and anterior segment in newborns, infants, and young children should be entirely normal and no different from that of a normal young adult except for size. Visualization of these structures, however, may be difficult because of the degree of compliance or cooperation. In infants and newborns, eye opening often can be achieved by holding the child in an upright position. To obtain magnification, one can look through the direct ophthalmoscope, using it as a hand-held magnifier by dialing in the black or green "plus" numbers and getting progressively closer to the child. With the 3 to 5 year old, this can be turned into a "peak-a-boo" game to allow the examiner to get close enough to visualize the front of the eye with magnification.

If more magnification is desired, the adult slit lamp can be used even for the small infant by holding the child in a horizontal position as the chin is placed on the chin rest. When doing this, it is important that the examiner be "in position," with all the necessary adjustments to the slit lamp already made for proper visualization, because the child may quickly become uncomfortable and tearful. A hand-held slit lamp also is available for the examination of infants and small children (Fig. 23-7).

Pupils

The examination of a child's pupils is conducted in the same way as for adults. It is sometimes difficult, however, to obtain the distant fixation required to eliminate the normal miosis that occurs when a person focuses at a near target. To do this, many pediatric ophthalmologists have animated toys in their offices that can be controlled by a foot pedal. This distracts the child to the distant target while the pupils are being tested. One can even play a "magic game" by turning the child's nose while secretly stepping on the pedal that activates the toy. Children then think that they can control the toy with their nose. This keeps them sufficiently amused while the examination continues. This device also is useful for the examination of ocular motility and alignment.

The pupil should normally respond to light at birth although the pupillary light reaction may be sluggish until the baby is 1 to 2 months of age. The pupils of infants are relatively small as compared with those of adults. In addition, because the eye examination of an infant may at times be conducted while the infant is asleep, it should be noted that during sleep, pupils are physiologically constricted. The concentual pupillary reactions are present at birth.

INSTILLATION OF EYE DROPS

Eye drops are feared by most children with the same vigor that they object to receiving injections. In fact, some children will immediately ask, "Am I getting eye drops?" when they walk into the room for their eye examination. Although one should never lie to a child, one might defer the answer to that question by saying, "Let's talk first and then decide." Once the time comes for the instillation of eye drops, the child must be informed, but it is preferable to do so as the child is getting positioned for this procedure. The child can be held securely in the parent's arms in a cradled position as if they were going to receive a bottle- or breast-feeding. The parent should be responsible for restraining the child's hands while the examiner controls the child's head and eyes. A child must always be told that the drops are going to sting. Well-meaning attempts by parents to alleviate a child's fears by indicating that "this won't hurt" should be corrected by saying that the drops might be painful for approximately 15 to 20 seconds. Before eye drops are instilled, the parents should be informed about the number of drops that are to be given and their purpose. To accomplish this goal, it may be helpful to instill first a drop of topical anesthetic (proparacaine or tetracaine), immediately followed by the dilating drops. The onset of action of these topical anesthetics is quite rapid, which helps to lessen the painful sting of the mydriatic agents.

Relaxation of the pupillary sphincter and the ciliary muscles that govern accommodation can be much more difficult in infants and small children, particularly if they have heavily pigmented brown irides. Although different examiners may vary in their selection of mydriatic agents, it is safe to use some combination of phenylephrine 2.5%, tropicamide 1%, and cyclopentolate 1% in all children except premature babies. Children who are born before 36 weeks' gestation, or children who are born small for gestational age at full-term, may require more dilute solutions of mydriatic agents, in particular cyclopentolate 0.5%. It is helpful to check for pupillary dilation and reactivity 15 minutes after the first instillation of eye drops to see if adequate mydriasis is occurring. A repeat instillation of drops may be necessary, particularly in premature babies and darkly pigmented children. A full 30 minutes should be given for adequate paralysis of accommodation to occur. If there is any concern on the part of the ophthalmic assistant that a given child should not receive the standard eye-drop regimen, then instillation of drops should be deferred until consultation with the ophthalmologist or pediatrician is sought. In particular, newborns and infants with hypertension, seizures, or respiratory problems may require an alteration in the usual regimen.

Some children will not respond adequately to the eye drops used in a routine eye examination, or they may require stronger cycloplegic agents for the assessment of farsightedness as it relates to esotropia. In these situations a prescription may be given by the physician for atropine drops (0.5% for children younger than 1 year of age, 1% for children older than 1 year of age) to be used twice daily for 3 days before a repeat examination. Parents should be cautioned to monitor their child for signs of atropine toxicity such as a fever and redness (flushing). Although this protocol generally is quite safe, parents must be cautioned to keep this medication locked away because ingestion by a toddler or small child could be fatal.

When the child returns to the examination room for dilated eye examination, it is often helpful to begin that segment of the examination first by announcing that no more drops will be necessary. However, one must be prepared to defer the examination should the discovery be made later that additional eye drops are in fact needed. The examiner must always adhere to the basic principle of being honest with pediatric patients.

REFRACTION

Newborns, infants, and small children cannot participate in analysis and refinement of their refractions by sitting behind the phoropter and indicating which

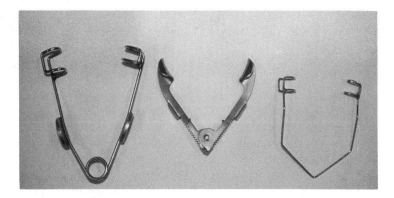

Fig. 23-8 Pediatric eyelid speculums.

lenses give them better vision. Rather, the examiner simply uses the retinoscope and hand-held lenses, as described elsewhere in this book, to determine the child's refractive error. Most infants and small children are farsighted, although glasses usually are not required because the strong accommodative power of their eyeballs allows them to "self-correct" for their hyperopia. Higher degrees of farsightedness, however, can lead to esotropia and amblyopia. Likewise, myopia in the newborn and infant may be quite functional as their visual world is almost completely at near. Higher degrees of nearsightedness, however, also may lead to strabismus and amblyopia. Different ophthalmologists have different thresholds for the prescription of glasses. Contact lens may be used in babies and small children with extremely high refractive errors or surgical aphakia after cataract extraction.

RETINA AND OPTIC NERVE EXAMINATION

Examination of the posterior segment of the eyeball through the dilated pupil in an infant or young child is essentially identical to that for an adult and requires the use of an indirect ophthalmoscope. In certain situations, however, it may be difficult to open the eyelids sufficiently to allow an adequate view. This may be best accomplished by the use of pediatric speculums, which are commercially available (Fig. 23-8). They are placed after the child has been restrained and a topical anesthetic applied. Al-

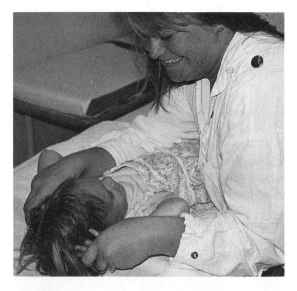

Fig. 23-9 Technique for restraining a small child. Parent assists by leaning over the child's abdomen while holding the child's hands next to the temples to immobilize the head.

though various commercially available papoose boards can be used, it usually is most reassuring and comfortable for the child to be restrained by having an adult, preferably the parent, lie comfortably across the child's chest while holding the child's hands on either temple to keep the head still (Fig. 23-9). The reassuring voice of a parent often can be quite helpful. Newborns and infants can be re-

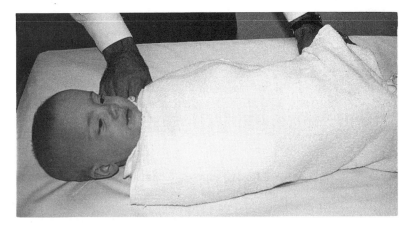

Fig. 23-10 Technique for restraining an infant. Child is wrapped in towel with arms at sides. Parent or assistant can then lie over the child's abdomen while controlling the child's head at the temples.

strained by wrapping a towel or blanket around the child's arms and trunk simultaneously (Fig. 23-10). The parent must be informed about the nature of this procedure because some adults feel quite uncomfortable about watching a speculum being placed into the eye. The examination is painless but quite scary for a small child. Immediately after the examination is complete, the child should be allowed to seek solace in the parent's arms.

For older children who may sit cooperatively in their parent's lap, the introduction of a large and unusual headpiece can be frightening. The ophthalmic assistant or examiner might reassure the child by giving this hat a silly name such as a "space hat" or allow the parent to be examined first. Once the child knows that this imposing instrument is "safe," cooperation may be enhanced.

Although the macula may not be completely developed in the first few months of life, the intraocular anatomy of a newborn and infant is otherwise identical to that of an adult.

QUESTIONS FOR REVIEW AND THOUGHT

1. What techniques can you use to reassure a frightened child during their examination?
2. What are the normal developmental visual milestones for a newborn and infant?
3. What factors should you use when deciding which chart is most appropriate for testing vision in a child?
4. What is the red reflex?
5. How do the pupils of a baby differ from that of an adult?
6. What might happen to a baby who is severely farsighted if glasses are not prescribed?
7. What tests are available to quantify vision in the preverbal child?
8. What drops usually are used to dilate a newborn baby's eyes for examination?

SELF-EVALUATION QUESTIONS

True-false statements

Directions: Indicate whether the statement is true (T) or false (F).

T or F   1. Atropine 1% eye drops should be used to dilate the pupils of newborn babies.

T or F   2. Most babies are nearsighted.

T or F   3. Children with nystagmus see better when one eye is covered.

Missing words

Directions: Write in the missing word in the following sentences.

4. The type of strabismus associated with hyperopia is _____.

5. The abbreviation used to record the visual assessment of a preverbal child with nystagmus who has good fixation with the right eye in the straight-ahead position is _____.

6. Two tests that are useful in assessing visual acuity when a child is just learning letters are the _____ and _____ test.

Choice-completion questions

Directions: Select the one best answer in each case.

7. Before instilling eye drops in a child, the parent should be informed that:
   a. The drops will sting
   b. A certain number of drops will be given
   c. The drops are given to make the pupils dilate
   d. The child should be cradled securely and lovingly in the parent's arms
   e. All of the above

8. Quantitative tests of visual acuity include all of the following except:
   a. Snellen letters
   b. VEP
   c. ERG
   d. Allen pictures
   e. Preferential looking

9. All of the following statements about the newborn are true *except:*
   a. Visual fixation is present.
   b. Intermittent strabismus may be present.
   c. Hyperopia may be present.
   d. The pupils do not react to light.
   e. An equal and symmetric red reflex is present.

10. The blind or very poorly sighted infant:
    a. May have wandering eye movements
    b. May have nystagmus
    c. May have dysconjugate eye movements
    d. May still show normal "eye-popping reflex"
    e. All of the above

ANSWERS, NOTES, AND EXPLANATIONS

1. **False.** Atropine 0.5% eye drops should be used in children younger than 1 year old to avoid systemic complications such as irritability, flushing, bradycardia, and fever.

2. **False.** Most babies are hyperopic in the first few years of life. Myopia becomes more common after the age of 5 or 6 years.

3. **False.** When one eye of a child with nystagmus is covered, the amplitude of the nystagmus in the uncovered eye may increase. This is called *latent nystagmus*. Visual acuity may worsen. It is preferable to test the visual acuity of children with nystagmus by fogging the untested eye with a +5.00 sphere. This prevents the development of latent nystagmus. Visual acuity with both eyes open, while allowing the child to adopt any preferred anomalous head position, also is important.

4. **Accommodative esotropia.** When children use their inherent mechanisms of accommodation to correct for their hyperopic refractive error, a "reflex" crossing of the eyes may occur. By giving hyperopic spectacles to "do the work" instead of the eyeball, this esotropia may be abolished.

5. **CNSM or CUSM (central, not steady/unsteady, maintained).** This child fixates in the straight-ahead position (central), with an eye that has nystagmus (not steady), but with apparently good vision relative to the other eye (maintained).

6. **Sheridan Gardiner test and HOTV matching game.** In both tests, the child is holding a cue card that allows the youngster to match projected letters or letters hand-held by the examiner, thus providing some extra support if the child is not completely comfortable with letter recognition by name.

7. **e. All of the above.** The parent must be completely informed about the instillation of eye drops. The drops are painful for only 15 to 20 seconds, particularly if a topical anesthetic is given before the mydriatic agents. Each ophthalmologist may have an individual regimen of dilating drops. However, that regimen should be explained to the parent who can then provide support by restraining the child in a comfortable fashion.

8. **c. ERG (electroretinogram).** The ERG is a quantitative and qualitative test of retinal function, but it does not give information about visual acuity. Visual acuity is a foveal function. The ERG is a test of the entire retina, which does not allow for specific testing of the small foveal area.

9. **d. The pupils do not react to light.** Although the pupillary reactions of a neonate may be sluggish, constriction to a bright light normally should be observed at birth. At birth some visual fixation to a large object or light should be present, although the eyes may be intermittently misaligned. Intermittent exotropia is the most common form of strabismus in neonates. Most newborn babies are hyperopic. In all babies an equal and symmetric red reflex should be seen, although the relatively miotic newborn pupil may make this test difficult.

10. **e. All of the above.** Infants who are blind or very poorly sighted often manifest wandering purposeless, dysconjugate eye movements, or true nystagmus. The presence of nystagmus, however, does not necessarily indicate that the child is blind. Some children with congenital nystagmus may have surprisingly good vision. The "eye-popping reflex" may still be seen in poorly sighted children, although it will be absent in children who are completely blind.

CHAPTER 24

Maintenance of ophthalmic equipment and instruments

- Applanation tonometer
- Noncontact tonometer
- Keratometer
- Slit-lamp biomicroscope
- Phoropter
- Projector

The maintenance of ophthalmic equipment and instruments often becomes the responsibility of the ophthalmic assistant. Certain measures may be delegated, such as replacement of bulbs, dusting, and other measures that may reduce the amount of time that the equipment is out of service. In some cases more complicated repairs may be required.

It is important that adequate supplies of replacement bulbs be maintained and that the ophthalmic assistant be familiar with the different bulbs that are required for each of the available pieces of equipment. Lists of the required bulb for each piece of equipment should be made and posted. If batteries are required, a suitable battery supply should also be maintained. If the batteries are the rechargeable type, they should be charged fully the first time. They can be recharged to the same full capacity on each recharging. They should be recharged on a regular basis. Handles usually contain rechargeable batteries that require nightly recharging. All instruments should be kept covered with dust covers that are supplied.

APPLANATION TONOMETER

Calibration of the applanation tonometer is important and should be checked approximately every 2

months, or sooner with regular use. Tonometers always are supplied with a calibration bar. The most common applanation tonometer is the Goldmann tonometer. Applanation tonometers may be checked for accuracy by the use of a central weight. For the Goldmann tonometer, a short rod of measured weight is attached to the balancing arm of the tonometer and the rod set at 0, 2, and 6, respectively. At each measure, the measuring drum should be placed at the corresponding stop. At each stop, the tonometer head should move only plus or minus 0.05 to 0.1 g of these settings (Fig. 24-1).

To be specific, follow these guidelines.

1. To check at drum position 0 (zero), insert the measuring prism at measuring position −0.05. The zero mark on the measuring drum is set one line width below the index. When the pressure arm—with prism in position—is gently pushed, it should move freely between the two stops and return toward the stop on the examiner's side (Fig. 24-2). At measuring position +0.05, the zero mark on the measuring drum is set one line width above the index. As this procedure is followed, the pressure arm should move toward the patient's side.

2. Check at drum position 2. For this check the control weight is used. Five circles are engraved on

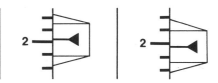

Fig. 24-3 Calibration with larger weight toward the examiner. Balance should show scale variation no greater than ±0.05 g.

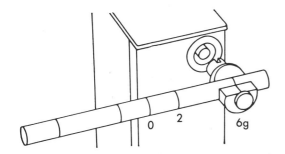

Fig. 24-1 Calibration bar for calibrating the Goldmann applanation tonometer.

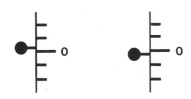

Fig. 24-2 Calibrating Goldmann applanation tonometer at position 2. The tonometer head should move only 0.05 to 0.1 g from zero.

the weight bar. The middle one corresponds to drum position 0, the two immediately to the left and right are position 2, and the outer ones are position 6. One of the marks on the weight corresponding to drum position 2 is set precisely on the index mark of the weight holder. Holder and weight are then fitted over the axis of the tonometer so that the longer part of the weight points toward the examiner (Fig. 24-3).

At drum positions 1.95 and 2.05 (graduation mark 2 on measuring drum set one line-width below/ above the index, respectively), the pressure arm should return from the area of free movement to the corresponding stop.

The check at drum position 2 is the most important and should be carried out frequently, because the measurement of intraocular pressure in this range is of particular importance.

3. Check at drum position 6. In the same manner the tonometer may be checked at drum position 6. The corresponding checking points are 5.9 and 6.1. The graduation mark 6 on the drum is offset by half an interval below or above the index.

The applanation tonometer consists of a plastic prism with a flat anterior surface and a diameter of 7 mm. This prism is brought into contact with a fluorescein-stained tear film of the cornea, which it displaces to the periphery of the contact zone until a surface of known and constant size of 3.06 mm is flattened. The inner border of the ring represents the line of demarcation between the cornea flattened by applanation and the cornea not flattened. The measuring drum can regulate the tension to produce a force between 0 and 8 g.

NONCONTACT TONOMETER

Calibration of the noncontact tonometer is important. The use of the logic circuits in the instrument, which are necessary to measure and record intraocular pressure, enables the operator to check the calibration of the pneumatic-electronic network in the following procedure.

1. Turn instrument to *on* (red dot).
2. Remove objective cap and wait 30 seconds for warm-up.
3. Depress the trigger switch—display at 68.
4. Push power switch knob and set it at *D*.
5. Depress trigger switch—display at 47 + 1.

Triggering is repeated several times 8 to 10 seconds apart. The display must not change more than +1 count. There must be no SLI light in any of the tests. During the check of calibration, the display number has no quantitative significance; its repeatability must be the concern. The number displayed is a specially selected equivalent to a critical check at approximately 20 mm Hg, with twice the resolution that is used in the actual intraocular pressure (IOP) measurement.

The noncontact tonometer is sturdily constructed

and normally will require little care to keep it operationally perfect. Protecting the equipment against dust is important to maintain it in good working order. It is recommended that the supplied dust covers be used.

Bulb replacement

Target illuminator bulb

1. Always disconnect instrument from its source of electrical power.
2. Remove instrument top by unscrewing two screws with a $\frac{3}{32}$ hex wrench.
3. Free bulb holder by loosening set screw, marked *B,* with a $\frac{1}{16}$ hex wrench.
4. Pull out bulb holder.
5. Remove bulb by unscrewing knurled retainer ring.
6. Replace bulb with No. 12419 bulb, and wipe bulb clean of fingerprints.
7. To adjust for maximum and even target illumination, view red dot target through the objective orifice and adjust bulb holder on axis with power *on*. Tighten set screw.
8. Replace and secure instrument cover to protect against dust.

SLI light. If replacement is ever necessary, it should be made only by a qualified service technician. An authorized American Optical distributor should be contacted.

Fixation lamp. To replace fixation bulb, the center joint is separated by pulling apart. The screw base bulb (No. 11583) is exposed for replacement.

Chin rest

The chin rest is easily removed by twisting 90 degrees, then pulling up. It is made of a durable material that can be sterilized (maximum 250° F [121° C]) or washed in soap and water or alcohol.

Headrest cushions

Headrest cushions are wiped clean with alcohol. They also may be replaced.

Eyepiece and objective

1. The exposed surfaces of the eyepiece and objective should be kept free of dust, fingerprints, and smudges. The lens surfaces should be dusted occasionally with a camel-hair brush.
2. The alignment target, as viewed by the operator, may become blurred by accumulation of grease from eyelashes on the annular aperture of the objective. Clean the annulus with a dry, cotton-tipped stick.
3. After prolonged service or use in a dusty or humid environment, the inside surface of the objective should be cleaned. Remove the objective by unscrewing counterclockwise, and dust the surface with a brush or, if necessary, wipe it clean with a dampened tissue paper before reassembly.

Lensmeter

1. The lensmeter requires little maintenance. The eyepiece should always be adjusted for each technician using this instrument. Operators should focus or adjust the eyepiece to their eye.
2. If the lensmeter has a prism compensator, which is located just under the eyepiece, the compensator should always be set on zero to ensure obtaining the correct reading.

KERATOMETER

We shall use the Bausch & Lomb keratometer as an example. When not in use, the keratometer should be kept covered with the dust cover supplied with the instrument.

1. Dirt on the daylight-blue filter sometimes will cause smudges in the mire imagery. The filter can easily be removed and cleaned by removing the two screws that hold the lamp housing to the body of the instrument.
2. When carbon deposits begin to form on the lamp bulb, the mire imagery will be diminished. If this occurs, a new bulb should be used in the instrument.
3. The lower part of the lamp housing is easily removed for the insertion of a new bulb. To replace the bulb, rotate the instrument by turning *B* until the lamp housing is away from the central carriage. The base can be removed by loosening the two screws on the sides of the lamp housing. In replacing the base, care must be taken to see that the base rests squarely on the shoulder of the

housing; otherwise that part will not clear the carriage when it is rotated back into position.

4. There is also an attachment that can be used for checking keratometer measurements. This attachment comes complete with bracket and three test ball bearings with specific radii. To calibrate, use a spherical test ball of known radius of curvature inserted in a holder. When the correct radius of curvature of the test ball is obtained, the accuracy of the keratometer can be confirmed. If the keratometer is out of alignment, it should be repaired by a trained professional.

SLIT-LAMP BIOMICROSCOPE

The slit lamp is an important instrument. All personnel who use it should make a habit of keeping it covered with a dust cover when it is not in use.

1. When changing bulbs, always be sure the instrument is unplugged. Also, always remember to wipe off all fingerprints on the bulb to extend its life.

2. If the slit lamp will not operate, replace bulbs even if they appear to be in good condition. If the slit lamp does not light when a new main bulb is installed, check contacts on the bulb cap and remove any dirt with a small file or knife. If the instrument still does not operate, check all electrical connections to be sure that all wires are plugged into the transformer and that the main power cord is plugged in. Also check for a faulty fuse in the transformer.

3. The Haag Streit and copies are the only slit lamps that contain mirrors which require cleaning. Removal of the mirror is easiest when the microscope and illuminator are well separated and the latter is inclined by approximately 10 degrees or more. Grasp the narrow shank of the long mirror and pull upward. The small mirror, which has no shank, is more difficult to grasp; therefore the point of a pencil should be used to get the mirror started on its way out. The mirror should then be dusted and sprayed with a glass cleaner. Wipe clean with cotton balls or some other material that will not scratch the surface, using a downward stroke. Repeat until dry.

4. If the slit lamp becomes difficult to move with the joy stick, clean the joy-stick pad with a cleaning solution. If slit-lamp movement still continues to be difficult, apply a thin coat of three-in-one oil or sewing machine oil to the pad.

PHOROPTER
American Optical Ultramatic Phoropter

All personnel should make it a habit to keep the American Optical Ultramatic Phoropter protected with a dust cover when not in use. Alcohol should not be used on any part of the phoropter.

1. The semipermanent face shields furnished with the phoropter are made of white nylon. This material can be washed with soap and water, soaked in alcohol, or boiled in water.

2. All lenses should be kept clean and free of dust and fingerprints. Do not put a finger in the sight aperture to check lens placement. Fingerprints on the lenses make refracting difficult. Cleaning of dust on enclosed lenses can be done with an ear syringe. The back lenses are the retinoscopy lens, polarizing lens, red lens, and Maddox rod. These are the only lenses that may be cleaned by office personnel; a glass cleaner and cotton-tipped swabs are used. The phoropter should be sent to an authorized repair shop every 2 years for preventive maintenance and lens cleaning.

3. Because the cross cylinder and the rotary prism are not enclosed, it is advisable occasionally to wipe each one carefully with lens tissue to remove dust.

Green's refractor

The Green's refractor should be protected with a dust cover when not in use. Alcohol should not be used on any part of the refractor.

1. Face shields, which can be purchased from a local supplier, should be replaced after each patient use.

2. The only lenses that can be cleaned in the office are the retinoscopy lens and the +0.12-diopter lens. These are located in the shutter disc and may be cleaned with a glass cleaner and cotton-tipped swabs. These two lenses become dirty because they are in the back of the refractor where patients' eyelashes can touch them.

3. Because the cross cylinder and the rotary prism are not enclosed, it is advisable occasionally to wipe each one carefully with lens tissue to remove dust.
4. Do not put a finger in the sight aperture to check lens placement. Fingerprints on the lenses make refracting difficult.
5. Removing dust from the internal lens may be done with an ear syringe. It is not recommended, however, for self-cleaning of the internal lens.
6. The Green's refractor should be sent to an authorized repair department for preventive maintenance and lens cleaning every 2 years.

PROJECTOR

The projector requires little care. Occasionally the glass slides and the lenses in the focusing tube should be wiped with a soft clean cloth. Best results are obtained if the cloth is dry because any moisture can cause streaks that will be projected onto the screen.

1. *Do not remove lenses from the objective barrels.* The refractor can be easily cleaned because the entire inner lamp house is removable.
2. When it is not in use, switch off the instrument to conserve the life of the lamp and to prevent burning it out prematurely. It is desirable to keep several spare bulbs on hand to ensure always having a lamp of correct voltage and proper filament center.

Projection slide

Water or any other substance should not be sprayed on the slide. Wet substances can slip between the lenses and destroy the slide. Only the slide is cleaned by rubbing lightly with a lens tissue.

Cleaning the projector screen

The projector screen has a high reflectance characteristic. It is, however, susceptible to abrasive scratches and fingerprints.

1. Periodic cleaning of the screen is advised. Simply use a mild detergent solution, wiping screen surface gently with dampened absorbent cotton.
2. Fingerprints normally will be removed by the recommended cleaning procedure. Scratches, however, cannot be removed, and the screen does not lend itself to refinishing.

Replacing the lamp

Warning: Projector must be off before proceeding with lamp replacement!

- To replace the lamp, push the small aluminum button on the side of the instrument. This will release the catch and allow the outer lamp house to swing back, exposing the inner lamp house. To remove the inner lamp house, pull top back until spring clips have disengaged, then lift out. The lamp is then entirely exposed and can easily be removed from the socket by a downward pressure and at the same time turning the lamp until it is free of the bayonet slide.

Caution: The lamp socket and reflector are factory adjusted and should not be disassembled.

Projection front-surface mirrors

Front-surface mirrors have silvering on the first or front surface. They are cleaned by spraying a glass cleaner in small amounts on the mirror, stroking downward with a cotton ball *(do not rub back and forth)*, and disposing of cotton ball. The process is repeated until the mirror is dry.

Patient viewing mirror

The patient viewing mirror is cleaned like any other mirror (except the front-surface mirror). Most viewing mirrors are not front surface; they are plate glass with rear silvering. A front-surface mirror is identified by touching the mirror surface with an object such as a pen or pencil. If the end of the object touches the reflection in the mirror, it is first surface.

PART THREE

Assisting the surgeon

CHAPTER 25 Aseptic technique and minor office surgery

- Aseptic technique
- Minor office surgery
- Complications during and after office surgery

ASEPTIC TECHNIQUE

Aseptic technique in the office or hospital is an attempt to prevent infection by the elimination of microorganisms. Ophthalmic surgery demands maximum asepsis, particularly in operations involving the globe itself. Microorganisms that gain access to the interior of the eye can multiply and cause irreparable damage, often resulting in blindness. Aseptic technique demands (1) proper sterilization of all instruments, (2) sterilization of the skin adjacent to the operative site, (3) sterilization of the hands of both the operator and the assistant, and (4) use of sterile solutions and ointments during and after the operation. For the most part the following discussion of aseptic technique will be oriented toward ophthalmic surgery in the office.

Disinfection of eyelid skin

Office surgery for conditions involving eyelid skin requires carefully applied skin antiseptics (Table 25-1). (Spray packs of antiseptics are contraindicated.) Care must be taken that none of the antiseptic material enters the eye. This may be done with careful application by cotton applicators soaked in such solutions as (1) tincture of iodine, 2%, (2) povidone-iodine (Betadine), (3) Ioprep, (4) alcohol, and (5) cetrimonium bromide. It also may be done by scrupulous scrubbing of the area with pHisoHex or green soap.

Scrubbing (degerming of hands). For many minor office procedures scrubbing may be unnecessary if both the operator and the assistant adhere to a "no-touch" technique. In this technique the tops of the sterile instruments are never touched by hands or laid down in a nonsterile area.

The skin of the hands contains normal bacterial inhabitants, as well as many transient microorganisms with which the individual may recently have come in contact. It is virtually impossible to scrub the hands sufficiently to get rid of all normal inhabitants, but the use of rubber gloves overcomes this handicap.

Scrubbing with a brush degerms the hands by (1) the removal of bacteria, (2) the dilution of the bacteria content by rinses, and (3) the use of antiseptic skin agents that are bactericidal. Before scrubbing, the fingernails should be cleansed with an orange-wood stick. The various antiseptic agents available have their own scrubbing time, which should be followed rigidly. The fingers and nails should be carefully scrubbed and all hidden recesses of the hands scrupulously cleansed.

Instillation of eye medication

Eye medication may easily become contaminated by improper instillation. There is a right and a wrong way to instill eye medication both before and after minor office surgery (Fig. 25-1). With the patient's head tilted back, the dropper, dropper bottle, or oint-

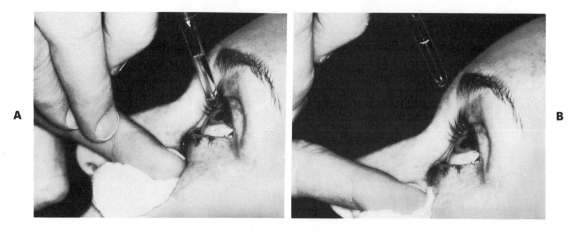

Fig. 25-1 Instillation of eye drops. **A,** Incorrect method. Note contamination of dropper by lashes. **B,** Correct method. Note tip of dropper held free of globe and lashes.

Table 25-1 Skin preparations

Skin preparation or trade name	Manufacturer	Type of bactericide
Tinctures		
Tincture of iodine, 2%		Iodine-alcohol
Alcohol, 70%		Alcohol
Zephiran Chloride	Winthrop	Quaternary ammonium compound + alcohol
Merthiolate	Eli Lilly & Co.	Sodium ethylmercurithiosalicylate + alcohol
Aqueous preparations		
Aqueous Merthiolate	Eli Lilly & Co.	Sodium ethylmercurithiosalicylate
Aqueous Zephiran Chloride	Winthrop	Quaternary ammonium compound
Hexachlorophene scrubs		
Gamophen	Arwood	Hexachlorophene
Septisol	Vestal	Hexachlorophene
pHisoHex	Winthrop	Hexachlorophene
Iodophors		
Ioprep	Johnson & Johnson	Iodophor
Wescodyne	West	Iodophor
Betadine	British Drug Houses	Iodophor
Virac	Ruson	Iodophor

ment tube should be held about ½ inch from the eye before the release of medication. When corneal anesthesia is required, the patient should be asked to look down so that the cornea will be completely covered by the medication. It is important that the tip of the dropper or dropper bottle *never touch* the eye or eyelid. Contamination will result, in which case the dropper and medication should be discarded.

Sterility of ophthalmic solutions

The sterility of eye solutions is desirable not only because of the obvious danger of ocular infection but also because contaminated solutions may prove

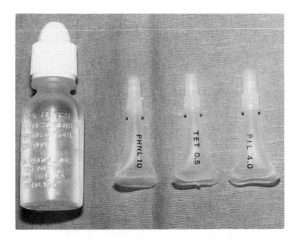

Fig. 25-2 Disposable sterile solutions.

toxic and irritating to the eye. The sterilization of ophthalmic solutions may be performed effectively by filtration through bacterial filters. The addition of a preservative, such as chlorobutanol, or benzalkonium chloride, aids in preventing contamination.

The ophthalmologist's office should contain solutions that are well prepared and that contain an added preservative. They should be bottled in small bottles and never in large stock sizes. Individual-dose sizes are commercially available in disposable plastic containers (Fig. 25-2). In addition, the ophthalmic assistant must be careful about contamination of the eyedropper, particularly if it has touched an infected eye. If contamination is suspected, the solution should be discarded. One solution notorious for harboring microorganisms, particularly *Pseudomonas aeruginosa,* is fluorescein. However, fluorescein is available in dried sterile strips that are safe to use.

Sterilization of tonometer

Ideally every tonometer should be sterilized before use. The main purpose of sterilization of the tonometer is prevention of the spread of infection from patient to patient, especially of the viruses that cause epidemic keratoconjunctivitis and acquired immunodeficiency syndrome (AIDS). Most attention has been directed toward the sterilization of the Schiøtz tonometer. There are three main methods for ster-

ilizing this instrument: (1) by heating the base of the instrument with a flame from an alcohol lamp for 10 seconds (sufficient time must be allowed for cooling before the instrument is deposited in the cornea), (2) by cleaning the base of the tonometer with alcohol or ether (sufficient time should be permitted for the chemical to dry or evaporate), and (3) ultraviolet radiation. These methods of sterilizing the tonometer are unsatisfactory, however, because sterility is not achieved in all areas of the tonometer. Pipe cleaners are useful in cleaning the inside of the barrel. If the plunger does not slide smoothly in the barrel, erroneous readings will result. Some ophthalmologists employ a disposable sterile cap, a Tonofilm, on the base of the tonometer to ensure complete protection.

The Goldmann applanation tonometer is cleaned best by wiping the contact surface with alcohol ether or hydrogen peroxide. The latter has proved effective against the human immunodeficiency virus (HIV) if the tonometer head also is soaked in hydrogen peroxide.

After use of either the Schiøtz or Goldmann tonometer, the contact surface should remain clean and dry, which in itself will prevent organisms from multiplying.

MINOR OFFICE SURGERY

Ophthalmologists vary in the amount and type of office surgery they perform. Such factors as the availability of outpatient facilities in a nearby hospital, the time spent at the hospital by the physician, the physical layout of the physician's office, and the presence of a trained and efficient ophthalmic assistant will influence the decision to perform surgical procedures in the office or in the outpatient department of the hospital. When adequate physical facilities and a trained assistant are available, many minor procedures can be performed in the ophthalmic office.

Of fundamental importance is the general sterility of the area in which the surgical procedure is to be performed. Maintaining adequate cleanliness and dusting of the surgical area should be a daily duty of the ophthalmic assistant. The area should be segregated from the routine patient flow as much as

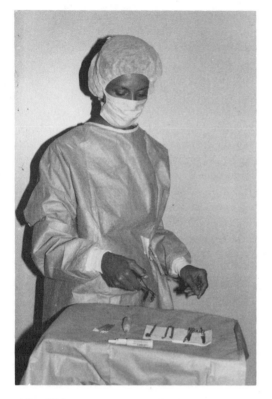

Fig. 25-3 Preparation of sterile instrument tray.

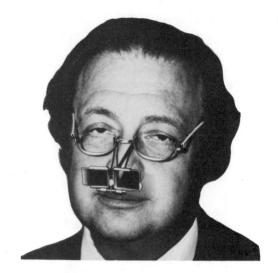

Fig. 25-4 Beebe loupe for stereoscopic magnification in performing office surgery.

possible. It should be noted that an office operating room will not achieve the same high standard of sterility that is found in the operating room of a hospital. Such factors as a separate scrub area, elimination of all street clothing, shoe covers, air filtration, and positive-pressure operating rooms are not generally found in the office operating room. In an office that one enters without a mask, airborne bacteria may remain active for hours. In all offices emphasis must be placed on adequate sterilization of instruments, combined with personal measures to ensure that there is reasonable cleanliness and sterility in the surgical area.

Careful and complete *cleanliness of instruments* must precede all efforts at sterilization. It is useless to place a blood-stained curet into an antiseptic solution, heat oven, or autoclave, because these dirty instruments can never be thoroughly sterilized. Scrupulous cleansing with a fine brush and careful in-

spection of the instruments are essential. This inspection is done most efficiently under magnification with magnifying lenses or loupes. The cleansing may be done in soapy water or with one of the many detergents available. To remove blood and tissue debris from the instruments, enzyme solutions are available. Instruments with moving parts should be lubricated periodically or dipped into surgical Instrument-Milk. After these instruments are carefully rinsed, they are sterilized (Fig. 25-3).

Sterilization of the instruments may be performed by one of the methods outlined previously. Small autoclaves are available for office use. They have their own time devices and will sterilize within 5 minutes. Disinfection of the patient's skin is performed for many lid procedures by applying an antiseptic solution such as iodine, povidone-iodine, or benzyl ammonium chloride.

The surgeon and the ophthalmic assistant should observe all rules of cleanliness, particularly for the more advanced procedures that may be performed in the office. Before handling sterilized instruments, the ophthalmic assistant should scrub, preferably with hexachlorophene soap. Gloves may be required for some of the minor operations performed. The ophthalmic assistant should never use nail polish or wear hand or wrist jewelry when assisting during minor office procedures. Masks and caps are often not necessary for most minor office procedures. More extensive operations, however, such as pterygium removal and plastic eyelid surgery, may require surgical care comparable to the standards used in a first-class operating room of a hospital. Minor surgery should be performed under magnification with loupes (Fig. 25-4).

Instruments and surgical materials for ophthalmic procedures

The following surgical instruments may be required in minor office surgery. These include forceps, scissors, needle holders, clamps, curets, scalpels and blades, and lacrimal instruments and cannulas. The numerous individual variations of these instruments depend on the surgeon's choice.

Forceps. Forceps are used to grasp small tissues for either removal or suture insertion. The teeth of these instruments vary from 0.12 to 0.5 mm. The jaws may be rounded, flat, or serrated. Some forceps, called *tying forceps,* have no teeth. Other forceps, called *epilation forceps,* also have no teeth and are used to remove lashes. Thus both tooth and non-tooth tine forceps often are available in the office (Fig. 25-5).

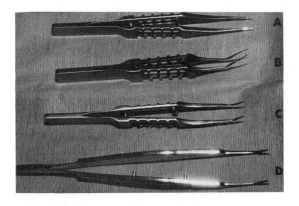

Fig. 25-5 Forceps: **A,** Colibri 0.12 mm. **B,** Capsular-hesus. **C,** Tying. **D,** 0.5 mm.

Scissors. Scissors may be blunt or sharp, curved or straight. They may have spring action or direct action.

Needle holders. Needle holders hold suture needles and provide good control for inserting needles. Some of these instruments are nonlocking, some locking; some handles are spring-loaded. Some needle holders have a thumb release (Fig. 25-6).

Clamps. Clamps used in ophthalmic surgery may be round, with a guarded plate behind to provide

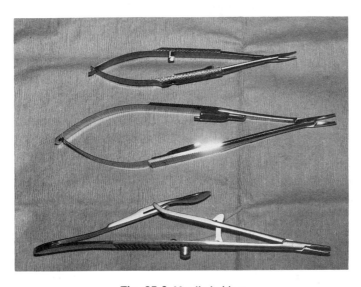

Fig. 25-6 Needle holders.

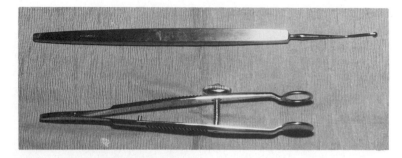

Fig. 25-7 Curet and chalazion clamp.

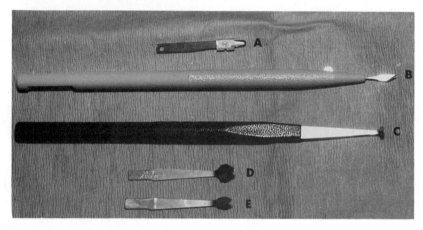

Fig. 25-8 Disposable blades: **A,** Guarded incision blade. **B,** Superblade. **C,** Spatula-angled keratectomy blade. **D,** 5.2 mm keratome. **E,** 3.2 mm keratome.

hemostasis during removal of chalazions. Other clamps are used to hold eyelids during eyelid surgery, as well as to create hemostasis.

Curets. Curets are slim-handled and have a bowl-shaped end. The ends are either round or serrated and are used to remove chalazions and other small cystic material (Fig. 25-7).

Scalpels and blades. Scalpels used by the physician depend on preference. Commonly used instruments are disposable small blades and the Bard-Parker scalpel (Fig. 25-8). The latter may be used for removing sutures.

Lacrimal instruments. A lacrimal set consists of a punctum dilator, which enlarges the punctum, a sterile medicine glass to hold sterile saline solution or an antibiotic solution, and a disposable syringe

with a blunt lacrimal cannula. The last introduces a solution into the canaliculus (Figs. 25-9 and 25-10).

Corrosion of stainless steel instruments

A wide range of metals constitute what is known as stainless steel. These metals have iron and chromium in common but may also contain carbon, nickel, sulfur, tungsten, manganese, molybdenum, and other elements. Chromium imparts the stainless quality to the metal, and the more chromium present, the more resistant it is to corrosion. Carbon provides hardness to the metal but also reduces the corrosion-resistant effect of chromium. Special hardening processes are undertaken by different manufacturers to try to produce a hardened instrument with low corrosion properties. Polishing also reduces the corro-

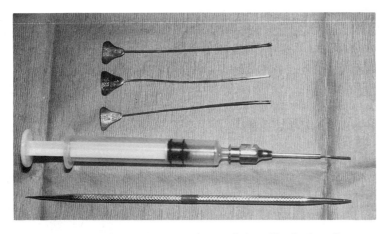

Fig. 25-9 Lacrimal probing and irrigating set: probes, syringe and lacrimal needle, punctum dilator.

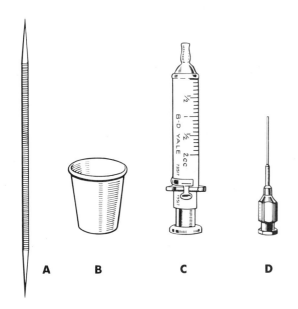

Fig. 25-10 Lacrimal set. **A,** Punctum dilator; **B,** sterile medicine glass to contain either sterile normal saline solution or an antibiotic solution; **C,** syringe; **D,** lacrimal needle.

sive effect, but some areas such as the knurled handles cannot be polished very well and consequently are the first to suffer corrosion.

The most common causes of corrosion are inadequate cleaning and drying after use, too long ex-

posure to sterilizing solutions, or too corrosive a sterilizing solution. The most important factor that causes corrosion is inadequate cleaning so that particles of material remain on the surface.

Fortunately, many sharp instruments today are available in disposable form. Where available, these usually are preferred because a sharp instrument is guaranteed every time.

Procedures

Chalazion surgery. This condition is caused by an obstruction of a meibomian gland of the eyelid. Because of this blockage, the gland becomes distended and ruptures, the oily contents being liberated into the substance of the lid. This results in a granulomatous inflammatory reaction that subsides spontaneously in some cases but in other cases appears to remain as a chronic nodule on the eyelid (Fig. 25-11). The nodule may be removed under the eyelid through a vertical conjunctival incision or, occasionally, externally through the skin.

The ophthalmic assistant's help is essential in (1) arranging the patient comfortably in the operating chair, (2) adequately anesthetizing the eye with topical anesthetic drops, (3) setting out the syringe and needle with the local anesthetic for infiltration into the eyelid, (4) setting out a sterile towel with the instruments required, (5) securing hemostasis by application of pressure directly at the operative site

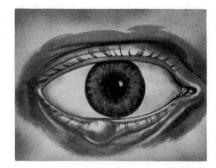

Fig. 25-11 Chalazion of the lower eyelid.

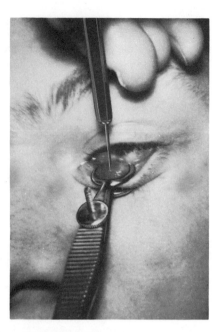

Fig. 25-13 Removal of a chalazion.

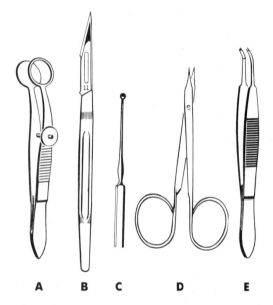

A B C D E

Fig. 25-12 Chalazion set. **A,** Chalazion clamp; **B,** scalpel; **C,** curet; **D,** fine scissors; **E,** fine forceps.

after chalazion removal, and (6) preparing the dressing, which usually consists of an antibiotic ointment and a firmly-applied eye pad. The instruments required for the chalazion operation are shown in Figs. 25-12 and 25-13.

Eye patch application. An eye patch must be applied correctly if it is to perform the necessary function of preventing further bleeding and an accumulation of lid edema (Fig. 25-14). After the instillation of an antibiotic ointment, a recommended method

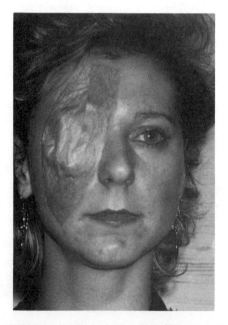

Fig. 25-14 Eye patch. Note that the patch is angled away from the mouth to prevent interference with eating.

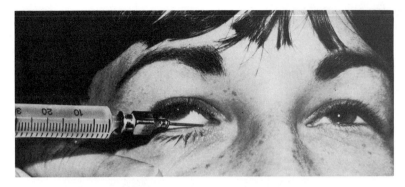

Fig. 25-15 Irrigation of nasolacrimal duct.

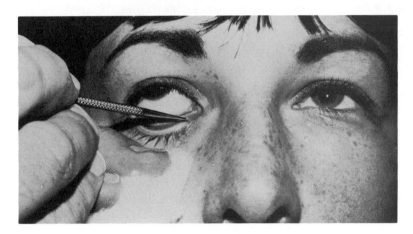

Fig. 25-16 Dilation of the punctum.

is to immobilize the eyelid through pressure by (1) applying an eye pad doubled in half over the site of the chalazion, (2) applying a second eye pad over this pad, and (3) fixing the pad firmly by small ½-inch strips of adhesive tape in an overlapping fashion, taking care that the hair is not involved in any way in the adhesive.

Tear duct irrigation. Epiphora, or watering of the eye, is a common condition, especially affecting older patients. This condition may result from a blockage of the nasolacrimal passage. One important test to determine the site of blockage is washing out or irrigating the nasolacrimal passageway (Fig. 25-15). Instruments required for irrigation of the tear duct are shown in Fig. 25-10.

In most cases, disposable syringes are used. However, carefully cleaned and sterilized reusable syringes may be used and are used in many parts of the world where cost is a factor and labor is inexpensive. Lacrimal instruments are best sterilized by using the dry-heat oven.

Normally the upper and lower punctum are quite small and will not admit a lacrimal needle or probe. The punctum dilator is employed to enlarge the orifice of the punctum to permit the lacrimal needle to enter the lacrimal canaliculus (Fig. 25-16). Many ophthalmologists prefer to use an antibiotic solution for irrigation in case the lacrimal passageways are traumatized.

Fluorescein test to determine lacrimal function.

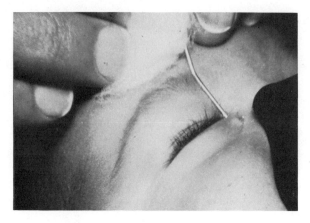

Fig. 25-17 Probing of tear duct with patient under general anesthesia. The probe is passed through the punctum and canaliculus into the nasolacrimal duct.

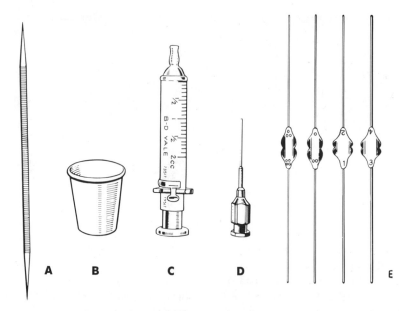

Fig. 25-18 Tear duct probing set. **A,** Punctum dilator; **B,** medicine glass; **C,** syringe; **D,** lacrimal needle; **E,** series of probes usually ranging from 00 to 2 wire size.

A simple test to determine the patency of the lacrimal passageway is performed by placing one or two drops of fluorescein into the conjunctival sac, with the patient's head bent forward. If there is no obstruction to flow, then the fluorescein will drain into the nose within 30 seconds. A test that indicates good patency consists of placing a dried cotton swab in the nose to see if the stain is present. Occasionally the fluorescein will drain to the back of the throat, and the stain can be found by having the patient cough and deposit the stained sputum into a tissue. The fellow eye can be checked at the same time with use of rose bengal stain.

Tear duct probing. In cases of complete blockage

of the nasolacrimal passage, there results either constant watering (epiphora) or sometimes a combination of watering with an infection of the lacrimal sac (dacryocystitis). This is particularly common among newborn infants.

Many ophthalmologists prefer to perform this procedure at the hospital with the patient under general anesthesia (Fig. 25-17). When a general anesthetic is used, the anesthesia should be just sufficient to allow the patient to retain the swallowing reflex. The ophthalmologist can observe if the irrigation is successful, and it prevents fluid from entering the patient's lungs.

With adults, the probing of tear ducts may be performed with the use of a topical anesthetic (such as proparacaine or tetracaine) combined with local infiltration of anesthetic. The injectable anesthetic may be combined with some *hyaluronidase* to increase the spreading effect throughout the tissues. Further anesthesia may be achieved by irrigating a small amount of proparacaine or tetracaine through the punctum. It is important that the patient be relaxed and comfortable because sudden movement of the head may cause damage to the eye or produce a false passage in the lacrimal apparatus. The instruments required for probing are shown in Fig. 25-18.

Ziegler cautery. Ziegler cautery refers to thermal, or heat, cauterizing of the lower eyelid to either

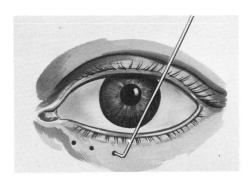

Fig. 25-19 Correction of entropion by Ziegler cautery.

invert or evert the lower lid (Fig. 25-19). This procedure is used more commonly for spastic senile entropion (turning inward of the eyelid), but it also may be used for ectropion (turning outward of the eyelid). This operation has particular value for the elderly patient with a spastic entropion. The instruments used are shown in Fig. 25-20.

Electrolysis. A method used to permanently remove lashes from the eyelid margin by applying heat to the base of the hair follicle is known as *electrolysis*. It is employed in the treatment of congenitally aberrant lashes, trichiasis, and postoperative and posttraumatic conditions that result in the turning of the lashes toward the cornea.

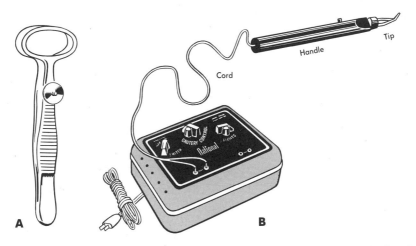

Fig. 25-20 Instruments for Ziegler cautery. **A,** Large chalazion or lid clamp; **B,** fine thermal cautery.

Anesthesia is performed by direct infiltration of the base of the lash. The Hyfrecator with a fine needle is inserted along the pathway to the root of the lash. Magnification is essential in this procedure to see the tiny orifices through which the hairs emerge. Epilation is complete after the Hyfrecator has been turned on for a few seconds and the lash can be removed without pulling.

Electrosurgery. Electrosurgery is based on the principles of diathermy. Diathermy is the amplication of high-frequency alternating currents. This diathermy produces heat as a result of the resistance of the tissues. Frequencies employed are between 2 and 4 MHz, which includes part of the radio-frequency spectrum. Because of this, as a precaution these currents should not be used with individuals who have pacemakers or in the presence of any flammable or explosive gases or liquids.

A number of modes of electrosurgery are available for use in ophthalmology. The most familiar mode is that of wet-field cautery. This is a bipolar cautery in which electrical current passes between two points in a wet field of saline and creates hemostasis. The two points are usually the two tips of a forceps. This is one of the methods of coagulating bleeding vessels during ocular surgery.

Fulguration or *spark gap* current is a form of electric current. Fulguration current produces a potent dehydrating effect on tissues that is destructive and self-limiting. The spark must jump across to the tissues, thereby producing a charring or carbon effect on the tissues. This procedure can coagulate heavy bleeders or destroy bases of tissue to prevent such things as recurrences of carcinoma.

A fully filtered current is a continuous flow of a high-frequency current that results in a nonpulsating flow of current. This produces a smooth cutting flow with a minimal amount of heat and tissue destruction. This type of current is ideal for cutting.

Fully rectified current produces a minute but perceptible pulsating effect that can, under certain conditions, reduce the efficiency of the cutting while producing some lateral heat. A benefit is that this heat can produce coagulation of the tissue surfaces and provide effective hemostasis.

Partially rectified current is an intermittent flow of high-frequency current. Because it is partially rectified, it produces more hemostasis and seals off bleeders. This type of current commonly is used in eyelid surgery.

Eyelid growth removal. Patients with large growths of the eyelid will require hospitalization and removal of the growth under adequate operating room conditions. However, many small papillomas, benign melanomas, verrucae, and other small lesions of the eyelids may be carefully and safely removed in the office. Specimen bottles that contain formaldehyde should be available from the local pathology laboratory so that the specimens may be microscopically examined. Many of these lesions on the eyelid may be removed and the base cauterized. Others may require sutures. Fig. 25-21 shows the instruments that are required and that should be available when eyelid procedures are performed.

Pterygium removal. A pterygium is a fibrovascular membrane that extends from the medial aspect of the bulbar conjunctiva and invades the cornea (Fig. 25-22). It tends to be progressive and in time can make its way to the central portion of the cornea and interfere with vision. Pterygia are most common in southern climates where people have greater exposure to ultraviolet light, which appears to promote growth. In northern areas, people who have outdoor vocations, such as farmers, sailors, and postal workers, are most prone to develop this growth.

The purpose of pterygium removal is to excise the membrane before it can significantly interfere with vision. Because this operation requires incision into the cornea as well as the conjunctiva, scrupulous cleanliness, disinfection of the patient's skin and the surgeon's hands, and sterilization of the instruments are required. The anesthesia usually is provided by topical anesthetic drops or combined with subconjunctival injection. Placing the patient in a horizontal position is the preferred method for the surgical removal of the pterygium. Adequate light is important. The instruments for a pterygium procedure are shown in Fig. 25-23.

Xanthelasma lesion removal. Xanthelasma lesions are yellowish and subcutaneous, and they are found on the inner aspect of the upper and lower

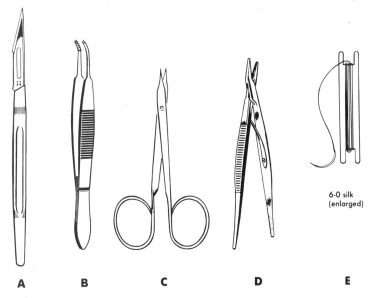

Fig. 25-21 Eyelid growth removal set. **A,** Scalpel; **B,** fine forceps; **C,** fine scissors; **D,** needle holder; **E,** fine suture.

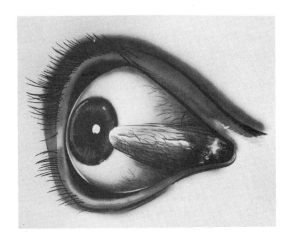

Fig. 25-22 Pterygium.

eyelids (Fig. 25-24). Normally they are bilateral and progress slowly. These lesions tend to form an arc in both the upper and lower eyelids and are often associated with high serum cholesterol levels. Xanthelasma lesions are removed for cosmetic purposes only, because these deposits have no invasive properties. Despite removal, however, they tend to recur.

Smaller lesions may be removed by the application of a chemical such as trichloroacetic acid. Larger xanthelasma deposits require surgical removal. Excision usually is quite simple, requiring excision of the skin and the underlying subcutaneous tissue. Instruments required for removal of xanthelasma lesions are shown in Fig. 25-25.

COMPLICATIONS DURING AND AFTER OFFICE SURGERY

The ophthalmic assistant must be alert for complications that may arise after surgery. The assistant may be the closest at hand and in a position to render immediate first aid for the following conditions that may arise: (1) fainting, (2) central nervous system stimulation, (3) respiratory emergencies, (4) allergic reaction, and (5) drug reaction.

Fainting

Fainting is a common occurrence in office surgery. The patient who faints should be placed in a head-down position, with the head lower than the heart. This may be done by tilting the head forward between the knees or tilting back the operating table

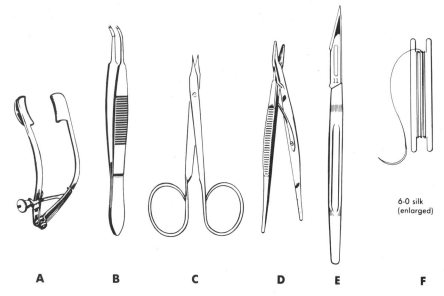

6-0 silk
(enlarged)

A   B   C   D   E   F

Fig. 25-23 Pterygium set. **A,** Eyelid speculum; **B,** fine forceps; **C,** fine scissors; **D,** needle holder; **E,** Bard-Parker scalpel; **F,** fine suture.

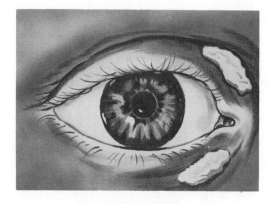

Fig. 25-24 Xanthelasma.

or chair. Ophthalmic personnel should be sure that there is an adequate airway present and that a tight collar is loosened. Aromatic spirits of ammonia or smelling salts may be administered to encourage breathing by reflex stimulation.

Central nervous system stimulation

A patient may show signs of great excitability, tremors, or even convulsions. This may be the result of cocaine toxicity. The patient should be placed head down, ensuring that the airway is not restricted by collars or ties, and given reassurance. The ophthalmologist should be contacted immediately if not already available. He or she may consider giving intravenous sedation.

Respiratory emergencies

If any difficulties arise in breathing, such as shallowness or decreased respirations, the patient must be watched carefully. Oxygen may be administered by a small portable oxygen unit that is readily available. If artificial resuscitation becomes necessary, mouth-to-mouth resuscitation is the treatment of choice. See Chapter 38 on cardiopulmonary resuscitation for more detailed information.

Allergic reaction

Severe allergic reactions or idiosyncrasies to drugs may occur in which there is a resultant edema of the respiratory passages. This may require mouth-to-mouth resuscitation, oxygen therapy, and intravenous cortisone.

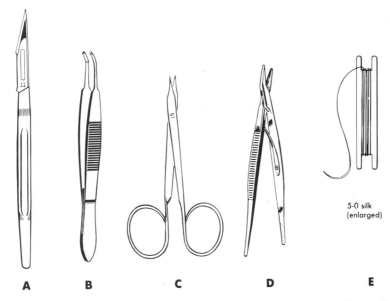

5-0 silk
(enlarged)

A   B   C   D   E

Fig. 25-25 Xanthelasma set. **A,** Scalpel; **B,** fine forceps; **C,** fine scissors; **D,** needle holder; **E,** silk suture.

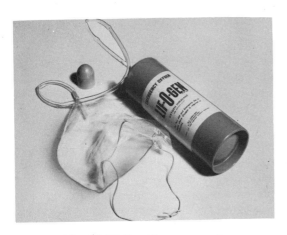

Fig. 25-26 Portable oxygen unit.

Drug reaction

The ophthalmologist should be immediately alerted to any signs of a drug reaction. He or she may elect to control the reaction by the use of drugs such as epinephrine (Adrenalin) or cortisone.

An important rule for the ophthalmic assistant is to have available at all times (1) oxygen (Fig. 25-26), (2) epinephrine, (3) syringes with needles, (4) meperidine (Demerol), (5) barbiturates, (6) intravenous cortisone, (7) spirits of ammonia or smelling salts, and (8) scalpel. The assistant should periodically check for current dating on supplies.

SUMMARY

An outline of effective aseptic technique and methods of dealing with instruments and layouts for office surgical procedure has been presented. The ophthalmic assistant who has been given this challenging responsibility must become familiar with the basic routine of the ophthalmologist. The assistant will then become a necessary and invaluable aid in the smooth performance of these minor surgical procedures and will derive a great deal of personal satisfaction from the work.

QUESTIONS FOR REVIEW AND THOUGHT

1. What is meant by asepsis? When is aseptic technique of particular importance in eye surgery?
2. Outline ways in which the operative field may be contaminated at the time of surgery.
3. Outline ways in which wound contamination may be prevented.
4. Discuss the methods by which skin may be prepared for surgery.
5. How are tonometers sterilized?
6. How are eye medications rendered sterile, and how is contamination of such medications avoided?
7. What are the main functions of the ophthalmic assistant with respect to minor office surgery?
8. List several minor ophthalmic procedures commonly performed in the office.
9. Discuss the procedure for nasolacrimal irrigation in an adult.
10. What instruments should be set out for the surgical removal of a chalazion?
11. What are general complications that may result from minor office surgery?
12. What emergency supplies should be on hand to deal with such complications?
13. How would you handle a patient who faints in the office?
14. What instruments are available for removing a corneal foreign body?
15. What is the purpose of an eye patch after a corneal abrasion?
16. What is the advantage of fluorescein strips over solutions?
17. What reactions may occur after injection of a local anesthetic?

SELF-EVALUATION QUESTIONS

True-false statements

Directions: Indicate whether the statement is true (T) or false (F).

T or F
1. In office practice, fluorescein in paper strip form is preferable to the large solution form of 2% fluorescein.

T or F
2. Ophthalmic solutions are always sterile.

Missing words

Directions: Write in the missing word in the following sentences.
3. A technique that results in absence of microorganisms is called _____ technique.
4. Excitability, tremors, and convulsions are indications of _____ stimulation.
5. An agent that may be used to relieve immediate serious allergic reactions to drugs is _____.

Choice-completion questions

Directions: Select the one best answer in each case.
6. Which of the following is not necessary for a chalazion procedure?
   a. Scalpel blade
   b. Curet
   c. Forceps
   d. Speculum
   e. Clamp

7. Which of the following is incorrect? Tear duct irrigation for epiphora may be used to identify:
   a. Blockage of the punctum
   b. Stenosis of the canaliculus
   c. Blockage of the nasolacrimal duct
   d. Ectropion
   e. Presence of a stone in the lacrimal sac

ANSWERS, NOTES, AND EXPLANATIONS

1. **True.** Fluorescein in large bottle solutions can easily become contaminated, particularly with *Pseudomonas aeruginosa,* and consequently one may be introducing a new organism into the eye. Paper strips are far safer for office use. However, individual sterile dropper units are available, and although these are relatively expensive, they also may be used.

   The technique of applying fluorescein paper is to wet the fluorescein strip with saline solution or touch the wet conjunctiva so that a thin film of fluorescein will spread over the corneal surface. Any defect in the epithelial cells will be stained by fluorescein and become more easily visualized. It is advisable in record keeping to make a sketch of the staining area on the patient's record for later comparison and also to follow the progress of healing. This may become important in recurrent corneal abrasion to identify the site of initial injury.

2. **False.** Although manufacturers provide preservatives such as chlorobutanol, thimerosal, EDTA, and benzalkonium chloride to prevent the solutions from contamination, nevertheless there is no fail-safe method. Once a bottle has been opened and used on any patient, organisms can enter the solution and not be destroyed by the preservative. The longer the bottle remains on the shelf of the ophthalmic office, the more likely is this to occur.

   As a consequence, safeguards for ophthalmic drugs should be put into action once the bottle has been opened. These bottles should not remain for any length of time on the shelf. Second, when introducing drops into the eye, one should avoid contaminating the tip of the bottle or the tip of the eye dropper by touching the lashes or eyelid of the individual receiving the drops. If contamination is suspected, the solution should be discarded.

3. **Aseptic.** Aseptic technique refers to a technique of surgery in which there is an absence of all living microorganisms. This technique involves sterilization of instruments, disinfecting the skin of patient and hands of the operator, and the use of sterile solutions, drapes, and medications so that nothing that reaches the operative site has any microorganisms that will cause contamination.

4. **Central nervous system.** Some drugs reach the central nervous system and induce this type of excitability, tremors, or convulsions. Cocaine may be such an offending agent.

5. **Epinephrine (Adrenalin)** or **cortisone.** Both agents may be used in certain situations to relieve an acute anaphylactic reaction in which the body responds adversely to some drug. Both of these agents should be kept on hand and be readily available for such emergencies.

6. **d. Speculum.** A chalazion clamp usually is satisfactory for holding the lid and creating hemostasis during the procedure. Chalazion clamps can be small or large and can be selected to suit the size of the chalazion.

7. **d. Ectropion.** The diagnosis of ectropion usually is made from external examination and does not require probing or tear duct irrigation to identify the problem. However, if the latter were the chief complaint, these procedures might then be done to identify if any stenosis of the canaliculus has occurred as a result of the ectropion.

   In other situations, such as occlusion, stenosis, or presence of a stone of the lacrimal sac, there will be a resistance on irrigation of the nasolacrimal system.

CHAPTER 26

The operative patient

- Arrangements for bed and operating privileges
- Preparing the child and parent for surgery
- Preparing the adult for major ocular surgery
- Eye surgery
- Types of anesthesia

The ophthalmic assistant must be familiar with the preoperative and postoperative routines for the management of the operative patient. Such a patient must feel secure that the case is being dealt with competently from the time the decision is made to have surgery until the final postoperative management is complete. A single error, such as giving the patient the wrong date of surgery, will only increase the patient's anxiety and undermine the patient's confidence in the physician. Operative routines should be well set, so that at each phase the patient knows exactly what to expect.

This chapter deals with the total management of the patient's care before hospitalization and during the postoperative period.

ARRANGEMENTS FOR BED AND OPERATING PRIVILEGES

The ophthalmic assistant who makes the booking and arrangement of admission to the appropriate hospital or surgical center has been delegated a great deal of responsibility (Fig. 26-1). Each operative procedure involves a dislocation in the patient's life. The patient may be required to take time off from work, school, or homemaking and to make arrangements for someone to fill his or her place in the performance of regular duties. Therefore it is helpful if the patient is asked beforehand which date is most

convenient to schedule the necessary surgery.

In addition to scheduling time for surgery according to the convenience of the patient, the ophthalmic assistant should prepare the surgical schedule according to the convenience of the surgeon. The assistant must know the duration of each operative procedure so that a surgical schedule will not be unreasonably crowded, as well as the number of surgeries the ophthalmologist can perform and follow each week without creating a strain.

There are three types of operative bookings that require attention: (1) emergency admission, (2) urgent admission, and (3) elective admission.

Emergency admission

The emergency patient is one who experiences a serious ocular calamity and because of the nature of the condition must be treated by surgery without delay. This type of patient does not have the time to adjust psychologically to the onset of the illness or to the necessary treatment. This patient usually is anxious, agitated, often confused, and commonly in a great deal of pain, as well as emotionally disturbed because of the loss of vision. Inasmuch as the patient cannot be psychologically prepared for surgery, prime attention is focused on the orderly transfer of the patient from the office to the emergency room of the hospital. None of the details of

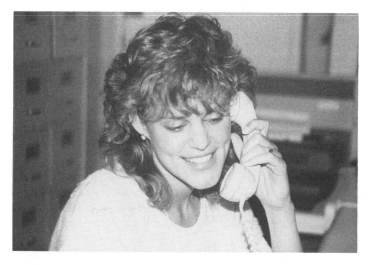

Fig. 26-1 Correct bookings are important to patient, hospital, and surgeon.

the transfer should ever be left to the patient. Relatives or friends should be called and the transportation to the hospital arranged through them. They can also, at a later date, bring the patient's personal articles to the hospital and take care of the patient's personal commitments. The emergency room of the hospital should be called in advance to anticipate the patient's arrival so that delay will not be incurred because of the number of routine admissions. It is helpful to note the patient's room number and visiting hours for family and friends. Each hospital has its own regulations regarding visiting time, duration of visits, the number of relatives admitted per visit, and visiting by children. Thus the ophthalmic assistant should understand the rules for visitors.

The most common ocular emergencies that require surgical intervention are lacerated globes and eyelids, intraocular foreign bodies, acute glaucoma, and intraocular hemorrhage.

Urgent admission

The urgent patient is one whose problem requires special consideration because of the patient's condition. Such a patient requires priority hospital admission because the problem cannot be tolerated for an unlimited period of time. For example, the patient

with a retinal detachment is best treated as soon as the detachment is discovered. If, however, the hospital is overcrowded and immediate admission is not possible, the patient should be placed on the hospital urgent list on a day-to-day basis.

The patient with an urgent problem should always be available and prepared to enter the hospital on a day-to-day basis. Patients in this category should be called regularly so that they do not feel they are languishing at home, forgotten.

Other conditions that may be classified as urgent disorders are chronic glaucoma, orbital tumors, dislocated lenses, uveitis, and temporal arteritis.

Elective admission

The patient with an elective problem has an ocular disorder that is chronic, slowly progressive, and that will not significantly deteriorate by a delay in admission to a hospital or surgical center. The patient has ample time to be fully briefed on the duration of the hospital stay and the expected postoperative convalescence. It is helpful if patients of this type are prepared for surgery by giving them some of the available literature on their particular condition. Pamphlets and videotapes on glaucoma, strabismus, and cataracts explain the nature of these disorders and the purpose of operative therapy.

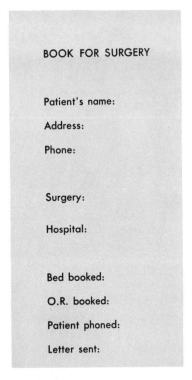

BOOK FOR SURGERY

Patient's name:

Address:

Phone:

Surgery:

Hospital:

Bed booked:

O.R. booked:

Patient phoned:

Letter sent:

Fig. 26-2 Record of surgical booking.

Operative booking schedule

To ensure that all arrangements with the patient and the hospital are secure, the ophthalmic assistant should have a plan to follow on each operative case.

Our plan has been for the ophthalmic assistant to record a number of essential points before a patient is considered to be booked and awaiting surgery (Fig. 26-2). These points are (1) date of admission, (2) type of bed if any is required, (3) date and time of operation, with type of anesthesia, (4) date the patient was notified by telephone, (5) date of letter sent requiring confirmation, and (6) confirmation by the patient. A reminder slip in bright red is affixed to the front of every surgical chart.

The *date of admission* often will be the day of surgery if the surgery is outpatient. It may, however, be the evening before surgery if the patient requires hospitalization. If such a condition is not under complete control, surgery may be hazardous to the patient. A medical consultation may be necessary to ensure that the patient does not have any infections,

cardiac irregularities, uncontrolled diabetes, hypertension, or other medical disorders.

Operative time and date must be carefully integrated with the surgeon's schedule so that there is no duplication of this time by office appointments or other commitments. The decision as to *local or general anesthesia* is most important in booking the operating room. It is preferable if procedures that require general anesthesia are scheduled to follow each other so that the anesthetist's time is more efficiently utilized. Patients with infection such as dacryocystitis always should be placed last on the operative schedule. The ophthalmic assistant should be familiar with the length of time it requires the surgeon to complete a procedure. Additional time should be set aside during the time of surgery for changeover of instruments and materials between patients.

As soon as arrangements for the operative time and date have been completed, the patient should be notified by *telephone* to be sure that the time is suitable. Occasional adjustments may have to be made for illness, holidays, work, and special requests of the patient. A well-run ophthalmic practice, emphasizing good will, permits some latitude in this direction, depending on the urgency of the problem.

Our practice has been to follow up the telephone call with a *confirming letter* outlining the date and time of admission to the hospital and requesting confirmation by return call or letter (Fig. 26-3). The purpose of having the patient provide a return call or letter is to ensure that the date of surgery is agreeable to the patient and that the patient's schedule has been altered accordingly.

The *confirmation* should always be double-checked, and those patients who have not confirmed should be contacted.

A simplification of this routine may be followed when the patient has outpatient surgery. With outpatient surgery today, blood tests and physical examinations are arranged ahead of time. The patient may be asked to return to the office to pick up blood test forms. In addition, intraocular lens implant power will be required for all cataract procedures. The A-scan may be performed at this particular time if it has not been performed before. An A-scan is

Dear Mrs. White

Dr. Jones has made arrangements for your eye operation to be performed at The Central Hospital on Tuesday, March 24th.

It will be necessary for you to enter the hospital on Tuesday, March 23rd at 7:00 AM.

Kindly confirm these arrangements as soon as possible by calling the office at 111-2020 or by letter.

Sincerely yours,

Miss L. Jordan
for Dr. H. Jones

Fig. 26-3 Sample operation letter.

usually performed on both eyes at the same time. In some cases a B-scan may be required if the cataract is dense and the practitioner wishes to view the vitreous cavity and the status of the retina. Other investigational tests may be performed.

PREPARING THE CHILD AND PARENT FOR SURGERY

The child who is about to enter the hospital will have a great deal of apprehension. If this is the second or third hospital visit, the child's apprehension may have been increased by previous experiences. For many children this will be the first experience away from their parents in strange surroundings.

Some hospitals have facilities for admission of the mother to the same room so that she may stay with the child the night before surgery and the night after. This is good practice because it diminishes the child's sense of insecurity and abandonment. If dual admissions are not possible, the child should be admitted to a room with other children where the child would feel more comfortable. The child may be terrified if placed with a sick adult given to groaning or erratic behavior.

It is important that the child be given some explanation about the purpose of the visit to the hospital and the routines to be expected. Virtually every hospital requires some preliminary investigations, including a chest x-ray examination, urinalysis, hemoglobin determination, and temperature. The child should be told that a few simple painless tests will be performed the day before surgery. The child should be informed by the parent that he or she will be put to sleep and, on awakening, will find a bandage over one eye.

The parent should be instructed as to the time of discharge and the necessary office visits that may be required afterward. A fully-informed parent will be a cooperative parent after surgery.

PREPARING THE ADULT FOR MAJOR OCULAR SURGERY

It is necessary to have the patient who will be undergoing surgery in the best physical and emotional condition to avoid any preventable complications. The ophthalmic assistant should endeavor, where possible, to relieve the patient's anxiety and apprehension. Fostering cooperation and confidence is all-important in the patient's psychologic approach to the operation.

The patient should be told how to find the admitting department of the hospital and what documents may be required for entry. The patient should leave all valuables at home. The ophthalmic assistant should call the hospital before the patient's admission to ensure that the accommodation the patient desires is available. If changes are necessary, the patient should be told beforehand, rather than at the admitting desk.

Alterations in the patient's personal habits may be necessary in the postoperative period. The patient who is a heavy smoker should be asked to abstain for at least 1 week preoperatively and during the immediate postoperative period, because a smoker's cough can easily cause disruption of the delicate operative wound. The patient who is taking aspirin should be asked to refrain from doing so for 1 week before surgery to avoid excessive bleeding.

On discharge from the hospital the patient will require instillation of medication. If the patient is unable to perform the task personally, prior arrangements should be made for a homemaker, nurse, or a member of the family to instill the medication.

Restrictions have gradually been lightened in the past few years as a result of the advent of smaller-incision surgery and better wound architecture. Thus today the patient may even return home immediately and carry on normal activities with little restriction.

EYE SURGERY

The patient contemplating surgery of the eyes is beset with many misgivings and fears about the amount of suffering that will be endured and the possibility of losing sight permanently. As opposed to the internal organs of the body, the patient has some concept of the eye and therefore is more likely to develop anxieties. The patient knows where they are, what they are used for, and that they are extremely painful to touch with a hair, let alone a sharp scalpel. On the other hand, a patient who is going to have a gallbladder removed usually has, at best, a remote idea of the location of this structure and certainly no concept of its function, because the body appears to carry on with or without a gallbladder. The patient with an ocular problem that requires surgery consciously fears damage to the eye and knows full well the consequences of removal. Because ocular surgery is often dramatic, in that blind people are given sight, it is often the subject of much

attention in the popular and lay press, in current magazines, and on television. Much of this medical information fed to the public is boiled down in the interests of simplicity so that the patient often has a naive concept of the function and mechanics of ocular surgery or, even worse, a totally distorted view of it. The ophthalmic assistant should be able to intelligently handle many of the general questions regarding ophthalmic surgery and be able to relate to the patient a simple but accurate account of what is to be expected during the procedure.

Some questions and misconceptions commonly asked by patients regarding ophthalmic surgery are discussed next.

Can an eye be transplanted?

Only the cornea can be transplanted; the entire eye cannot. The cornea was one of the first structures of the body to be replaced with tissues from another body. The body was found to be able to accept a transplanted cornea because of the lack of blood vessels in this structure and the inability of the immune mechanisms of the body to reach the transplanted tissue and reject it. Every ophthalmologist experiences the necessity of having to tell a blind patient, with perhaps absolute glaucoma or retinitis pigmentosa, that the patient's blindness cannot be cured by one of the "new transplant procedures." Not every eye is suitable for a transplant.

Is the eye taken out for surgery?

The eye is never removed from its socket unless, of course, an enucleation actually was intended. Some patients think that the ophthalmologist takes the eye out, places it in some kind of vise on a workbench, completes the surgery, and then merely pops the eye back into place.

Are sutures placed in the eye?

Every time a surgeon makes a wound over 1 or 2 mm in length, the wound must be closed with sutures. In many instances, however, the sutures are composed of catgut, which dissolves by itself after the tissues have been united and thus does not require removal. Other sutures, such as the virgin-silk suture or 10-0 nylon, are so fine and nonirritating that they can be left in the eye permanently. Some sutures— especially those employed for skin closure, some forms of cataract surgery, and corneal surgery— must be removed. Suture removal for skin surgery usually is carried out 5 or 6 days after surgery, whereas corneal sutures usually are not removed before 2 to 4 weeks.

The removal of sutures from the eye is completed with use of a local anesthetic. This procedure is painless and merely requires that the patient keep the eyes still and look straight ahead. Removal of the sutures from the eye can cause serious complications to the eye if they are not removed by an expert. Needless to say, the *ophthalmic assistant should never take out ocular sutures.*

Will there be any unsightly scars on the eye after surgery?

Ophthalmic surgeons are very much aware of the cosmetic importance of the eyes and usually leave no trace of their incisions with respect to the naked eye. This is particularly true of cataract and strabismus procedures. After fistulization procedures for the treatment of glaucoma, the patient may develop a soft bulge above the cornea, but it usually is well hidden by the upper eyelid.

Will both eyes be patched after surgery?

With the exception perhaps of retinal detachment surgery, both eyes are not patched after surgery. Even after bilateral strabismus surgery, one patch usually is removed shortly so that the child will not feel blinded after the operation.

Is there a great deal of pain after ocular surgery?

The pain is minimal. It is controlled by medications freely available to the patient in the immediate postoperative period so that the patient's discomfort is comparatively insignificant.

Must the head be placed between heavy sandbags after surgery?

In the early days of ophthalmic surgery, before the development of good sutures, needles, and instruments, the wound was not apposed with sutures so that the patient's head had to be held rigid and the eyes immobilized until healing took place. Almost all patients today, with only few exceptions, are allowed up and around, with minimal restrictions, on the day after surgery.

TYPES OF ANESTHESIA

General anesthesia is used for all children's surgery, most strabismus procedures, retinal detachments, enucleations, and removal of orbital tumors. Local anesthesia often is preferred for adults undergoing other types of eye surgery, such as cataracts or glaucoma. Local anesthesia can be achieved by a combination of topical anesthetic drops instilled in the eye and infiltration anesthesia. There are four main methods of infiltration anesthesia: (1) nerve block, (2) direct infiltration subcutaneously, (3) retrobulbar anesthesia, and (4) peribulbar anesthesia.

In a *nerve block* the anesthetic is directed at the site of the emerging nerve, and the area supplied by that nerve is affected.

Direct infiltration subcutaneously facilitates surface anesthesia of the skin and paralyzes the underlying musculature. In Fig. 26-4 the purpose of the subcutaneous infiltration of the local anesthetic is to inactivate the orbicularis oculi muscle, which closes the eye. This muscle always is inactivated before intraocular surgery.

Retrobulbar anesthesia provides complete anesthesia of the globe and paralysis temporarily to the muscles attached to the globe so that unwanted eye

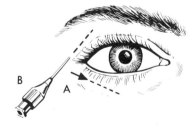

Fig. 26-4 Infiltration anesthesia. The needle is pointed under the skin along the lower eyelid (**A**) and along the upper eyelid (**B**) to anesthetize the skin and inactivate the orbicularis oculi muscle. (Modified from Berens C, King JH: *An atlas of ophthalmic surgery,* Philadelphia, 1961, JB Lippincott Co.)

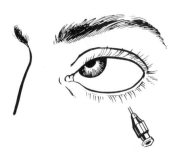

Fig. 26-5 Retrobulbar anesthesia through skin of the lower eyelid. The patient is asked to look up and away from the site of penetration of the needle. The needle penetrates into the muscle cone behind the eye to paralyze the intraocular and extraocular muscles. (Modified from Berens C, King JH: *An atlas of ophthalmic surgery,* Philadelphia, 1961, JB Lippincott Co.)

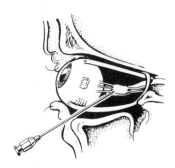

Fig. 26-7 Point of destination of the retrobulbar injection. Note the needle point is in the muscle cone and amid the delicate nerves extending toward the eye. Injection of the anesthetic at this point paralyzes the muscles of the eye. (Modified from Berens C, King JH: *An atlas of ophthalmic surgery,* Philadelphia, 1961, JB Lippincott Co.)

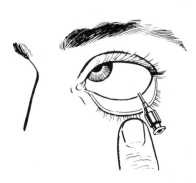

Fig. 26-6 Retrobulbar anesthesia through the conjunctiva. (Modified from Berens C, King JH: *An atlas of ophthalmic surgery,* Philadelphia, 1961, JB Lippincott Co.)

movements cannot occur during the procedure. The site of the penetration can be through either the skin (Fig. 26-5) or the conjunctiva (Fig. 26-6), the needle coursing under the globe itself and the point of the needle emerging in the muscle cone of the eye (Fig. 26-7).

Peribulbar anesthesia has gained widespread popularity as a result of an occasional compression damage to the optic nerve caused by retrobulbar injections. In peribulbar anesthesia a needle is directed down to the floor of the socket (or to the roof of the orbit) so that the anesthetic surrounds the soft tissue of the globe rather than being placed in the muscle cone itself.

QUESTIONS FOR REVIEW AND THOUGHT

1. Outline a routine to be followed in hospital booking when a patient requires surgery.
2. Discuss the psychologic handling of a child who has to enter the hospital for strabismus surgery.
3. What forewarnings should be given to the adult patient before admission for major ocular surgery?
4. Discuss various types of anesthesia for ocular surgery.
5. What are the advantages of a local anesthetic over general anesthesia for cataract surgery?
6. What types of sutures need not be removed?

SELF-EVALUATION QUESTIONS

True-false statements

Directions: Indicate whether the statement is true (T) or false (F).

T or F   1. An important factor in scheduling patients for surgery is the length of the surgical procedure.

T or F   2. An individual requests a certain date for surgery because of a forthcoming wedding in the family. This is considered an urgent booking.

T or F   3. In advanced glaucoma, corneal transplantation may offer some hope in restoring vision.

Missing words

Directions: Write in the missing word in the following sentences.

4. A lacerated globe is considered an _____ operation.

5. Children's surgery most often is performed under _____ anesthesia.

6. Anesthetic drops instilled in the eye are called _____ anesthesia.

Choice-completion questions

Directions: Select the one best answer in each case.

7. Retrobulbar anesthesia consists of placing an anesthetic agent in:
   a. The lower fornix
   b. The muscle cone behind the eye
   c. The peribulbar space
   d. The preauricular space
   e. The subcutaneous space

8. Which of the following methods is not considered local anesthesia?
   a. Infiltration anesthesia
   b. Intubation
   c. Retrobulbar
   d. Peribulbar
   e. Systemic

9. Which of the following is not required in scheduling major surgery?
   a. Phoning the patient
   b. Confirming the letter
   c. Assisting at surgery
   d. Identifying the date of surgery
   e. The time required for the operation

ANSWERS, NOTES AND EXPLANATIONS

1. **True.** Individual ophthalmic surgeons vary in the time they require for different procedures. A dacryocystorhinostomy by one surgeon may take only 1 hour whereas another surgeon may take 3 hours. Similarly, this can occur in cataract surgery. This is an important variable in determining the overall time required for the operating room.

2. **False.** An urgent booking is one in which the nature of the ocular problem requires very special consideration in getting the patient in as soon as possible. Social reasons are not considered urgent. However, accommodation often is made to provide convenient times to the individual.

3. **False.** In advanced glaucoma corneal transplantation is not indicated. Corneal transplantation is indicated only for diseases and disorders affecting the cornea. In this procedure a hazy cornea can be replaced with a clear transparent cornea from donor tissue. Because of the avascular nature of the cornea, there is a minimal amount of antibody response. This will permit the donor cornea to survive.

4. **Emergency.** Any laceration of the globe, eyelid, or adjacent area that requires surgical repair is considered an emergency admission. Although the patient may not necessarily have to stay overnight in the hospital or surgical center, the patient is admitted with proper documentation of the details of the injury. This detailed admission has medical/legal implications in case a lawsuit arises at a later date.

5. **General.** Almost all children's surgery is performed with the child under a general anesthesia. The psychologic trauma of instruments appearing close to the eye can be devastating to children. Consequently, they should be completely asleep and their eye movements controlled.

6. **Topical.** Applying drops directly to the eye is considered topical anesthesia. This can be highly effective and is used primarily in adults in combination with infiltration anesthesia.

7. **b. The muscle cone behind the eye.** By directly penetrating into the muscle cone there is an effective anesthesia of the ciliary ganglion. There has in recent years, however, been some concern about the compression of the optic nerve or the possible perforation of the globe itself.

8. **b. Intubation.** In intubation anesthesia a tube is inserted into the trachea and the patient's complete anesthesia is controlled through gaseous vapors that are absorbed in the lung.

9. **c. Assisting at surgery.** Although this is an important act, it is not part of the routine in scheduling surgery. In the scheduling of surgery, it is very important that all the details are fully understood by the patient and that there is an accuracy in both time and place for the surgery.

CHAPTER 27 Highlights of ocular surgery

- Strabismus surgery
- Cataract surgery
- Glaucoma surgery
- Retinal detachment surgery
- Vitreous surgery
- Laser surgery
- Corneal transplantation
- Eyelid surgery
- Pterygium removal
- Dacryocystorhinostomy
- Enucleation and evisceration
- Eye dressings

Many surgical procedures are performed to cure eye disorders, restore vision, prevent blindness, correct congenital abnormalities, or cosmetically improve the area in and about the eye. For each eye condition, various surgical procedures—sometimes ingenious—have been devised.

To familiarize the ophthalmic assistant with some of the highlights of ocular surgery, the most commonly performed ocular procedures are outlined in this chapter.

STRABISMUS SURGERY
Preparation

When having strabismus surgery, children may be admitted to the hospital the afternoon before the day of surgery or on the day of surgery. Often surgery is performed on an outpatient basis. The child is more comfortable at home with his or her parents at night. Unless there is some adverse medical problem such as asthma, this seems to be a safe procedure. Parents often are encouraged to remain with the chil-

dren to alleviate fears and dilute the child's feeling of abandonment. Older children are told that they may expect a bandage on one or both eyes after surgery but that at least one bandage will be removed before they are sent home.

Surgery

In strabismus surgery, the four recti muscles insert close to the limbus, the medial rectus muscle being the closest (approximately 5.5 mm, whereas the lateral rectus muscle is 7 mm). The rectus muscles would be easily visible if they were not covered with the conjunctiva and subconjunctival tissue. To isolate these muscles, the surgeon must cut through the conjunctiva and place a muscle hook under the muscle. The oblique muscles insert at the back of the globe, so that muscle surgery on these muscles is not performed at their insertions.

Muscle surgery involves weakening or strengthening of the muscles to improve the alignment of the eyes.

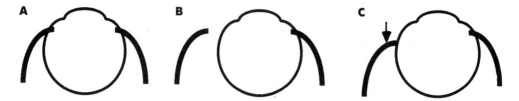

Fig. 27-1 Recession operation. **A,** Preoperative position of muscles. **B,** Muscle detached from globe. **C,** Muscle reattachment to sclera at a point further back from its original insertion. (From Stein HA, Slatt BJ, Stein RM: *Ophthalmic terminology: speller and vocabulary builder,* ed 3, St Louis, 1992, Mosby.)

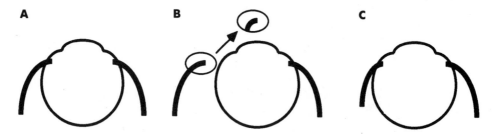

Fig. 27-2 Resection operation. **A,** Preoperative position of muscles. **B,** Muscle detached from globe and an anterior portion of muscle cut away. **C,** Muscle resutured to sclera at original insertion point. (From Stein HA, Slatt BJ, Stein RM: *Ophthalmic terminology: speller and vocabulary builder,* ed 3, St Louis, 1992, Mosby.)

The following procedures *weaken* the extraocular muscles:

1. *Recession* (Fig. 27-1). The muscle is removed from its original insertion and repositioned farther back on the sclera. This loosens the grip the muscle has on the globe.

2. *Transverse margin myotomy.* Overlapping cuts are made on each side of the muscle to lengthen it. No change is made in the insertion.

3. *Complete tenotomy.* The muscle or tendon is severed completely and allowed to retract.

The following procedures *strengthen* an extraocular muscle:

1. *Resection* (Fig. 27-2). A section of the muscle is removed from its insertion, and the muscle is reattached to its original position. A resection shortens a muscle, thereby increasing its effective tension and pull.

2. *Advancement.* This procedure usually is combined with a resection. After the resection has been completed, the muscle is repositioned ahead of, or anterior to, its original insertion. An advancement increases the arc of contact of the muscle with the globe, thereby enhancing its effective pull.

Postoperative routine

After strabismus surgery, the child usually is allowed up as soon as the effects of the anesthetic have disappeared. Normally, the child is able to resume school activities almost immediately and sports within 2 weeks. The parents are informed that the eye operated on may be red in the immediate postoperative period but that gradually the redness will fade until the eye looks normal again. In some cases, the eyes are not straight in the immediate postoperative period because of swelling, hemorrhage, and trauma to the muscles, all of which check eye movements. The parents are told of these postoperative variations so that they do not become upset if the eyes are not straight on removal of the bandages. Occasionally a child will show an allergic response to the sutures used. This is likely to occur 2 or even

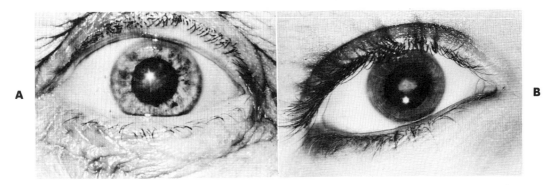

Fig. 27-3 A, Senile cataract. **B,** Posterior polar cataract.

3 weeks after surgery, during a period when recovery is virtually complete. The lids suddenly swell, the conjunctiva balloons out, and the child's eyes generally look dreadful. This is a rather innocuous event, which subsides within 3 or 4 days without causing any complications.

Questions often asked about muscle surgery include the following.

1. *Can vision be lost because of muscle surgery?* No. Because the muscles are attached on the surface of the globe, the eye itself is never opened.

2. *Are the eyes usually straight after one procedure?* Yes, in most cases. However, undercorrections and overcorrections do occur, and no ophthalmic surgeon can say with certainty which patient will require further surgery. Therefore parents generally are informed that two procedures may be necessary to straighten the eyes. With this approach, parents are not disappointed or bitter if reoperation becomes necessary, and they are extremely happy if surgery results in a complete success after the first procedure.

3. *Can muscle surgery improve the vision of an adult who has a turned eye that is amblyopic?* No. Strabismus surgery on an adult is strictly cosmetic. The turn can be corrected so that the position of the eyes appears normal, but the vision is not affected for better or worse.

4. *Can the eyes of an adult with strabismus be straightened?* Yes. Age is no barrier to a cosmetic strabismus procedure.

5. *Can the eyes be straightened with orthoptic exercises to avoid surgery?* Usually orthoptics is an adjunct to ophthalmic surgery and not a substitute for it. Strabismus may be corrected with the use of glasses, eye drops, or orthoptic exercises in some selected patients. Where possible, nonsurgical methods are employed first and, in small degrees of strabismus, may result in a correction.

CATARACT SURGERY

A cataract is an opacity of the lens of the eye (Figs. 27-3 and 27-4). The opacity may be minimal in size and faint in density so that the transmission of light is not appreciably affected, or it may be large and opaque so that light cannot gain entry into the interior of the eye. When the cataract is pronounced, the examiner cannot see the interior of the patient's eye with any clarity, and conversely the patient cannot see the examiner very clearly.

A cataract is removed if it endangers the health of the eye or interferes with the patient's ability to function. No visual level can be identified on the Snellen chart because contrast sensitivity, glare, pupillary constriction, and ambient lighting may significantly affect a person's functioning ability, even with an early cataract.

Preoperative evaluation

The cataract, when it becomes mature, obscures all details of the fundus. When this occurs, efforts should be made to evaluate the health of the interior

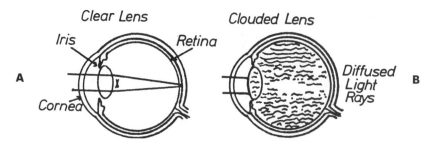

Fig. 27-4 A, Normal eye, clear lens. **B,** Eye with cataract.

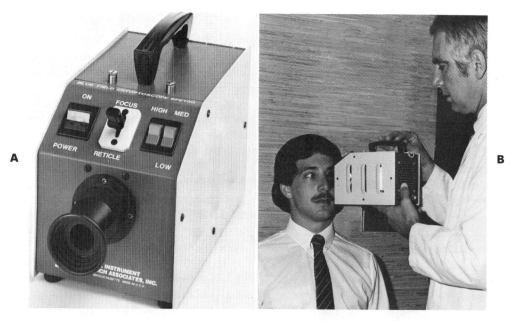

Fig. 27-5 A, Blue field entoptoscope. **B,** Blue field entoptoscope in use.

of the eye before cataract surgery. This evaluation has important prognostic importance. It can be performed by the following methods:

1. *Two-point light discrimination test.* Two lights are held a measured distance (60 cm) from the affected eye—the fellow eye being firmly covered—and are gradually separated until they can be identified as two lights. These measurements are recorded. The normal separable amount that two lights can be identified will vary with the preoperative acu-

ity. For visions reduced to hand movements, the lights should be identified about 12.5 cm apart. For visions better than 20/400, they should be identified about 5 cm apart.

2. *Light projection in all quadrants.* An assessment of active sensory retina in all quadrants should be performed by asking the patient to determine the position of a small transilluminator light.

3. *Ultrasound.* Ultrasound, or high-frequency waves, passes through the dense cataract and iden-

tifies any interference between the lens and the retina by rebounding off any firm obstruction. Abnormalities in the ultrasonogram can confirm the presence of a tumor mass, hemorrhage, or detached retina behind the lens. The B-scan is the main method of evaluating the area behind the lens. However, A-scan measurements may detect defects in the central pathway.

4. *Blue field entoptoscope* (Fig. 27-5). This device permits the patient to observe his or her own white blood cells flowing in the retinal capillaries in the macular area. This flow is visible even with a dense cataract. This entopic phenomenon is created by an intense blue light that the patient views. With normal retinal function the patient will describe "flying corpuscles" moving in the entire field. If the macula is not functioning, no flying corpuscles will be seen.

This phenomenon occurs because the blue light is strongly absorbed by the hemoglobin and red blood cells, which results in the photoreceptors behind the capillaries becoming relatively dark-adapted. When a white blood cell moves through the capillary, the blue light passes through it and excites the photoreceptors behind it. Thus the passage of a leukocyte is perceived as a moving bright dot or a "flying corpuscle." The intensity of the blue light can be adjusted so that sufficient light reaches the retina in cases of media opacities.

Abnormalities in perception of the corpuscles are the result of changes in the perifoveal circulation or functional impairment of the neural elements in the retina, or both. Differentiation between the two is possible in conjunction with other tests such as those based on fluorescein angiography and electrophysiology.

Abnormal entoptoscopic findings include one or more of the following:

- Total or partial absence of corpuscle perception in one or both eyes
- Absence of pulsatile motion
- Fewer corpuscles in one eye
- Lower corpuscle speed in one eye

Clinical experience with cataract patients has shown that a positive response to the blue field entoptic test indicates a 98% probability of good postoperative macular function (visual acuity 20/40 or better). The test is especially useful when a direct view of the fundus is obscured in cases of corneal edema or scarring; hyphema; cataract; and vitreous hemorrhage, membranes, or exudates.

5. *Brightness acuity tester (BAT)*. This instrument, devised by Dr. Jack Halliday, can determine a significant visual loss attributed to a bright light's creating a small pupil and glare. The excess light is the normal light that a person may experience when outdoors in bright sunshine. An individual with a small central cataract may be seriously affected in driving and participating in sports when the pupil contracts.

Another important aspect of evaluation is to determine the required dioptric power of the intraocular lens to be chosen. A-scan measurements are used to determine the axial length of the eye. By use of the keratometric values of the cornea and an A-scan constant value for specific lenses, the exact dioptric power required for an intraocular lens can be determined (Figs. 27-6 and 27-7).

6. *Prediction of potential acuities*. Interferometers and potential acuity meters (PAM) are used in office tests to predict potential acuities in patients with cataracts and those with hazy posterior capsules after cataract extractions. This allows realistic expectations on the part of the surgeon and patient before cataract surgery or a neodymium YAG posterior capsulotomy. The interferometers pass two beams of laser light through the pupil, producing a three-dimensional interference pattern within the retina. This allows the ophthalmologist to bypass problems with most opacities of the media, as well as refractive errors. If the patient can see the interference pattern, which will appear as bands in a specific direction, this is evidence of macular function. The narrower the bands that are projected and seen, the higher the degree of macular function.

The potential acuity meter is basically a pinpoint light source, a transilluminated visual acuity chart, and a lens (Fig. 27-8). It projects a brightly illuminated Snellen acuity chart through an area approximately 0.15 mm in diameter. It can be used to test approximate acuities through mildly dense media because of the brightness of the stimulus and the

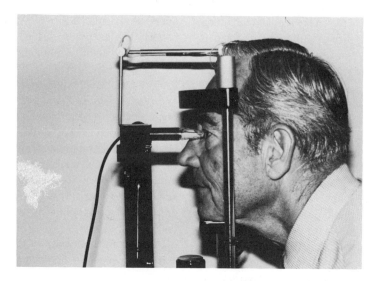

Fig. 27-6 A-scan measurement used to determine the axial length and the power required for an intraocular lens.

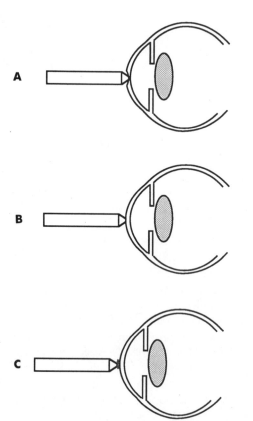

Fig. 27-7 Errors in A-scan measurements. **A,** Too much pressure with probe indents cornea and may cause excessive shallowness of the anterior chamber and a shorter axial length. **B,** Correct pressure. **C,** Too little pressure may leave a thick tear layer between the probe and cornea, resulting in a longer axial length.

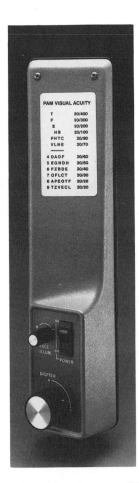

Fig. 27-8 The potential acuity meter (PAM) is attached to the slit lamp.

tiny diameter of the beam being used for the examination.

In the clinical application of these tests, the following guidelines should be used.

a. Do not shine lights into the patient's eyes before testing, because this may decrease the acuity readings.

b. Have the pupil well dilated.

c. PAM testing: Drop chin rest to enable patient to talk without moving the head so that the acuity chart will remain visible to the patient.

d. Interferometer testing: Stress that "background noise" will be seen (swirls of light, dots, wavy lines, half lines) but that the patient should ignore these and indicate only the direction of the lines of light seen.

e. Focus the beam in the center of the pupil at the plane of the iris; then scan the pupil until best responses are obtained.

f. With the interferometers, first use horizontal and vertical bands until the best acuity has been reached and then use oblique lines to verify this.

g. With the PAM, start with large letters and ask the patient to read only the first two or three letters in each line. If at any time two or more letters are identified in a given line, that line, if it is the smallest read, is the end point even though the patient may not be able to detect that line again.

h. Never tell patients they should see letters or lines, because this tends to upset the patient. Simply ask, "What do you see?" If they see letters, they will say so. With the interferometer, ask "What do you see?" If they begin to see something, ask if there are any lines as you make them larger and larger until they see them.

7. *Endothelial cell function.* Although specular microscopic examination is the standard method of evaluating the functioning reserve of the endothelial cells, the use of slit-lamp biomicroscopy can aid the clinical observation. With use of a 16x objective lens in the slit lamp and careful positioning of the slit light, the endothelial mosaic may be viewed. By use of the Endo lens designed by Tomey Corporation, the image may be enhanced 22x. The image may be compared with a grid (Fig. 27-9) that can be placed in the objective lens assembly.

Preparation

Each patient should be seen by the family physician at least 1 week before cataract surgery to ensure that medical conditions such as diabetes and hypertension are under control. Also, the ophthalmic surgeon should be provided with the names and dosages of the medications the patient may be taking.

Patients should be instructed to wash their hair before entering the hospital because hair washing is avoided during the first few postoperative days to prevent contamination of the wound by dirty rinse

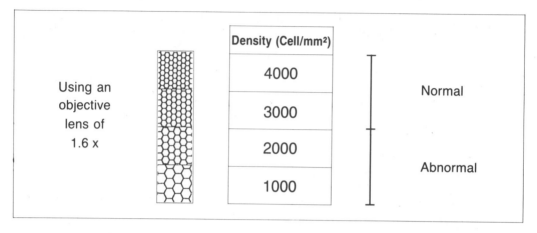

Using an objective lens of 1.6 x		Density (Cell/mm²)	
		4000	Normal
		3000	
		2000	Abnormal
		1000	

Fig. 27-9 The slit lamp may be used for evaluation of cell density.

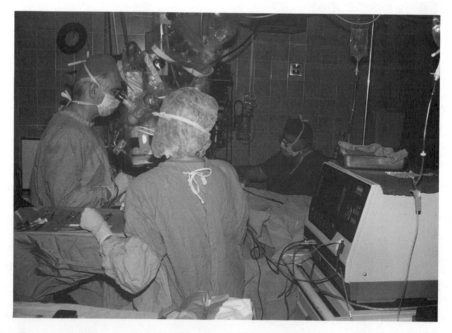

Fig. 27-10 The operating microscope provides magnification during surgery. The automated machine at the right provides phacoemulsification, irrigation, and aspiration of the nucleus and cortex of the lens.

water. Smoking, of course, should be discouraged inasmuch as a heavy cough can easily disrupt a fresh wound or initiate bleeding. Because aspirin may cause bleeding, it should be eliminated at least 1 week before surgery.

Surgery

The object of cataract surgery is to remove the crystalline lens of the eye that has become cloudy. This usually is performed under an operating microscope that permits magnification (Fig. 27-10).

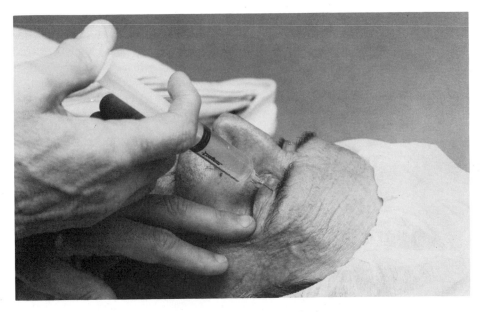

Fig. 27-11 Peribulbar anesthesia.

Fig. 27-12 Honan intraocular pressure reducer.

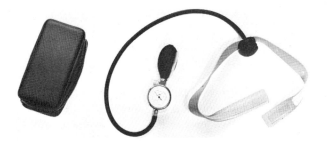

The three methods used for cataract surgery are the extracapsular procedure, the intracapsular procedure, and phacoemulsification. The extracapsular procedure is protected by the majority of the world's ophthalmologists at the time of this writing. Intracapsular surgery is rarely performed except for dislocated lenses. Of increasing importance is phacoemulsification, particularly in the posterior chamber. The latter advantage results from the retention of the posterior capsule of the lens, impeding unwanted ultraviolet light and maintaining the vitreous space intact and thus eliminating vitreous turbulence. It is small-incision surgery, with the incision size reduced from 10 mm for extracapsular surgery to 4 to 5 mm for phacoemulsification. Often only one stitch or no

stitches are required in the latter procedure, which results in minimal astigmatism and rapid recovery. Most surgeons today are performing cataract surgery in freestanding surgical centers on an outpatient basis. (See Chapter 30.)

Extracapsular cataract surgery. Before surgery, the skin around the eyelids is prepared with an antiseptic, usually iodine-based. The eye is irrigated free of debris and normal bacterial flora. A topical anesthetic may be used, along with either a retrobulbar anesthetic or a peribulbar anesthetic (Fig. 27-11). Facial nerve paralysis may be produced by an O'Brien, Van Lint, or Nadblath anesthetic. The Honan intraocular pressure reducer (Fig. 27-12) or the superpinky ball, championed by Dr. James Gills,

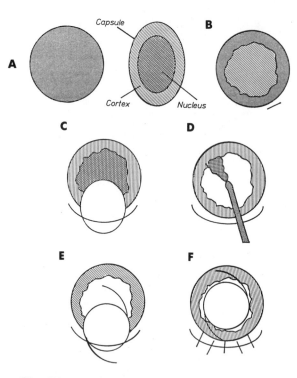

Fig. 27-13 Extracapsular cataract extraction. **A,** Cataract. **B,** Can-opener capsulotomy. **C,** Removal of nucleus. **D,** Cortex aspiration and enlargement of incision. **E,** Insertion of intraocular lens. **F,** Wound closure.

significantly lowers the intraocular pressure before surgery. Hand massage also may be used, but one should guard against excessive massage because of the possibility of central retinal artery or vein obstruction.

An incision is made at the superior limbus and a small opening is made into the anterior chamber. A viscoelastic substance is introduced. A small bent needle or cystotome is introduced, and a cut is made

into the anterior capsule in a circular can-opener, triangular, or D-shaped fashion (anterior capsulotomy) (Fig. 27-13). The wound is enlarged in extracapsular surgery to a chord diameter of 10 to 11 mm (approximately a 150-degree arc) to allow removal of the cataractous nucleus.

The nucleus is then expressed or looped out of the eye. Sutures are inserted to maintain the anterior chamber so that the remaining cortex can be removed. The cortex may be removed by a manual method (for example, Simcoe or McIntyre needle) or by an automated system. There are many automated systems on the market. These are sometimes referred to as *I/A units* (irrigating/aspirating units). These instruments irrigate balanced salt into the eye in proportion to the amount of aspiration that is occurring. The automated systems are foot-controlled.

Once all of the cortex is removed from the capsular bag, the posterior capsule may be "polished" to remove any residual plaques. An intraocular lens is then inserted into the posterior chamber. This lens may be positioned either into the capsular bag (Fig. 27-14, *A*) or into the sulcus (Fig. 27-14, *B*). The former site is preferred.

To prevent the complication of pupillary block glaucoma from occurring, a peripheral iridectomy or iridotomy may be performed to ensure the flow of aqueous fluid from the posterior chamber to the anterior chamber. Some surgeons prefer to omit an iridectomy.

Sutures are then placed in the cornea or corneoscleral wound. These may be radial interrupted sutures, a continuous suture, or a combination of the two (Fig. 27-15). At the end of the procedure, an antibiotic or antibiotic-steroid combination injection may be given subconjunctivally. (See box.)

This operation has become almost obsolete for

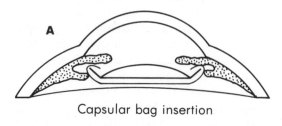

Capsular bag insertion

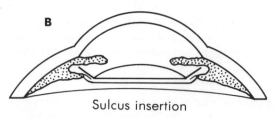

Sulcus insertion

Fig. 27-14 Posterior chamber intraocular lens. **A,** Capsular bag insertion. **B,** Sulcus insertion.

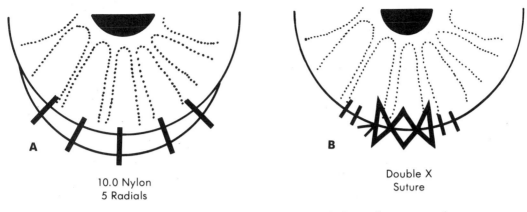

**10.0 Nylon
5 Radials**

**Double X
Suture**

Fig. 27-15 Each surgeon has a preferred method of wound closure for extracapsular surgery. **A,** Radial sutures. **B,** Combination radial sutures and double-x sutures.

EXTRACAPSULAR SURGERY
STEP BY STEP

1. Draping and speculum insertion
2. Bridle suture for superior rectus
3. Conjunctival incision
4. Cauterization of bleeders
5. Scleral or corneoscleral incision
6. Viscoelastic substance introduced
7. Capsulotomy or capsulorrhexis
8. Nucleus expression
9. Cortical cleanup
10. Intraocular lens (IOL) insertion
11. Suture placement
12. Conjunctival reapproximation
13. Injections—subconjunctival
14. Instillation of medication and patching of the eye

PHACOEMULSIFICATION

ADVANTAGES	**DISADVANTAGES**
Small incision	Machine-dependent
Less wound problems	Longer learning period
Less astigmatism	Complications while
More rapid physical reha-	learning
bilitation	Expensive equipment
Less risk of expulsive hem-	Difficult with hard nucleus
orrhage	Need good pupil dilation

---

routine cataracts except for cases of dislocated or partially dislocated lenses. The essential difference between intracapsular surgery and extracapsular surgery is that in intracapsular surgery the entire lens and capsule are removed from the eye, while in the latter, the posterior capsule remains intact, permitting a pocket for an intraocular lens. This usually is performed with a cryoprobe, which forms an iceball on the lens and facilitates removal. If a cryoprobe is unavailable, a capsular forceps may be used.

Phacoemulsification. In 1963 Dr. Charles Kelman commenced research to ascertain the possibility of removing a cataract through a small incision. After attempting many preliminary techniques, including crushing the lens, cutting the lens, and drilling it, he finally perfected an apparatus and tip that he used to apply oscillating and ultrasonic frequency to emulsify the cataract. He was attempting to improve on the system of cataract surgery by freezing with a cryoprobe or by using a capsule forceps. A major flaw of these two methods, however, was that they required an incision of almost 180 degrees at the limbus to facilitate the lens removal. With the phacoemulsifier, a tiny incision of only 1.5 mm is required. This means less tissue destruction, less wound reaction, less chance of wound disruption and its attendant complications, less astigmatism, and earlier ambulation. (See box.) In most cases, the

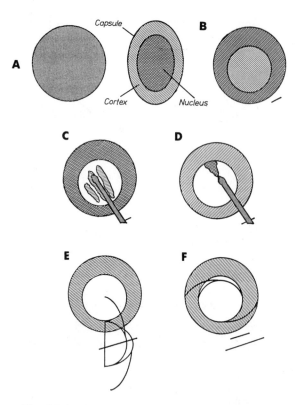

Fig. 27-16 Phacoemulsifaction. **A,** Cataract. **B,** Small incision and capsulorhexis. **C,** Phacoemulsification of lens. **D,** Cortex aspiration. **E,** Insertion of folded lens. **F,** Rotation of lens in capsule.

patient is able to resume normal activities immediately after the operation.

The technique involves making a small opening in the limbus and introducing a cystotome to cut a large opening in the anterior capsule of the lens (Fig. 27-16). The lens mass is then prolapsed into the anterior chamber through a widely dilated pupil; the emulsifier with aspirator is put in place; and the lens is removed over a 1- to 3-minute period. The small incision is closed with a single suture or even no suture at all. Special wound construction is required to perform this type of small-stitch incision. The induced astigmatism is minimal, and the limbus area superiorly is quite smooth because very little of it has been disturbed by the procedure.

There has been a rebirth of interest in phacoemulsification because of the minimal amount of

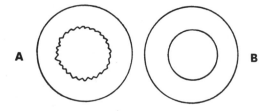

Fig. 27-17 A, Can-opener capsulotomy. **B,** Continuous curve capsulorhexis.

astigmatism, the minimal disability, and the immediate return of function. This interest has been furthered by the development of soft implant and small phacointraocular lenses that are now available. These can be inserted through a very small wound with only a very slight enlargement to 4 mm. Clever injectors and folders have been designed that aid the surgeon in the placement of these lenses. The techniques and variations of insertion devices are beyond the scope of this text.

Until recently the opening into the anterior capsule was made with a capsulotomy needle by a series of jagged punctures that converted the central capsule into a series of postage-stamp cuttings. Currently, for phacoemulsification a continuous tear opening, often called *continuous curve capsulorhexis* (CCC), is made by tearing the capsule so that the edges remain sharp, well-demarcated, and very strong. This prevents extension into the periphery of tears of the capsule and permits the capsule to hold the lens implant securely (Fig. 27-17).

Sutures. The sutureless, or one-suture, closure has resulted in more rapid rehabilitation after cataract surgery. The basic principle of sutureless incision is the creation of a valvelike self-sealing wound that is relatively small. The valve permits the incision to withstand unusual stress or intermittent raised intraocular pressure that may follow in the postoperative period. Various shapes of design (Fig. 27-18) have been advocated that lessen the degree of induced astigmatism. These include variations of straight incisions or a curvilinear incision, which is sometimes labeled the "frown and smile" incision. These styles are outlined in Fig. 27-19.

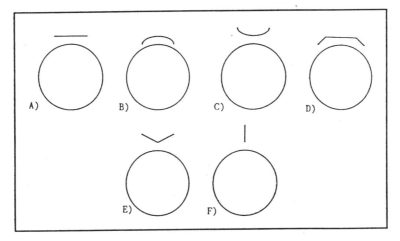

Fig. 27-18 Incision variations, including the "frown" and "smile."

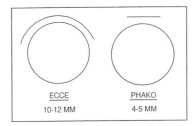

Fig. 27-19 A, Incision used for extracapsular surgery. **B,** Incision used for phacoemulsification.

Postoperative care

The patient, who is usually ambulatory right away, may be warned, however, to avoid bending, stooping, lifting, straining, or sleeping on the side of the operated eye. If the patient lives alone or has no assistance, arrangements may be made for someone to do such household chores as cooking and cleaning.

While convalescing, the patient is more comfortable wearing dark glasses with ultraviolet protection. Protection in the form of a metal or plastic eye shield need be worn to shield the eye from the patient's own hands only during periods of sleep. Reading, watching television, and walking are not restricted. There are no dietary limitations.

Usually it is safe for a patient to return to work soon after surgery depending on occupational requirements and the need to use the operated eye for visual function.

The ophthalmic assistant should always keep in mind the patient's dependency after cataract surgery. Such a patient is handicapped because of a cataract in one eye and a fresh wound in the other. Fears increase in the postoperative period, and the person is frightened of doing anything that might jar the eye. The inability to see, however, prevents the person from taking precautions to avoid bumping into things. The postoperative patient should be given every consideration. In the ophthalmologist's office, the patient should be helped off and on with his or her coat, assisted in and out of the examining chair, and given explicit verbal and written instructions about repeat visits and the time and methods of instilling medication into the eye.

Intraocular lenses

One of the major problems after cataract surgery has been the use of aphakic spectacles. Elderly patients have to bear the attendant magnifications and distortions by spectacles to replace their own lens that has now been removed (Fig. 27-20). A search for a better solution has been directed in two main areas. One is the use of contact lenses, especially those

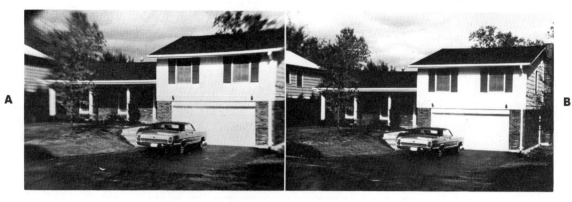

Fig. 27-20 A, Aphakic spectacles produce peripheral distortion. **B,** The same picture as it would be seen by a patient with successful cataract and lens implant operation. (Courtesy Mr. Kenneth Swanson.)

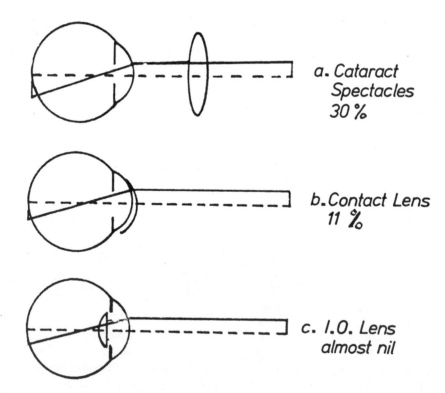

Fig. 27-21 Magnification induced by aphakic spectacles, contact lenses, and intraocular lenses.

that can be worn overnight to avoid the handling difficulties of insertion and removal, which are a constant hazard to the insecure elderly aphakic patient. The other solution has been in the direction of intraocular lens implants, which Ridley introduced in 1949. Today, through the pioneering efforts of Cornelium Binkhorst of Holland, Peter Choyce of England, and Edward Epstein of South Africa, the intraocular lens has become the major form of visual rehabilitation after cataract surgery. With the use of Healon (sodium hyaluronate) and other viscoelastic substances, endothelial damage is minimized during implant surgery. Magnification induced by spectacles and contact lenses has been reduced to zero with intraocular lenses (Fig. 27-21).

Present-day success of intraocular lenses is due to more skillful microsurgery, as well as better design, finish, and fixation of the lenses. In addition, a better understanding of positioning of the lenses within the capsular bag, the use of the YAG laser for capsular opacification, and the better management and minimization of complications have led to significant success with intraocular lenses. Their use is indicated in virtually all patients undergoing cataract surgery.

Lens materials and design. Intraocular lenses are composed of an optical portion called the "optics" of the lens and the "haptics" (Fig. 27-22). The optics portion has a dioptric power that permits the focusing of light onto the retina. The "size" of the optics varies from 5 to 7 mm in diameter. The term *haptics* is from the Greek word *haptesthai* meaning "to lay hold of." The haptics refers to the method of holding the optical portion in place in the human eye. The haptics consist of loops that are made of either polymethylmethacrylate or prolene. Polymethylmethacrylate is noteworthy as a hard, firm, inert material that has been singled out for the manufacture of quality intraocular lens optics that are inert in the human body. Loops made of this material are commonly used instead of prolene. Prolene is a suture material that is also relatively inert in the human body and provides a softness and pliability that permit its support of the optical portion of the lens. Tantalum and metal loops have disappeared in the manufacture of intraocular lenses because of the adverse reaction

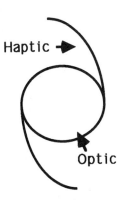

Fig. 27-22 Intraocular lenses. (From Stein HA, Slatt BJ, Stein RM: *A primer in ophthalmology: a textbook for students,* St Louis, 1992, Mosby.)

they produce on the human retina. Loop designs are now made more flexible to permit greater adjustments within the structure of the eye itself to variations of the ocular changes that occur with each blink and contraction of the rectus muscles. This in itself has been a major step forward in the design of intraocular lenses.

The shape of the optical portion may be *planoconvex*, in which case the anterior portion of the lens is *convex*, whereas the back surface is flat. They may have reverse optics, in which the back surface of the lens is convex and the front surface is flat. They also may be *biconvex*, in which both sides of the optical portion are convex. Some lenses are made *aspheric*, in which there is an alteration in power from the center of the lens to the periphery.

Designs incorporate an ultraviolet filter into the optical portion of the lens. This eliminates wavelengths in the ultraviolet spectrum below 400 nm. Some designs also incorporate a *laser ridge*. This is a ridge placed on the back surface of the lens to minimize damage to the lens that may occur when the neodymium-YAG laser is used to open a posterior capsular membrane.

Optical portions may have fenestrations, in which one or more small openings are made in the lens periphery to facilitate the technical movement of the lens within the eye.

The power of the intraocular lenses varies from

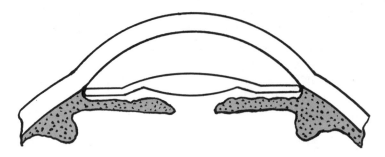

Fig. 27-23 Anterior chamber, angle-fixated intraocular lens.

Fig. 27-24 Posterior chamber intraocular lens placed in the ciliary sulcus.

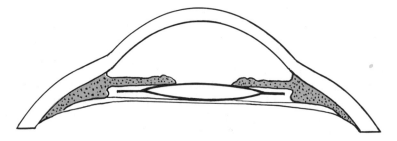

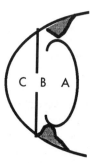

Fig. 27-25 Most common positions of intraocular lenses. **A,** Capsular bag. **B,** Ciliary sulcus. **C,** Anterior chamber. (From Stein HA, Slatt BJ, Stein RM: *A primer in ophthalmology: a textbook for students,* St Louis, 1992, Mosby.)

eye to eye. The use of A-scan or biometry with ultrasound allows the examiner to measure the axial length of the human eye and to determine exactly the required power of the implant. The more common powers are about +18.00 to +20.00 diopters, but lenses are available for any power.

Intraocular lenses may be classified according to their position and their method of fixation. Anterior chamber lenses (Fig. 27-23) include lenses that lie in the anterior chamber of the eye. These may be angle-supported, in which case they are supported in the angle of the anterior chamber, or they may be iris-supported, in which case they may be attached with or without sutures to the iris. These lenses are fast becoming obsolete. Lenses may lie in the posterior chamber, and they may be supported by capsular support, in which case they may be called *in-the-bag lenses* because they are fitted directly into the capsular bag that contained the former crystalline lens, or they may be sulcus-supported (Fig. 27-24), in which case they lie in front of the remainder of the anterior capsule and are supported in the sulcus of the eye (Fig. 27-25).

New developments in soft implants composed of silicone and hydrogels have heralded a new generation of implants, which may be folded and inserted into a much smaller incision. The development of endocapsular surgery with lens placement into the capsular bag has now become state of the art.

Multifocal lenses (bifocal intraocular lenses) are another attempt to replace the human crystalline lens with an exact duplicate in function. Bifocal intraocular lenses, which are sometimes referred to as *multifocal intraocular* lenses because they focus at many distances, have been introduced to try to eliminate spectacles entirely for the patient who has had a cataract removed. The advantage of multifocal lenses is simply that the patient does not require spectacles for most activities. Spectacles are not effective if an uninduced astigmatism follows surgery. In addition, even at best a decrease in contrast sensitivity often occurs.

A current design is the diffractive lens by 3M (similar to the Echelon contact lens bifocal). Data show that 65% of patients obtain functional vision for both distance and near with this implant, whereas most of the others first require glasses for either distance or near. Another bifocal lens is the True Vista bifocal manufactured by Storz. It has a central distance zone (1.5 mm wide), a peripheral near zone (2.6 mm wide), and an outer distance zone. The lens is pupillary-dependent as compared with the 3M lens which is pupillary-independent. Thus a dilated or constricted pupil may have a negative effect on the functional results of this intraocular lens. The aspheric intraocular lens also is available as a multifocal lens.

Patient selection and expectations are critical to the acceptance of multifocal lenses. In addition, exact biometric readings and exact placement centrally and in the bag are critical for success. Low induced astigmatism error also is critical.

Early complications after cataract surgery

Hyphema. If blood is present in the eye when the first postoperative dressing is changed, the surgeon should be notified.

Raised intraocular pressure. This may occur within the first 24 to 48 hours as a result of the blockage of outflow chambers by the viscoelastic substance used at surgery. Pressure also may rise because of the trauma of surgery. Pain and corneal edema are common features of raised intraocular pressure.

Corneal edema. This appears as a central clouding of the cornea. It may result from trauma at surgery or from high postoperative pressure in the eye.

Shallow anterior chamber. This temporary condition may be due to inhibition of aqueous production by acetazolamide (Diamox) or beta-blocker drops. It must be observed carefully because pupillary-block glaucoma may occur.

The endothelial cells (innermost layer of the cornea) function to keep the cornea transparent by maintaining it in a state of relative dehydration by means of turgescence, that is, pumping water constantly out of it. With anterior chamber lenses, even the slight touch of endothelial cells by an intraocular lens causes the cells to be stripped off the cornea. The risk of endothelial cell damage by a touch can be reduced by the use of Healon before lens insertion.

Flat anterior chamber. The surgeon must be notified of this problem *immediately*. Allowing corneal endothelial touch to occur can result in permanent corneal decompensation. See the preceding discussion of shallow anterior chamber.

The postoperative loss of the anterior chamber may result from any of the following events:

1. Leaking wound diagnosed by Seidel test, that is, observing the escaping aqueous wash away fluorescein from the leak in the wound. The wound requires resuturing.
2. Inhibition of aqueous secretion in the treatment of glaucoma by acetazolamide and timolol drops.
3. Postoperative ocular trauma. Patients should wear protective shields while asleep.
4. Pupillary block (raised intraocular pressure). Treat by immediate dilation and/or peripheral iridectomy.

Iritis. In its mildest form, iritis may manifest as broad, thin, gray or brown deposits on the intraocular lens precipitates, sometimes with cells in the anterior chamber, or aqueous flare. The goal of treatment of iritis is to prevent synechiae (adhesions of the iris) to the vitreous face or implant feet, inasmuch as they may be the precursors of retrolenticular membrane formation and glaucoma.

It is advisable to use mydriatic agents to promote

gentle dilation and pupillary motion. However, with iris-fixed lenses this is not possible because pupil dilation tends to cause dislocation of the lens. Therapy therefore depends more on topical steroids (such as prednisone or cortisone drops) to control the inflammation.

Retinal detachment. This occurs more frequently after cataract surgery and YAG laser treatment. A sudden loss of full or half vision is an important symptom.

Cystoid macula edema (CME). This condition can be defined as an extracellular, intraretinal edema at the macula, which may be demonstrated by fluorescein angiography. Clinically the patient manifests a reduction in visual acuity that may disappear over a period of time with restoration of vision.

Extracapsular extraction of the lens seems to result in a lower incidence of CME and retinal detachment than the intracapsular procedure. Loss of vitreous and bright sunshine can be contributing factors.

Questions often asked about cataract surgery

1. *Is a cataract a film that grows over the eye?* No. It is not a growth of any kind. It is a haziness that occurs in the lens of the eye and interferes with sight.

2. *Can cataracts grow back once removed?* No. However, secondary membranes may form from opacities in the posterior capsule or from Elschnig's pearls that appear.

3. *If the cataract is removed completely, does this guarantee sight?* No. The recovery of vision depends on two factors: the provision of clear optic media and the integrity of the retina and macula. Because the surgeon often cannot see the fundus preoperatively, recovery of vision cannot be guaranteed despite a superb surgical result. If the patient's macula has been damaged, a successful cataract extraction will improve side vision only and not central vision.

4. *Does a cataract have to be "ripe" before it is removed?* No. In the early days of cataract surgery a completely opaque, or mature, lens was easier to deliver, and therefore surgery often was delayed until the lens became mature. The patient often thought

of the cataract as a fruit that had to ripen before it could be picked. In addition, physicians were reluctant to operate on one eye in cataract patients because of the troublesome double vision that could develop if the other eye was normal.

With the surgical techniques available today, any cataracts can be removed. The disability of the patient, rather than the maturity of the lens, has become the prime consideration regarding a decision for lens extraction.

5. *How important is ultraviolet (UV) light?* Ultraviolet light can be classified as follows:
- UVA contains wavelengths from 400 to 320 nm.
- UVB contains wavelengths from 320 to 280 nm.
- UVC contains wavelengths from 280 nm.

The ozone layer of the atmosphere absorbs all UVC from the sun. However, other sources of UVC include welding arcs and germicidal lamps. Of the total solar radiation that reaches the Earth about 90% is UVA and 10% is UVB.

Ultraviolet light varies with the season, being greatest in summer and near the equator. It is also more intense at high noon and in high mountains. Fresh snow reflects about 68% of the incident light whereas sandy beaches reflect about 15% and water reflects about 5% of the incident light. Some laboratory experiments have shown that ultraviolet light can damage human tissues. The details may take many years to unfold and often are difficult to prove. Ultraviolet light has been implicated in both cataract production and macular degeneration. Study results are inconclusive at present.

Ultraviolet filters can be incorporated into intraocular lenses. When a cataract is removed, the ultraviolet filtering mechanism is removed; thus an ultraviolet filter in the intraocular lens is valuable.

GLAUCOMA SURGERY

The glaucoma procedure most often performed is called an *iridectomy*. In this operation a small incision is made either directly through the cornea at the upper limbus or under a flap of conjunctival tissue. The iris is grasped with a small forceps and pulled out of the eye and partially excised. The excision of the iris may involve a sector down to the

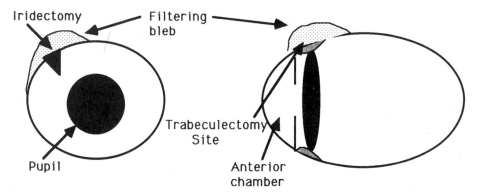

Fig. 27-26 Filtering procedure. Aqueous fluid flows from anterior chamber through opening in sclera (trabeculectomy site) to subconjunctival space where a filtering bleb is formed. (From Stein HA, Slatt BJ, Stein RM: *Ophthalmic terminology: speller and vocabulary builder,* ed 3, St Louis, 1992, Mosby.)

pupillary area *(sector iridectomy)* or only a peripheral area near the root of the iris *(peripheral iridectomy).* The cornea is sutured and the eye bandaged.

At this time, a *trabeculectomy* is the most popular glaucoma operation. In this procedure a small portion of the trabecular meshwork is surgically removed, permitting the aqueous to filter out of the anterior chamber (Fig. 27-26).

Laser trabeculoplasty has become a principal strategy to reduce intraocular pressure on a permanent basis. This is a procedure in which the argon laser is used to produce mild burns in the trabecular meshwork, causing mild shrinkage of the trabeculum, which in turn opens up the interspaces in the meshwork. This permits an increased outflow of aqueous from the anterior chamber. It is useful for mild rises of pressure in open-angle glaucoma in which peripheral synechiae are absent or minimal, with a good exposure of the trabecular meshwork.

The holium laser is rapidly becoming of interest in the management of glaucoma. This technique produces subconjunctival filtration and offers great hope in the management of glaucoma.

In some cases a *sclerectomy* may be performed. This procedure is similar to an iridectomy except that an additional small button of the sclera is removed, usually at the superior junction of the cornea and sclera. The scleral button may be removed with

scissors or by a small punch. The sclerectomy provides for a permanent drainage of aqueous fluid from the anterior chamber of the eye to an area underlying the conjunctiva.

Another glaucoma operation, called an *iridencleisis,* is a filtration procedure. A flap of conjunctiva is elevated, and the anterior chamber is entered with a superblade knife. The iris is then grasped with forceps, and a segment is cut with scissors. One portion of the cut iris is allowed to fall back into the eye, while the other portion is drawn into the incision and left there to act as a wick to maintain permanent filtration from the anterior chamber to an area under the conjunctiva.

Occasionally, glaucoma is seen at birth or in infancy (congenital glaucoma). A procedure that requires a small gonioknife has been devised for this condition. The gonioknife is passed across the limbus of one eye to the opposite area, and a sweep is made to open the angle of the opposite portion of the eye *(goniotomy).* In some cases the knife is passed under the opposing conjunctiva as well, which allows fluid to pass through this channel *(goniopuncture).*

RETINAL DETACHMENT SURGERY

When looking in the normal eye with an ophthalmoscope, the examiner can see the retina lying

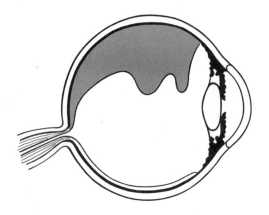

Fig. 27-27 Retinal detachment superiorly.

against the choroidal layer, from which it receives part of its blood supply and nourishment. Normally the retina is loosely attached to the choroid, but when it becomes separated from the choroid, it flaps loosely within the vitreous fluid of the eye (Fig. 27-27). Naturally, retinal detachment leads to poor nutrition and function of the retina and eventually to loss of vision. Many things predispose to retinal detachments, such as injury, myopia, and previous surgery. Often there is a tear or hole present that permits fluid to collect under the retina. This is called a *rhegmatogenous retinal detachment* (Fig. 27-28).

Correction of a retinal detachment is accomplished either by bringing the retina back to the choroid or by pushing the choroid up to the retina. To bring the retina back to the choroid, scleral punctures are made in attempts to surgically drain some of the fluid that

lies between the retina and the choroid. If the retina is lying against the choroid at this stage, either electrocoagulation or cryotherapy with a cold probe against the sclera will unite the retina to the choroid. The choroid and retina are brought together by placing a buckling band of silicone on the overlying sclera and choroid, which exerts inward pressure. If the retina is not attached at this stage, air, special gases, or oil may be injected into the vitreous to push the retina back against the choroid.

In retinal detachment surgery, cryotherapy is useful because it can create a firm adhesion of the tissues so that retinal breaks and holes can be sealed. Before the development of cryotherapy, retinal surgeons used diathermy, which created a firm bond in the retinal tissues by heat coagulation. Cold treatment was found superior to heat treatment because it did not damage large blood vessels, with the attendant risk of thrombosis or hemorrhage in these vessels. Also, the cold seal was effected without damaging other tissues, such as the sclera. With diathermy the sclera had to be moved aside surgically before the diathermy current could be applied. In many instances cryotherapy has reduced the need for implants and buckles, which may give rise to infection and may even extrude at a late postoperative date. Cryotherapy has not rendered obsolete other methods of treatment for retinal disease but has merely added to the surgeon's versatility in approaching the general problem. Retinal surgery has always been difficult, but now the ophthalmic surgeon has a number of tools in the handling of this problem.

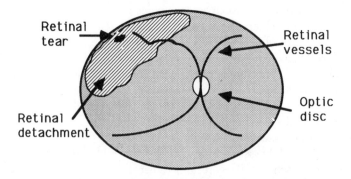

Fig. 27-28 Rhegmatogenous retinal detachment with associated retinal tear. (From Stein HA, Slatt BJ, Stein RM: *A primer in ophthalmology: a textbook for students,* St Louis, 1992, Mosby.)

Today, with modern techniques, the outlook for reattachment of the retina and restoration of sight is excellent.

VITREOUS SURGERY

The vitreous infusion suction cutter (VISC) represents a major milestone in ophthalmology. This instrument can be used to treat disorders of the vitreous that were considered inoperable until its development in the early 1970s. This instrument performs three major functions within the vitreous cavity of the eye: it is able to cut the vitreous, remove the debris from the eye by suction, and replace the aspirate with an infusion of Ringer's solution.

The VISC is introduced into the vitreous cavity anywhere over the pars plana 4 to 7 mm from the corneal limbus. In this position it is possible to avoid hitting the lens of the eye, as well as to avoid stripping the retina itself. In some cases in which a cataract obscures the view of the vitreous, the instrument with its cutting action can be employed to remove the cataractous lens material itself.

The results of vitrectomy surgery in many instances have been astonishing. When it is effective, visual acuity can be improved from hand movements to 20/30. Despite preselection of cases, not all results are successful, and the visual improvement in some instances is not so dramatic. However, when we remember that these cases were previously thought to be hopeless, any improvement is gratifying.

The most common indication for a vitrectomy is a nonclearing vitreous hemorrhage in a patient with diabetes. With removal of the blood-filled vitreous, light is able to reach the retina and therefore improve the level of visual acuity (Fig. 27-29).

Vitrectomy also has been used to handle cases of retinal detachment to eliminate the traction on the retina. In such instances there are usually strong vitreous bands, contracting and pulling on the retina and preventing it from being returned mechanically. In cataract extraction there sometimes is vitreous loss, and with the loss of vitreous the retina can become detached. Detachment is largely the result of shrinkage of the trapped vitreous, which is attached at the wound site of the cataract extraction. Again, the vitrectomy instrument has been effective in cutting and eliminating these traction bands, which can produce complications such as retinal detachment, macular cysts, macular holes, macular edema, and retinal holes.

The vitrectomy instrument also has been employed in cases with heavy intraocular connective tissue formation after foreign body injuries. Vitrectomy is the only way of removing severe scar formation in the vitreous cavity. It also has been useful in cases of severe inflammatory reaction in the vitreous.

In some instances, vitrectomy is not effective. It has had poor results in eyes with massive preretinal retraction. At times vitreous hemorrhage may occur, which will lead to a poor result.

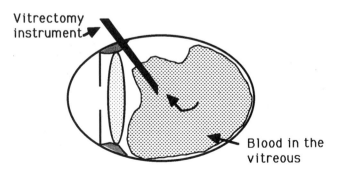

Fig. 27-29 Vitrectomy performed to remove vitreous that is mixed with blood. (From Stein HA, Slatt BJ, Stein RM: *Ophthalmic terminology: speller and vocabulary builder,* ed 3, St Louis, 1992, Mosby.)

LASER SURGERY

The principle of lasers was predicted by Albert Einstein in 1917. During the 1950s, Townes and Schawlow at Columbia University and Vasov and Prokhorov at the Lebeder Institute, working independently in the field of microwave physics, demonstrated that simulated emission of radiation could be made available for practical use. The researchers received a Nobel Prize for this work in 1964.

Lasers are now being employed in a growing number of medical procedures that permit surgeons to perform noninvasive surgery. Diseased tissue can be cut away or vaporized by lasers with less damage or trauma to neighboring healthy tissues. Surgery also can be accomplished in inaccessible parts of the body by transmitting laser beams to those parts through fiberoptics, transmission cables, and other innovative delivery systems. In ophthalmology, the delivery system is usually a slit-lamp microscope, but new laser cutting instruments are being studied.

In ophthalmology, the argon laser can alter the trabecular meshwork and increase outflow of aqueous. It can be used for gonioplasty and for iridotomy because it can coagulate, retard, or destroy new vessel growth in the anterior and posterior segments of the eye. The neodymium YAG laser also has a wide variety of uses in ophthalmology, but its most popular use has been that of opening the posterior capsule when it has become opacified.

The YAG laser is widely used today. Contrary to popular belief, this laser does not remove cataracts. Within months or years after a cataract has been removed, eye surgeons frequently use the YAG laser to clear cloudy and secondary membranes. This results in restoration of vision by a noninvasive method of opening these membranes. The procedure is nonpainful and requires no hospitalization. The YAG laser is a "cold" type of laser and uses quick pulses of laser energy on clear tissues within the eye. It also is used for performing an iris iridotomy in cases of narrow-angle glaucoma.

CORNEAL TRANSPLANTATION

The cornea is the clear portion in the front part of the eye that is similar to the transparent covering on a watch. When injury, degeneration, or infection occurs that causes the cornea to become cloudy, vision will be disrupted. Only by replacing a portion of the cornea with a clear window taken from a donor eye can vision be restored.

Not everyone with a corneal disease can be helped by corneal transplantation.

The cornea, because it is devoid of blood vessels, is one of the few tissues in the human body that may be transplanted from one human being to another with a large degree of success. The absence of blood vessels in both the donor and host cornea reduces the allergic reaction, in which reactive immunoglobulins are carried through blood flow, and permits the body to retain and not reject the "foreign" cornea. Thus only conditions in which the cornea is free of blood vessels are suitable for transplantation.

Two basic types of corneal transplantation are performed. One is the *lamellar* or *partial penetrating* procedure, in which a half thickness of cornea is transferred from the eye of a donor to that of the host (Fig. 27-30, *A*). In this procedure the anterior chamber of the eye is not entered, and only the outer half or two thirds of the cornea is transplanted. Union is made of the donor cornea with the host cornea by means of several interrupted fine sutures or a continuous suture around the periphery of the donor button. The donor button will vary anywhere from 6 to 10 mm in diameter, depending on the extent of the disease involved. The second type of transplant operation is the *penetrating* or *full-thickness* corneal transplant (Fig. 27-30, *B*). In this operation, the full thickness of the cornea is removed from the donor eye and replaces the full thickness of the central portion of the host cornea. The surgery involves entering the anterior chamber, inserting the donor cornea, and establishing a tight fit by direct suture closure or a continuous suture (Figs. 27-31 and 27-32). Healon often is used to minimize endothelial damage.

In the postoperative period the most common complications include a wound leak, suture breakage and wound dehiscence, infection, and graft rejec-

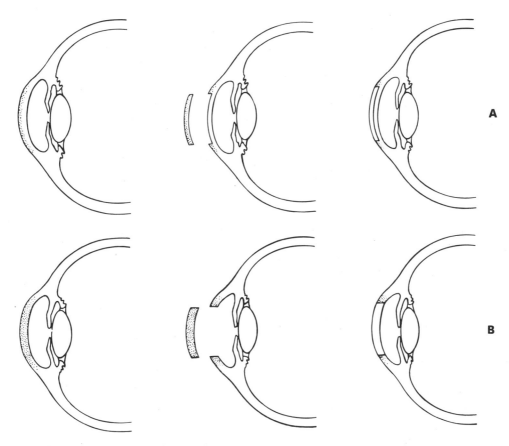

Fig. 27-30 Corneal transplant. **A,** Lamellar, or partial penetrating, corneal transplant. The clouded outer portion of the cornea is removed and replaced with clear donor cornea. **B,** Penetrating, or full-thickness, corneal transplant. The entire central portion of clouded cornea is removed and replaced with clear donor cornea.

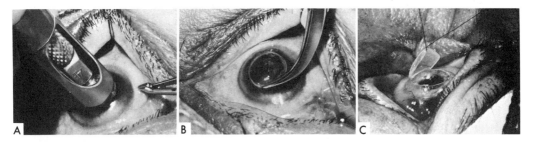

Fig. 27-31 Corneal transplant surgery. **A,** Trephining the host cornea. **B,** Excising the host cornea. **C,** Inserting the donor cornea.

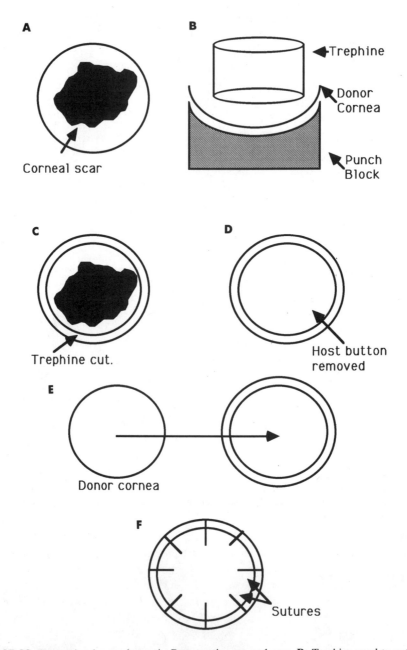

Fig. 27-32 Penetrating keratoplasty. **A,** Preoperative corneal scar. **B,** Trephine used to cut donor cornea. **C,** Trephine used to cut patient's cornea. **D,** Cut cornea of patient is removed. **E,** Donor cornea is placed in opening of patient's cornea. **F,** Donor cornea is sutured into position. (From Stein HA, Slatt BJ, Stein RM: *Ophthalmic terminology: speller and vocabulary builder,* ed 3, St Louis, 1992, Mosby.)

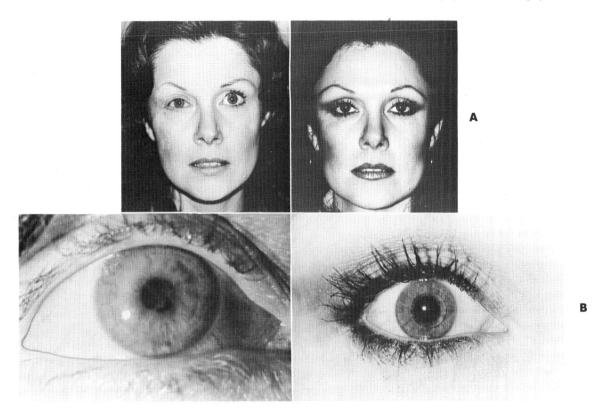

Fig. 27-33 A, Recurrent corneal ulceration after herpes simplex virus with visual loss. **B,** After corneal transplantation.

tion. If detected early and managed appropriately, these complications can be controlled or eliminated, enabling a high level of success for the operation. Thus, careful monitoring by the doctor, nurse, or ophthalmic assistant is required.

In both the lamellar and full-thickness corneal transplant, the donor and the host buttons are trephined with a round cutting trephine, which cleanly and sharply removes the affected part. The cornea taken from a recently deceased person is then carefully sutured in place (Fig. 27-33).

EYELID SURGERY

Entropion is a condition in which the eyelashes roll in and rub against the cornea. Numerous types of eyelid operations are performed for the correction of this condition. One of the simplest types is Ziegler cautery, in which the cautery is applied to the area just below the eyelashes.

Other procedures include tightening of the underlying muscles of the eyelid or removal of a wedge of tarsus from the inner aspect of the eyelid.

Ectropion occurs when the eyelid rolls outward. This may be the result of scarring from burns, and insertion of grafts of skin taken elsewhere will be required to reduce the pull frrom the scar tissue. Grafts of skin for the eyelids may be taken from upper eyelids or from behind the ears. In some cases, ectropion results from a laxity of the skin and underlying structures. This requires surgical removal of these tissues to properly evert the lid so that the lid margin lies in its correct position against the globe.

Ptosis occurs when the eyelid droops to cover the

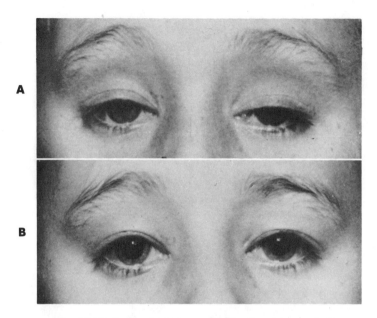

Fig. 27-34 Ptosis. **A,** Uncorrected. **B,** Corrected surgically.

upper portion of the pupil (Fig. 27-34). Investigation in the adult should rule out medical causes before surgery is undertaken. If the levator muscle still functions, a resection of this muscle will be performed— either from the undersurface of the eyelid or through the eyelid skin. In this procedure the muscle is identified and shortened a measured amount of millimeters. When the levator muscle is completely paralyzed, the eyelid may be suspended from the brow muscles to the tarsal plate by use of fascia lata taken from the thigh or from cadavers, by collagen tapes, or by white silk sutures.

PTERYGIUM REMOVAL (Fig. 27-35)

Pterygium is a growth of the conjunctiva that invades a portion of the cornea. It is usually vascular when active. With a knife or superblade, the pterygium is completely excised from the cornea and adjacent conjunctiva or is transplanted to another position to redirect its growth.

DACRYOCYSTORHINOSTOMY

Blockage of the tear canal may result from obstructions arising anywhere, beginning at the small punctum on the eyelid margin and extending to the na-

solacrimal duct. Obstructions involving the lacrimal sac and nasolacrimal duct require correction by dacryocystorhinostomy.

In this procedure a large opening, approximately 8 to 10 mm in size, is made in the wall of the nose, and a union is created between the mucosal lining of the nose in this area and the lacrimal sac. Thus the lacrimal sac opens directly into the nose through this large opening. The operation usually ensures relatively good success in curing tearing and infection problems that arise from stagnation in the lacrimal sac.

ENUCLEATION AND EVISCERATION

An eye may be removed because of tumor, injury, or severe pain combined with dysfunction. Enucleation usually is performed with the patient under general anesthesia because of the psychologic impact of removing an eye.

The conjunctiva is opened around the limbus, and the four rectus muscles are identified and severed from the globe. An enucleation scissors is passed behind the globe, and the optic nerve is severed. The oblique muscles are then severed from the globe, and the globe is removed from the socket. Pressure

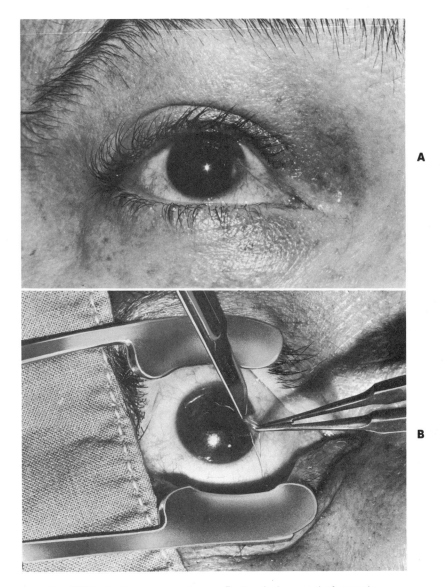

Fig. 27-35 A, Pterygium, right eye. **B,** Surgical removal of pterygium.

is applied until bleeding has stopped. An implant of glass, plastic, or silicone is placed in the socket to fill the defect. The muscles or tissues are sewn over the implant in a way that permits movement of the implant. When healing has occurred, the patient will be directed to an artificial-eye maker *(ocularist)*, who will fashion a cosmetic shell with a built-in painted iris and pupil to match the fellow eye. Some-

times only the contents of the globe are removed, leaving the outer shell. This procedure is called an *evisceration*.

EYE DRESSINGS

Eye patches are usually used postoperatively to prevent infection and absorb discharge. They also immobilize the eyes and protect them from accidental trauma. Most eye pads have a cotton center and a fine mesh surface to prevent the cotton from being absorbed into the discharge and wound.

An eye pad is secured in place with the application of three or four strips of adhesive or cellophane tape. The strips are directed on an angle from the cheek to the forehead, away from the margins of the mouth so that eating will not be hampered. A shield of metal or plastic is commonly applied over the eye pad to protect the eye from undue external pressure or injury.

SUMMARY

The ophthalmic assistant should maintain routines that can be adapted for every surgical patient. The management of a surgical patient involves attention to the mechanical details of surgery, as well as to education of the patient regarding the nature of the hospital stay.

QUESTIONS FOR REVIEW AND THOUGHT

1. Outline an operative technique for strabismus surgery, cataract surgery, and glaucoma surgery.
2. What are the principles behind cataract surgery? Corneal transplant surgery? Muscle surgery?
3. What is the cryophake?
4. What is the most common major ocular surgical procedure performed?
5. Name some complications that can occur after cataract surgery.
6. How can a patient's general health affect the outcome of surgery?
7. Identify the use of drugs during cataract surgery.
8. Identify the difference between phacoemulsification and extracapsular cataract surgery.
9. Describe the steps of the cataract phacoemulsification procedure.

SELF-EVALUATION QUESTIONS

True-false statements

Directions: Indicate whether the statement is true (T) or false (F).

T or F   1. In muscle surgery, recession of a muscle involves moving it from its attachment and placing it at a point closer to the cornea.

T or F   2. Cryosurgery refers to any surgical procedure involving cold temperatures during surgery.

T or F   3. Phacoemulsification is removal of a cataract through the use of ultrasound.

Missing words

Directions: Write in the missing word in the following sentences.

4. Removal of an eye is called _____.
5. Removal of a portion of the trabeculum for glaucoma is called _____.
6. An out-turning of the eyelid is called _____.

Choice-completion questions

Directions: Select the one best answer in each case.

7. In strabismus surgery, which procedure is not considered a normal surgical practice?
    a. Uncovering the eye the day after surgery
    b. Patching the unoperated eye preoperatively
    c. Giving systemic antibiotics

d. Letting the patient go home the day after surgery

e. Utilizing orthoptic exercises soon after surgery

8. Which of the following is not a surgical procedure for glaucoma?

a. Laser iridectomy

b. Trabeculectomy

c. Sclerectomy

d. Cryotherapy

e. Ziegler cautery

9. Corneal transplantation is utilized as a surgical procedure for which of the following conditions?

a. Cataracts

b. Advanced glaucoma

c. Toxic keratitis

d. Keratoconus

e. Keratoconjunctivitis sicca

ANSWERS, NOTES, AND EXPLANATIONS

1. **False.** In recession of a muscle, the reattachment is made at a point toward the posterior portion of the eye and away from the cornea. This in effect weakens the pull of the muscle so that it has a less effective contraction. In convergent strabismus, the medial rectus may be recessed, whereas in divergent strabismus the lateral rectus is recessed.

2. **True.** Cryosurgery involves the use of a probe cooled by liquid nitrogen, carbon dioxide, or Freon, so that the temperature ranges anywhere from $-20°$ to $-70°C$. By so lowering the temperature, a small probe can be applied to the lens of the eye to create an iceball formation and adhesion of the lens to the probe. This forms a bond that is useful in extracting the cataract. Cryotherapy also is used to destroy lashes and hair follicles. It is used in retinal detachment repair to create adhesions of the tissues themselves. It may be used in glaucoma to shrink the vascular coat of the eye.

3. **True.** In this procedure, which has gained widespread acceptance throughout the world, ultrasound is employed in a small probe that enters the eye. By means of high-frequency sound waves, the cutting edge impinges on the cataractous lens and emulsifies it so it can be easily removed by aspiration.

4. **Enucleation.** Enucleation is performed whenever an eye is diseased and painful or whenever a malignant tumor is present. During enucleation, all muscles are severed from the globe, and then the optic nerve is severed and the globe is removed. An implant of plastic, glass, or silicone is placed in the socket to fill the defect left by removal of the eye. An artificial eye is then fashioned that moves with the implant and simulates the appearance of a normal eyeball.

5. **Trabeculectomy.** Trabeculectomy is the removal of a portion of the trabeculum to improve the outflow of fluid from the eye. It thereby reduces the devastating destructive effect that the elevated intraocular pressure of glaucoma creates.

6. **Ectropion.** An eyelid that turns out is called an *ectropion,* from *ec-,* meaning out. This may occur as the result of scarring of the overlying eyelid tissue (cicatricial ectropion), or it may occur from the laxity of the muscles (senile ectropion) as occurs in elderly persons. Surgical correction is the only means to repair an ectropion.

7. **c. Giving systemic antibiotics.** An operation such as strabismus surgery performed in a sterile environment requires no systemic antibiotics. Topical antibiotics may be given at the time of surgery and may even be given by some ophthalmologists in the postoperative period. This is usually satisfactory to overcome any invading organism. The rich blood supply of both the

vascular coat and the muscles of the eye is usually sufficient to take care of any inflammation that may arise.

This situation, however, may not be true for intraocular surgery when there is an absence of blood vessels and thus an absence of the vascular response to an invading microbacterial organism. In these intraocular cases, antibiotics may be preferred to raise the intraocular level of the antibiotics to prevent infection.

8. **e. Ziegler cautery.** All the procedures except Ziegler cautery are used for either narrow-angle or wide-angle glaucoma. Ziegler cautery is used to correct a spastic entropion of the eyelid.

9. **d. Keratoconus.** Keratoconus is a progressive outpouching and thinning of the cornea with rupturing and scar formation. A corneal transplant is required when the cone has reached the point at which contact lenses or spectacles can no longer satisfactorily correct vision. The cornea eventually may become extremely thin, in which case a penetrating corneal transplant is required.

CHAPTER 28

The surgical ophthalmic assistant

- Bedside ophthalmic assistant
- Operating room assistant
- Amoric environment
- Care and handling of surgical instruments
- Operating room microscope
- Ethical behavior of the ophthalmic assistant
- Medicolegal tips

Most surgical procedures for the eye are performed on an outpatient basis (see Chapter 30). However, some procedures are performed in the hospital on an inpatient basis, e.g., corneal transplants, retinal surgery, etc. This chapter will highlight those patients who are admitted.

BEDSIDE OPHTHALMIC ASSISTANT

One of our most important senses is that of sight. A blind or partially sighted individual is considerably impaired in the ability to move about freely, perform work, and function effectively. Daily living is seriously jeopardized. Consequently, any threat of loss or impairment of these abilities is a threat against an individual's independence.

Without sight, no longer can drivers drive their cars, pilots fly their planes, or surgeons perform their work. Because of the consequences of blindness and the fear associated with this threat, the nursing care of patients with eye disorders is challenging and demands extraordinary skill.

The background for ophthalmic nursing requires a good understanding of people and their management. Psychologic problems induced by the emotional havoc created by the threat of losing one's vision must be dealt with effectively. Ophthalmic assistants who are interested in eye nursing will become involved in these emotional reactions.

Nurses are expected to increase their knowledge of the eye and eye disorders. They must become familiar with the terminology and acquainted with various diagnostic tests and surgical procedures. They also must become aware of the relationship between disease of the eye and disease of the body. A gentle touch and fine dexterity are prerequisites in caring for patients, particularly in the administration of eye medications and treatment to eyes that have undergone recent surgery. Nurses must move about quietly in the rooms of such patients—not dash into the room, bump into beds, or in any way startle patients who could become alarmed because they cannot see anyone's movements. Ophthalmic nursing is essentially "quiet" nursing. The successful restoration or, indeed, improvement in eyesight often provides a stimulating and rewarding experience for ophthalmic nurses.

The visually impaired patient

Blindness is considered total lack of vision, or vision insufficient to conduct the ordinary activities in life. Blindness is defined as a central visual acuity of 20/200 or less in the better eye with corrective glasses, or a field defect in which the peripheral field is contracted to such an extent that the widest diameter of the visual field subtends an angle not greater than 20 degrees.

599

With both these limitations, a person is *economically* blind. A vast majority of the blind are in the group just below this threshold. Some are able to read newspaper headlines, and some can identify distant objects. They may see light in various directions—in the corridors and the windows and in the streets. Only in the most severe form is the blind person completely devoid of any light sensation.

Some blind patients often live in false hope of a possible cure and refuse to adjust to their decrease in vision. Others withdraw from society and lean heavily on their visual defect. They no longer face the normal problems of daily living and become dependent on others to relieve them of their responsibilities. These blind individuals find comfort, because they do no encounter failures and disappointments and are free from judgment and condemnation by others.

Others recognize that their visual impairment imposes limitations in their way of life. They have difficulty in accepting their disability and become aggressive in their behavior and angered, and this anger often is reflected toward others. Some adjust realistically; they measure what assets they have and use their resources positively, thereby maintaining an ultimate degree of independence. They constantly work toward making life worthwhile for themselves and those with whom they are in contact.

When a patient who has poor vision arrives in the hospital, the nurse must evaluate the patient's degree of acceptance of visual impairment in terms of the person's physical ability and psychologic dependence. The patient who denies existence of the disability and withdraws from society needs to be brought back to reality and to develop meaningful relationships with others. Gradual motivation can be instilled so that the patient eventually will assume a degree of responsibility for self-care. When confronting a patient who is aggressive and hostile because of the impairment, the nurse should establish communication so that the patient feels free to voice negative feelings about his or her limitations.

Patient orientation

When a partially sighted or a blind patient has to be admitted to a hospital, there should be a structured system of orienting the patient to the environment.

The nurse should greet the patient warmly, addressing the person by name, and rapidly clarify the nurse's position in the hospital setting. It is important that patients know to whom they are talking, who will take care of them, and what hospital personnel will do for them. Often shaking the patient's hand and touching an arm provide a feeling of welcome. The ophthalmic nurse should observe the patient's movements to decide what type of help the individual will require. Patients who walk slowly and hesitantly, with the body bent forward and arms extended to find certain guiding objects, may require a great deal of assistance and orientation.

Patients with vision that is normal in one eye but impaired in the other eye will have little difficulty in adjusting to the hospital environment and will need little orientation. Partially sighted persons with impaired vision usually are aided by bright lights, such as the corridor and window lights. Consequently, rooms and corridors should be kept well-lighted before eye surgery, and hospital design should allow for this level of increased illumination.

The partially sighted individual who is being escorted should be permitted to take the assistant's arm lightly above the elbow. This automatically places the patient a step behind the guide, which provides protection and the ability to feel slight movements, as well as anticipate directional changes. An individual should never be pushed or steered. Any stairs, ramps, or surface changes should be indicated and described so that footing adjustments can be made. While walking with the patient, the assistant should engage in conversation and give a description of the surroundings. A blind person should be oriented to the room and the bathroom by having the person move about, touch the furniture and equipment, and become familiar with their location. These objects should be kept in a fixed location so that the patient may use them as landmarks.

Many patients and parents of children undergoing surgery will ask the hospital assistant questions they have been hesitant to ask the ophthalmologist. The assistant must be sure to say the right thing with tact and diplomacy and in a quiet authoritative manner, speaking in lay terms that are readily understandable and not shocking. For example, the parents should not be told that their child is cross-eyed and requires sight-saving surgery. It is more tactful to state that the child requires the surgery to correct the eyes' tendency to turn and that surgery offers the best treatment for a permanent correction. It even helps to reassure the parents by telling them that the procedure is simple and painless and requires only a short recuperation period.

Children in particular enter the hospital with a fair degree of apprehension. Basically they want to like and trust the people they meet, but they are afraid of the unknown, of the atmosphere, of the strange white uniforms, of the instruments, and of the worry about needles. Usually a sincere smile, a soft voice, and a warm greeting will "break the ice."

Preoperative preparation

Before surgery, the ophthalmic nurse should review with the patient the type of surgery that is about to be performed and what is expected of the patient to promote the success of the operation. This approach will considerably lessen the patient's anxieties and will elicit postoperative cooperation. Even though basic information has been given to the patient by the ophthalmologist, securing the confidence of the patient will develop a good nurse-patient relationship, which will promote the patient's recovery.

For those procedures that are performed with the patient under local anesthesia, the patient should be instructed in deep breathing and movement of the limbs to encourage circulation. Elderly persons tend to lie rigidly in the same position for prolonged periods, fearful of movement. The voluntary movement of limbs and chest muscles will greatly lessen respiratory difficulties that may ensue postoperatively.

Patients also should be instructed that coughing, sneezing, and squeezing of the eyelids will have a detrimental effect on the operation. Bowel evacuants are commonly used the night before surgery so that abdominal discomfort is relieved and harmful straining after surgery is eliminated.

If the patient has never had eye drops instilled, it is appropriate for the ophthalmic nurse to provide instructions regarding the procedure and the purpose of medication before surgery so that undue squeezing of the eyes after medication will be avoided. Oph-

thalmic nurses will probably be responsible for administration of eye ointments and solutions, and it is important that they take extreme care in administering these medications. The eyes are especially sensitive after surgery, and any abrupt manipulation will cause discomfort and squeezing, which will endanger the eye. Hands should be washed before instilling drops. The dropper tip should not touch the eyelashes. The head should be tilted back, the patient asked to look up, and the lower eyelid pulled down. The drop is then instilled in the lower fornix (Fig. 28-1). Topical anesthetic drops, however, are placed in the eye with the patient looking down and the solution directed to the 12 o'clock area of the sclera near the limbus. This permits the drop to run down over the cornea, where it produces maximal anesthesia.

Patients should be advised that whether they have local or general anesthesia, they will feel little discomfort during or after surgery. Some patients are very concerned that they will see everything during the operation and must be reassured that this is not so.

Postoperative care

When the patient has returned from the operating room to bed or chair, gentleness is of utmost importance. In intraocular procedures the patient should exercise caution and avoid rapid head movements. To prevent dislodging the eye dressing or pressing the eye bandage into the pillow and thereby injuring the eye, the patient should avoid lying on the side that has had surgery. The patient must be reminded to refrain from touching or disturbing the eye dressings to prevent any self-inflicted injury or infection. With very elderly persons, during sleep, the assistant may put loose restraints on the wrists as a reminder for the sleeping patient not to touch the eye dressing. After retinal detachment operations the head of the bed will often be placed in the position that is most beneficial for securing the reattachment. For some of these patients a considerable amount of encouragement is necessary, and every effort should be made to ensure that the patient avoids exertion or strain in the immediate postoperative period. For surgery that is not intraocular, such as for strabismus or eyelid repair, limitations

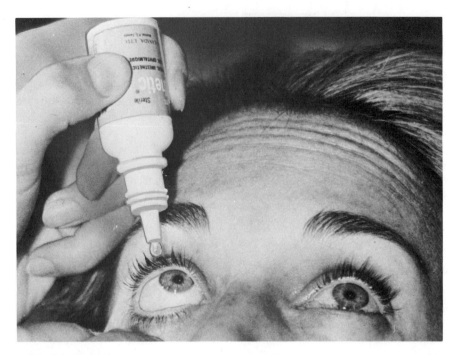

Fig. 28-1 Instilling eye drops. Avoid any pressure on the eye or contamination of the dropper bottle by the eyelashes.

seldom are placed on the patient's activity. For small-incision intraocular surgery, many of the safeguards are being abandoned.

The hospital atmosphere should be quiet and subdued. We recommend blackout drapes in each room so that the drapes may be drawn if the patient is photosensitive, as so often occurs after an eye operation. The nurse should be on guard for signs of restlessness or confusion in the patient. Some patients undergo behavioral changes and even have hallucinations. We are all dependent on sensory input from exposure to the world about us. The patient who suddenly loses the sense of sight because of a bandage often feels isolated from his or her environment and becomes disoriented. This creates a state of confusion, and disturbing illusions may occur. Any changes of this sort require a watchful nurse who constantly communicates with the patient and tries to effect relaxation and a return to reality. Radios may help in giving the patient this touch of reality through the auditory sense.

If nausea or vomiting occurs in the immediate postoperative period, adequate medication must be given immediately for relief. Usually a light, often liquid, diet is ordered for the day of surgery as a prevention. Foods should be sufficiently low in residue so that they require only a minimum amount of chewing and are not constipating. The physician's orders must be carefully followed, and order abbreviations must be well known (Table 28-1).

Some eye patients require special assistance at meal times. They will have both eyes bandaged or will have their only good eye bandaged. When the meal tray is being served, its arrival should be announced to the patient and the food described in an appetizing way. It is helpful to describe the location of the various items of food by using the numbers of the clock as a guide. The patient can be instructed to locate the food by using the back of the hand to find the coffee cup, the soup bowl, and similar items. This helps avoid spills and wet fingers. For a person who has little vision in the postoperative period, all food should be ready to eat—milk cartons opened,

Table 28-1   Hospital abbreviations

Abbreviation	Meaning
a̅a̅	of each
ac	before meals
ad lib	as desired
amp	ampule
bid	twice a day
c̅ or cum	with
caps	capsule
cc	cubic centimeter
collyr	eyewash
dr	dram
g	gram
gr	grain
gt	drop
hs	at bedtime
ic	between meals
IM	intramuscularly
IV	intravenously
lot	lotion
mg	milligram
non rep	do not repeat
ocul	eye
od	right eye
os	left eye
ou	each eye
pc	after meals
PO	by mouth
prn	as needed
qh	every hour
qid	four times a day
qs	sufficient quantity
s̅	without
s̅s̅	half
stat	immediately
tab	tablet
tid	three times a day
ung	ointment

meat cut, salt and pepper added as the patient desires, and the coffee poured.

The person feeding a patient should explain what the food is, ask what the patient prefers to eat first and how he or she likes to eat, attempt to make the person comfortable and relaxed, and offer finger foods that can be managed without difficulty. Patients should be encouraged to visit and talk with other patients after the first 2 or 3 days following surgery. Conversation is a good social outlet and helps pass the time.

It is important that the patient be advised to wear slippers that are easy to slide into and that have a firm sole with a good grip to avoid slipping during movement.

Sometime before the first eye dressing, the patient should be made aware that removal of the bandage will not immediately result in clear vision. No matter what the surgery, it will require time for the process of healing to occur and for the final vision to be obtained.

Alarming postoperative signs and symptoms

The ophthalmic nurse who has been designated to undertake the immediate postoperative treatments for eye patients should be on the watch for unusual eye signs that indicate untoward complications. Any hemorrhage present in the anterior chamber should be noted and the attending physician informed. Unusual pain may be accompanied by a prolapse of the iris, in which a knuckle of iris protrudes from the wound incision; this is an alarming sign and requires immediate attention. The presence of a flat anterior chamber that has not reformed or that has suddenly occurred should be noted. Any evidence of small whitish material present in the lower portion of the anterior chamber is an ominous sign and should be brought to the attention of the ophthalmologist immediately. It indicates a developing hypopyon, which may indicate an intraocular infection. If accompanied by severe pain, it is even more ominous. Marked swelling of the eyelids combined with excoriation of the skin should be noted, because this is a common sign of allergy to the medication that is being introduced or of an infection that may be starting. Unusual complaints of pain in the immediate postoperative period should be brought to the attention of the ophthalmologist because occasionally wound rupture does occur, which is marked by severe pain. Evidence of a purulent discharge postoperatively is an ominous sign.

Instructions to patient on discharge

When the patient is about to be discharged from the hospital, instructions should be given that will ensure the continuing success of the eye surgery. Eyes that have had surgery require cautious care for the first few weeks after operation (see the box on p. 604).

DIRECTIONS FOR PATIENTS LEAVING THE HOSPITAL AFTER CATARACT SURGERY

Your wound is healing, but it will not be firm enough to stand much pressure for 2 months. You may feel that something is in your eye. This is because of the stitches. This feeling will go away.

1. Continue to be careful.
2. Avoid closing the eyes tightly. One often closes the eyes tightly when laughing, talking, sneezing, coughing, yawning, or if irritated. At these times you should be particularly careful not to close your eyes tightly. Never *rub* or *touch* the eye.
3. Avoid stooping, straining, lifting, and particularly, bending over.
4. If there is much secretion, wipe off the lids with cotton, but *avoid exerting pressure* on the eye, particularly the upper lid.
5. You will be given drops to use in your eye. Please follow these directions carefully. When the drops are finished, use the prescribed drops.
   HOW TO INSTILL DROPS
   a. Wash your hands thoroughly before and after putting in eye drops and ointments.
   b. Clean the edges of your eyelids, using a clean cotton ball or washcloth that has been moistened with tap water. Do not press on the upper lid.
   c. Pull your lower lid down with one hand, forming a "pouch." Look up.

   d. Put one drop of medicine in the pouch. Do not touch the tip of the bottle to your lid, eyelashes, or any other place.
   e. Close your eye for one full minute after each drop.
   f. If you find the preceding difficult, lie on the bed and repeat above instructions while looking up at the dropper.
   g. Never use eye drops that are over 2 months old. Discard them.
6. You may watch television and read.
7. You may go outdoors for a walk or drive. It is not necessary to cover the eye, but it is preferable to shield it from bright sunlight by sunglasses with ultraviolet protection.
8. If necessary, take a mild laxative.
9. You may wash your hair 2 weeks after surgery, but do not get soapy water in your eye.
10. Mild pain and discomfort may be relieved by aspirin. If there is more severe pain, please contact us.
11. You may have the feeling of something in the eye because of the incision, but do not close it tightly. This feeling may persist for a few weeks.
12. Glasses or contact lens will be prescribed when the eye is fully healed and the prescription is stable.

Each ophthalmologist has specific individual methods of dealing with patients. The physician's input is most important in giving directions to patients.

OPERATING ROOM ASSISTANT

Many ophthalmic assistants working in offices and clinics have the privilege of accompanying the ophthalmologist to the operating room. Here a new challenge awaits.

The drama of the operating room, the exactness, care, and detail required in eye surgery, and the satisfaction resulting from a successful procedure instill a sense of accomplishment in the assistant at the end of each operating period. Here the operating room assistant is expected to fulfil his or her role with the utmost gentleness, care, and attention.

The ophthalmic assistant probably will be responsible for the selection, care, handling, and sterilization of the many ophthalmic instruments required. A meticulous scrub and gown routine must be adhered to. One should be exceptionally careful that the exact sterile technique in scrubbing, gowning, and draping in the eye operating room is not broken by any member of the team, lest an infection develop that not only may cause irreparable damage but also may result in blindness and even removal of the eye itself (Fig. 28-2).

The operating room must be quiet except for background music. Sudden loud noises might make the patient move unexpectedly and endanger the eye.

All those who assist the ophthalmologist must ensure that the environment is pleasant and quiet from the time the patient is brought into the room until he or she leaves.

Aseptic technique in the operating room

Although surgery has been practiced since ancient times, the practice of a sepsis is recent. As long ago as 3000 BC, Egyptians bored holes in skulls to let evil spirits out. Even in 700 BC, the Hindus performed cataract and eyelid surgery. Those who performed the surgery learned to keep their fingernails short, take daily baths, and wear white clothing. It was only in the nineteenth century that Joseph Lister introduced modern surgical aseptic techniques. Lister recognized that results of surgery improved tenfold if microorganisms could be kept out of the wound. Thus many methods of sterilization of instruments and preparations for cleansing and disinfecting the skin came into being, until today's modern methods were attained. Aseptic technique is discussed in Chapter 24. Strict adherence to the principles of instrument sterilization, skin disinfection, and eye preparation is essential to eliminate ocular infections, which can be visually devastating (see box below).

Routine procedure for the operating room assistant

Before scrubbing. Assistants must know the operative procedure well, even if it requires additional reading to become familiar with the technique. There should be an updated card or page listing the surgeon's preferences in instruments, sutures, and preparation of the patient. Assistants should question other operating room personnel who have worked with the surgeon to understand his or her special variations. If all are unfamiliar with the procedure, assistants should not hesitate to contact the surgeon

---

SOME COMMON ERRORS IN ASEPTIC SURGICAL TECHNIQUES (Fig. 28-2)

Masks and caps
1. Mask covering only the mouth and not the nose
2. Mask tied too loosely
3. Hair permitted to protrude from the cap

Scrub
1. Fingernails too long (should not exceed 1 mm)
2. Allowing the runoff to drip from the hands, thus contaminating them (runoff should be from the elbow)
3. Too short a scrub time
4. Failing to develop a systematic scrub routine and thus leaving bare spots
5. Splashing the clothes, thus contaminating sterile gown later

Drying
1. Using wet section of towel to dry upper arms, thus contaminating dry fingers
2. Allowing towel to touch unsterile clothing

Gowning
1. Allowing gown to become contaminated by the hands or other unsterile objects
2. Allowing gown to touch unsterile objects by walking about the room

Powdering hands
1. Dispensing powder from the hands into the air
2. Not carefully cleansing powder from outside of gloves

Gloves
1. Touching outer portion of glove
2. Failing to detect perforations or breaks in the glove
3. Holding hands against the body while waiting

Skin preparation
1. Believing in the manufacturer's claim for the product; check it out
2. Relying on aqueous antiseptics
3. Failing to realize that quarternary ammonium compounds (Zephiran) may be neutralized by even small traces of soap
4. In applying antiseptics, going back and forth from clean to contaminated areas and back to the clean area again (instead, ever-widening circles should be made, starting from the eyelid margin)
5. Forgetting to prepare the eyelashes, the eyelid margin, or the eyebrows

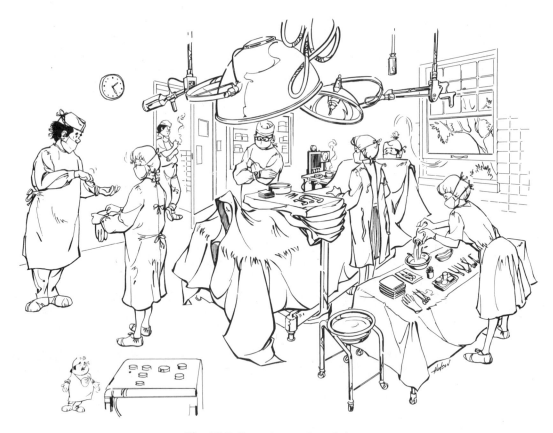

Fig. 28-2 Errors in aseptic techniques.

a day or two before surgery to ensure that all necessary equipment is available.

Bringing the patient to surgery. The patient should be as relaxed as possible. A cheerful but quiet manner will provide an atmosphere of relaxation. Assistants should try to instill optimism and confidence in patients and should be particular to point out that everything will go well. They should always express confidence in the skill of the operating surgeon. It has been our habit to employ soft music in the eye operating room throughout the procedure to ensure relaxation. Coming to the operating room for surgery is a unique and often terrifying experience to the patient. Each patient should be treated as if he or she were the only one and not one of many who pass through each day.

Cutting the eyelashes is not routinely performed for all procedures and may be abandoned by some

surgeons. However, when it is necessary, the eyelashes should be cut before skin preparation. A thin film of ointment is placed on the cutting edge of an eyelash scissor so that the free lashes will adhere to the blades and be prevented from falling into the eye (Fig. 28-3). The patient should be reassured that the lashes will rapidly regrow.

Scrubbing. Assistants should carefully clean the area under their nails with a nail file or orangewood stick before scrubbing. The water should be turned on so that it is at a comfortable temperature. Many sinks have elbow, knee, or foot controls provided for this so that adjustments can be made during the scrub technique. Assistants should adhere to the required time and the antiseptics used in any given hospital. They must be sure to follow a definite scrub routine so that no bare areas or blind spots occur on the sides of fingers, back of hands, or back of arms.

There should be at least 20 to 30 brush strokes for every portion of skin. The water and the debris should always be allowed to run down from the elbows into the sink and never to run back down over the hands, which have been scrubbed.

Gowning. The gown must be folded so that the scrub assistant can unfold and put the gown on without touching the outer side with the bare hands. A towel placed on top of the gown should be used for careful drying of the hands before taking up the gown.

Gowns should be of sufficient thickness to provide protection from contamination by underclothing. Each sleeve should have a fitting wristlet. Many gowns now have wraparound backs to prevent the back area from contaminating instrument tables.

Gloving. Several techniques are available for putting on gloves under sterile operating room conditions. The closed gloving technique represents perhaps the best method available for the scrub assistant. Some of the advantages of the closed gloving technique are reduction of possible contamination of the gloves from the hands and minimizing of the use of free glove powder, which scatters in an operating room.

In the closed gloving technique (Fig. 28-4), the scrub assistant puts on the gown but slides his or her hands into the sleeves only until the sleeve cuff seams can be grasped between the fingers and thumbs. The hands do not protrude beyond the seam of the gown. The gloves are then laid out with the gown-covered hand. The glove is placed in the sleeve thumb down, with the fingers pointing toward the shoulder, and the wrist edge of the glove is level with the sleeve cuff seam. The cuff of the glove is then grasped against the sleeve with the thumb and forefinger, which are inside the sleeve. The upper edge of the glove cuff is grasped with the sleeve-covered fingers of the opposite hand, and the glove opening is pulled down completely over the gown cuff of the hand being gloved. If the glove is being placed on the left hand, the glove cuff and the stockinette cuff are grasped with the right hand, and both the cuff and the glove are pulled on at the same time. With the gloved hand the other glove is now picked up, and the same procedure is followed for gloving the other hand. Using this technique, the gloves are never touched with the bare hands.

Arranging the preparation table. A small preparation table should be arranged to provide all the necessary solutions and supplies for preparing the skin and giving local anesthetic. These will include

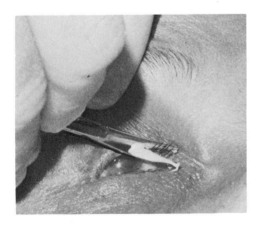

Fig. 28-3 Cutting eyelashes.

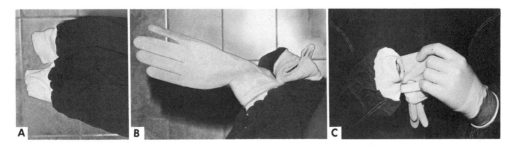

Fig. 28-4 Closed gloving technique.

antiseptic solutions, irrigation solutions, applicators, gauze, and local anesthetic solutions, as well as suitable syringes and needles. It is desirable that the sterile table be kept separate from the main instrument table and be removed once the eye and eyelid have been prepared.

Arranging the back table. The back table should be laid out in a definite order of use to provide necessary towels, gowns, and gloves for the surgeons, as well as drapes for the patient. Supplies such as gauze and applicators should be placed here. The back table should include basins for solutions and basins for waste, in addition to required syringes for mixing and drawing up special solutions. Care must always be taken that solutions are never mixed or confused. Instruments will be placed on the back of the table, leaving work space in front. Additional instruments that are seldom used but occasionally required may remain on the back table and not be transferred to the instrument, or Mayo, stand.

Arranging the instrument stand. (Fig. 28-5) The instrument, or Mayo, stand should be arranged according to a consistent pattern. Forceps will be placed in one area, scissors in another, and needle drivers in still another area. Irrigating solutions, applicators, gauze, and so on will have their own place on the instrument stand.

Most ophthalmic surgical procedures can be classified in two main sections: (1) intraocular, which includes cataract extractions, corneal transplants, and corneal or scleral lacerations, and (2) extraocular, which includes correction of strabismus and eyelid surgery. Each surgeon uses different instruments that he or she is comfortable with.

Instruments for basic intraocular set

1 right and 1 left corneal section scissors
1 pair Stevens scissors, curved
1 pair spring scissors
1 superblade or diamond blade
1 pair iris scissors
1 pair Vannas scissors
1 straight and 1 angled fixation forceps (0.12 teeth)
2 fine-tying forceps
1 anterior chamber irrigating cannula
1 Sinskey hook
1 eye speculum
2 straight and 2 curved fine hemostats

1 muscle hook
1 iris spatula
1 synechia spatula or cyclodialysis spatula
1 lens loop
2 needle drivers, finely curved
1 Kalt needle driver
3 anterior chamber irrigating tips (19, 27, and 30 gauge)
1 irrigating cannula
Series of irrigating aspiration probes
Series of phacoemulsification tips and handpieces
Cautery cord and tip
1 Hershman spatula
1 intraocular lens-holding forceps

Instruments for extraocular procedures

1 No. 3 Bard-Parker knife handle
1 pair Stevens scissors
1 pair spring scissors
1 straight and 1 angled fixation forceps
1 double-pronged scleral forceps
2 muscle hooks
1 caliper
1 right and 1 left muscle clamp
2 straight and 2 curved fine hemostats
2 towel clips
2 skin hooks, fine
1 anterior chamber irrigating tip, 19 gauge
1 speculum

Special instruments for procedures such as intraocular lens implants, corneal transplants, enucleation, and so on may be sterilized in separate packages and dispensed as necessary in addition to the basic instrument tray. This method avoids unnecessary handling and sterilization of instruments not needed for routine surgery. It applies specifically to the delicate, and expensive, microsurgical instruments.

Demagnetization. Poor and frustrating surgical technique may be brought about by magnetization of microsurgical instruments, which in turn will magnetize the fine needles commonly used today. This magnetization may occur in the operating room or may occur by exposure to larger surgical instruments while being sterilized with ethylene oxide. It is most frustrating to have to dislodge a fine needle from a needle driver during a critical point in a delicate eye operation.

A number of inexpensive demagnetizing instru-

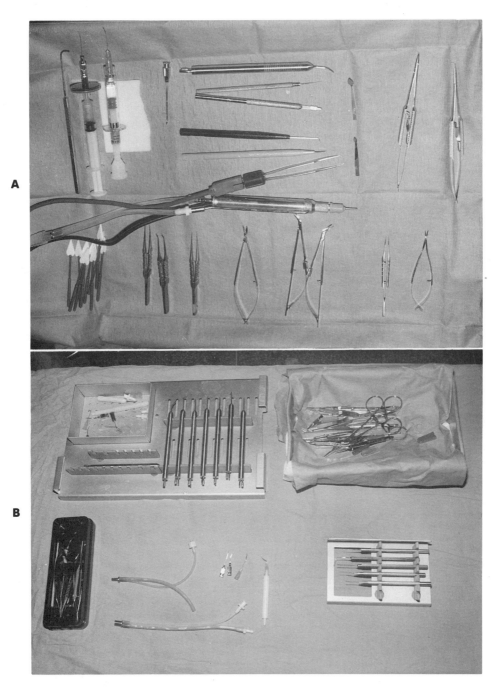

Fig. 28-5 A, Typical instrument table for intraocular surgery. **B,** Backup table for additional instruments.

ments are available for demagnetization of both instruments and needles (Fig. 28-6).

Diamond knives. The diamond blade is made from a gem-quality diamond, which is the hardest element known. Diamond knives are used in ocular surgery because of their extreme sharpness and ability to make a corneal or corneoscleral incision with ease and without tissue destruction. The use of diamond blades in radial or astigmatic keratotomy has been shown by electron microscopic examinations of the wound to be far superior to steel blades (Fig. 28-7, *A*). In radial keratotomy a guarded diamond knife is usually used. This extension of the knife may be measured by the caliper on the handle but should also be checked against a coin gauge (Fig. 28-7, *B*),

a ruler, or micronscope. Diamond knives used for cataract surgery are usually unguarded.

Because the edges of a diamond knife are extremely thin, they can be damaged easily and should never make contact with any metal or wood object. One must be careful not to chip or damage the edges because the sharpening of these knives is expensive.

To care for the diamond knife, one should use the following procedure.

1. Immediately after surgery, advance the knife blade sufficiently to be exposed, but not beyond the feet, and rinse thoroughly with sterile distilled water squirted with force through a syringe.

2. Visually examine the blade under a microscope for possible dirt or residue, which can be removed

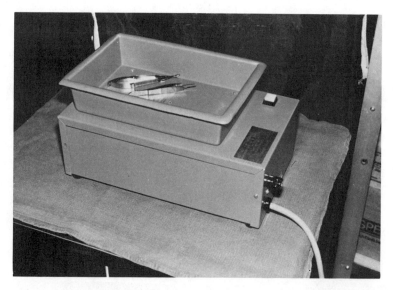

Fig. 28-6 Demagnetizing tray used to demagnetize microsurgical instruments and needles. (Courtesy Keeler/Diversatronics, Inc., Broomall, Penn.)

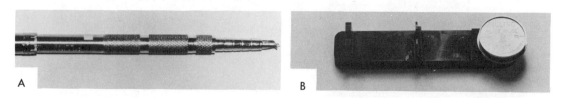

A

B

Fig. 28-7 A, Diamond knife with guarded handle. **B,** Coin gauge used to check calibration of the diamond knife.

by extending the diamond beyond the feet and lightly plunging the blade into Styrofoam. *Caution:* Cleaning should always be done by making fresh insertions into the Styrofoam. Never apply excessive side motion to the diamond. Rinse thoroughly.

3. Visually examine the blade under a microscope for any remaining dirt or residue. If there is residue, repeat steps 1 and 2.

4. Retract the diamond blade.

5. Proceed with any method of sterilization normally used; 275° F (135° C) as maximum temperature for 3 to 5 minutes is an acceptable sterilization method for diamond knives and coin gauges. Try not to let blood, tissue, or saline solution dry on the blade, which causes susceptibility to cracking and edge chipping when the blade is autoclaved. After extended use a film may be noted, and the diamond blade should be cleaned by immersing it in a pan of distilled water with one tablet of an enzyme cleaner used for contact lenses. This proteolytic enzyme cleaner will remove the protein that adheres to the surface of the diamond. Then rinse with distilled water and repeat the cleaning procedure.

Sapphire blade. The sapphire blade is made of crystal sapphire and is extremely sharp and delicate. Like the diamond blade, it is subject to chipping. The same requirements for cleaning with distilled water and an enzyme for film apply. Before the film develops, it may be appropriate to insert both the diamond blade and the sapphire blade into a wet sponge or fiberglass packing material. One should not expose the sapphire blade to ultrasound cleaning. It may be sterilized by means of steam autoclave, ethylene oxide gas, or dry heat.

Ruby blade. The ruby blade should be stored in a retracted position until it is used. Any wiping motion against the blade will dull the cutting edge. The blade should be flushed with distilled water squirted with force through a syringe. Blood, saline, or tissue should not be allowed to dry on the blade. The blade may be cleaned with contact lens enzyme cleaner. It also may be cleaned in an ultrasonic cleaner.

Special care of gem blades. The following procedure should be used to care for gem blades.

1. Always protect the tip of the blade and store it in a retracted position.

2. Use a rest when laying an extended blade on a Mayo stand.

3. Observe the blade under high magnification with retroillumination for cleanliness and chips.

4. Immediately after use, flush the blade with a steady stream of distilled water with a syringe and needle.

5. The surgeon may gently wipe the side of the blade with a wet merocel sponge.

6. Diamond and ruby blades can be cleaned after each use by ultrasound with hydrogen peroxide. Rinse thoroughly.

7. Clean baked-on protein:
- Expose blades as far as possible.
- Use a soft wet Styrofoam packing peanut. Stab the blade and work it through incisions for 20 to 30 seconds in the direction it is designed to cut.
- Rinse thoroughly with distilled water.

8. Inspect with a calibration scope.

9. Instruments should be dried immediately with a hot air blower. Blow drying removes excess moisture from hard to dry areas that are most susceptible to rust. It is a preferred method over towel drying because it prevents lint, keeps edges and tips sharp, and prevents accidental breakage or bending of delicate tips. Drying is not necessary if it is immediately followed by steam sterilization.

10. Avoid sudden hot or cold changes. Always allow the knife from the autoclave to cool in the air. Do not put in a basin of water if in a hurry, because blade damage can result.

Sutures. Sutures are available from the manufacturer in packets consisting of two parts: a primary packet enclosing the suture and a peel-apart overwrap enclosing the inner sterile packet. The inside packet is sterile as long as the overwrap remains intact and undamaged. The circulating nurse must deliver the sterile inner packet to the sterile field without touching it or permitting the inner packet to touch unsterile surfaces. The circulating nurse may use one of three methods to accomplish this:

1. The two flaps of the overwrap may be grasped between the thumbs and forefingers and peeled back to offer the packet to the scrub assistant, who may remove it with a sterile instrument (Fig. 28-8).

2. The inner packet may be flipped out onto the sterile table.

3. After the outer packet is opened, a transfer forceps may be used to place the inner packet on the instrument table.

The scrub assistant will then take the suture packet and open it. Many absorbable sutures contain a preservative, which must be carefully rinsed before the suture can be used. The suture should then be laid out on the tray in preparation for use.

Types of ophthalmic sutures. Ophthalmic sutures are made of a variety of materials, each material having specific advantages that can be chosen and tailored to the individual surgeon's likes (Table 28-2). The broad categories include the following:

1. *Plain surgical gut,* commonly referred to as *plain catgut,* a term believed to have originated from the Arabic word "kitgut" or "kitstring," signifying a fiddle string. The Arabian dancing masters used a three-string violin called a *kit,* and ancient instrument makers created these strings from the intestines

of a variety of animals. This material is absorbable. It eliminates the need for suture removal, which is of prime importance in children and uncooperative individuals. The disadvantages are, in time, variability of loss of tensile strength, as well as on absorption, an increased tendency to neovascularization, and some reaction to the material with granuloma formation.

2. *Chromic surgical gut,* which is gut that is chromicized to retard the tensile strength loss and lengthen the time of absorption. The disadvantage is that, like any natural suture, it causes some moderate tissue reaction.

3. *Vicryl* or *Dexon,* a synthetic suture that is absorbable, has strong tensile strength, elicits less tissue reaction than gut, and provides excellent knot security. Because of the hydrolytic absorption process, it is more predictable in terms of tensile strength retention and absorption than are the natural absorbable sutures. There is significant absorption in 30 days and maximum absorption in 60 to 90 days. These synthetic absorbable sutures, in sizes 4/0 through 8/0, are of a braided construction to maximize the handling properties. To further improve the passage through tissue and knot-tying characteristics, an absorbable coating has been added to Vicryl sutures. The coating affects neither the absorption nor the degree of tissue reactivity elicited by the suture.

4. *Nylon,* a synthetic monofilament suture commonly used in anterior segment ophthalmic surgery. It maintains its tensile strength and does not irritate the tissues or support bacterial growth. The suture degrades, however, losing approximately 10% to 15% of its strength yearly and is more difficult to

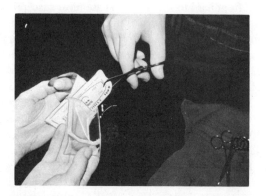

Fig. 28-8 Removing suture from sterile packet.

Table 28-2   Origin of suture materials used in ophthalmology

Suture	Raw materials
Surgical silk	Raw silk spun by silkworm
Catgut (plain or chromic)	Submucosa of sheep intestine or serosa of beef intestine
Collagen (plain or chromic)	Flexor tendon of beef
Nylon	Polymeric amide derived by chemical synthesis
Mersilene (polyester fiber)	Polymer of terephthalic acid and polyethylene

tie than silk. It is available in a variety of sizes for ophthalmic use (Fig. 28-9).

5. *Silk,* a natural protein material derived from the silkworm but treated with resins and waxes. This handles the best of all sutures and has excellent knot-tying security. It evokes a slight tissue reaction.

6. *Polypropylene* (Prolene), a strong, inert suture that ties well and does not degrade with time. This suture causes minimal inflammatory reaction, is not absorbed, and is not subject to biodegradation or weakening by the actions of tissue enzyme. Because of its relative biologic inertness, there are no known contraindications. This suture is pigmented with copper phthalocyanine blue. It has more elongation than nylon, and because of its hydrophobic nature and inertness in the eye it has become increasingly useful in suturing intraocular lenses and in iris repair surgery, as well as in anterior segment wound closure.

7. *PDS* (Polydioxanone) suture, a monofilament absorbable suture for corneoscleral closure. Wound-holding tensile strength is 56 days. The monofilament nature of this suture allows for easy passage through ocular tissue. Available in size 9/0, it is attached to a wide range of fine ophthalmic needles.

8. *Mersilene* polyester fiber suture, a monofilament polyester suture for corneoscleral closure. This suture is nonbiodegradable and has 50% more tensile strength than nylon suture. Mersilene suture is 20% less elastic than nylon; therefore it is said to create less suture-induced astigmatism. Available in size 10/0, it is attached to a wide range of fine ophthalmic needles.

Suture evaluation. Uniform standards are required in sutures for microsurgery. The *needles* should be sharp and should not dull easily with repeated passage. They must be securely swaged onto the suture. The *appearance* is important because colored sutures are more easily seen. The suture should be reasonably *pliable* to permit ease of handling. The *tensile strength* should be adequate for the area and should not crack or break with normal handling. The *pull-through* effect should be smooth and should not drag tissue. *Tying* should be performed simply. The knots should remain secure and the suture should not *fray.*

Postoperatively the knots should remain secure. There should not be a marked reaction to the suture, although a minimal reaction may accelerate wound healing. With absorbable sutures, the absorption time should be sufficient to maintain closure until wound healing is secure.

Ophthalmic needles. Needles have a variety of shapes, points, and curvature, each designed to perform a special task and each related to the type of material that the suture will be required to track through.

Preparing the patient's eyelids. In ophthalmic surgery, skin antiseptic agents should be carefully applied, beginning at the lash margin and carefully including the lashes (Fig. 28-10). Ophthalmic personnel should avoid having any of the solution enter the eye. A dry applicator is preferred for skin prep-

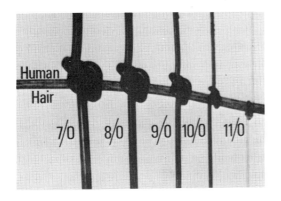

Fig. 28-9 Comparison of sizes 7/0 to 11/0 nylon suture with the human hair. (Courtesy Ethicon, Inc.)

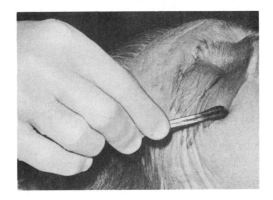

Fig. 28-10 Preparing skin of the surgical patient.

aration. Beginning in increasing circles from the eyelid margin, a large area above the eye is prepared. Special care must be taken that the eyebrow and underlying skin be adequately prepared with the antiseptic solution. The eye should then be flushed with saline or self-sterilizing aqueous antiseptic solution by use of an irrigating bulb or an Asepto syringe.

Draping the patient. A large folded sheet is used to cover the patient's body. The head is commonly draped with a double-thickness sheet or double towels. An eye sheet, preferably with a small opening, or a disposable eye sheet is then placed over the operative site.

AMORIC ENVIRONMENT

The room for operating must be amoric (Greek *a* means no; *morion* means particle). This term was coined by Jose Barraquer to indicate that particular matter can be as devastating to the visual performance of an eye as infected material. To obtain this amoric environment it is ideal if the operating room is limited to eye surgery only and the room has positive pressure. The number of personnel in the operating room should be minimized, as well as movements in and out. All talcum powder should be eliminated. All cotton balls should be eliminated. All syringes, cannulas, needles, and Petri dishes should be washed at least five times. Ideally, Millipore filters should be used for any solution irrigated into the anterior chamber. A lint-free type of drapes, such as plastic or paper, should be used. Instrument tips must be examined under the microscope and, if particulate matter is present, cleaned with a lint-free wipe. After any instrument has been used, it should be rinsed in saline and wiped well.

CARE AND HANDLING OF SURGICAL INSTRUMENTS

Manufacturers of quality stainless steel instruments (both in the United States and in Germany) have always done their best to produce surgical instruments that are extremely resistant to rust or corrosion. The stainless alloys that are used in the manufacturing are subject to strict industry and government standards. Their composition may vary to enhance certain desired qualities in the final product;

for instance, to guarantee an extra hard cutting edge in scissors, the manufacturer will select a type of stainless steel that contains a higher percentage of carbon molecules, thus making the steel extra hard after hardening and tempering. For some eye instruments that need to be nonmagnetic, in which hardness is not of prime importance, the stainless steel selected will contain little carbon and more chromium and nickel. As a general rule, the more carbon content, the harder the steel can be made by the instrument maker. However, it is exactly the carbon content of the stainless steel that can later present a corrosion or rusting problem if the instrument was not properly manufactured or is improperly used by the consumer.

To increase its corrosion resistance, a properly manufactured surgical instrument will have passed through two special processing steps. The first of these steps is called *passivation*. The instrument is treated with an electrochemical process to thoroughly clean its surfaces, thereby reducing its tendency to corrode. The same process can be achieved through a bath in a heated aqueous solution of 30% nitric acid.

The second special processing step is polishing. Polishing creates an extremely smooth surface that removes areas of possible corrosive action. It actually builds a fine layer of chromium oxide on the instrument. This chromium oxide layer is highly resistant to corrosion and will actually continue to build up with regular handling and sterilizing of the item. Naturally, improper cleaning and handling may cause this layer to become damaged or disappear, thus increasing the possibility of corrosion problems.

Surfaces that cannot be effectively polished, such as knurled or serrated handles and glare-reducing satin finishes, are more prone to corrosive attack. Because this corrosion does not penetrate deeply, it may be removed by scrubbing with a brush or detergent. As an alternative, the instrument can be returned to new condition by passivation and repolishing by the manufacturer or a professional instrument repair service.

Use of shortcuts in instrument care can lead to rust, corrosion, stains, and spotting. Corrosion, the gradual wearing away of material, eventually will impair the function of an instrument. The most common causes are linked to (1) inadequate cleaning and drying after use, (2) corrosive chemicals or sterilizing solutions, (3) use of ordinary tap water rather than distilled or softened water in the cleaning process, (4) laundry detergent residue remaining in operating room linens, (5) harsh detergents, and (6) a malfunctioning autoclave.

Cleanliness, lubrication, and correct handling and storage procedures will ensure an instrument's proper performance. In addition, inspection, troubleshooting, and a professional instrument maintenance program can actually lengthen the serviceable life of surgical instruments. To that end, the following instrument care habits are recommended.

Rust

If the problem is one of real rust (which is rare), it is necessary to determine whether the rust originated from the instrument itself or whether the rust was transferred from another source. To check whether the item itself is rusting, a pencil eraser is used to remove the rust; then the surface beneath the rust is checked to see if it is pitted. A pitted and rusting instrument must be taken out of a set of instruments immediately because it can cause a rust problem for the entire set. The item is returned to the manufacturer (provided it is not too old), and in many cases, the manufacturer will replace it at no charge.

If the instrument is not actually rusting but shows some rust deposits, it must be refinished by the manufacturer or a competent repair facility. An attempt should then be made to find the source of the rust. There are several possibilities, the most common one being that one or more instruments in the set are rusting because they are old and of the chrome or nickle-plated type. When this plating wears off through use or sharpening, the carbon steel below it becomes exposed and is subject to immediate corrosion during autoclaving or immersing in cold sterilization solutions.

Inexpensive instruments sometimes rust because they have not undergone the passivation process; thus the surfaces will contain carbon molecules. High-quality stainless steel instruments will pass certain tests (boiling, copper sulfate), whereas some of the lesser-grade instruments will not. It is these that can cause a problem. The fact that these instruments were stamped "stainless" will not always guarantee that they were made corrosion resistant by the manufacturer. The buyer must be aware of this.

Another source of rust can be the water used in the autoclave. It is recommended that a distilled, deionized water be used because this has been stripped of all minerals and metals. Please note that distilled water alone may not be pure enough, because many marketed distilled waters still contain many essential minerals for plant growth or human consumption. These minerals will sometimes tend to stain the instrument. Thus deionized distilled water is best.

How to avoid a stained appearance

Stains are deposited onto the instrument's surface, plated on, or in the case of rusting, develop from the instrument itself. The most common discoloration is a result of deposit stains, and these commonly occur during autoclaving. Instrument stains appear in a variety of colors and in most cases the colors can depict the origin of the stain.

Brown/orange stain. The most common stain is also the one that is the most often mistaken for rust. After erasing the stain with an eraser, which usually is not difficult, the ophthalmic assistant should check the surface of the instrument for porous signs (pits). If none are found under the stained area (usually the instrument surface will be smooth), proceed to locate the cause of the staining.

With the brown/orange stain, the problem is most often a phosphate layer (brown to light orange) on the instrument, which develops as a result of the following causes:

1. *Detergents used to wash and clean instruments.* Many of the detergents sold are highly alkaline and contain polyphosphates that aid in the breaking down of fats and blood. Hands are also left softer after prolonged use. However, it is this high alkaline content that develops the brown or orange stain during the autoclave cycle. The best detergents for instrument washing are those that are neutral pH 7 (on a pH scale of 0 to 14). They are available from hospitals and surgical suppliers

and do not cost much more than regular detergents. Also, often the instruments are not rinsed long enough to neutralize the detergents. A thorough rinsing will ensure that the detergent is no longer on the instrument.

2. *Water source*. Traces of minerals or metals (or both) may be contained in the tap water in a particular geographic area. The best way to check whether the water is the cause of the staining is to take a clean (or new) instrument that has no staining on it, wash it thoroughly in distilled deionized water with neutral pH detergent, rinse it thoroughly in distilled deionized water, and put it through a sterilization cycle. Follow the same procedure with another clean instrument, but this time wash and rinse with tap water. If the second instrument shows staining, it could reasonably be assumed that the tap water contains elements that stain the instrument. If both instruments still show stains, then a check of the autoclave will be necessary. In this case, clean the autoclave according to manufacturer's instructions, and also run one or two cleaning cycles with a recommended cleaner.

3. *Dried blood*. This usually results in a dark-brown stain that can be rubbed off. Blood should be removed from the instrument surface as soon as possible because it will break down the surface by chemical reaction.

4. *Surgical wrappings*. If the laundry uses too much detergent or detergents that contain a lot of phosphates (which are the less expensive ones available), surgical wrappings may contain enough remaining detergents to cause a reaction during autoclaving. A tell-tale sign is the brown stain on the towel (the outline of the instrument in an orange stain on the towel may even be visible). This type of stain is difficult to remove, and many times the instrument will have to be refinished by the manufacturer.

5. *Cold-sterilization solutions*. Many times, these are high in pH (like detergents), and need to be rinsed off thoroughly before storing instruments or before autoclaving.

6. *Foreign matter inside steam pipes*. Rust-colored film is particularly prevalent in new hospitals as a result of foreign matter inside steam pipes during installation. Unfortunately, nothing can be done, but the situation is only temporary.

Light- and dark-colored spots. Light- and dark-colored spots are caused by the slow evaporation of condensation of instruments. Traced to mineral residue, such spots can be prevented by following the autoclave manufacturer's directions carefully and using distilled or demineralized water for all cleaning procedures and solution preparation.

Purplish-black stains. Purplish-black stains indicate exposure to ammonia; thorough rinsing after use and cleaning in the usual manner should eliminate this stain.

Bluish-black stains. These are usually a result of plating and are extremely hard to remove from the instrument's surface. The surface beneath the stain is always smooth, but the instrument may have to be refinished by the manufacturer to obtain good results. The cause for this staining is mixing of dissimilar metals in ultrasonic cleaners and during autoclaving.

Multicolor stains. These are caused mostly by excessive heat (chromium oxide stains) and actually show rainbow colors with a blue or brown overtone. When the instrument shows these heat stains, it may have lost part of the original hardness and may not perform as well (especially in scissors, which need the extra hardness on their edges for cutting performance). Such instruments usually can be refinished by the manufacturer, and the hardness can be tested. The staining can be polished off.

Black stains. The most common black stains are caused by an acid reaction. The eraser will minimize the stain, but the surface beneath will remain slightly rougher than that of a normal instrument. Black stains may result from the detergents used. Similar to the brown stain caused by high pH in detergents, the black acid–type stain can be caused by low pH (less than 6) during autoclaving. The autoclaving temperature and pressure magnify the chemical effects of acid on steel many times, so the neutrality of the pH in the autoclave environment is of great importance.

Bluish-gray stains. Bluish-gray stains are indicative of cold sterilizing solutions. Following a manufacturer's directions explicitly will remedy the solution.

•   •   •

As described, stains are deposited onto the instrument surface, plated onto it, or in the case of rusting, develop from the instrument itself.

The most common discoloration results from deposit stains that commonly occur during autoclaving. To minimize such staining, it is important that the autoclave run perfectly and that it have a well-functioning drying cycle. The instruments should come out bone dry, whether in wrappers or loose on a tray. If any moisture is left in the pack or on the instruments, it will result in tiny water droplets that will leave a circular stain on the instrument surface after drying.

An interesting fact in regard to plating stains, or the stains that are a result of metal deposits, is that the area of staining is always near the most magnetic parts of the instrument. New instruments are often highly magnetic in the locks, serrations, and ratchets because the carbon steel tools used to work on the instruments during production are highly magnetic themselves. This magnetism wears off gradually during handling and sterilization. This is the reason the newer instruments tend to stain more visibly, thus causing the complaint that new instruments are showing stains but not the old ones.

If there is any suspicion as to what might cause a staining problem, one clean instrument should be processed in the manner that is suspected of causing the problem and then autoclaved. A control instrument should then be processed, which of course must be clean, by washing and rinsing it in distilled and deionized water only. This instrument should process without problems, whereas the first instrument will show the stain. All types of stains can be tested for in this manner, including water, detergent, wrapping, and cold sterilization solution left on the instrument.

Meticulous care during surgery will also prolong the life of surgical instruments. Although blood and saline are the most common causes of corrosion and pitting, instrument contact with the following solutions should be avoided if possible:

Aluminum chloride
Barium chloride
Carbolic acid
Chlorinated lime
Dakin's solution
Ferrous chloride
Lysol
Mercury bichloride
Mercury salts
Phenol
Potassium permaganate
Potassium thiocyanate
Sodium hypochlorite
Stannous chloride
Tartaric acid

Exposure to the following solutions is extremely detrimental:

Aqua regia (a mixture of nitric and hydrochloric acids)
Ferric chloride
Diluted sulfuric acid
Hydrochloric acid
Iodine (not to exceed 1 hour)

Another point to consider is that instrument counts guard both patients and instruments and reduce the instrument's chance of an unnecessary trip to the laundry.

Steps in cleaning and sterilization

Cleaning. All instruments should be thoroughly cleaned immediately after use. Blood or debris should never be allowed to dry on the instruments. Baked-on blood in a box lock or crevice can result in corrosion and subsequent cracking under stress. Therefore box locks should be opened, and instruments with removable parts should be disassembled.

Cleaning solutions with a neutral pH level (7.0 to 8.5) are recommended. An extremely alkaline detergent (higher than 9.0) may stain and might cause breaks, and an extremely acid detergent (lower than 6.0) may cause an instrument to pit.

After cleaning, the instruments should be dried quickly to avoid water stains. Of course, if they are to be autoclaved immediately, it is not necessary to dry them first.

Washer-sterilizers are ideally suited for washing

and terminally sterilizing soiled instruments. However, it is imperative that the sterilizer itself be clean and functioning properly. Hospitals in hard-water areas should implement a water-softening or demineralizing system. Surgical wrappings must be free of any laundry detergent residue.

A helpful machine is the ultrasonic cleaner. For most offices, the medium-sized unit, 10 inches by 4 inches (6 to 8 inches deep) is usually adequate (Fig. 28-11). Ultrasound is a form of acoustic vibration occurring at frequencies too high to be perceived by the human ear, usually above 20,000 Hz (20,000 cyles per second). Ultrasonic cleaning uses acoustic vibration at high frequencies through a liquid medium. The vibration of the fluid is so rapid that it forms bubbles. This process is known as *cavitation*. The bubbles "adhere" to and collapse on the surfaces of instruments, causing the foreign matter on the surface to be dislodged gently but totally. Millions of microscopic bubbles or "vacuum cleaners," therefore, dislodge the foreign matter from the surfaces, blind holes, pores, tight joints, and places that cannot be reached by lengthy soaking and scrubbing. Ultrasonic cleaning accomplishes this in minutes and is so gentle it will not etch glass. The instruments are thoroughly cleaned and ready for sterilization, eliminating the possibility of "disinfected dirt." The minivacuum created by the exploding bubbles removes up to 90% of all foreign matter from the instrument, particularly in the hard-to-reach areas, like the box locks, scissor locks, and other crevicelike areas.

Although an ultrasonic cleaner removes up to 90% of the soil, it does not preempt the need for sterilization. *Caution: Microsurgical instruments must not come in contact with one another during ultrasonic cleaning.* The unit's vibrations may cause premature wear on their precision tips.

Lubrication. Ultrasonic cleaners remove all lubrication from instruments; therefore all clean instruments should be bathed in instrument milk or a similar product after ultrasonic cleaning. Instruments should be lubricated after every five procedures. It is also recommended that instruments be lubricated after every cleaning process to guard against mineral deposits and other water-system impurities that can lead to stains, rust, and corrosion. Also, previous vigorous cleaning removes all lubrication and may result in "frozen" lock boxes. To impede the growth of bacteria in the lubricant wash, only antimicrobial water-soluble lubricants are recommended. The manufacturer's instructions should be followed carefully.

Inspection. In addition to being completely clean and free-moving to ensure proper function and sterilization, instruments must be inspected before packaging for reuse.

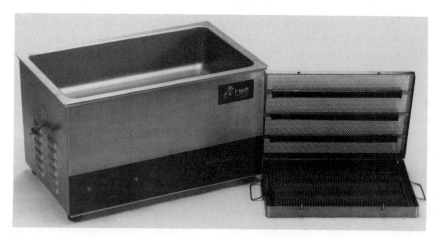

Fig. 28-11 Ultrasonic cleaning system designed for small eye instrument trays. (Courtesy I-Tech Industries, Addison, Ill.)

Hinged instruments should be inspected for alignment of jaws, meshing of teeth, and stiff or cracked joints. Ratchets should close easily and firmly. To test ratchets, clamp the instrument on the first tooth. Holding the instrument at the box, tap the ratchet end against a solid object. Repair is required if the instrument springs open. Close instrument to test its tension; when jaws touch, a space of $\frac{1}{16}$ inch to $\frac{1}{18}$ inch should exist between the ratchet teeth of each shank.

Ring-handled instruments can be tested by holding one handle in each hand. Open the instrument and try to wiggle it. If the box lock is loose, jaw misalignment will occur.

Large scissors should cut four layers of gauze at the tip of the blade. Smaller scissors (less than 4 inches in overall length) should cut at least two gauze layers. Blades should be inspected for burs.

If a needle that is clamped in the jaws of a needle holder locked on the second ratchet tooth can easily be turned by hand, the instrument should be tagged for repair.

Finally, elevated heat temperatures weaken stress points and can actually change molecular structures of the metal. This change weakens and dulls instruments, resulting in their continual diminished performance. Be on the lookout for weakened stress points.

Preparing a set of instruments. Instruments made from differing alloys should be sterilized separately. Place all sharps (such as scissors, knives, skin hooks) individually, so that they do not touch each other at the sharp areas during autoclaving. The tips of sharps can be protected with either small corks or tygon tubing that can be slipped over the area. Cotton or gauze also can be used to protect some of the smaller instruments. Special trays are available to keep small and microinstruments in place, so that they cannot move during autoclaving or storage. An extra towel can be folded to a strip and wound around the critical areas of several cutting instruments in a set.

Make sure that all instruments are in an open position. Instruments autoclaved in a closed position (especially those with ratchet locking devices) may spring the box lock because of the increased tension during the heat and pressure in the autoclave. Also,

in cases of metal-to-metal contact in a closed instrument, such as near the tips and the ratchets, make sure that the steam reaches these areas. Otherwise, the instruments may not be sterile.

Do not overload trays. Try to standardize with as few instruments as are commonly used in the particular procedure, and keep all other instruments set up separately to be available as they are required. Overloading causes unnecessary handling and sterilization, which not only creates extra work but also shortens the life of the instrument.

Sterilization. Sterilization is the complete destruction of all microorganisms within or about an object. Articles are either *sterile* or *unsterile;* there is no middle ground. Essentially, sterilization is accomplished by subjecting all material to either physical or chemical treatment to destroy all microorganisms. Careful sterilization must be carried out not only to avoid infection of wounds but to prevent the transmission of organisms from patient to patient. The bacterial spore is the most stubborn of all living organisms in its capacity to withstand destruction. Therefore standards of effectiveness of sterilization are based on the destruction of these bacterial spores.

The following methods are most commonly used in ophthalmology for sterilizing instruments and material:

1. Boiling
2. Dry heat (hot oven)
3. Moist heat (autoclave)
4. Chemical disinfectants (germicides)
5. Gas
6. Radiation
7. Ultraviolet

Boiling. By subjecting instruments to boiling water for 20 minutes, most microorganisms are destroyed. However, it may take several hours of boiling to kill some resistant spores and encapsulated bacteria. A timer should be available so that ineffective sterilization does not result from removing the instruments too early. Instruments with sharp points or blades rarely are boiled because this process dulls the cutting edges. Some instruments will rust after sterilization in boiling water if they are not properly dried or if they are allowed to remain in the water. It is important to use distilled water because this prevents minerals from precipitating on the instruments and walls of the sterilizer (Fig. 28-12). It is recommended that the water sterilizer be emptied, washed, rinsed well, and dried thoroughly at the end of each day.

Dry heat (oven). Several types of dry-heat ovens are available for the sterilization of instruments. Run by electricity, these ovens provide a constant and controlled amount of heat to instruments, drapes, gowns, and gloves for a given time. Temperature should be maintained at 320° F (160° C) for a period of 60 minutes. The disadvantage of this method is the long period of time required for the sterilization of instruments and packs (Fig. 28-13).

Moist heat (autoclave). The most common and practical form of sterilizing instruments is steam sterilization. The autoclave is designed to use steam under pressure in the destruction of microorganisms. Moist heat has a greater destructive effect on bacteria than heat alone (Fig. 28-14).

In autoclaving, the higher the temperature or pressure obtained, the shorter the time required to sterilize. For instance, instruments under 15 pounds of pressure at 250° F (121° C) are effectively sterilized in 15 minutes. Under the same pressure at 270° F (132° C), they are effectively sterilized in 3 minutes.

The time of effective sterilization varies with the type of material being autoclaved. For example, cloth (gauze) takes longer to sterilize than steel (instruments). Autoclaving may be used for a wide range of items of different materials, such as towels, sponges, rubber gloves, and masks. These items may be wrapped in special packages, and they will remain sterile for some time after removal from the autoclave.

When ovens and autoclaves are loaded, it is important to prepare all the packs and to arrange the instruments in a way that will permit proper permeation of the materials by the moisture and heat. Crowding must be avoided. All oil and grease must

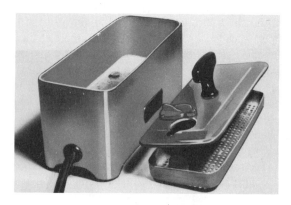

Fig. 28-12 Water sterilizer.

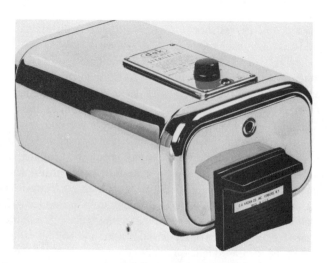

Fig. 28-13 Dry-heat oven.

be removed from instruments before autoclaving because steam will not penetrate through oil.

The autoclave has to be in good working order and operating perfectly in both steam and drying cycles. Commercially available autoclave tapes and chemical indicators may serve as controls to show that the autoclave is functioning properly.

Instruments loaded into the autoclave chamber should not be too cold, because they can cause steam condensation and staining. In some instances it may be advisable to heat the load (by using the drying cycle) to warm up the instruments before sterilization. This should be tried first whenever water stains are encountered after sterilization. Also, it is important not to open the chamber immediately after sterilization, but rather to crack the door for a few minutes (7 to 10 minutes, as per manufacturer's recommendations) while the drying cycle is on. In any case, the instruments should come out bone dry, without any condensation moisture anywhere in the packs. To minimize steam staining, only distilled, deionized water should be used in the autoclave. Also, all autoclaves should be flushed according to manufacturer's time schedules and recommendations. Iron, sodium, calcium, magnesium, or copper in hard water can cause spotting, staining, or corrosion to occur.

Chemical. Chemicals should be used when heat would dull the sharp cutting edges or would destroy the object to be sterilized (such as plastic). These chemicals that are used on instruments and plastics are called *germicides*. (Chemicals that are used on living tissues are called antiseptics.) The process of chemical sterilization with germicides is commonly referred to as *cold sterilization* (Fig. 28-15).

Cold sterilization (germicidal solution bath). Contrary to popular opinion, cold sterilization is not better for instruments than steam sterilization. Remember, with cold sterilization most professional offices leave the instrument in germicide for hours and even days at a time. Even though the germicides are only slightly corrosive, this extra long time of immersion takes its toll on the instrument surface. A short (20 to 30 minute) steam exposure is much less corrosive and also less dulling to sharp edges of scissors and knives than is long exposure to cold sterilization. Also, some of the cold sterilization solutions are either highly alkaline (high pH—more than 7), or

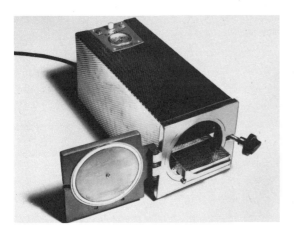

Fig. 28-14 Small autoclave.

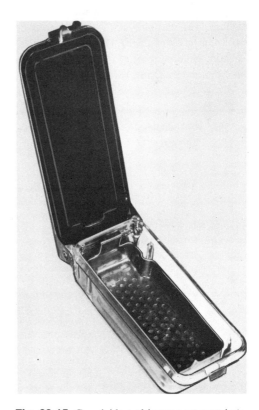

Fig. 28-15 Germicide and instrument container.

highly caustic (low pH—less than 7), and can cause staining and corrosion when autoclaved after a germicidal bath. Make sure to rinse the instruments thoroughly after taking them out of the germicidal bath. Do not leave instruments in the following solutions for extended periods, because corrosion can result: aluminum, barium, calcium, ferrous, or stannous chloride; phenol, lysol, or iodine; benzalkonium chloride (Zephiran); and any acid, mercury, or potassium solution.

The minimum time for chemical sterilization is 20 minutes. The pan in which the instruments are placed for sterilization should be padded with soft material to prevent the tips of the instruments from becoming damaged. In some of the commercial germicides, rust inhibitors are often added to prevent instruments from rusting. The following germicides are commonly used: (1) ethyl alcohol, 70%, (2) benzalkonium chloride (Zephiran), (3) mercury cyanide solution (1:1000), (4) formaldehyde germicides (Bard-Parker solution), (5) cetrimonium bromide (Cetavlon), (6) carbolic acid, (7) aqueous nitromersol solution (Metaphen), (8) phenol derivatives, (9) alkaline glutaraldehyde, (10) hydrochloride solution (sodium or calcium), (11) benzyl ammonium chloride (Germiphene), and (12) acetone (Table 28-3).

Gas and radiation. Ethylene oxide is an effective gas for sterilizing instruments and materials (Fig. 28-16). It is useful in sterilizing articles that would be damaged by heat or by exposure to strong liquid disinfectants. It is the method of choice in sterilizing intraocular lens implants. Some of the advantages of gas sterilization are that it (1) can be used on most materials, (2) can sterilize materials that cannot be sterilized by other means, (3) is effective against all organisms, and (4) achieves good penetration. The disadvantages of gas are that it is slow, costly, flammable, and toxic, and it requires special equipment.

Electron beam irradiation may be applied to articles completely sealed, such as sutures.

Acetone sterilization. Concentrated acetone is used by some practitioners for its rapid bacteriocidal effect. It has a 50-year track record and is inexpensive, readily available, and evaporates rapidly at room temperature, thus eliminating residual activity. Drs. Robert Drews and Jan Worst were the first to draw the attention of ophthalmologists to its disinfecting qualities in concentrated form. It is rapidly effective

Table 28-3   Advantages and disadvantages of germicides

Germicide	Advantages	Disadvantages
Ethyl alcohol	Good bactericidal and virucidal activity in the presence of protein; reduced toxicity; not harmful to instruments, lenses, or plastics; inexpensive	No sporicidal activity
Benzalkonium chloride (Zephiran)	Controversial bactericidal activity; low toxicity	Reduced bactericidal activity against *Proteus* and *Pseudomonas* organisms; no sporicidal activity
Phenol derivatives (Staphene)	Good bactericidal activity	Poor sporicidal activity; toxic
Alkaline glutaraldehyde (Cidex)	Good sporicidal and bactericidal activity in presence of protein; rapidly effective but instruments should be soaked 3-10 hours and rinsed well; low toxicity; not harmful to lensed instruments	Three hours required to kill some spores; before the product is effective, it must be activated with sodium bicarbonate
Benzyl ammonium chloride (Germiphene)	Rapid bactericidal activity within 30 seconds; no toxicity; not harmful to plastic, instruments, or rubber	Poor sporicidal activity

against bacteria, but it is only sporistatic rather than sporacidal against spores.

Acetone in 100% concentration may be used to disinfect instruments that have become contaminated in surgery. A 1-minute dip is sufficient for disinfection of minor surgical instruments for chalazions, foreign bodies, and eyelids. It should be remembered that acetone will not kill some spores and may not be effective against the virus of serum hepatitis. It is not nearly as reliable as autoclaving. Acetone will neither corrode instruments nor damage sharp edges. It will not pass biologic tests for sterility, but it is a practical effective solution for minor nonintraocular surgical procedures.

Alcohol disinfection. Like acetone, alcohol is rapidly effective against vegetative bacteria and mycobacteria. Its action against fungi (30 to 60 minutes) is slower, and virucidal activity is highly erratic. An ophthalmologist has to decide whether an item should be sterile or simply clean. If the item need only be clean, then the disinfection process of alcohol should destroy most microorganisms known to cause disease in that situation.

Effectiveness. To test the efficacy of sterilization methods, one may attempt to culture organisms from the instruments after obtaining what is considered proper sterilization. If any organisms are cultured, the method and solution used must be reevaluated. In standard tests, specific organisms may be placed in the sterilizing apparatus and cultures analyzed to test effectiveness.

Sterile packs. Many microsurgical instruments and supplies are provided as disposables in sterile packs. Single-use instruments such as blades, injection needles, trephines, and suture needles should conform to standards established and described in the manufacturer's promotional material.

A potential problem in shipping, storage, and use of sterile packs is the possibility of contamination or loss of sterility, or both. A sterile pack should contain an indicator to confirm maintained sterility and freedom from exposure to ambient air and possible contamination through cracks, tears, or perforations in packs sterilized by heat, ethylene oxide, or radiation.

OPERATING ROOM MICROSCOPE

Ophthalmic surgery has become microsurgery. The operating room microscope is the most important piece of equipment in ophthalmic surgery. Zeiss designed the first microscope so well that Zeiss operating microscope equipment is the kind most commonly used in operating rooms. Other brands such as Mueller, Olympus, Weck, and Wild are also available throughout North America, with minor improvements over the more common Zeiss equipment. An advantage of Zeiss microscopes is that they are interchangeable with existing components and accessories.

The modern operating room microscope supplies the surgeon with illumination, magnification, and controlled poisoning. Equipment is designed to minimize the clutter and to place it in the most accessible part of the operating room. Because of the magnification involved, a minimal amount of vibration is tolerated, and therefore heavy bases or ceiling

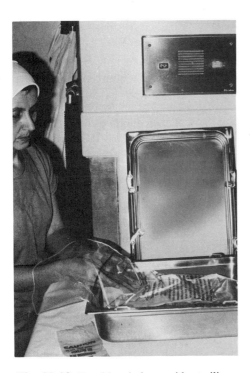

Fig. 28-16 Portable ethylene oxide sterilizer.

mounts are required. A lightweight microscope beside the table stand is inconvenient and commonly causes vibration that can be troublesome to the operating surgeon. Heavy-weighted instrument tables or ceiling mounts are preferred. Dr. David McIntyre has designed a combination microscope and chair that minimizes vibration to make the unit more compact. It is the same system that is used on the airplane *Orbis*.

The first Zeiss microscope was the Omni One, developed in 1956, and has been improved to create the currently used Omni Six S series. Its microscope provides motorized zoom and focus capability in a short body, in addition to zoom capability that allows greater magnification and fine focusing adjustments. Also available is a movement attachment in two planes called the *XY movement*, which provides smooth, controlled movement in repositioning the microscope. The oculars of the microscopes are usually $12.5 \times$ and may be increased to $16 \times$. The objective lens of the microscope, found under the microscope, should be suitable for a definite working distance that is compatible with the surgeon's requirements. The focal length of the objective can be interchangeable. Most surgeons use a 200 or 175 mm objective lens.

A number of accessories can be obtained for most microscopes. These include (1) observer systems, (2) accessory lights, (3) ultraviolet filter, (4) occluder filter, (5) accessory lights, (6) photo/video adapters, (7) XY coupling to include alignment and self-centering devices, (8) pupillary distance adjustment, (9) foot-control switch, (10) hand-control switch, (11) voice activation, and (12) Retrolux fit that will move the fixation beam so it is coaxial with the microscope light.

A beam splitter is required to provide accessories such as the observer system and the photo/video adapter. Additional lights may provide slit view or diffuse side lighting.

The microscope may be covered by (1) a microscope drape, (2) knob covers, or (3) light plastic sterile drapes.

Adjustment knob covers that can be readily sterilized between cases and applied at the beginning of the surgery are available from Zeiss.

Troubleshooting

Lamp failure. If the microscope lamp fails to go on at the outset or goes off during the procedure, it may not always be the bulb. The main power to the operating room may fail, of course. On the other hand, microscopes have fuses in a variety of locations. Replacement fuses should always be available. Microscope lamps may fail, and additional lamps must be available. Newer microscopes have a double system of lamps so that easy interchange into another box unit is possible. The personnel in the operating room should be familiar with the method of reinstituting the light in cases of failure.

Failure of the zoom operation. The zoom operation is powered by a small motor. This motor may become wet, in which case it may not function properly. As the microscope ages, it also may fail. Professional maintenance may be required.

Power focus. The most common failure of the Zeiss Omni Six S series of microscopes is jamming in the down position of the power focus. If this should occur, jiggling of the up focus switch while tapping on the microscope body may cause the clutch to engage. Again, professional maintenance is required.

Failure of foot switch. The foot switch may be dampened by balance salt that flows from the incision into the mechanisms of the foot control. Corrosive change may reach the electrical contacts, causing the foot switch to become unreliable and to perform intermittently. This requires professional servicing. Covering the foot controls in a light plastic bag will often prevent this problem.

Blurred image. Blurred images may occur if breath fogs the surface of the oculars. It may require skin taping of the mask to prevent breath from appearing from the upper portion of the mask. Blurring also may occur if eyelashes smear skin oil on the glass surface. Periodically, outer surfaces should be cleaned carefully with lens cleaner to prevent fogging. In humid rooms, moisture condensation may occur on the optical surface of the microscope.

Filters. Ultraviolet filters can be placed within the system of the microscope to impede ultraviolet from entering the eye. This is important because ultraviolet may have an injurious effect on the macular area. This is more important if there has been a break in the capsule. An eclipse filter is available that can be added to the microscope by turning a knob to bring it into position. This feature may be valuable in occluding light rays from entering the eye while suturing is occurring.

ETHICAL BEHAVIOR OF THE OPHTHALMIC ASSISTANT

1. Never betray a patient's confidence. During this trying period, patients may take you into their confidence and tell you details about their personal lives that they do not wish communicated to others.

2. You may learn things from observations, or from co-workers, that are highly private—for example, that someone wears a wig or a person's real age is revealed. These must be kept private.

3. Persons in public life, or well-known personalities, may come under your care and wish to remain anonymous.

4. Do not discuss any surgical case or complication of a patient with anyone outside the hospital environment.

5. Respect the confidence of your co-workers. If you cannot respect their abilities, do not gossip about them. Some of your co-workers may have personal problems that should not be relayed to others.

6. Develop a sense of loyalty to your co-workers.

7. Do not overstep the limits of your legal responsibility. There will be some restrictions placed on you in many areas, and these restrictions are for your own protection. The minute you overstep these limitations, you are placing yourself in legal jeopardy.

MEDICOLEGAL TIPS

1. Ensure the identification of the correct patient and the correct side for any surgical procedure.

2. Establish good rapport with the patient. The patient who likes the physician and the environment in which surgery is performed is less likely to sue. Some lawsuits evolve from a patient's vindictiveness even if the physician is not at fault. A practitioner whom the patient views as compassionate and understanding has already acquired some protection against legal actions.

3. Operative notes should be made soon after surgery, not weeks or months later.

4. Be sure there is a good consent form that is well-outlined to the patient. Effective personnel communication with the patient concerning risks, benefits, and alternatives is extremely valuable.

5. Maintain good records in the office and the hospital. The quality and legibility of one's records affect the quality of one's practice. It is important to attach to the records a log of telephone advice. Cursory, sloppy, or nonexistent notes call the practitioner's credibility and standards of practice into question. The physician should initial all laboratory and x-ray reports before they are filed.

QUESTIONS FOR REVIEW AND THOUGHT

1. In a 5-minute period identify as many errors as you can in Fig. 28-2.
2. What are some fears a patient may have who is admitted to the hospital for eye surgery?
3. What are some of the problems facing the almost-blind patient?
4. How should you go about orienting a partially blind patient who is admitted to the hospital?
5. Delicate handling of eye patients after intraocular surgery is important. Outline what measures you would take to ensure a smooth postoperative course.
6. What significant postoperative signs and symptoms should be brought to the attention of the ophthalmologist? After cataract surgery?
7. Outline a routine for postoperative care that cataract patients could follow after discharge from the hospital.
8. How would you prepare a child for strabismus surgery?
9. When should skin sutures be removed after a blepharoplasty?

10. What instructions should be given to a patient for a retinal detachment?
11. Describe the function and care of cataract instruments.
12. Describe the rationale for proper technique of scrubbing, gowning, gloving, preparation, and draping.
13. Outline the components of the operating microscope.

SELF-EVALUATION QUESTIONS

True-false statements

Directions: Indicate whether the statement is true (T) or false (F).

T or F   1. The hospital ophthalmic assistant is commonly a nurse.
T or F   2. Blind or partially sighted individuals should take the assistant's arm and follow.
T or F   3. Preoperative orientation is not a function of the hospital ophthalmic assistant.

Missing words

Directions: Write in the missing word in the following sentences.

4. An environment that is free of particles is called _____.
5. Sterilization of the operator's skin is called _____.
6. A technique of putting on gloves by not hand touching the cuffs of the gloves is called _____ glove technique.

Choice-completion questions

Directions: Select the one best answer in each case.

7. Which is not an alarming immediate postoperative sign after cataract surgery?
   a. Blood in the anterior chamber
   b. Severe pain
   c. Photophobia
   d. Pus in the anterior chamber
   e. Prolapse of the iris
8. Which is an incorrect postoperative instruction?
   a. Avoid heavy lifting
   b. Avoid straining at bowel movement
   c. Keep hands and face clean
   d. Avoid car rides
   e. Wear sunglasses outdoors
9. Which is not an error in surgical technique?
   a. Splashing the surgical gown
   b. Permitting hair to protrude from cap
   c. Cleaning nails in scrub sink before scrubbing
   d. Mask not covering the nose
   e. Leaving skip spots while scrubbing

ANSWERS, NOTES, AND EXPLANATIONS

1. **True.** Most often the nurse, when employed by a hospital or employed by the ophthalmologist, is the individual who assists in the care of eye patients. A nurse is usually the individual in the operating room who by training and experience can quickly learn the skills of assisting, aseptic technique, and microsurgery. At the bedside, the nurse can follow the progress of a patient, identify abnormal signs and symptoms, and report progress to the ophthalmologist. However, in many states someone who is not a nurse but who is well trained in these functions may accompany the ophthalmologist and assist with preoperative, operative, and postoperative care of the patients. In surgicenters, a trained layperson is taking on increasing importance in this role.

2. **True.** By taking the assistant's arm just below the elbow, the partially sighted individual will be protected from interfering objects in the pathway and also will be able to anticipate directional changes. In this way the person will feel a better sense of security in walking. A blind person should never be steered. The assistant should engage in conversation and provide information on the patient's surroundings.

3. **False.** No matter how well the patient has been oriented to any particular surgery by the office personnel of the ophthalmologist, the person is still apprehensive on the night before surgery. The evening before, the hospital ophthalmic assistant should review the routines that will occur before the surgery and the convalescent care that may be required. The patient should be given necessary cautions that are routine at the hospital. The patient should be forewarned as to what to expect from the type of anesthetic to be given, be it local, intravenous, or general.

4. **Amoric.** Creating an amoric or particle-free environment is as important as creating a sterile environment for ocular surgery. Fine particles of dust, debris, or powder can be devastating if they enter an eye.

5. **Scrubbing.** By vigorous scrubbing with a scrub brush soaked in antiseptic solution, the skin of the operator may be temporarily rendered safe. However, bacterial flora rapidly return to the skin within minutes, and so the skin does not remain sterile. However, pathogenic microorganisms will be permanently destroyed. Thus, whereas scrubbing does not produce sterility, it does produce a considerably decreased risk of transferring pathogenic organisms.

6. **Closed.** This is the most sterile way of putting on gloves. Here the hands enter the sleeves of the gown only down to the cuffs, and then the gloves are grasped with the sterile gown cuffs until the hands enter the gloves. The advantage of this technique is to minimize bacterial recovery on the scrubbed hands from the outside of the glove.

7. **c. Photophobia.** Generally, because of a traumatic iritis with cells on the anterior chamber, most eyes are light-sensitive after cataract surgery. A darkened room or sunglasses may be comforting for the first few days. A dilated pupil will often contribute to the photophobia.

8. **d. Avoid car rides.** As long as the driver is careful to avoid bumps and jars, there is no reason that an individual cannot ride in a car, go for walks, or lead a reasonably normal life during the postoperative period. Today's modern suturing techniques avoid the one major complication of wound rupturing with iris prolapse that was seen in the past. However, excessive straining can raise thoracic pressure and secondarily the venous return. This may give rise to intraocular hemorrhaging on relatively fragile vessels.

9. **c. Cleaning nails in scrub sink before scrubbing.** This is a correct and important part of achieving cleanliness before scrubbing. All of the other activities are serious breaks in surgical technique. For sterility and cleanliness attention must be paid to three participants in the operation: (a) the operator and assistants, (b) the patient, and (c) the instruments, drapes, and surgical accessories that are used. All must be carefully cleaned and sterilized or disinfected.

CHAPTER 29 Lasers in ophthalmology

E. R. SIMPSON

- Laser theory
- Pumping and spontaneous emission
- Stimulated emission
- Types of lasers and their clinical use
- Safety in the laser clinic
- Future applications of laser technology

Perhaps more than any other recent advance in medical science, the advent of laser technology has produced a major impact on clinical ophthalmology. The effect of solar radiation was well-known in ancient times; the first description of a central scotoma after a solar burn of the retina was reported in the mid-seventeenth century. Although Albert Einstein described the concept of stimulated emission of light in 1917, it was not until 1960 that the first laser was produced, by T.H. Maiman.

Medical applications of this new energy were explored at an early stage, but the first experiments were poorly controlled and commonly produced unsatisfactory results. Some of these early investigators used effects of the sun or the carbon arc to produce a lesion in the retina. In 1927 Maggiore focused sunlight on two eyes that were later enucleated. These eyes showed a significant reaction in the retina as a result of this focused energy. In 1949 Dr. Meyer-Schwickerath focused light from the sun through a rudimentary optical instrument and successfully photocoagulated the human retina with a retinal hole. In 1960, the first optical *laser*—standing for *l*ight *a*mplification by *s*timulated *e*mission of *r*adiation— as it was eventually called, was produced, which provided the ophthalmologist with an intense, pure beam of light that could produce extremely small burns of varying intensities. The use of the argon ion laser for the treatment of various retinal vascular diseases was first considered in 1965, and in 1971 clinical trials concerning the photocoagulation potential of the krypton laser, as well as the neodymium YAG laser, were begun and shortly thereafter, this equipment became available commercially.

Several external ocular growths were removed by a carbon dioxide laser in 1971. Various glaucoma conditions became treatable in 1973 with high-powered laser; and in the last 15 years the neodymium YAG laser has been used extensively to cut membranes and persistent capsular material in the human eye after cataract extraction. As an investigative tool, laser light is being used to treat sensitized malignant ocular tumors and to produce highly accurate incisions in corneal tissue to correct refractive errors.

LASER THEORY

A laser is a source of extremely intense monochromatic coherent light. The electromagnetic spectrum is composed of radiant energy that ranges from short cosmic waves (10 nm) to the longest radiowaves (1000 m). Laser light is basically the same as light from the sun or a household light bulb. It is formed by photons and, like any other form of light, is propagated in an electromagnetic wave form. In the visible portion of the electromagnetic spectrum, the radiation with the shortest wavelength is in the violet region. These wavelengths are in the region of 400 nm (nanometers; a nanometer is 1 millionth of a meter). The visible radiation with the longest wavelength is red light.

Red light waves may be up to 70 nm long. Lasers can produce light energy with wavelengths shorter than the visible spectrum (ultraviolet) or longer than the visible spectrum (infrared), each one causing different forms of tissue destruction in the eye (Fig. 29-1).

Three basic conditions must be met for most lasers to operate (Fig. 29-2).

1. There must be an active medium, that is, a material such as a gas or solid in which the atoms, molecules, or ions will emit optical radiation when properly stimulated.
2. There must be a suitable energy source that can pump the atoms, molecules, or ions in the active medium, producing the emission of photons of radiation.
3. There must be some form of optical feedback or gain, which usually is provided by mirrors or other reflecting surfaces in the laser's optical cavity.

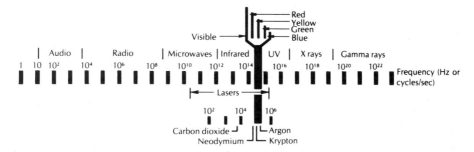

Fig. 29-1 Positions of lasers in the electromagnetic spectrum. (From L'Esperance FA Jr: *Ophthalmic lasers: photocoagulation, photoradiation, and surgery,* ed 3, St Louis, 1989, Mosby.)

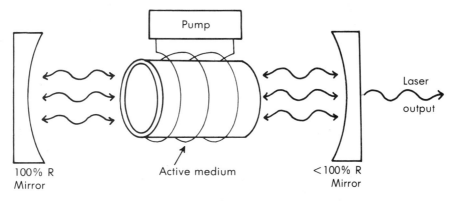

Fig. 29-2 Elementary laser scheme that illustrates the active medium within the optical resonant cavity formed by the mirrors and the pump, which creates a population inversion in the active medium. (From Steinert RF, Puliafito CA: *The Nd-YAG laser in ophthalmology: principles and clinical applications of photodisruption,* Philadelphia, 1985, WB Saunders Co.)

Argon, krypton, carbon dioxide, helium-neon, various liquids (dyes) and solids, such as neodymium supported by yttrium-aluminum-garnet (YAG), as well as many other types of semiconductors, are all in use as lasing media. The active medium in the neodymium YAG laser, for instance, consists of an insulating crystal fabricated from yttrium, aluminum, and garnet and doped with the rare earth neodymium (Nd) ion. The energy source used to pump or excite the neodymium ions is typically a quartz body or flashlamp for pulsed applications, or a direct current arc lamp when continuous laser output is desired. Optical gain is provided by placing mirrors at each end of the Nd YAG rod in this type of laser to reflect the light back and forth through the crystal. Alternatively, the ends of the laser rod can be coated with reflective material and thereby serve as the laser mirrors.

PUMPING AND SPONTANEOUS EMISSION

When photons of light from the pumping lamp collide with the active lasering medium, they often impart enough energy to raise some of their orbiting electrons to higher-than-usual energy levels. This is referred to as *optical pumping*. These electrons remain at the higher energy levels for varying periods of time, dropping back to lower energy levels randomly and spontaneously. When they drop from a higher to a lower level, they in turn emit energy in the form of photons of radiation. This phenomenon is called *spontaneous emission*. The wavelength of the radiation emitted depends on the difference in the potential energy of the two levels.

STIMULATED EMISSION

If a photon strikes an electron that is in a high (or pumped) energy level, the electron will instantaneously drop back to a lower energy level only if the triggering photon is of the same wavelength or frequency as the one that will be emitted when the electron falls to the lower energy level. When an electron is stimulated to give off a photon of radiation, the photon emitted will travel in exactly the same direction as the photon that triggered it. Therefore the laser light will be reflected back and forth

along the axis. In a short period of time, many identical photons will form in a standing wave (all of them in phase), producing coherent radiation. This standing wave, which has now become a beam of laser radiation, will continue to be amplified as it passes back and forth through the laser rod cavity between the two mirrors. This process is referred to as *stimulated emission*.

Spontaneous emission, therefore, occurs randomly without any need for external intervention, whereas stimulated emission occurs when an ion, in its excited state, interacts with a photon of the proper wavelength. To achieve release of the stimulated emission, one of the mirrors is made fully reflective and the other only partially reflective. The portion of the light wave striking the second mirror leaves the cavity as the emitted laser beam, and the reflectivity of the mirror is selected to satisfy the requirements for efficient application in a particular system of reflecting mirrors, which are then fitted to either a slit lamp or other delivery system.

TYPES OF LASERS AND THEIR CLINICAL USE

Each lasing medium produces a different wavelength with a selective absorption effect in tissue. Tunable dye lasers have been produced that are capable of providing a broad range of wavelengths and a wide range of tissue responses. The most powerful lasers generally are used in industrial applications; although such lasers may generate many kilowatts of energy, those used in medicine require much less, generally no more than 100 W.

Many factors other than power levels determine a laser's effectiveness as a medical instrument. The characteristics of both the target tissue and the laser source determine the biologic consequences of laser radiation. This fit, between the laser light and its target, is what allows for selective damage or alteration of ocular tissue. For example, red objects strongly absorb green or blue light but reflect most red light. Thus the argon laser, with its blue-green light, is used for many procedures that involve coagulating blood or sealing off blood vessels. In general, longer wavelengths penetrate tissue more deeply than do shorter wavelengths, and that is why krypton red laser light produces damage at a deeper level in tissue than argon green light. Carbon dioxide laser light, at 10,600 nm, is absorbed completely by water in tissue and is therefore effective in cutting tissue with a high water content. The medical lasers produce tissue damage by three basic mechanisms: thermal, ionizing (photodisruptive), and photochemical.

Thermal mechanism

The human eye transmits light between wavelengths of 380 and 1400 nm. In principle, light throughout this interval may be used to treat intraocular structures by delivery through the pupil. At wavelengths shorter than 380 nm, the ultraviolet-absorbing properties of the lens and cornea limit the exposure to the retina. At wavelengths longer than 1400 nm, water absorption sharply limits this transmission. Because laser light is monochromatic, highly columnated, and intense, and because the eye is an optically open system, laser irradiation is well-suited to produce thermal effects resulting in photocoagulation. When absorbed by tissue, laser light is transformed to heat energy, causing a thermal response.

Absorption of laser light is related to wavelength and absorption characteristics of the tissue. When light strikes a tissue surface, part of this light is reflected, part is absorbed by various cells or cell layers, and part is transmitted inward until the energy is depleted. The absorption of laser light depends on the chromophore content of the tissues. Tissue chromophores include hemoglobin (present in blood vessels), melanin (present in the retinal pigment epithelium, iris pigment, epithelium, uvea, and trabecular meshwork), and xanthophyll (present in the inner and outer plexiform layers of the retina in the macula) (Fig. 29-3). When these tissues absorb light, the light is transformed into heat energy, a thermal reaction occurs, and photocoagulation results with surrounding tissue destruction. Argon blue-green (composed primarily of the 488 and 514.5 nm emission lines), argon monochromatic green (514.5 nm), and krypton red (647 nm), are commonly employed in ocular photocoagulation to induce thermal effects. Krypton yellow (568 nm) and continuous wave and long-pulsed neodymium YAG (1064 nm) sources also have been used for thermal photocoagulation.

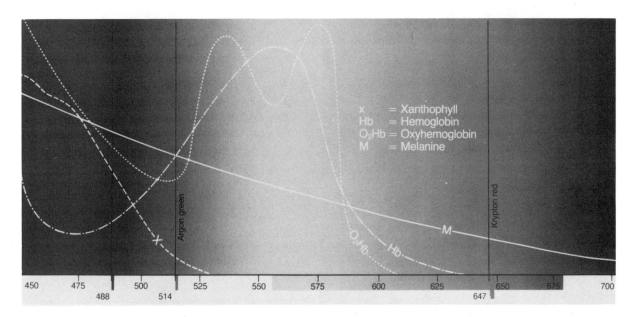

Fig. 29-3 Light wavelength absorption in certain tissue chromophores.

Thermal photocoagulation (Fig. 29-4) is used extensively in the treatment of diabetic retinopathy, branch or central retinal venous occlusion, retinal telangiectasia, closure of retinal holes, and certain varieties of localized retinal detachment without traction. Choroidal neovascular membranes (200 to 2500 nm from the center of the foveal avascular zone) also may be treated with thermal photocoagulation. The target ocular chromophores for producing the desired effects in this type of treatment are melanin in the retinal pigment epithelium and hemoglobin in the retinal and choroidal vessels. Central venous retinopathy with active leakage also can benefit from thermal photocoagulation.

Tunable dye laser systems (Fig. 29-5)

Although there is an advantage to a laser system that offers a wide selection of wavelengths to interact with different tissue chromophores in the eye, the absorption characteristics of melanin is the single most important consideration in applying laser energy to melanin-containing ocular tissue to produce a thermal effect.

Dye lasers, which have become important in treating vasculopathy in tissue of low melanin content, have permitted new approaches in treatment through photosensitization. In the anterior segment of the eye, thermal photocoagulation can be used to (1) produce an iridotomy in the treatment of angle-closure glaucoma, (2) improve trabecular meshwork function in the treatment of open-angle glaucoma (trabeculoplasty), and (3) produce alterations in pupil size and shape (iridoplasty).

Most of these procedures just take several minutes to perform under local anesthesia and usually require a contact lens to focus the energy in the desired

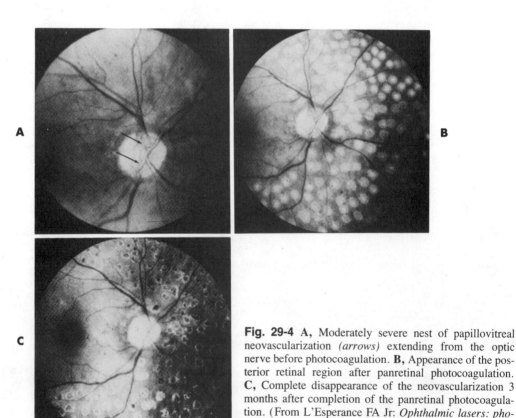

Fig. 29-4 A, Moderately severe nest of papillovitreal neovascularization *(arrows)* extending from the optic nerve before photocoagulation. **B,** Appearance of the posterior retinal region after panretinal photocoagulation. **C,** Complete disappearance of the neovascularization 3 months after completion of the panretinal photocoagulation. (From L'Esperance FA Jr: *Ophthalmic lasers: photocoagulation, photoradiation, and surgery,* ed 3, 1989, Mosby.)

location. Patients usually are seated during the procedure and most require topical anesthetic only. In some instances, where extensive procedures are required, retrobulbar anesthesia is accomplished so that the procedure is relatively pain-free.

Laser light from a carbon dioxide source is absorbed by water, and inasmuch as a high percentage of cellular content is water, this laser is effective in cutting tissue because it can be focused to vaporize cells in a very fine line. Its use in ophthalmology is reserved primarily for removal of skin lesions and production of fine skin incisions for various forms of lid surgery (Fig. 29-6). The neodymium YAG laser in a continuous waveform is only partially absorbed by hemoglobin or water and penetrates much more deeply than the argon laser. Although the neodymium YAG laser can be used for thermal photocoagulation, its main use employs the principle of photodisruption.

Diodes. Diode lasers that use gallium-arsenide plates to induce rapid electron transfer have been developed to induce thermal photocoagulation.

These systems are efficient and cost-effective but lack wavelength flexibility.

Photodisruptive (ionizing) mechanism

If the power of laser energy is released over an extremely short period of time (1-billionth or 1-quadrillionth of a second), tissue ionization or complete ablation results, giving rise to local intense heating and generation of mechanical and acoustic shock waves in tissue. This form of laser tissue destruction is known as *photodisruption* and can be accomplished by the neodymium YAG laser. The laser beam itself is invisible, having a wavelength of 1064 nm, and focusing is therefore accomplished by placing a red helium-neon laser in the beam path. The laser energy is "q switched" (quality switched) or "mode locked" and is delivered in a single pulse or train of pulses over an extremely short time interval of nanoseconds (q switched) or picoseconds (mode locked). The energy is supplied to the tissue so quickly that damage is produced by a microexplosion rather than by a heating effect, as in thermal pho-

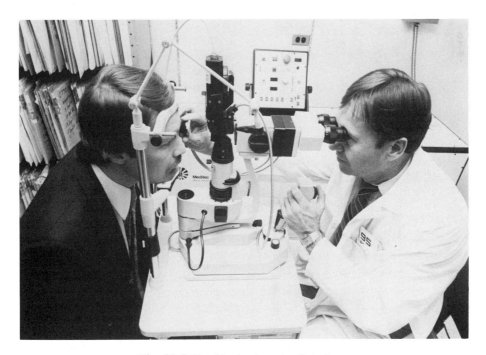

Fig. 29-5 Tunable dye laser in clinical use.

tocoagulation. It is critical that this laser be focused with extreme accuracy, with the minimum power and the minimum number of shots to achieve the desired effect. An appropriate contact lens usually is used because it forms part of the optical focusing system in the laser beam path. This improves accuracy and allows a higher power density, thus minimizing the total energy required to accomplish a given task such as opening a posterior capsule after cataract surgery (Fig. 29-7). Vision can be immediately improved as soon as the small opening is produced. Patients with thick capsules or secondary cataracts occasionally may be treated with this form of laser surgery. Cyclitic membranes that form after trauma to the eye, surgery, or uveitis occasionally can be treated in this manner. High laser energies usually are required, and generally it is safer to use multiple treatment sessions. Iridotomies for the treatment of angle-closure glaucoma are accomplished with this form of laser application. Infrared laser systems that use short pulses are being evaluated in a number of clinical settings, including the production of a fistula as a filtering mechanism in the treatment of glaucoma. Most of these procedures can be carried out with use of a topical anesthetic, as in the case of thermal photocoagulation. Occasionally, however, local anesthesia is required.

Photochemical mechanism

When certain wavelengths of laser light interact with a photosensitizing agent, the absorbed light energy is converted into a highly reactive oxidative process that can bring about cell death. Therapeutic use of laser-induced photochemical damage in ophthalmology has been limited. Recent attempts have been made to treat cancer in the eye by shining red laser light at a photosensitizing agent known as *hematoporphyrin derivative,* which is preferentially localized in cancerous eye tissue. Cancer cell death has been achieved by this form of therapy, although results remain preliminary.

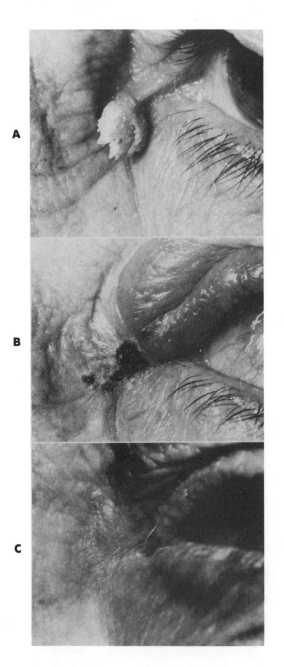

A

B

C

Fig. 29-6 A, Keratic growth near the inner canthus before CO_2 laser photovaporization. **B,** Appearance of the keratotic area immediately after CO_2 laser photovaporization. **C,** Appearance of the area of photovaporization of the keratotic growth three weeks after CO_2 laser photovaporization. (From L'Esperance FA Jr: *Ophthalmic lasers: photocoagulation, photoradiation, and surgery,* ed 3, 1989, Mosby.)

Photorefractive and phototherapeutic keratotomy

The development of short wavelength lasers called *excimer* (*exc*ited di*mer*) lasers, which can efficiently generate high-power ultraviolet light, has prompted the use of short-pulsed ultraviolet radiation for tissue destruction. Clinical trials currently are under way to establish the efficacy and safety of excimer corneal ablation for the correction of refractive errors and removal of superficial corneal scarring.

Pulsed 193-nm light is used to ablate a small amount of corneal stroma (30 to 100 μg) to induce corneal flattening in a spherical or cylindric manner. Early results indicate that the procedure is safe and generally stable. Predictability for correction of myopia varies with the degree of refractive error correction required.

SAFETY IN THE LASER CLINIC

Safety features that protect the operator and the patient from accidental laser exposure have been incorporated into most laser systems, and each product should be carefully scrutinized with these features in mind. It is difficult to formulate mandatory safety rules for an ophthalmic laser clinic because of lack of extensive clinical experience. It is possible, however, to suggest a list of precautions to be followed in the use of such an instrument.

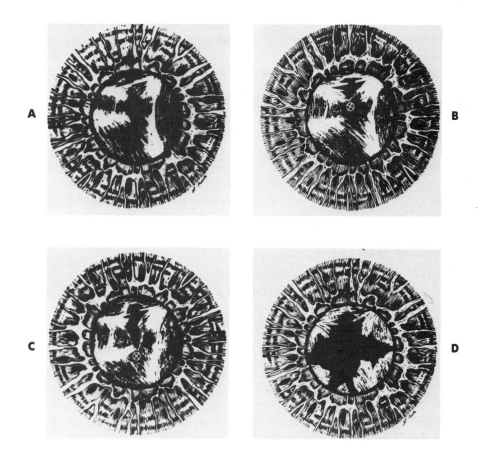

Fig. 29-7 Progressive opening of a posterior capsule with Nd-YAG laser photodisruption. (Modified from Steinert R, Puliafito CA: *The Nd-YAG laser in ophthalmology: principles and clinical applications of photodisruption,* Philadelphia, 1985, WB Saunders Co.)

1. Insist that all onlookers wear appropriate laser eye protection.
2. Keep all delivery optical equipment, including contact lenses, clean.
3. After extensive maintenance or unusual jolting of the instrumentation, check the laser beam alignment by firing the beam at a sample target. A sudden change in laser output for the same setting can indicate problems with the laser energy monitor.
4. Always use the lowest energy to accomplish the task.
5. In the case of neodymium YAG lasers, avoid procedures close to the retina, and cease laser use if the plasma formation becomes sporadic, which implies malfunction or lowered energy output.
6. Position laser to avoid accidental exposure either directly or indirectly to laser light.
7. Use appropriate signs or indicators to prevent direct viewing of the operating laser by a person entering the room.

FUTURE APPLICATIONS OF LASER TECHNOLOGY

As experience with laser energy increases in the field of ophthalmology, other forms of therapy are being investigated. Noninvasive glaucoma-filtering procedures using neodymium YAG laser energy are currently under study. Neodymium YAG laser disruption of vitreous opacities and retinal traction bands has been accomplished. Ciliary body ablation procedures to control end-stage glaucoma and methods to emulsify and ultimately remove cataractous lenses with laser energy in a noninvasive manner have met with some success in both animals and humans. Photochemical interaction between laser light and specific sensitizers continues to show promise in producing selective tissue damage (see Fig. 29-7). The excimer laser, at wavelength of 193 nanometers, has had a remarkable effect on tissue ablation, which can flatten the central portion of the cornea and eliminate refractive errors. This has improved the lifestyle of many.

Today the laser shares space in the clinic and operating room with many other types of medical instrumentation. The capability of this new mode of therapy in ophthalmology has been substantial in treating many of the more challenging forms of ophthalmic disease, and we can look forward to further advances in this technology in the years to come.

QUESTIONS FOR REVIEW AND THOUGHT

1. What are the different types of lasers used in ophthalmology?
2. What are the indications for laser use?
3. What anatomic structures must the argon laser light pass through before being absorbed by the pigment epithelium of the retina?
4. What safety precautions should be employed when lasers are used?

SELF-EVALUATION QUESTIONS

True-false statements

Directions: Indicate whether the statement is true (T) or false (F).

T or F   1. Laser application to the eye requires the patient to undergo general anesthesia.

T or F   2. The argon and krypton lasers work on the principle of thermal photocoagulation.

T or F 3. The neodymium YAG laser works on the mechanism of photodisruption.

Missing words

Directions: Write in the missing word in the following sentences.

4. The letters of the word laser stand for _____.
5. The lasers that use ultraviolet radiation for tissue destruction are referred to as _____.
6. The letters of the word YAG stand for _____.

Choice-completion questions

Directions: Select the one best answer in each case.

7. Laser light is consistent with which of the following?
   a. Monochromatism
   b. Coherence
   c. Low divergence
   d. Brightness
   e. All of the above
8. Of the following lasers, which has the shortest wavelength?
   a. Argon
   b. Krypton
   c. Neodymium YAG
   d. Carbon dioxide
   e. Excimer
9. The argon laser is not used to
   a. Ablate ischemic retina in proliferative diabetic retinopathy
   b. Produce a full-thickness iris hole (iridotomy) in angle-closure glaucoma
   c. Create burns to the trabecular meshwork in patients with open-angle glaucoma
   d. Create a central opening in an opacified posterior capsule after cataract surgery
   e. Ablate ischemic retina in central vein occlusions

ANSWERS, NOTES, AND EXPLANATIONS

1. **False.** Laser surgery can be performed under local anesthesia. If a specialized contact lens is used to focus the laser light, topical anesthesia is used. If the surgery involves coagulating the retina, for example, panphotocoagulation, then in addition to topical anesthesia, a retrobulbar block often will make the patient more comfortable.
2. **True.** The light from argon and krypton lasers is absorbed by tissues, resulting in sufficient heat energy so that the surrounding tissue is coagulated.
3. **True.** Unlike the argon and krypton lasers, the neodymium YAG laser uses high energy and an extremely short period of light exposure that results in vaporization of tissue.
4. *Light amplification by stimulated emission of radiation.*
5. **Excimer lasers.** Inasmuch as the laser light has a wavelength less than 380 nm, this light will not penetrate to the back of the eye because it will be completely absorbed by the cornea and lens. It is for this reason that the laser can be used to produce fine cuts in the cornea to change the refractive error of the eye.
6. **Yttrium-aluminum-garnet.** These are the components (in addition to neodymium ions, an energy source that can excite the molecules, and an optical feedback mechanism) that comprise the neodymium YAG laser.

7. **e. All of the above.** Lasers are composed of monochromatic light in that one or more specific wavelength is characteristic of each type of laser medium. Coherence refers to the light waves traveling in perfect step. The low divergence means that as light rays leave the laser cavity, they are nearly parallel. The brightness of laser light exceeds all known man-made and natural light sources.

8. **e. Excimer.** The excimer laser has the shortest wavelength at 193 nm. The other lasers in increasing order of wavelength are argon (488 and 514.5 nm), krypton (568 and 647 nm), and neodymium YAG (1064 nm), and carbon dioxide laser (10,600 nm).

9. **d. Create a central opening in an opacified posterior capsule after cataract surgery.** The neodymium YAG laser, unlike the argon, acts to vaporize tissue, and it is for this reason that an opening in an opacified posterior capsule can be made. All the other answers are appropriate indications for use of the argon laser, which acts by photocoagulation.

CHAPTER 30 Ambulatory surgery

- Ambulatory surgery centers
- Tips on medical/legal protection
- Preparation for admission
- Admission for surgery
- Postoperative recovery

Ambulatory surgery is one of the most dramatic changes in ophthalmic practice in recent years. In contrast to the previous patterns of hospitalization and restricted activity, most types of ophthalmic surgery, including cataract and intraocular surgery, are now performed on an ambulatory, outpatient basis. For example, whereas 85% of cataract surgery used to be performed on an inpatient basis, now over 85% of cataract surgery is performed on an ambulatory, outpatient basis in one of three specially designed ophthalmic surgery areas: (1) hospital-based facilities, (2) free-standing surgical centers, and (3) office surgical suites.

Several factors have influenced this dramatic change. The shift from intracapsular surgery to extracapsular ophthalmic surgery has contributed to the safety of cataract surgery performed on an ambulatory basis. Wounds have become smaller and the capsule has remained in place to prevent vitreous herniation. Suture material has improved with increased tensile strength, and there is now a greater knowledge about better wound closure. Valvelike wound architecture is now possible.

AMBULATORY SURGERY CENTERS

The development of ambulatory surgical centers (surgicenters) throughout North America has contributed significantly to the changes in ophthalmic

surgery. The overall emphasis of surgery is now placed on keeping hospital inpatient beds reserved for ill patients who require acute or prolonged care and attention. Thus significant financial savings can be realized by the public, the insuring agent, and the government.

Economics, however, was not the primary motivating factor for the directional change toward ambulatory surgery. Progressive ophthalmologists have long questioned the medical necessity of keeping patients immobilized for 24 hours after surgery, with gradual ambulation over several days. Dr. Norval Christie, in Pakistan, was a pioneer in this area, having operated on thousands of cataract patients annually on an outpatient basis. Other leading surgeons in the world followed with ambulatory surgery and immediate ambulation for their patients. Phacoemulsification surgery, with its small wound opening, gave impetus to this approach to surgery. Thus ambulatory surgery was ushered in, and the Outpatient Ophthalmic Surgery Society (OOSS) was created.

Reports by Dr. Galin of New York and Dr. Williamson of Florida, and others, have clearly shown that there is no statistical difference in either the short- or long-term complications in patients discharged shortly after cataract surgery compared with those who are hospitalized for 7 to 10 days after cataract surgery. The most important factor is meticulous surgery and particular emphasis on wound closure.

One major value of an office-based or a freestanding surgical facility is that there is continuity of patient care. The same people are involved from the initial work-up to the final discharge. This continuity with familiar faces, combined with trained personnel who care, eases the patient's anxiety.

The OOSS has established standards for surgical ophthalmic centers that address the areas of construction, asepsis, and record keeping. These standards provide for the safety of patients, as well as the legal responsibility of the surgicenter for monitoring and maintaining continuous self-assessment programs for quality control. Periodic site reviews are carried out. Equipment standards also are required.

To be eligible to receive Medicare payments, ambulatory surgical centers (ASC) must be inspected by state Medicare agencies and certified that they meet federal standards. These standards require the ASC:

1. To comply with state licensure requirements
2. To name a governing board that assumes full legal responsibility for the ASC's policies
3. To have an effective procedure for the immediate transfer to a hospital for emergencies, as well as a written transfer agreement with the hospital; all of the ASC's physicians must have privileges at the hospital
4. To have policies relating to surgical procedures and ASC privileges for qualified physicians, including examination of the patient by the physician before and after anesthesia
5. To have policies on the discharge of patients, including who should be discharged in the company of a responsible adult
6. To have procedures for ongoing, comprehensive self-assessment of the quality and necessity of care
7. To have a safe and sanitary environment
8. To be accountable to the ASC governing board, and policies must be established for granting clinical privileges, periodic reappraisal, and supervision of the nonphysician staff
9. To direct and staff nursing services to ensure that the nursing needs of all the patients are met
10. To maintain complete, comprehensive, and accurate medical records to ensure adequate care
11. To provide drugs and biologic agents in a safe and effective manner, according to accepted professional practice, and under the direction of a responsible designated individual
12. To have arrangements for obtaining routine and emergency laboratory and radiologic services from Medicare-approved facilities

The advantages of a surgical facility have been pointed out by Dr. Sanford Severin of Albany, California. These advantages include:

1. *Patient acceptance*. A more pleasant and comforting environment is provided with ready access to familiar faces.
2. *Cost effectiveness*. There is a major savings for the patient and the government or insurance company. The government can save over $1 billion per year if the 800,000 cataract extractions in the United States are charged a small facility fee instead of the $1,500 to $2,500 required for an individual to enter a hospital and have eye surgery.
3. *Complete control of the operating room*. Personnel can be chosen who work well together and are effective, not only in knowing the surgeon's routines and the purchasing and replacement of equipment and supplies but in maintaining good public relations with the patients and answering questions in a meaningful way, allaying the fears of the patients. Thus a surgical team is evolved that relates to both the surgeon's and the patient's wishes.
4. *Scheduling*. Scheduling is at the convenience of the surgeon. There is no waiting for surgical time or being bumped for emergencies of other surgeons.
5. *True effectiveness*. There is a better efficiency of time for the surgeon and the patient. There is less travel time for the surgeon, less waiting time for surgery for the patient, and the wait between

cases can be reduced for maximum utilization of the operating room and the staff's time.

The disadvantages of a free-standing ophthalmic surgical center or an office surgical center include the following.

1. The surgeon and staff must assume more responsibility in maintaining adequate stock, equipment, and sterility.
2. Medical/legal responsibilities increase. If a patient should become seriously ill during surgery, the ASC staff is responsible for the care of the patient and the transfer to a general hospital.
3. The need for ongoing interaction with agencies for payment reimbursement and peer review for certification standards.
4. Expenses can be greater than the reimbursement

rate unless a large number of procedures are being performed. The center may not be cost effective.

5. The ambulatory center as a major financial commitment is threatened in the case of sickness of the primary surgeon or key staff members or the reduction in surgical volume.
6. There may be a lack of patient compliance with the postoperative regimen after the patient is discharged from the surgical center.

TIPS ON MEDICAL/LEGAL PROTECTION

About 1 in 10 physicians will be sued at some time during their average 30-year medical career. Approximately 75% of these claims result from surgical procedures. Ophthalmologists, fortunately, have the lowest malpractice/litigation in the medical profes-

---

WAYS TO AVOID A LAWSUIT

1. Ensure that you identify the correct patient and the correct side for any surgical procedure.
2. Establish good rapport with the patient. The patient who likes his or her physician and the environment where surgery is performed is less likely to sue. Some lawsuits are started because of the patient's vindictiveness, even if the physician is fault-free. A doctor whom the patient views as compassionate and understanding has already acquired some protection against legal actions.
3. Discharge the patient into the care of a competent adult—one who will take care of the patient at home. The name of this individual should be recorded on the chart.
4. Provide written, easy-to-understand directions for the follow-up care and return visits. These should be read and explained to the patient or relative and all questions answered.
5. Include in the list potential problems or symptoms that may arise at home and what to do if they occur.
6. Provide in the instructions directions for obtaining an appropriate physician for medical problems. Telephone numbers of the physician, ophthalmologist, and a nearby hospital emergency room should be given.
7. Arrange for a nurse to telephone that evening or the next day to check on the patient's condition if the situ-

ation warrants, and record this on the chart.
8. Make operative notes soon after surgery, not weeks or months later.
9. Instruct patients to leave valuables at home, or arrange some system for safekeeping of the patient's valuables during surgery. Often lockers are provided.
10. Make sure that life-sustaining equipment is available and in good working order (Fig. 30-1).
11. Be sure there is an adequate consent form that is well-outlined to the patient. Good personal communication with the patient as to risks, benefits, and alternatives is highly valuable. An informed consent for major surgery is mandatory. These consent forms can range from a simple page or two to an elaborate 12-page document with video viewing and the patient's response questionnaire. Each physician determines his or her own comfort level. Appendix 16 contains the principles of informed consent.
12. Maintain good records in the office and the hospital. The quality and legibility of your records affect the quality of your practice. It is important to attach to the records a log of telephone advice. Cursory, sloppy, or nonexistent notes call the physician's credibility and standards of practice into question. The practitioner should initial all laboratory and x-ray reports before they are filed.

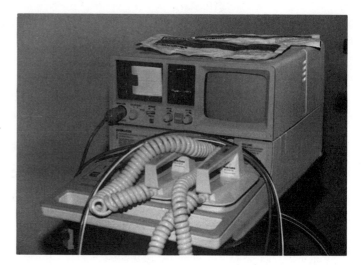

Fig. 30-1 Electrocardiograph monitor and defibrillator.

sion. Only about 2.5% of practicing ophthalmologists claim to have been sued. The most common suits are negligent performance of cataract surgery, negligent treatment of ophthalmic conditions, failure to diagnose ophthalmic conditions, postoperative vision loss, and complications as a result of negligent surgery or follow-up (see box, p. 641).

PREPARATION FOR ADMISSION

In preparation for admission to an ambulatory surgery center, each patient should have a careful medical evaluation before surgery by the family physician or internist. A checklist should be made of such events as routine laboratory tests and electrocardiograms. (See box, p. 645.) A complete eye work-up should be performed. A-scan measurements should be determined. If the power of the intraocular lens is beyond the range of stock maintained, then a correct dioptric power intraocular lens should be obtained from the manufacturer. An additional visit may be required for the patient to consult with the anesthesiologist, who can review the laboratory results and the work-up of the family physician (see box, p. 643). All surgical patients should be given extensive education concerning their problem. Videotapes may be shown and visual aid instructions may be given. Every effort should be made to have the family present at the teaching session. Providing

written handouts also can be of some value (see box, p. 644.)

ADMISSION FOR SURGERY

Each surgicenter has its own specific requirements for admission for cataract surgery. We arrange to have our patients report 1½ hours before surgery. This is to ensure adequate dilation of the pupil before surgery. Vital signs are recorded. The patient is free to move around and sit with relatives. Preoperative intramuscular sedation may be given to the nervous patient. Local anesthesia is administered by way of topical drops and peribulbar or retrobulbar injection. Some surgeons prefer to give an injection of IV Brevital or Pentothal during this latter procedure to reduce any awareness of this injection. Compression either by the Honan balloon or by super pinky is performed. Some patients are given intravenous medication for sedation. The patient is then led into the operating room and helped onto the operating table and made comfortable. The electrocardiograph leads and blood pressure cuffs are put in place. The eye is prepared with antiseptic solution. The nurse explains these procedures as they are being performed. The specialized ophthalmic assistant often participates actively in the surgery in an outpatient facility where a medical assistant may not be available (Figs. 30-2 through 30-6).

PATIENT QUESTIONNAIRE: DAY SURGERY

The following set of questions have been designed for use by the department of anesthesiology. They are to be completed before your operation. Please answer each question carefully. Bring the completed form to the preadmittance laboratory.

Name				
Address				
Phone	Age	Sex	Health Card No.	

	Answer (√)	Yes	No	Do not know
1. What is your approximate weight? _____ (pounds)?				
2. Did you ever take any medicine or pills for your heart?				
3. Did you ever have trouble with your heart?				
4. Did you ever take any medicine or pills for your blood pressure?				
5. Did you ever have high or low blood pressure?				
6. Did you ever take any medicine or pills for your breathing?				
7. Did you ever have any trouble with your breathing?				
8. Did a doctor ever tell you you had asthma?				
9. Do you take any medicine, pills, or injections of any type regularly while you are not in the hospital?				
10. Within the last year, have you taken any medicine for rheumatism, arthritis, or allergies?				
11. Have you taken a drug called **cortisone** or **prednisone** within the last year?				
12. Have you taken any tranquilizers or nerve pills within the last 2 weeks?				
13. Have you been pregnant within the last 3 months?				
14. Do you have any bleeding or bruising tendencies?				
15. Do you take pills for thinning your blood?				
16. Have you had a general anesthetic within the last 3 months?				
17. Were you ever told that you were unusually sick after a previous general anesthetic?				
18. Have you ever been jaundiced or had liver trouble?				
19. Do you have a family history of problems with anesthesia or of malignant hyperthermia?				
20. Do you have loose, false, or capped teeth?				
21. Do you wear contact lenses?				
22. Do you have glaucoma or use eye drops regularly?				
23. To the best of your knowledge, are you allergic to anything?				

Continued.

24. If so, to what are you allergic?

25. Please list below the operations you have had during your life:

26. Please list below the illnesses you have had during your life:

27. Please list below the names of the medicines you have taken regularly and the reasons for taking them:

Anesthetist's Comments:

_____
Signature of Patient

PATIENT INSTRUCTION FOR AMBULATORY SURGERY

Your procedure is scheduled for: _____
(Date to be inserted by surgeon's office)

1. Come to the admitting office at: _____
(Time to be inserted by surgeon's office)

2. Bring this form with you.

3. *You must not eat or drink anything after 11:30 PM* on the evening before your procedure.

4. Leave valuables at home. Your stay will be short. You will *not* be staying overnight.

5. Remove make-up and nail polish before coming to hospital.

6. If you have a *cough or cold,* whether taking medication or not, *please call your surgeon* as soon as possible, because your operation may have to be rescheduled.

7. You must not drive a motor vehicle for 24 hours after surgery. You must arrange for a responsible person to pick you up and accompany you from the hospital as soon as you are able to go home. Please arrange to have this person call _____ approximately 3 hours after you arrive at the hospital to establish the time of pick-up.

8. Male and female patients will be prepared for procedures in the Ambulatory Procedure Unit on the third floor. After surgery, you will be taken from the operating room recovery room to the ambulatory surgery recovery room, and then be discharged to go home.

9. It is expected that a parent will stay with children younger than 10 years of age until time of discharge.

10. You must not take any drugs or alcohol 24 hours after surgery unless prescribed by a physician.

SURGICAL CHECKLIST

CAT/IOL   OD/OS   PATIENT _____
CAT ONLY   _____ ADDRESS _____
SECONDARY IOL DATE OF SURGERY PHONE NO. _____
OTHER _____   RELATIVE'S NAME _____
                     PHONE _____

PREOPERATIVE VISIT
_____ Preoperative booklet given
_____ Operative instructions given
_____ History and physical form given
_____ Laboratory tests arranged
_____ Appointment scheduled with Dr. _____ for _____
_____ A-Scan scheduled for _____
_____ A-scan result: Lens style _____
        Diameter _____
_____ Endothelial studies
_____ Financial planning
_____ Insurance
_____ Surgery scheduled: Date _____
SURGERY DAY
_____ Operative consent reviewed and signed
_____ Premedication given
_____ Postoperative instructions given
_____ Postoperative appointment made for _____
_____ Responsible home person: _____
_____ Medication given
_____ UV glasses given or ordered

POSTOPERATIVE RECOVERY

The patient's family is invited to wait in the waiting room during surgery. After surgery they are invited to be with the patient in the recovery area. Here, vital signs are checked regularly. The patient may sit up and be served juice, coffee, tea, or light refreshments. The patient is given counseling in postoperative care. The patient is discharged shortly after surgery, and an appointment is arranged for the following day for examination. The only restriction is to avoid excessive exertion. The total time spent in the surgical center is minimal. The patch is removed the following day, eye drops are prescribed, printed instructions are given, and a pair of dark glasses are provided.

SUMMARY

In ambulatory surgical centers, the operation is performed in a friendly environment that is familiar to the patient and relatives. Each step from check-in before surgery to check-out after surgery is designed to allay fears and make the patient as relaxed as possible. It is important that the center have caring dedicated personnel, with compassion and a real willingness to cater to the needs of elderly persons, who are the typical eye patients. In addition, they must be well-trained and competent.

 Outpatient ambulatory surgery is based on the fact that with currently available techniques, complications are no greater than with inpatient cataract surgery in hospitals. The patient's acceptance is, how-

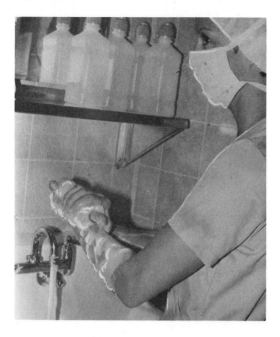

Fig. 30-2 Careful and meticulous scrubbing is required.

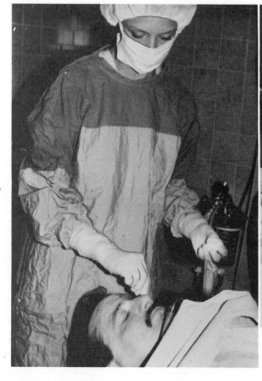

A

B

Fig. 30-3 A, Preparation of the skin with Betadine before draping. **B,** Double-glove technique in which outer gloves are removed.

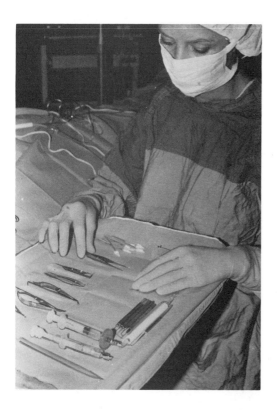

Fig. 30-4 Preparing the Mayo stand with appropriate instruments from the back table.

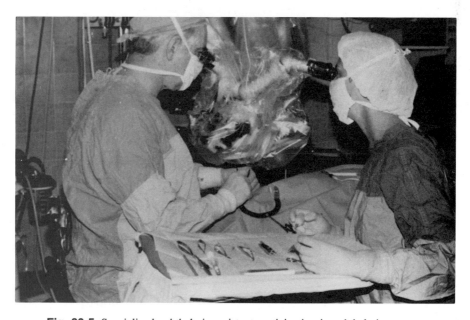

Fig. 30-5 Specialized ophthalmic assistant participating in ophthalmic surgery.

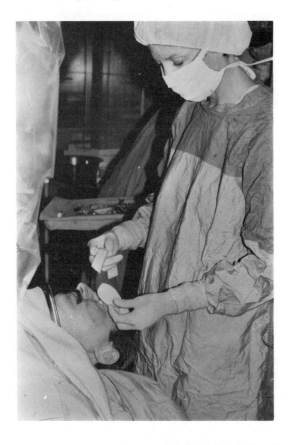

Fig. 30-6 Instilling medication and bandaging after surgery.

ever, much greater with ambulatory surgery. In the United States, outpatient cataract surgery has become the rule rather than the exception. Federally certified ambulatory surgical centers have created centers that are as high in quality as major hospital operating rooms.

QUESTIONS FOR REVIEW AND THOUGHT

1. List the significant advantages of ambulatory surgery.
2. List the possible disadvantages of ambulatory surgery.
3. Outline safety standards in a free-standing surgical facility.
4. What are the operative routines followed in your practice?
5. What are the preoperative testing routines before major surgery?
6. What medication, both ocular and systemic, is given before a cataract operation by your ophthalmologist?
7. What is the role of the ophthalmic medical assistant in the care of patients before and after cataract surgery?
8. What is the medical/legal responsibility of the ophthalmic assistant?

SELF-EVALUATION QUESTIONS

True-false statements

Directions: Indicate whether the statement is true (T) or false (F).

T or F 1. Operative notes must be detailed in a free-standing surgical facility.

T or F 2. A consent form is required only in some major eye operations.

T or F 3. Drugs and biological agents can be administered only by a physician.

Missing words

Directions: Write in the missing word in the following sentences.

4. A _____ list is used to record that all necessary preoperative and postoperative evaluations have been ordered.

5. The abbreviated form for medication given by injection in the muscle is called _____.

6. _____ is the Latin term for medication taken by mouth.

Choice-completion questions

Directions: Select the one best answer in each case.

7. Which is not true?
   1. Ambulatory cataract surgery may be performed in:
      a. Hospital-based facility
      b. Office treatment rooms
      c. Free-standing surgical centers
      d. Office surgical suites
      e. Hospital emergency operating rooms

8. Which condition is least likely to be performed as ambulatory surgery?
   a. Cataract with IOL
   b. Orbital tumor
   c. Strabismus surgery
   d. Glaucoma surgery
   e. Pterygium surgery

9. Standards for an ambulatory surgical center involve a number of requirements. Which of the following is not required?
   a. A governing body responsible for policies
   b. A mechanism for transfer to a hospital for emergencies
   c. A mechanism for ongoing care
   d. An attending nurse at all times
   e. Maintenance of complete records

ANSWERS, NOTES, AND EXPLANATIONS

1. **True.** The requirements for an ambulatory surgical center are as rigid as those of major hospital operating rooms. The details of the surgical procedure must be outlined in a standard operative report attached to the records.

2. **False.** All major surgery requires an informed consent form.

3. **False.** Drugs and biologic agents can be given orally or by eye drops by allied health personnel who have been trained to do this. Intramuscular or subcutaneous injections must be given either by a physician or someone licensed in the state to invade tissue. This may be a registered nurse.

4. **Surgical checklist.** Checklists are important to jog one's memory that all items necessary for preoperative and postoperative evaluations are conducted and the results tabulated. Such information as A-scan measurements may be critical when the time comes for surgery. A checklist is vital.

5. **IM.** The injection is given into the muscle mass.

6. **Per os.** When medication is given orally, it is often written per os, meaning through the mouth.

7. **b. Office treatment rooms.** Office treatment rooms usually do not have the sterility required for major surgery. They also are not adequately equipped for respiratory or cardiovascular emergencies that potentially could occur.

8. **b. Orbital tumor.** Orbital tumors may result in bleeding postoperatively, which may require blood transfusions. There also is a possible danger that there could be an invasion in adjacent tissue or some unusual tumor found that requires more extensive dissection.

9. **d. An attending nurse at all times.** An attending nurse is not required at all times. Often the physician may supervise a great deal of the ambulatory surgery personally. Often the ophthalmic medical assistant can be trained to be responsible for a great deal of the patient's care.

CHAPTER 31 Refractive Surgery

- Basic principles of refractive surgery
- Radial keratotomy
- The excimer laser
- Radial keratotomy and excimer laser surgery: a comparison
- Additional procedures

The 1990s are the decade of refractive surgery. The ophthalmic assistant should have a basic understanding of this new and exciting technology. Refractive surgery is rapidly changing. No sooner does one put pen to paper and there is new information that changes old concepts of ophthalmology and challenges practitioners to develop new procedures. The old saying, "If it works, make it better," applies to refractive surgery.

A large segment (20%-25%) of the world's population is myopic. There are 75 million people in the U.S. who require some form of refractive correction.

Refractive surgery is an elective procedure that is performed for relief of myopia, hyperopia, and astigmatism, with the goal of eliminating the need for glasses and contact lenses. It also had been found to be effective in correcting surgically induced refractive errors after cataract surgery and corneal transplantation. Because refractive surgery, with a track record of more than 20 years, has had few complications and a level of predictability that rivals that of intraocular lens implantation, many ophthalmologists are adding it to their routine surgical practice. The lay press also has awakened the general public's interest in refractive surgery. For many oc-

cupations good vision unencumbered by spectacles or contact lenses is important for safety reasons. In addition, many performers and professional athletes want to be free of spectacles and contact lenses. For some spectacle and contact lens wearers, it may be a lifestyle change.

The cornea is the most refractive component of the eye, accounting for more than 70% of the eye's refractive ability. In addition, over 70% of the outside world is introduced to us from the visual senses. Therefore most of the procedures in refractive surgery involve the cornea. The development of equipment for corneal topography has significantly improved our understanding of the cornea before and after surgery. Corneal topography equipment (see Chapter 34) provides a colored picture of corneal curvature taken from several thousand points from the center of the cornea (Fig. 31-1).

Two of the most common procedures for refractive surgery are discussed in detail, radial keratotomy (RK) and excimer laser surgery, commonly known as photorefractive keratectomy (PRK). Other less commonly performed procedures also are discussed, such as lamellar corneal implants, keratomileusis, epikeratoplasty, clear lens removal, corneal rings, and intraocular lenses for phakic persons.

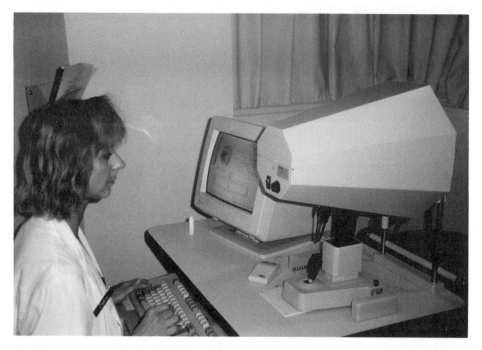

Fig. 31-1 Corneal topography provides corneal curvature radii. at a few thousand points on the cornea.

BASIC PRINCIPLES OF REFRACTIVE SURGERY

The cornea's function is to maintain the integrity of the eye and the transparency of the anterior surface of the globe so that light can pass through to the retina. Most important, this anterior surface is responsible for 70% of the refraction of light entering the eye. In myopia, either the cornea may be too convex or the axial length of the eye may be too long, causing light to converge at a focal point anterior to the retina. Corneal reshaping is an important concept in refractive surgery, and is the procedure most commonly used. The surgery aims to flatten the center of the cornea so that light will focus more posteriorly (Fig. 31-2).

Radial keratotomy achieves the reshaping by radial incisions made with a diamond knife (Fig. 31-3). This weakens the periphery of the cornea, so the normal intraocular pressure pushes the center of the cornea outward, thus flattening the central cornea. Unlike radial keratotomy, laser surgery or PRK tends to remove the superficial layers of the center of the cornea. The total amount of tissue that is removed or ablated usually is less than one tenth of the full thickness of the cornea (about 50-100 microns).

RADIAL KERATOTOMY
History

Interest in correction of myopia by means of radial keratotomy began in 1953 when Sato of Japan reported that he had obtained 3 diopters of correction in patients with -1.50 to -7.00 diopters of myopia by making as many as 32 posterior cuts in the cornea in a radial fashion, leaving a clear optical zone of 5 to 6 mm. Because of a high complication rate, this procedure was abandoned. The endothelium had been violated in the procedure, causing late complications.

Twenty years later in 1973 radial keratotomy was initiated and popularized by Svyatoslav N. Fyodorov at the Moscow Institute of Clinical Eye Surgery. Fyodorov noted that a teenager who had injured his

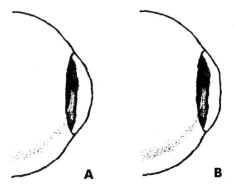

Fig. 31-2 A, Normal, smoothly contoured cornea. **B,** Flattened, central cornea after radial keratotomy or laser surgery.

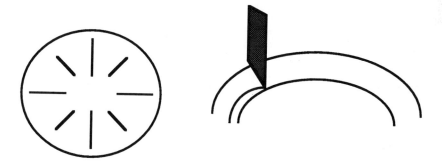

Fig. 31-3 Corneal incisions are produced with a diamond blade in radial keratotomy.

cornea with spectacle glass had marked reduction in his nearsightedness after the cornea healed. After performing thousands of radial keratotomy operations, Fyodorov reported a success rate of more than 85%. Later, surgery for hyperopia and astigmatism was developed. Leo Bores brought radial keratotomy to North America in 1978. In the next 16 years, several hundred thousand operations were performed in North America and more than one million in Russia.

To evaluate the effectiveness of radial keratotomy, a multicenter study called *the PERK study* (PERK stands for *Prospective Evaluation of Radial Keratotomy*) was undertaken in the United States under the sponsorship of the National Eye Institute and chaired by George Waring. Initial results released in 1984 indicated that corrected visual acuity of 20/40 or better was found in 78% of the eyes studied.

The procedure

Radial keratotomy is performed under the operating microscope. Radial incisions made in the periphery of the cornea with a guarded diamond knife tend to weaken the periphery and alter its shape, making the center flatter and the periphery steeper. This eliminates or reduces nearsightedness by permitting the light rays to focus on the retina. Incisions usually do not perforate the cornea, nor do they affect the central portion of the cornea.

Local topical anesthesia is used, with proparacaine 0.5% or lidocaine 4% used to anesthetize the eye. The central optical zone is identified first so that a central area ranging from 3 to 4.5 mm is spared from any incisions (Fig. 31-4). The depth of the incision is usually 90% to 95% of the corneal thickness, with a guard preventing the diamond blade from cutting deeper. Depth measures have become more precise.

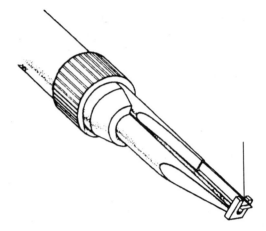

Fig. 31-5 Diamond knife with guarded blade.

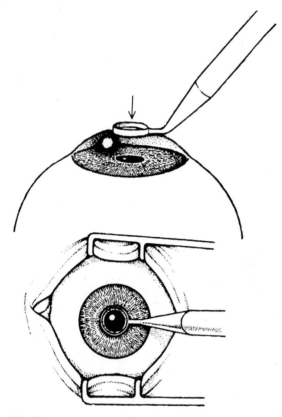

Fig. 31-4 Optical zone size is determined, and a marking device is placed on cornea.

New microgauges with $100\times$ magnification have been developed to set exquisitely thin diamond knives. No longer are metal blades used. Footplates on the blades act as guards and prevent penetration of the diamond below the deepest layer (Fig. 31-5). This gauge is set according to the depth of the area of the cornea as identified by a pachymeter. The incisions may be made from the central portion toward the periphery (American style) or from the periphery to the central portion (Russian or reverse style). The operation takes about 5 minutes, after which a patch or contact lens is often applied to the eye overnight. The operation is performed on an outpatient basis, and the patient may leave shortly after the procedure. There is mild discomfort for a few hours. The bandage or contact lens is usually removed the following day, and the patient may return to work the day of or the day after the procedure. The pain is minimal because only linear cuts are made, which do not produce a true corneal abrasion.

The improvement in vision is dramatic and usually begins the day after the procedure. Vision continues to improve for the next several weeks. Fluctuation in vision may occur during the first few months of healing. This usually levels off between 4 and 6 months but may persist for a few months longer. Some patients report postoperative glare and starbursts, especially at night. This usually diminishes relatively rapidly. Rare cases of infection have been reported. The structural integrity of the eye has been found to be weaker at least temporarily, after radial keratotomy.

Guidelines

Guidelines and nomograms (Table 31-1) by Spencer Thornton, Casbeer, and others have provided increased predictability for the procedure for myopia and astigmatism. A relatively good method for correcting hyperopia with the incisional procedures still has not been developed. In general, there is an 85% to 90% chance of achieving good vision if lower degrees of myopia less than 6.00 diopters is considered. Some studies have shown the presence of a continuing progressive hyperopia or reduction in the myopia some 1 to 4 years later.

Table 31-1 Thornton nomogram for radial keratotomy incisions

Theoretic working sphere (range of myopic power)*	Optical zone (No. of incisions)
0.75-1.12	5.00 (8)
	4.75 (4)
1.13-1.49	4.75 (8)
	4.50 (4)
1.50-2.11	4.50 (8)
	4.25 (4)
2.12-2.61	4.25 (8)
	4.00 (4)
2.62-3.11	4.00 (8)
	3.75 (4)
3.12-3.73	3.75 (8)
	3.50 (4)
3.75-4.36	3.50 (8)
	3.25 (4)
4.37-5.11	3.25 (8)
	3.00 (4)
5.12-6.11	3.00 (8)
6.12-7.50	3.00 (8 and redeepen to 98% from 5 mm OZ)
7.51-8.00 or more	3.00 (8 and redeepen to 98% from 5 and 7 mm OZ)

*Factors considered: refractive error, age, sex, intraocular pressure (IOP), corneal thickness, corneal diameter and keratometry. The sum of all these factors equals the working sphere (theoretic).

Age: For every year below age 30 add 2% to the myopic error. For every year above age 30 subtract 2% from the myopic error to age 50, then 1% per year thereafter to age 75.

Sex: Subtract 3 years from age for premenopausal females to age 40.

IOP: For every mm IOP below 12 add 2% to the myopic refractive error. For every mm IOP above 15, subtract 2% from the myopic refractive error.

Corneal thickness: For central corneal thickness less than 490 μg, add 10% to the myopia. From 490 to 510, add 5%. From 510 to 580 make no change. From 580 to 600, subtract 5%, and above 600 subtract 10% from the myopia.

Corneal diameter: If the corneal diameter is less than 11.5 mm, add 10% to the myopic error. If the corneal diameter is greater than 12.5 mm, subtract 10% from the myopic error.

Keratometry: If the average K is 42.75 or less, add 10% to the myopia. From 42.75 to 43.50, add 5%. From 43.50 to 46.00, make no change. From 46.00 to 46.75, subtract 5%. If the average K is 46.75 or more, subtract 10% from the myopia.

(Courtesy of Dr. Spencer Thornton, Nashville, Tenn.)

Results

Risks and complications. Visual complications have included increased astigmatism, irregular astigmatism, light sensitivity, and glare and starbursts.

Monocular diplopia has been reported. There have been some reports of increased vascularization of the RK lines, particularly if soft lenses are worn. Recurrent corneal erosion may occur as a result of perforations and intersection of incisions.

A great deal of data have been collected during the past 20 years on radial keratotomy, providing a long track record and a relatively safe procedure. It is important to realize that radial keratotomy has some risks, and the eye is at least temporarily structurally weaker. In comparison with other procedures, it is dramatic and quick to heal. The patient can return almost immediately to work.

How does it work? Radial keratotomy works by weakening the peripheral portion of the corneal so that the normal intraocular pressure will increase pressure against the periphery of the corneal, stretching it for a short time while the incisions heal, thus flattening the central portion of the cornea.

How long does it last? After the initial 6-month stabilization process, the procedure should last a lifetime. There are some reports of a progressive hyperopia occurring (or decrease in residual myopia). There also may be some increase in astigmatism as time goes on as a result of the contracture of the incisions.

What are the drawbacks? It is important that the patient does not have undue expectations of seeing perfectly for distance. Glare from headlights and fluctuation of vision often occur in some patients and may last longer than the 6-month period. Eventually these symptoms disappear.

THE EXCIMER LASER

Excimer laser corneal surgery may be divided into phototherapeutic keratectomy (PTK) or photorefractive keratectomy (PRK). PTK is the removal of tissue from the cornea to correct a medical problem with the eye; PRK is the removal of tissue from the cornea to correct a refractive problem of the eye (nearsightedness or farsightedness). Both procedures are performed with an excimer laser beam.

The word *excimer* is a contraction of "excited" and "dimer." The laser is a product of a reaction between a rare gas (argon) and a hologen (fluorine)

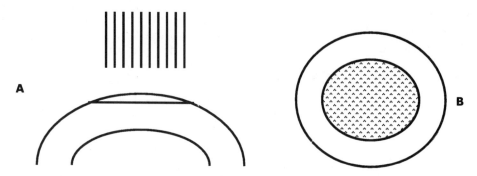

Fig. 31-6 Excimer laser vaporizes a thin layer from the surface of the cornea. **A,** Cross-section of cornea. **B,** Direct view of cornea.

in the presence of a strong electrical discharge. This reaction creates short-lived molecules (excited dimers) that emit strong pulses of light in the form of ultraviolet radiation at 193 nm. When precisely focused on the cornea, this pulse of light can remove tissue from the cornea in a manner that is cleaner and more controlled than any diamond knife. It can remove tissue to within a fraction of a micrometer (Fig. 31-6). The excimer laser energy is almost totally absorbed by the epithelial cells, Bowman's layer, and the stroma as the energy is pulsed onto the cornea at a 0.25-μm depth per pulse. Ablation of the corneal layers results in a flattening and a reduction of the myopic error.

History

Excimer laser was first developed by IBM in 1975 for etching microchips. In 1981, Toboada and Archibald investigated the clinical aspects of the excimer. Stephen Trokel and Charles Mulleryn saw its clinical application to the cornea and became involved. Trokel, Pulofito, Hanna, MacDonald, and others began the process of scientifically studying the procedure in the laboratory and later in blind human eyes.

Procedure

The procedure, which is performed using a topical anesthetic such as proparacaine 0.5% drops, takes anywhere from 15 seconds to 2 minutes, depending on the degree of myopia and astigmatism. A mechanical shutter controlled by a computer program is used to regulate the laser beam. It can be opened and closed to a desired size depending on the strength of correction required (Fig. 31-7). The beam is set for a period of time, and the shutter is programmed to slowly open from center outward during this period. The epithelium is removed by scraping or by using the laser to reveal Bowman's membrane. Centration is critical through either a holding device or self-fixation on a red light. The laser beam is turned on by a foot control, and the ablation process on Bowman's membrane and the anterior 50 to 100 μm of stroma occurs after the procedure. A contact lens is inserted for 24 to 48 hours, and medication is given.

In refractive surgery (PRK), more tissue is removed from the center than the periphery so that flattening of the cornea can occur.

Results

The results of excimer laser surgery have been extremely good. A majority of patients (90% to 95%) have had success with the procedure, having achieved 20/40 vision or better within 1.00 to 2.00 diopters of emmetropia. The downside risk has been negligible; less than 1% of patients having lost one or two lines of best corrected vision.

The risk. On the basis of available data, there appears to be minimal risk associated with excimer laser surgery on the cornea of the eye. However, a number of side effects can occur.

1. *Delayed epithelial healing.* The outer layer of the cornea is removed before excimer laser surgery.

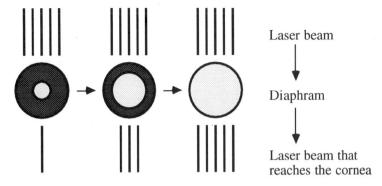

Fig. 31-7 Size of laser beam that reaches the cornea depends on size of diaphragm. The diaphragm opens gradually from the center and then becomes fully open at the end of the procedure.

Normally this layer replaces itself within 2 or 3 days. However, topical steroids or nonsteroidal antiinflammatory drops are required to minimize the epithelial thickening that can occur. Medication may be required for 6 months to avoid a regression.

2. *Light sensitivity.* Because of temporary disturbance of tissues, sunglasses probably should be worn in sunlight for at least the first week. This is not a major factor.

3. *Corneal haze.* This occurs in most cases. However, it usually does not interfere significantly with vision. The patient may possibly notice some glare. The haze is a result of keratocytes that enter the cornea to react to the ablation process and begin the healing process. Eventually they disappear, but they may persist and cause impaired vision.

4. *Overcorrection.* Overcorrection of the myopia or induced hyperopia may occur as the cornea reshapes itself. The hyperopia usually regresses. This presents an inconvenience to the person who wishes to return to work quickly. The eye may take a few months to regain its clarity.

5. *Undercorrection.* Small amounts of undercorrection do not seriously affect vision, particularly if the person is young and has a large accommodative reserve. Repeat ablation can be performed for undercorrections.

How it works

The excimer laser uses a mixture of argon and fluorine gases in a mirrored tube to produce a cold,

ultraviolet beam of light that vaporizes tissue by breaking molecular bonds a few molecular layers at a time. This process allows for vaporization or ablation of tissue without burning or disturbing the underlying tissue. Ultraviolet laser beams break up tissue by excitation of the atomic links—a photochemical process. The result is a precise cut with very straight edges and no discoloration or dehydration of surrounding tissue. The excimer laser is so precise that it can remove tissue 0.25 μm at a time (1 micron = $\frac{1}{1000}$ of a millimeter). The treated area of the cornea is so smooth and the ablation amount is so accurate that very precise modification of the corneal curvature is possible. In addition, higher myopic and astigmatic errors are treated.

Before excimer laser surgery was performed on humans, a wealth of information on the procedure was gathered from testing performed first on animal eyes and later on blind eyes.

In addition to its use in eye surgery, the excimer laser is being tested by heart specialists as a way of clearing out clogged coronary arteries; it is also being studied for use as a better way to remove kidney stones.

RADIAL KERATOTOMY AND EXCIMER LASER SURGERY: A COMPARISON
Radial keratotomy

Radial keratotomy offers two main features over laser surgery. First, it is quite dramatic in ridding the patient of spectacle or contact lens dependency within a very short period. Second, the side effects are not major and the complications are minimal. The central optical zone is not invaded. Although there is always the danger of a surgical misadventure, it is rare. The negative aspects are that the procedure still lacks predictability, even with the newer diamond blades and the microgauges, and the operator component remains a factor. Radial keratotomy is not as effective in higher degrees of myopia. The eye is structurally weaker, making it more susceptible to direct injuries.

Excimer laser surgery

The advantage of excimer laser surgery is that it is computer-driven and is more reproducible than a hand-held surgical knife. Excimer laser removes tissue by ablation. Usually neither deformation of the cornea nor induced astigmatism occurs. The sculpting is computer-programmed, leaving room for very few human-generated variables. In addition, the procedure is quick.

With the excimer laser, incision problems are avoided because the surgery ablates only a very thin layer of the cornea. Anatomically the eye is almost unaffected because laser surgery does not cause detectable weakening of the cornea, and susceptibility to injury is prevented.

Other advantages of excimer laser surgery are:
- Surgery with the excimer laser is more reproducible than a hand-held surgical knife.
- The speed with which the laser sculpts minimizes the variability as a result of corneal dehydration during the course of surgery, hence accuracy is much more complete.
- The laser is capable of creating a variety of patterns currently not practical with the hand-held knife.
- The laser procedure can be performed on a topically anesthetized patients, reducing both the patient's anxiety and the cost of the surgical procedure.
- With the excimer laser there are no incision-healing problems because the surgery removes a very thin layer of the cornea, less than $\frac{1}{10}$ the thickness of the cornea. In radial keratotomy, the cornea is permanently weakened as the cuts have to be more

than $\frac{9}{10}$ the thickness of the cornea to achieve the flattening effect required.
- There is no detectable weakening of the cornea with laser surgery, therefore there is no increased susceptibility to injury.
- Because a very small amount of the cornea is affected (microscopic layers on the surface of the cornea) the eye is almost unaffected anatomically.
- Excimer laser surgery is extremely accurate—the sculpting is computer programmed, leaving very few human-related variables. In addition, the procedure is very fast.

The disadvantage of PRK is that the procedure lacks the long-term follow-up available for radial keratotomy. Currently it appears to be safe, predictable, and readily rehabilitative. Because the ablation process is performed in the central 5 to 6 mm of the cornea, the procedure carries some risks. The depth is usually not more than 50 to 80 μm, or 10% of the corneal thickness. However, software has been designed to provide a sculpting of the borders and a blending of the curves to reduce the greater ablation process and depth in the cornea that is required in high myopia. The danger of too deep an ablation may result in a weakening of the entire cornea, which may lead to a central desmetocele. After the ablation process is performed by use of the excimer laser, the epithelium slides in and covers the denuded area. This may take 48 to 72 hours. Meanwhile the patient is often very uncomfortable during this time. Recently, pain has been minimized by the use of a contact lens and nonsteroidal anti-inflammatory drops.

Therapeutic corneal surgery (PTK). The excimer laser for therapeutic use offers tremendous potential for improving sight to literally millions of persons affected by corneal scars or corneal dystrophy. Superficial ablation of the stroma 50 to 80 μm in depth can remove scars and permit normal regularly aligned stromal fibers to be covered by regenerated epithelial cells. Astigmatism that may follow implant cataract surgery may be corrected by the excimer laser with the astigmatic module available with the VISX 20/20 laser.

The use of the excimer in corneal surgery enables

doctors to treat a number of corneal injuries, scars, and diseases without having to go to the extreme of a corneal transplant.

Therapeutic areas in which the excimer laser has been very useful are: removal of shallow and superficial scars and irregularities on the cornea as a result of trauma and infections; removal of corneal ulcers; removal of corneal dystrophies; removal of fungal corneal ulcers (to allow for deeper penetration of topical antimycotic medications); smoothing of corneal surface after excision of a neoplasm (e.g., squamous cell carcinoma); smoothing out irregularities (pterygium); and treatment of pathological corneal disease. In other words, the excimer laser is useful in removing any opacifications of the superficial layers of the cornea with retention of the health and clarity of the deeper layers.

New lasers are fast-appearing on the market. The intrastromal laser for intrastromal photokeratectomy has been developed; it is a picosecond YAG laser at 1053 nm. It is still in the investigational stage for corneal sculpting. This laser offers a tracking device that can place the beam to any point within the cornea or even the eye, e.g., the crystalline lens.

ADDITIONAL PROCEDURES
Keratomileusis

Jose Barraquer first described the procedure of keratomileusis in the early 1960s. In this procedure, lamella of the patient's own cornea are removed and lathed on a cryolathe in a frozen state and resutured back to the cornea in a flattened condition centrally. The cornea can be either steepened or flattened. This procedure requires a sophisticated cryolathe and a well-trained cryolathe technician. It can be used after cataract operations and can correct up to 12 diopters of hyperopia. Complications involve undercorrection and overcorrection. It is a sophisticated procedure that requires an experienced surgeon and an experienced technician for precise measurement. It is not user friendly.

Automated lamellar keratoplasty (ALK)

A more user friendly, nonfreeze method has recently been developed. The patient's own cornea is removed with an electric microkeratome, the cornea

is reshaped in a flattened state, and then the anterior layer is simply placed on the eye. New modifications of reshaping this lenticule on the patient's own stroma with excimer laser are being developed.

Epikeratoplasty

Epikeratoplasty comes from the Greek word *epi* (on top of) and *kerato* (cornea) (Fig. 31-8). Epikeratoplasty was developed at Louisiana State University by Herbert Kaufman, Marguerite MacDonald, and Theodore Werblin. It has recently become more simplified and safer. This procedure is most useful for pediatric aphakia, keratoconus, and high myopia. When performed after cataract surgery, it is called *epikeratophakia* (Fig. 31-9). In this procedure a precarved corneal donor button is rehydrated at the time of surgery when the surgeon sews it into a recipient bed in the peripheral cornea of the host.

Intraocular lens implantation

The intraocular lens (IOL) can be used to reduce myopia or hyperopia in a patient without cataracts. The IOL, which is placed in the anterior chamber of the eye in front of the iris and the crystalline lens, does not correct astigmatism. Complications are such that the lens may produce a cataract with time.

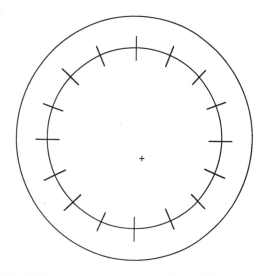

Fig. 31-8 Epikeratoplasty. A lamellar graft is sutured in place.

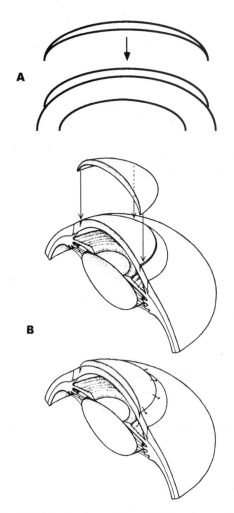

Fig. 31-9 A, Epikeratoplasty. **B,** In epikeratophakia a donor lenticule is sutured to surface of the cornea after the peripheral epithelium is removed.

Also, the depth of the anterior chamber is critical in the insertion of this particular lens. It shows promise, particularly with children.

Lensectomy

Lensectomy (lens removal) is being performed along with an intraocular implant at time of surgery. Through removal of the clear crystalline lens and insertion of an appropriate IOL power according to axial length measurements, the total new refractive error can be significantly reduced. This procedure is being performed in patients with clear crystalline lenses.

Corneal implants

Corneal implants, which are still being investigated, have not been used in North America for human beings. A small incision is made into the corneal stroma, and an implant of collagen or polysulfone is inserted, which alters the refractive component of the cornea (Fig. 31-10).

Peripheral ring implants

Peripheral ring implants currently are being investigated by David Shanzlin and co-workers. In this process a small band of silicone is inserted in the periphery through a circumferential stromal incision. These bands, which vary in size, steepen the peripheral contour and thus diminish the central contour to correct myopia (Fig. 31-11).

Holmium laser for hyperopia

The holmium laser currently is being developed to correct hyperopia by shrinking the periphery of the cornea, permitting the central part of the cornea to steepen and thus reduce hyperopia.

Thermokeratoplasty

Developed by Fydorov, radial heat is used in the periphery to shrink the collagen of the cornea and produce a central steepening. This results in a reduction of hyperopia. Regression is common and at this time its effect not predictable.

SUMMARY

Patients who desire to have refractive surgery should be aware of all the inherent risks of these procedures. As with any new procedure in medicine, there is a certain amount of positive and negative criticism from within the medical profession. Reputable ophthalmologists and optometrists may disagree concerning the safety and efficacy of radial keratotomy, laser surgery or other procedures for nearsightedness. Their scepticism is probably based on the concept of operating on an essentially healthy eye and putting it at risk. It is important to know that re-

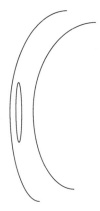

Fig. 31-10 Corneal implant.

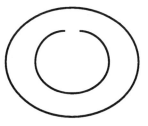

Fig. 31-11 A ring can be inserted in the cornea to flatten the central portion and thus reduce myopia.

fractive surgery procedures, whether it is radial keratotomy or excimer laser, or other procedures have been developed to correct refractive errors. Refractive surgery does not treat glaucoma, cataracts, or other disorders that affect and damage vision. It cannot make a blind eye see.

A person who is happy with his or her present method of correction (glasses or contact lenses) should by all means continue with it and *not have surgery.* Before refractive surgery is performed, a clinical evaluation is necessary to determine the patient's suitability for either radial keratotomy or ex-

cimer laser. Corneal topography has proved most valuable in this evaluation. It is important that the proper information be given to the patient. An informed consent means that the physician has outlined the risks and complications of the procedures so that the person can make an informed decision as to whether to proceed.

We are looking forward to developments in refractive surgery that will improve its predictability and results. The computerized accuracy of lasers may eliminate human variables. There is, however, a biologic variability to healing. Whether regression or visual decompensation occurs will require more long-term results and a larger patient base than is currently available. The FDA currently is monitoring events to prevent surprises down the road.

PART FOUR

Special procedures

CHAPTER 32   Ocular motility and binocular vision

- Evaluation of strabismus
- Retinal correspondence
- Amblyopia
- Eccentric fixation
- Treatment of strabismus

Ocular motility refers to the movements of the eye in all directions of gaze and to its relationship in movement with its fellow eye. Strabismus is failure of the eyes to spontaneously direct their gaze at the same object because of muscular imbalance (such as crossed eyes). Orthoptics is a paramedical specialty that investigates the motor and sensory adaptations to strabismus and deals with nonsurgical treatments to help patients regain the ability to use both eyes together normally to obtain comfortable, binocular single vision. Orthoptics originates from the Greek words *orthos* (meaning straight) and *ops* (meaning eye).

In the investigation of strabismus, the orthoptist is required to assess the vision or fixation of each eye, the alignment of both eyes in all directions of gaze, and the ability of the two eyes to work together binocularly. Orthoptic therapy is directed toward the elimination of suppression and amblyopia and toward the correction of anomalies in binocular vision. Therapy includes prescription glasses, optical correction with prisms, eye exercises, patching, and recommending drugs that modify the focusing power of the eye. The work of the orthoptist is an adjunct to that done by the ophthalmologist, not a substitute for it.

Because the brain controls visual sensation and ocular muscle coordination, orthoptic practice must involve a process of mental retraining. In terms of vision, the eye is not strengthened by the amblyopia therapy; rather, the brain becomes readapted so that it can accept, receive, and store all the visual imagery received by the eye. Because therapy is directed toward the higher centers of the brain controlling all visual responses, the child receiving orthoptic therapy must be alert, cooperative, and properly motivated. The age of the patient controls the approach the orthoptist takes and largely determines the success of the entire program. Younger children have visual patterns that are not well established. Therefore abnormal patterns can be restored to normal by vigorous retraining. After the age of 6 or 7 years, the vision and ocular motor control and the reflexes governing these areas become more difficult to change. The older patient, being more mature, may be easier to work with, but established visual patterns are much more difficult to disrupt.

Ultimate responsibility for every stage in the treatment of all patients with strabismus rests with the ophthalmic surgeon. Orthoptic assessment and treatment are carried out by a well-trained orthoptist. An understanding of what techniques are available is important to the ophthalmic assistant. Thus a brief

The authors wish to thank Stephen P. Kraft, M.D., for his review of this chapter.

outline of some of these tests is presented to familiarize the assistant with the more commonly used orthoptic instruments and methods.

EVALUATION OF STRABISMUS
History

When the history of a child with strabismus is documented, the following points should be noted: (1) age at onset and type of onset (rapid or slow), (2) whether turn is intermittent or constant, (3) whether one eye turns at all times or whether either eye alternately turns, (4) whether it is more apparent with close work or when looking in the distance, (5) precipitating causes before onset of squint (illness, trauma, and so forth), (6) previous family history of strabismus, (7) previous therapy for treatment of strabismus, (8) birth history, and (9) general health and past health.

Vision testing

Vision is tested by using the conventional Snellen chart, the illiterate E chart, Landolt's broken-ring chart, the picture chart, the Allen cards, Sjögren's hands, and more recently and effectively, the Sheridan-Gardiner (see Chapter 8). If the child is too young to be tested, some statement should be made of the child's fixation. This can be accomplished by means of the central, steady, and maintained classification. *Central* indicates that the corneal reflex is the same in both eyes; *steady* means that fixation is not wandering (common with amblyopia) and nystagmus is not present; and *maintained* denotes that fixation is sustained by a given eye through a blink or through an induced smooth pursuit movement. This method for testing a young child can be accomplished by holding an interesting toy nearby.

The visual acuity of an infant is much poorer than that of an older child. The orderly improvement of visual acuity is greatest in the first few months of life. Normal adult vision (20/20) is achieved somewhere after 6 months of age depending on the method of testing used to assess vision. Vision tests based on preferential looking techniques, such as Teller acuity cards, are helpful in assessing vision in a clinical setting.

Hirschberg's test

Hirschberg's test is a rather gross method of determining the presence or absence of strabismus and its magnitude. The examiner shines a light in the child's eyes and notes the position of the reflex of light, which normally falls centrally on the cornea or on a slightly nasal spot off the center of the pupil of each eye. If this reflex is temporally placed in one eye and is normal in the other eye, the child obviously has an esotropia. Each millimeter of deviation from the normal position of the light reflex represents 7 degrees. To be displaced 3 mm from its normal position on the temporal side, the magnitude of the esotropia would be grossly judged at approximately 20 degrees. The corneal reflection test is not sensitive enough for the detection of small-angled strabismus. However, Hirschberg's test is commonly used as a preliminary assessment to determine the magnitude of deviation in an older child and may be the easiest method of assessing the amount of strabismus in an infant.

Another method for measuring angle of strabismus that is more accurate than Hirschberg's test is named after Krimsky, who first described it. This test is used on infants or those with deep amblyopia. Prisms are placed in front of the fixating eye to force it to move over. This draws the fellow (deviated) eye to a straighter position so that its corneal reflex is centered. The strength of the prism required to center the corneal reflection in the strabismic eye is equal to the amount of deviation present.

Cover test

The cover test is perhaps the one most widely used by ophthalmologists for the detection and measurement of a strabismus angle. It is reliable, easy to perform, and requires no particular equipment. This test is conventionally performed at both distance and near, with and without glasses, the eyes being examined in the primary position. To ensure fixation in very young children, the fixation object should be an interesting and detailed article, such as a brightly colored toy or a toy with a squealer. A flashing clown or dog in the distance is quite useful for fixation. A strabismus misalignment is called *heterotropia* or *tropia*.

Once the examiner is sure that the child is looking at the fixation object, an occluder is interposed in front of one eye. If the child has a strabismus of the right eye and the left eye is occluded, the following possibilities may ensue. (1) The right eye, which is deviating, may move horizontally (esotropia: moves from an inward position to take up fixation; exotropia: moves from an outward position to take up fixation) or vertically (hypertropia: moves from an upward position to pick up fixation; hypotropia: moves from a downward position to pick up fixation), indicating that the child has a manifest strabismus. (2) The right eye may wander, indicating that the fixation of the eye is defective or absent, as may occur with gross amblyopia. (3) There may be no movement of the right eye, indicating that this eye is straight. The procedure is then repeated, this time covering the right eye, without allowing the patient to become binocular during testing.

A manifest strabismus tropia is revealed by observation of any eye movements of the uncovered eye to take up fixation when the cover is placed before the fellow eye. In addition to the *primary* straight-ahead position of gaze, the cover test may be executed in each of the eight *cardinal* or *diagnostic* positions of gaze (Fig. 32-1).

On occasion, a child will be referred who appears to have an ocular deviation but has no detectable strabismus. This condition is called *pseudostrabismus* (Fig. 32-2). In most instances, the appearance of a strabismus is caused by the presence of prominent epicanthal folds that extend from the upper lid, cover the inner canthal region, and blend into the medial aspect of the lower lid. The child's eyes commonly appear to be turned in because a minimal amount of the "white of the eye" shows medially and a normal amount laterally. Furthermore, this false impression of a turn inward (esotropia) is augmented when the child looks to either side. The adducting eye commonly slips under the epicanthal fold that bridges the corner of the eye. Parents, when commenting on this phenomenon, commonly state that the turn is so severe when the child is looking to the side that the eye almost disappears from view.

Pseudostrabismus can be differentiated from *true strabismus* by means of the cover test. With pseudostrabismus, neither eye has to move to pick up fixation with alternate occlusion if the eyes are straight. Once pseudostrabismus has been detected, the parents can be reassured that even the appearance of a turn will disappear with growth. This occurs because the growth of the root of the nose displaces these epicanthal folds medially and eventually eliminates them so that the amount of white of the eye visible on the medial aspect is in proportion to that found on the lateral aspect.

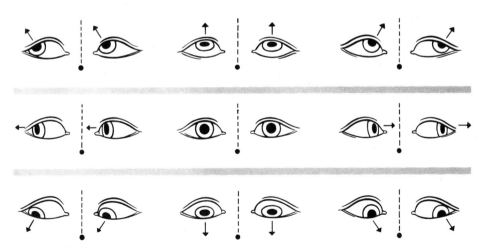

Fig. 32-1 Eye rotations: the primary and eight cardinal positions of gaze that should be tested to detect weakness of an extraocular muscle.

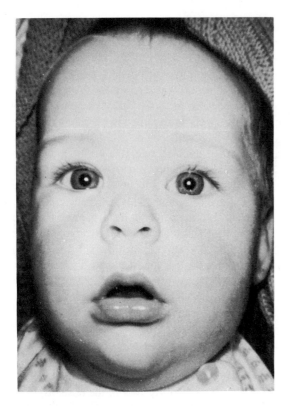

Fig. 32-2 Pseudostrabismus. The right eye appears to turn in because of a wide nasal bridge and epicanthal fold.

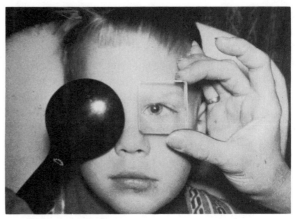

Fig. 32-3 Measurement of degree of strabismus by a prism.

The measurement of the magnitude of a true strabismus is carried out by means of a prism (Fig. 32-3) and an alternating cover test, whereby the cover is shifted back and forth between the two eyes. The apex of a prism is placed in the direction of the eye turn. The purpose of the prism is to displace the image of the object of regard onto the fovea of the turned eye so that on alternating cover there is no movement of either eye to take up fixation. Prisms of gradually increasing magnitude are introduced before one eye, the other being occluded. The magnitude of the deviation with use of prisms is indicated by the prism that, when placed before a deviated eye, allows no movement of either eye with alternating cover test. Fixation on a suitable accommodative target, such as a letter or number for an older child or an interesting toy for a young child, must be maintained by the patient. If the patient is too young to cooperate, the examiner must exercise ingenuity to attract the patient's attention and to maintain his or her interest on a particular fixation target.

Eye rotations (versions)

Weakness of an extraocular muscle is detected by simple observation of the two eyes as they track together in the different directions of gaze. One looks for defects in ocular movement in one or both eyes. The positions of gaze that should be tested are along the horizontal and vertical meridians and the oblique positions between them (see Fig. 32-1). Versions are commonly designated *dextroversion* (right gaze), *levoversion* (left gaze), *supraversion* (straight-up gaze), and *infraversion* (straight-down gaze). The eyes also should be examined in the four oblique positions. Versions are binocular eye movements in which both eyes move in the *same* direction, such as both eyes moving into left gaze (levoversion) or both eyes into right gaze (dextroversion).

Vergence movements are also binocular movements in which both eyes move in *opposite* directions in an effort to attain and maintain fusion, such as convergence and divergence that are required when changing fixation distance.

Electrooculography (Fig. 32-4) assists in the understanding of the function of the eye muscles in normal and pathologic states. It can detect various

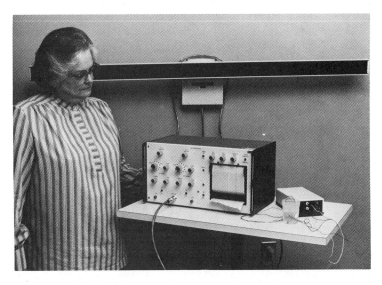

Fig. 32-4 Electrooculogram recorder and electrodes.

types of nystagmus and can determine velocities of eye movements.

Measurement of a heterophoria

A heterophoria (or phoria) is a latent ocular deviation kept in check by the power of fusion and made intermittent by disrupting fusion. A heterophoria must be differentiated from a heterotropia, which is a constant manifest ocular deviation.

Heterophorias are classified in a similar fashion to heterotropias: *esophoria* is the tendency of the eyes to turn in; *exophoria* is the tendency of the eyes to turn out; and *hyperphoria* is the tendency of one eye to turn up. Any of these conditions may occur normally when fusion is disrupted.

The prism and alternating cover test is the most useful test for measuring a phoria (as with a tropia). The Maddox rod is sometimes used; however, it is not as accurate.

The *cover-uncover* test is similar to the alternate cover test, but attention is focused on the covered eye as the cover is removed. The cover disrupts fusion, and any latent tendency of the eye to turn is revealed by the deviation of the eye under cover. For example, if the eye moves from an inturned position outward to fixate when the cover is removed, then esophoria is present. The alternate cover test, com-bined with prisms, provides a measurement of the deviation.

The Maddox rod has a series of red cylinders that distort a point of light into a fine red band, thereby changing the size, shape, and color of an image before one eye. Thus as the patient views a fixation light, one eye sees the light while the other sees a fine red line. Because these images cannot be fused, the eyes take up the fusion-free position.

The direction of the red line is perpendicular to the direction of the red cylinders. If the Maddox rod is held horizontally before one eye, the red line will appear either through the light (orthophoria) or to one side of the light (esophoria or exophoria). Mea-surement of the magnitude of the phoria is deter-mined by the amount of prism required to displace the red line so that the patient sees it running through the muscle light. If the Maddox rod is held so that the red cylinders are running vertically, the red line will appear as a horizontal band either through the light (orthophoria), above it (hypophoria), or below it (hyperphoria). Again, prisms are used to measure the magnitude of the deviation.

The Maddox rod test can be used to measure the magnitude of both vertical and horizontal phorias at either distance or near.

Hess screen test, Lees screen test, and Lancaster screen test

The Hess, the Lees, and the Lancaster screen tests are similar in principle and purpose. The difference among the tests is in the type of screen employed and the method of charting.

For the Hess and the Lancaster screen tests, the patient wears red-and-green goggles. The patient is given a flashlight that projects a green light, and the examiner holds a flashlight that projects a red light. In the Hess test, the examiner places his or her light at the indicated dots on the chart, and the patient tries to place his or her light over that of the examiner (Fig. 32-5). The patient fixates on the examiner's red light with the eye covered by the red lens and projects the green light in the direction toward which the eye under the green lens is pointing. If the eyes are not straight, the displacement of the green light in relation to the red light is a measure of the deviation.

The Lees screen test is plotted in the same way as the Hess: however, it is not as dissociating a test because the patient does not wear red-and-green glasses. The patient sits approximately 1 m away from two screens that are at right angles to one another. A two-sided mirror with an attached chin rest bisects the junction of the two screens. The patient is shown targets on one screen and is asked to point with his or her light to localize the points on the second screen while looking into the mirror. The displacements of the patient's perceived points from their true locations are proportionate to the muscle imbalances.

The Lancaster screen test is similar to the Hess test except that the examiner usually begins at the zero position and then moves his or her light to the cardinal positions of gaze. These tests are useful in the detection of paretic ocular muscle palsies and of strabismus. Both tests are based on the fact that foveae of straight eyes project to the same point in space. In patients with strabismus, the foveae do not project to the same point in space. The measurement of this difference is a measure of the deviation.

RETINAL CORRESPONDENCE

Normally images from the foveas of the two eyes project in the same visual direction. This is known as *normal retinal correspondence*. Anomalous retinal correspondence is another faulty sensory adaptation to a strabismus in which the fovea of one

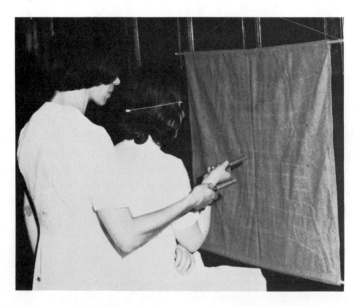

Fig. 32-5 Hess screen test used to measure the magnitude of a muscle imbalance.

eye projects to the same point in space as an extra-foveal point on the retina of the other eye. Conversely, the definition may be stated as a condition in which the foveae of both eyes do not point in the same visual direction. Anomalous retina correspondence develops most commonly in relatively long-standing monocular strabismus. It is a sensory adjustment on the part of the turned eye. The fovea of the turned eye is suppressed to avoid confusion of images and diplopia, but a nonfoveal point on the retina takes up the function of the fovea so that its projection comes in line with the projection of the fovea of the other eye. In a sense the patient does develop binocular vision but of a gross form.

Worth four-dot test

The Worth four-dot test is a gross test employed to detect the presence of fusion or the suppression of one eye. It consists of an illuminated panel of lights in diamond formation. It is housed for near-vision testing in a flashlight and in a panel for distance testing. In this apparatus the two lateral lights are green, the upper is red, and the lower is white (Fig. 32-6). The patient wears red-and-green glasses and is merely asked to note the number and color of the lights. The white light usually is described either as a combination of red and green in the presence of fusion or as changing from red to green. When one eye is definitely dominant, the light is either red or green, depending on the dominant eye. If the patient has single binocular vision, four lights will be seen:

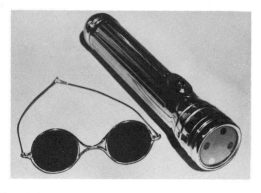

Fig. 32-6 Worth four-dot test used to detect suppression and diplopia.

the red above, the two greens at the side, and a pale pink or green below, depending on which eye is dominant. If the patient has diplopia, five lights will be noted: three green and two red. If the patient is suppressing, only the colored lights observed by one eye will be seen; that is, either two red lights or three green lights will be seen. The patient may have one response for distance and an entirely different response for near.

Bagolini striated-glasses test

Bagolini striated-glasses test is the least dissociative of the three most common tests for determining the presence of anomalous retinal correspondence. In the Bagolini striated glasses test, patients wear two lenses (one over each eye) with striations placed at 90-degree angles to each other. The responses are interpreted as follows.

Normal retinal correspondence (NRC) exists if the patient has no manifest deviation on cover test and sees a perfect cross.

Abnormal (anomalous) *retinal correspondence* (ARC) exists if the patient has a manifest deviation on cover test and sees a perfect cross. A streak with a gap indicates suppression with abnormal retinal correspondence. Two separate streaks (not in the form of a cross) indicates diplopia with normal retinal correspondence (see below).

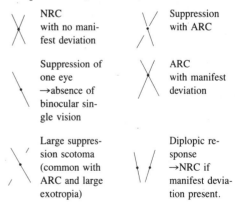

Afterimage test (Fig. 32-7)

In the afterimage test the patient fixates with one eye occluded for 10 seconds on a dot on a bulb containing an electrical filament. During this time the electrical filament is held vertically and flashed. This imprints a vertical afterimage across the macula of the fixating eye. Then the eye is covered, and a horizontal flash of light is presented to the fovea of the other eye. If the patient has normal retinal correspondence, the afterimages are seen as a perfect cross. If the patient has anomalous retinal correspondence, the position of the two bars will be displaced. For example, if the patient has a right esotropia, and if the vertical bar is presented to the right eye and the horizontal bar is presented to the left eye, the afterimage would consist of a vertical line to the left of the horizontal line (Fig. 32-8).

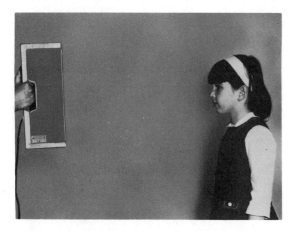

Fig. 32-7 Afterimage test used to detect anomalous retinal correspondence.

Major amblyoscope

The major amblyoscope is a device for the measurement of strabismus and the assessment of binocular vision. In the past it was used as a treatment of suppression and amblyopia (Fig. 32-9).

The instrument itself has two viewing tubes so that each eye can be presented with a picture. The instrument can be adjusted to each patient's interpupillary distance and chin level. The tubes can be moved horizontally to neutralize a horizontal deviation (main purpose) or to create a demand for convergence or divergence. They also can be moved vertically to neutralize a vertical deviation or to create a demand for a vertical vergence movement, or they can be displaced vertically. Cyclotorsion also can be measured subjectively. Each optical tube contains a slide carrier, a low-intensity light source for the illumination of the slides, and a high-intensity light source for creating after-images. Some of the amblyoscopes also contain a device called *Haidinger's brushes,* which is employed to test macular function and projection. A 6.50-diopter lens is placed in front of each tube to eliminate the accommodation required for viewing through a short tube that is only about 6 inches in length.

To assess the grades of binocular vision, different targets are presented to the eye.

Grade 1 binocular vision requires simultaneous perception. (Parafoveal, foveal, or macular slides may be used; this choice depends on visual acuity.) Dissimilar targets, such as a lion and a cage, are presented to each eye. The patient who sees the lion

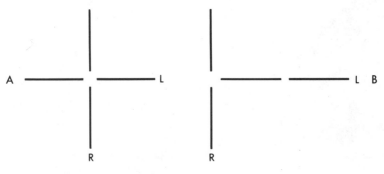

Fig. 32-8 A, Normal retinal correspondence. **B,** Right esotropia with abnormal retinal correspondence *(crossed images).*

in the cage is seeing with each eye simultaneously and has grade 1 binocular vision (Fig. 32-10). If suppression is present, one image disappears intermittently. The "jump" is caused by the disappearance of an image and therefore is repetitious.

Grade 2 binocular vision requires fusional ability. Similar targets presented to each eye must be fused before a complete picture is identified. A grade 2 target may present to one eye a picture of a rabbit with no tail, clutching flowers (Fig. 32-11); the other eye would be presented with a picture of the same rabbit, but it would have a tail, and held in its hand would be a stem without flowers. Grade 2 binocular vision is present if the patient fuses these images and reports seeing a tailed rabbit clutching a group of flowers by a stem. If the patient has suppression, one of the controls (the tail or the flowers) will disappear. With grade 2 targets, fusional reserves can be measured by moving the arms of the instrument in or out (fusional convergence and divergence) until a point is reached where the patient complains of diplopia (sees two rabbits) or suppression (flowers or tail disappear) at the break point.

Grade 3 binocular vision requires the coordinate use of the two eyes together to yield the sensation of stereopis (depth perception). Grade 3 slides present to the viewer pictures that are not quite superimposable. The fusion of these slightly dispa-

rate images by the brain creates the sensation of depth, or stereopis (Fig. 32-12). If fused correctly, one of the seahorses will appear distinctly in front of the others.

Clinical measurements of strabismus using the major amblyoscope. The patient is placed before the amblyoscope, chin on the chin rest, which has been adjusted so that each eye looks straight through the

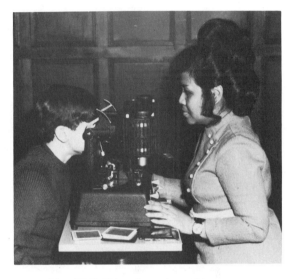

Fig. 32-9 Using the major amblyoscope.

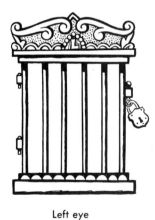

Left eye

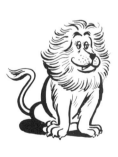

Right eye

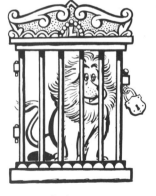

Both eyes

Fig. 32-10 Grade 1 targets used for determining simultaneous macular perception. Targets are dissimilar and cannot be fused, but the brain superimposes the images when slides are brought together.

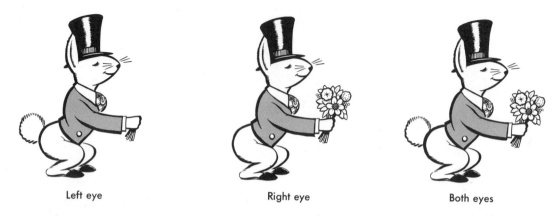

Left eye   Right eye   Both eyes

Fig. 32-11 Grade 2 targets used for determining simultaneous macular perception plus fusion. The targets are similar and when fused present a complete picture.

lenses. All the readings on the amblyoscope are set at zero.

Consider a patient with a left esotropia. Grade 1 targets are placed in the tube; the patient will be looking with one eye through the right tube, and the left eye will be turned in. The targets are presented alternately, first to one eye and then to the other. To take up fixation the turned eye will move. The arms of the tube on the left side are moved in the direction of the deviation until no movement occurs on flashing. This measurement is called the *objective measurement* and corresponds to the amount of manifest deviation.

If the patient fuses images when the angle of strabismus is corrected, then the patient is said to have *normal retinal correspondence*. When *abnormal retinal correspondence* is present, the patient fuses even if the angle is only partially corrected (subjective angle). A difference between the two angles is referred to as the *angle of anomaly*. If the angle of anomaly is the same as the objective measurement of the deviation, the abnormal retinal correspondence is called *harmonious*. If the angle of anomaly is less than the objective measurement of the deviation, retinal correspondence is called *unharmonious*.

Detection and treatment of suppression

Theoretically any child whose eyes are crossed and whose foveae are not pointed to the same position in space would be expected to see double. The reason

that children do not see double or have diplopia awareness is that they are capable of suppressing an area of the retina to avoid double vision and confusion of images. It is the constant habit of continuous suppression that eventually leads to loss of binocular visual function and to strabismic amblyopia. In the past, antisuppression devices were used to make the patient aware of diplopia and to try to overcome suppression. Some examples of these devices (which no longer are in active use) are the stereoscope, the Tibbs binocular trainer, the amblyoscope, red-and-green glasses, and the reading bar.

AMBLYOPIA

Amblyopia is a term for loss of vision in one or both eyes in which no organic pathologic condition is seen in the eyes or optic nerves. The incidence is approximately 2.5% of the population. Vision is reduced in the affected eye to 6/12 (20/40) or worse.

Unilateral amblyopia is caused by conditions that affect vision in one eye only. The most common cause is a manifest strabismus of one eye, and suppression often is associated with it. Other causes include a significant refractive error of one eye and conditions of stimulus deprivation that block or blur images to the retina, such as ptosis, cataract, or corneal opacities. Thus unilateral amblyopia can occur in conditions other than strabismus, in which the eyes may be straight.

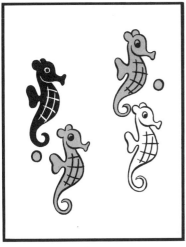

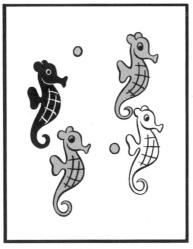

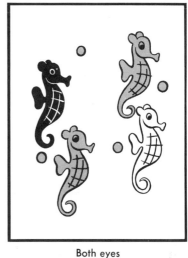

Left eye · Right eye · Both eyes

Fig. 32-12 Grade 3 targets used for determining stereopsis. The targets are similar but viewed at a slightly different angle so that a sensation of depth occurs.
(Courtesy M. Blair, American Orthoptic Council.)

Bilateral amblyopia is caused by symmetric abnormalities of the two eyes, causing blurring of retinal images. These conditions include bilateral significant refractive errors and bilateral stimulus deprivation, such as in bilateral cataracts or corneal scars.

Amblyopia caused by refractive errors or strabismus usually responds well to treatment in children younger than the age of 6 or 7, after which the success rate declines with age. This interval of reversibility is known as the *critical period*. Although the critical period for reversing amblyopia caused by refractive error or strabismus is the first few years of life, such is not the case for stimulus-deprivation amblyopia caused by congenital cataracts or corneal scars. These disorders must be treated within the first few weeks of life, or the visual deficits may be permanent and irreversible. Thus, fundamental to the treatment of amblyopia is early detection and therapy.

The treatment of amblyopia depends on the cause. Any causes of stimulus deprivation such as cataracts must be removed and appropriate refractive correction instituted. Significant refractive errors in one or both eyes are corrected by glasses or contact lenses.

A unilateral amblyopia caused by strabismus is treated by patching the sound eye to force the amblyopic eye to work harder for most of the child's waking hours.

The most common amblyopia therapy is occlusion of the good eye and use of the amblyopic, or lazy, eye. Occlusion, to be effective, is maintained constantly during all waking hours until visual acuity is equal and voluntary alternation is attained.

Many types of occluders are available. The Elastoplast occluder is an extremely effective one that seals off the eye and prevents peeking in any direction (Fig. 32-13). However, this type of occluder is uncomfortable in hot weather, often tends to slip off, and may cause contact dermatitis with prolonged wear. An alternate patch presently used is micropore tape and tissue. This tape is hypoallergenic, fully adhesive, and nonirritating to the skin during removal. The tissue is cut into the appropriate shape and size and is placed in the center of the tape and positioned over the eye. The Opticlude is a hypoallergenic type of occluder patch. Another type is the rubber suction-cup occluder,which is applied to the posterior lens surface and totally occludes the eye because of a temporal extension that prevents peeking (Fig. 32-14). Frosted lenses and clip-on occluders are not satisfactory inasmuch as the patient tends to peek over, under, or around the occluder.

If the child is uncooperative and tears off patch after patch, occlusion can be provided by placing atropine ointment in the fixating eye. Atropine has the outstanding merit that, once instilled in the eye, the child cannot remove it. It can be extremely effective in a child who is hyperopic, because the

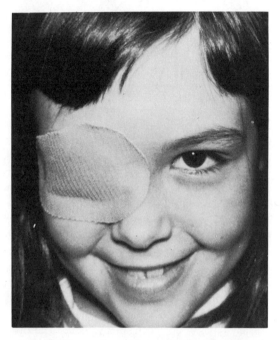

Fig. 32-13 Elastoplast occluder.

atropine paralyzes the child's ability to compensate for the hyperopia by eliminating accommodation. The atropine ointment is preferred because it is less apt to produce systemic reactions (fever and flushing) and is also easier to instill.

Once the child has accepted the occlusion therapy and the performance of the amblyopic eye has improved to 20/25 or 20/30, occlusion of the dominant eye can be maintained by painting the front and back surfaces of the lens with two or three coats of clear nail polish. The only advantage of this method of occlusion is that it is less noticeable and psychologically easier for the patient to accept.

Children between the ages of 1 and 3 years respond quickly to occlusion therapy and are seen weekly to avoid occlusion amblyopia. Because conventional visual acuity tests cannot be performed on this age-group, the children's response to occlusion therapy is estimated by their fixation pattern. With a successful result, the child should be able to maintain fixation on a target steadily and centrally with the affected eye. If no improvement occurs after 3 months, occlusion therapy usually is discontinued.

The older child, between the ages of 4 and 7 years, usually requires a much longer period of therapy to produce improvement in visual acuity. Although older children are more resistant to therapy, they are easier to work with because conventional vision tests can be used. If improvement in vision does not occur after 3 months of constant effort, amblyopia therapy usually is discontinued. Occlusion is maintained until the vision in the affected eye is brought up to 20/

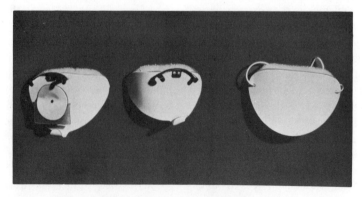

Fig. 32-14 Types of occluders: suction, clip-on, and pirate patch.

25 or 20/20, or until vision no longer improves. Then the daily hours of patching are tapered over several weeks as long as visual improvement is maintained.

The success of occlusion therapy often depends on the child's cooperation and enforcement of the regimen. Some parents become terrified at the thought of a patch on their child's good eye, believing that the child will become accident prone and be in physical danger. Parents should be reassured about such fears, because patching the good eye does not produce a blind child and accidents in the home as a result of patching are rare. Also, some parents will regard the patch as a stigma of weakness in their child and will remove it when the child is playing with friends at school or is seen by adults. It is vital that the parents be informed about the principles of amblyopia therapy and the necessity for total occlusion. It should be impressed on them that neglect of total occlusion only prolongs the duration of amblyopia therapy and that failure to achieve significant gains in visual acuity by the age of 6 or 7 years usually results in a defective eye and an absence of stereopsis for the rest of the child's life.

With older children, amblyopia therapy can be enhanced by encouraging the child to enter into activities involving eye-hand coordination. Such home games include tracing, coloring, cutting out patterns, threading beads, watching television, and putting models together. All these games are performed, of course, with the use of the amblyopic eye. Visual games can be played in the automobile or out walking by having the child attempt to read street signs, billboards, license plates, and so forth.

Before one discontinues any amblyopia program as a total failure, it is important to reassess (1) the method of occlusion (ensuring that the occluder completely covered the eye and prevented the dominant eye from being used) and (2) the duration of occlusion (ensuring that the supervision of the child was close and that occlusion was maintained fully). Finally, any child with amblyopia should be given the opportunity for a patching trial, even one who is older than 7 years of age. Some children will respond well beyond age 7 into the teen-age years.

ECCENTRIC FIXATION

Eccentric fixation is the culmination of damaging sensory habits in strabismus—primarily suppression and amblyopia. With eccentric fixation the vision loss in the affected eye usually is profound because an area other than the fovea is used for fixation. Visual acuity often is less than 20/200, and the patient is unable to gaze directly at an object when the sound eye is covered.

Eccentric fixation may be detected by the visuscope, combined with a reduction in visual acuity. An abnormal position on the corneal reflex may be a clue to eccentric fixation.

TREATMENT OF STRABISMUS

The first concern in treating strabismus is the elimination of any coexisting amblyopia. Some forms of strabismus can be corrected by improving the vision in the amblyopic eye inasmuch as the eye muscle control may improve at the same time. In addition, the eyes may straighten in some patients with strabismus who require glasses to correct vision or amblyopia.

Patients with heterophorias that are well controlled or who have small heterotropias may need no treatment at all. Some forms of strabismus, such as nerve palsies, are temporary and will subside with time. Other forms, such as convergence problems that cause reading difficulties, will respond to orthoptic exercises.

Patients who have diplopia may experience relief of the double vision and regain fusion through the use of prisms. Both permanent and temporary types of prisms are available. Sometimes eye drops that constrict the pupil (miotics) aid in straightening eyes with certain forms of esotropia.

If none of these treatments are indicated or are not successful in straightening the eyes, then two options are available. One is eye muscle surgery, which involves the strengthening of weak eye muscles and weakening of overactive or tight muscles. In adults this can be performed by means of an adjustable suture technique whereby the alignment of the eye can be altered on the same day as the surgery while the patient is awake. The techniques of eye muscle surgery are described in more detail in the chapter on extraocular surgery. The other option is the injection of botulinum toxin into eye muscles, which paralyzes them and straightens the eyes with certain forms of strabismus.

SUMMARY

The main function of an orthoptist is to evaluate muscle imbalances and to promote binocular cooperation between the patient's two eyes by a reeducation process. It is not a cure for a strabismus but is an excellent adjunct in the preoperative and postoperative management of patients who can cooperate for the required procedures. Orthoptic training attempts to improve the quality of fusion and to break down faulty adaptive sensory habits of strabismus, such as suppression, and abnormal retinal correspondences.

The role of the ophthalmic assistant is to assist either the ophthalmologist or the orthoptist in the practical diagnosis and therapy of strabismus. Participation by the ophthalmic assistant in orthoptics will depend on the enthusiasm and knowledge of the assistant and the facilities available in a given office or clinic.

QUESTIONS FOR REVIEW AND THOUGHT

1. Many patients, particularly infants, have facial features that make them appear to have strabismus although their eyes are orthophoric. What is this condition called?
2. When an eye truly deviates outward, what is it called?
3. If the eye has a tendency to turn in, the condition is called *esophoria*. What is it called when there is a tendency to turn up?
4. Vision is depressed in one eye and the eye obviously appears to turn in. However, when the fellow eye is covered, the eye does not take up fixation on a muscle light. What type of fixation is said to exist?
5. How does amblyopia come about? What are some of its causes?
6. The light reflex demonstrated by the Hirschberg test is centered on one pupil but falls to the outer portion of the cornea on the fellow eye in a given patient. What condition exists?
7. A patient complains of double vision. Outline a method of detecting which muscle or muscles are at fault.
8. Outline a method of measuring the amount of strabismus present in a patient.
9. The Worth four-dot test is used to detect suppression of one eye, the presence of fusion, or diplopia. How is this test performed?
10. Discuss the treatment of amblyopia.

SELF-EVALUATION QUESTIONS

True-false statements

Directions: Indicate whether the statement is true (T) or false (F).

T or F   1. The *primary* difference between the alternate cover test and the cover-uncover test is the use of prisms.

T or F   2. Abnormal retinal correspondence is a monocular adaptation to strabismus.

T or F   3. To neutralize an exodeviation with prisms, the base of the prism is held toward the nose.

Missing words

Directions: Write in the missing word in the following sentences.

4. A term synonomous with *binocular single vision* is _____.

5. An alternating deviation is usually indicative of _____ visual acuity .

6. _____ are conjugate eye movements, and _____ are disconjugate eye movements.

Choice-completion questions

Directions: Select the one best answer in each case.

7. When performing the alternate cover test:
   a. Use a light for fixation
   b. Allow the patient to be binocular
   c. Observe the occluded eye only
   d. Never have the patient wear his or her glasses
   e. Never allow the patient to be binocular

8. When a constant monocular deviation is present, the patient:
   a. May have anisometropia
   b. May have fusion ability
   c. Has a deviation that cannot be neutralized
   d. Never demonstrates suppression
   e. Has an esodeviation

9. Strabismus:
   a. Is only monocular in nature
   b. Has motor and sensory adaptations
   c. Is always present when the corneal reflexes are not properly positioned
   d. Indicates the visual acuity is always lower in both eyes
   e. Requires surgical correction

10. The Worth four-dot test:
   a. Is used to quantitate a deviation
   b. Is a test for color blindness
   c. Detects the presence and type of diplopia
   d. Detects the presence of amblyopia
   e. Is used to evaluate fusional amplitudes

ANSWERS, NOTES, AND EXPLANATIONS

1. **False.** The primary difference between the alternate cover test and the cover-uncover test is binocularity. During the alternate cover test, the patient is *never* allowed to become binocular. While the cover-uncover test is performed, the patient must be allowed to become binocular between the occlusion of each eye.

2. **False.** Abnormal retinal correspondence is a *binocular* adaptation to strabismus. By definition, it is an abnormal relationship that develops between retinal elements in each eye.

3. **True.** To neutralize an exodeviation with prisms, the base of the prism is held toward the nose. In an exodeviation the object of fixation stimulates the temporal retina and is therefore projected nasally. A prism displaces an image toward its apex. Therefore when a prism is held base in front of an eye, the object of fixation appears to the temporal side, and thus the deviation can be neutralized.

4. **Fusion.** Fusion is the unification of visual impressions by the brain into a single visual image, received as the result of stimulation of corresponding retinal elements.

5. **Equal.** An alternating deviation is a condition in which first one eye and then the other fixates.

Both eyes are used, which assists in providing good visual acuity in both eyes. Monocular fixators develop amblyopia.

6. **Versions, vergences.** Versions are binocular eye movements in which both eyes move in the *same* direction, such as both eyes moving into left gaze (levoversion) or both eyes into right gaze (dextroversion).

   Vergence movements are also binocular movements in which both eyes move in *opposite* directions in an effort to attain and maintain fusion, such as convergence and divergence that are required when changing fixation distance.

7. **e. Never allow the patient to be binocular.** The alternate cover test is performed to provide an accurate determination of the amount of deviation present. One essential factor to eliminate is motor fusion. The motor fusion mechanism is sufficient to keep the eyes aligned. Therefore the patient is constantly dissociated by occlusion and is never allowed to become binocular to eliminate any attempt to fuse.

8. **a. May have anisometropia.** Anisometropia is a condition in which the refractive error is unequal in the two eyes. Therefore one eye perceives an image that is much clearer than the other eye, an obstacle to fusion. Anisometropia may be a precipitating factor to amblyopia and strabismus.

9. **b. Has motor and sensory adaptations.** Strabismus is an abnormal condition in which there is a misalignment of the visual axes. Motor fusion is inadequate to maintain a proper alignment of the eyes; therefore a new position is adapted. Corresponding retinal elements are no longer simultaneously stimulated, and a comfortable sensory adaptation, providing single vision, must be made, such as suppression or abnormal retinal correspondence.

10. **c. Detects the presence and type of diplopia.** An evaluation of the patient's peripheral fusion status can be ascertained with the Worth four-dot test. It is a subjective test used to determine the presence or absence of fusion, suppression, alternation, or diplopia. If diplopia is present, the type (homonymous or heteronymous) can be established by the position of the lights in relation to the position of the filters in the goggles.

CHAPTER 33

Ophthalmic photography

CSABA L. MARTONYI, C.O.P.R.A., F.O.P.S.

- Photographic terms
- Film
- External photography
- Photo slit-lamp biomicrography
- Goniography
- Endothelial specular photomicrography
- Fundus photography
- Fluorescein angiography
- Cinematography and video recording
- Slides

In 1960, Novotny and Alvis performed the first successful fluorescein angiogram on a human being. That event marked the advent of modern ophthalmic photography. Subsequent development of sophisticated instrumentation has made it possible to consistently produce precise documentation of subtle changes within the eye. Intravenous fluorescence angiography has contributed greatly to a better understanding of the posterior segment of the eye and continues to be of particular importance in the diagnosis and treatment of many of the diverse disease processes that affect it. Since 1976, endothelial specular photomicrography has made possible the documentation of the cell density of the posterior layer of the cornea of the living eye. Moreover, photography plays an indispensable role in many areas of research and teaching. With the techniques of external photography, photo slit-lamp biomicrography,

fundus photography, fluorescein angiophotography of both the posterior and anterior segments, motion picture and video recording, and endothelial specular photomicrography, ophthalmic photography today is a vital, well-established adjunct to ophthalmology.

Although this chapter cannot treat the full scope of ophthalmic photography, it provides an overview and an introduction to its most practical applications.

PHOTOGRAPHIC TERMS

Standard, hand-held 35-mm cameras are of two basic types: single-lens reflex and those using a range finder or a viewfinder. (The latter type is not recommended unless specifically designed for eye photography.) Numerous lenses are available, and their important characteristics include focal length, lens speed, depth of field, and resolution. Exposure is determined with an exposure meter and regulated by means of an adjustable diaphragm, or "f" stops, and shutter speeds.

Associate Professor and Director of Ophthalmic Photography, W.K. Kellogg Eye Center, Department of Ophthalmology, The University of Michigan Medical School, Ann Arbor, Michigan.

Focal length

The focal length of a lens is the distance between the lens and the film plane in the camera (actually measured from the principal plane of the lens when focused at infinity). The focal length, expressed in millimeters, is engraved on most lens systems along with the serial number and trade name. The normal, or standard, camera lens is that which will produce an image of a scene in the same perspective as seen by the unaided eye. The normal focal length for a camera is roughly equivalent to the diagonal measurement of the film size used. For a 35-mm (film size) camera, the standard lens is 50 mm in focal length and has approximately a 45- to 55-degree angle of view. A wide-angle lens, such as a 35 mm (focal length), has a short focal length with an angle of view of about 62 degrees; a telephoto lens, such as a 135 mm, has a long focal length and is restricted to an angle of 18 degrees.

Lens speed

Lens "speed," or widest aperture, refers to the maximum light-gathering power of the lens. It is expressed in the form of an "f number," which represents the ratio of the diameter of the lens to the focal length. Engraved on the lens system, it may appear as f2.5, or f1:2.5 (or merely 1:2.5). The diameter of an f1 lens is equal to its focal length and is termed a *fast* lens because it permits a great amount of light to reach the film. Such a lens would be well suited for photography in available light. Most lenses have adjustable f stops, operated by a diaphragm between lens elements.

Depth of field

The distance within which all objects closer to and farther from the camera are acceptably sharp is called the *depth of field*. As a general rule, one third of the total depth of field will fall in front of the point at which the camera is focused and two thirds beyond that point. For instance, if the depth of field covers a distance of 3 feet when the camera is focused at 15 feet, all objects that are between 14 and 17 feet from the camera will appear sharp on the photograph. (Depth of focus is the same phenomenon occurring at the film plane.)

Depth of field is a function of focal length and f number. It increases with the use of larger f numbers (smaller apertures) and decreases with smaller f numbers (larger apertures). Depth of field is also greater for a wide-angle lens (short focal length) and less for a telephoto lens (long focal length) when both are set at the same f number. Depth of field is further affected by the camera-to-subject distance. The effective distance covered by the depth of field when a lens is focused at or near infinity is far greater than that of the same lens focused on a very near object. The closer a lens is focused, the more "shallow" becomes the depth of field. Because most photography in ophthalmology is done at high magnifications with a short distance between the camera and the subject, natural limitations in depth of field must be compensated for by using the highest possible f number (referred to as *stopping down*) and by using a light source that is sufficiently bright to provide the necessary exposure.

Resolution

Resolution, or resolving power, is the ability of a lens, film, or the eye to distinguish fine detail. This resolving ability of films and lenses is measured by the highest number of lines per millimeter that they are still able to define clearly without blurring together.

Shutter speed

Shutter speed is measured by fractions of a second, indicated by numbers such as 30, 60, and 125, which stand for $\frac{1}{30}$, $\frac{1}{60}$, and $\frac{1}{125}$ of a second. These numbers represent the length of time the shutter is open when the shutter release is activated—the interval during which the light passes through the lens and strikes the film.

Shutters may also have a "B" or "T" setting for time exposures. These are impractical for patient photography because a blurred image will result. Time exposures are useful in photographing nonmoving objects in dim light, when the camera is mounted on a tripod.

Setting

A specific area should be set aside for ophthalmic photography if possible. The photographic environment, including background and room lighting, can thus be better controlled, providing more consistent results. A degree of privacy, an important courtesy to the patient, also will be ensured.

FILM

Although film comes in many sizes, the one most commonly used in eye photography is the full-frame 35 mm, which yields transparencies with the dimensions of 24 × 35 mm (⅞ × 1⅜ inches). These are mounted into 2 × 2 inch cardboard mounts, from which their name *two-by-two slide* is derived.

Speed and types

The *speed* of a film refers to its sensitivity to light, expressed in International Standards Organization (ISO) numbers (formerly: American Standards Association [ASA] numbers). The higher the number, the more sensitive, or "faster," the film. Standard color films range from 25 to 1000 ISO (up to 3200 available with push processing), and black and white films for general use range from 25 to 400 ISO, or greater. Films having low ISO numbers will have fine-grained patterns on the film emulsion and higher resolution. The sharp detail offered by slower films (color or black and white) makes them valuable to scientific or diagnostic study, particularly when large prints are to be made from the slides or negatives.

There are two types of color film: positive transparency and negative. The name of each film indicates its type. Names ending in "-chrome" (for example, Kodachrome, Ektachrome, Anscochrome) signify positive transparency films that produce color slides. Names ending in the word "color" (for example, Kodacolor, Ektacolor, Fujicolor) refer to films that produce negatives from which prints are made. When desired, the preparation of *internegatives* will permit prints to be made from slides. Black and white negatives and subsequent prints can also be made from color slides for publication purposes.

Color films are designated *daylight* or *tungsten,* which refers to the lighting conditions under which the film must be used. All lighting sources have a *color temperature,* which is expressed in degrees Kelvin (K). Normal daylight, around midday, has a color temperature of approximately 5400° K. The light produced by an electronic flash, blue flashbulbs, or a blue filter over white bulbs has the same color temperature and requires the use of daylight film. Photo floods and other sources of tungsten illumination have a much lower color temperature and require the use of tungsten film. Tungsten films were designed to be used with lamps that produce 3200° K.

The use of daylight film under tungsten illumination will result in pictures having a yellow-orange or "warm" cast; the use of tungsten film outdoors, or with electronic flash or blue bulbs, will result in a decidedly blue, or "cold"-appearing, picture, inappropriate for patient photography. If a single type of film must be used under both lighting conditions, conversion filters can be placed over the lens, but an increase in exposure is required.

In general, daylight films have a higher ISO rating than comparable tungsten films.

Exposure

Exposure is the total volume of light that strikes the film. It is the *sum* of light *intensity* and *duration* of exposure. Correct exposure is achieved through the balanced interaction of film sensitivity, brightness of illumination, f stop, and shutter speed.

With the use of available light, the shutter speed is used to control the duration of the exposure and the f stop is used to regulate the intensity of the light striking the film. Each full f stop setting (f8, f11, f16, and so on) and each shutter speed setting (30, 60, 125, and so forth) affects the total exposure by a factor of two. For example, if the camera were set at a correct exposure of $\frac{1}{60}$ of a second at f11, and then the lens were opened to f8, twice as much light would reach the film and the image would be overexposed. Conversely, if the lens aperture were closed down to f16, only half the needed light would reach the film and the image would be underexposed. Likewise, if the f stop remained constant and the shutter speed varied, the same alteration in total exposure would result. By decreasing the shutter speed from $\frac{1}{60}$ to $\frac{1}{30}$ of a second, the exposure would be doubled; by increasing the shutter speed from $\frac{1}{60}$ of a second to $\frac{1}{125}$ of a second, the exposure would be halved. Correct settings, therefore, are vital to correct exposure. If either f stop or shutter speed is off by just one setting, a serious overexposure or underexposure may result on the film.

Exposure meters

Whenever a light source other than a flash is used, the correct exposure must be determined with a light meter. All modern light meters are marked in ISO numbers that correspond with the ISO ratings of available films. Before a reading is taken, the light meter must be set to the ISO of the film being used. With the use of a hand-held exposure meter, care should be taken to read the average intensity of light reflected from the subject. If the light meter is allowed to respond to an area that is either much brighter or much darker than average, a proportionate underexposure or overexposure will result. Also, to prevent underexposure the sensing element of the meter should be shielded from sources of light that do not strike the subject itself. Another manner of determining exposure is to take an incident reading. Rather than measuring the light being reflected by the subject, a special filter is placed over the sensor of the light meter, and then the light source itself is measured from the position of the subject to be photographed.

The newest single-lens reflex cameras have built-in exposure meters that offer automated exposure control when set to correspond to the ISO rating of the film being used.

Flash illumination

With the use of electronic flash, the *duration of the exposure* usually is determined by the *duration of the flash*. Inasmuch as most modern electronic flash units have a duration of approximately $\frac{1}{1000}$ of a second, the length of the exposure will be $\frac{1}{1000}$ of a second. This very short, motion-stopping duration makes the electronic flash ideally suited for eye photography. Because the duration of the exposure is now essentially beyond our control, correct exposure is achieved by regulating the *intensity* of the light, either at its source or when it passes through the lens, or both. In most cases, the intensity of the flash source itself need not be altered. In fact, it is desirable to have ample light to guarantee a good exposure at very high f stops, thereby ensuring the greatest possible depth of field at close working distances, especially with the use of slower, fine-grained film. Should it be impossible to stop down sufficiently to compensate for flash intensity, a diffuser can be used over the flash source itself.

All flash sources (electronic or flashbulb) are assigned a *guide number,* which is a numeric representation of the intensity of that particular flash source when used with a specific sensitivity (ISO) of film. The correct exposure is determined by dividing the guide number by the number of feet between the camera and subject. For instance, a guide number of 40 used with 25 ISO film, at a camera-to-subject distance of 5 feet, requires a lens aperture of f8 or at 10 feet, a lens aperture of f4. That same light source would have a guide number of 55 when used with a film rated at 50 ISO, requiring an aperture of f11 at 5 feet and of f8 at 10 feet. As one can see, doubling the ISO rating influences the exposure again by a factor of two. The use of film with an ISO rating twice as great, under the same lighting conditions, requires a reduction of exposure by one half.

Although no longer a variable with the use of electronic flash illumination, the shutter speed *must* be set at the speed prescribed by the manufacturer to provide proper *synchronization* (maximum light output coincident with a fully open shutter). In addition, the synchronization cord of the flash unit must always be connected to the *X* outlet on the camera. Incorrect shutter speed settings, or use of the wrong synchronization connector, can result in the loss of part or all of the picture. For electronic flash, *only* the X outlet may be used.

With the use of flashbulbs, the synchronization selector (when available) is set to *M* and the synchronization cord attached to the M outlet. When flash bulbs are used with a camera equipped with a focal plane shutter, the synchronization cord must be attached to the *FP* outlet, and only FP type flashbulbs are used.

Processing

Kodachrome film must be returned to a major processing plant for developing, but some films, such as Ektachrome, can be processed by local photofinishers with little delay. If local services are unavailable, special mailers may be purchased and film sent for processing elsewhere.

Black and white processing, although much simpler, should be carried out in a suitably equipped darkroom. Fluorescein angiograms can be made into positive transparencies by "proof" printing onto 8 × 10 inch graphic arts film. After processing, the angiogram can be studied on a light table with a suitable magnifier. When desired, individual frames can be cut from the sheet, mounted into 2 × 2 inch mounts, and projected. Enlargements, or paper prints, also can be made from selected frames.

EXTERNAL PHOTOGRAPHY

A 35-mm single-lens reflex camera with interchangeable lenses is recommended for external eye photography. The single-lens reflex feature permits viewing and photography through the same lens system. Composition and sharp focus are thus made easy because the image being photographed is seen in the viewfinder exactly as it will appear on film. To achieve the necessary magnification, a macrolens (specially designed to permit focusing on very near objects) is recommended. Macrolenses for 35-mm cameras are available from approximately 50 to 200 mm in focal length. The advantage of a longer (100 mm and over) focal length macrolens is that it permits a greater working distance between camera and subject and will produce less perspective distortion. (An extreme example of perspective distortion is that which results from the use of a very wide lens, such as a "fish-eye" lens.) Photography of an intraoperative procedure, for example, would dictate the use of a longer focal length lens to provide a suitable working distance–to-magnification ratio.

The close focus range capabilities of a macrolens can be further extended with the use of an *extension ring* or *tube,* which merely extends the lens further from the camera, enabling one to focus on an even closer object. Similarly, lenses designed for normal photographic use also can be extended for close focus applications. Varying lengths of rigid extension tubes may be used on the same camera interchangeably to provide an extended range of magnifications. Another method of extending lenses is the use of a bellows-focusing device between the camera body and the lens. Effectively a variable extension tube, it allows for continuous adjustment over a wide range

when used with the appropriate focal length of lens (Fig. 33-1). A good, practical magnification-to–working distance ratio can be achieved with the use of a 100- or 135-mm lens.

If only a fixed (noninterchangeable) lens camera is available, an add-on portrait lens can be used; however, whereas it is seemingly simple and inexpensive, it may provide limited magnification and resolution. Whenever its use is elected, it must be with a single-lens reflex camera to ensure proper framing and focus.

Illumination

For illuminating external photographs, an electronic flash device is recommended. Problems created by rapid eye movements or blinking are eliminated by the extremely short duration of the flash. Many inexpensive flash units are available today, some with automatic exposure control, eliminating the need to change f stops while providing the ability to alter the distance between camera and subject over a given range. If such a flash is being contemplated, its ability to function in the automatic mode at such close distances must be ensured. Not all have that capability.

A flash source should always be positioned to provide even, diffuse illumination over the area being photographed. The bridge of the nose, prominent brows, and so forth should never be allowed to cast a shadow onto the area of interest. For making photographs of a single eye area, the light should be positioned on the patient's temporal side. For taking a two-eye view or full-face photograph, the light should be positioned directly above the lens. The resulting photograph will show uniform illumination over the subject area, with shadows falling directly behind and below the patient. The use of a lens of 100 mm or more in focal length will considerably lessen the problems attendant with use of sharply oblique illumination, which results from working at too close a range to the subject.

A suitable background should be provided. A simple solution is to obtain several large (30 × 40 inches) matte boards available in a variety of pleasing colors. Fairly light, warm colors, such as yellow or light orange, are best. Greens and especially blues

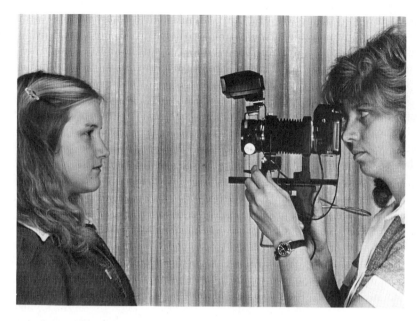

Fig. 33-1 Contax RTS Camera, Contax Auto Bellows, 100-mm Yashica Bellow Lens, and pistol grip.

are seldom complimentary to flesh tones. As a general rule, the lighter the subject, the darker should be the background, and vice versa. Patients with oculocutaneous albinism, for instance, might be best photographed in front of a dark background, whereas a lighter background must be used for darkly pigmented persons. Another point to keep in mind is that in photographing dark subjects, it is advisable to make additional, lighter exposures by "opening up" half an f stop (half the distance to the next smaller f number).

For persons not familiar with photography, the Lester A. Dine system (Fig. 33-2), which incorportes a Polaroid camera, is most useful. It is supplied with a color-coded series of lenses and frames to establish framing and camera-to-subject distance, and a flash source preset to provide correct exposure.

Whenever flashbulbs are used for patient photography, a clear protective shield must be placed over the bulb; this will prevent the possibility of injury should a bulb explode during the photographic session.

PHOTO SLIT-LAMP BIOMICROGRAPHY

Many conditions affecting the anterior segment of the eye—especially the transparent cornea, anterior chamber, and lens—are of such a subtle nature that they defy detection by any means other than *slit-lamp biomicroscopy*. Because the adverse conditions occurring in these transparent or translucent structures are themselves commonly transparent, conventional, diffuse illumination is unsuitable for their visualization. Only the specialized "optic sectioning" ability of the slit-beam illumination and high magnification of the slit-lamp biomicroscope provide an adequate view of subtle changes of interest to the ophthalmologist.

Fundamental to producing consistently useful photo slit-lamp documentation is a thorough knowledge of (1) the structures of the eye, (2) the location and general appearance of the diverse conditions affecting the eye, and (3) the basic forms of illumination and their application to these conditions. Basic illumination techniques include direct focal, tangential, direct and indirect retroillumination from

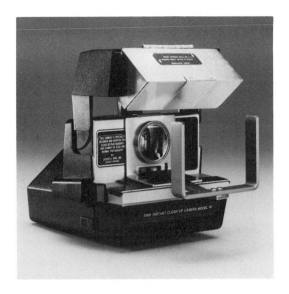

Fig. 33-2 Dine instant (Polaroid) camera with close-up lens and built-in flash. (Courtesy Lester Dine Co.)

the iris; retroillumination from the fundus; transillumination; sclerotic scatter; proximal illumination; and Tyndall's phenomenon for aqueous cells and flare.

A slit-lamp biomicroscopic examination is a dynamic process. With the use of a narrow slit beam to provide optic sectioning, transparent structures, such as those in the cornea, can be examined in minute detail, a small section at a time. The result is, in essence, a composite image of the entire cornea. In slit-lamp photography, however, each photograph is restricted to a single moment in that examination. To overcome this limitation, some slit lamps are equipped with a diffuse illuminator as well. When used in conjunction with the slit illuminator, the result can be a pleasingly subdued image of the overall eye with a superimposed narrow slit beam to provide specific information about that section of the structure that it isolates (Fig. 33-3). Whereas diffuse illumination will cause some fine detail to become obscured through the scattering of light, it is useful to provide general, introductory photographs. With these as a basis, additional photographs can illuminate areas of more precise inter-

est, further isolated through increased magnification. The result then will be a series of slides that leads the viewer through a logical progression from an overview to the most subtle detail. Fig. 33-4, *A* through *L,* shows some of the forms of illumination, along with recommended exposures as used on the Zeiss photo slit lamp. For other photo slit lamps, exposures should be established by exposing test films based on the manufacturer's recommendations.

Several photo slit lamps are available today. Desirable features include coaxial viewing (viewing and photography through the same lens system) and a flash source for both the slit and diffuse illuminators. Slit lamps not designed for photography may, on occasion, produce satisfactory photographs with the appropriate attachments. Of these attachments, electronic flash illumination is the most essential to provide the short exposures necessary to "freeze" eye movements and provide the correct color temperature of light for daylight film. Most tungsten bulbs used in slit-lamp biomicroscopes do not produce the exact color temperature required by available films. Another important attachment for a nonphotographic slit lamp is a diffuse illuminator to provide the overviews mentioned earlier.

Beyond the mastery of the mechanics of a photo slit lamp, the diligent practice of slit-lamp biomicroscopy is important to gain experience in disease entity recognition and light source manipulation to achieve maximum detail enhancement.

GONIOGRAPHY

Certain important structures of the anterior segment of the eye, such as the filtration angle, cannot be seen directly. To obtain a view of the angle, a gonioscopic lens (contact lens, some containing mirrors) is placed on the eye. With use of a moderate beam from the slit-lamp illuminator and the standard exposure for that slit width, excellent photographs are obtainable (Fig. 33-5). Diffuse illumination is not used in goniography because of the increase in light scatter within the gonioscopic lens.

Before the placement of the lens on the eye, a topical application of proparacaine hydrochloride, 0.5%, is used to anesthetize the corneal surface. The

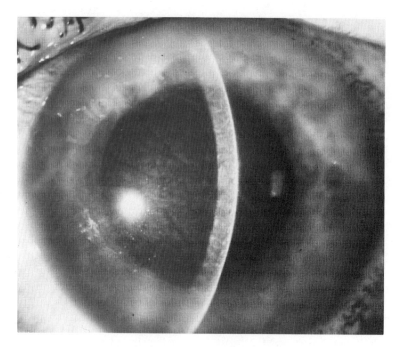

Fig. 33-3 Slit-lamp photograph showing diffuse, overall illumination with a superimposed narrow slit beam.

concave, contact end of the lens is filled with a viscous solution of methylcellulose to provide the necessary optical medium and a cushion between the lens and the eye. Once on the eye, the lens is rotated to place the desired mirror *opposite* the area to be viewed and photographed (see Fig. 33-4). (Goldmann and Haag-Streit lenses are available with three mirrors set at varying angles to facilitate a view of the angle, anterior vitreous, and retina.) Care should be taken to position the lens to eliminate reflections from its flat, rear surface. A three-mirror Haag-Streit lens with a special antireflection coating (similar to coatings on photographic lenses) is available from Ocular Instruments, Inc., Redmond, Washington. This coating, as on photographic lenses, permits a more efficient passage of light and contributes to the quality of the photographs. Another type of goniolens, the Koeppe, not containing mirrors, is ideal for examining or photographing patients in the supine position or children under anesthesia. In this case a hand-held fundus camera, such as a Kowa,

is used instead of the slit lamp and produces excellent results.

When desired, slit-lamp photographs of the fundus can be obtained through the center of the Goldmann type of contact lenses (Figs. 33-6 and 33-7). The slit-lamp illuminator must be placed in a fairly coaxial position with the microscope to provide adequate illumination through the relatively small aperture of the pupil.

All contact lenses, especially those used for photography, must be carefully maintained. By rinsing with running warm water immediately after each use, the methylcellulose is easily removed and will prevent the formation of a crusty residue that can easily scratch the surface of the lens if one attempts to wipe it away. Following standard procedures for decontamination, the lens should again be rinsed, be carefully dried with a soft cloth or tissue to remove droplets (which may leave precipitates behind), and stored in a sturdy, dust-free container.

To ensure the quality of goniographs, new lenses

Text continued on p. 696.

All exposures listed assume the use of 2× magnifiers on the side arms. When 2× magnifiers are not used, increase magnification or f-stop.

ISO 200
Diffuse illum. open
Slit 9   10×
Side arm f16

ISO 200
No diffuse illum.
Slit 9   16×
Side arm f32-44

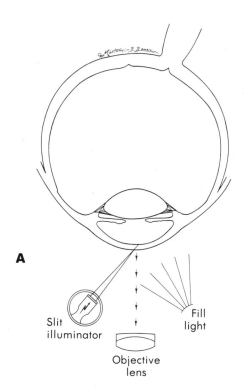

A

Slit
illuminator

Objective
lens

Fill
light

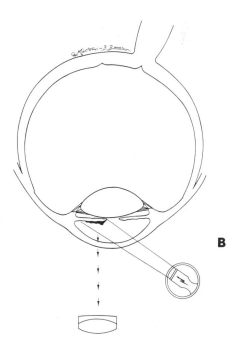

B

Fig. 33-4 A, Optical sectioning with fill illumination. Overall, diffuse illumination *(fill light)* provides a view of the entire eye, and the superimposed, direct focal illumination of the narrow slit beam provides specific information about the area that it isolates. Direct focal illumination in the form of a very narrow slit beam, without overall, diffuse illumination, is the most selective, direct method of examining the structures of the eye.

Fig. 33-4 B, Tangential illumination. A moderate to wide slit beam is projected onto the area of interest at a sharply oblique angle to produce clearly defined highlights and shadow areas, greatly enhancing topographic detail.

Continued.

ISO 800 or greater
No diffuse illum.
Slit 9
Side arm f16

16×

ISO 200
No diffuse illum.
Slit 9
Side arm f44

16×

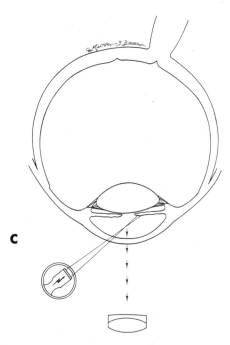

C

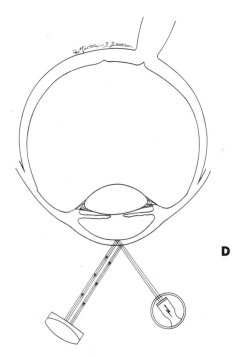

D

Fig. 33-4 C, Pinpoint illumination. Pinpoint illumination, based on Tyndall's phenomenon, is used to visualize and photograph aqueous cells and flare. The smallest circle beam is directed through the anterior chamber at an oblique angle. If the aqueous is turbid with cells and protein, the small cone of light will be visible to a variable degree depending on the amount of abnormal material it contains, demonstrating anywhere from "one" to "four-plus" aqueous cells and/or flare.

Fig. 33-4 D, Specular reflection. A moderate slit beam is projected onto the surface of interest (the corneal endothelial surface in this example) and viewed at an angle from the perpendicular that is equal to the angle of incidence. An area of nonreflectance from normally flat, reflective surfaces indicates an abnormality.

ISO 200
No diffuse illum.
Slit 9
Side arm f16-22   16-25 ×

ISO 400
No diffuse illum.
Slit 9
Side arm f16   16 ×

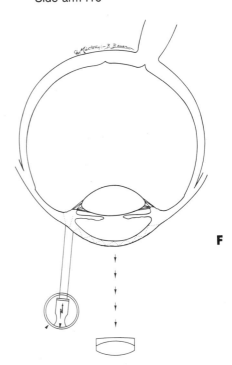

E

F

Fig. 33-4 E, Proximal illumination. A moderately narrow slit of light is directed to strike an area just adjacent to the area of interest. The light is absorbed by the surrounding tissue and scattered behind the abnormality, outlining it in relief against a now lighter background. This is an especially useful technique for delineating the general size and shape of an opaque object obscured by overlying soft tissue (such as an imbedded foreign body).

Fig. 33-4 F, Sclerotic scatter. A wide slit beam is directed to strike the limbal area where the light is absorbed and "piped" throughout the cornea. When corneal changes are present, they become visible by reflecting a small portion of the light passing through the cornea.

Continued.

ISO 200
No diffuse illum.
Slit 9
Side arm f22-32   16-25×

ISO 200 to 400
No diffuse illum.
Slit 9
Side arm f16   16-25×

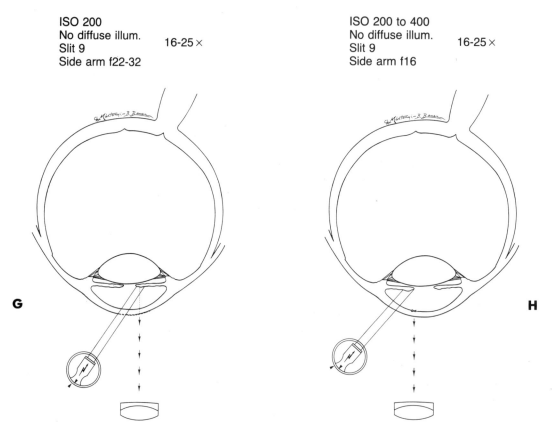

Fig. 33-4 G, Direct retroillumination from the iris. A moderate slit beam is directed onto the iris surface behind the corneal abnormality. (The slit beam must not strike the corneal changes directly.) The corneal abnormality is then examined or photographed in silhouette against the light background of the illuminated iris. The slit illuminator is rotated from its normally isocentric position to permit centration of the principal subject area in the final photograph.

Fig. 33-4 H, Indirect retroillumination from the iris. A moderate slit beam is directed to strike the iris just adjacent to the area that lies directly behind the corneal abnormality. The light striking the iris will be reflected in all directions and the subtle corneal changes can be seen, diffusely retroilluminated, against the dark background of the unilluminated iris and even darker pupil. The most useful zone of information will often be at the interface of light and dark backgrounds at the pupillary margin. The slit illuminator is rotated from its normally isocentric position to permit centration of the principal subject area.

ISO 200
No diffuse illum.
Slit 9
Side arm f32

10-16×

ISO 200
No diffuse illum.
Slit 9
Side arm f14

16×

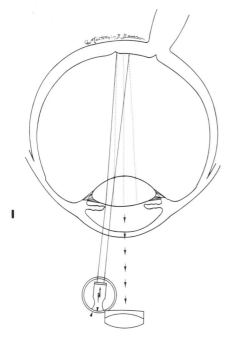

I

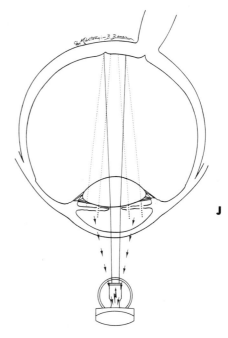

J

Fig. 33-4 I, Retroillumination from the fundus. A moderate slit beam is projected through the dilated pupil to strike the fundus in an area behind the abnormality to be examined or photographed. The slit illuminator must be brought into a nearly coaxial position with the biomicroscope and the slit beam decentered to enter at the pupillary margin. Through careful positioning of the slit illuminator and the slit beam in the pupillary area, the red reflex will be seen, against which subtle corneal and lenticular changes will be outlined. Considerably greater levels of illumination may be achieved by rotating the subject eye to position the optic nerve head to provide a much brighter background. This is an especially useful technique in photographing patients with dark fundi.

Fig. 33-4 J, Iris transillumination. Photographs should be taken with the pupil only partly dilated (3 to 4 mm when light stimulated). With the slit illuminator in a coaxial position with the biomicroscope, a small, full circle beam of light is projected through the pupil into the eye. Defects in the iris will be visible by transmission of the orange light reflected from the fundus.

Continued.

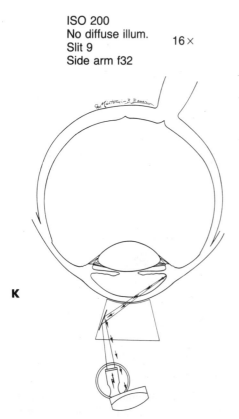

ISO 200
No diffuse illum.
Slit 9
Side arm f32

16 ×

K

Fig. 33-4 K, Goniography. After placement on the eye, the goniolens is rotated to bring the desired mirror into position opposite the area to be examined or photographed. A slit beam of moderate width, made parallel with the angle, usually is used. The same basic technique is used for the study and documentation of peripheral vitreal and retinal conditions, through a well-dilated pupil.

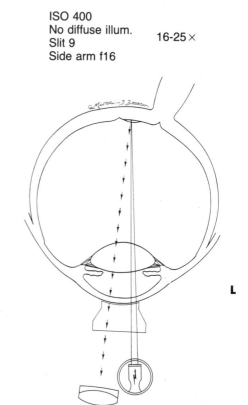

ISO 400
No diffuse illum.
Slit 9
Side arm f16

16-25 ×

L

Fig. 33-4 L, Photography of the posterior pole through a fundus lens. A contact lens is placed on the eye, which permits a view of the fundus with the biomicroscope. With a narrow or moderate slit beam, the structures of the posterior fundus can be examined in minute detail. The slit illuminator must be placed in a relatively coaxial position with the biomicroscope; the larger the pupil, the better the opportunity for oblique sectioning.

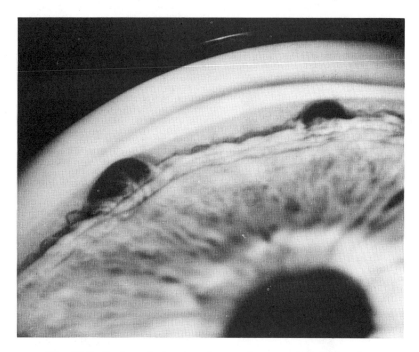

Fig. 33-5 Goniograph showing pigmented cysts and angle recession.

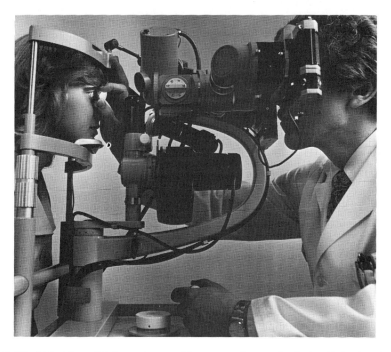

Fig. 33-6 The Zeiss Photo Slit Lamp in use with a contact lens to obtain the slit fundus photograph shown in Fig. 33-7.

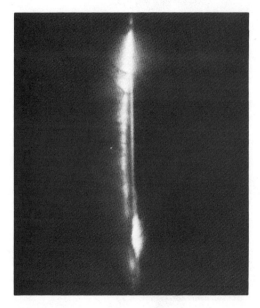

Fig. 33-7 The double slit indicates a shallow detachment of the sensory retina.

should be purchased and their use restricted for photographic purposes only.

Goniography, like all slit-lamp biomicroscopy, should be practiced as often as possible under the direction of the ophthalmologist.

ENDOTHELIAL SPECULAR PHOTOMICROGRAPHY

Specular micrography is a method of photographing and evaluating the endothelial surface of the cornea. As its name implies, specular micrography is based on a system of projecting a light onto the endothelial surface and photographing the information contained within the *specular reflection* of that light source. *Specular,* from the latin *specularis,* means "mirror-like." A specular reflection can be obtained from any relatively smooth surface. To be visible, however, it must be viewed at an angle from the perpendicular directly proportionate to the angle of incidence. The glossy surface of the endothelial cells will reflect a considerable amount of light, whereas their borders, not being smooth and flat, will absorb the light, thus providing a discrete "negative" outline of the cells (Fig. 33-8).

Although endothelial cells play a critical role in maintaining corneal clarity, they are of a finite number and do not regenerate. Several conditions, including age, can contribute to their compromise, and an assessment of their density and general health can be of significant value in the consideration of such procedures as cataract extraction or intraocular lens implantation.

Two types of endothelial microscopes, contact and noncontact, are available. The former requires direct contact with the patient's cornea. Before use of the contact microscope, the patient's cornea must be anesthetized and extreme care taken during the procedure to avoid inadvertent, excessive pressure on the eye. To this end the patient must be positioned in the head-rest assembly so as to be able to maintain steady, gentle pressure against the chin rest and, most important, the forehead stabilizing bar. If the patient's forehead is allowed to move away from the camera, there is the risk of the patient moving abruptly forward and applying excessive pressure to the eye. The slight amount of pressure required for photography is no more than that needed to slightly flatten the cornea against the applanator surface. Contact microscopes help minimize the normal movements of the eye. Appropriate cleaning and disinfection procedures should be followed between patients. Noncontact types may be extremely useful when direct contact with the patient's cornea is contraindicated.

FUNDUS PHOTOGRAPHY

The modern fundus camera, equipped with rapid recycling flash illumination, has vastly simplified photographic documentation of the posterior segment of the eye. Viewing and photography are done through a single-lens system, and correct exposures are ensured by predetermined flash intensity settings. With a little practice, even the novice can produce consistently acceptable photographs of the posterior pole.

The fundus camera system consists of a camera mounted on a specially designed instrument table equipped with a chin rest assembly to provide a comfortable and steady support for the patient's head. A power supply provides viewing illumina-

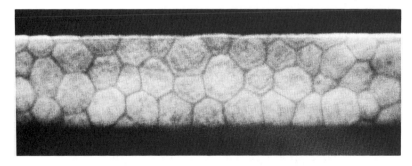

Fig. 33-8 Mosiac pattern of corneal endothelial cells.

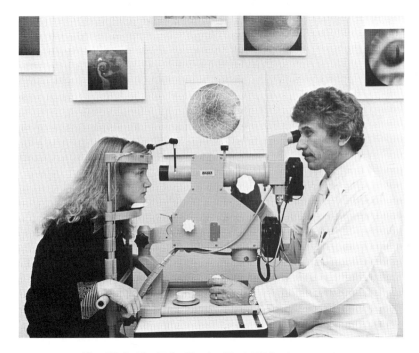

Fig. 33-9 The Zeiss Fundus Flash III fundus camera.

tion, rapid recycling flash illumination (up to three flashes per second), motor-driven film transport systems, and data imprint (identification number and elapsed time readings for rapid sequence fluorescein angiography) (Fig. 33-9).

The fundus camera, like the slit-lamp biomicroscope, utilizes an aerial image system of focusing. Unlike the single-lens reflex camera in which the image is projected onto a ground-glass surface, the aerial image is projected into space. This space is,

in fact, a well-defined plane designated by a "cross-hair" reticule. With use of this system, the only means of ensuring a sharp image at the film plane is to maintain the cross-hair reticule and the fundus detail in sharp focus simultaneously. Because accommodation on the part of the photographer can result in a dramatic shift of the aerial image away from its intended plane, neglect of the cross-hair reticule can result in unsharp photographs. The eyepiece of the fundus camera has an adjustable diopter range to correct for the photographer's refractive error. To establish the correct eyepiece setting, the eyepiece must be turned to its maximum up, or "plus," position. Then, while the examiner looks through the camera at some distant object with both eyes open, he or she slowly rotates the eyepiece downward toward the "minus" side, until the crosshair reticle is sharply seen. The examiner should *stop at this point*. This procedure should be repeated several times, or until the photographer's accommodation is relaxed and the same setting is consistently arrived at. When no refractive error exists, the eyepiece setting should be near zero. Accommodation can be more easily controlled if the examiner works in a darkened room with both eyes open while viewing through the fundus camera.

Before fundus photography is attempted, the patient's pupils must be dilated. The minimum pupil size through which acceptable photographs are achievable will vary from one fundus camera to another. Wide-angle cameras (45 to 60 degrees) generally require a proportionately larger pupil for acceptable results. The larger the pupil, the easier it will be to obtain good photographs. (If there is an opacity, such as a central cataract, a poor image of the fundus will result when the camera is properly centered. If the pupil is large enough, however, the camera can be placed off center, resulting in a much clearer photograph.) The use of a cycloplegic is also recommended to minimize the *patient's* accommodation. Inasmuch as the optic components of the eye—the lens and cornea—become part of the total optic system of the fundus camera, continued, active accommodation by the patient will result in an image that will drift in and out of focus.

By following a set routine, the editing of processed materials will be simplified. Before the patient is seated in front of the camera, it is a good practice to take a photograph of a standard form containing the patient's name, identification number, date of photography, and so on to positively identify the photographs to follow. If numbered forms are used and each roll is marked with the form number at its completion, identification of each patient's slides will be a simple matter.

The photographic sequence should begin with the posterior pole of the right eye and should include the disc and macula for positive identification of the eye being photographed. Stereo photographs of macula and disc can be taken at the same time. When a fundus "map" is required, following a routine sequence will aid in reconstruction of the photographic map after processing (Fig. 33-10).

When fundus photography is attempted for the first time, or when a new camera is being tried, careful documentation of exposures and procedures will provide a baseline from which appropriate adjustments can be made.

After seating the patient comfortably, the examiner should position the camera to produce a well-delineated circular image of the viewing bulb filament on the cornea or, if not well visualized there, on the closed eyelid (Fig. 33-11). With the camera aligned at this distance on the center of the pupil, a good view of the fundus should be attained. Without alteration of the camera position, the image should be sharply focused, after which final adjustments in camera position can be made.

To achieve a view of the desired area of the fundus, the patient's eye should be rotated by moving the fixation target, and the camera is moved to again line up on the center of the dilated pupil. Correct *saturation,* or maximum intensity of the correct color of the fundus, is achieved by moving the camera toward or away from the eye. When the camera is too far from the eye, a blue-gray halo will form around the image. As the camera moves forward, the color will become more saturated. When camera is placed slightly off center and moved closer to the eye, an orange to bright yellow crescent will appear on one side. This crescent signals maximum saturation beyond which the examiner should not go. By moving the camera laterally away from the crescent, it will disappear, but by moving too far in that direction, the crescent will reappear on the opposite side. A crescent appearing on the top of the picture is eliminated by moving the camera down; moving the camera up eliminates an inferior crescent. In attempting photography through a small pupil or other medial opacity, it may be impossible to avoid the bluish haze or crescent, but both should be minimized as much as possible. When a view of

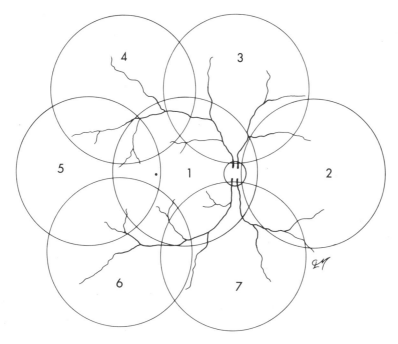

Fig. 33-10 Suggested format of successive fields to provide a composite of the posterior fundus. Proceed counterclockwise in the right eye and clockwise in the left.

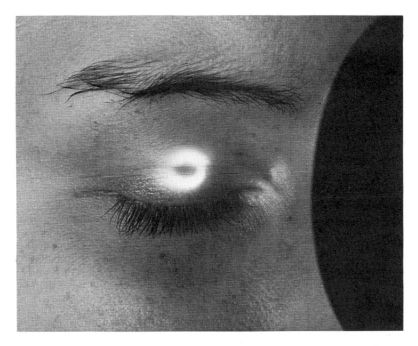

Fig. 33-11 The appearance of a correctly focused image of the viewing lamp filament on the closed eyelid.

the fundus is so dark it requires an increase in the viewing illumination intensity, a proportionate increase in the flash intensity must be made to ensure correct exposure. Conversely, for extremely light fundi, both viewing and flash intensities may be proportionately reduced.

Stereofundus photography

Sequential stereofundus photography is achieved by aligning the camera initially as described, then moving the camera laterally from one side of the dilated pupil to the other, taking a photograph in each position to provide the three-dimensional effect. When crescents are encountered, the camera should continue in the *direction of the crescent,* which should cause it to disappear. If a crescent persists, the camera should be moved slightly back from the eye. By previewing the area to be photographed in stereo while moving the camera briskly between the two laterally displaced positions, the examiner can get an excellent appreciation for the elevation or depression of the structure or lesion being viewed. Optimum camera position for each side of the stereo pair can thus be appraised before making the actual exposures. The greater the *stereo base* (distance between the two camera positions), the greater the three-dimensional effect. Because stereo photography requires using the camera in a drastically off-center position, it may not be possible to eliminate all artifacts; and at times, especially when the patient's pupil size is relatively small, stereo photography may involve a compromise to the quality of the individual frames. However, the two frames will reinforce one another considerably in addition to providing the three-dimensional effect so vital to the evaluation of many disease entities. Whereas a mechanical device called a stereo separator is available for some fundus cameras, the manual displacement method of obtaining stereo photographs described previously will provide the greatest degree of flexibility.

A wide range of fundus cameras is available today. Both table-mounted and hand-held instruments are obtainable. Some table-mounted systems produce a single, fixed angle of view, and others may be variable through a range of 60 to 15 degrees. A camera capable of photographing 180 degrees of the fundus on a single slide (using a special objective lens placed in contact with the patient's eye) also has been developed. Hand-held fundus cameras (Fig. 33-12) are excellent for photographing children under anesthesia or other patients who are unable to sit at a table-mounted system. The hand-held fundus camera also can serve as an excellent external camera—for example, for goniography with a Koeppe lens.

Most fundus cameras provide sufficient illumination to allow the use of fine-grained color films such as Kodachrome 25 and 64. When rapid processing is required, Ektachrome film can be used and processed locally. Polaroid camera backs are available for most systems, providing immediate records, when desired.

FLUORESCEIN ANGIOGRAPHY

For fluorescein angiography a fundus camera must be equipped with a rapid-recycling, high-output power supply and an *exciter* and *barrier* filter combination. The exciter filter is placed in the path of the light and allows only a specific wavelength of blue light (approximately 490 nm) to strike the fundus. When fluorescein is introduced into the circulation of the eye, the blue light excites the fluorescein molecules to a higher state of activity causing them to emit a greenish-yellow light of a higher wavelength (approximately 520 nm), creating the "fluorescence" that we are able to record on film. The barrier filter is positioned to filter out the blue exciter light and allow only the excited yellow-green light of actual fluorescence to strike the film. Most modern filter combinations are so efficient that they permit the recording of true fluorescence only. Older filter combinations, however, are less efficient and commonly produce a dim, but discernible, image of light structures within the eye, such as the optic nerve head, even without the injection of fluorescein. This level of exposure of light objects *without* fluorescein is generally referred to as *pseudofluorescence.* As a means of dealing with pseudofluorescence, a "control" photograph of the area to be documented should be taken. The exposure is made before the injection of fluorescein, with the exciter and barrier

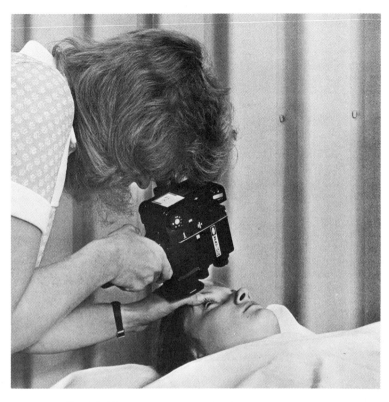

Fig. 33-12 The Kowa hand-held fundus camera in use.

filters in place and the flash intensity set at the level for fluorescein angiography. When this procedure produces an image, it is generally indicative of filter failure, perhaps requiring filter replacement.

Before fluorescein angiography is undertaken, the patient should be informed of the procedure and its implications, and consent is obtained. (Laws and regulations for obtaining consent vary among states and institutions.)

To produce an angiogram (Fig. 33-13) the following steps are recommended.

1. Load the camera back with 400 ISO black and white film. (A fresh roll of 36 exposures should be used for each patient.)
2. Set the flash intensity to the level used for color photography or, if possible, one step lower.
3. Introduce the green or "red-free" filter into the light path.

4. Expose the patient's name and identification (as described for fundus photography).
5. Position the patient at the camera, and take a stereo photograph of the area to be studied with the green filter in place, at the *low* power setting previously used (step 2).
6. *Increase* the flash output to the level required for fluorescein angiography, check *focus* and *alignment,* and then immediately place the blue exciter filter and the yellow barrier filter into the light path and expose the "control" photograph.
7. Remove the exciter filter from the light path, and prepare for the injection of sodium fluorescein.
8. When the needle is correctly set in an appropriate vein, check the patient's head position and, viewing through the green filter, *again ensure proper alignment and focus.*

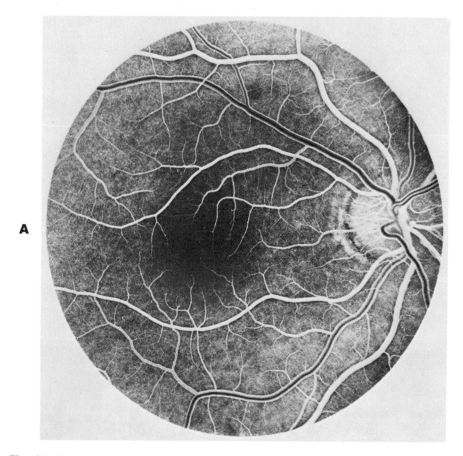

Fig. 33-13 A, Normal angiogram showing the early venous "laminar" or "lamellar" stage of circulation.

9. Initiate the rapid injection of the fluorescein with a *predetermined signal,* and *simultaneously activate* the data-imprinting device.

10. At 5 to 7 seconds following the start of the injection, the exciter filter should be placed into the light path, the viewing illumination increased, and the exposure sequence commenced. The average arm-to-eye circulation time in an adult is between 8 and 15 seconds and in a child, it can occur within 4 to 7 seconds.

11. After the rapid-sequence documentation of the initial circulation of fluorescein through the full arteriovenous phase, the frequency of exposures may be reduced considerably in-

asmuch as further development in the angiographic pattern will occur much more slowly beyond this point. (An understanding of the hemodynamics of the choroidal and retinal circulation, as well as the appearance of fluorescein angiographic characteristics of the various lesions studied, will improve judgment in sequencing and will aid in the conservation of film for later phases when required.)

12. Intermediate, or recirculation phase, photographs should be taken at approximately 1 to 3 minutes after injection.

13. A late photograph, approximately 20 minutes after injection, is also recommended. Certain

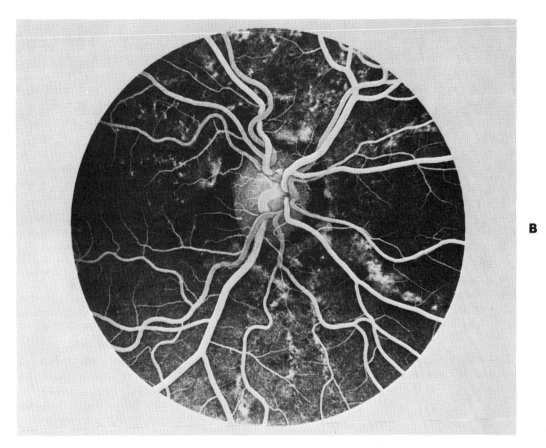

Fig. 33-13, cont'd B, Angiogram in the full arteriovenous stage of circulation in an eye affected with angioid streaks.

conditions are not delineated until this point, and the time interval can be used to monitor the patient for any signs of possible side effects from the fluorescein angiographic procedure. Stereo fluorescein photography can be incorporated at any stage of the angiogram by use of the procedure described for stereo photography.

CINEMATOGRAPHY AND VIDEO RECORDING

Both forms of motion recording have advantages and disadvantages. The foremost advantage of cinematography over video recording is its ability to produce finer detail—crucial if duplication for wide distri-

bution is anticipated. The "original" film can be completely edited, then reproduced many times, either onto film or video cassettes, without an excessive loss of information and without a striking increase in contrast. Among the disadvantages of cinematography, however, are the high cost of film and processing, the time required for processing, and the time lost reshooting because of poor exposure or other technical problems.

Major advantages of video recording are the relatively low cost of tape and our ability to monitor and make immediate adjustments when necessary. Sound may be recorded simultaneously or narrated after the video portion has been recorded. Playback is instantaneous and duplication is simple and relatively inexpensive. Video's major disadvantage is its relatively poor resolution. An *edited master* is in fact a copy of the original, and subsequent copies tend to further increase in contrast with a proportionate degradation of image quality.

Requests for motion recording may be made for patient eye movements and intraoperative procedures. Extraocular motility studies are most easily recorded on videotape but can, of course, be recorded on motion picture film as well. Macrolenses are available for both television cameras and motion picture cameras, but standard lenses may be extended for close-up applications in the manner described under External Photography. The television camera should always be used with a monitor (built-in or accessory), and the motion picture camera should be of the reflex type to ensure correct framing and focus. When television is used to document a patient's eye movements, instructions to the patient can be recorded simultaneously with the video to positively identify the direction of gaze being attempted. If desired, the sound portion can be eliminated or recorded over at another time. Videotapes may be completely erased and reused.

For much of the intraoperative recording of surgical procedures today, both motion picture film and television cameras are mounted on the operating microscope and may be coaxial with the surgeon's view (necessary for documenting intraocular procedures such as vitrectomies, and so on).

A video system is generally left on for an entire procedure. When using a motion picture camera, however, the surgeon usually activates the system to document selected portions of the operation. A major limitation of microscope-mounted motion picture cameras is their limited film capacity. A video system can record almost indefinitely, and even while a completed tape is being replaced with a fresh one, monitor display of the procedure can usually continue. A major, obvious benefit is the teaching value of such a system, which allows a number of observers to benefit from the view normally seen only through the microscope oculars (Fig. 33-14).

For documenting procedures not requiring an operating microscope, a system as described for ocular motility may be used. A long focal-length macrolens

is recommended to provide a suitable magnification-to–working distance ratio. Regular lenses also may be used by extending with extension rings or spacers. The camera must be placed on a sturdy tripod of sufficient height to provide the desired angle of view. The photographer may have to be positioned on a short stepladder to provide a comfortable stance.

Whereas the color temperature of light sources, such as the operating field lights, is of importance to both video and motion picture photography, it is much more important for the latter. The operating light may be used with a tungsten type of film, and the slight shift to the warm tones can be corrected, when desired, with the use of color correction filters.

In cinematography, titles may be superimposed over scenes by (1) shooting the scene, (2) rewinding the film in the camera, and (3) reexposing that section of film by photographing titles made of white or colored letters on a pure, nonreflective black background. Only the letters are thus recorded, and the result will be letters superimposed over the scene previously photographed. Titles may be faded in by initially stopping the lens down completely and as the camera is running, slowly (over a 1- to 2-second period) opening the lens to the f number required for correct exposure. The process is reversed to fade off the titles. Titles for videotapes are most easily obtained with the use of two cameras, one recording the scene and the other recording the title simultaneously onto the same tape. Titles can be prepared and faded on and off as with cinematography. Some video cameras have character generations built in, which can create titles electronically.

SLIDES
Cataloging

It is essential to establish an editing and filing system that will guarantee positive identification and ready retrieval of all patient photographs.

As already mentioned, the maintenance of the photographic log should include patient name, date of photography, medical identification number (when used), eye being photographed (OD/OS), types of photographs requested (stereo, fundus map,

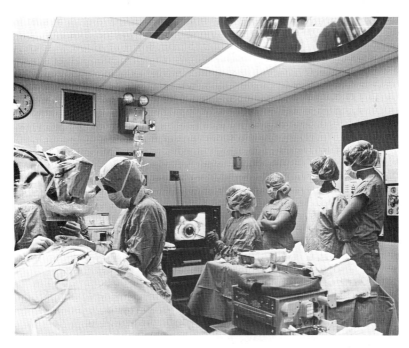

Fig. 33-14 Operating room personnel observe a surgical procedure on closed-circuit television.

fluorescein angiogram, and so on), and provisional diagnosis. A separate log should be kept for each camera to avoid confusion. If a photograph is taken of the patient's data first, all photographs after the identification slide will belong to that patient. When processed slides are kept in order and consecutively numbered (as they are when processed by Kodak), they are simple to identify even when several rolls of film are involved.

Upon receipt from the processor, slides should be grouped by patient, sorted for quality, properly labeled with the patient's name and number and date of photography, and identified as a right or left eye. The inclusion of the patient's age and diagnosis also is recommended, because this will facilitate use of the slides for future lecture or research purposes.

Stereo pairs may be mounted either in stereo glass mounts or simple aluminum frames covered by a protective plastic shield. Correct orientation of stereo pairs can easily be determined by use of a light table and a stereo map viewer. When right and left sides are interposed, a reverse stereo effect will be seen.

When mounting is not desired, the slides should be marked as being a stereo pair, left and right sides identified, and placed side by side into plastic loose-leaf sheets for filing.

Photographic records can be filed either alphabetically or by patient registration number. Perhaps the simplest method is to place 2 × 2 inch slides into readily available plastic loose-leaf pages accommodating 20 slides each. Fluorescein angiographic negatives should always be stored in sleeves designed for that purpose. Both the negatives and the prints may then be placed into an 8 ½ × 11 inch envelope and filed along with the slides, Polaroid prints, and so on in a letter-size drawer file. Pendaflex folders may be used in conjunction with steel-case type of files.

Because most photographic files eventually are used for teaching or lecturing, it is wise to initiate at the onset a cross-indexing system to permit retrieval by disease entity. Whereas several methods have been tried and are in use across the United States, it is difficult to establish a card file system that is both complete and manageable. Whenever the resources are available, a computer program,* with its inherent ability to handle considerable data with speed and accuracy, should be established. At the minimum, the photographer should maintain a listing of those patients and cases that the photographer or the ophthalmologist find to be of special interest or teaching value.

Whenever a photographic procedure is carried out, a notation indicating date, type and extent of photography, and signature or initials of the photographer should be entered into the patient's records.

Presentation

Projection slides in the most commonly used 2 × 2 inch format can be made easily with a minimum of equipment.

A 35-mm single-lens reflex camera equipped with a close focusing lens (macrolens or normal lens extended with bellows or extension rings) can be mounted on an inexpensive copy device consisting of a platform, a movable (up and down) stand for the camera, and four lights for illumination. Printed materials can then be copied from a book or manuscript, or the desired information can be typed onto white paper with a carbon-ribbon typewriter. Capital letters and adequate spacing are helpful, and the number of lines should be restricted to 12 or less.

---

*Montague PR, Weingeist TA, Eichmann DA: *Iowa data retrieval system: computers in ophthalmology,* New York, 1979, (University of Iowa Press, 1983).

To liven up the presentation, the information can be typed onto colored paper or a color filter placed over the lens and exposed on color film. A film from Polaroid (PolaBlue) is now available that will produce white (clear) letters on a blue background, and it can be processed in 6 minutes in a desk-top processor.

A number of programs are available for generating slides on a computer. They can be quite flexible and fairly easily learned. Several printing devices are also available with excellent resolution and speed. For projection, slides must be placed in the projector upside down. To simplify loading, the standard marking system should be used: the slide should be placed on a light table in its correct position and the lower left-hand corner of each slide marked with a red dot. (Self-adhering labels are not recommended because they may separate from the mount and cause the slide to jam.) The slides should be loaded with the red dot in the upper right-hand corner.

SUMMARY

In ophthalmology, a picture can truly be "worth a thousand words," and ophthalmic photography has indeed become an indispensible adjunct to the eye care profession.

To provide this vital service, the ophthalmic photographer must learn proved methods and stay abreast of new developments in technique and instrumentation. The success of each individual hinges primarily on his or her interest in photography, as well as in ophthalmology, along with a keen desire to excel in this challenging specialty.

QUESTIONS FOR REVIEW AND THOUGHT

1. The aperture of a camera refers to the size of opening that permits light to enter the camera. Is an f16 opening a large or small opening?
2. The depth of field indicates how much of the picture will come into sharp focus. Does an f2.6 opening have a large or small depth of field?
3. A fast film is used when there is insufficient light available. Name a film and film speed that are relatively fast.
4. What are the chief sources of lighting for external photographs of the eyelid and cornea?
5. How can you obtain steadiness of the patient and the camera during photography?

6. Fundus photographs may be taken with special cameras designed for this purpose. Name the camera type that you are familiar with, and outline a routine of photographing the fundus.
7. Outline a method of performing fluorescein angiography and photography.

SELF-EVALUATION QUESTIONS

True-false statements

Directions: Indicate whether the statement is true (T) or false (F).

T or F   1. A longer than normal focal length lens tends to reduce perspective distortion.
T or F   2. Fluorescein angiography should be recorded on Panatomic-X film.
T or F   3. The normal average arm-to-retina circulation time is in the range of 8 to 15 seconds.

Missing words

Directions: Write in the missing word in the following sentences.

4. The sensitivity, or "speed," of a film is expressed in _____ numbers.
5. Normal daylight has a color temperature of _____ degrees Kelvin.
6. Before attempting contact endothelial specular photomicrography, a drop of _____ must be instilled in the eye.

Choice-completion questions

Directions: Select the one best answer in each case.

7. When using electronic flash, the synchronization cord must be plugged into the outlet marked:
   a. M
   b. X
   c. FP
   d. B
   e. E
8. The ability of a lens to discriminate fine detail is called:
   a. Speed
   b. Angle of acceptance
   c. Focal length
   d. Resolution
   e. Depth of field
9. When an exposure is adjusted from $\frac{1}{30}$ of a second at f16 to $\frac{1}{60}$ of a second at f5.6, the total volume of light striking the film:
   a. Becomes one half as much
   b. Remains the same
   c. Becomes twice as much
   d. Becomes four times as much
   e. Becomes one third as much

ANSWERS, NOTES, AND EXPLANATIONS

1. **True.** A lens of a wide angle of acceptance must be used close to the subject with a resultant overemphasis of things nearest the camera. With a long-focus lens, the camera is used farther from the subject, resulting in more normal-appearing perspective.

2. **False.** Most modern fundus cameras still require the use of a high-speed film such as Tri-X or T-Max 400 for adequate exposures. The slow speed (ISO 32) of Panatomic-X makes it unusable for angiography in normal situations. Panatomic-X requires a nearly four-stop increase in exposure, amounting to nearly 16 times the light needed to expose Tri-X or T-Max 400.

3. **True.** Arm-to-retina circulation time for the average adult is approximately 12 seconds. A child's will be from 5 to 8 seconds, and in individuals with certain problems the dye will circulate much more slowly. It is important to be prepared for this factor to ensure correct sequencing during the initial phase of the angiogram.

4. **Formerly ASA, or American Standards Association, now ISO, or International Standards Organization.** The sensitivity of each film is designated by a numeric value, its ISO number, which must be calculated into the exposure for that film. The ISO number for the film being used is simply set on the exposure meter, and the reading will be correct for that film. If, however, the photographer neglects to change the ISO setting after changing to a different sensitivity of film, proportionate overexposure or underexposure will result. If, for instance, a meter had been set to 100 ISO and then a film of only 25 ISO was substituted without resetting the meter, the 25 ISO film would be underexposed by two full stops and would in most cases be unusable.

5. **5400° K.** The color temperature of fluorescent lights is approximately 3700° K, photofloods are 3400° K, and ordinary household light bulbs are approximately 2700° K. Care must be taken to use the type of film best suited for the lighting conditions under which it will be used. If accurate color reproduction is essential and the correct film and lighting combination is not available, correction filters can be used. Consult your local photographic retailer about your specific needs.

6. **Proparacaine hydrochloride, 0.5%.** The surface of the cornea must be anesthetized before placing the applanator in contact with it.

7. **b. X.** Only the X synchronization mode will provide proper synchronization for electronic flash. The duration of electronic flash is approximately 1 millisecond ($\frac{1}{1000}$ second), and the electronic contact to fire the flash *must* occur at the moment when the shutter is fully open. The shutter must also be set to the speed recommended by the manufacturer for use with electronic flash. If the flash is fired when one of the shutter curtains is in front of the film plane, the portion of the film that the curtain is obscuring will not be exposed.

8. **d. Resolution.** The resolution of a lens is measured by its ability to discriminate the maximum number of lines per millimeter. In other words, if a lens can produce a negative of a 1-mm area containing 200 line pairs so that those lines can be counted on the negative, but in an attempt to record 200 line pairs, the lines become blurred together and cannot be counted, that lens has a resolving capability of line pair lines per millimeter.

9. **d. Becomes four times as much.** The basic exposure is $\frac{1}{30}$ of a second at f16. Each setting of either shutter speed or f stop influences the total exposure by a factor of two. Changing the shutter speed from $\frac{1}{30}$ to $\frac{1}{60}$ of a second cuts the exposure in half. By "opening up" from f16 to f11, that half is again increased by two to the original total exposure of "one." One sixtieth of a second at f11 equals $\frac{1}{30}$ of a second at f16. By opening up to f8, the exposure is doubled, and is doubled again, or increased to four times, at f5.6.

CHAPTER 34 Advances in diagnostic testing

- Fluorescein angiography
- Computed tomography
- Magnetic resonance imaging
- Dacryocystography/lacrimal scan
- Computerized corneal topographic analysis

Specific tests are available to provide diagnostic information relevant to the clinical situation. This information will enable the clinician to make sound decisions regarding the most appropriate patient management. The ophthalmic assistant often is involved in reviewing the results of these tests with the ophthalmologist. A general understanding of the nature of these tests, as well as the appropriate indications, will create a more interesting and challenging work environment.

FLUORESCEIN ANGIOGRAPHY

Fluorescein angiography has become a widely used technique to study retinal circulation and diseases involving the retina and choroid. Although the retina is readily available for study by direct and indirect ophthalmoscopy, fluorescein angiography is a valuable adjunct to these methods of clinical examination. It is not intended to replace these methods but only to amplify some of the findings obtained by their use.

Fluorescein angiography is made possible by the unique chemical and physical properties of fluorescein. Fluorescein is an inexpensive, nontoxic, highly fluorescent compound. It absorbs blue light and emits yellow-green light, and therefore only relatively simple modification of existing fundus cameras is necessary to perform angiography. The test

can be performed with minimum discomfort to the patient.

Fundus photography in rapid sequence after intravenous injection of fluorescent dye provides information on the flow characteristics in the blood vessels, as well as fine details of the retina and choroid that may not be appreciated by other means. These details depend on anatomic features of the retinal and choroidal vessels and retinal pigment epithelium. Normal retinal vessels are impermeable to the dye. This characteristic allows a clear picture of the retinal vessels and assessment of their functional integrity inasmuch as leakage from any retinal vessel is abnormal. Because the fine vessels of the choroid (the choriocapillaris) leak fluorescein dye and the normal retinal pigment epithelium is a barrier to both the passage of the dye and its fluorescence, it is possible to use the technique of fluorescein angiography to study diseases that affect the retinal pigment epithelium.

The technique of dye administration is as follows.
1. The patient is seated comfortably at the fundus camera with one arm extended and the forearm exposed.
2. Fluorescein dye is drawn into a 10-ml syringe. A 21-gauge needle is then used to enter a vein in the arm. Care should be taken to ensure that the needle is in the vein by drawing back blood

and injecting just a slight amount of dye. It is important to make sure that the dye will not extravasate from the vein because this may be painful.

3. Before injection of the main bolus of dye, red-free photographs usually are taken. This can be done with the appropriate filter in the fundus camera.

4. The dye is injected into the patient's arm fairly rapidly so that the entire volume of dye is injected in about 2 seconds.

5. Photographs are taken at moderately rapid intervals (about one each second) immediately following injection of the dye. After the dye has filled the retinal vessels in one eye, pictures are taken of the fellow eye. In most instances it is helpful to photograph both eyes so that the fellow eye can be used for comparison and as a control.

There is a mild degree of morbidity inherent in this method. Some patients will have transient nausea and occasional vomiting 30 to 60 seconds after the injection of the dye. Vomiting usually can be avoided by reassuring the patient. Hives and asthmatic symptoms occasionally may develop. These symptoms can be treated by oral or intravenous administration of diphenhydramine hydrochloride (Benadryl) or cortisone.

A number of fluorescein angiographic phases are recognized (Fig. 34-1). About 10 to 15 seconds after injection into the antecubital vein, the dye reaches the ocular circulation. In the prearterial phase, the choroidal vessels fill and one can discern a patchy hyperfluorescent "choroidal flush." In the arterial phase, which is 1 second later, the retinal arterioles fill. The dye then flows into the capillaries and then into the veins. When there is partial venous filling, that is, *laminar flow,* the arteriovenous phase is recognized. When the veins are filled with fluorescein, this is the venous phase. The dye is distributed throughout the blood (recirculation phase) 3 to 5 minutes after injection, and early leakage and staining occur during this period. The elimination phase can be observed between 30 to 60 minutes after injection.

Damage to the endothelium of retinal capillaries or the retinal pigment epithelium causes leakage into and beneath the retina. Diagnostic patterns include defects of the pigment epithelium (which act as windows to the underlying choroidal fluorescence), accumulation of dye between choroid and retina (for example, serous detachment), staining within the retina (secondary to leakage from retinal capillaries), interference with visualization of choroidal fluorescence (by exudates, pigment, hemorrhage), obstruction to filling (arteriole or venous occlusion), and abnormal vessels (for example, neovascularization).

Fig. 34-2 shows the presence of dye leakage into the macula. This is associated with a decrease in vision and is consistent with the diagnosis of cystoid macular edema. This condition may be seen after any type of intraocular surgery, most commonly after cataract extraction, or it may be a consequence of an inflammatory condition of the posterior segment that causes leakage of the macular vessels.

Fig. 34-3, *A,* shows a diabetic fundus with microaneurysms, which appear as punctate areas of hyperfluorescence. A later stage of the angiogram (Fig. 34-3, *B*) shows significant leakage of dye into the macula, which accounts for the decrease in vision.

Fig. 34-4 is an angiogram of a central retinal vein occlusion. One can appreciate the tortuous retinal veins, hypofluorescent areas that represent scattered hemorrhages, and hyperfluorescent areas that are a result of leakage from the vessels. This is in contrast to Fig. 34-5, which is an angiogram of a branch retinal vein occlusion that shows blockage of the choroidal fluorescein by blood in a sector distribution. The patient has decreased vision as a result of macular edema from vessel leakage. Laser photocoagulation can be performed to improve the visual prognosis.

COMPUTED TOMOGRAPHY

Computed tomography (CT) scanners, which were developed in Great Britain in 1972, convert x-ray pictures into digital computer codes to make high-resolution video images. The computer graphics employed are similar to those used to reassemble pictures transmitted from distant space probes. Depicting bone structures in fine detail, CT scans also can show small differences between normal and ab-

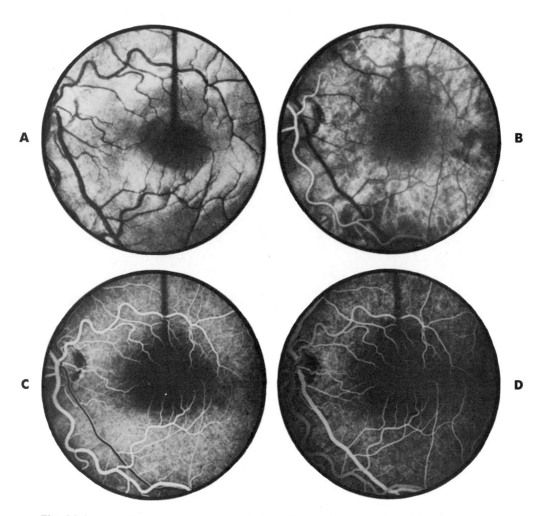

Fig. 34-1 Normal fluorescein angiogram. **A,** A red-free photograph of the ophthalmoscopic view of the left macula. **B,** In this retinal arterial filling phase of the fluorescein angiogram, there is patchy filling of the choroid. Large choroid vessels can be seen in some areas. The central retinal artery has begun to fill. **C,** In the early retinal arteriovenous phase, the choroid has completely filled with a diffuse and even fluorescence. The retinal arteries fluoresce; the retinal veins show laminar flow. **D,** In the later arteriovenous phase or recirculation phase, fluorescence has begun to fade from the choroidal and retinal vascular circulations. (From Schatz H, et al: *Interpretation of fundus fluorescein angiography,* St Louis, 1978, Mosby.)

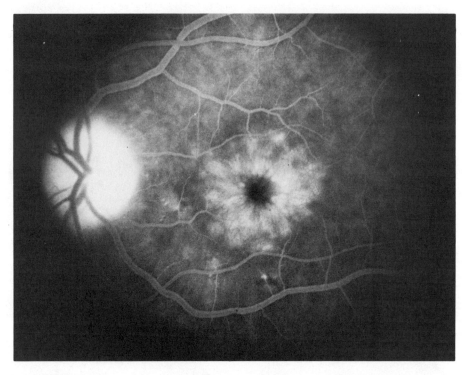

Fig. 34-2 Fluorescein angiogram that demonstrates cystoid macular edema.

normal tissues. CT scans are used for diagnostic purposes in the detection of orbital and lacrimal gland masses and of intraocular and orbital foreign bodies, as well as excluding fractures of the orbital bones.

Malignant melanoma of the choroid, when advanced, will extend into the eye in a mushroom shape and cause an overlying retinal detachment. A CT scan (Fig. 34-6) shows these features, as well as the lack of obvious orbital invasion by the tumor.

Lacrimal gland masses can be benign or malignant. Malignant lesions, such as the adenoid cystic tumor, often are associated with a more rapid onset of painful symptoms, as well as evidence on CT scan of erosion of bone. Fig. 34-7 shows lacrimal gland enlargement on the left side without bone erosion. This picture is consistent with the benign mixed tumor or the result of a lymphoproliferative disorder.

An intraocular mass lesion in an infant is most commonly a result of a retinoblastoma. The patient often will exhibit leukokoria (a white pupil). Fig.

34-8 shows a CT scan of a 4-month-old with bilateral calcified masses within the globes consistent with retinoblastomas.

Orbital lesions can cause proptosis, which is a forward protrusion of the globe; displacement, which is a deviation of the globe in an up-down or side-to-side shift; or a restriction in motility. Mass lesions of the orbit may originate within the confines of the orbit or may spread from another source—most commonly the breast or lung. Fig. 34-9 shows a CT scan of the orbits with a mass lesion that on biopsy was found to be a lymphoma. This is a tumor of abnormal lymphocyte cells that can be localized to the globe or can involve multiple organs.

Tumors of the optic nerve can involve the nerve substance proper, such as a glioma, or can affect the covering of the nerve, such as a meningioma. Both optic nerve tumors are associated with poor vision and the presence of pallor of the optic disc. Fig. 34-10 shows a CT scan that demonstrates an optic nerve sheath meningioma.

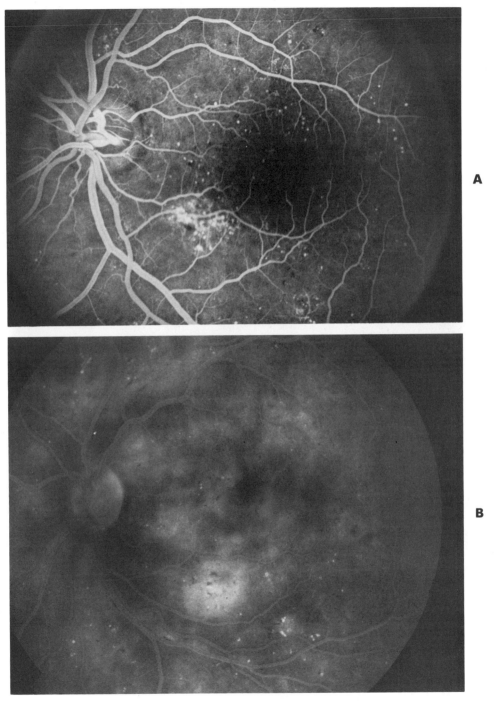

Fig. 34-3 A, Fluorescein angiogram of a diabetic fundus. **B,** Later angiogram phase of the same diabetic fundus as in **A.** Areas of hyperfluorescence represent leakage of fluid into the macula.

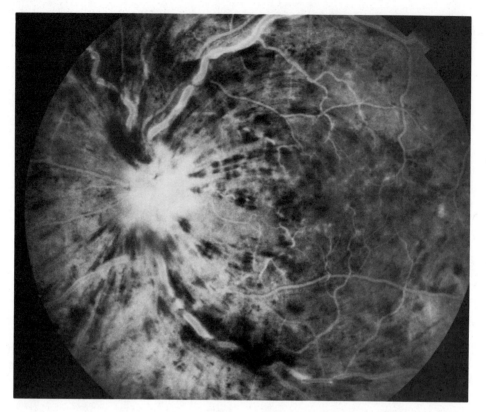

Fig. 34-4 Fluorescein angiogram of a central retinal vein occlusion.

Foreign body injuries often result in a blood-filled eye that does not permit ophthalmoscopic viewing. Plain x-ray studies will demonstrate only iron-containing foreign bodies and will not allow the physician to determine whether the foreign body is within or behind the globe. CT scan will demonstrate most foreign objects, which will enable the examiner to accurately localize the foreign body. Fig. 34-11 shows a CT scan that demonstrates a foreign body, as well as air and a vitreous hemorrhage in the left globe.

After a blow to the eye, patients can have diplopia and a restriction in motility because of an orbital bone fracture. The most common bone to be fractured is the orbital floor. Fig. 34-12 shows a CT scan with a coronal view that demonstrates an orbital floor fracture with herniation of the inferior rectus into the underlying maxillary sinus.

MAGNETIC RESONANCE IMAGING

Magnetic resonance imaging (MRI) is a revolutionary diagnostic imaging technique that uses a strong magnetic field, a radio-frequency pulse, and the energy emission of hydrogen nuclei (protons). Unlike x-ray studies and CT scans, MRI does not employ ionizing radiation; therefore patients are free from the dangers of radiation exposure.

MRI often will detect subtle differences between tissue structures. This will be represented on film as a change in black and white density. Unlike CT scanners, bone does not appear in MRI; therefore the detection of orbital fractures would not be an indication for its use. Also, because of the strong magnetic field, patients with intraocular foreign bodies should not have MRI scans performed for fear that the foreign bodies may be magnetic. This can result in significant ocular injury if the foreign

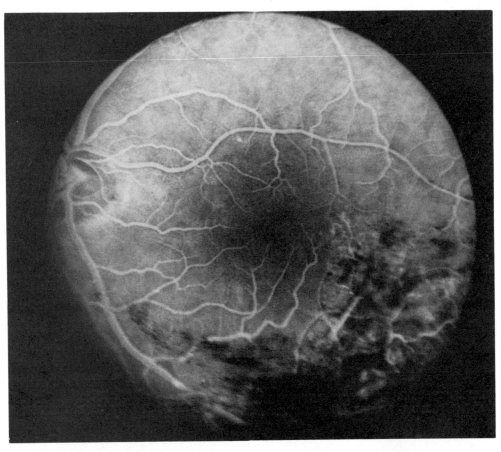

Fig. 34-5 Fluorescein angiogram of a branch retinal vein occlusion.

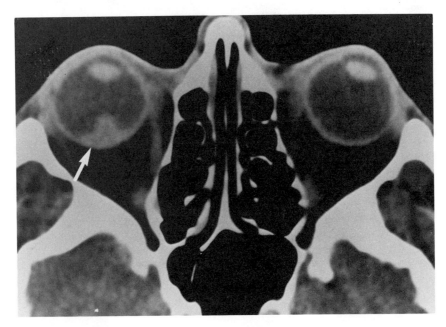

Fig. 34-6 CT scan of a malignant melanoma of the left globe.

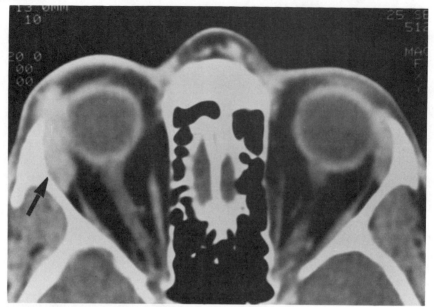

Fig. 34-7 CT scan that demonstrates enlargement of the left lacrimal gland.

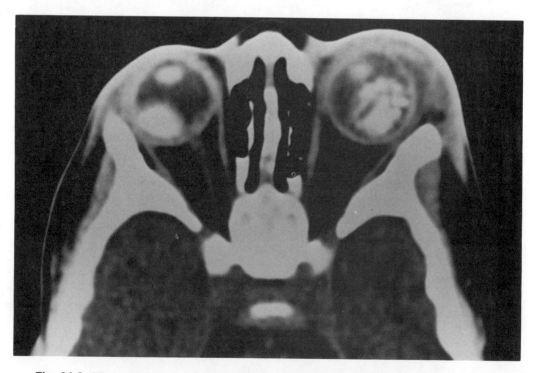

Fig. 34-8 CT scan that shows bilateral calcified masses consistent with retinoblastomas, an intraocular tumor of infancy.

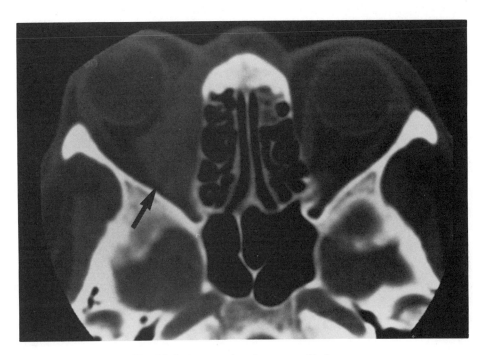

Fig. 34-9 CT scan that shows an orbital tumor.

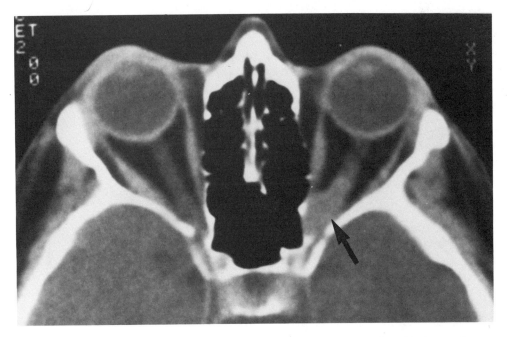

Fig. 34-10 CT scan that shows enlargement of the optic nerve near the orbital apex due to meningioma.

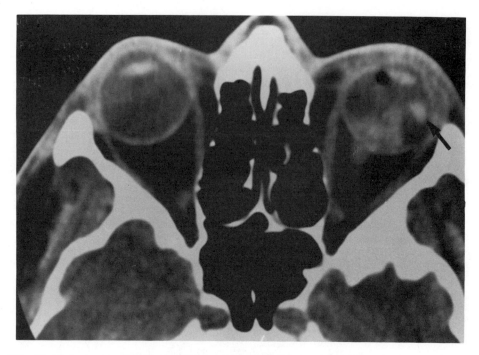

Fig. 34-11 Intraocular foreign body demonstrated on CT scan. The black area within the eye represents air that entered the eye at the time of penetration by the intraocular foreign body.

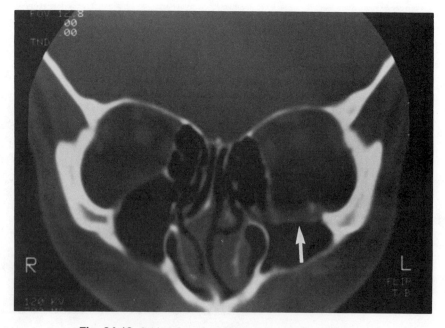

Fig. 34-12 Orbital floor fracture demonstrated on CT scan.

body is pulled through ocular structures, such as the retina or lens. Because of the ability of MRI to depict soft tissues in high contrast, it has proved effective in ophthalmology for the imaging of orbital and lacrimal gland lesions.

Although MRI is an exciting field, it also is an expensive one. The equipment, which consists of a huge electromagnet, a radiofrequency generator, and a computer for evaluation, costs about $2 million. The equipment must be kept in a room completely insulated from external radio frequencies, adding another three quarters of a million dollars to the cost. MRI has become a major part of the imaging armamentarium. MRI has proven to be as great a tool to modern medicine as the x-ray, discovered by the German physicist Wilhelm Konrad Röntgen in 1895.

Fig. 34-13 depicts an MRI scan that demonstrates the normal anatomy of the brain and eye. The various structures of the brain can be appreciated in exquisite detail. Fig. 34-14 demonstrates an enlarged lateral rectus muscle of the right eye. The patient was found to have an inflammatory condition that resolved rapidly with a short course of systemic steroids.

DACRYOCYSTOGRAPHY/LACRIMAL SCAN

Dacryocystography (DCG) and lacrimal scan are imaging techniques that occasionally are used to evaluate the lacrimal outflow system in patients who report persistent tearing. DCG is the best anatomic test for determining the actual site of obstruction in the lacrimal outflow system. With the patient lying down, a drop of topical anesthetic is placed in the palpebral aperture. Both lower puncta are simultaneously intubated and injected with a low-viscosity oil. Serial radiographs are taken during injection.

The lacrimal scan is the most physiologic test to date. It simulates passage of the tears through the lacrimal excretory passages without the use of invasive instruments. The test, however, does not give the same detail as the DCG in determining the actual obstruction site. The lacrimal scan determines whether the tearing is caused by the inability of the lids to promote tear flow into the lacrimal passages or by an obstruction of the outflow system. A drop

of technetium sulfur colloid is placed on the marginal tear strip of each lower lid while the patient is sitting upright. No anesthetic is necessary because the drop is nonirritating and has the same pH and osmolarity as tears. Pictures are taken by a specialized gamma camera that uses less than 2% of the radioactivity of routine x-ray studies. The photographs are taken every 10 seconds for the first minute and then every minute for 20 minutes after which time the patient's eyes are wiped and a final picture is taken.

COMPUTERIZED CORNEAL TOPOGRAPHIC ANALYSIS*

During the past several years there has been increased research and growing interest in the field of corneal topography, that is, measurement of the curvature of the anterior corneal surface. With the capabilities of modern computers and software technology it has become feasible and practical to precisely analyze the radius of curvature (millimeters) and corresponding refractive power (diopters) at thousands of points across the corneal surface. Computerized corneal topography is a logical advance from the basic principles of keratometry and photokeratoscopy developed during the past century. Photokeratoscopy provides the user with only qualitative information about the curvature of the cornea and changes that accompany surgery, contact lens wear, and progressive corneal abnormalities. The keratometer yields quantitative data, but only at four points. These points are located at approximately the 3-mm optic zone along two perpendicular meridians. One pair of points is aligned along the steepest axis of the corneal surface, with the second pair 90 degrees away. Each pair of points is averaged across its respective meridian to yield two k values, which approximate the cornea's central refractive power. The keratometer has fundamental limitations in that it is able only to measure points along the annulus of the 3-mm optic zone and it assumes orthogonal symmetry of the flat and steep axis of the cornea. In contrast, systems such as the EyeSys Corneal

---

*Contributed by T.D. Padrick and J.S. Wakil EyeSys Laboratories.

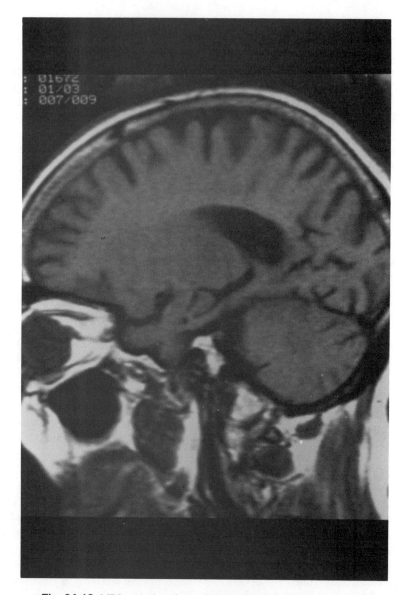

Fig. 34-13 MRI scan that shows fine details of the brain and orbit.

Analysis System measure the corneal refractive power at 6000 to 8000 points on the corneal surface from inside the 1-mm optic zone to outside the 9-mm optic zone. This information provides a complete color-coded representation of the cornea's shape and the ability to monitor corneal curvature changes from the apex to the periphery.

To understand how this additional information about the corneal surface helps the eye-care professional, one must understand the function of the cornea in the visual process. First, it is important to note that the cornea, more specifically the anterior tear film surface, provides most of the refractive (light bending) power of the eye. Approximately 75% of the overall focusing or refractive power of the normal adult eye is provided by this air/tear film

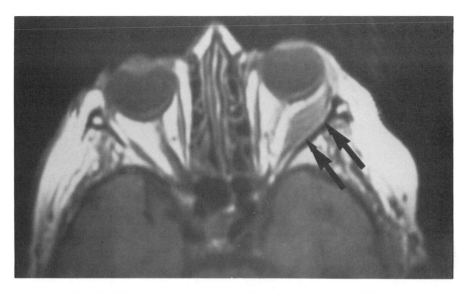

Fig. 34-14 Enlargement of the lateral rectus muscle on an MRI scan.

interface on the cornea (Fig. 34-15). The remaining 20% to 25% of the eye's focusing power, which is provided by the lens, is needed primarily for near-vision focusing or accommodation of the eye. The corneal curvature provided to the anterior tear film is truly the "lens" of the eye. From a strictly optical perspective, the cornea must provide two functions for good vision: (1) it must be transparent and (2) it must provide the proper curvature to the tear film. Thus it is important that the eye-care professional understand the importance of the corneal tear film as the primary refractive element in vision.

Having the ability to measure refractive power across the corneal surface and to follow corneal shape changes induced by corneal pathology and surgery provide a much greater understanding of the refractive complaints a patient may have. In other words, the subtleties of a patient's refraction may be elucidated through corneal topography.

Instrument design

Basic design features. Today's computer-assisted corneal topography systems are based on a concept developed in 1880 by A. Placido. He placed a planar concentric ring target with alternating black and white rings in front of a patient's eye and then ob-

served the shape of the rings in the virtual image of that target created from the reflection off the patient's cornea. If the cornea is spherical, the rings appear circular and concentric. Deviations of the corneal shape appear as either distortions in shape or concentricity of the rings. This method provides the observer with qualitative information about the patient's corneal curvature.

Modern computerized corneal topography systems utilize personal computers to qualify the data obtained from reflected Placido disk images. The EyeSys Corneal Analysis System uses a back-lit conical dish as its Placido target; other systems use a cylindric light cone as the Placido target. With either a conical dish or a cylindric light cone, a Placido ring image is produced on the cornea. With today's instruments the video camera (the observer) visualizes the virtual image of the black and white Placido ring pattern on the eye. The computer then analyzes this digitized video image and displays the data in a variety of useful formats.

Working distance. The working distance of the Placido source is a fundamental and important design difference between the EyeSys Corneal Analysis System and other systems. Fig. 34-16 illustrates this design difference. A ray from either source reflects

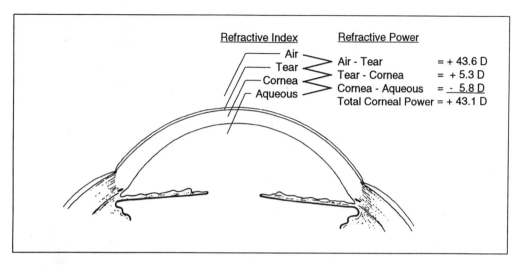

Fig. 34-15 Refractive power of corneal surfaces. (Courtesy EyeSys Laboratories, Houston, Tex.)

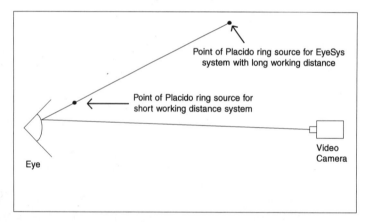

Fig. 34-16 To achieve the same corneal coverage, a longer working distance requires a larger-diameter Placido ring source. (Courtesy EyeSys Laboratories, Houston, Tex.)

from the surface of the eye to a given point on the video camera. The location of this point on the video camera determines the measured radius of curvature at the point of reflection. If the location of the ring in the video image is displaced, a different radius of curvature is measured. In systems using a short working distance (see Fig. 34-16), slight displacement of the video camera results in changes to the angle of reflection, which correspond to larger displacements of reflected Placido ring points in the video image. EyeSys utilizes a long working dis-

tance (approximately 8 cm from the surface of the eye to the effective plane of the Placido source compared with approximately 2 cm for other systems) to minimize these displacement errors and the resulting differences in measured radius of curvature data (Fig. 34-17). Thus, long working–distance systems provide greater reproducibility as a result of reduced sensitivity to focus and alignment errors. The errors associated with a short working distance affect the overall performance of the system despite any other potential short working–distance advan-

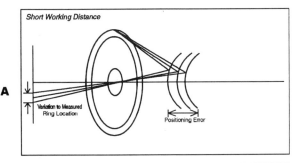

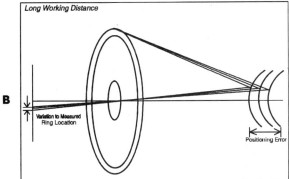

Fig. 34-17 Comparison of ring displacement errors for short (**A**) and long (**B**) working distance. (Courtesy EyeSys Laboratories, Houston, Tex.)

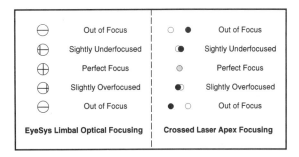

Fig. 34-18 Two types of focusing methods. (Courtesy EyeSys Laboratories, Houston, Tex.)

tages. A working distance similar to that used by EyeSys is common to most ophthalmic diagnostic instruments, including slit lamps, keratometers, autorefractors, and fundus cameras. The high level of reproducibility achieved with the longer working–lens system provides confidence in the results.

Focusing methods. In every computerized videokeratoscopy system there is a means of establishing the appropriate distance between the eye and the video camera to ensure that the Placido rings are in proper focus. Most corneal topography systems are aligned by manually maneuvering the Placido source on a joy-stick base. The main difference between the focusing methods is in the manner of visualizing the proper focus point. One system uses two laser sources which produce light spots that blur slightly from scattering within the stroma of the cornea; these two light spots must be precisely overlapped to achieve proper focus. The degree of fine adjustment is still limited by the ability of the operator to control

the joy stick and to discern proper overlap of the two laser spots as shown in Fig. 34-18. EyeSys users visualize proper focus by positioning cross hairs within a lighted circle on the temporal limbus. The focusing and positioning of these cross hairs are illustrated in Fig. 34-18. Note that in both the slightly underfocused and slightly overfocused positions of the crossed laser system, the user would see oval patterns that are indistinguishable from each other. This leads to a wider range of acceptability and resulting error. With the optical cross-hair system, the operator can distinguish each focus position and use this information to critique examination acceptability and to improve reproducibility.

The use of the limbus as the focal reference point provides two secondary benefits.

1. The focus information (vertical line in small white circle) is outside the Placido ring pattern and does not interfere with the image processing; therefore it can be saved along with the eye image to become a permanent verification of the focus quality of the examination. With an apex laser–focusing system, the lasers must be turned off just before saving the eye image. If left on, the laser lights would produce spots in the center of the Placido ring pattern that would prevent proper image processing. Therefore laser focusing systems provide no record of proper focusing for subsequent clinical reference.

2. EyeSys designed a focus system that utilizes the stable cornea periphery as the point for focus visualization. This is the most stable region on the corneal surface, which is especially important

with the increased emphasis on refractive surgery that purposely alters the corneal apex.

Other considerations

Tear film. The reflected ring image captured by the video camera in every corneal topography system actually is generated from the anterior tear film, the first surface of the eye that the light strikes. The tear film has important properties that must be taken into account in evaluating corneal topography systems. Because of its surface tension properties, the tear film smoothes irregularities on the corneal surface. This is nature's way of providing the best available "polished" refractive surface for vision. This fact is illustrated by patients with dry eyes who have poor vision as a result of an unstable tear film. The design of the EyeSys system takes into account the physical properties of the tear film, thus providing an instrument that yields the required corneal curvature information in a maximum number of situations. From the center to the periphery, EyeSys edge-detection image processing algorithms yield 16 radial data points that are approximately 0.25 mm apart on a 42.5-diopter surface. Because of the physiologic smoothing effect of the tear film, this spacing of data points more than adequately detects curvature changes in the corneal tear film. In cases of steep curvature in which more closely spaced rings would tend to blend together and become undetectable, the EyeSys optimal ring spacing still allows the edges to be detected, permitting analysis of these surfaces.

Corneal coverage. The area of corneal coverage claimed by any manufacturer must be carefully evaluated inasmuch as the actual amount of coverage achieved with any system depends on the curvature of the surface under investigation. Each company has its own range of coverage, with the EyeSys system being one of the larger.

Edge detection. Another important consideration is the image processing performed by the computer on the digitized video image. Placido-based computerized videokeratographs function by locating a specific point on or within a ring that can be referenced to or calculated from a similar point in a calibration file. Because of the nature of the detector arrays in video cameras, it is necessary to locate these points to subpixel resolution. Thus it is critical that the image processing be capable of measuring to this degree of accuracy. EyeSys has chosen to design a keratoscopy target with wide white and black rings and to use a sophisticated edge-detection algorithm. It is more precise to find the location of the ring edge (sharp black/white transitions) than it is to locate the center of smaller width rings (where the ring is the brightest) as is done in other systems.

Because the computer processing in topography systems is not infallible, EyeSys provides the capability to edit the processed eye image. This highly beneficial feature is absent on other systems, which occasionally exhibit processing inaccuracies. Without editing capabilities, these processing errors cannot be corrected. Thus the clinician who did not actually acquire the image would be unaware of the error if an inaccurate color map was placed in a patient's file.

Scaling. If topography information is to be beneficial to the clinician, it must be displayed in a clinically relevant manner. The most common way to view corneal topography data is on an isodioptric color-coded display. For most systems the scaled color range is normalized; that is, the central value of the range of colors and/or the step size of the individual colors will be scaled to the examination under consideration. Caution must be used in viewing these color-coded maps (whether singularly, in multiple-display format, or as difference maps) to be certain that one is aware of the step size. In some situations the steps may be unreasonably *small*, making a normal cornea surface appear abnormal. Likewise, in some cases the step sizes may be too *large*, masking clinically significant corneal irregularities or differences from one examination to the next. To minimize the risk of misreading these color-coded maps, EyeSys has made two significant improvements. First, to avoid overinterpretation of topography maps the EyeSys model normalizes scale defaults to 0.3- or 1.0-diopter step sizes, depending on the total range of values for the examination under consideration. Second, EyeSys has introduced a high-resolution absolute scale that covers a range of 35 to 52 diopters in clinically significant 0.5-diopter steps to provide true color-coded diagnoses of the cornea. The colors and patterns assigned to each dioptric range remain fixed for all examinations and do not scale to the examination under consideration. By use of this dynamic scale for printing or reviewing patient records, it is quite simple to observe changes from one examination to the next. Isodioptric contour lines that differentiate each dioptric range allow the user to quickly assess the amount of astigmatism simply by counting the lines across one quadrant.

Calibration. To determine the radius of curvature for a specific point on the corneal surface, the location of that point must be referenced to a calibration file. Minute changes in the location of that point, especially if located in the central area of the cornea, can result in significant changes in the measured radius of curvature. Therefore it is imperative that corneal topography systems be carefully calibrated. Proper calibration in the field is fundamental to the design of any medical device. Products that depend strictly on factory calibration and that do not allow for users to verify this calibration or recalibrate the

instrument are unacceptable to most medical professionals. Jostling during shipping and handling or exchanging system components could alter a factory calibration. The EyeSys Corneal Analysis System provides its users with a set of calibrated surfaces that can be used to easily verify the calibration of the system and, if necessary, easily and quickly recalibrate the system in the field. It is suggested that calibration be verified at least on a monthly basis.

Clinical uses

Of primary importance is the use of corneal mapping in keratoconus (Fig. 34-19), irregular corneal surfaces, and particularly elevated lesions of the cornea. Two significant advantages of corneal mapping are its use in preventing surgical intervention such as refractive surgery in the patient with keratoconus and in designing a contact lens that will fit the cornea.

The image reflects 6000 points of the entire corneal surface into a form that can be analyzed. A simple button can detect what changes have occurred

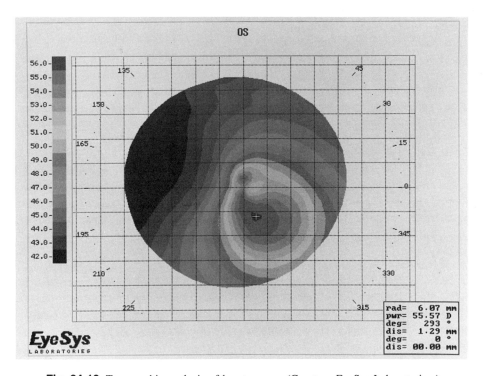

Fig. 34-19 Topographic analysis of keratoconus. (Courtesy EyeSys Laboratories.)

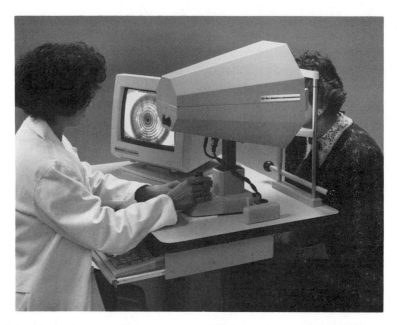

Fig. 34-20 Computer-assisted topographic analysis system for the cornea. (Courtesy EyeSys Laboratories, Houston, Tex.)

after any refractive surgery. This gives one significant input into the effectiveness of the radial keratotomy, corneal transplant, or excimer laser procedure.

It is important to recognize hot colors—such as red, orange, and yellow—as being steeper and cool colors such as green, blue, and purple as being flatter. It is important to look at the color scale on the left, which corresponds to the dioptric powers that determine the optic intervals between color changes. One can increase the sensitivity for detecting these smaller and more subtle corneal changes.

Computer-assisted corneal mapping aids us in analyzing the corneal shape after refractive and transplant surgery, in the study of corneal diseases such as pellucid marginal degeneration, and in contact lens compression. Of utmost importance is the use of centering analysis after corneal surgical procedures such as occurs in refractive surgery and corneal transplantation. The ablated zone in excimer laser can be readily detected on the video keratoscope and thus provide an explanation of compli-

cations that may occur if the ablated zone is off center. Off-center ablations can result in glare or monocular diplopia, especially at night with pupillary dilation. It also can result in suboptimal image clarity and decreased contrast sensitivity.

Computerized corneal topographic analysis (Fig. 34-20) can serve as a useful guide in postoperative management of astigmatism (Fig. 34-21), with selective removal of sutures after penetrating or lamellar keratoplasty. The computerized videograph also can assist the surgeon in choosing the optical incision site for cataract surgery or secondary implant to minimize the degree of postoperative astigmatism.

The future of computer-assisted photokeratoscopy may include the following advantages:

1. Operative topography that would permit the surgeon to adjust suture tension at the time of surgery and to assess the effect of astigmatic keratotomy.
2. Custom contact lenses. Instrument makers are trying to design information that can be generated

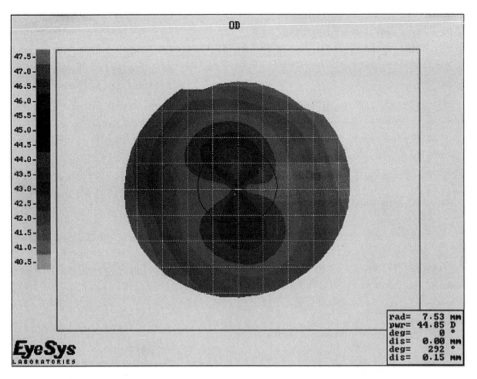

Fig. 34-21 Topographic analysis of astigmatism. (Courtesy EyeSys Laboratories, Houston, Tex.)

and sent directly to a manufacturing laboratory by modem for manufacturing contact lenses. This would have exciting clinical implications for patients who have previously been unable to wear contact lenses with comfort and would substantially reduce the number of visits required to achieve adequate fitting of lenses in particularly difficult cases.

3. Ray tracing analysis. Corneal topography is able to identify off-center laser ablations and radial keratotomy procedures in those with moderate degrees of irregular astigmatism.

QUESTIONS FOR REVIEW AND THOUGHT

1. What are the most common indications for ordering a computed tomography scan?
2. What are the basic anatomic structures visible on a CT scan of the orbits?
3. Name at least three indications for fluorescein angiography.
4. What are the most common complications of fluorescein angiography?

SELF-EVALUATION QUESTIONS

True-false statements

Directions: Indicate whether the statement is true (T) or false (F).

T or F   1. Computed tomography is not as useful as routine x-ray studies in determining the presence of an intraocular foreign body.

T or F   2. Magnetic resonance imaging is superior to computed tomography in demonstrating blow-out fractures of the orbital floor.

T or F   3. Fluorescein in molecules usually is unable to pass out of the retinal blood vessels or across the retinal pigment epithelium.

Missing words

Directions: Write the missing word in the following sentences.

4. The best test for determining the actual site of obstruction in the lacrimal outflow system is called _____.

5. The best test for determining whether tearing is caused by a lid malfunction versus a problem with the lacrimal outflow system is called a _____.

6. The fluorescein angiographic phase that occurs when dye is partially filling the veins is called the _____.

Choice-completion questions

Directions: Select the one best answer in each case.

7. Which of the following is not an indication for computed tomography:
   a. Proptosis
   b. Ptosis with a palpable mass of the suprolateral orbit
   c. Diplopia on upward gaze after a blow to the eye and periorbital structures
   d. Significant increase in hyperopia over a 6-month period
   e. Corneal foreign body

8. Leakage of fluorescein dye can be seen in all of the following conditions except:
   a. Neovascular tufts of the disc or retina as seen in diabetes
   b. Subretinal neovascular membranes as seen in macular degeneration or presumed ocular histoplasmosis
   c. Central retinal artery occlusion
   d. Central retinal vein occlusion
   e. Cystoid macular edema

9. Blockage of the choroidal fluorescence can be seen in all of the following conditions except:
   a. Pigmented choroidal nevus
   b. Retinal hemorrhages such as in diabetes, hypertension, or central retina vein occlusion
   c. Atrophy of the pigment epithelium as seen in macular degeneration
   d. Vitreous hemorrhage
   e. Retinal exudates as seen in diabetes or hypertension

ANSWERS, NOTES, AND EXPLANATIONS

1. **False.** Computed tomography is the most accurate method of localizing foreign bodies. Unlike routine x-ray studies, CT will show whether the foreign body is located within or behind the

eye. The appropriate management of the patient depends on the location of the foreign body. An intraocular foreign body usually is removed surgically in contrast to an orbital foreign body, which usually is left alone.

2. **False.** Magnetic resonance imaging will not show bony details. Computed tomography or routine x-ray studies will show the details of orbital bones. CT also has the advantage of being able to show soft tissue structures, so that in an orbital floor fracture, the ophthalmologist is able to determine if there is entrapment of muscle within the fracture that is responsible for the diplopia. Surgical correction usually is the procedure of choice.

3. **True.** The diagnostic features of fluorescein angiography depend on basic anatomic principles. Normally the fluorescein molecules are unable to pass out of the retinal blood vessels or through the pigment epithelium. Vessels with microaneurysms or neovascularization, such as seen in diabetes, will cause leakage of fluorescein as evidenced by areas of hyperfluorescence. Defects in the pigment epithelium, such as seen in central serous chorioretinopathy, will be evidenced by leakage of fluorescein through the pigment epithelium and into a subretinal location.

4. **Dacryocystography.** This is the procedure of choice in determining the site of obstruction in the lacrimal outflow system.

5. **Lacrimal scan.** This is the procedure of choice in determining whether tearing is caused by poor lid function or by an obstruction of the lacrimal outflow system.

6. **Arteriovenous phase.** The phases in order of appearance are prearterial, arterial, arteriovenous, venous, recirculation, and elimination. Because fluorescein angiographic photographs are taken sequentially from just after dye injection to several minutes later, all these phases may be appreciated. Certain disease entities have characteristic angiographic features with respect to phases. Subretinal neovascular membranes, as seen in macular degeneration and histoplasmosis, fill by the choroidal circulation, and hence these vessels are seen early in the angiogram, often in the prearteriole phase. Neovascularization of the disc or retina appears later in the angiogram because this follows filling of the retinal blood vessels. The details of central serous chorioretinopathy often are best appreciated later in the angiogram after the fluorescein has found its way through the pigment epithelium to a subretinal location.

7. **e. Corneal foreign body.** A corneal foreign body is easy to diagnose with the slit lamp, and therefore more elaborate tests are not indicated. A CT scan may be indicated in patients who exhibit the following symptoms: proptosis, because this may be a result of an orbital mass; ptosis with a palpable mass of the suprolateral orbit, because this may be caused by a lacrimal gland tumor; diplopia after blunt trauma to the eye and periorbital, because this may represent a blow-out fracture; and increase in hyperopia associated with the ophthalmoscopic finding of folds in the choroid, because this may be caused by an orbital tumor pushing on the posterior orbital structures.

8. **c. Central retinal artery occlusion.** In an acute central retinal artery occlusion there is absence of retinal blood flow and hence no fluorescein is seen in the retinal vessels. With the passage of time, recannulization of the blocked vessel occurs and blood will flow to supply the retina, but long after the ischemic damage has occurred. Although leakage of fluorescein will not occur in central retinal artery occlusions, it will occur in neovascular tufts of the retina or disc, in subretinal neovascular membranes, in central retinal vein occlusions, and in cystoid macular edema.

9. **c. Atrophy of the pigment epithelium as seen in macular degeneration.** Atrophy of the retinal pigment epithelium results in an increased transmission of fluorescein leakage that normally occurs in the choroid from the choriocapillaris. Blockage of choroidal fluorescence can be a result of pigment, as seen with a choroidal nevus; from blood, as seen with a vitreous hemorrhage or retinal hemorrhage; or from exudates, as most commonly seen in diabetes or severe hypertension.

CHAPTER 35 Visual aids for the partially sighted

- Factor of age
- Optical aids
- Types of magnifying devices
- Lighting
- Nonoptical visual aids
- The partially sighted child
- Understanding the patient
- Selection of a visual aid

The partially sighted comprise that group of individuals whose vision is not sufficient for ordinary reading or ambulation despite correction with conventional glasses. Normally, a person is not incapacitated until the vision in the best eye has deteriorated to at least 20/50. The partially sighted person has only 20/60 vision or worse in the best corrected eye. Included in the classification of the partially sighted are persons deemed legally blind—who have a visual acuity of 20/200 or worse in the better eye—and persons with a field restriction of 20 degrees or less. Not usually included in this classification are persons whose near vision remains normal or near normal although their distant vision may have worsened; this often is the case with nuclear sclerosis and early myopic retinal degeneration.

Most persons with subnormal vision can be assisted by properly selected optical aids. The assistance does not mean restoration of vision but rather use of available vision to restore the person's sense of self-sufficiency. To an adult this may mean opportunity for employment. In industries in which the partially sighted have been employed, their work output has been as good as that of fellow workers

or often better, and their safety record usually is superior. Children can be given the opportunity to obtain an education, instead of becoming wards of the state. For the elderly person, visual assistance may provide a new lease on life, preventing the insidious decline to a state of mental lethargy because of inability to read, write, or maintain hobbies. The rehabilitation of the partially sighted is extremely gratifying, especially because patients have been told that their vision cannot be improved, which has caused them to believe that they probably have to abandon their work or hobbies, or both. Witnessing a partially sighted individual reading for the first time in years is a more dramatic event than seeing a postoperative cataract patient read the 20/20 line, because the first person often is in despair and expects nothing, whereas the second usually is confident that vision will be restored.

FACTOR OF AGE

Management of the partially sighted varies with the age of the patient. Affected children comprise a small but important group, because if they are not assisted with their disability, they may fall behind their peers and eventually fail to achieve a level of education that will allow them to live an independent and satisfying life. They have the longest period to live with their disability and have had so little time to acquire knowledge to sustain them. Yet it is in this group that motivation, a necessary factor in learning to use an optical aid, is likely to be high, whereas it may be lacking in elderly persons. Also, children are assisted by possessing an excellent range of accommodation, which enables them to perform visual feats at near despite poor distance vision. Many children with distance vision of 20/200 have excellent reading vision. In this group are children who have congenital nystagmus, high myopia, albinism, or congenital chorioretinitis. In the early grades children often require no special optical aids, because they either have normal reading acuity or can compensate for the disability by holding the print quite close. Also, children's books are printed in rather large type. For children aged 7 to 8 years, the size of the print is conventionally about 18 points (requiring 20/100 vision), whereas for ages 9 to 12 years it is 12 points (requiring 20/80 vision). As the child progresses into the higher grades, the print in the textbooks invariably becomes smaller. It usually is at about the seventh-grade level that the child, who has been able to get along previously in a school for the sighted, becomes unable to keep up and must obtain special assistance from visual aids and from the teaching staff. At this point optical aids become important because they may enable many of these children to continue with their sighted classmates.

Young adults actually constitute the smallest group of those becoming partially sighted, inasmuch as the adult usually experiences the onset of loss of vision because of injury or disease. The situation of young adults often is difficult because their livelihood depends on successful rehabilitation. Although motivation should be high, young adults tend to experience depression, apathy, despair, and even bitterness concerning their recently acquired visual disability, and this reaction, of course, retards effective visual retraining.

Elderly persons constitute the largest group of the visually handicapped, principally because they often suffer from the diseases of aging. The group is often difficult to assist because of other physical infirmities, which may include senility, tremors, defective hearing, and diminished vigor. Although a proportion of patients in this age-group is slow to accept the necessary changes in learning to cope with their new disability (and in fact, some of them never adjust), a larger proportion is, or can be, motivated to make the adjustments necessary to achieve some useful vision.

Assistance for patients with subnormal vision is provided through (1) a careful eye examination, (2) a good history from the patient, including an assessment of the reaction to vision loss, the degree of adjustment made, and a survey of the patient's interests, education, and visual needs, and (3) the provision of optical and nonoptical aids.

It is important in the eye examination to accurately test visual acuity for distance. The partially sighted patient therefore should be tested at 10 feet rather than at 20 feet. Most projectors or charts have no test print beyond 20/200, and if a patient is tested at 10 feet, this deficiency is remedied.

To convert to standard notations, the results are multiplied by 2; for example, 10/70 = 20/140. To test vision less than 10/200, the patient is instructed to walk closer to the chart, and the visual acuity is recorded in terms of the distance the patient can stand before the chart and read the 20/200 letter; for example, 7/200, 3/200. It also is important to obtain a careful refraction because correction of the basic refractive error sometimes may be all that is necessary.

A good history provides many essential details. The patient who has not accepted the visual loss is not a good candidate for optical aids, nor is the individual who recently has experienced visual loss. Many patients have discovered some sort of visual aid, and they are good candidates for more sophisticated aids. Some individuals are content to be able to read hockey scores and manage their shopping and personal mail, whereas with others, reading may play a much larger part in their daily life, whether for personal pleasure or in earning a living. Many young people need the assistance of visual aids to finish school.

OPTICAL AIDS

Optical aids are divided into (1) conventional lenses (strong minus lenses for high myopes, and scleral and corneal contact lenses for those with corneal scars, keratoconus, high myopia, and so forth) and (2) magnifying lenses.

The patient often can see details only if they are magnified. Magnification devices are available for both distance and near vision. The degree of magnification required will, of course, depend on the patient's visual acuity and age, and the work for which the optical aid is designed. In terms of visual acuity alone, the Kestenbaum rule is commonly helpful. The numerator of the patient's distance visual acuity is divided into the denominator; the result should approximately equal the magnification required for seeing Jaeger's test type 5 (J5) on the near vision chart. This figure is divided to achieve J1, for example:

20/100 = +5.00 for J5, +10.00 for J1
20/200 = +10.00 for J5, +20.00 for J1
20/400 = +20.00 for J5, +40.00 for J1

An adult patient with 10/100 would require a +5.00 lens in addition to his or her ordinary spectacle correction for seeing print of this size. This may be used as a rule of thumb, with trial and error methods carried on from this point for further refinement. A young person, especially a child, would need less than a +5.00 lens because of accommodation, and usually the addition to the ordinary spectacle correction would be the weakest lens that would enable reading of J5 on the near vision chart. In addition, word charts are available that assist in assessing magnification requirements of partially sighted patients.

For viewing distant objects, telescopes or binoculars sometimes can be useful, and although Kestenbaum's rule is helpful, the patient often will have to try two or three aids before deciding which is best.

All magnifying devices function by effectively enlarging the size of the retinal image (Fig. 35-1). A similar effect can be produced by bringing the object closer to the eye, because an object viewed at 10 inches has a retinal image twice the size of the same object viewed at 20 inches. However, only in children is the range of accommodation sufficient to

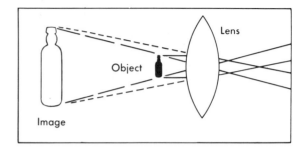

Fig. 35-1 Magnification by a convex lens is obtained by bringing the object within the focal distance of the convex lens. An erect magnified image is obtained.

provide exceptionally close viewing. The clarity of distant objects often can be improved by walking closer to them or sitting closer, and this is useful, for example, in watching television.

TYPES OF MAGNIFYING DEVICES
Hand readers and stand magnifiers
(Figs. 35-2 to 35-5)

The dioptric strength of most hand magnifiers already owned by most patients can be checked on a lensmeter. Some hand magnifiers are of a power greater than the range of a lensmeter. A rough test is set out here to determine the magnification of any hand magnifier.

1. Use a magnifying lens to form an image, on a piece of paper, of a distant object. Measure the distance from the image to the lens in inches, and divide this distance into 10. This gives the magnifying power of the lens (for example, a lens that focuses at 2 inches is a ×5 magnifier). NOTE: Those who prefer to work in centimeters will arrive at the same answer by dividing the measurement in centimeters into 25.

2. The magnification of the lens multiplied by 4 equals the approximate plus dioptric power of the lens.

The advantage of a hand magnifier is that it is small and inexpensive and can be carried in the pocket. Its greatest limitation is the fact that it is usually of low power, the average lens offering magnification of only between 1.0 and 2.5, or between 4.0 and 10.0 diopters. The *aspheric* lens has been developed now for hand and stand readers and is a

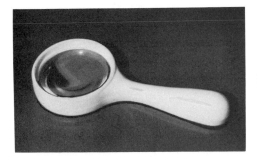

Fig. 35-2 Hand magnifier, ×5.

Fig. 35-3 Stand magnifier, ×5.

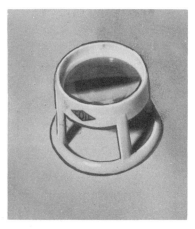

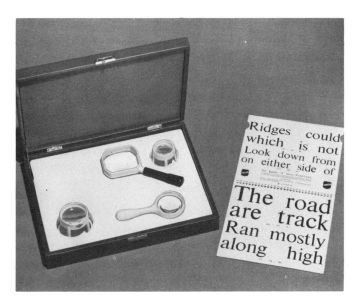

Fig. 35-4 Assorted selection of hand and stand magnifiers, with Keeler low visual acuity word chart.

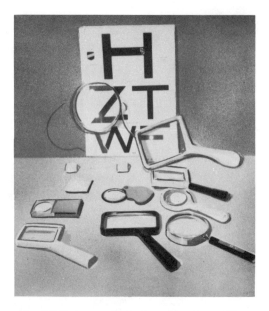

Fig. 35-5 Assorted selection of hand magnifiers.

considerable improvement over the old glass magnifiers inasmuch as it effectively reduces the distortion found at the edge of the field.

Most patients, when buying magnifiers, believe the larger the glass area, the greater the magnification. Exactly the reverse is true. A large plus lens cannot be a strong plus lens, or, conversely, a high plus dioptric lens with its short radius of curvature is too small for a large area magnifier. Many patients relate large-sized devices with high power and are discouraged when none of the physically large magnifying glasses are suitable for them.

Projection devices

Projection devices include movie screens, television and slide projectors, and so forth. These devices are not too popular today because of their bulk, cost, and lack of portability and versatility. Also, the illumination of these devices is relatively poor so that what is gained by enlargement is lost to a certain extent by lack of contrast.

Closed-circuit television has been used in limited areas, with the camera scanning the reading material as a low visual aid. The justification for such an elaborate device is that the magnification is almost unlimited, and the contrast and brightness can be adjusted. In addition, a negative image can be projected onto the television screen so that black letters printed on a white paper may be seen as white letters on a black background.

A number of companies have introduced scanners to see text such as a book or newspaper (Fig. 35-6). These scanners can increase the magnification 35 times and also can permit viewing of a single line of text. The text can be viewed at the reader's desired speed and allows hands-free operation. The smearing qualities associated with camera-based systems have been eliminated.

Readers can copy virtually any text up to legal-sized documents into the memory of the system. They also can select three different reading modules, including full-page, column, and single-line modules, as well as choose black letters on a white background or white letters on a black background. The instrument is user-friendly; the user places material on the scanner and reads it into the system by pushing a button similar to that of a photocopier. The system captures the page image and finds the lines and columns of text on it, and readers can then display the entire page of the text and identify their position on the whole page with a single press of a button. Of interest is that even if the book is crooked when it is placed on the scanner, it automatically centers the page. The system provides the highest possible contrast and smooths the contours of the characters. No adjustment of focus contrast or lighting is required.

Strong convex lenses

The use of strong convex lenses (that is, $+4.00$ to $+6.00$ diopters or more) is the most popular method today of providing magnification. The strong convex lens has a short focal distance so that reading material can be brought close to the eye. For example, with spectacles of $+5.00$ diopters, print is held about 9 inches away, whereas with a $+20.00$-diopter lens, the reading distance is only about 2 inches from the spectacles. Cosmetically, they are no more unsightly than cataract lenses. Anything over 10.00 diopters ($\times 2.5$), however, cannot be fitted binocularly. These high plus lenses may be made up in forms quite similar to cataract glasses, in lenticular form to re-

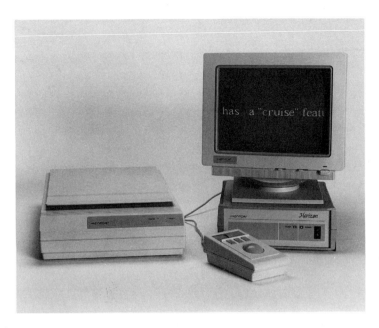

Fig. 35-6 Computerized low vision scanner permits magnification to 35 times and one lens display. (Courtesy Mentor O and O, Inc., Norwell, Mass.)

duce weight, in bifocal form, or in plastic. Important considerations in the spectacle reading aid are freedom from aberrations, its light weight, and a relatively wide field of view. Spectacles also allow both hands to be used for holding the reading material so that reading often is faster than with a magnifying glass. A major disadvantage of spectacle lenses is that the reading material must be held quite still in the hand at the critical focal point. With elderly persons, early fatigue occurs in maintaining this fixed posture. Also, the hands may be tremorous, making reading at a fixed distance an impossibility. At the higher power corrections the reading material is so close to the face that it often cuts out a great deal of the light that normally would fall on the type. Despite these disadvantages the high-powered spectacle lens remains the most widely used and popular aid employed today for the partially sighted.

In addition to the Kestenbaum rule as a method of determining how much magnification a patient needs to read, there is a Keeler low-vision acuity word chart. The patient should be wearing correction spectacles to focus on print held at 25 cm (10 inches) in good light. The chart will then indicate the magnification required to read small print. The patient should be prevented from trying to move the chart closer than 10 inches. Devices with the indicated magnification are then tried. Children (or adults who have not read for many years) are asked to spell the letters rather than read words—or to spell words backward.

If a patient is a high myope, merely removing the glasses and reading without them may produce sufficient magnification. If, however, the patient with low visual acuity has had a cataract operation and is wearing aphakic eyeglasses, the extra lens needed to provide the required magnification for reading may result in a very strong lens. As an example, an aphakic eyeglass of +12.00 diopters, combined with a ×7 reading addition, would mean a reading eyeglass lens of 40.00 diopters.

Finally, children can acquire large powers of accommodation and can achieve excellent reading ability by holding their reading material in focus close to their eyes. This is not harmful, and parents and teachers may need to be reassured on this point.

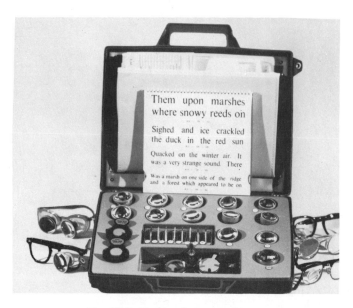

Fig. 35-7 Keeler telescopic trial set.

Distance magnifiers

Distance magnifiers seldom are worn permanently by the partially sighted. For the partially sighted to travel alone safely and efficiently, a wide field of vision is of more importance than good central visual acuity. Telescopes that magnify distant objects cannot be tolerated for long periods of time, because they seriously reduce the field of vision, interfere with correct judgments of distance, and magnify lateral motions. For occasional use, however, such as identifying bus numbers, street signs, or faces, *telescopic lenses* can be useful (Fig. 35-7). These devices include binoculars, ordinary field glasses, and telescopes. For sustained reading at a distance, such as from a blackboard, a monocular telescope that hooks over the spectacle lens often is quite useful (Fig. 35-8).

Monocular telescopes are preferred to the binocular ones because they are lighter in weight and can be placed over the better-seeing eye with ease. Some individuals sever an ordinary binocular or opera glass in two and use one half as a monocular telescope (Fig. 35-9). Also, a variety of light small monocular telescopes are readily available in strengths from $2\frac{1}{2}\times$ to $10\times$.

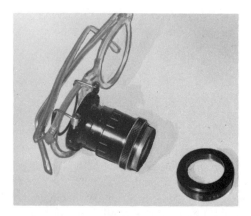

Fig. 35-8 Monocular telescope.

Telescopes generally have limited usefulness. They are quite conspicuous and if worn continuously, are a hazard to both the patient and persons in the vicinity. Their prime function is for occasional use outdoors and for watching a stationary scene, such as a theater performance or a television screen.

Some telescopes are constructed so that in addition to viewing distant objects, they can be focused to reading distances. Some telescopes designed for distances will accept reading caps of various strengths.

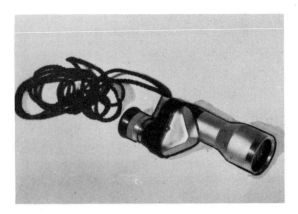

Fig. 35-9 Half of miniature binocular used as a visual aid.

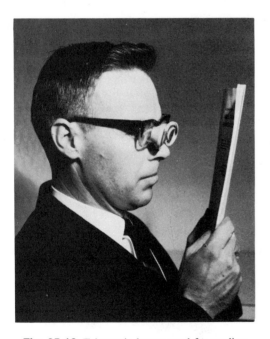

Fig. 35-10 Telescopic lenses used for reading.

Finally, some telescopes are designed only for reading and are mounted in an eyeglass frame (Fig. 35-10). The advantage of a reading telescope is that the reading distance is increased, but because the increase in reading distance becomes less and less with stronger telescopic readers, the advantage is significant only with the weaker telescopic readers.

The small field of view, the increased "motion" of print as the head is moved in reading, and the limited depth of field are significant deterrents to the use of telescopic readers.

LIGHTING

Good lighting is an important visual aid for everyone, but it is particularly important for partially sighted patients. What is good light for normal vision may be inadequate for the partially sighted. Lighting increases contrast between print and the background, thereby making details more legible. The best contrast is achieved by good type with black print on a white or near-white background.

Valuable improvement in lighting often can be achieved by having the patient simply alter the position of existing lamps or their shades, or even by altering the strength of the bulbs used. The patient soon will realize the benefits, and even those who may have mild photophobia usually can obtain some benefit.

A valuable lamp is one that uses a 40- or 60-watt bulb, with a metal reflecting shade and adjustable metal spring-mounted extendable arms, which can bring light efficiently onto such things as reading material, sewing, and hobbies. This type of light is readily available in lighting stores in a variety of mountings.

Another light source, a *tensor lamp,* can be useful. It usually is a smaller lamp with a bright light and an extendable arm; however, it is somewhat more expensive to purchase and operate, and it may be too warm (Fig. 35-11).

The failure of an optical or nonoptical visual aid to work in the patient's home when success was indicated in office testing often means that the home setting has inadequate lighting available for the visual aid to be of assistance.

NONOPTICAL VISUAL AIDS

Several accessory, nonoptical visual aids are available that are commonly helpful to the patient with subnormal vision. These devices operate mainly by providing fixation guides, achieving magnification through the use of large print, and giving special lighting effects. Some of these devices include the reading rectangle, large type, filters, writing guides, and marking pens.

Reading rectangle

The reading rectangle is a device in which its rectangular opening shows only a few lines of type (Fig. 35-12). Squaring off the reading material often can produce improvement in the vision of patients with incipient cataracts or corneal opacities by cutting off the reflected light from the reading page. It also is a useful means of finding the beginning of the next line of print to be read. This feature is particularly helpful with high magnification aids, through which only a few words or even a few letters of print are discernible.

Large type

Large-type visual aids include telephone dials with large numbers (Fig. 35-13), playing cards with large figures, and school textbooks. The use of large print is somewhat limited because the patient's reading activity is restricted to material available in large form. Most patients are far better off with some optical device to provide the magnification so that the range of reading, both for pleasure and work, is unrestricted. However, convention name-plate typewriters (speech writers), which use large capital letters (bulletin type), may be helpful for some.

A yellow filter

In some cases in which a patient reports fuzzy vision, yellow light will improve the contrast between the dark letters and the white paper. Yellow light can be provided by dark-yellow clip-ons, the coating of the lenses with dark yellow, or the use of a dark yellow light bulb in the reading lamp or a yellow cellophane sheet laid on the page.

Writing guides

Often the partially sighted patient cannot use an ordinary magnifier to write, because the field of vision

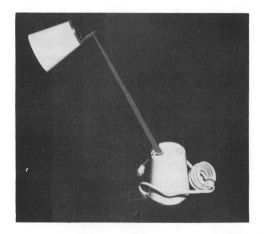

Fig. 35-11 High-intensity lamp.

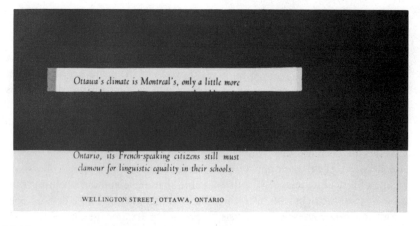

Fig. 35-12 Reading rectangle to provide a guide in reading. All but the line to be read is blocked out.

is not large enough to encompass a line. The writing guide gives direction, which could not be accomplished otherwise, and so may be useful for this purpose.

Marking pens

Marking pens are nylon-tipped or felt-tipped pens that write or print in different widths so that a partially sighted person can read his or her own writing or printing with greater ease. The partially sighted person chooses a pen with the width of mark most easily recognized and then writes or prints as large as is needed to be able to read the writing. These pens are readily available in all stationery stores.

THE PARTIALLY SIGHTED CHILD

A question commonly posed to the ophthalmologist is "Should the child with partial sight be allowed to continue in regular grade school?" There are no hard and fast rules, because so many factors are involved besides those attributable to loss of sight. Of great importance are the child's intelligence, motivation, and ability to cope emotionally with the handicap among regular schoolchildren. If a particular child

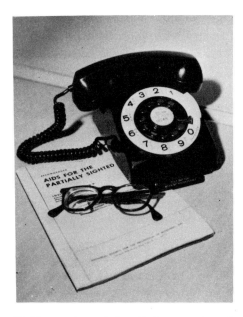

Fig. 35-13 Telephone dials with large numbers for the partially sighted.

is bright, alert, competitive, and capable of maintaining grades at a level commensurate with age, attending a regular school is to be encouraged. In effect, a child who can carry on such a program despite the handicap must have superior ability. Certainly the early experience of competing with normal children will better prepare the child for future life. On the other hand, if the child experiences nothing but frustration and defeat in the environment of the sighted, it might be better in the long run to acquire basic educational skills at a school where children can proceed at their own pace and obtain the individual attention needed. However, even in this setting it is best for the child to learn to use regular textbooks and materials as long as possible, rather than employ large-print books and braille.

If the child with a visual handicap is excluded from ordinary children's games, such as marbles, throwing a ball and catching it, and baseball, the loss of position in the social community can be just as discouraging as failure at school. Such a child requires guidance even in choice of play. This youngster can be encouraged to participate in team activities in the capacity of manager, coach, and so forth to feel included in the group or can be encouraged to develop skills in sports not requiring visual accuracy, such as track and field, wrestling, and weight lifting.

UNDERSTANDING THE PATIENT

Partially sighted persons use their other senses, such as touch and hearing, to the full extent. There is no evidence in favor of the belief that the blind or partially sighted develop greater acuteness than others can achieve. They undoubtedly use their other senses to the maximum of efficiency, but not beyond the ordinary range of variation. Certainly they do not develop any form of extrasensory perception. If partially sighted patients can be given a good optical aid to enable them to function with their disability, their chances of effecting a complete rehabilitation are enhanced.

SELECTION OF A VISUAL AID

No single visual aid is best, because each patient must be considered in terms of age, interests, motivation, and the type of activity for which the aid is intended. For example, an elderly individual with a shaky hand would be better off with a stand magnifier; a hand-held magnifier would be almost useless. Other patients will have to see to make their living, and they will have to read. It is therefore necessary to discover the amount of reading required for a given patient and to consider the distance at which work must be carried out. In this context, the general rule is to give patients the weakest magnification that will enable them to function, because as the magnification is increased, so is the difficulty in working and reading. Children, especially those in the early grades, because they have a large range of accommodation and because their texts usually are printed in rather large type, often require no visual aids until they reach grade 6 or 7.

Patients who have recently lost vision often are poor candidates for visual aids. Many of them have not learned to accept their handicap, and they secretly harbor a notion that their vision may return. Also, the emotional upheaval in reaction to sensory deprivation may be so great that the factor of motivation is either nil or even minus in quality in the early period of visual loss. A period of incubation— which varies, of course, with each patient—usually must pass before the patient accepts the fact that the disability is permanent. Acceptance of this handicap is the first step toward reentering the active community.

The partially sighted person who has been allowed to vegetate for many years without a remedial education program also requires specific consideration. Such persons may have accepted their disability with resignation and be too dispirited to try to learn to read again. In addition, they may have been unable to read for such a long period that their ability to read has decreased. In a sense they have forgotten how and need a period of practice.

The important single goal to keep in mind is that even a small visual improvement often can ease a person's problems, allowing a greater chance for education and employment, or ameliorating a tedious and frustrating existence.

QUESTIONS FOR REVIEW AND THOUGHT

1. Most persons with reduced vision can be assisted by proper optical devices. What are the simplest devices that they can use?
2. Although a patient with subnormal vision is handicapped at both distance and near, which of these two is the most important for most patients? Which is easier to correct optically?
3. Why can children with subnormal vision in the early grades of school manage in the normal classroom, whereas as they progress in school they often require optical aids?
4. Often partially sighted persons will have tried some optical aid on their own. What types of optical aids are readily available? Discuss different types of these optical aids as to the value of size and shape.
5. Discuss the effect of lighting on the world of the partially sighted.
6. Jewelers and other specialized workers may require magnification for their work. Discuss how you would incorporate magnification for their work and how you would assess their requirement.
7. The magnification of a lens is stated as $\times 5$. What is the approximate dioptic power?
8. A lens has a back focal length of 25 mm. How much magnification would this give?
9. Why do large-diameter hand readers fail as an aid for the patient with low visual acuity?

SELF-EVALUATION QUESTIONS

True-false statements

Directions: Indicate whether the statement is true (T) or false (F)

T or F   1. Many people who are legally blind are able to see well enough to work for a living and read normal-sized print.

T or F   2. Patients should be given the weakest aid in terms of magnification.

T or F   3. Children require the same magnification as adults.

Missing words

Directions: Write in the missing word in the following sentences.

4. Equally important to the power of the lens is _____.
5. The best form of "eye exercise" for a partially sighted person is _____.
6. If there is a gross difference between the two eyes, a _____ correction should be made.

Choice-completion questions

Directions: Select the one best answer in each case.

7. Magnification of a lens is determined by:
   a. The reading of a lensometer
   b. The neutralization by another lens.
   c. Taking the focal distance in inches and dividing this number into 10
   d. The lighting present
   e. All of the above

8. The problems with spectacle magnifying devices are:
   a. They cannot be worn for distance
   b. Cosmetically they are unsightly and draw attention to the defect
   c. They are tedious to use
   d. The reading material must be held close at a precise reading distance
   e. All of the above

9. The use of strong convex lenses creates which of the following:
   a. Aberrations similar to those of highly myopic spectacle lenses
   b. An exceptionally close near point—for example, 20.00 diopters has a focal point of 2 inches
   c. Distortions that are best controlled with a single-cut lens
   d. Headaches if the correction is not bilateral
   e. All of the above

ANSWERS, NOTES, AND EXPLANATIONS

1. **True.** One of the greatest handicaps of being legally blind is the common notion that such people are sightless and no longer can render a service to society. This is simply not true. Being legally blind with vision of 20/200 or less is a disability but not a total handicap. Blind people have prospered through ingenuity, determination, and selected visual aids.

2. **True.** As the magnification of a device increases, so does its weight, its distortion, and the critical nature of its focal point. Rather than depend on magnification alone, the patient may

be better served by increasing illumination, which aids contrast. Also, with high-power magnification devices, a patient cannot read by scanning but must labor like a child, going from word to word.

3. **False.** Children who are partially sighted can achieve better magnification by simply holding the book or paper a little closer to their eyes. Adults, especially those over 45, have virtually depleted the accommodation ability and cannot naturally hold things close. A child may have an accommodative reserve of 14 diopters, whereas an adult counterpart may not have more than 2 diopters.

4. **Illumination.** Good lighting can make the difference between comfortable reading and labored reading. Tensor lamps, yellow light, and focal lighting each has its advocates. It is important to remember that the best light is that of the sun.

5. **Reading.** Many partially sighted people feel that their eyes are like tires—that if they are used too much, they will wear out. This is a myth. Whereas reading is not an ocular exercise per se, it should be encouraged. It gives the person more contact with his or her world and helps destroy that psychologic feeling of being different and handicapped. If a person can read, most of the visual handicap is gone.

6. **Monocular.** If a patient has 20/60 vision in one eye and 20/400 vision in the other eye, only the 20/60 eye should be treated. Attempts at providing balance are useless and confusing. A partially sighted person does not have binocular vision. To improve the worst eye only adds confusion and, at times, diplopia.

7. **c. Taking the focal distance in inches and dividing this number into 10.** A lens that focuses at 2 inches has a magnification of 10/2, or 5. In centimeters the correct answer will be present by dividing the measurement in centimeters into 25. On the other hand, magnification times 4 equals the dioptic power of the lens. Aspheric magnifiers for lens +10.00 or over (magnification of ×25) should be ordered, because of the enlargement and the relative lack of distortion of the peripheral field.

8. **e. All of the above.** Many blind people have excellent peripheral vision and, because of this wide field of vision, can walk comfortably with no or minimal assistance. They may not see a road sign, but they will see cars, people, and obstructions through their peripheral vision and move about without a distance aid. The major problem is reading. For young people the best device is a spectacle device that frees the hands, allowing a partially sighted person to work or gain employment.

9. **b. An exceptionally close near point—for example, 20.00 diopters has a focal point of 2 inches.** A magnifying lens is alway convex: +10.00-diopter to +20.00-diopter lenses are in the most utilized range. Lenticular lenses were popular to reduce weight and distortion, but Welch's four-drop lens, popularized for the correction of aphakia, is an excellent low visual aid lens. It is lighter, offers less distortion, looks better cosmetically, and can be fitted in attractive frames.

PART FIVE

Community ocular programs

CHAPTER 36

Blind persons in the modern world

- Blindness defined
- The recently blinded person
- Ophthalmic assistant's role
- The blind child
- Rehabilitation
- Available aids

BLINDNESS DEFINED

The most widely accepted definition of blindness considers an individual blind whose central visual acuity does not exceed 20/200 in the better eye with a correcting lens, or whose visual acuity, if better than 20/200, has a limit to the central field of vision to such a degree that its widest diameter subtends an angle no greater than 20 degrees. Thus many legally blind persons have sight of varying degrees. Some can distinguish only the difference between light and darkness. Others see vague shapes and patterns as if a thick fog were always in front of their eyes. Still others have peripheral sight and see the world around the edges of a great dark mass in the center of their eyes; they never see the whole shape of anything but only the top and bottom or the ends. In the partially sighted population the different ways people see are almost as varied as the people themselves. It is estimated that among blind persons in the United States and Canada, only one quarter are actually totally blind (no light perception).

Partial sight and blindness

It must be remembered that most persons who are legally classified as blind have some sight. Psycho-logically, the individual has a better regard for himself and his capacities if he thinks of himself as partially sighted rather than as blind. For this reason a patient should not be advised to learn to read braille if he can read type, even though he is classified as legally blind. About two thirds of the legally blind children between 7 and 17 years of age are attending regular school. Low-vision aids that give intense magnification are of great assistance to these children.

Braille is probably indicated when the distance vision is 20/200 or less and at near when a patient cannot read smaller type than Jaeger 13 or 18 point at a distance of 1 to 5 inches from the eye.

THE RECENTLY BLINDED PERSON

In most instances it is the ophthalmologist who is faced with the responsibility of telling the blind person that he or she has a permanent loss of vision. Most authorities in the field of rehabilitation believe the blind person should be informed as early as possible once the diagnosis has been made. The sooner the person understands his disability and accepts its reality as a permanent state, the sooner he will become effective in dealing with the realities of his visual loss. The practice of prolonging the blind person's hope of restoring vision only serves to impede effective rehabilitation and eventually invites a bitter confrontation with reality.

Although it is important for the ophthalmologist to present the diagnosis in a candid and factual manner, it is just as essential for the practitioner to appreciate the emotional impact of such information. A supportive environment in which the blind person is allowed time to ask questions, as well as hear about community resources available to help him deal with his vision loss, is imperative.

For most individuals, loss of vision arouses a deep emotional response—usually fear. Others may become hopelessly depressed. They may feel completely dependent and unable to care for themselves. They may feel worthless and of no use to themselves or society. They may be afraid to carry on their accustomed way of life, and they may be afraid of financial dependence, isolation, and loss of social status.

Myriad repeated frustrations occur in the daily lives of the totally blind that accentuate the dependency of the condition. Maintaining their personal life becomes a feat in itself. The routines that the sighted do automatically and without thought must be deliberately learned, step by step, by the blind. For example, the blind person must learn how to eat all over again. If the portions on a plate are not placed in a certain location, the blind person must explore the plate with a fork to discover where the portions of food are placed. Cutting meat can be so difficult that in many instances a blind person requires having his meat cut into bite-sized portions for him. Simple tasks can arouse feelings of insecurity, fear, and anxiety, especially when they have to be performed in public. The blind person is afraid of mistakes and of being clumsy and awkward for fear that he will become an object of attention. It is these little things, such as dining, combing the hair, lighting a cigarette, or setting down a glass of water, that the blind person must train himself to do with confidence before he can join the sighted as an active member of the community.

The blind person may withdraw into a familiar and unchanging environment that can be controlled with his visual incapacity. If he withdraws, he will be safe from physical harm and public ridicule but limited in his thoughts and actions like a child in a playpen. The other extreme is to tackle the problem head on—that is, to ignore the disability and continue with life despite the inconveniences, dangers, and hardships—functioning as best he can. The most desirable reaction is the one that balances the disability with new ability and redirects interests, skills, and strengths so that the visual need in selected activities is minimized. It is toward this reorientation both physical and psychologic, that the physician and trained rehabilitation personnel attempt to direct blind patients.

OPHTHALMIC ASSISTANT'S ROLE

The ophthalmic assistant will encounter in his or her daily work individuals who have little or no vision. The assistant should be familiar with the methods currently employed to provide orientation to those with visual disabilities and to facilitate their mobility.

On first meeting a blind person, the ophthalmic assistant should take his hand and touch his arm. This physical contact gives the person some sense of the assistant's interest in him. The assistant should speak directly to him but not shout because the blind person receives impressions through hearing and learns to use his ears more efficiently. Shouting or talking in a loud voice embarrasses the blind individual because it attracts unnecessary attention and focuses on a hearing disability that does not exist. The sense of touch is developed through necessity and may become unusually acute. The sense of smell, although usually underrated, is also important. All three sensations—hearing, touch, and smell—are used in combination to develop orientation. In talking to a blind person, the assistant must remember that he cannot see a smile, but he can hear it in a voice. The conversation should be kept natural. It is quite in order for the ophthalmic assistant to ask the blind person how much he sees. In this way the assistant can judge the amount of help the patient will require. A blind person with guiding sight does not need as much help as someone who is totally blind. If he needs assistance to get about in the office, the assistant can give him verbal instructions or let him touch the assistant's elbow. The blind person should not be pushed ahead of the assistant or pushed along; he should be told where the chair is or his hand put on the back of it.

Naturalness, kindness, and inherent human respect will result in the most successful relationships and will avoid an overdose of assistance, which makes a handicap more noticeable and damages the value of the assistant's contact. The assistant should always offer his or her arm to the blind person. With his hand lightly on the arm, the patient feels the movement of the assistant's body, and because the assistant will be slightly ahead of him, he will have a feeling of confidence with each step. To be propelled from behind can be most awkward and unnerving. The assistant should be sure to ask a blind person if he needs help; assistance should not be forced on him.

If a blind person has been guided to a place and left by himself, he should be told about the nature of his surroundings. It is desirable, under such circumstances, to establish some position of safety and orientation, such as a table, chair, or wall.

The blind person should always be informed of movements when one leaves his presence or returns to him. The assistant should never leave the patient who is talking alone. When a patient is directed through a room, the assistant should attempt to be precise and accurate; mixing the left or right side is a frequent mistake and occurs especially when one is facing the patient. Directions should always be given in terms of the blind person's right or left.

The ophthalmic assistant should be aware of the thin line between giving someone assistance and making him feel helpless. Many blind people are quite proud of the many functions they can perform for themselves. They do not like their disability emphasized and their dependency magnified. The assistant can ask the patient, in a quiet voice, if he or she can help him with this or that, and let the patient make the decision about the degree of assistance wanted.

The ophthalmic assistant should never discuss with the patient the status of his eyes, the compensation the patient can expect, or the facilities available for him. Each of these areas must be handled by trained professionals working in their fields. The assistant should avoid giving false hope to a patient by casually mentioning the miracles being rendered every day in the fight for sight.

Finally, a blind person should not be regarded as witless. The patient should be asked questions directly, not through a second party. Conversation should never be allowed to flow around or through him as though he did not exist. He should be treated as an individual without sight, not as one without insight.

THE BLIND CHILD

The congenitally blind child, unlike some of his adult counterparts, has no recollection of the visual world to assist him. Without this visual memory the blind child must learn about the world by being exposed to his environment and provided with the opportunity to concretely explore it through his other sensory systems. Although parents know their child best, early intervention by child development specialists who have training in visual impairment can offer additional support to parents and assist them with encouraging their child's normal development. Other professionals who can offer support with the habilitation needs of the blind child are orientation and mobility specialists and life skill instructors. These personnel are trained to assist blind children and their families with the development of daily living skills and the attainment of safe independent travel skills.

The young child who does not have a visual memory may have to be physically shown and encouraged to develop some skills such as creeping, walking, holding a spoon, and drinking from a cup. The blind child who has never seen these activities cannot rely on visual modeling as a learning tool. Parents of blind children must be patient and firm, allowing their child the opportunity to succeed by independently doing a task, as well as permitting the child an opportunity to fail at times and learn from his mistakes. It is important that some routine be established in the home to assist the blind child with understanding his environment. For example, it is easy for a totally blind child to confuse day with night; thus the routine of going to bed is important. Because bedtime is not accompanied by a change of light, a preliminary quiet period can be substituted. The blind child's language and concept development can be facilitated by bringing the child into direct association with the object or action while the appropriate words are being used. This helps the child to acquire a meaningful conceptual base.

Some blind children may develop mannerisms such as rocking, touching, and rubbing their eyes or waving their hands. These and other repetitive motions are known as *blindisms*. Early intervention with blind children focuses on trying to prevent these blindisms from developing. Once the blindisms are established, diminishing them may take attention and correction over a period of years.

It is currently being estimated that up to 60% of young blind infants and preschool children in North America have additional disabilities. One reason for this is the greater capabilities of modern medicine to save premature infants. Although many of these infants may be perfectly normal, premature infants with very low birth weights (less than 750 grams) do have a greater incidence of disability. The blind child with additional disabilities requires a transdisciplinary team approach to effectively meet his diverse and unique habilitation needs.

Today most blind children receive their education through local schools in an integrated educational setting. Although educational integration legislation varies by region the totally blind child usually requires some form of educational support services to assist with meaningful learning in the integrated classroom. Residential schools for blind children still exist in some areas, thus allowing families and school placement personnel choices and options to best meet the educational needs of the individual child.

One form of written communication the blind child may use is braille, a system of raised dots on paper read by touching them with the ends of the fingers (Fig. 36-1). Although modern technology presents blind children with more communication options, the importance of braille has not diminished as a tool for literacy. The braille system was developed by Louis Braille, a blind student who in 1824 developed a six-dot raised code. The braille alphabet consists of combinations of one or more raised dots

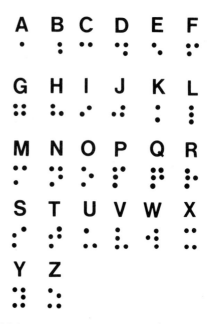

Fig. 36-1 Braille alphabet based on the six-dot system.

in a six-dot square known as the *braille cell*, which is three dots high and two dots wide. There are 63 possible combinations of dots; after the letters of the alphabet are arranged, the remaining signs are used for punctuation, music, codes, and mathematics. Braille can be written through the aid of a slate, a braille writer, or a computer system employing a braille printer. To facilitate the development of later braille skills, young children are introduced early to activities to assist with the development of tactual sensitivity, manual dexterity, and fine motor development. Later the preschool blind child will receive training and materials that focus on prebraille readiness skills. The reading and writing of braille is taught to blind children in the early years.

Braille libraries are available from which the blind student can obtain books. To supply textbooks for blind students in higher education in Canada, the Canadian National Institute for the Blind has developed a large group of volunteers who have learned to write the braille system and spend many hours each week transferring printed pages into braille. In other countries, similar organizations provide this service. Many popular magazines, trade journals, and periodicals are available in braille.

Blind children may use a variety of forms of written communication. The proliferation of communication technology has made it possible for blind students to gain access to print information by computer through synthesized speech, large print, or braille access modes. The combined use of these devices makes possible a scenario in which a blind student can access a print exercise through synthesized speech or braille modes, respond to the exercise in his chosen medium of braille, and then make a print copy of his answers for the sighted teacher and a braille copy of the answers for his own files. Although communication technology provides amazing possibilities to assist the blind child with learning, unfortunately not all blind children are able to receive funding for equipment and training to use the equipment in the school and home setting.

Some blind persons may find it difficult to read in an efficient manner with their fingers. To help these individuals the talking book was developed. Books are recorded on tape and fitted into a cassette. The blind person places the tape cassette into a device similar to a tape recorder, which is called a talking book machine.

With the right support and appropriate early intervention for families, the capabilities of the blind child are limitless. Blind persons today are independently employed successfully in an astounding variety of work roles. If society does not limit its expectations of the blind child, these children will be allowed to live normal and fulfilling lives.

Ophthalmic assistant's role

The orientation of the blind child in an office or any situation is similar to that of an adult, with one exception; with small children, the ophthalmic assistant can simply take their hand. With older children, the assistant can offer an arm, as for an adult. The child should be warned in advance about the general geography of a room and the location of steps as he comes to them. In the ophthalmologist's office, the assistant should lead the child to a chair, gently turn him, and place his hand on the arm of the chair; he or she should also tell the child on which side the seat is located. Again, the right and left side should always be designated with reference to the position of the blind person. A blind child should be spoken to in a friendly, natural manner; these children become very skilled in assessing people by the tone of their voice, just as a sighted child would assess a stranger by the person's facial expression.

REHABILITATION

Rehabilitation assists a blind person to acquire the practical skills and outlook to minimize the effects of disability and lead to increased self-esteem, independence, and social competence.

Rehabilitation programs are often essential for working-age blind persons to regain basic independent living skills that make possible further educational training or gainful employment. More than 70% of blind and visually impaired persons are older than 65 years of age. For those individuals a rehabilitation program can contribute substantially to their quality of life and assist them with continuing to live in as independent an environment as possible.

Rehabilitation programs usually are staffed by a multidisciplinary team of professionals. The rehabilitation team will assess specific learning needs, develop a training program to meet the needs, and evaluate the blind person's progress in achieving established goals. Services include counseling, daily living skills instruction, orientation and mobility training, braille and tape library services, sight-enhancement services, and concept and sensory development, as well as the provision of consultation and educational information to caregivers, family members, and the general public.

Career development and employment

The goal of rehabilitation for working-age blind persons is competitive employment. Barriers faced by blind persons seeking employment are related to both information and to attitudes.

In making an occupational choice, blind persons must have information to make meaningful decisions. They need information about their own skills and interests, various occupations that they might find suitable, the technologic knowledge that would qualify them for the job, and how other blind persons have adapted various job tasks.

Occupations pursued by blind and visually impaired persons cover the whole range of occupational categories; thus there need be very few limits placed on their career aspirations. Obtaining the necessary information is still a problem for many blind and visually impaired persons. Expertise related to the disability and employment opportunities is often hard to find inasmuch as mainstream employment services possess little knowledge or expertise on blindness and visual impairment, and the specialized employment services for blind persons are thinly spread.

The attitudinal barrier is formidable. Prevailing public perceptions of the potential of blind persons tend to inhibit the hiring practices of employers. Blind and visually impaired persons may be placed in the position of having to defend themselves from a variety of popular misconceptions held by job interviewers. For this reason the public education function of agencies for the blind is of critical importance. So too is the outreach function of specialized employment services for blind and visually impaired job seekers, in which employment counselors perform a marketing function on behalf of their clients.

The greatest single factor in employment of blind persons over the last 20 years is the emergence of information technology. Blindness is handicapping in terms of availability of information; thus access to information is of the utmost importance. Part of the prevocational education component of blind and visually impaired persons, whether they are children or newly blinded adults, will in future be in the field of electronic communications.

Vocations

Most rehabilitation programs culminate in placing the blind person in a job within the sighted community. Job placements require, of course, that special safeguards be made available for the blind worker. It has been shown conclusively that the output of the blind worker in assembly work may be equal in both quantity and quality to that of sighted colleagues if the work is suitably chosen. However, only a limited number of industries have special facilities for the blind worker. Many workshops are run under the auspices of blind institutions and are geared to obviate the blind person's disability. Many blind people actually prefer working under these conditions because of the protections afforded them both physically and psychologically.

The active rehabilitation of blind persons depends on many individual factors, such as aptitudes, skills, native intelligence, and previous training. Blind people have gone on to attain degrees in law, social work, and economics. Many musicians are blind, and some have achieved a great measure of fame; pianist George Shearing is an excellent example.

Vocational teaching

The key figure in the rehabilitation of the blind is the rehabilitation teacher. These teachers, because they are blind, are inspirational figures to an individual who has recently lost his sight and feels his life is over. Such teachers understand very well the many tiny frustrations that accumulate daily and reduce the morale of the blind trainee. Their understanding of these frustrations and their own unwillingness to be defeated by such problems serve as an excellent example to the individual who has recently lost his sight. Rehabilitation teachers teach braille reading and handicrafts such as knitting, mat making, and leather work. The function of the teacher is to show the newly blind person that he can still learn and acquire skills despite his handicap. The teacher is fundamentally a builder of confidence and self-esteem.

AVAILABLE AIDS

Many ingenious devices have been designed to assist the blind person to cope with everyday living. Among these devices are braille or talking watches and clocks (Fig. 36-2). Braille watches typically have a spring catch that, when pressed, causes the watch glass to open, allowing the user to read the location of the raised hands on the braille face of the watch. Talking watches announce the time aloud at the press of a button, and many also include auditory alarms. These watches are available in various designs, including both pocket and wrist types.

The Optacon was one of the first electronic aids for blind persons (Fig. 36-3). It changes visual print into touch type for reading by fingers. A small scan-

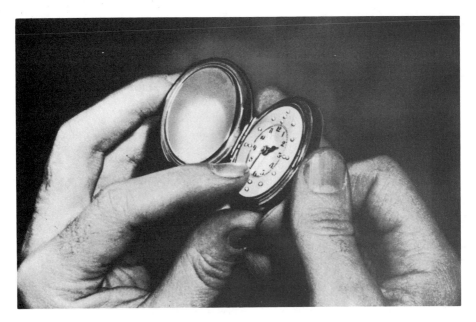

Fig. 36-2 Braille watch.

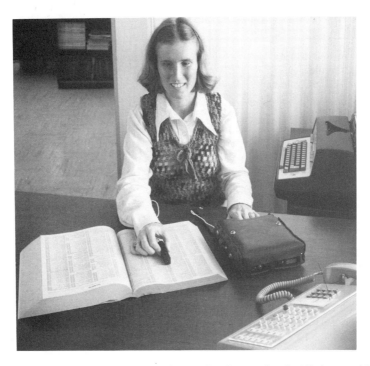

Fig. 36-3 Optacon. The miniature camera activates vibrations so that the blind can use their tactile sensation to read regular print.

ner is tracked across a line of print that is transferred electronically by vibrating raised type, letter by letter. This has since evolved into today's talking optical character recognition, which scans print on a small photocopy type scanner and converts it into speech. In addition, many computer-based technologic aids are available that provide audible access to information or braille displays. Small portable devices such as the Braille 'n Speak, which has a braille input keyboard and speech output, allow the user to access a note taker, calculator, and appointment book, all in a device that weighs less than two pounds.

Kitchen aids available for the blind homemaker include pressure cookers with braille timers and controls, liquid level indicators, and triangular pie cutters. There are self-threading needles that consist of a groove at the back of the needle before the actual eye of the needle. The thread is positioned into this

groove, and a small tug pulls the thread into the eye of the needle. Measurements can be made with a tape measure with inches marked off in elevated markings.

Among the medical aids are talking thermometers. Talking thermometers announce aloud the temperature. For the blind diabetic patient, insulin needle guides enable the person to locate the center of the rubber cap over the insulin bottle. There are also tactile raised markings on the syringe itself to measure the amount of insulin drawn up.

Recreation is a vital part of everyone's life in today's modern world. Tactile games have been developed by adapting standard games such as bingo, chess, Scrabble, Monopoly, dominoes, and playing cards. For more vigorous exercise and recreation, blind persons participate in all sports, including swimming, track, bowling, horseback riding, golf, and wrestling.

QUESTIONS FOR REVIEW AND THOUGHT

1. In your area what level of vision qualifies an individual to be considered as legally blind?
2. Imagine yourself having both eyes bandaged for 24 hours. Outline the inconvenience and problems you may be confronted with in your normal living.
3. Cover both eyes during a meal period and try to cope with the problems of finding your silverware and eating.
4. What is the basis of the braille system?
5. Name the agency or agencies in your area that help blind persons.
6. What aids are available to help blind people?
7. Spend half a day touring your nearest institute for blind persons. Outline your impressions and the facilities available.

SELF-EVALUATION QUESTIONS

True-false statements

Directions: Indicate whether the statement is true (T) or false (F).

T or F   1. A legally blind person cannot read.

T or F   2. The Braille system was developed by Louis Braille, a blind student who in 1824 developed a six-dot raised code.

T or F   3. There is an association between blindness and mental retardation in the adult.

Missing words

Directions: Write in the missing word in the following sentences.

4. The mannerisms of blind children, such as walking in circles and rubbing their hands, are called

    _____.

5. Blindness is defined in most places in the world as vision of _____ or less in the best eye and a peripheral field no greater than _____.

6. The ultimate solution to relieve permanent blindness is to implant _____.

Choice-completion questions

Directions: Select the one best answer in each case.

7. The blind person can:
    a. Ski
    b. Go to a university and become a doctor or Ph.D.
    c. Be employed, with better records for safety, productivity, and punctuality than his sighted counterparts
    d. Play golf
    e. All of the above

8. Braille should be taught:
    a. To every blind person
    b. Only to the young blind person
    c. To a person recently blinded
    d. Only to those who cannot possibly read with visual aids
    e. To people going blind

9. In North America the leading cause(s) of blindness is (are):
    a. Cataracts
    b. Corneal disease
    c. Retinal disease
    d. Diseases of the vitreous
    e. Diseases relating to dryness of the eyes

ANSWERS, NOTES, AND EXPLANATIONS

1. **False.** A legally blind person may have 20/200 vision and with adequate visual aids and good lighting can read normal-size print. The ability to compensate depends on the person's drive, determination, and intelligence. The worst handicap a blind person has is acceptance of his blindness as a totally incapacitating event. Only 25% of blind people have no light perception and are truly blind.

2. **True.** The braille cell is three dots high and two dots wide. Most popular books are available in braille. Also, many magazines, such as *Reader's Digest,* have a braille edition. Textbooks in braille are also available, and blind students have been graduated in medicine, law, accounting, and other demanding courses of study.

3. **False.** People who are blind may have macular degeneration, diabetes, or glaucoma, none of which is associated with mental deterioration. In developing countries trachoma can cause blindness because of corneal scarring. Simple cataracts, undetected and untreated, are a common source of blindness. Whatever the cause, the blind person commonly is treated with pity as though not only can he not see but cannot think properly.

4. **Blindisms.** These habit spasms are difficult to eradicate, but with trained help, they can be. They should be removed, as such traits remain an obvious stigma of a person's blindness.

5. **20/200, 20 degrees.** Blindness is not the absence of light perception. A person is considered blind only if he cannot function in the ordinary world. With this definition there are many legally blind people who do not consider themselves blind nor are they considered blind by others. In a sense, it is a state of mind.

6. **An artificial eye.** The artificial eye is not the pipe dream of science fiction writers. Blind people can "see" through a television monitor that is hooked up to implants placed on the surface of the occipital lobe. The eye cameras have to be miniaturized so the blind person can function with movement. The basic apparatus, however, is available now.

7. **e. All of the above.** A protected environment is not needed for an ambitious, hard-working blind person. Blind people cannot fly a plane, drive a car, or play baseball. However, they can do many things at home, at work, or in sports without special assistance.

8. **d. Only to those who cannot possibly read with visual aids.** Although braille has served the blind well for 150 years (through braille watches, typewriters, and so on), it does narrow the range of options for the blind. Only a small segment of the world's literature is turned into braille symbols. The options for learning and promotion are far greater if the blind person can stay in the sighted world even if it means a constant struggle. It is better to have a handicap than to be handicapped.

9. **c. Retinal disease.** Fortunately, cataracts and most forms of corneal disease can be treated surgically with great success. Diseases of the vitreous are usually secondary to retinal or ciliary body disorders. Whereas great advancement has been made in retinal disease, there are no replacement parts for a sick macula or optic nerve. When the macula is injured by disease or trauma, the effects are permanent. The optic nerve, the victim of such common disorders as temporal arteritis, glaucoma, and arteriosclerosis, cannot be helped once damaged. The retina and optic nerve play a major role in creating blindness simply because there is no therapy for these problems. Years ago, the same could be said for diseases of the cornea or lens.

CHAPTER 37 Reading problems in children

The child with a reading problem has a disability as incapacitating as any physical infirmity. Bascially, the poor reader is thwarted in the attempt to acquire knowledge. Just like children with a physical deformity, poor readers cannot effectively compete with their classmates because of a handicap. However, unlike the physically handicapped child whose deformity is obvious, the poor reader is difficult to distinguish from others as having a special problem. This child usually passes all preschool medical examinations and is declared healthy and able to meet the challenge of early grade school. Of course, the youngster does poorly and either suffers a major failure at a young age or is carried by the current of regular promotion to higher grades, insecure, unprepared, and destined to become an early school dropout. It is estimated that from 10% to 20% of the school population has some form of reading disability.

There are many reasons for poor achievement at school. The operative factors include immaturity, cultural deprivation, discord in the home (divorce, separation, or inadequate or hostile parents), poor health, and mental retardation. The child with a reading problem does not necessarily have any cultural, social, or intellectual failings. In many cases the youngster does poorly in spite of being gifted with every tangible advantage both at home and at school.

WHOSE PROBLEM IS IT?

Because many children with a reading disability become juvenile delinquents, marginal unskilled laborers, or severely emotionally disturbed adults, the problem is obviously a matter of public health and welfare, with major responsibility directed toward both federal and local government bodies. Many heterogeneous groups have or should have a vested interest in this disability. These groups include departments of education and more specifically subdepartments of special education; the medical schools, in particular departments of ophthalmology, neurology, psychology, psychiatry, and pediatrics and schools of social work; and the paramedical groups, such as optometrists, orthoptists, ophthalmic assistants, and technicians. Obviously, with such a large number of subsidiary groups, there is plenty of room for each to avoid or ignore its responsibility toward the entire subject. Thus instead of disciplined group responsibility, the situation has deteriorated to the point of undisciplined group evasion. For example, many poor readers are incorrectly assumed to have poor vision. The ophthalmologist, after careful examination, usually will find that vision is 20/20 in each eye and will reassure the parents that there is no ocular pathologic condition present. The ophthalmologist's responsibility toward that patient usually ends at that point. Unfortunately, the problem does not.

Many of these children develop behavioral problems. They are listless or hyperactive and cannot concentrate on their lessons at school. Their failure at school and subsequent admonishment both at school and at home lead to acts of rebelliousness, disregard of authority, and, of course, further failure. Often the secondary behavior problem overshadows the primary problem, and many are sent for psychiatric evaluation as emotionally disturbed children. The psychologist may be consulted to conduct a battery of tests to determine the child's IQ, verbal and nonverbal skills, and abilities. Other areas of nonperformance may become apparent. The child may have difficulty with speech and with coordination of fine motor skills (writing, tying shoe laces, throwing a ball) or may show faulty spatial orientation. Many questions are raised, and a pediatric or neurologic consultation may become desirable and helpful. Some children show faulty development patterns (for example, in crawling and walking) during the formative years, whereas others reveal clinical and electrophysiologic evidence of minimal brain dysfunction.

A brief glance at the subject of reading disabilites indicates that many different professions and groups have a stake in the diagnostic and therapeutic aspects of this disorder. A multidisciplinary approach is mandatory. Until teams of effective and interested specialists are mustered and captains of the teams chosen to administrate their productive efforts, the problem of the poor reader will remain a conundrum tackled by anyone who shows an interest in the subject, regardless of qualification. In the partial vacuum of any treatment center, some good work has been done by interested persons, but the need for treatment also has been exploited by quacks, charlatans, and the demigods of truth who, in effect, make a cult of their beliefs.

TERMINOLOGY

Dyslexia is the inability or reduced ability to read, and *developmental dyslexia* refers to the presence of that condition from childhood and the first attempts to read. This is different from the dyslexia occurring in an adult who formerly read but who has lost the ability because of brain damage. *Agraphia* is the inability to write. The ability to read and the ability to write are not mutually dependent, because a person can have difficulty with reading but none with writing.

Inability to recognize an object or a written or auditory symbol is called *agnosia*. Inability to correlate verbal information into meaningful terms by means of sensory organs is called *aphasia*. The individual, then, who cannot recognize a spoon or fork has agnosia, but the one who can state what it is but has forgotten its function has aphasia.

Apraxia is inability to perform a previously learned task in spite of an intact sensory and motor system. In terms of reading, apraxia may be applied to the child who cannot recall what has been previously assimilated, so that errors of reading are repetitiously made.

The terms *agnosia, aphasia,* and *apraxia* belong to the neurologic jargon used to describe organic lesions of the parietal and temporal lobes. Because many children with general perceptual motor defects have signs and symptoms that are similar to acquired organic disturbances of the parietal and temporal lobes, the terminology used to describe their symptoms is most easily understood in the context of organic lesions.

ACT OF READING

The ability to read depends on different overlapping cerebral mechanisms, each functioning independently, and yet totally dependent on the other. These overlapping processes include visual sensation, recognition, and comprehension.

Visual sensation begins with visual experience, which depends on the penetration of an adequate amount of light through the clear optical media of the eye. This stimulates the retina with the relay of visual information mediated through an intact afferent visual pathway from the optic nerve to the visual striate area of the cerebral cortex.

Vision in human beings can be either monocular (employing one eye) or binocular (employing both eyes). Binocular vision occurs when the images from both eyes are fused into a single mental impression. Binocularity depends, then, on strict anatomic alignment of the eyes and the ability of the eyes to project to the same point in space at a given distance. Stereopsis, a higher aspect of binocular vision, features the ability not only to form a single visual picture but to perceive depth by parallax.

Adequate visual sensation per se is not defective in most children with reading problems. They can see with the uncorrected eye or with properly prescribed spectacles, and they have 20/20 vision in each eye when tested with the Snellen chart. There is no dispute on this point. Contention arises on the subject of binocular vision. Some persons believe that the harmonious act of binocular coordination is faulty in the perceptually handicapped child. They find difficulties in eye muscle balance, abnormal ocular movements, and faulty sensory fusion, and they actively treat these disabilities. Other workers cite the lack of harmony between ocular and hand dominance as a paramount problem in the perceptually handicapped. Although many points are still unsettled, most ophthalmologists believe that disorders of ocular motility have little to do with perception or comprehension.

Recognition involves the ability to correctly ascribe a given name to a given set of visual symbols. The child must be able not only to see the particular letter or word but also to correctly identify those letters or words. The child should be able to recognize shapes such as squares, rectangles, or triangles.

Comprehension involves assimilating visual information with material learned previously and deriving some meaning from a particular visual symbol. In short, comprehension involves understanding what is read. English, like all European languages, is written phonetically. Groups of letters are assembled into words that are expressed phonetically. In learning, the written word must become the spoken word almost automatically. However, this is a highly complex act because our words are not written with exact phonetic correlation. For example, the words "bed" and "lead" have the same phonetic vowel but are represented symbolically quite differently. Words such as "fight," "foreign," and "fought" have noncontributing consonants or vowel combinations that defy phonetic exactitude. Difficulties also arise in differentiating the singular from the plural (for example, sheep versus sheep), because some words sound and look the same but have different meanings. In view of the inherent difficulties in understanding the English language, most children make mistakes in learning how to read and write. These errors, which may include *writing letters backward* and *reading backward,* may be quite normal in a 6-year-old but become symptomatic of a learning disability if perpetuated until the age of 8 or 9 years.

In the child with a reading disability no single defect is present. All factors mentioned contribute to this pathologic state, with the least emphasis being placed on perception.

TYPES OF SLOW READERS

The term *perceptual handicap* has become a familiar diagnosis. Not only educational authorities and other professional groups have become interested in this field but also parent groups and the popular press have stressed its existence and pressed for its treatment, almost to the neglect of other causes—social, environmental, and psychologic—of reading failure. Although readers of this text will tend to think of *perception* as mainly a visual experience, perception is an operative function related to all sensory modalities. Sometimes, forgetting that reading is a language experience, current writers seem to overlook the necessary part that auditory-verbal perception and kinesthetic-tactile perception play in dealing with the written word. They tend to concentrate their efforts on visual perception or, at best, on the association between visual perception as a base and the other sensory and cognitive factors. Similar to other changing terminology, the term *perceptually handicapped* is rapidly giving way to the term *learning disabled*.

Slow readers may be grouped into five categories. In the first group are children who suffer from simple mental retardation and who thus learn all skills later and less well. Those who lack a sensory capacity, including blind or deaf children, make up the second group. In the third group are those who have not had a reasonable opportunity to learn because of the limitations imposed by their socioeconomic level, a limited language experience, or a lack of appropriate and consistent instruction. Those in the fourth group suffer from some degree of emotional barrier in the form of primary mental and emotional disturbance, or less dramatically, from simple emotional immaturity that makes them relatively unfit for taking on the responsiblity of the task involved in learning to read.

Most of the children in these four groups may be identified readily, and treatment procedures are fairly obvious, although circumstances may make them hard to indicate. The fifth group is much more difficult to diagnose and to treat. It is made up of those who have, as it were, "everything going for them" but who nevertheless do not respond to reasonably adequate classroom instruction. To these children the term *congenital dyslexia* or *learning disability* may be applied, with the understanding that the condition is seen in every degree from a complete inability to learn to read to a much slowed-down speed of learning in that particular skill.

It should be added that the school system in itself imposed some limitations on certain individuals. Generally, children are placed in first grade, the class in which formal reading instruction begins, at the chronologic age of 6 years; that is, children born between January 1, 1986, and December 31, 1986,

began reading instruction in September 1993. Approximately one fifth of the total maturity reached by 6 years of age accrues in that final year before the sixth birthday; therefore youngsters born in October, November, and December start out with a considerable handicap compared with those born early in the year, and yet they are expected to learn from the same program, begin at the same level, and carry on at the very same pace.

During the early years, boys mature at a notably slower rate than do girls, and at age 6 years they generally are considered to be about 1 year behind girls on the average, in fine-motor and language development, two very important skills in learning to read and write. It is therefore possible for a boy born in late December to be in the same class as a girl born at the beginning of January and to be 2 years behind her in reading readiness because of a slower maturity rate.

It also should be mentioned that first grade classes offer widely differing amounts of structured assistance for learning to read. The progressive, child-centered, discovery- and experience-oriented class may offer little until the child spontaneously wants to become involved in reading, whereas the more traditional curriculum-centered class may start the first sight words, a few initial sounds, or both, as well as other beginning phonetic concepts in the first month of the school year for all children.

The classification of causes of dyslexia is by no means simple, nor is there any one particular type that seems to predominate. Dr. Arthur Keeney, a noted authority in this field, has outlined one useful type of classification*:

A. Specific (primary) developmental dyslexia (strephosymbolia or dyssymbolia): inability or difficulty in the cortical process of symbol interpretation appearing in individuals of average to high performance IQ and with functionally adequate sensory input mechanisms; appears predominantly in males and has a dominant genetic inheritance

B. Symptomatic (secondary) dyslexia (secondary reading retardation)

---

*From Keeney, AH: *Ocular examination: basis and technique,* ed 2, St Louis, 1976, CV Mosby, p. 264.

1. Secondary to organic brain pathology (brain damage, cerebral dysfunction, other encephalopathy, cerebral palsy, mental retardation, low IQ, visual agnosia, anomia, soft neurologic stigmata)
   a. Genetically determined
   b. Posttraumatic (prenatal, natal, postnatal)
   c. Postinflammatory (intrauterine or extrauterine encephalitis, meningitis)
   d. Asphyxic (intrauterine, extrauterine)
   e. Prematurity
   f. Other specific brain lesion (aneurysm, meningioma, porencephalic cyst, others)
2. Secondary to slow maturation (late bloomer, developmental delay)
3. Secondary to emotional disturbances (hyperactivity, depression, anxiety)
4. Secondary to uncontrolled seizure states
5. Secondary to environmental disturbances (cultural deprivation, poor motivation, poor instruction)

C. Slow reading (handicap without symbolic confusion)
   1. Ocular impediment to sustained visual use (hyperopia, heterophoria, astigmatism, partial cataracts, retinal and macular abiotrophies)
   2. Auditory impairment
   3. Hypothyroid state
D. Alexia or acquired dyslexia: lesions usually in the region of the angular gyrus of the dominant hemisphere
E. Mixed types

CHARACTERISTICS OF THE CHILD WITH A READING DISABILITY

Sex. Of the children with reading disabilities, boys are affected more commonly than girls, the ratio varying from 4:1 to 10:1. The great preponderance of males is related to their physiologic maturation lag. Boys acquire neuromuscular coordinating abilities more slowly than do girls. In early grade school they tend to be more awkward in writing, art, and even dressing themselves. Thus any specific disability related to a perceptual motor deficit is increased in the boy in the formative years.

Behavior. Children with reading disabilities sometimes tend to be very distractable and possess a short attention span. They daydream in the clasroom, especially when abstract material is being considered. If their interest is aroused, they may show a longer attention span, but this does not last longer than a period or two. They sometimes tend to be hyper-

active in the sense of being restless rather than busy at their work. They appear to be in constant motion, shifting from one object or activity to another, and concerned with everything in general but nothing in particular. Children cannot keep from touching and handling objects, especially in a strange or over-stimulating environment.

Often these children have conflicts with their teachers and schoolmates. They may display an emotional lability that may vary from placid behavior to violent temper tantrums. Commonly they become hostile and aggressive with seemingly minimal provocation. Later this errant behavior can become disturbingly pathologic, with a child committing crimes such as fire setting and stealing. These children often are impulsive and appear to be unable to thwart a sudden desire regardless of the situation or consequences. This impulsiveness may show itself in continual punching, pushing, or pulling of others whenever the child comes in contact with them or by a desire for immediate recognition by others.

Often the children show a lack of propriety and are quite uninhibited. For example, they may show no regard for carrying on at school or in games with obviously soiled trousers.

Learning disability. Reading skill is profoundly retarded and is not appropriate for the child's age or grade. The reading disability increases under stress, such as when the child is asked to read before the class. Some of the reading disabilities found include (1) failure to see likenesses and differences in the form of words—for example, musician and magician; (2) reversal in writing or reading certain words—for example, stop and pots (Fig. 37-1); (3) failure to keep one's place; (4) failure to read from left to right; (5) mirror writing or backward reading—for example, writing number 7 backward, or writing capital D backward; (6) omissions and deletions of words and letters; and (7) distortion of words—for example, cloud instead of could.

In addition to poor reading, the child fails at those subjects that primarily depend on reading skills. Spelling, written composition, and writing also are poorly done. Yet the child may reveal a visual imagination, excel in oral composition, and appear bright when spoken to in a casual conversation. It is this

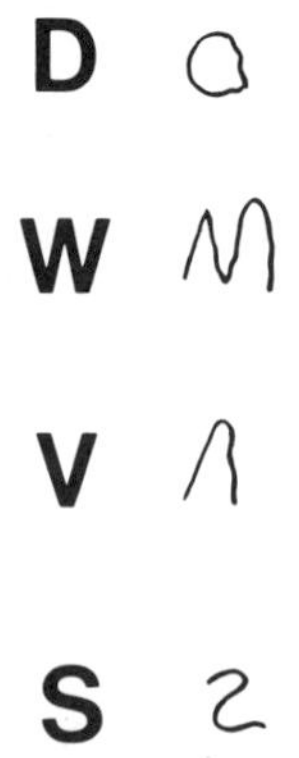

D ◌

W ʍ

V ʌ

S ↄ

Fig. 37-1 Copying of a 6-year-old dyslexic child. Note the mirror writing and reversals of letters.

ability that parents see at home, and therefore they often blame the schools or the teachers for the child's lack of achievement.

Perceptual motor defects. Children with perceptual motor defects commonly are described as awkward and clumsy. Any skill that requires finely coordinated motor ability is performed poorly (Fig. 37-2). In the early grades, when copying from the board or from visual aid posters is vital, these children are inordinately handicapped. They cannot trace a figure, copy a geometric form either from memory or directly, draw, or even print in neat fashion between two lines (Figs. 37-3 to 37-5). This gross failure to complete the simplest tasks in the classroom is augmented outside the classroom. Success eludes them in this setting as well; they perform poorly in athletics because they are unable to throw or catch a ball with any degree of constancy.

The characteristics of the perceptually handicapped child are not uniform. They vary in accordance with the child's level of intelligence, disposition, cultural environment at home, and the integrity of the family unit. These modulating factors will influence the child's adaptation to the disability and to a great extent determine behavior patterns.

The natural course of a child with a reading problem is in an interruption of learning. The child falls farther and farther behind in reading ability, becomes increasingly frustrated in academic areas that require reading, and so as a rule comes to dislike school. Consequently the youngster does not rely on

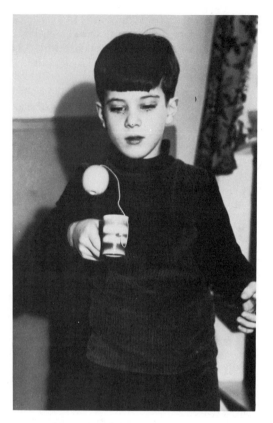

Fig. 37-2 Game to test coordination.

reading for information or pleasure. Without practice, the student actually regresses. Thus begins the vicious circle—lack of progress, frustration, dislike for reading, and avoidance of tasks, leading to further failure in related areas.

ROLE OF BRAIN AND EYE DOMINANCE

It has been estimated that 65% of patients with reading difficulty have some conflict in establishing laterality. These patients show right-left confusion and are ambidextrous; they fail to establish a cerebral dominance, often until the age or 8 or 9 years. Also, it has been shown that these children commonly fail to show harmony between their dominant hand and dominant eye. The view, championed by Orton—that inability to establish a synchronous complex between hand and eye coordination is paramount in

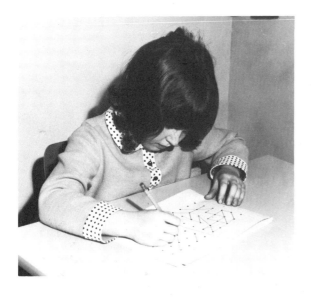

Fig. 37-3 Child is asked to connect dots to improve hand-eye coordination. This is part of the Marianne Frostig test of visual perception.

Fig. 37-4 Building blocks used to improve fine muscle coordination.

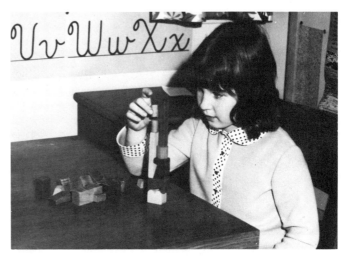

causing reading disabilities—has many advocates in both Canada and the United States. Acting on this premise, the disciples of this belief have set up schools, training centers, and remedial reading centers with the singular objective of establishing a dominance in the perceptually handicapped child. The most vigorous of these theorists train the children to relearn every motor act acquired since birth (including reaching, creeping, and crawling) and claim success in their efforts to overcome reading problems, difficulties in motor coordination, and even strabis-

mus. The object of these programs is to establish well-defined cerebral dominance.

In literature on the topic, little attention or credibility is placed on the role of ocular dominance. Good readers are found among children who do not have well-established motor laterality (for example, Leonardo da Vinci wrote with his left hand and did mirror writing).

Many centers use extensive visual exercises. These eye exercises are designed to establish harmonious eye-hand dominance, improve defects in

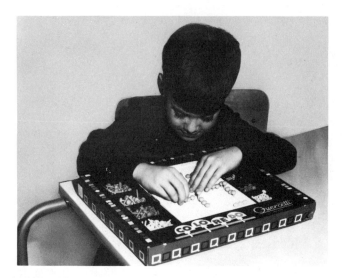

Fig. 37-5 Child's ability to reproduce designs on a pegboard is tested.

binocularity, or help overcome faulty visual spatial projection disorders. The exercises themselves are usually quite simple and designed to hold the child's interest. They may include, for example, following a pendulum, copying blocks, and tracing figures and designs. The eye exercises are regarded by most ophthalmologists as of no value in terms of the major problem.

NEUROLOGIC FACTORS

Many perceptually handicapped children are regarded as having minimal brain dysfunction. However, this is only by definition. It has not been demonstrated neurologically that minimal clinical signs are in fact related to minimal brain abnormalities. Minimal signs may be concomitant with significant lesions of the brain. Of course, the converse also holds true. To complicate the situation further, many neurologically impaired children do not present any specific learning problem in the classroom, whereas children without brain injury but with supposedly aberrant behavior do have difficulty.

EDUCATIONAL CONSIDERATIONS

Probably the greatest problem in this area lies in the identification of the child with a specific learning disability. In most schools there are no formal

screening tests to detect overt or latent perceptual inadequacies in children, and the diagnosis initially rests with the teacher. Dyslexia first becomes evident as the child reaches kindergarten and first grade, although it is often not recognized until much later and indeed is commonly never recognized for what it is (Fig. 37-6).

Teachers of an early grade have two roles to fill. They must teach the group as a whole a task for which the teachers are prepared by virtue of their training, and they must sort out and refer for special instruction the child who fails to progress at the expected rate. It is the second role in which teachers may fail because of the inadequacy of their training. Teachers, like general practitioners of medicine, are the first line of defense before the specialist takes over. Unlike their medical counterparts, however, their training primarily is concerned with teaching methods rather than diagnostics.

Ideally, the dyslexic child's learning program takes into account the handicap and tries to surmount it. Physically the classroom should be geared to this child's distractibility, the main stumbling block to learning. The desk position—the child's place in the class—is designed to shut out many of the distractions that divert the youngster from the lesson. Also, the material is presented so that these children

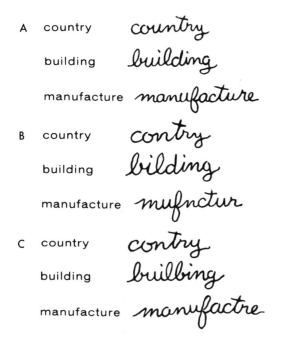

A country *country*

  building *building*

  manufacture *manufacture*

B country *contry*

  building *bilding*

  manufacture *mufnctur*

C country *contry*

  building *briilbing*

  manufacture *manufactre*

Fig. 37-6 Writing of a 9-year-old boy. **A,** Words dictated one syllable at a time. **B,** Words dictated at normal speed. **C,** Words copied from blackboard.

learn at their own pace either in a special classroom or in a special place in the ordinary classroom. If they are forced to compete with their classmates, as opposed to themselves, they struggle and usually fail to make much progress.

In some areas that are equipped with special classrooms and highly specialized teachers, children with perceptual problems have been isolated for periods of 1 to 3 years and then successfully returned to their regular classes. With special training, they not only make academic progress but show remarkable changes in behavior.

PROBLEMS AT HOME

Children with a learning disability, although failing at school, often appear quite bright to their parents. Indeed, most of these children are alert, possess a vivid imagination, and do well on intelligence tests that avoid their particular disability. The parent usually is perplexed by the inability of the child to learn to read and may regard the whole business as a temporary aberration. Eventually, consistently poor achievement drives parents to find a rationale for it. Slightly bewildered and somewhat angry, parents may blame the child's teacher or the school system. Later, as they attempt to correct these injustices by home tutorials and fail miserably in teaching their own child to read, parents may accuse the child of laziness, lack of ambition, truancy, or just plain stupidity. Needless to say, the loss of parental regard is only the prelude to the child's own loss of self-esteem.

In the neighborhood the child's unpredictable and sometimes negative or hostile behavior leads to rejection by other children. Such children do not stay with group games very long because they do not possess the motor skills needed to play effectively and often cannot understand the basic organization of the game.

The child who finds rejection at school, rebuff in the neighborhood play group, and criticism at home is bound to develop feelings of intense hostility and rebellion. The child may become totally unmanageable. Being impulsive, hyperactive, and emotionally labile, the child with a severe emotional crisis augments these tendencies, and behavior problems soon eclipse the initial one.

Parental reaction can vary from frank hostility to bland indifference or indulgence. Sympathetic parents who understand the nature of the child's problem probably are the most frustrated. Desiring a solution they first attempt to discover whether a physical disability is present. The investigation may trail through an array of professionals, including general practitioners, pediatricians, ophthalmologists, neurologists, and psychiatrists, only to reveal that the child has no gross physical disability. The quest for a solution carries them to the schools. If the school has facilities for psychologic testing and the waiting list for such tests is not interminably long, the child may be assessed and assigned to special classes. Most schools, however, do not have enough classrooms for the regular students, let alone facilities for special students. Even if enough physical space could be found and structured to meet the needs of the distractible child, there would be difficulty in finding a sufficient number of teachers with special training to meet the demand. In some instances, parents have reacted to this void by sending their children to private remedial reading schools, optometrists or small centers for the learning disabled. Some of these private agencies and individuals obtain good results because of their knowledge, enthusiasm, and general integrity. Their facilities, however, are not subject to inspection by any government department, and their abilities are not tested by any particular credentials committee. Thus it is found that among the available therapists, many will alleviate the problem, whereas others will exploit it.

Isolated groups of frustrated parents have formed associations for the child with a learning disability. The function of these lay bodies is to disseminate information on the subject and to encourage the professions of medicine, psychology, and pedagogy to take a more active interest in the child with a perceptual motor disorder. These groups acknowledge the isolated efforts of interested therapists but have concentrated their efforts on bridging the gap among the various professions so that a multidisciplinary approach can be offered to each child.

CONDITIONS THAT ARE CONFUSED WITH A LEARNING DISABILITY

Hearing deficit. Many learning-disabled children have some defect in hearing. Some cannot differentiate sounds, as opposed to differentiating visual symbols, and they do not respond well to hearing test situations. Hearing ability, therefore, is difficult to determine, and some children are mistakenly placed in classes for deaf children. Others may appear to hear properly, but they do not understand and are considered to be mentally retarded.

Mental retardation. In many respects learning-disabled children and mentally retarded children are very much alike. Both groups fail to progress at a rate appropriate for their age. Both may have difficulty caring for themselves and may be late in becoming toilet trained and in dressing and feeding themselves. Both fail to establish good personal relationships with other children. The retarded child commonly does not even make an effort to be part of the group, whereas the learning-disabled child may try and fail miserably. The fundamental difference between the two children is that the latter does not have a low intelligence quotient. The child's interest can be aroused, but it is difficult to sustain. Also, this child does not necessarily underachieve in all subjects and may even show brilliance in some courses of study while doing poorly in others.

Childhood schizophrenia versus autism. Autistic children live in their own world of social isolation and often behave in the same manner toward most people, be they strangers or members of their own family. Learning-disabled children do not behave as though the outside world were of little importance. They not only know the difference among people but will adjust their behavior to individuals according to their importance. They can be diverted from undesirable social behavior when pride and interest in accomplishment are established through proper teaching; the autistic child cannot be diverted.

Emotional disturbance. There is often great difficulty in differentiating the truly emotionally disturbed child from the child whose behavior is the result of frustration caused by inability to communicate orally and to understand language. There are no easy methods of distinguishing the two groups, and this task must be left in the hands of professional psychologists and psychiatrists.

TREATMENT

The treatment of learning-disabled children has followed three general patterns, the emphasis varying with the individual therapist and the particular needs of the child.

One approach is to reorient the teaching program to suit the particular handicap of the child. This program usually is devised by the department of special education of large school boards. In ideal situations extra classrooms are built in such a manner as to aid the student to focus attention on school material. These rooms are located at the end of corridors, out of range of other children passing back and forth. The walls are built of sound-absorbing materials, and the windows are made translucent to reduce distracting visual stimuli coming in from the outside. The number of children in a class is small, and eight in a group usually is regarded as a high optimum number. The teachers, the focal point of the entire operation, are specially trained in both special teaching methods and psychology. It is desirable that they be warm, friendly, and patient, and some authorities even believe that such teachers also should undergo psychotherapy to understand themselves in their relationship to their students. Of utmost importance is that the teachers be given extensive opportunity to evaluate the case records and to talk with the psychiatrist, neurologist, and psychologist, because the teachers are an integral part of the team.

When the learning disability is more circumscribed and behavior problems are not dominant, the child can be left in the ordinary classroom while receiving special attention. This type of child may need a more phonetic approach to reading and should not be required to compete with the other children. If the teacher is made aware of the child's problem, the little extras—extra help, extra understanding, extra tutorials, and extra inducement—may be of great value.

Another method of treatment is to approach the child as a whole and concentrate on rehabilitating the child in all aspects—visual, auditory, kinesthetic, and motor. The practical implications of this method are rather vague and broad. The Frostig method tries to encompass visual perceptual training and sensory-motor training concurrently with language training. The training in sensory-motor function includes four areas: (1) general training of movement skills through a program of physical education, (2) development of body awareness, (3) training in eye-hand coordination and manipulation skills, and (4) training in eye movement through tracking exercises.

Other groups have emphasized the difficulty of establishing lateral dominance as the major cause of a child's problem and have relegated their efforts in this regard. The exercises are fundamental initially, and the child is retrained in hand reaching, creeping, crawling, and even in sleeping posture.

A more segmental approach is taken by optometrists who deemphasize the emotional and neurologic aspects of the learning-disabled child and focus only on supposed errors of binocular function, ocular motor coordination, and ocular dominance. In regard to ocular motor coordination, the theory is that children, to complete or trace an oblique line, must be able to nimbly perform oblique movements of their eyes. Therefore, they are started on tracking exercises with pendulum-gazing devices, projection exercises, and so forth.

In most large training centers, therapy is broadly approached, with several therapists working with problems of speech, motor skills, penmanship, verbal formulation, auditory and visual perception, visual memory, and directional confusion.

Regardless of the treatment initiated, it is essential that each child have a complete diagnostic evaluation to discover both weaknesses and strengths. The work-up should include a medical evaluation and a behavioral assessment. The medical evaluation is essential to prevent the development or continuation of unsuspected disease processes. The behavior assessment provides the basis for a logical management and education program.

CLINICAL TESTS

Vision. Each child's vision should be fully evaluated to ensure that each eye is seeing normally. Refraction with a cycloplegic agent should be performed to detect any latent refractive error.

Letter reversal. When the child is given standard test letters to read at either distance or near, the examiner should be alert for letter reversals such as *b* for *d,* or *d* for *p,* or *p* for *q.* The examiner also should observe whether the child reads from right to left instead of from left to right. Occasionally a child will read vertically when asked to read across.

Color vision. Commonly, defects in color vision are detected among children with a reading disability. Color vision should be tested by the colored yarn test when the child is small or by pseudoisochromatic plates in the older child.

Dominance test. Although the relationship of the dominant eye to perceptual motor difficulties is still questionable, it may prove of interest for research projects. To identify the dominant eye, the child is asked to point to a distant object. By first covering one eye and then the other eye, the examiner can identify the dominant eye as the one that, when left uncovered, does not require a shift of the finger to the target.

Line drawings. The child should be asked to draw a clock complete with numbers. Children with normal spatial relationship usually will space the numbers evenly around the circle; those who do not will crowd them on one side.

Visual perception and comprehension tests. The child is asked to read a standard paragraph geared to his or her approximate grade level while the examiner notes the number and type of errors that the child makes. The examiner then asks a few pertinent questions about the paragraph just read to detect lack of comprehension.

Auditory perception test. The examiner can test auditory perception by dictating a simple sentence, preferably using words with *b, d,* and *p,* and asking the child to write out the sentence. The child with dyslexia will be unable to transfer the spoken word to the written word. It is important that these children have an audiogram to rule out primary hearing defects.

SUMMARY

Children with a reading disability can function efficiently and effectively in a calm emotional climate if they are allowed to compete only with students of their own caliber. These children require custom-designed educational facilities so that the sensory input, or information, does not come through a system that is blocked.

Children with a reading disability suffer from lack of simple identification. They do not possess a gross physical disability that can be easily pictured or publicly championed to elicit funds and facilities. Because their handicap is broad and subtle, it is poorly comprehended, and it does not receive the allowance due it. If these children were deaf or blind or had crippled hands, they would be spared the necessity of functioning in the areas in which they are crippled.

The prognosis depends on the age at which the handicap is identified, the family background, the presence or absence of severe secondary emotional reactions, and the magnitude of the disability. The earlier children with a handicap are discovered, the less apt they are to become a behavior problem. By the time they are 8 or 9 years of age, they have already developed a dislike of reading and learning that eventually spills over in hostility toward those who teach them. Before long, their hostility is directed at all persons of authority, including parents.

It has been estimated that about three out of four of the mildly affected children with a reading disability will learn to read well if presented, on a group basis, with modifications of current teaching methods. Of the remainder, about two thirds, if they are given enough time and protected from emotional stresses, improve through remedial teaching techniques applied on an individual basis. The remaining one third, who are the "hard core" of children with reading disability, eventually are forced to join the ranks of the school dropouts and usually lead a marginal existence in the unskilled labor pool.

QUESTIONS FOR REVIEW AND THOUGHT

1. Record the names of members in your community who can be of aid to the child with a reading problem.
2. Eye disorders play what factor in learning disability?
3. What exercises are available for the slow reader?
4. Outline the characteristics of children with a reading disability.
5. What conditions are often confused with a learning disability?
6. Do eye exercises help remedy the learning disabled?
7. Do children with reading problems usually have impaired vision?
8. Do children with perceptive difficulties have a low IQ?

9. Are children with learning disabilities likely to be (a) placid or (b) emotionally disturbed, with hostile behavior? Explain.
10. Does reading take place (a) when the eye moves or (b) when the eye pauses?
11. Are reading glasses of value in remedying learning disabilities?
12. Do some children have minimal brain dysfunction?
13. Do children with strabismus have greater problems with reading? Explain why or why not.

SELF-EVALUATION QUESTIONS

True-false statements

Directions: Indicate whether the statement is true (T) or false (F).

T or F   1. The child with a reading problem is usually of normal intelligence.
T or F   2. Reading problems are often the cause of abnormal ocular movements or faulty sensory function.
T or F   3. Eye exercises help remedy learning disabilities.

Missing words

Directions: Write the missing words in the following sentences.

4. The inability or reduced ability to read is called *dyslexia*. The presence of that condition from the first attempts to read is called _____.
5. Among children with reading disabilities, there is a great preponderance of _____.
6. Reading problems are a subgroup of a more general classification called _____.

Choice-completion questions

Directions: Select the one best answer in each case.

7. The child with a learning disability often has:
   a. Reading problems
   b. Visual perceptual problems
   c. Auditory perceptual problems
   d. a or c
   e. a, b, or c
8. The treatment of a reading disability is primarily the work of the:
   a. Optometrist
   b. Pediatrician
   c. Psychologist
   d. Special education teacher
   e. Psychiatrist
9. One of the most serious resultant side effects of a reading disability is:
   a. Minimal brain dysfunction
   b. Right-left confusion
   c. Poor self-image
   d. Eye muscle imbalance
   e. Hyperactivity

ANSWERS, NOTES, AND EXPLANATIONS

1. **True.** Although reading problems in children can occur in many different kinds of populations—for example, in the mentally retarded—the one kind of reading problem that is of particular interest to educators at this time is a reading problem that occurs in children who are of normal intelligence or above normal intelligence. The child of average intelligence with a reading problem has difficulty reading for a variety of reasons. Some have difficulty with language generally, and because reading is a language process, they cannot comprehend what they read. Other children, however, have good oral language skills but cannot grasp the mechanics of reading. Because a child's intelligence is normal, the expectation is that with the appropriate remedial help the child can begin to read. Of course, this often depends on the severity of the learning disability. It is noteworthy that the better a child's overall language is, the more he or she is able to compensate for the reading problem.

2. **False.** Although some people blame reading problems on abnormal ocular movements or faulty sensory fusion, studies show that reading problems occur because of difficulties at a higher level of cortical functioning. In other words, there is nothing wrong with the peripheral ocular mechanism. The difficulty is the result of the brain's inability to integrate and deal with some of this information. Reading problems do not occur only because of visual processing difficulties. As was pointed out previously, reading problems also can occur because of difficulties with auditory processing and with general language difficulties. The examiner should avoid the mistake of interpreting the cause of reading problems as a difficulty with the external eye mechanism, because this certainly affects how he or she goes about helping these children. Those professionals who try to correct ocular movements or faulty sensory fusion are wasting precious time that would be better spent in remedying reading problems in the more traditional ways. Traditional methods of remediation usually are best carried out by a teacher who has been well trained in special education.

3. **False.** This statement obviously follows from the incorrect premise that it is the external eye that is causing the child to be learning disabled. As was pointed out previously, the difficulties occur at a different level of functioning, namely at the cortical level, and eye exercises certainly cannot help remedy this problem. The best kind of remedial intervention not only deals with the areas of difficulty but also helps the child to compensate by using some of his or her strengths. The magic ingredient in all of this, of course, is to build up the child's self-image and feeling of self-worth as a learner.

4. **Dyslexia and developmental dyslexia.** The term *dyslexia* has been traditionally used to describe an individual, usually an adult, who formerly read but lost the ability to read because of brain damage. This word also has been applied to the inability to learn to read from childhood and often has been referred to as *developmental dyslexia*. (The term has not been used as readily in the field.) People generally use the term *learning disabilities* to describe many different kinds of difficulties with learning. Learning to read is one of them. It is rare to find a child who has only an inability to learn to read and no other problems. Often these children also show difficulties with visual or auditory processing. Often these children also are characterized by specific kinds of behaviors or learning styles; some have a poor attention span, are impulsive, are emotionally labile, or show a combination of all of these.

5. **Males.** Boys are affected more commonly than girls, the ratio varying from 4:1 to 10:1, although a ratio of 5:1 usually is given. It is difficult to know for certain why there is a great preponderance of males, although it has been suggested that this is related to their general physiologic maturation lag. It is interesting to note that this condition also is familial, although

how it is carried from one generation to another is unknown at this point. It is not uncommon to find on questioning the father of a learning-disabled boy that the father had similar problems when he was a youngster.

6. **Learning disabilities.** To understand the field it is important to think of reading problems as a subgroup of the more general classification of "learning disabilities." A learning disability has been defined as a disorder in one or more of the basic psychologic processes involved in the understanding or use of spoken or written language. It may manifest in disorders of listening, understanding, speaking, reading, writing, spelling, or computation. It has been variously referred to as a *perceptual handicap, minimal brain dysfunction,* and *dyslexia.* Learning disabilities do not include learning problems that are due primarily to visual, hearing, or motor handicap; mental retardation; emotional disturbance; or environmental disadvantage.

It is sometimes beneficial to think of learning disabilities as two types: (a) developmental learning disabilities and (b) academic disabilities. The developmental disabilities include such factors as difficulties in visual processing, auditory processing, kinesthetic functions, integration of modalities, language, and attention. The academic disabilities often are the result of some of the developmental learning disabilities, and they show up as difficulties in reading, writing, spelling, mathematics, and written expression. The assumption, then, is that developmental learning disabilities are the forerunners of academic learning disabilities.

7. **e. a, b, and c.** As was mentioned in the explanation for No. 6, the child with a learning disability often has reading problems as well as visual- and auditory-perceptual problems. All of these difficulties can exist in one child, and often the visual- and auditory-perceptual problems are the main contributors to the reading problem.

8. **d. Special education teacher.** It has been found that the treatment of a reading disability is best done by the special education teacher who uses his or her knowledge in remedying this kind of disability. Other professionals should certainly be involved in dealing with the problem of the learning-disabled child.

The best kind of remediation is done by the teacher who has a full and complete psychologic and educational assessment of the child. This assessment must outline the child's strengths and weakneses and the areas in which help is needed. The pediatrician who is the child's primary care physician certainly has an involvement with the child and family and should be involved in knowing what is going on with the individual child. Sometimes the emotional difficulties secondary to the problem are great enough to warrant some kind of psychiatric involvement as well. Other professionals such as occupational therapists, speech and language therapists, and ophthalmologists have a role to play in dealing with the child and family and sometimes even in helping to remedy specific problems. The best kind of treatment is carried out by a multi-disciplinary team that deals with all of the difficulties. There is great need for open communication among parents, teachers, and other professionals so that each individual who is helping the child knows what the goals are and what the other people are doing.

9. **c. Poor self-image.** There is no doubt among those who have worked with children with reading disabilities that one of the most serious side effects of a reading disability or learning disability is the child's poor self-image. Building up a child's self-image and helping the youngster gain confidence are among the primary goals of treatment of these children. It sometimes is more difficult to deal with this aspect of the problem than it is to deal with the remediation of specific difficulties in the areas of visual processing or auditory processing, or even in teaching the child to read. Good remedial therapists will begin the remediation by attempting to build a solid and warm relationship with the child and in this way give the child confidence that is lacking. It also is important, because of the pervasiveness of this poor self-image, that a parent be involved in helping build up the child's confidence.

CHAPTER 38 Cardiopulmonary resuscitation

- Basic life-support methods
- CPR procedures
- Obstructed airway procedures
- CPR for infants and small children
- Obstructed airway procedures for infants and children

A cardiopulmonary arrest is the gravest of all emergencies. Cardiovascular patients are at particularly high risk for developing a cardiopulmonary arrest as a result of primary cardiac causes. When breathing and circulation are absent, clinical death occurs. Unless effective cardiopulmonary resuscitation (CPR) is administered immediately, biologic death or brain death usually will occur within 4 to 6 minutes.

CPR consists of basic life support and advanced cardiac life support. Successful resuscitation depends on the application of precisely performed basic and advanced life support skills. The standards and guidelines concerning basic life support are described in this chapter.

Basic life support (BLS) involves recognizing and treating a patient with an obstructed airway or a

Information for this chapter from Guzzetta, CE: The person requiring cardiopulmonary resuscitation. In Guzzetta CE, Dossey BM: *Cardiovascular nursing: holistic practice,* St Louis, 1992, Mosby. Heart and Stroke Foundation of Ontario: Revisions in basic cardiac life support from 1985 National Conference on Standards and Guidelines for Cardiopulmonary Resuscitation and Emergency Cardiac Care and Heart and Stroke Foundation of Canada: *Cardiopulmonary resuscitation basic rescuer manual,* Canadian Heart Foundation, Toronto, 1987. Unless credited otherwise, illustrations from Guzzetta CE, Dossey BM: *Cardiovascular nursing: holistic practice,* St Louis, 1992, Mosby.

respiratory or cardiac arrest by administering CPR. CPR involves the classic *ABCs* of resuscitation: *airway, breathing,* and *circulation.*

BASIC LIFE-SUPPORT METHODS
Assessing unconsciousness

Any person found unconscious can be considered to have suffered a respiratory or cardiopulmonary arrest. Assessing unconsciousness is accomplished using the shake and shout technique—tapping and gently shaking the patient's shoulder while shouting "Hey! Are you okay?" Some people who appear unconscious may simply be sleeping, deaf, or intoxicated. The diagnosis of unconsciousness is confirmed if the patient does not respond.

Call for help

After the diagnosis of unconsciousness is confirmed, one should shout for help even if no one is in sight in the hope that someone will hear the call. The assistant should not leave the patient.

Positioning the patient

The patient is then positioned so that CPR can begin. A prone patient is log-rolled onto the back by raising the person's arm above his or her head and rolling him or her to a supine position to prevent aggravation of back, neck, or other injuries.

Establishing an airway

It is important to quickly establish an airway. In the unconscious patient, the head is flexed on the cervical vertebral column, the jaw muscles are relaxed, and the tongue falls back against the pharynx, thereby obstructing airflow into the trachea (Fig. 38-1, *A*). Establishing an airway can be accomplished without any adjunct equipment.

Head tilt–chin lift maneuver

The head tilt–chin lift maneuver is currently the preferred method of opening the airway. To perform this maneuver, place the fingers of one hand under the patient's lower jaw (on the bony part) and lift the chin forward, being careful not to obstruct the trachea by compressing the soft tissues under the jaw. Lift the chin so that the upper and lower teeth are brought almost together, but ensure that the mouth is not completely closed. The thumb should not be used for lifting the chin but may be used to slightly lower the patient's lower lip or hold loose

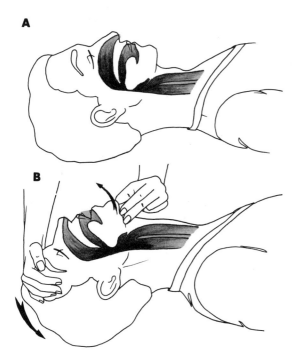

Fig. 38-1 A, Airway obstruction. **B,** Head tilt–chin lift maneuver.

dentures in place. Place the other hand on the forehead, using firm pressure to tilt the patient's head back *maximally* (Fig. 38-1, *B*). The head tilt–chin lift maneuver may establish spontaneous respirations in some patients.

The head tilt–chin lift maneuver is advantageous for an unconscious patient who is making inadequate respiratory movements. In such a case the negative pressure created in the airways causes the tongue to act as a valve and occlude the airway.

Assessing breathlessness

Before administering artificial ventilation, check for breathlessness. While maintaining an open airway, look, feel, and listen for breathing for 3 to 5 seconds. Place an ear over the patient's mouth (with eyes facing chest) *looking* for the rise and fall of the patient's chest, *feeling* for air movement against your cheek, and *listening* for exchange of air (Fig. 38-2, *A*).

If the patient is breathing spontaneously, maintain the airway until help arrives or until the patient becomes conscious. In some cases the patient may be making respiratory movements but not actually exchanging any air. If the patient is not adequately ventilating, begin artificial ventilation.

Administering artificial ventilation

Mouth-to-mouth ventilation. After diagnosing breathlessness, begin mouth-to-mouth ventilation immediately. While maintaining an open airway, gently pinch the patient's nostrils with the thumb and index finger of the hand on the forehead. Take in a deep breath and establish a tight seal over the patient's mouth (Fig. 38-2, *B*) while delivering two initial ventilations at 1.5 seconds per breath within the span of 4 to 7 seconds without allowing time for the patient to completely exhale between ventilations.

To determine if artificial ventilation is effective, assess these three parameters: (1) note whether the patient's chest rises and falls; (2) listen and feel for air escaping during exhalation; and (3) feel the patient's airway resistance and compliance during ventilations.

Artificial ventilation should never be delayed

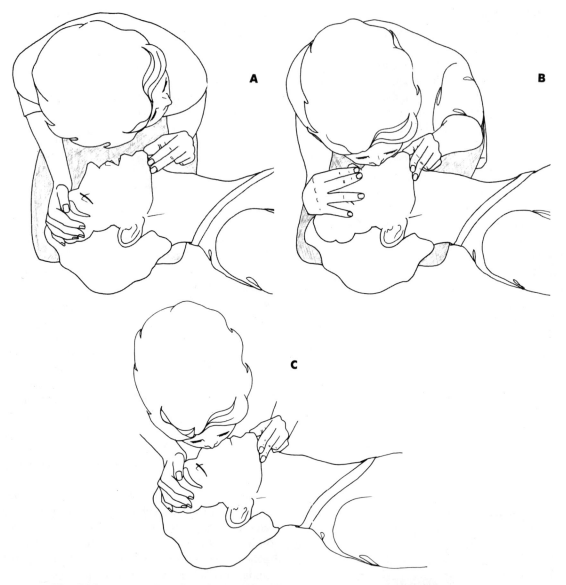

Fig. 38-2 A, Look, feel, listen for breathing. **B,** Mouth-to-mouth ventilation. **C,** Mouth-to-nose ventilation.

while waiting for adjunct ventilatory equipment. It is not essential for effective CPR.

If the patient has a strong carotid pulse, artificial ventilation is continued 12 times per minute, or once every 5 seconds, until the patient resumes spontaneous ventilation. The carotid pulse should be rechecked after 12 ventilations or after the end of each minute.

Following the two slow full breaths for one-person rescue CPR, two slow full breaths are delivered after each 15 chest compressions. For two-person rescue CPR, one breath is delivered after every fifth chest compression.

Dentures should be left in place, if possible, because they maintain the shape of the mouth, making it easier to establish a tight seal. If loose dentures are a problem when administering artificial ventilation, try the head tilt–chin lift maneuver or remove the dentures.

Mouth-to-nose ventilation

Mouth-to-nose ventilation may be used in the following circumstances: (1) when the mouth is seriously injured, (2) when a tight seal cannot be established around the mouth, (3) when the mouth cannot be opened, or (4) when it is impossible to ventilate through the mouth.

Mouth-to-nose ventilation is accomplished by tilting the patient's head back with one hand while lifting the lower jaw with the other hand to seal the mouth and lips. Seal your lips around the patient's nose, and deliver artificial ventilation (Fig. 38-2, *C*). The patient's lungs should be allowed to deflate passively. Because the soft palate may produce nasopharyngeal occlusion during exhalation, it may be necessary to open the patient's mouth to allow air to escape during exhalation.

Absent pulse

Assess the pulse after artificial ventilation is delivered. To check for pulselessness, maintain the patient's airway by keeping one hand on the forehead while using the other hand to locate the carotid pulse. Locate the patient's trachea, and slide your fingers laterally into the groove between the trachea and the sternocleiodomastoid muscle. Palpate the carotid artery closest to you by using gentle pressure (Fig. 38-3). Begin artificial circulation if pulselessness is observed for 5 to 10 seconds.

Activating the emergency medical service system

If you are outside the hospital and pulselessness is confirmed, activate the Emergency Medical Service (EMS) system by phoning 911 or the appropriate local emergency number. Within the hospital, activate the emergency response ("code blue") system. The EMS system is activated *after* the check for breathlessness and pulselessness; thus this vital information is available to the dispatcher. If you are not alone, send a bystander to relay the location and condition of the patient to the EMS. If you are alone, administer CPR for 1 minute before quickly tele-

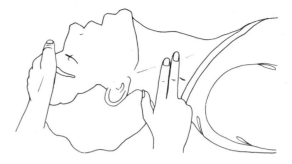

Fig. 38-3 Assessing the carotid pulse.

phoning for help, and then resume CPR as quickly as possible. If a telephone is not available, usually your only option is to continue CPR.

Performing external cardiac chest compression

External cardiac chest compression raises the intrathoracic pressure and produces a cardiac output and an artificial, pulsatile blood flow. External chest compressions always must be given with the patient in the supine position on a flat, hard surface. The floor provides firm support and is an ideal place for performing CPR. The patient who is in a chair must be placed in a horizontal position before chest compression is begun. Venous return and artificial circulation may be augmented during CPR by elevating the patient's lower extremities while keeping the rest of the body horizontal.

To perform external chest compression, position yourself close to the patient's side. Locate the tip of the patient's xiphoid process with the middle finger of the hand closest to the feet, and place the index finger beside it (Fig. 38-4, *A*). Place the heel of the other hand (closest to the head) on the long axis on the lower half of the sternum next to the index finger (Fig. 38-4, *B*). Place the heel of the hand locating the xiphoid process directly over the heel of the hand on the sternum so that both hands are parallel and the fingers straight away from you. Only the heel of the hand should be touching the patient's chest (Fig. 38-4, *C*). Some people prefer to interlock the fingers of both hands as a method for keeping the fingers off the chest (Fig. 38-4, *D*).

If arthritic hands and wrists are a problem, grasp the wrist of the hand on the sternum. The hands,

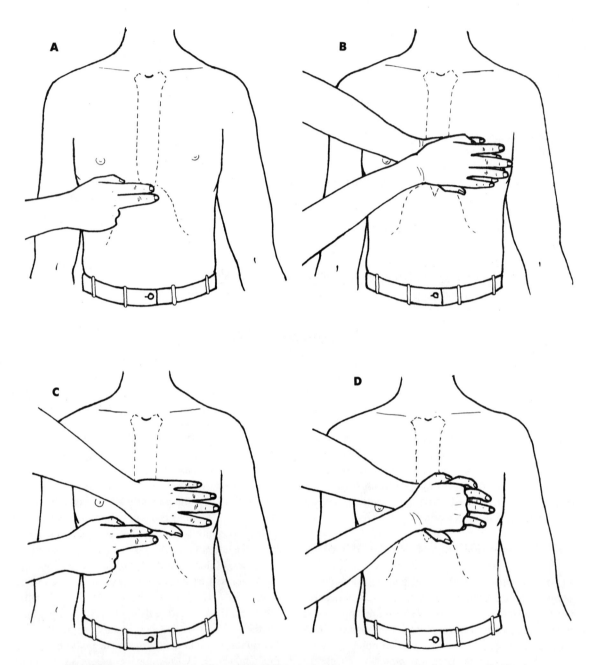

Fig. 38-4 A, Locating xiphoid process. **B,** Hand placement on lower half of sternum. **C,** Hand position for chest compression. **D,** Alternate hand position with interlocking fingers.　*Continued.*

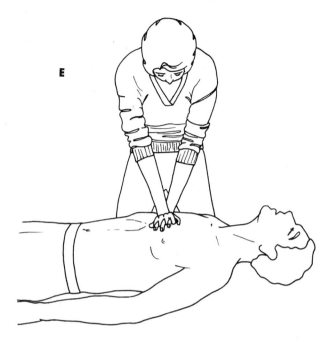

Fig. 38-4, cont'd. E, Body position for chest compression.

however, should not be crisscrossed over each other; this can cause unequal downward pressure during compression, resulting in rib fracture.

To maintain the correct body position, keep your shoulders directly over the patient's sternum: keep your elbows locked while exerting downward vertical pressure to depress the sternum 4 to 5 cm (1 ½ to 2 inches) (Fig. 38-4, *E*). The compressions are smooth and regular, without bouncing or jabbing movements and without interruption. Half the cycle is used for compression and half is used for relaxation. Do not lift the heel of your hand off the chest during the upstroke of the compression, and do not change your hand position in any way. Completely release pressure on the sternum before the next downstroke, allowing the chest to return to its normal position and the heart to refill with blood. The chest compressions are performed at a rate of 80 to 100 times per minute.

Assessing the effectiveness of CPR

During CPR, palpate the carotid pulse to check the effectiveness of the external cardiac compression and to reconfirm pulselessness. Palpate the carotid artery

after the first full minute of CPR and every few minutes thereafter.

The *pupillary reaction* also can be checked periodically to assess the effectiveness of CPR. The pupils will constrict when they are exposed to light if there is adequate oxygenation to the brain. Serious cerebral damage may be indicated by persistently dilated, nonreactive pupils. Widely dilated pupils that react to light, on the other hand, may indicate cerebral hypoxia without serious cerebral damage. Pupillary reactions, however, commonly do not reflect the patient's condition and the effectiveness of CPR. Drugs such as atropine and narcotics and conditions such as glaucoma and cataracts alter the pupillary reaction. Therefore assessing the pupillary reaction is optional during CPR.

Interrupting CPR

Except during endotracheal intubation or when the patient must be carried up or down stairs, CPR should not be interrupted for more than *5 seconds*. During intubation or transportation, interruption of CPR may extend to 30 seconds.

Complications of CPR

Gastric distention occurs commonly during CPR, particularly in infants and small children. Excessive tidal volumes commonly are given during ventilation or when the airway is partially or completely obstructed. Severe gastric distention can elevate the diaphragm, thereby reducing the ventilatory capacity of the lungs, and it can induce regurgitation and aspiration.

Gastric distention can be prevented or reduced by limiting the artificial ventilatory volumes to the point at which the chest wall rises so that the esophageal opening pressures will not be exceeded. If gastric distention occurs, you should *recheck* and *reposition* the airway, assess how great a volume of air is needed to raise the chest wall, and avoid excessive airway pressures. Artificial ventilation should be continued without an attempt to relieve the gastric distention, because manual pressure applied to the patient's epigastrium usually provokes regurgitation and increases the complication of aspiration. Manual pressure should be used *only* if artificial ventilation is severely restricted by gastric distention. To apply manual pressure, turn the patient on his or her side, press over the epigastrium, wipe out any vomitus from the mouth, and continue CPR. If vomiting should occur at any time during CPR, turn the patient on the side, wipe out the mouth, and continue administering the CPR.

Rib fracture is a common complication of CPR. It generally occurs because of improper hand positioning, although it may occur even during proper performance of chest compressions. Other complications of CPR include sternal fracture, liver lacerations, costochondral separation, cardiac or lung contusions, pneumothorax, hemothorax, and fat embolization.

CPR PROCEDURES
One-person CPR

If you are alone, perform one-person CPR by administering external chest compressions and artificial ventilations at a ratio of 15:2. After performing steps 1 to 9 shown in the box at right, administer 15 compressions, then lean over from the waist, keeping the knees in place, and administer two slow (1.5

PROCEDURE FOR ONE-PERSON CPR (LAYPERSON OR HEALTH PROFESSIONAL)

1. Tap, shake shoulder gently, and shout "Are you OK?"
2. Shout for help.
3. Position the victim, turning if necessary.
4. Open an airway using head tilt/chin lift.
5. Assess breathing (3 to 5 seconds). If no breathing:
6. Give two slow, full breaths (4 to 7 seconds).
7. Assess the carotid pulse (5 to 10 seconds). If no pulse:
8. Instruct bystander to activate the EMS system.*
9. Locate the sternal landmarks and position hands.
10. Do compression at the rate of 80 to 100 per minute (while counting aloud "one-and, two-and...").
11. Do 15 compressions; 2 breaths.
12. Assess for the return of spontaneous ventilations and pulse after the first minute and every few minutes thereafter. Checking the pupils is optional. When assessing ventilations and pulse, use the following sequence:
    a. 15 compressions
    b. 2 ventilations
    c. Assess ventilation and pulse
    d. 2 ventilations
    e. 15 compressions
    f. 2 ventilations
    g. Repeat sequence

*If you are alone, complete approximately 1 minute of CPR, then activate the EMS system yourself.

seconds), full breaths (Fig. 38-5). The two breaths are delivered in succession and within 4 to 7 seconds of each other. The chest compressions are performed at a rate of 80 to 100 times per minute. This rate allows an overall compression rate of approximately 80 to 100 per minute because of the interruption during artificial ventilation. For timing purposes, the chest compressions should be performed while counting aloud, "1-and, 2-and, 3-and, 4-and, 5-and; 1-and . . . 10-and; 1-and . . . 15-and."

To maintain the correct timing for the compressions in one-person CPR, a mnemonic or memory device is used that consists of counting aloud. A count of "1-and, 2-and, 3-and . . . " helps you keep

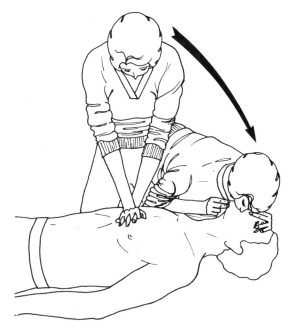

Fig. 38-5 One-person CPR. After administering 15 external chest compressions, the rescuer administers two slow, full breaths.

your place and your timing. The *number* is the downstroke of your compression, and the *and* is the upstroke each time. Equal time is given to compression and release.

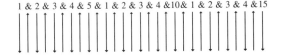

Fifteen compressions are given before you pause to give two slow breaths. Counting from 1 to 5 allows you to use numbers with just one syllable for best control and a smooth rhythm. Any counting sequence is acceptable as long as the compressions are given smoothly.

Done perfectly, cardiac compression can achieve approximately 25% to 35% of the body's needs in terms of arterial blood flow.

Check the patient for the return of spontaneous ventilation and circulation after 1 full minute of CPR. After delivering two slow breaths, assess for breathlessness and pulselessness. If ventilation and

pulse are absent, continue CPR. Give two slow breaths before continuing the 15:2 cycle again (see box at left). Checking the pupils at this time is optional. Assess the patient for breathlessness and pulselessness every few minutes thereafter if CPR is continued alone.

Two-person CPR

Two-person CPR is taught only to health care professionals and professional rescuers. The most effective means of CPR is with a two-person rescue team to ensure that there are no interruptions between compressions and ventilation. The compression rate for two-person CPR is 80 to 100 per minute with a compression-to-ventilation ratio of 5:1. For timing purposes, the person administering the chest compressions (the *Compressor*) counts aloud, "1-and, 2-and, 3-and, 4-and, 5-and" and pauses for ventilation. The person performing the ventilation (the *Ventilator*) ventilates once every 5 seconds between compressions (Fig. 38-6).

The technique for two-person CPR by health care professionals is outlined in the box on p. 778.

When a second rescuer becomes available to assist, that person should inform the first rescuer that he is willing to help and is qualified to perform CPR by saying "I know CPR. Can I help?" The first rescuer should inform the second rescuer that she does need help and is ready to begin a two-person rescue by saying "Check the pulse." The second rescuer kneels down next to the patient in the position for artificial ventilation and opposite the first rescuer. While the Compressor continues the compressions, the second rescuer palpates the carotid artery to check the effectiveness of the compressions. If a pulse is not felt, the Compressor's technique should be reevaluated. As soon as the pulse is palpated, the second rescuer calls out, "Stop compression," and then checks for the return of the patient's spontaneous pulse for 5 seconds.

If pulselessness is reconfirmed, the second rescuer informs the Compressor of the findings by saying, "No pulse, continue CPR." The second rescuer then gives a full, deep breath, which is the signal for the Compressor to change to a compression ratio of 80 to 100 times per minute. The technique for changing

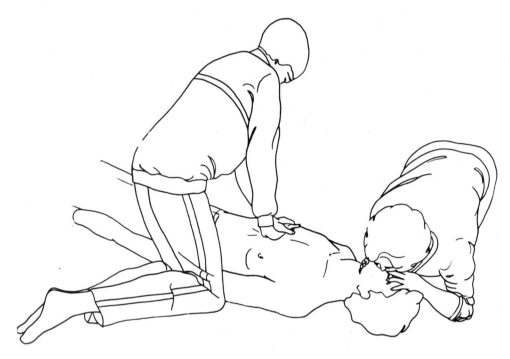

Fig. 38-6 Two-person CPR.

PROCEDURE FOR TWO-PERSON CPR (PERFORMED BY HEALTH PROFESSIONALS ONLY)

1. Tap, shake shoulder gently, and shout.
2. Call for help.
3. Position the patient.
4. Establish an airway.
5. Assess breathing (3 to 5 seconds). If no breathing:
6. Give two slow, full breaths (4 to 7 seconds).
7. Assess the carotid pulse (5 to 10 seconds). If no pulse:
8. Activate the EMS system.
9. Locate the sternal landmarks and position hands.
10. Do compressions at the rate of 80 per minute (while counting aloud "one and, two and, three and, four and, five . . .").
11. Do 5 compressions; 1 breath.
12. Compressor assesses pulselessness every few minutes during the switch technique. Checking the pupils is optional. The Ventilator palpates the carotid pulse frequently during chest compressions to evaluate the effectiveness of the Compressor.

---

from one-person to two-person CPR is outlined in the box on p. 779. If both rescuers are lay persons who have taken a basic cardiac life support (BCLS) course, they will know to perform one- and two-person CPR. If both rescuers have taken only Heart Saver, they will know only one-person CPR and choking; therefore, the second person, in taking over the CPR, will do one-person CPR.

Switch technique

During a two-person rescue, the Compressor and Ventilator exchange positions every few minutes to prevent Compressor fatigue and to monitor vital signs. To prevent unnecessary interruption, the rescuers are positioned on opposite sides of the patient. The Compressor is in control of two-person CPR and therefore is responsible for calling the switch, assessing pulselessness after the fifth compression when the switch occurs, and then administering artificial ventilation.

To accomplish the switch technique, the Compressor states that the switch will take place at the end of the 5:1 sequence. The Compressor calls out

PROCEDURE FOR CHANGING FROM ONE-PERSON TO TWO-PERSON CPR (TWO HEALTH PROFESSIONALS ONLY)

1. Follow procedure for one-person CPR.
2. Second rescuer arrives and states, "I know CPR. Can I help?"
3. First rescuer accepts help by saying, "Check the pulse."
4. Second rescuer:
   a. Kneels down near patient's head opposite first rescuer.
   b. Palpates the carotid artery (5 seconds).
   c. Calls out "Stop compressions."
   d. Assesses return of spontaneous pulse (5 seconds).
   e. If no pulse, states, "No pulse, continue CPR."
   f. Gives a full, deep breath 1 to 1.5 seconds.
5. First rescuer continues compressions at a rate of 80 to 100 per minute in 5 compressions/1 ventilation sequence.

PROCEDURE FOR OBSTRUCTED AIRWAY IN AN UNCONSCIOUS PATIENT

1. Tap, shake shoulder gently, and shout "Are you OK?"
2. Shout for help.
3. Position the victim, turning if necessary.
4. Open an airway using head tilt/chin lift.
5. Assess breathing.
6. Attempt to ventilate. Seal mouth and nose. If unable to ventilate the patient:
7. Reposition the head using head tilt/chin lift.
8. Reattempt to ventilate. If still unable to ventilate:
9. Activate EMS.
10. Administer 6 to 10 abdominal (or chest) thrusts.
11. Open the patient's mouth with the tongue-jaw lift technique. Do the finger-sweep technique to clear the airway of any foreign body.
12. Establish an airway.
13. Reattempt to ventilate using head tilt/chin lift.
14. If still unable to ventilate the patient, repeat steps 9 to 14. If able to ventilate patient, continue with steps 15 to 18.
15. Palpate the carotid pulse. If no pulse:
16. Locate the sternal landmarks.
17. Do cardiac compression and ventilation.
18. Check for the return of spontaneous respiration and pulse after the first minute and every few minutes thereafter.

"Change-one and, 2-and, 3-and, 4-and, 5-and." The Ventilator gives the patient a breath and moves into the position to give compressions. After giving the fifth compression, the Compressor moves to the patient's head and checks the pulse for 5 seconds. If pulselessness is reconfirmed, the person in position near the patient's head tells the new Compressor "No pulse, continue CPR" and gives a breath. This is the signal for the Compressor to begin compressions in the 5:1 sequence. If there is a pulse but no breathing, the rescuer should say so and continue artificial ventilation.

OBSTRUCTED AIRWAY PROCEDURES
Unconscious patient

An *upper airway obstruction* can produce unconsciousness and cardiopulmonary arrest. Airway obstructions caused by foreign bodies and those associated with eating occur at a rate of approximately 3000 per year. An airway obstruction caused by food (commonly steak) often is mistaken for a heart attack, giving rise to the name *café coronary*. Choking can be caused by dentures, poor mastication, and intoxication. Other causes of airway obstruction include tracheal trauma, tracheal edema caused by infection, burns, gas or smoke inhalation, anaphylactic reactions, bilateral vocal cord paralysis, strangulation, and drowning. The most common circumstance in an unconscious patient, however, is an inadequately opened airway during cardiac arrest.

It is commonly difficult to determine initially if unconsciousness is a result of an airway obstruction or other causes. Therefore any person discovered unconscious must be considered in a state of cardiopulmonary arrest. The technique for managing an airway obstruction is used only if the patient cannot be ventilated and if the diagnosis of airway obstruction has been made. Administer abdominal thrusts and use the finger-sweep technique to alleviate the obstruction. The box above outlines the procedure for an unconscious patient.

To manage an upper airway obstruction, begin by following the basic steps of CPR. Tap and gently shake, asking, "Are you okay?" Call for help, establish an airway, assess breathlessness, and attempt to ventilate. If the patient cannnot be ventilated, *reposition* the head using the head tilt–chin lift maneuver and attempt to ventilate a second time. Repositioning the head is essential because the most common cause of an inability to ventilate a patient is improper head-tilt positioning, allowing the tongue to block the airway. If the patient cannot be ventilated after the second attempt, the diagnosis of upper airway obstruction is made. It is essential that the obstruction be removed before you can go on to the remaining steps of CPR. If a second rescuer is available, he or she should activate the EMS system.

Manual thrusts

Abdominal thrusts. To administer abdominal thrusts to an unconscious patient, place the person in the supine position, turning his or her head up while positioning your knees close to the victim's hips. Place the heel of one hand against the patient's abdomen in the midline between the umbilicus and the xiphoid process, with the fingers toward the patient's head. Place the other hand on top of the first with the fingers pointing toward the patient's head. To prevent complications, neither hand should be touching the patient's sternum or ribs. Position your shoulders directly over the patient's abdomen while administering 6 to 10 quick inward and upward thrusts. Abdominal thrusts also may be performed while astride the unconscious patient. This position is particularly useful for a small rescuer administering abdominal thrusts to a large patient. While astride, the rescuer can use total body weight to ensure effective abdominal thrusts. This position also helps prevent misdirected thrusts that could cause liver or spleen injury (Fig. 38-7).

Chest thrusts. (Table 38-1). To administer chest thrusts, position yourself at the patient's side with the patient supine. Position your hands as for external cardiac chest compression (see Fig. 38-4, *C* and *D*) and compress the chest four times quickly. Chest thrusts are recommended for obese or pregnant adults and infant CPR only.

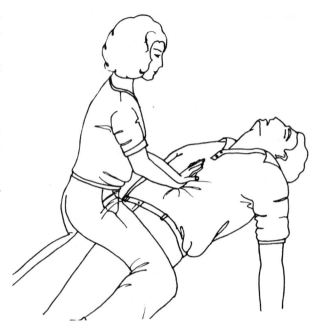

Fig. 38-7 Abdominal thrust for the unconscious patient with rescuer astride.

Finger sweep

If the manual thrusts have successfully dislodged the foreign body, then it must be removed. To remove a foreign body, use the *tongue-jaw lift*. Open the patient's mouth by grasping both the tongue and lower jaw between the thumb and fingers and lifting the patient's head up (Fig. 38-8). This maneuver alone may be useful in partially relieving the obstruction because it draws the tongue away from the pharynx.

The finger-sweep technique is done by inserting the index finger of the other hand down the side of the cheek and deeply toward the base of the tongue. Using a hooking action, sweep any debris out of the mouth. Occasionally it is necessary to push the foreign body to the opposite side of the throat to dislodge and remove it.

Conscious patient

It is important that an upper airway obstruction caused by a foreign body be differentiated from other conditions that may mimic it, such as a heart attack,

Table 38-1	Guidelines for the use of the abdominal and chest thrusts	
	Indication	**Complications**
Abdominal thrusts	Elderly patients with brittle ribs	Gastric regurgitation
	Most other patients	Internal organ injury, laceration, rupture
	Children	Rib fracture if any portion of the hand is allowed to touch the patient's lower rib cage
Chest thrusts	Obese patients	Rib fracture
	Patients in advanced stage of pregnancy	Internal organ injury, laceration, or rupture
	Infants	

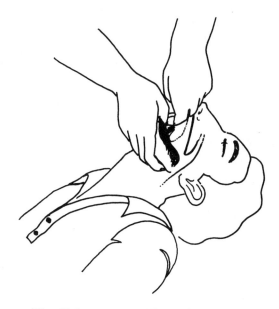

Fig. 38-8 Tongue-jaw lift and finger sweep.

stroke, and drug or alcohol ingestion. The general public is being taught, therefore, to use the distress signal for choking, that is, clutching the neck between the thumb and index fingers of both hands (Fig. 38-9).

Partial airway obstruction with good air exchange

Most persons have, at some time in their lives, experienced a partial airway obstruction by choking on food. In such a situation the individual has good air exchange with a forceful, spontaneous cough and good color. The treatment of choice for such an individual is continual assessment without interference to his or her own attempts to repel the foreign body. The individual usually is able to use protective physiologic mechanisms to relieve the obstruction (Table 38-2).

Partial airway obstruction with poor air exchange and complete airway obstruction

The person with a partial airway obstruction may progress to a situation of poor air exchange. This condition is characterized by increasing respiratory distress (stridor), crowing noises, cyanosis, and a weak, ineffective cough. In some cases the patient may progress to complete airway obstruction, characterized by an inability to breathe, cough, or speak. These conditions must be treated immediately by manual thrusts known as Heimlich maneuver, preferably while the patient is still conscious (see Table 38-2). Complete airway obstruction is evident by the patient's inability to breathe, and partial airway obstruction manifests with poor airway exchange by the patient's color and inability to cough productively.

Manual thrusts. One of two types of manual thrusts is used. The indications for and complications of each maneuver are provided in Table 38-1.

Abdominal thrusts. To administer abdominal thrusts to a seated or standing conscious patient, stand behind the patient and wrap your arms around the person's waist. Place the fist of one hand against the patient's abdomen between the umbilicus and the xiphoid process. With the other hand grab the fist positioned on the abdomen. Then give 6 to 10 quick inward and upward thrusts by pressing your fists into the patient's abdomen (Fig. 38-10, *A*).

Chest thrusts for overweight or pregnant patients. An alternate maneuver to the abdominal thrust is the chest thrust. Stand behind the patient who is sitting or standing and wrap your arms under the person's arms to encircle the chest. The thumb side of one fist is placed against the lower sternum above the xiphoid process and away from the ribs. The other hand is used to grasp the fist to deliver quick backward thrusts (Fig. 38-10, *B*). As with abdominal thrusts, this maneuver should be continued until the obstruction is relieved or the victim becomes unconscious.

Conscious patient who is later unconscious

The patient may lose consciousness if the airway obstruction cannot be relieved in a short time. The management of such a patient involves a combination of the techniques used for conscious and unconscious patients, as outlined in the box at right. In this procedure, repositioning the head and attempting to ventilate a second time is not done because the diagnosis of an airway dysfunction has already been confirmed.

CPR FOR INFANTS AND SMALL CHILDREN

Infants and small children rarely suffer cardiopulmonary arrest from primary cardiac causes. Respiratory arrest is more commonly seen in this group, followed by severe hypoxemia leading to cardiac

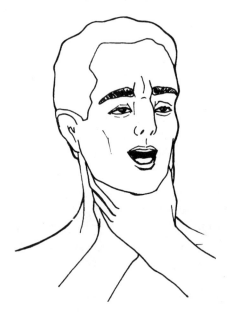

Fig. 38-9 Universal distress signal for choking.

Table 38-2	Procedures for obstructed airway in the conscious patient
Situation	**Procedure**

Partial airway obstruction with good air exchange	1. Assessment
	  a. Ask "Are you choking?"
	  b. Observe for good air exchange, forceful, spontaneous cough, and good color.
	2. Management
	  a. Do nothing; do not interfere with the patient's efforts to expel the foreign object.
	  b. Observe the patient closely for any signs and symptoms of complete obstruction.

Partial airway obstruction with poor air exchange; complete airway obstruction	1. Assessment
	  a. Ask "Are you choking?"
	  b. Observe for poor air exchange (respiratory distress, weak, ineffective cough, stridor, cyanosis).
	2. Management
	  a. Administer Heimlich maneuver (or chest thrusts) until your efforts are successful. If the patient becomes unconscious, follow the procedures for obstructed airway on p. 783.

arrest. Thus establishing an airway and providing artificial ventilation are essential for infants and small children. Other resuscitative steps usually are not necessary.

The major causes of cardiopulmonary arrest in infants and small children include (1) suffocation caused by objects such as toys, peanuts, plastic bags, (2) near drowning, (3) automobile or other accidents, (4) poisoning by drugs or chemicals, (5) sudden infant death syndrome, and (6) airway infections (for example, croup, epiglottitis).

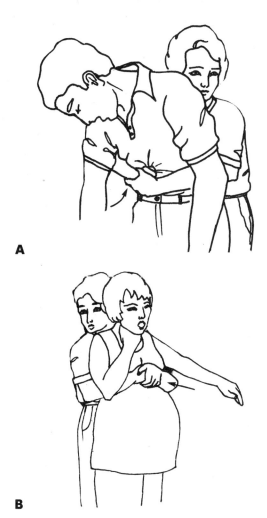

Fig. 38-10 A, Abdominal thrusts for the conscious patient. **B,** Chest thrusts for the pregnant or obese patient.

For the purposes of performing CPR an *infant* is defined as being up to 1 year of age and a *child* as ages 1 to 8 years. A child older than 8 years of age is resuscitated as for an adult.

The principles for performing the *ABCs* of CPR are the same for infants and children as they are for adults, with a few minor variations (see box, p. 784). If you discover an unconscious child, rap and gently shake the shoulder and observe if the child responds. Then call for help and place the child in a supine position. To open the airway use the head tilt–chin lift maneuver.

To perform the head tilt–chin lift maneuver, extend the head by placing one hand on the forehead. Lift the mandible forward with the fingertips of the

---

PROCEDURES FOR OBSTRUCTED AIRWAY IN A CONSCIOUS PATIENT WHO IS LATER UNCONSCIOUS

1. Assess the patient (see Table 38-2).
   a. Ask "Are you choking?"
   b. Observe for poor air exchange.
   c. Observe for no air exchange.
2. Administer 6 to 10 abdominal (or chest) thrusts until successful or until patient becomes unconscious.
3. If patient becomes unconscious, call for help.
4. Position the patient.
5. Establish an airway.
6. Attempt to ventilate. If unable to ventilate the patient:
   a. Activate the EMS system.
   b. Administer 6 to 10 abdominal (or chest) thrusts.
   c. Do the finger sweep technique to clear the airway of any foreign body.
7. Establish an airway.
8. Attempt to ventilate.
9. If still unable to ventilate the patient, repeat steps 6 to 9. If able to ventilate, continue with step 10.
10. Assess the carotid pulse. If no pulse:
    a. Locate the sternal landmarks and position hands.
    b. Do cardiac compression and ventilations.
    c. Assess for the return of spontaneous ventilations and pulse after the first minute and every few minutes thereafter.

CPR PROCEDURE FOR INFANTS AND CHILDREN

1. Tap, shake shoulder gently, and observe if child responds.
2. Shout for help.
3. Position the patient, turning if necessary.
4. Establish an airway using head tilt/chin lift.
5. Assess breathing. If no breathing:
6. Give two slow (1 to 1.5 seconds), gentle puffs of air if infant; two slow breaths if child.
7. Assess pulse. If no pulse:
   a. Infants: check brachial pulse.
   b. Children: check carotid pulse.
8. Instruct bystander to activate EMS system.*
9. Locate sternal landmark and position hand.
   a. Infants: place index and middle fingers on mid-sternum.
   b. Children: place heel of one hand on lower sternum.
10. Administer chest compressions.
    a. Infants: compress 1.3 to 2.5 cm (½ to 1 inch) with tips of fingers at rate of 100 per minute (counting aloud "one, two, three...") and a ratio of five compressions to one breath.
    b. Children: compress 2.5 to 3.8 cm (1 to 1½ inches) with heel of one hand at a rate of 80 to 100 per minute (counting aloud "one-and, two-and...") and a ratio of five compressions to one breath.
11. Assess for return of spontaneous ventilations and pulse after the first minute and every few minutes thereafter.

*If you are alone, complete 1 minute of CPR and then activate the EMS system yourself.

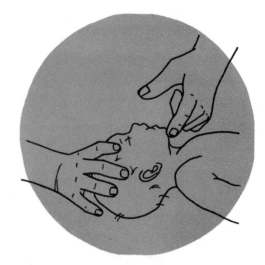

Fig. 38-11 Head tilt–chin lift for infants.

artificial ventilation. Occasionally you may need to decide if artificial ventilation should be administered to an infant who is gasping or making respiratory efforts. If there is effective air exchange, the infant's color will be pink. If respiratory efforts are ineffective, the infant's lips will be cyanotic and artificial ventilation should be started.

For an infant, make a tight seal around the mouth and nose and administer two gentle puffs of air. In a young child administer two slow breaths of air. If the child is too large to make a tight seal around the mouth and nose, then mouth-to-mouth ventilation is used as for an adult, but with smaller tidal volumes. Because the child's lung capacity is smaller than the adult's, artificial ventilatory volumes should be limited to the amount of air needed to raise the chest. Because resistance to airflow is greater in a child than in an adult, a sufficient amount of ventilatory pressure is needed to adequately inflate the lungs.

If the infant or child can be easily ventilated, proceed with the next step in CPR—assessing pulselessness. For a child, check the *carotid artery,* as for an adult. Assessing the pulse in an infant is done by checking the *brachial artery* (Fig. 38-12, *A*). The carotid pulse is not used because of the short and commonly fat necks of infants. The precordial impulse is no longer used because precordial activity

other hand, making sure that the mouth is not closed completely and that the fingers under the jaw are not obstructing the trachea (Fig. 38-11). This maneuver draws the tongue away from the back of the throat. Occasionally, opening the airway is all that is necessary to reestablish spontaneous ventilations. Use caution to prevent overexaggeration of the head-tilt position. An infant's head should be tilted only to a neutral or "sniffing" position.

After establishing the airway, look, feel, and listen for breathing. If the patient is not breathing, begin

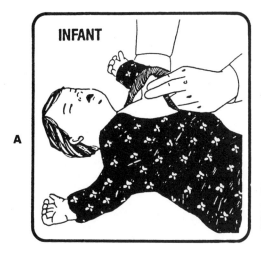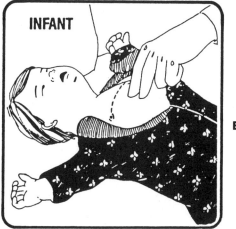

Fig. 38-12 A, Checking for brachial pulse in infants. **B,** Performing external chest compression for infants. (From Heart and Stroke Foundation of Canada: *Cardiopulmonary resuscitation basic rescuer manual,* Copyright Canadian Heart Foundation, Toronto, 1987.)

may be absent, even though the infant may have adequate cardiac functioning, leading the rescuer to wrongly conclude that chest compressions are needed.

When a pulse is present and breathing is not, administer artificial ventilation once every 3 seconds, or 20 times a minute, for an infant and once every 4 seconds, or 15 times a minute, for a child.

If the patient is pulseless, begin artificial circulation. Because the ventricles of infants lie higher in the chest than do those of an adult, external chest compression is performed over the *midsternum* (Fig. 38-12, *B*). For infants, use the tips of the index and middle fingers to depress the sternum (1.3 to 2.5 cm, or ½ to 1 inch) at a rate of 100 compressions per minute. Each chest compression should produce a palpable pulse. Infants usually are resuscitated by one-person CPR. The ratio of compressions to ventilations is 5:1. Because you do not need to move your body to administer artificial ventilation and circulation to infants, you can maintain the head-tilt position with one hand and administer chest compressions with the other (see Fig. 38-12, *B*)

Chest compressions for a child are applied to the lower half of the sternum, as for an adult, using the heel of one hand to depress the sternum 2.5 to 3.8 cm (1 to 1½ inches) at a rate of 80 to 100 compres-

sions per minute. with a ratio of 5:1 compressions to ventilations. The procedure for CPR for infants and children is provided on p. 784.

OBSTRUCTED AIRWAY PROCEDURES FOR INFANTS AND CHILDREN

An airway obstruction can occur in infants and small children because of a foreign body or some other cause, such as infection or inflammation of the airways. It is important to differentiate between an airway obstruction caused by a foreign body and that caused by some other fact; the procedure to dislodge a foreign body will not be helpful if the obstruction is the result of inflammation or infection.

The same principles and sequence of techniques used for adults are used for infants with foreign body airway obstruction. If the patient has poor air exchange (characterized by respiratory difficulty, ineffective cough, and cyanosis) or no air exchange, a combination of back blows and chest thrusts is used. Because of the possibility of injuring internal organs, abdominal thrusts are not recommended for infants.

If the patient is an infant, place the baby's face down over your forearm with the head and chest in the dependent position. Support the head by placing your hand on the patient's jaw and chest and resting

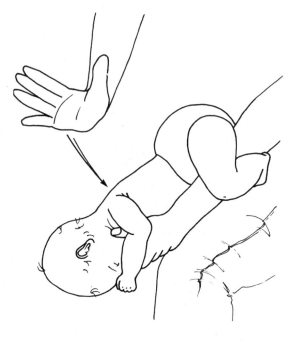

Fig. 38-13 Back blows for infants with foreign body airway obstruction.

your forearm on your thigh. Deliver four quick back blows between the infant's scapulae with the heel of your hand, taking care that the force is not excessive (Fig. 38-13). Then turn the infant on the back by using your free hand to support the back while leaving the other hand in place to support the chest and head. While supporting the head, neck and back, turn and place the infant against your thigh with the baby's head lower than the body. Deliver four chest thrusts rapidly, using the technique for external chest compressions in the infant.

QUESTIONS FOR REVIEW AND THOUGHT

1. What are the major causes requiring CPR?
2. Outline your procedure for performing one-person CPR.
3. What are the differences between one-person and two-person CPR?
4. What are the various procedures to deal with obstructed airways?

SELF-EVALUATION QUESTIONS

True-false statements

Directions: Indicate whether the statement is true (T) or false (F).

T or F   1. Establishing an airway is accomplished by performing a combination of head-tilt and chin-lift maneuvers.

T or F   2. Mouth-to-mouth ventilation is an effective method of providing oxygen.

T or F   3. CPR should rarely be interrupted for longer than 5 seconds.

Missing words

Directions: Write in the missing word in the following sentences.

4. The ABCs of CPR are _____.
5. In the absence of CPR, brain death usually will occur within _____.
6. The most common complication of CPR is _____.

Choice-completion questions

Directions: Select the one best answer in each case.

7. External cardiac compression should not be performed:
   a. With the patient in a supine position
   b. On a flat, hard surface
   c. With pressure exerted on the xiphoid process
   d. With depression of the sternum 4 to 5 cm (1½ to 2 inches)
   e. Without interruption
8. Two-person CPR does not involve:
   a. Establishing an airway
   b. Assessing breathing
   c. Evaluating the carotid pulse
   d. Compressions at a rate of 80 to 100 per minute
   e. Ratio of 5 compressions per 2 breaths
9. One-person CPR does not include:
   a. Positioning the patient
   b. Compressions at a rate of 80 to 100 per minute
   c. Ratio of 15 compressions per 1 breath
   d. Counting aloud "one-and, two-and, three-and . . . " to improve the timing of cardiac compression
   e. Assessing for the return to spontaneous ventilations and pulse after four complete cycles of compressions and ventilations

ANSWERS, NOTES, AND EXPLANATIONS

1. **True.** The preferred method to establish an airway is to lift the patient's chin with one hand and at the same time to exert pressure on the patient's forehead to tilt the head back maximally.
2. **True.** Artificial ventilation can be an effective method of delivering oxygen to the patient. The oxygen concentration delivered during mouth-to-mouth ventilation is approximately 16%, which is enough to sustain life.
3. **True.** The vital oxygen supply and circulation is completely dependent on CPR. It is therefore apparent that CPR should not be interrupted for more than 5 seconds except during endotracheal intubation or when the patient must be carried up or down stairs.
4. **Airway, breathing, circulation.**
5. **4 to 6 minutes.**
6. **Gastric distention.** If severe, this can elevate the diaphragm, thereby reducing the ventilatory capacity of the lungs and possibly inducing regurgitation and aspiration.
7. **c. With pressure exerted on the xiphoid process.** The rescuer must be aware of the xiphoid process at all times and should not be performing cardiac compression over this site. Complications that can occur from pressure exerted over the xiphoid process or other improper hand positions include liver lacerations, lung or cardiac contusions, pneumothorax, hemothorax, and sternal fracture.

8. **e. Ratio of 5 compressions per 2 breaths.** For two-person CPR, the compression rate is 80 to 100 per minute with a compression-to-ventilation ratio of 5:1. After 5 compressions, there is a pause for 1 to 1½ seconds, during which time ventilation is performed.

9. **c. Ratio of 15 compressions per 1 breath.** In one-person CPR the compression rate should be 80 to 100 per minute, with a ratio of 15 ventilations to two breaths. The chest compressions should be performed while counting aloud "one-and, two-and, three-and . . . ." This mnemonic is a valuable aid to more precise timing of cardiac compressions.

PART SIX

Expanded roles of the ophthalmic assistant

CHAPTER 39

Computers in an ophthalmic practice

GERALD E. MELTZER

- Computer basics
- Types of computers
- Components of a computer
- What do computers do?
- Computer-controlled ophthalmologic equipment
- Special ophthalmologic applications software

Although computer technology is quite young (the first computer, as we know it, was built in 1939), computers have an enormous effect on the way ophthalmology is practiced every day. It is now estimated that at least 50% of all ophthalmologic offices now use computers on a daily basis for tasks such as word processing and billing, and their use continues to increase significantly. By 2000 it is estimated that more than 95% of all ophthalmologic offices will be using computers for such tasks as insurance billing, practice management, sending recall notices, and calling patients automatically to remind them of missed appointments or to notify them that their contact lenses have arrived, as well as controlling many of the instruments in daily office use, such as the telephone, lensometer, keratometer, perimeter, ultrasound, and the copy machine. Thus computers will contribute significantly to better patient care as well as increased office productivity.

The impact of computers in the field of ophthalmology is a reflection of many trends in office automation. Universal acceptance of computer technology by worldwide industries, coupled with markedly decreased cost and widespread availability of inexpensive programs for use throughout both the business and medical communities, has created a mushrooming demand for computer technology. It is estimated that by 2000, 50% of all employees will have their own computer terminals. A well-chosen computer system integrated into an efficient, well-run office will greatly improve office productivity and management of patient information (both medical and financial), as well as the quality of life of both office and medical staff members by relieving them of many mundane, repetitive tasks.

This chapter is designed to teach the ophthalmic assistant about computers, how they work, what they can do for an ophthalmologic office and its personnel, and how to use them efficiently.

COMPUTER BASICS

A computer can be defined as a "device capable of accepting, storing, retrieving and manipulating or processing information automatically at high speeds by applying a sequence of logical arithmetic or textual operations that follow instructions provided through a prearranged program." In simpler terms a computer is able to execute a series of instructions that allows the user to ask questions such as, "What does Fred Smith owe on his account?" or "Who is his insurance carrier?" or even "List all names of patients who have astigmatism and are candidates for fitting with toric soft lenses." Computers can even make some intelligent decisions through the use of artificial intelligence techniques. By reviewing a medical record and then comparing it with a list of preprogrammed rules, computers are now able to interpret visual fields, suggest appropriate therapy for glaucoma, or even propose additional diagnoses that physicians might not yet have considered.

TYPES OF COMPUTERS

Analog computers were the first computers manufactured. They are designed to deal with physical interrelationships. Examples of an analog computer include a car speedometer and a clock dial. Analog computers are especially useful in many types of engineering research.

Digital computers

Digital computers, the type we will be discussing, solve problems that use numbers or symbols by applying rules of logic to arithmetic operations (for example, if this number is greater than that number, then . . .).

Microcomputers, which make up the majority of all computers used in medical offices, are identified by their central processing unit (386, 486, etc.), the amount of memory they have, the capacity of their disk drive, and their operating systems.

Mainframe computers

Mainframe computers are large, expensive machines that are able to store enormous amounts of information and to communicate with hundreds if not thousands of individuals simultaneously. In general, most medical offices will use smaller computers such as microcomputers or even small minicomputers for daily work. However, they will be dependent on large mainframes for insurance processing because major insurance carriers such as Blue Cross and Medicare use them to process insurance data and to communicate directly with medical offices.

COMPONENTS OF A COMPUTER

The physical components of a computer are referred to as *hardware*. Computer hardware includes four major computer parts: (1) the central processing unit, (2) input devices, (3) output devices, and (4) storage devices.

Central processing unit

The central processing unit (CPU) is the heart of the computer. It performs logical and mathematic functions such as addition and subtraction, as well as comparing numbers or names. Newer CPUs are capable of executing 30 or 40 million instructions each second. The CPU also controls the flow of information within the computer, retrieving and storing information at the same time it is processing data.

Input devices

The most common computer input device is the keyboard. Keyboards generally are arranged with keys in the traditional QWERTY format, names for the first six letters of the top row of this type of keyboard. This keyboard has been in use for the past 90 years and was designed to keep typists from typing too fast and jamming keys rather than to increase productivity. Recently newer keyboard layouts, such as the DVORAK, allow good typists to increase their output as much as 20% to 30%. The keyboard layouts are not in common use today because of the retraining required.

Other significant variations in keyboards used in medical offices include function keys that are either on the left side or at the top of the keyboard. Keys that move the cursor (the flashing light on the screen) usually are placed in a distinct location and are separate from the numeric keypad, but in some older designs they may be part of the keypad. Some numeric keypads do not have an enter key—a significant inconvenience for a 10-key accounting operator using the numeric keypad to enter financial data.

Recently a number of cases of carpal tunnel syndrome have been associated with the use of a keyboard. This painful affliction of the wrist seems to be associated with hand position and frequent use of a computer keyboard. A number of wrist rests are now available that may alleviate or prevent this problem.

Many other forms of input devices are now available. Mice have become quite popular in the past few years. They are used to manipulate data on the computer screen, move paragraphs around, and delete words in word processing and graphics programs, as well as to control the operation of many new windows programs. Also, some offices and hospitals use light pens, touch screens, and bar codes to enter data into the computer and control its operation. Ophthalmic assistants can now enter the output of devices such as an automated lensometer, visual field machine, or corneal mapping devices directly into the computer by using sophisticated circuitry built into these devices.

Voice-recognition technology, presently in its infancy, is now being used regularly in emergency rooms and radiology offices to enter patient clinical data directly into the computer, thus bypassing the handwritten clinical record. It will be only a few years until ophthalmologic offices will be dictating the entire medical record directly into the computer for storage and future retrieval, thus ushering in the age of the paperless office.

Output devices

The two main output devices of a computer are video display terminals and printers.

Video display terminals. Video display terminals (VDTs), also called *monitors,* are the operator's main link to the computer (Fig. 39-1). A good monitor with a high resolution screen is essential for the computer operator's comfort. Glare can be a significant factor in causing visual fatigue. If this is a problem, there are a number of glare filters that can be installed directly over the front of the monitor

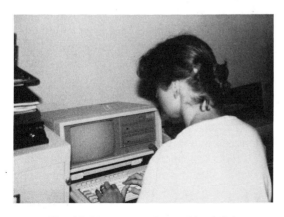

Fig. 39-1 Video monitor and hard disk.

that will reduce glare significantly and thereby increase operator comfort.

Color monitors. Color monitors are now becoming the accepted standard for most ophthalmic offices. Although somewhat more expensive than monochrome (green or yellow) monitors, color monitors can significantly increase operator efficiency by calling attention to important details in a patient's record through the discriminating use of different colors.

Printers. Printers are available in several varieties: (1) daisy wheel, such as that in most electric typewriters, (2) dot matrix, which uses a series of very small dots to form characters, (3) ink-jet printers, which use a small ink cartridge to print with, and (4) laser printers, which use the same technology as a copy machine to produce an image on the paper. There are significant differences in speed, quality of output, and noise among the various types of printers. There also are some differences in cost, but as technology improves, these cost factors are becoming less a consideration in printer selection.

Daisy wheel printers. Letter-quality, or daisy wheel, printers produce letters that are indistinguishable from an average typewriter. Slow, noisy, and expensive, they gradually are being phased out in favor of the new ink-jet and laser printers.

Dot matrix printers. Dot matrix printers constitute the workhorse of most medical offices; they combine good quality printing and speed with inexpensive operating costs and high reliability. Newer dot matrix printers produce a quality of print that is virtually indistinguishable from an electric typewriter.

Ink-jet printers. These recent additions offer the same high-quality print output as a laser printer at about one half the cost. Their main disadvantage is that they are significantly slower than laser printers.

Laser printers. The most expensive and quietest of all printers, the laser printer has the advantage of providing the highest output (6 to 12 pages per minute) and the highest quality of print. Unfortunately, their cost is two to four times that of the average dot matrix printer.

Storage devices (memory)

The last part of the computer is memory. Information entered into the computer needs to be stored for later use. A patient record most likely will be stored in random access memory (RAM) where the CPU can look up the information in a few microseconds. RAM has the significant disadvantage of being volatile—that is, if the computer loses power for even an instant, the information will be lost. To store information permanently, it is written on a hard disk—a series of magnetized platters spinning at 360 RPM—that can hold many millions of pieces of information for later retrieval.

Backups

It is critical that hard disks have a backup on a regular basis. Backups can be provided by use of diskettes or cassette tape. These tapes are now capable of storing several gigabytes (billions of data words) of information. Slower than other forms of archival devices, they nonetheless are critical when it comes to storing or backing up data. Further, they are crucial for restoring lost data if the computer crashes.

WHAT DO COMPUTERS DO?
Applications software

Computers can perform a variety of tasks in an ophthalmic office, including billing patients, scheduling appointments, keeping medical records, and sending insurance forms to Medicare and other insurance companies. Computers aid physicians in managing their finances, writing journal articles, or doing literature searches.

The program that allows the computer hardware to do these tasks is called *software*. Without the appropriate software, even the world's most expensive computer is useless. Most of the software used in a physician's office is known as *applications software*. Computerization of business-oriented tasks can increase the efficiency and productivity of the average physician's office, thus making the ophthalmic assistant more productive. Properly designed and installed computer hardware and software should make the ophthalmic assistant's task of seeing and treating patients easier and more rewarding. Software packages are available today that are specifically written for an ophthalmic office. There is even software for special interest areas such as contact lenses.

Word processing. Learning to use word processing programs takes some time and practice to get the most out of them, but they eventually allow even nontypists to turn out perfect letters and reports. These programs may be simple, designed to type short letters, or complex programs that have built-in spelling checkers. There also are programs that have canned, preformatted letters to cover many different subjects, such as how to write to delinquent accounts and how to write a letter to a supplier about defective merchandise.

Mail-merge. Mail-merge is a process whereby data, such as names and addresses, are intertwined (merged) with a prewritten letter, resulting in the printing of a personalized form letter. This feature can allow the ophthalmic assistant to send personalized form letters to all delinquent accounts automatically. It also can send insurance forms with a cover letter to all insurance companies that are late in paying their claims.

To help build a practice, mail-merge also allows the ophthalmic assistant to send letters announcing a new contact lens to all patients selected (assuming that that information is already part of the computer's base of data). For example, if the ophthalmic assistant wanted to send a letter about a new contact lens insurance program being started, all contact lens wearers between the ages of 16 and 60 who live in a specific zip code area and have not been seen in the office for 6 months might be selected to receive a letter.

Billing. Accounts receivable software allows an office to easily prepare bills, convert codes for services into statements, produce reminder letters for delinquent accounts, and analyze accounts and referral sources. As most ophthalmic assistants know, insurance billing is probably the most boring job in an office to do manually. Even with universal claim forms, this is tedious and time-consuming, and insurance clerks are prone to making errors.

Because most patients have some form of insurance, however, it is imperative to have a way to properly complete an insurance form, send it to the appropriate insurance company, and alert the office staff if it is not paid promptly. A good billing package will do all of this and more, keeping close watch on the lifeblood of any medical office—its accounts receivables.

Accounting. In addition to billing patients, many

medical billing packages include software to write checks and do payroll, as well as keeping the general ledger. Again, if an ophthalmic assistant or secretary writes a large number of checks each month to the same people, this can save a lot of tedious work and, in the long run, can save many dollars by automating the monthly posting functions.

Medical records

Increasingly offices are beginning to computerize their medical records. Physicians or scribes now type directly into the computer the patient's medical record as the patient is examined. Advantages of computerizing the medical record include better legibility, no lost records, less paper and clutter around the office, and usually better patient care. Computerized medical records also make it possible to automate clinical data research inasmuch as all records have been stored on the computer, to find and correlate disease entities, and even to critique quality of care given.

Once the patient record is entered into the computer, consultation letters can be automatically sent to referring physicians. In addition, research reports can be printed that inform pharmaceutical and contact lens companies of patients who are eligible for studies or research projects, and these companies can track the progress of ongoing clinical research studies.

Management reports

The main reward of computerizing a medical office is that of more efficient use of the data collected daily in the office, such as patient names, diagnosis, zip code, referring sources, and procedures done. Thus computers make it possible for the office manager to determine easily where patients are coming from, whether a marketing program is successful, and how well office costs are being controlled.

Computers make it relatively easy to produce a report showing all delinquent accounts so that a staff member can begin calling them to find out when these patients intend to pay their bills. Monitoring insurance receivables is becoming important as offices process and collect directly from many more insurers, health maintenance organizations (HMOs), and preferred provider organizations (PPOs). Pro-

grams exist that rebill the insurer automatically after a specified number of days or that produce a list of patients whose insurance payment is in arrears.

Another advantage of computerized management reports is that they can be easily changed if new or different information is needed. If the information is in the computer, it can be easily obtained without having to go through all of the medical records again.

Appointment scheduling

Larger practices with several offices and many physicians find it almost mandatory to utilize the computer's ability to centralize appointment scheduling. In addition, the computer can be programmed to produce patient reminders, keep clinical records, and keep track of drugs or contact lenses, as well as notify office personnel of patients who repeatedly miss appointments. Computers also can call attention to patients who are receiving critically needed drugs and fail to return for routine follow-up visits.

COMPUTER-CONTROLLED OPHTHALMOLOGIC EQUIPMENT
Visual field testers

Automated visual field testers are now controlled by the use of computers. The order and size of stimuli presented, the timing, and even the monitoring of patient eye movement are controlled by a small computer present in the perimeter. Results of periodic testing are now being computer-analyzed, with small differences in the test results being quantified to identify disease progression. Perimetric test results are stored on disks for storage and analysis in both the Humphrey and Octopus perimeters (Fig. 39-2).

Automated refractors

Small computers inside automated refractors control the placement of the infrared sensing beam that maintains correct placement of the light source. The computers then carefully analyze the readings, and an accurate reading of the patient's refractive status is ready within a few seconds (Fig. 39-3).

Automated keratometers

Keratometry is the measurement of the shape of the cornea. There are a number of instruments now being manufactured that calculate this information auto-

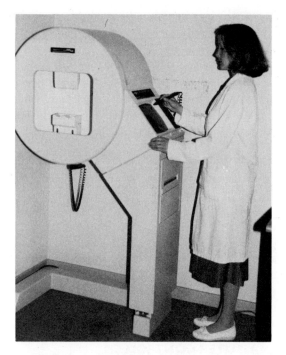

Fig. 39-2 Automated perimeter with computerized visual field plotter.

matically using microcomputers. In addition, corneal topographic measurements, as obtained by the photokeratoscope, can be analyzed and stored with the use of sophisticated computer programs.

Ultrasound

Microprocessor-controlled ultrasound equipment is used to determine the length of the eye for intraocular lens calculations. It also can be used to measure reflectance echoes of intraocular tumors to determine type, size, and location. The original A-scan equipment required the use of an oscilloscope, but today's computer-controlled equipment takes hundreds of measurements, discarding erroneous values and providing the ophthalmologist with an accurate measurement of globe length (Fig. 39-4).

Automated lensometers

Lensometry, the measurement of eyeglasses, can now be done automatically. The Humphrey Lens Analyzer, for example, makes many measurements

of the deviation of the light beam as it passes through a lens being measured. Multiple calculations are done by a small microprocessor in the lens analyzer to give the final accurate reading of sphere, cylinder, axis, and prism of the lens.

Corneal topographic analyzers

The placedo disk has been used to determine corneal shape for many years. It is used in automated keratometers not only to establish the shape of the cornea but to the amount of corneal astigmatism. Recently this concept has been improved amd expanded on, thanks to new computer hardware and software. EyeSys, Tomey, and Visioptic are three companies that use slightly different techniques to determine and plot a surface map with several thousand reference points of the entire cornea. This information is critical in planning and carrying out refractive surgery.

SPECIAL OPHTHALMOLOGIC APPLICATIONS SOFTWARE
Intraocular lens power programs

The power of the intraocular lens to be implanted at the time of cataract surgery was once a matter of guesswork. Now, various formulas can be used to determine the power of the lens to be implanted. These formulas can be calculated by built-in microprocessors in the ultrasound machine being used to measure the length of the eye or by using separate programs that can run on the office computer (see Fig. 39-4).

Contact lens program

There are several programs available to assist in selection of the proper contact lenses for difficult patient problems. In addition, Dr. Alan Mandelberg's contact lens tracker program can aid in inventory control, contact lens ordering, preparing yearly recall reminders, and service agreements.

Refraction software

Sims, McGowan, and Davidoff have all developed programs to calculate final refraction based on subjective overrefraction over the patient's old glasses. The end result is a more accurate refraction with a lower rate of dissatisfied patients.

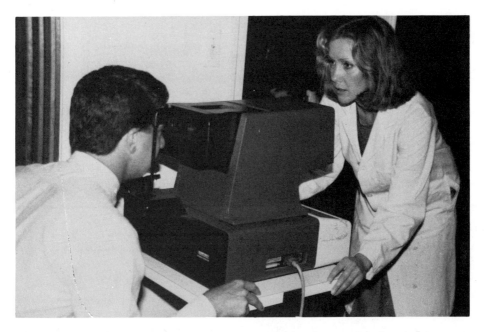

Fig. 39-3 Autorefractor with built-in computer mechanism for recording the refractive error.

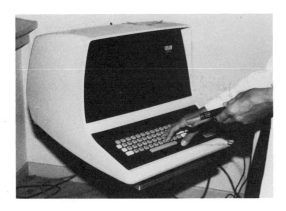

Fig. 39-4 Ultrasound using a computer mechanism to provide information on the axial length and power of the intraocular lens that will be required.

On-line databases

There are now over 200 medically related databases with an enormous range of information for sources such as state and specialty societies, The National Institute of Health, The National Library of Medicine, and the Centers for Disease Control. Any of these are accessible from a computer in the medical office and can be used to find information on almost any medical topic in current literature.

SUMMARY

Although the primary justification of any computer is financial, many physicians have been excited by the computer's clinical potential. Because the major activity in a physician's office is the processing of information for decision making, the attraction of a tool to help process this data is naturally appealing. As desk-top computers become more powerful, as electronic storage becomes less expensive, and as artificial intelligence techniques develop, much of the computer's clinical potential can be realized.

QUESTIONS FOR REVIEW AND THOUGHT

1. What are the major advantages of computerizing a medical office?
2. What are the major uses of computers in an ophthalmic practice?
3. List how computers can help the ophthalmic assistant in an ophthalmic practice.
4. How does a computer work in an autolensometer?
5. What types of printers are available for computers?
6. List the major types of microcomputers available and their advantages.
7. How can the ophthalmic assistant network several computers so that each computer has access to a data bank?

SELF-EVALUATION QUESTIONS

True-false statements

Directions: Indicate whether the statement is true (T) or false (F).

T or F   1. Dot matrix printers are the most common type of printers for office use.
T or F   2. Ophthalmologic equipment may be run by a computer.
T or F   3. A printout of a result obtained from ophthalmologic equipment is a computerized act.

Missing words

Directions: Write in the missing word in the following sentences.

4. The physical components of a computer are called _____ .
5. Typing manuscripts into a computer is performed on software packages called _____ .
6. An instrument that automatically measures the corneal curvature and provides a printout of the dioptric power of the cornea is called a(n) _____ .

Choice-completion questions

Directions: Select the one best answer in each case.

7. Which is not a use for a medical computer?
   a. Billing systems
   b. Word processor
   c. Patient records
   d. Game challenges
   e. Autoperimeter
8. Which is not computer-controlled ophthalmologic equipment?
   a. Autorefractor
   b. Autolensometer
   c. A-scan
   d. B-scan
   e. Indirect ophthalmoscope
9. Word processing software can help in which of the following ways?
   a. Providing laboratory results
   b. Producing reports and letters than can be word-perfect and recalled
   c. Providing A-scan results
   d. Providing access to literature reviews
   e. Having telephone modem access to a second office

ANSWERS, NOTES, AND EXPLANATIONS FOR SELF-EVALUATION QUESTIONS

---

1. **True.** Dot matrix printers are the most common type of printer in an ophthalmic office. These printers are also built into many of the ophthalmolic equipment that require printouts of measurements.
2. **True.** Microcomputers run many of the programs in ophthalmic equipment, particularly that for visual field analysis.
3. **True.** Printouts of test results are performed by a computer and a printer.
4. **Hardware.** Hardware is considered all of the physical components of the computer and consists of the monitor, disk drive, and the chips that run it.
5. **Word processing.** Almost all typewritten manuscripts are produced on a software program that is generically called *word processing*. There are many proprietary names for these software programs.
6. **Autokeratometer.** This instrument can automatically print out the corneal curvature in diopters or millimeters of radius.
7. **d. Game challenges.** Game challenge displays that are entertaining are not a use for a medical computer. Although all computers have a number of games available to them, they should not be incorporated into an ophthalmic practice because of the inordinate amount of time that may be spent in this area without patient benefit.
8. **e. Indirect ophthalmoscope.** The indirect ophthalmoscope that is currently in use has no computerized mechanism.
9. **b. Producing reports and letters that can be word-perfect and recalled.** The main function for word processing software is to type extensive letters and reports. By addition of a speller component to the software program, the letters can become word-perfect. The material can be easily corrected and recalled for future use.

CHAPTER 40   **The role of ophthalmic medical personnel in clinical ophthalmology practice**

BERNARD R. BLAIS, M.D., F.A.C.S.

- Definitions
- Contact lens technicians
- Ophthalmic photographers
- Ophthalmic registered nurses
- Opticians
- Orthoptists
- Ophthalmic medical personnel
- Programmatic and institutional accreditation
- The future of allied health personnel in ophthalmology

In 1973 Dr. Barnet Sakler, as President of the American Association of Ophthalmology, stated the goals of ophthalmologic care that have remained relevant for more than two decades: "The preservation of eye health requires complete eye care, which means comprehensive medical histories; examination of the eye; diagnosis of all eye conditions; prescribing of eye glasses; fitting of contact lenses and optical aids when indicated; prescribing of medications when needed; eye surgery when required; consultation with the eye specialist in all matters concerning vision and the eye as it relates to the whole body." The ophthalmologist, like all physicians, is assisted by ancillary personnel. In the armed forces, as well as in civilian life, the ophthalmologist has trained personnel working in the clinic and operating room and assisting in providing care for his or her patients. These personnel become members of the ophthalmology team in the management of the eye patient's care.

DEFINITIONS*
Allied health

Allied health includes a large cluster of health care–related professions and personnel whose functions include assisting, facilitating, or complementing the work of physicians and other specialists in the health care system and who choose to be identified as allied health personnel. Definitions of "allied health" vary because of its changing nature and the differing perspectives of those who attempt its definition. In ad-

Clinical Professor, Albany Medical College, Albany, New York, and Medical Director, General Electric, Niskayuna, New York.

*Information from *Allied health education directory:* ed 14, 1986, American Medical Association.

dition, professionals in certain medically related but traditionally parallel or independent occupations prefer identities independent of allied health, such as nursing, podiatry, pharmacy, and clinical psychology. Other professionals may or may not regard themselves as "allied," for example, nutritionists, speech pathologists, audiologists, public health specialists, licensed practical nurses, and medical research assistants.

Allied health care personnel

Allied health care personnel (allied medical personnel) include professional and skilled supporting persons in the field of patient care, public health, and health research who assist, supplement, or facilitate the work of other allied health care professionals—particularly the physician—and independent contractors in providing health services. They may use independent judgment within their areas of competence, as approved by the supervising physician.

The Allied Health Personnel in Ophthalmology (AHPO) includes the following:

Contact lens technicians
Ophthalmic photographers
Ophthalmic registered nurses
Opticians
Orthoptist
Ophthalmic medical personnel, for example, assistant, technician, technologist

Career ladder. This is a sequence of lateral or vertical steps that link jobs related in the same job family, permitting an employee to build from education and experience to move to an advanced position or to a related occupation.

Career mobility. This relates to the availability of opportunities for persons employed in a particular job to move without undo restrictions to (1) a similar job available in a different geographic location (geographical mobility), (2) a job with increased responsibility within the same or similar setting (vertical mobility), or (3) a job in a related occupation that requires similar knowledge and skills (lateral mobility).

Accreditation

Accreditation is a peer process whereby a private, nongovernmental agency or association grants public recognition to an institution or specialized program of study that meets or exceeds nationally established standards of acceptable educational quality. According to this concept, groups of educational institutions, professional practitioners, or educators form voluntary associations to encourage and assist institutions or programs in evaluating and improving the quality of their educational activities. For the institution or program the process generally includes (1) a clear statement of educational objectives, (2) a directed self-study focused on activities relating to these objectives, (3) an on-site visit by peers, and (4) a decision by an independent body that the institution or program does or does not meet its standards for accreditation.

Because this nongovernmental accreditation system is voluntary, review committees and the Committee on Allied Health Education and Accreditation (CAHEA) do not begin the process of program review until the chief executive officer of the institution sponsoring the program requests accreditation evaluation.

Certification

Certification is the process by which a nongovernmental agency or an association grants recognition to an individual who has met certain predetermined requirements specified by that agency or association and who voluntarily seeks such recognition.

CONTACT LENS TECHNICIANS

Contact lens technicians fabricate, polish, and fit contact lenses (Fig. 40-1). Their wide range of duties may include writing and transcribing contact lens prescriptions, selecting appropriate lens designs, and processing the materials to the desired prescription. In addition, the contact lens technician's duties may include contact with the patient and the professional, as well as with detail-oriented persons from ophthalmic supply firms.

The National Contact Lens Examiners, an association that is recognized by the National Commission on Allied Health Certifying Agencies as a "type A" member, provides the contact lens technician certification. In some states contact lens technicians are licensed by that state.

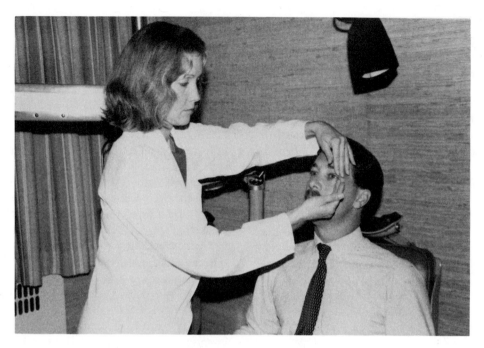

Fig. 40-1 Contact lens fitters play an important role in assisting in a medical contact lens practice.

OPHTHALMIC PHOTOGRAPHERS

The ophthalmic photographer is an individual who, either through a background in photography or as an ophthalmic medical photographer (OMP) becomes specialized in ophthalmic photography. This may entail either external photography or internal photography with or without use of contrast dyes. The ophthalmic photographer's professional organization, the Ophthalmic Photographers Society (OPS), encourages its members to provide the highest level of quality and service. The OPS certifies this highest level of ophthalmic photographer—including angiographers.

OPHTHALMIC REGISTERED NURSES*

The American Society of Ophthalmic Registered Nurses (ASORN) was organized in 1976 to unite registered professional nurses committed to provid-

ing quality eye care to ophthalmic patients. ASORN members are registered nurses (RNs) who currently practice ophthalmic nursing either on a full- or part-time basis. Members also may be RNs currently inactive in nursing but who were engaged in ophthalmic nursing immediately before becoming inactive. A category is also available for retired members. ASORN is accredited as both a provider and an approver of continuing education in nursing by the American Nurses Credentialing Center's Commission on Accreditation.

The National Certifying Board for Ophthalmic Registered Nurses (NCBORN) was organized in 1987 in response to an expressed need of ASORN members. NCBORN has been certifying registered nurses in ophthalmology since 1989. Individuals who successfully complete the examination are eligible to use the designation Certified Registered Nurse in Ophthalmology (CRNO) after their names. The examination is administered twice yearly at 20 sites throughout the United States.

---

*American Society of Ophthalmic Registered Nurses: Brochure, 1992, ASORN.

OPTICIANS

The U.S. Department of Health, Education and Welfare categorized opticians into two groups: (1) ophthalmic laboratory technicians and (2) ophthalmic dispensers.

Ophthalmic laboratory technicians are defined as those individuals who grind and polish lenses and fabricate eyewear by assembly of the various components. The technicians' wide range of duties may include writing and transcribing prescriptions, selecting appropriate lens forms, and processing the materials to the desired prescription. In addition, the technicians' duties may include contact with the patient and the professional, as well as persons from ophthalmic supplier firms.

Ophthalmic dispensers are broadly defined as those individuals who adapt and fit corrective eyewear as prescribed by the optometrist or ophthalmologist. The ophthalmic dispenser is an allied health technician with the proper training and proficiency to competently and accurately translate the written prescription into proper eyewear. The dispenser's wide range of duties include business-administrative functions relating to record maintenance, correspondence, purchasing, and maintenance of supplies and equipment. The dispenser's technical duties include patient occupational analysis, physiognomy measurement, preparation of laboratory job orders, verification of laboratory work, and the final adapting and fitting of eyewear. In some states, optical dispensing also includes contact lens dispensing, the fitting of artificial eyes, and the dispensing of subnormal vision aids.

The Commission on Opticians Accreditation, an autonomous organization that is recognized by United States Education Department (USED), accredits the training programs. The American Board of Opticians, which is recognized by the National Commission on Health Certifying Agencies as a "category A" member, provides the optician certification. In some states opticians are licensed by that state.

ORTHOPTISTS

The term *orthoptics* means straight eyes. This word comes from the two Greek words, *ortho* meaning straight and *optics* pertaining to eyes.

Orthoptics is the clinical science of ocular motility, binocular vision, and related disorders of the eyes. An orthoptist is an eye muscle specialist who works under the supervision of an ophthalmologist. In addition to diagnosis and treatment, the orthoptist assists the ophthalmologist with other professional ophthalmic tasks.

The American Orthoptic Council, composed of twelve ophthalmologists and four orthoptists, directs the practice of certified orthoptists in this country. Specifically the council (1) determines the qualifications necessary for candidates who wish to begin orthoptic training, (2) regulates the training and certification of orthoptist, and (3) supervises the practice of orthoptist after their certification.

After certification the orthoptist becomes eligible for membership in the *American Association of Certified Orthoptists*. In conjunction with the American Orthoptic Council, this association encourages the development and exchange of new ideas and techniques, stimulates professional growth by assisting in postgraduate instruction courses, and endeavors to advise individual orthoptists who have special or unusual problems.

OPHTHALMIC MEDICAL PERSONNEL*

Ophthalmic medical personnel (OMP) carry out a variety of duties assigned to them by the ophthalmologist with whom they work. However, they do not diagnose or treat eye disorders. They are not certified or licensed to be independent practitioners. They function in a professional setting similar to that in which an x-ray technician works with a physician radiologist or a medical technician supplies information to a physician treating a patient.

Ophthalmic medical personnel are certified at three levels of expertise by the Joint Commission on Allied Health Personnel in Ophthalmology (JCAHPO). In ascending order these are ophthalmic assistant, ophthalmic technician, and ophthalmic technologist. The certification is based on the career ladder con-

---

*Information from Joint Commission of Allied Health Personnel in Ophthalmology: *Criteria for certification and recertification of ophthalmic medical personnel,* ed 17 rev, June 1992, 40 M, JCAHPO.

cept. Even without major financial investments or additional college education, certified ophthalmic assistants and technicians can attain upward career mobility through the establishment of equivalent criteria (see box on p. 805-806). These criteria are detailed in the current edition of JCAHPO's *Blue Book.*

Criteria for certification and recertification of ophthalmic medical personnel

Candidates must pass a certifying examination before they can attain certification or advance in certification level. Examinations, which are held once a year, are administered at about 70 different examination sites in the United States and Canada.

Certification is maintained by earning the required number of JCAHPO-approved continuing education credits. The requirements for recertification vary according to the level of certification.

To be eligible for admission to the annual written certifying examination, applicants must meet specific requirements of education and training for the assistant and technician levels, in addition to an endorsement by the sponsoring ophthalmologist. Other criteria for admission to the written qualifying ex-

aminations at the technology level are established as alternate routes of advancement through equivalent criteria. Continuing education credits also are used in building the career ladder (see box on p. 809).

Categories of ophthalmic medical personnel

1. The certified ophthalmic assistant (COA) possesses skills and knowledge in the following:
- History taking
- Visual acuity testing in children and adults, color vision testing, lensometry
- Basic patient services
- Basic tonometry
- Basic instrument maintenance
- General medical knowledge and cardiopulmonary resuscitation (CPR)

2. The certified ophthalmic technician (COT) possesses skills and knowledge in the preceding and in the following additional areas:
- Refractometry
- Ocular motility testing
- Visual field testing
- Contact lens fitting assistance
- Advanced details of contact lens fitting
- Ocular pharmacology

ADVANTAGES OF JCAHPO

OPHTHALMIC MEDICAL PERSONNEL
- Increases office efficiency
- Demonstrates commitment to working in ophthalmology
- Improves the quality of patient care by allowing the ophthalmologist to see more patients and perform more time-consuming but important special tests
- Allows the ophthalmologist to concentrate specifically on the medical needs of the patient by delegating less-demanding tasks to skilled personnel
- Conveys to the patient the maintenance of high standards by the ophthalmologist in hiring personnel with credentials (the patient's favorable first impression can reinforce the doctor-patient relationship)
- Sets a standard of excellence through certain requirements of academic and clinical education and successful completion of appropriate written and practical examinations

OPHTHALMIC REGISTERED NURSES
- Formally recognizes those individuals who meet the eligibility requirements of the National Certifying Board for Ophthalmic Registered Nurses
- Encourages continued personal and professional growth in the practice of ophthalmic registered nursing
- Establishes and measures the level of knowledge required for certification in ophthalmic registered nursing
- Provides a standard of requisite knowledge required for certification, thereby assisting the employer, the public, and members of the health professions in the assessment of the ophthalmic registered nurse
- Recognizes professional qualifications and knowledge in ophthalmic nursing
- Demonstrates personal commitment to the improvement of ophthalmic nursing practice

SUMMARY OF CRITERIA FOR JCAHPO CERTIFICATION

REQUIREMENTS AT ALL SKILL LEVELS
- Evidence of successful completion of education and training
- Evidence of satisfactory work experience
- A current cardiopulmonary resuscitation (CPR) certificate
- Endorsement by the sponsoring ophthalmologist
- Successful completion of examination(s)

REQUIREMENTS AT SPECIFIC SKILL LEVELS

Assistant level

Education and Training	Work Experience
JRCOMP Approved educational program	One year
or	
Home study course	One year
or	
JRCOMP approved educational program (completed more than 3 years ago), plus 18 hours of JCAHPO approved continuing education credits (1:1)	One year

Technician Level

Education and Training	Work Experience
CAHEA accredited educational program	
or	
Certified ophthalmic assistant (COA) (active), plus 18 hours of JCAHPO approved continuing education credits (1:1)	One year as COA
or	
CAHEA accredited education program (completed more than 12 months ago), plus 18 hours of JCAHPO approved continuing education credits (1:1)	One year
or	
AOC or COC certified orthoptist, plus 12 hours of JCAHPO approved continuing education credits (1:1)	One year
plus	
Successful completion of skill evaluation	

Technologist Level

Education and Training	Work Experience
Four-year college degree in ophthalmic technology	
or	
Two years of college courses plus CAHEA accredited program for ophthalmic technologists	
or	
Less than 2 years (or no) college courses, but CAHEA accredited program for ophthalmic technologists, plus 12 hours of JCAHPO approved continuing education credits (1:1) for each year following graduation	Two additional years (within the last 5 years)
or	
Certified ophthalmic technician (active), plus 36 hours of JCAHPO approved continuing education credits (1:1)	Three years as COT
or	
AOC or COC certified orthoptist, plus 24 hours of JCAHPO approved continuing education credits (1:1)	Two years
plus	
Successful completion of the practical performance test	

Continued.

SUMMARY OF CRITERIA FOR JCAHPO CERTIFICATION—cont'd

Ophthalmic Surgical Assisting (OSA)

Education and Training	OSA Work Experience
CAHEA accredited educational program within last 12 months	
or	
CAHEA accredited educational program (completed more than 12 months ago), plus on-the-job training (no more than 3 years ago) in nationally accredited operating suite, plus current certification	6 months (within the last 12 months)
or	
Full-time academic year in hospital-based surgical technologist course in nationally accredited operating suite, plus current certification	6 months (within the last 12 months)
or	
On-the-job instruction and experience in a nationally accredited operating suite, plus current certification	18 months (within the last 3 years)

---

3. The certified ophthalmic medical technologist (COMT) is qualified to assist the ophthalmologist in all areas already listed and possesses skills and knowledge in the following additional areas:
- Advanced visual field testing
- Advanced ocular motility testing
- Advanced color vision testing
- Advanced clinical optics
- Ophthalmic photography
- Testing with special instruments and special diagnostic techniques
- Microbiology
- Advanced ocular pharmacology
- Advanced general medical knowledge

Ophthalmic surgical assisting

Ophthalmic surgical assisting (OSA) is a special content area in which the candidate may be examined and qualify for a certificate of proficiency. To qualify for the surgical assisting examination, candidates must be certified at one of the previously mentioned levels.

Certified ophthalmic medical assistants, technicians, and technologists with certification in ophthalmic surgical assisting are able to perform the following duties:
- Identification, selection, and maintenance of ophthalmic surgical instruments
- Sterilization and set-up of instruments for ophthalmic surgical procedures
- Assisting, scrubbing, or circulating as directed by the ophthalmic surgeon

The ophthalmic surgical assistant has knowledge of preoperative preparation of the ocular surgery patient and is able to perform the aforementioned tasks in assisting the surgeon, both in minor office surgery and in a hospital operating room.

Ophthalmic medical personnel job description*

Job descriptions for noncertified OMPs and certified assistants, technicians, and technologists were developed by examining the degree of correspondence between the amount of time the OMPs spend on various tasks and the amount of importance placed on these tasks by the ophthalmologist in the general practice of ophthalmology. Those tasks in which the OMPs estimated they spent most of their time and that the ophthalmologists rated as important to their practice were considered essential tasks for all or for one or more of the OMP levels of certification. These tasks, which are listed by the different levels of OMP certification and noncertification, are shown in Table 40-1.

---

*Joint Commission on Allied Health Personnel in Ophthalmology report: *Ophthalmic medical assistant job description,* 1986.

Table 40-1   Job description: ophthalmic medical assistant

	NC	AS	TC	TG
ADMINISTRATIVE AND CLERICAL DUTIES				
1. Perform receptionist or clerical procedures	+	+		
2. Carry out administrative, supervisory duties	+	+	+	+
3. Order and maintain inventory	+	+	+	+
COLOR VISION, BASIC SKILLS, PUPIL FUNCTION, HISTORY TAKING				
4. Obtain ocular, medical, and family history	+	+	+	+
5. Measure visual acuity	+	+	+	+
6. Measure, compare, and test pupils		+	+	+
7. Test color vision: Ishihara, HRR, Farnsworth, or other			+	+
OPHTHALMIC PATIENT SERVICES				
8. Instill ocular medications	+	+	+	+
9. Instruct concerning medicines, tests, surgical procedures	+	+	+	+
10. Apply eye dressings	+	+	+	+
11. Perform minor adjustment of spectacles	−	−	−	−
12. Clean, sterilize, and prepare instruments	+	+	+	
13. Assist with surgical procedures in office	+	+	+	+
OPTICS				
14. Neutralize lenses on a lensometer	+	+	+	+
15. Measure interpupillary distance				
16. Measure vertex distance with distometer	−	−	−	−
17. Perform retinoscopy			+	+
18. Refine refractive error using subjective response			+	+
19. Evaluate low vision aids for patients	−	−	−	−
OCULAR MOTILITY				
20. Identify version and duction anomalies				+
21. Measure near point of convergence				+
22. Perform cover-uncover test, alternate test			+	+
23. Measure stereoacuity				+
24. Measure deviations with prisms				+
25. Perform the Worth four-dot test				
26. Measure near point of accommodation				
TONOMETRY				
27. Measure pressure with Schiotz-type tonometer	−	−	−	−
28. Measure pressure with applanation tonometry			+	+
29. Measure pressure with probe or air puff tonometer	−	−	−	−
30. Perform and calculate tonography	−	−	−	−
31. Perform and record any provocative tests	−	−	−	−
VISUAL FIELDS				
32. Perform a confrontation field				
33. Use Goldmann-type perimeter	+	+	+	+
34. Calibrate a bowl-type perimeter				+
35. Perform tangent screen–type central field examination				
CONTACT LENSES				
36. Measure corneal diameter				
37. Measure corneal curvature with keratometer	+	+	+	+
38. Measure specifications of hard contact lens				
39. Instruct patient in insertion/removal of contact lenses			+	
40. Polish or modify hard contact lenses				
41. Perform a Schirmer tear test			+	+

NC, Noncertified; *AS,* assistant; *TC,* technician; *TG,* technologist.
ERG, Electroretinogram; *EOG,* electrooculogram; *VER,* visual evoked response; *VEP,* visual evoked potential.
HRR, Hardy, Rand, Rittler.

Continued.

Table 40-1	Job description: ophthalmic medical assistant—cont'd			
SPECIALIZED OPHTHALMIC TESTING					
42. Perform exophthalmometry		−	−	−	−
43. Assist in ophthalmodynamometry		−	−	−	−
44. Measure dark adaptation		−	−	−	−
45. Set up, assist with xenon arc or laser photography		−	−	−	−
46. Obtain A-scan measurement, calculate power of lens				+	+
47. Set up and perform B-scan		−	−	−	−
48. Measure and record results of ERG, EOG, or VER/VEP		−	−	−	−
OPHTHALMIC PHOTOGRAPHY					
49. Perform anterior segment photography					
50. Perform fundus photography				+	+
51. Perform fluorescein angiography					+
52. Perform corneal endothelial specular photography		−	−	−	−
53. Perform photographic dark-room procedures		−	−	−	−
MICROBIOLOGY AND PHARMACOLOGY					
54. Assist with conjunctival, corneal specimens					
55. Culture on plates using proper techniques		−	−	−	−
56. Perform a Gram or Giemsa stain		−	−	−	−
57. Identify bacteria or cells		−	−	−	−
58. Identify ocular medications		+	+	+	+
SURGICAL ASSISTING IN OPERATING ROOM					
59. Perform preoperative scrub, put on gown and gloves					
60. Perform accepted scrub nurse duties					
61. Maintain, operate equipment for surgeon					
62. Assist physician with surgical procedure					
63. Sterilize instruments and supplies					
MAINTENANCE AND REPAIR					
64. Change batteries, bulbs in instruments		+	+	+	+
65. Clean, assemble, and calibrate Schiotz-type tonometer					
66. Calibrate, adjust Goldmann tonometer					
67. Maintenance, minor repairs of instruments				+	

The duties of the OMP may be arranged under 13 major content areas:

1. Administrative and clerical duties
2. Color vision, basic skills, pupil function, and history taking
3. Ophthalmic patient services
4. Optics
5. Ocular motility
6. Tonometry
7. Visual field
8. Contact lens
9. Specialized ophthalmic testing
10. Ophthalmic photography
11. Microbiology and pharmacology
12. Surgical assisting in the operating room
13. Maintenance and repair

Education required for OMP certification

A high school diploma or equivalency certificate is required to enter training in ophthalmic medical assisting. Potential candidates also should possess scientific curiosity, sound judgment, cooperativeness, mature attitudes, and a basic aptitude for accuracy.

Two methods for achieving a career in ophthalmic medical assisting are through institutional programs and on-the-job experience.

Institutional programs. There are recognized formal institutional programs in the United States and Canada. Each program is geared toward one of the three certification levels; thus programs vary in intensity and duration. For more information on formal training programs, see the box on p. 811.

On-the-job experience. Certification also may be

EDUCATIONAL PROGRAMS FOR THE OPHTHALMIC MEDICAL ASSISTANT

A. Programs accredited by the AMA's Committee on Allied Health Education and Accreditation (CAHEA)
   1. Boston University Medical Center, Ophthalmic Technology Program, Boston, Mass. (24 mo, Tg)
   2. Detroit Institute of Ophthalmology, OMA Program, Grosse Point Park, Mich. (24 mo, Tg)
   3. Emory University School of Medicine, Orthoptic/Ophthalmic School, Atlanta, Ga. (27 mo, Tg, O)
   4. Georgetown University Medical Center, OMA Training Program, Washington, D.C. (2 yr, Tg)
   5. Medical University South Carolina, Ophthalmic Technician Program, Charleston, S.C. (24 mo, T)
   6. New York Eye and Ear Infirmary, Allied Health Program for OMAs, NY, N.Y. (24 mo, Tg, O)
   7. St. Paul Ramsey Medical Center, School for Ophthalmic Technicians, St. Paul, Minn. (21 mo, Tg)
   8. Schie Eye Institute, University of Pennsylvania, Ophthalmic Technology Program, Philadelphia, Penn. (2 yr, Tg)
   9. Triton College, Ophthalmic Technician Program, River Grove, Ill. (2 yr, T)
   10. University of Florida, Ophthalmic Technology Training Program, Gainesville, Fla. (2 yr, Tg)
B. Programs Reviewed by the Joint Review Committee for Ophthalmic Medical Assistants (JRCOMA) and the Committee on Allied Health Education and Accreditation (CAHEA) and accredited by the Canadian Medical Association (CMA)
   1. Stanton Yellowknife Hospital, OMA Program, Yellowknife, NWT, Canada (30 mo, T)
   2. Izaak Walton Hospital, OMA Program, Halifax, Nova Scotia, Canada (2 yr, Tg, O)
   3. National Defense Medical Center, Ophthalmic Technician Program, Ottawa, Ontario, Canada (24 mo, M, +)
C. Programs granted a "Letter of Review" by JRCOMA (recognition of programs that have not yet graduated their first class)
   1. ODU EVMS Program, Norfolk, Va. (24 mo, Tg)
D. Programs approved by the Joint Commission on Allied Health Personnel in Ophthalmology (JCAHPO)
   1. Academy of Health Sciences, Eye Specialist Course, Fort Sam Houston, Tex. (13 wk, A, M)
   2. Boston University Medical Center, Ophthalmic Assistant Program, Boston, Mass. (12 wk, A)
   3. Centennial College, Ophthalmic Assistant Program, Scarborough, Ontario, Canada (9 mo, A)
   4. Georgetown University Medical Center, OMA Training Program, Washington, D.C. (9 mo, A, T)
   5. Jules Stein Eye Program, Los Angeles, Calif. (6 mo, A)
   6. Mount Sinai Medical Center, Ophthalmic Assistant Training Program, Beachwood, Ohio (9 mo, A)
   7. Naval School of Health Sciences, Ocular Technician School (NEC 8445), San Diego, Calif. (22 wk, T)
   8. Tulane Medical Center, Department of Ophthalmology, OMA Course, New Orleans, La. (8 wk, A, T)
   9. University of Southern Florida, Department of Ophthalmology, OMA Course, Tampa, Fla. (6 wk, T)
   10. UMD–New Jersey Medical School, Ophthalmic Allied Health Program, Newark, N.J. (5 mo, A, T)
E. Home study courses approved by the JCAHPO
   1. Home Study Course for OMAs, American Academy of Ophthalmology, San Francisco, Calif.
   2. Ophthalmic Assistant Home Study Program, Canadian Ophthalmological Society, c/o Centennial College, Scarborough, Ontario, Canada

---

TG, Technologist level eligibility; *O,* program also meets criteria for certification as an orthoptist; *I,* technician level eligibility; *M,* program available for active, reserve, and national guard military personnel only; *A,* assistant level eligibility.

attained by working in the office of an ophthalmologist, successfully completing an approved home study course, and passing a certifying examination.

Professional organization of ophthalmic medical personnel

The Association of Technical Personnel in Ophthalmology (ATPO), formerly American Association of Certified Allied Health Personnel in Ophthalmology (AACAHPO), was established to represent *Allied Health Personnel in Ophthalmology (ATPO).* Its primary goals are continuing education, providing channels of communication among members, representation, and information dissemination. ATPO and JCAHPO conduct continuing education programs in conjunction with the annual meeting of the American Academy of Ophthalmology (AAO). ATPO is an organization of high standards and professional ethics dedicated to quality ophthalmic medical care.

PROGRAMMATIC AND INSTITUTIONAL ACCREDITATION

Joint Commission on Allied Health Personnel in Ophthalmology

The Joint Commission on Allied Health Personnel in Ophthalmology (JCAHPO) is a federation of twelve major professional ophthalmologic associations and societies throughout the United States and Canada (see box on p. 810). It was founded in 1969 for the purpose of facilitating eye care by the following objectives:

- Encouraging the establishment of medically oriented programs for training allied health personnel in ophthalmology
- Developing standards of education and training
- Examining, certifying, and recertifying
- Encouraging continuing occupational development

JCAHPO is a widely recognized organization because its certification provides a legally defensible credential during these times of rapidly changing laws concerning health care.

Educational programs for ophthalmic medical technicians and technologists, recognized as fulfilling the criteria of JCAHPO certification, are accredited by the Committee on Allied Health Education and Accreditation (CAHEA), and its program review committees are recognized by the Council on Postsecondary Accreditation (COPA) and the United States Education Department (USED).

The JCAHPO is recognized as a regular category A member of the National Commission for Health Certifying Agencies (NCHCA). The JCAHPO Education and Research Foundation, Inc., which is incorporated as a nonprofit organization, provides grants and scholarship awards for scholarships relating to ophthalmology and allied health personnel in ophthalmology, develops and provides educational materials and programs relating to ophthalmology and allied health personnel in ophthalmology, and conducts research relating to ophthalmology and allied health personnel in ophthalmology.

Joint Review Committee for Ophthalmic Medical Personnel

The Joint Review Committee for Ophthalmic Medical Personnel (JRCOMP), formally known as the Joint Review Committee for Ophthalmic Medical Assistants (JRCOMA), is a review committee for ophthalmic assistants and a member of the CAHEA umbrella. It is sponsored by three collaborating organizations: (1) ATPO, which represents the interests of allied health occupations, (2) JCAHPO, which represents the interests of ophthalmologic medicine, and (3) the Canadian Ophthalmological Association.

JRCOMP, in collaboration with CAHEA, has received recognition by COPA and USED for accreditation of educational programs of 6 months or longer for the ophthalmologic medical assistant. Thus JRCOMP is recognized by CAHEA, COPA, and USED. Schools accredited under this collaborative arrangement are now considered to have satisfied one of the statutory requirements for eligibility for participating in financial assistance programs administered by the U.S. Department of Education.

Accredited ophthalmic medical personnel programs located in hospitals or other non–degree-granting institutions should apply to the U.S. Department of Education if they desire to participate in any of its programs. Accredited ophthalmic medical assistant programs located in degree-granting

---

ORGANIZATIONS PARTICIPATING IN THE JOINT COMMISSION ON ALLIED HEALTH PERSONNEL IN OPHTHALMOLOGY

American Academy of Ophthalmology
Association of Technical Personnel in Ophthalmology
American Association of Certified Orthoptists
American Ophthalmological Society
American Orthoptic Council
American Society of Ophthalmic Registered Nurses
Association of University Professors in Ophthalmology
Canadian Ophthalmological Society
Canadian Orthoptic Society
Contact Lens Association of Ophthalmologists
Society of Military Ophthalmologists
Association of Veterans Administration Ophthalmologists

ACCREDITED PROGRAMS

**AMA'S COMMITTEE ON ALLIED HEALTH EDUCA-
TION AND ACCREDITATION (CAHEA)**

District of Columbia
Georgetown University Medical Center
Ophthalmic Medical Personnel Training Program
  Peter Y. Evans, MD, Medical Director
  Phyllis L. Fineberg, COMT, Program Director
  Department of Ophthalmology
  3800 Reservoir Road NW
  Washington, DC 20007
  (202) 687-4862 (2 years, T, Tg*)

Florida
University of Florida
Ophthalmic Technology Training Program
  Melvin Rubin, MD, Medical Director
  Barbara Cassin, CO, COMT, Program Director
  Department of Ophthalmology, College of Medicine
  Gainesville, FL 32610
  (904) 392-3111 (2 years, Tg, O)

Illinois
Triton College
Ophthalmic Technician Program
  Mary Dougal, MD, Medical Director
  Debra Baker, COMT, Program Director
  2000 N. Fifth Ave.
  River Grove, IL 60171
  (708) 456-0300 ext. 442 (2 years, T)

Massachusetts
Boston University Medical Center
Ophthalmic Medical Personnel Training Program
  Andre Quamina, MD, Medical Director
  Norma Garber, CO, COMT, Program Director
  Ophthalmology L907
  80 East Concord St.
  Boston, MA 02118
  (617) 534-4027 (24 months, T, Tg). In addition, an asso-
    ciate and a baccalaureate degree may be obtained.

Michigan
Detroit Institute of Ophthalmology
Ophthalmic Technology Program
  Philip C. Hessburg, MD, Medical Director
  Deanna Presnell, COMT, CST, Program Director
  15415 E. Jefferson Ave.
  Grosse Pointe Park, MI 48230
  (313) 824-4710 (24 months, T, Tg)

Minnesota
St. Paul Ramsey Medical Center
School of Ophthalmic Medical Technology
  J. Daniel Nelson, MD, FACS, Medical Director
  Richard J. Augustine, COMT, Program Director
  640 Jackson St.
  St. Paul, MN 55101
  (612) 221-3000 (21 months, T, Tg)

New York
New York Eye & Ear Infirmary
Allied Health Program in Ophthalmology
  Alan C. Weseley, MD, Medical Director
  Sara Shippman, CO, COMT, Program Director
  310 East 14th St.
  New York, NY 10003
  (212) 979-4375 (24 months, Tg, O)

North Carolina
Duke University
School for Ophthalmic Medical Technicians
  W. Banks Anderson, MD, Medical Director
  Judy H. Seaber, Ph.D., Program Director
  Box 3802
  Duke University Eye Center
  Durham, NC 27710
  (919) 684-6778 (1 year, T)

Puerto Rico
University of Puerto Rico
College of Health Related Professions
Ophthalmic Technicians' Program
  Muriel Rosa, MD, Medical Director
  Milagros C. Lopez, RN, Program Director
  Department of Ophthalmology
  Medical Sciences Campus—U.P.R.
  P.O. Box 5067, San Juan, Puerto Rico 00936
  (809) 756-7090 (2 years, T)

Virginia
Old Dominion University/Eastern Virginia Medical School
Ophthalmic Technology Program
  Ira Lederman, MD, Medical Director
  Kelley J. Fleming, CO, COMT, Program Director
  Norfolk General Hospital, Lions Sight and Hearing
  600 Gresham Drive
  Norfolk, VA 23507
  (804) 628-2100 (2 years, Tg). In addition, a four-year
    baccalaureate may be obtained.

Continued.

CANADIAN MEDICAL ASSOCIATION (CMA)

Northwest Territories

Stanton Yellowknife Hospital

Ophthalmic Medical Technician Training Program

 Leonard F. Smith, MD, FRCS, Medical Director

 Allen Knapp, COMT, Program Director

 c/o Department of Ophthalmology

 Box 10

 Yellowknife, NWT, Canada X1A 2N1

 (403) 873-3577 (24 months, T)

Nova Scotia

The Izaak Walton Killam Hospital for Children

School of Orthoptics/Ophthalmic Medical Technology

 E.V. Rafuse, MD, FRCS(C), Medical Director

 Heather Macpherson, OC(C), COMT, Program Director

 5850 University Ave.

 Box 3070

 Halifax, Nova Scotia, Canada B3J 3G9

 (902) 428-8021 (2 years, Tg, O)

APPROVED BY THE JOINT REVIEW COMMITTEE FOR OPHTHALMIC MEDICAL PERSONNEL (JR COMP)

Arizona

Pima Medical Institute

Ophthalmic Medical Assistant Program

 Robert M. Kershner, MD, Medical Director

 Maria Ojeda, COA, Acting Program Director

 3350 E. Grant Road

 Tucson, AZ 85716

 (602) 326-1600 (36 weeks, A)

California

Jules Stein Eye Institute

Ophthalmic Assistant Training Program

 Kenneth R. Diddie, MD, Medical Director

 Bobbi E. Shapiro, COT, Program Director

 100 Stein Plaza

 Los Angeles, CA 90024-1771

 (213) 825-4617 (6 months, A)

Naval School of Health Sciences

Ocular Technician School (NEC 8445)

 Capt. J.E. Sutphin, MC, USN, Medical Director

 Aurelio S. Esguerra, HMI, USN, Program Director

 San Diego, CA 92134-6000

 (619) 532-7831 (22 weeks, A, M)

District of Columbia

Georgetown University Medical Center

Ophthalmic Medical Personnel Training Program

 Peter Y. Evans, MD, Medical Director

 Phyllis L. Fineberg, COMT, Program Director

 Department of Ophthalmology

 3800 Reservoir Road NW

 Washington, DC 20007

 (202) 687-4862

 Two courses: (1) 5 weeks full time, A

 (2) 7 months part-time, at 3 hours per week, A

Illinois

Ophthalmic Medical Assistant Program

The Eye Center Carbondale/Marion

 Maqbool Ahmad, MD, Medical Director

 Michelle Pett Herrin, CO, COMT, Program Director

 1200 W. De Young

 Marion, IL 62959

 (618) 993-5686

Louisiana

Tulane University Medical Center

Department of Ophthalmology

Ophthalmic Assistant Course

 Delmar R. Caldwell, MD, Medical Director

 Donna George, RN, COT, Program Director

 1430 Tulane Ave.

 New Orleans, LA 70112

 (504) 588-5804 (8 weeks, A)

Massachusetts

Boston University Medical Center

Ophthalmic Assistant Program

 Andre Quamina, MD, Medical Director

 Norma Garber, CO, COMT, Program Director

 Ophthalmology L907

 80 East Concord St.

 Boston, MA 02118

 (617) 534-4027 (12 weeks, A)

New Jersey

UMD–New Jersey Medical School

Ophthalmic Allied Health Programs

 Alfonse A. Cinotti, MD, Medical Director

 Barbara F. Churchill, COT, Program Director

 Department of Ophthalmology

 Eye Institute of New Jersey

 15 S. 9th St.

 Newark, NJ 07107

 (201) 456-4625

 (201) 268-8051 (5 months, A)

New York

Ophthalmic Assistant Training Program

CMEOA, Inc. with Manhattan Eye, Ear and Throat Hospital

 Alexander Traykovski, MD, Medical Director

 Catherine Traykovski, RN, COA, Program Director

 46 West 86th St.

 New York, NY 10024

 (212) 877-7331 (A)

Ontario, Canada

Centennial College

Certificate of Achievement—Ophthalmic Assistant

 Harold A. Stein, MD, Medical Director

 Debby Kaplan, COA, Program Director

 Box 631, Station A

 Scarborough, Ontario, Canada M1K 5E9

 (416) 694-3241 (9 months, A)

ACCREDITED PROGRAMS—cont'd

Pennsylvania
Community College of Allegheny County
South Campus
Ophthalmic Medical Personnel Program
  John S. Kennerdell, MD, Medical Director
  Sherry Roisman, Coordinator
  1750 Clairton Road
  Route 885
  West Mifflin, PA 15122
  (412) 469-6310 (15 weeks, A)
Texas
Academy of Health Sciences
Eye Specialist Course
  Joe B. Hick, MD, Medical Director
  Major George L. Adams III, OD, Program Director
  Medicine and Surgery Division
  Ft. Sam Houston, TX 78234-6100
  (512) 221-1288 (13 weeks, A, M)
West Virginia
West Virginia University
Department of Ophthalmology
Ophthalmic Medical Assistant Program
  Judie F. Charlton, MD, Medical Director
  Michelle M. Michael, COT, Program Director
  Health Sciences Center North
  Morgantown, WV 26506
  (304) 293-3757 (1 year, A)

HOME STUDY COURSES APPROVED BY THE JOINT REVIEW COMMITTEE FOR OPHTHALMICMEDICAL PERSONNEL (JR COMP)
  Ophthalmic Medical Assisting: An Independent Study Course
  American Academy of Ophthalmology
  Box 7424
  San Francisco, CA 94120-7424
  (415) 561-8500
Ophthalmic Assistant Home Study Program
Canadian Ophthalmological Society
  Centennial College, Box 631, Station A
  Debby Kaplan, Chairperson, School of Continuing Education
  Scarborough, Ontario, Canada M1K 5E9
  (416) 694-3241, ext. 3404
Also available from:
  Southern Alberta Institute of Technology
  Gayla Gavan, COT, Coordinator
  1301 16th Ave. NW
  Calgary, Alberta, Canada T2M 0L4
  (403) 284-8456
  (403) 263-2123

---

institutions normally will not apply separately for eligibility, because the institution's accreditation by a regional or institutional accrediting body satisfies the accreditation element of the statutory requirements.

The JRCOMP recognition provides JRCOMP/CAHEA-accredited programs with benefits that otherwise would not be available had JRCOMP not pursued the detailed and rigorous request for recognition, including self-study and public hearings. Accredited OMP programs can be proud of this recognition by USED and COPA inasmuch as they are the only programs for allied health professionals in ophthalmology with this recognition.

In 1987 JRCOMP accepted the responsibility from JCAHPO for approving training programs of less than 6 months' duration. This process is compatible with the existing processes for accrediting programs of 6 months or longer by JRCOMP/CAHEA.

Accreditation in the United States

To ensure a basic level of quality, the evaluative practice of accreditation arose in the United States as a means of conducting nongovernmental, peer evaluation of educational institutions and programs. Private educational associations of regional or national scope have adopted criteria that reflect the qualities of a sound educational program and have developed procedures for evaluating institutions or programs to determine whether they are operating at basic level of quality.

Accrediting bodies vary greatly in sponsorship, organization, scope, and focus. They are regional and national in coverage and general, institutional, specialized, and programmatic in perspective. What they have in common is a commitment to the improvement of education through accreditation.

In the United States there are two bodies that nationally recognize accrediting agencies and associations: (1) the U.S. Education Department (USED) and (2) the Council on Postsecondary Accreditation (COPA). USED is required by statute to publish a list of nationally recognized accrediting agencies and associations that the Secretary of Education determines to be reliable authorities on the quality of training offered by educational institutions and programs. The Council on Postsecondary Accreditation (COPA) is a national, nonprofit organization. Its major purpose is to support, coordinate, and improve all nongovernmental accrediting activities conducted at the postsecondary educational level in the United States. In this role COPA assumes a unique "balance wheel" function in relation to the various groups involved in or affected by accreditation.

The American Medical Association. For the past 50 years the American Medical Association (AMA) has participated extensively in activities to promote quality in allied health education and accreditation review processes. In collaboration with the AMA, more than 40 allied health organizations and related medical specialty societies have collaborated with program review committees to develop educational standards for 25 allied health professions. Using these standards, the Committee on Allied Health Education and Accreditation (CAHEA), previously mentioned, accredits more than 3000 allied health educational programs in almost 1800 institutions, including hospitals and clinics, 2-year community colleges and universities, and other institutions throughout the United States. Since its organizational meeting in January of 1977, CAHEA has established its own priorities, as identified by CAHEA members and by groups with which CAHEA cooperates.

Joint review committees are developed for each allied health field under the CAHEA umbrella.

Programmatic accreditation in Canada

Canada also has no federal ministry for education or other centralized authority that exercises single, national control over educational institutions. The provinces assume varying degrees of control over education but, in general, institutions of postsecondary education are permitted to operate with considerable independence and autonomy. As a consequence, Canadian educational institutions can vary widely in the character and quality of their programs.

In Canada the allied health programs are accredited by the Canadian Medical Association (CMA). The Committee on Allied Health Personnel, Joint Review Committee Ophthalmic Medical Personnel (JRCOMP), and CAHEA work in collaboration with the CMA and the Canadian Ophthalmological Association (COA).

JRCOMP processes applications for accreditation, reviews statistics, and recommends all accreditation action to the CMA with a review process by CAHEA. The CMA provides the ultimate accreditation of the training program.

National Commission for Health Certifying Agencies (NCHCA)

This agency is an organization of organizations. Its members (in addition to professionals or associations and other groups with an interest in health occupational credentials) include voluntary certifying agencies that issue credentials attesting to the competence of individual health professionals in their field. To attain membership in the commission, these certifying agencies must meet lengthy and comprehensive criteria that cover such areas as examination, validity, and reliability. This process protects the public interest and the establishment of qualifications for certification appropriate to certified occupation. Certifying agencies that apply for admission to membership undergo an evaluation by experts with NCHCA membership.

THE FUTURE OF ALLIED HEALTH PERSONNEL IN OPHTHALMOLOGY

Certification of the OMP and accreditation/approval of training programs serve to maintain quality control and higher standards of patient care. The career ladder of upward mobility is another quality, rather than quantity, factor. The OMP is not, and should not be, expected to render medical judgment. Although 2-year training programs properly place ophthalmologic residents and OMPs-in-training side-by-side—thus educating the future ophthalmologist in the potential and efficient use of the OMP—their ability to perform such judgmental tasks as diagnosis and disposition, should not be equated.

P. Evans, M.D., Executive Director of JCAHPO, in his presentation to the AAO stated, "It is this speaker's conviction that OMPs are here to stay, that the quality is elevated by certification and continuing education, and that they will fulfill a most important supportive role in the comprehensive and effective professional team approach in rendering the highest level medical care to the public today and tomorrow."

PART SEVEN

Atlas of common eye disorders

Anomalies of the eyelids and extraocular muscles

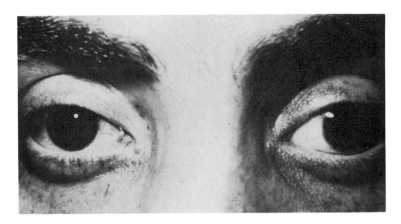

Fig. A-1 Left divergent strabismus.

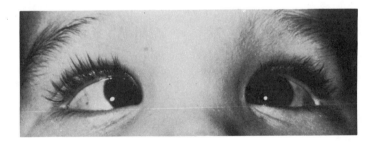

Fig. A-2 Right convergent strabismus.

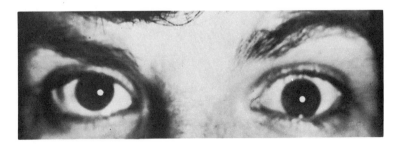

Fig. A-3 Right hypertropia.

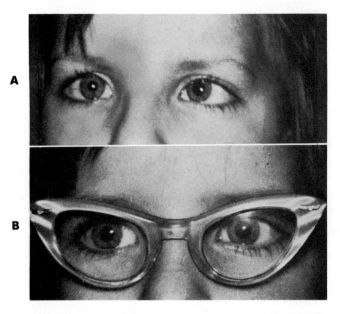

Fig. A-4 A, Accommodative left convergent strabismus. **B,** Strabismus corrected by glasses.

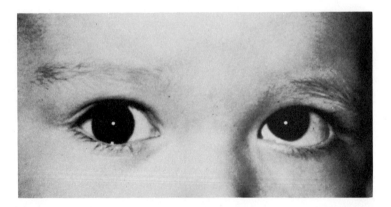

Fig. A-5 Vertical strabismus and head tilt due to underaction of left superior oblique muscle and overaction of left inferior oblique muscle.

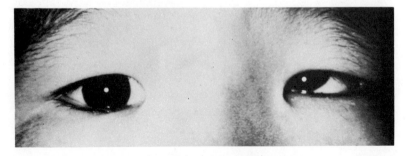

Fig. A-6 Epicanthal folds, wide nasal bridge, and overaction of left inferior oblique muscle.

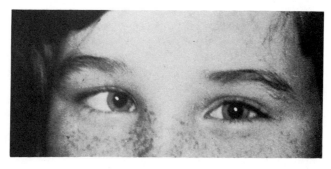

Fig. A-7 Duane's syndrome. There is inability of the left eye to look to the left when gaze is directed to the left and narrowing of the left palpebral fissure when gaze is directed to the light.

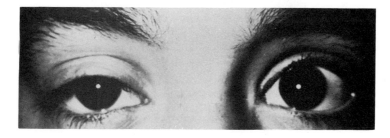

Fig. A-8 Congenital ptosis, unilateral.

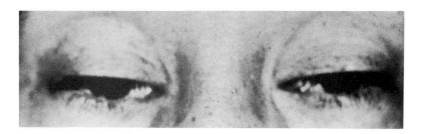

Fig. A-9 Congenital ptosis, bilateral.

Disorders of lid position

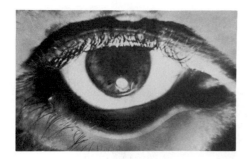

Fig. A-10 Ectropion.

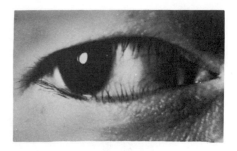

Fig. A-11 Entropion.

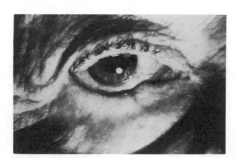

Fig. A-12 Radiation necrosis of lower eyelid with entropion.

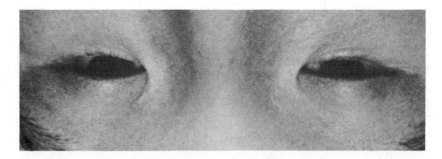

Fig. A-13 Epicanthal folds.

Disorders causing proptosis

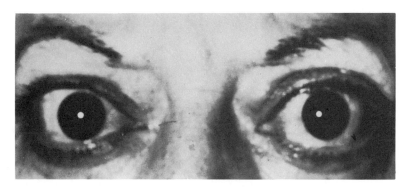

Fig. A-14 Exophthalmos of hyperthyroidism.

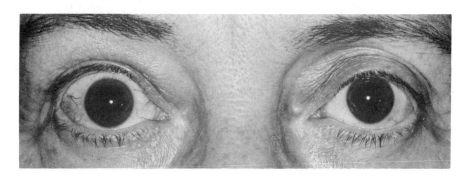

Fig. A-15 Unilateral exophthalmos and lid retraction in hyperthyroidism.

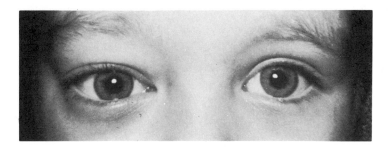

Fig. A-16 Sarcoma of right orbit.

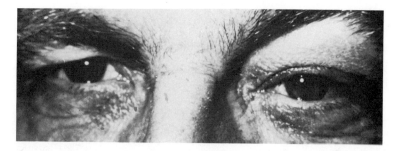

Fig. A-17 Lymphoma of left orbit.

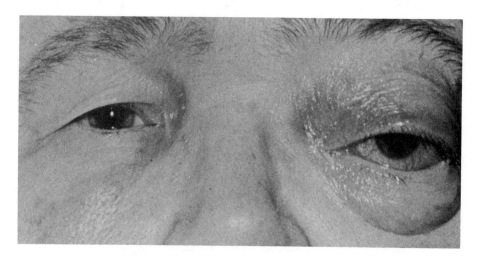

Fig. A-18 Proptosis secondary to sinus disease.

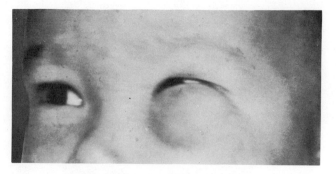

Fig. A-19 Hemangioma of left orbit.

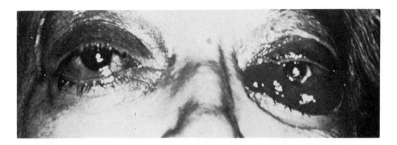

Fig. A-20 Pseudotumor of orbit with severe chemosis of conjunctiva.

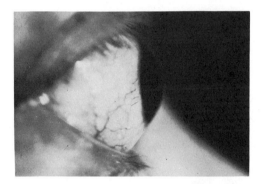

Fig. A-21 Endocrine exophthalmos.

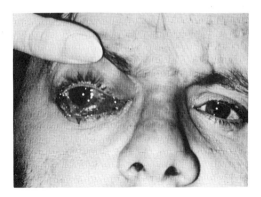

Fig. A-22 Proptosis and chemosis resulting from carotid-cavernous fistula following trauma.

Inflammation of the lids and lacrimal apparatus

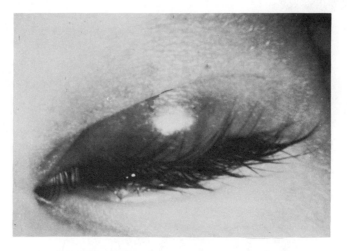

Fig. A-23 Acute internal hordeodum.

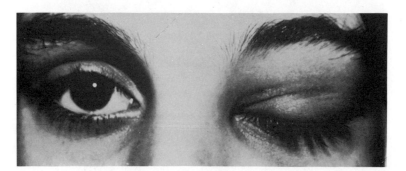

Fig. A-24 Allergic edema of upper eyelid due to insect bite.

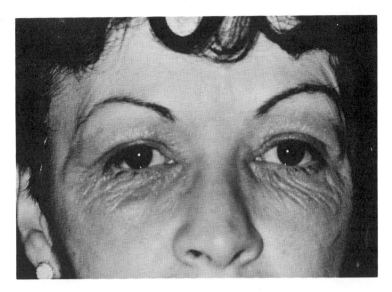

Fig. A-25 Contact dermatitis secondary to makeup.

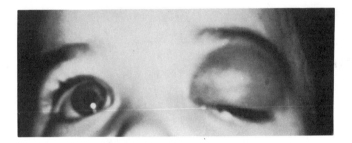

Fig. A-26 Orbital cellulitis secondary to ethmoiditis.

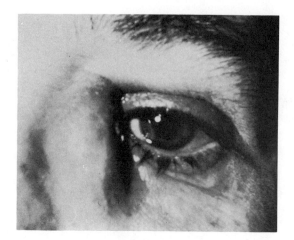

Fig. A-27 Dacryocystitis.

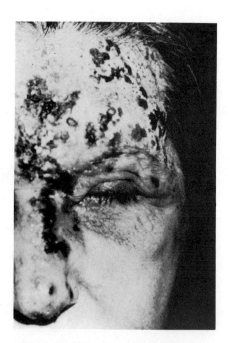

Fig. A-28 Herpes zoster ophthalmicus.

Disorders of the conjunctiva

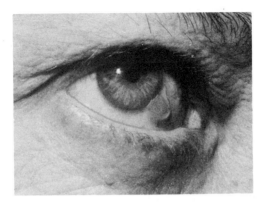

Fig. A-29 Tumor of the limbus.

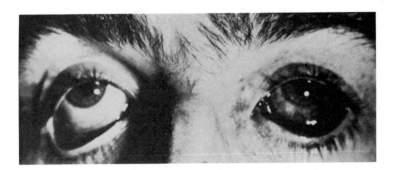

Fig. A-30 Conjunctivitis.

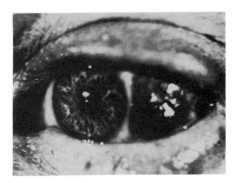

Fig. A-31 Subconjunctival hemorrhage.

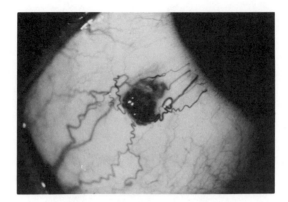

Fig. A-32 Vascular tumor of the conjunctiva.

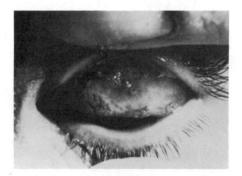

Fig. A-33 Acute meibomian cyst along with giant papules of the conjunctiva.

Benign and malignant tumors
of the eyelids

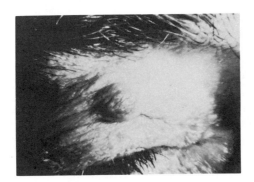

Fig. A-34 Sebaceous cyst of eyelid.

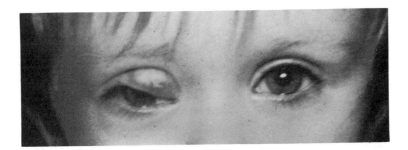

Fig. A-35 Hemangioma of eyelid.

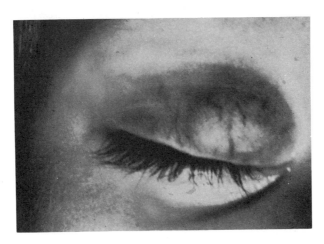

Fig. A-36 Hemangioma of eyelid.

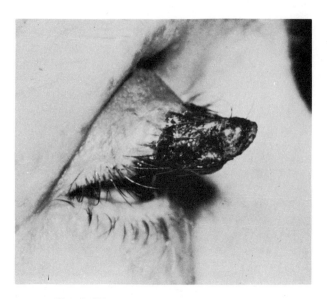

Fig. A-37 Keratoacanthoma of upper eyelid.

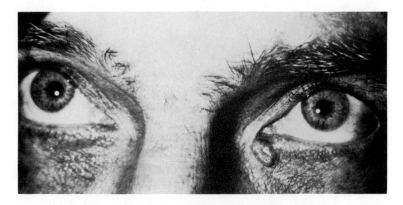

Fig. A-38 Basal cell carcinoma of skin of left eyelid.

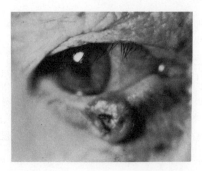

Fig. A-39 Basal cell carcinoma of lower eyelid margin.

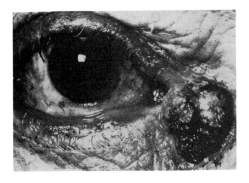

Fig. A-40 Squamous cell carcinoma of skin over lacrimal sac.

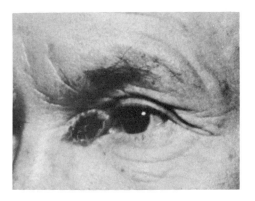

Fig. A-41 Basal cell carcinoma of inner canthus.

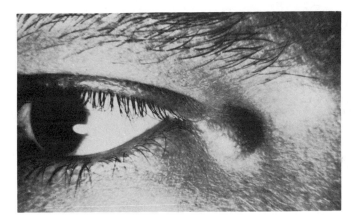

Fig. A-42 Angular dermoid cyst.

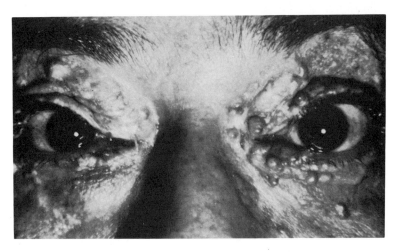

Fig. A-43 Multiple papillomas of eyelids.

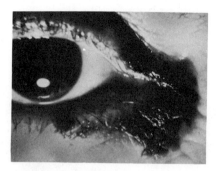

Fig. A-44 Melanoma of the skin.

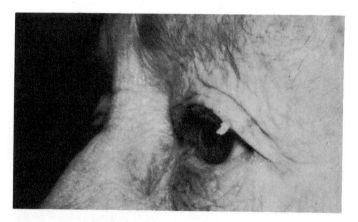

Fig. A-45 Cutaneous horn.

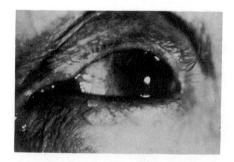

Fig. A-46 Verruca of lower eyelid.

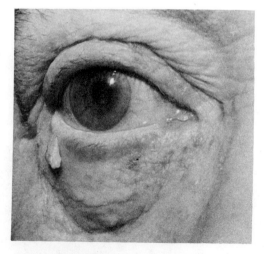

Fig. A-47 Papilloma of eyelid.

Disorders of the cornea

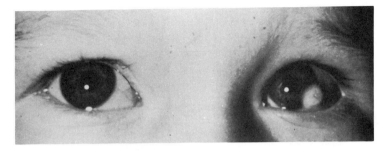

Fig. A-48 Congenital dermoid of the limbus.

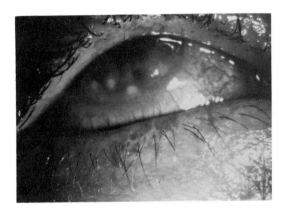

Fig. A-49 Marginal infiltrates secondary to staphyloccocus aureus.

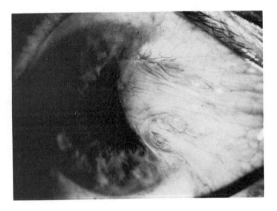

Fig. A-50 Active recurrent ptergium extending across cornea.

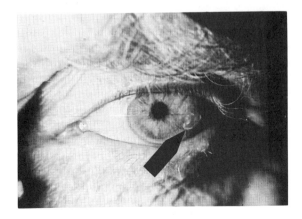

Fig. A-51 Bowen's disease. Carcinoma in situ at the limbus.

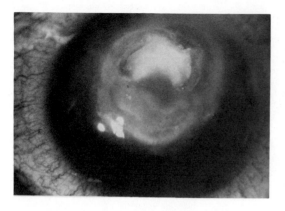

Fig. A-52 Corneal ulceration caused by pseudomonas.

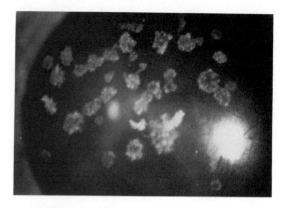

Fig. A-53 Granular dystrophy of the cornea.

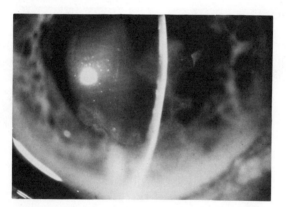

Fig. A-54 Geographic corneal ulcer due to herpes simplex virus.

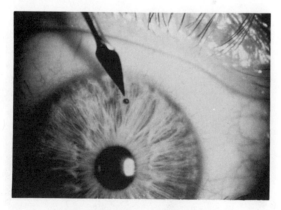

Fig. A-55 Corneal foreign body.

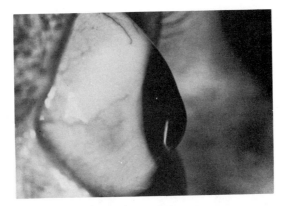

Fig. A-56 Keratoconus.

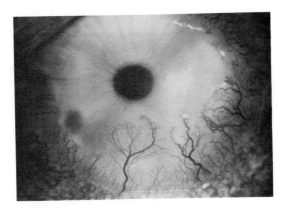

Fig. A-57 Corneal vascularization in a patient with severe blepharitis.

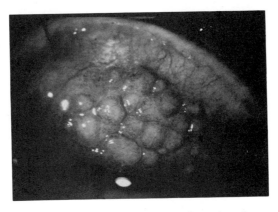

Fig. A-58 Vernal conjunctivitis-cobblestone formation of upper tarsus.

Disorders of the iris

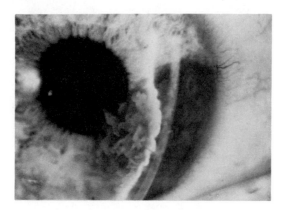

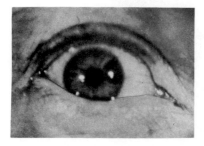

Fig. A-60 Cyst of the iris.

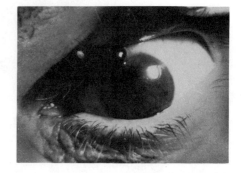

Fig. A-61 Prolapse of the iris at the 11 o'clock position due to trauma.

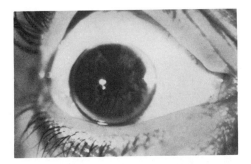

Fig. A-62 Peripheral iridectomy.

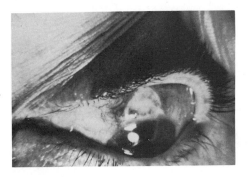

Fig. A-63 Filtering bleb after glaucoma surgery.

Disorders of the fundus

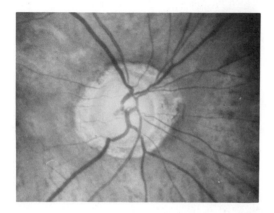

Fig. A-64 Glaucomatous disc cupping. Notice the inferotemporal vessel that is kinked at the disc margin.

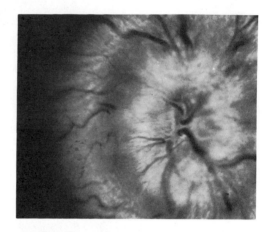

Fig. A-65 Papilledema of the optic disc.

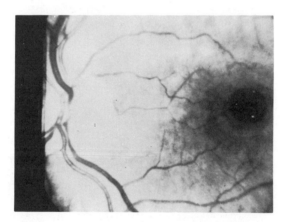

Fig. A-66 Hole in the macula.

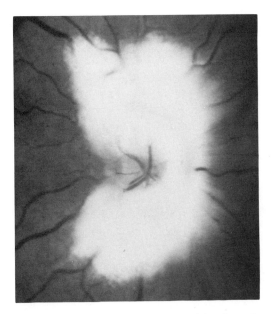

Fig. A-67 Myelinated nerve fibers arising from the optic disc.

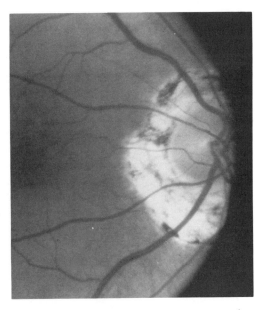

Fig. A-68 Presumed ocular histoplasmosis with peripapillary scarring and a few atrophic lesions of the macula.

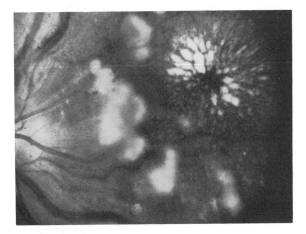

Fig. A-69 Hypertensive retinopathy advanced with cotton wool exudates and macular star.

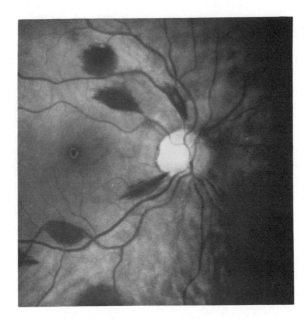

Fig. A-70 Retinopathy of acute leukemia.

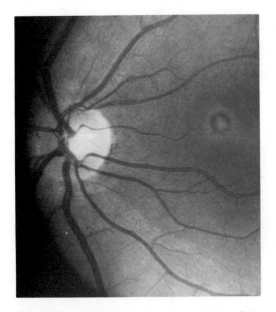

Fig. A-71 Subretinal neovascular membrane of the macula.

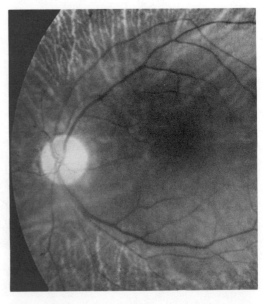

Fig. A-72 Retinitis pigmentosa with a waxy colored disc, narrowing of the arterioles, and midperipheral pigment clumping.

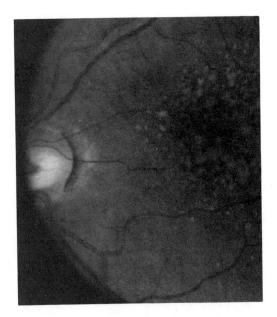

Fig. A-73 Macular degeneration.

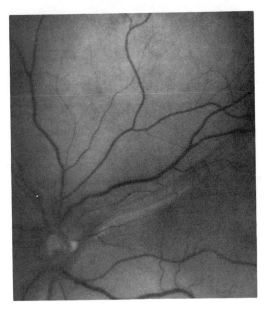

Fig. A-74 Metastatic lesions of the choroid from breast carcinoma.

Miscellaneous

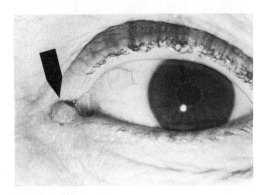

Fig. A-75 Syringoma of the caruncle.

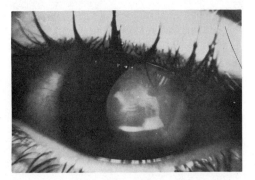

Fig. A-76 Dislocated cataractous lens into the anterior chamber

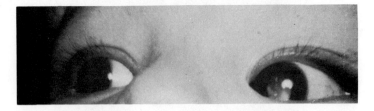

Fig. A-77 Retinoblastoma of left eye with white pupil.

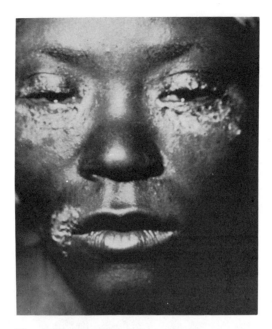

Fig. A-78 Vitamin deficiency—severe ulcerative blepharoconjunctivitis.

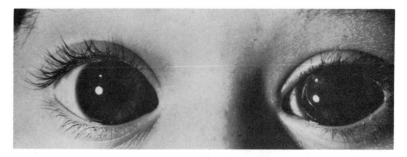

Fig. A-79 Congenital glaucoma (buphthalmos).

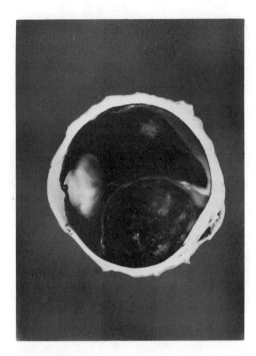

Fig. A-80 Malignant melanoma of the choroid.

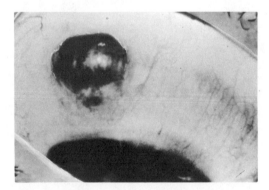

Fig. A-81 Staphyloma of the choroid in absolute glaucoma.

Appendixes

APPENDIX I Office supplies in common use

Cotton balls
Sterile eye pads
Adhesive tape (½ inch)
Cellophane tape
Nonallergenic tape
2 ml syringes
No. 27 or No. 30 needles
Bacteriological swabs
Specimen bottles, pathology and bacteriology
Towels
Cotton applicators
Eye shields
Bard-Parker blades
Penlights
Super blades
Assorted batteries

Assorted bulbs
Beaver blades (disposable)
Kidney basin
Smelling salts
Local anesthetics
Schirmer papers
Sterile fluorescein papers
Alcohol
Sterile saline solution
Sterile water (distilled)
Adhesive remover
Germicide solution
Sterile irrigating solution
Rose bengal solution
Fluorescein strips

APPENDIX 2 Estimating visual loss

Loss of central vision in one eye

Visual acuity for distance (Snellen)	Snellen	Meters (D)	Jaeger	Percent visual efficiency*	Percent visual loss
20/20	14/14	0.35	1−	100	0
20/25	14/18	0.44	2−	96	4
20/30	14/21	0.59	—	91	9
20/40	14/28	0.71	3	84	16
20/50	14/35	0.88	6	77	23
20/60	14/42	1.08	—	70	30
20/70	14/49	1.30	7	64	36
20/80	14/56	—	8	59	41
20/100	14/70	1.76	11−	49	51
20/160	14/112	—	14−	29	71
20/200	14/140	3.53	—	20	80
20/400	14/280	7.06	—	3	97

*The percentage of visual efficiency of the two eyes may be determined by the following formula:

$$\frac{(3 \times \%\text{Visual efficiency of better eye}) + \%\text{Visual efficiency of poorer eye}}{4} = \%\text{Binocular visual efficiency}$$

ESTIMATING LOSS OF VISUAL FIELD

A visual field test is performed on the perimeter with a 3-mm test object in each of the eight 45-degree meridians. The sum of each of these meridians is added and the percentage of visual efficiency arrived at by dividing by 485, the total of a normal field. For example:

Normal field	Degrees
Temporally	85
Down and temporally	85
Down	55
Nasally	55
Up and nasally	55
Down and nasally	50
Up	45
Up and temporally	55
TOTAL	485

Constricted field	Degrees
Temporally	45
Down and temporally	25
Down	30
Down and nasally	25
Nasally	25
Up and nasally	25
Up	25
Up and temporally	35
TOTAL	235

$$\%\text{Visual efficiency} \frac{235 \times 100}{485} = 46\%$$

APPENDIX 3 Short forms in clinical use

Acc	accommodation	RH	right hyperphoria
add	addition	LH	left hyperphoria
od	right eye *(oculus dexter)*	PD or IPD	interpupillary distance
os	left eye *(oculus sinister)*	NPA	near point of accommodation
ou	both eyes *(oculi unitas)*	NPC	near point of convergence
RE	right eye	MR	medial rectus (muscle)
LE	left eye	LR	lateral rectus (muscle)
NV	near vision	SR	superior rectus (muscle)
PH	pinhole	IR	inferior rectus (muscle)
V	vision or visual acuity	SO	superior oblique (muscle)
mm	millimeter	IO	inferior oblique (muscle)
mg	milligram	BO	base out
SC	without correction	BI	base in
CC	with correction	BD	base down
HM	hand movements	BU	base up
LP	light perception	NRC	normal retinal correspondence
MR	Maddox rod	ARC	abnormal retinal correspondence
L & A	light and accommodation	J1, J2, J3, etc	test types for reading vision
EOMB	extraocular muscle balance	N5, N6, etc	test types for near vision
EOM	extraocular movements	bid or bd	twice daily
CF	counting fingers	tid or td	three times daily
XP	exophoria	qid	four times daily
XT	exotropia	ac	before meals
W	wearing	pc	after meals
IOP	intraocular pressure	ic	between meals
T	tension	ne rep or non rep	do not repeat
ung	ointment		
A	applanation tensions	oculent	eye ointment
KP	keratic precipitates	per os	orally, by mouth
PSC	posterior subcapsular cataract	prn	when required, as necessary
ASC	anterior subcapsular cataract	qh	every hour
ET	esotropia	q2h	every 2 hours
°	degree	qs	quantity sufficient
Δ	prism diopter	stat	at once
D	diopter		

The following abbreviations may sometimes be found on ophthalmic charts:

VA	visual acuity	E_1	esophoria for distance
VAc or VAcc	visual acuity with correction	E^1	esophoria for near
VAs or VAsc	visual acuity without correction	ET_1	esotropia for distance
VA	visual acuity with the unaided	ET^1	esotropia for near
OT	eye	X_1	exophoria for distance
AT or Appl	ocular tension	X^1	exophoria for near
ST	applanation tension	$E(T)$	intermittent esotropia
EOM	Schiötz tension extraocular	$X(T)$	intermittent exotropia
	muscle	dd	disc diameters

APPENDIX 4 **Vision and driving**

Good vision is essential for the proper and safe operation of a motor vehicle. Generally, available vision-testing instruments can be used to ascertain if a person has adequate vision to meet specific standards set by the various state licensing jurisdictions. Because of the increasing injury and death toll resulting from traffic accidents, many of which may be related to visual impairment, physicians should consider it a medical obligation to diagnose visual deficiencies and to inform the patient of potential hazards involved in driving with such deficiencies.

There is no practical way of testing alertness or cerebral perception of what the eye focuses on, but it is important for drivers to have their eyes periodically examined for defects that can be evaluated. This is particularly important for those drivers with significant progressive visual deterioration.

In general, if any doubt exists about a person's visual ability to operate an automobile safely, the physician should not hesitate to recommend road tests for specific evaluation of visual skills.

Visual acuity. Automobile drivers with corrected central visual acuity of 20/40 or better generally read traffic signs and note obstructions, vehicles, and pedestrians while driving at usual speeds, whereas those with optimally corrected vision of 20/70 or less in the better eye have a serious limitation and should not drive.

Drivers with visual acuity between 20/40 and 20/70 should be referred to an ophthalmologist to ascertain if their vision can be improved. The physi-

cian, in serving the best interests of patients, should consider the conditions under which each patient drives and the presence or absence of associated defects. The physician is then in a position to advise the patient against driving under certain conditions, such as congested traffic, hazardous road conditions, bad weather, high speed, or at night. It is hoped that continuing research will more exactly define the criteria on which to advise patients.

One-eyed drivers and spectacle-corrected aphakic drivers have visual field limitations and present an increased risk of intersectional crashes. Most postoperative aphakic patients, particularly those in advanced years, also have increased difficulty with night vision and dynamic visual responses. They require special evaluation. Preoperative cataract patients, with early to moderate changes in the lenses of the eye, similarly have night-driving limitations (glare intolerance and reduced night vision) that generally preclude night driving. Patients requiring pupil-constricting medication, as in the control of chronic glaucoma, also have limitation for night operation.

Visual fields. Visual fields are obviously important for safe driving, since a driver must possess some breadth or lateral awareness to pass approaching vehicles safely and to be aware of vehicles or pedestrians approaching from the side.

Although visual form fields of 140 degrees generally are considered adequate for drivers of private motor vehicles, that figure should be considered as the absolute minimum for drivers of commercial and passenger-carrying vehicles. Such drivers also must have coordinate use of both eyes, as well as a corrected acuity of at least 20/30 in the better eye and

Adapted from the American Medical Association: *Physician's guide for determining driver limitation,* Chicago, 1968, The Association.

no worse than 20/40 in the poorer eye. Individuals with lesser fields have driver limitation and must be evaluated for the driving of private vehicles on the basis of the conditions under which they drive, the amount of lateral vision retained, and underlying ocular pathologic conditions.

Persons with markedly constricted fields, such as those from advanced glaucoma or retinitis pigmentosa, have distinct driver limitation and should be so advised.

Ocular muscle imbalance. Ocular muscle imbalance (heterophoria) is an indirect cause of automotive accidents in that it may cause driver fatigue. If sudden diplopia occurs, the accident may be directly attributable to the diplopia. Therefore, patients with uncontrolled or intermittent diplopia have definite driver limitation.

Color blindness. Impaired or defective color vision has been considered a potential cause of highway accidents. However, most traffic lights have been standardized, at least regionally; and it is doubtful if this deficiency is too hazardous, except in severe cases. A completely color-blind, or achromatic, person has very poor vision and should not drive under any circumstance. This also applies to the very limited number of persons who have severe protanopia, or red deficiency.

Dark adaptation. Dark adaptation and susceptibility to glare are of great importance in night driving, but testing procedures and standards are still largely empiric and not a component of routine eye tests. Dark glasses should never be worn for night driving, and the windshield tinting should be limited to the upper one third.

Depth perception. Current testing techniques in the near range do not have significant correlation with distance visual requirements in driving but are adequate for determining visual ability for such tasks as parking. The road test, however, is still the best and most practical guide in this area.

APPENDIX 5 Optical constants of the eye

Optical constants of the eye are summarized as follows:

1. The curvature of the anterior face of the cornea is 7.5 mm.
2. The index of refraction of the corneal tissue, the aqueous humor, and the vitreous equals 1.332.
3. The distance separating the anterior pole of the cornea from the posterior pole of the crystalline lens is 3.6 mm.
4. The curvature of the anterior face of the crystalline lens measures 10.0 mm.
5. The curvature of the posterior face of the crystalline lens is 6.0 mm.
6. The distance separating the anterior pole of the crystalline lens from the posterior pole of the crystalline lens is 4.0 mm.
7. The main refraction index of the crystalline lens equals 1.40.
8. The dioptric power of the cornea equals 44.26 D.
9. The dioptric power of the crystalline lens alone, when both of its surfaces are immersed in a medium having an index of 1.332, equals 17.82 D.
10. The total power of the eye equals 58.53 D.
11. The distance of the first principal plane of the crystalline lens back of the anterior pole of the crystalline lens is 2.4 mm.
12. The distance of the second principal plane of the crystalline lens ahead of the posterior pole of the crystalline lens is 1.4 mm.
13. The distance separating these two planes is 0.2 mm.
14. The distance of the principal plane of the whole eye behind the anterior pole of the whole cornea is 1.370 mm.
15. The distance of the second principal plane of the whole eye behind the anterior pole of the whole cornea is 1.664 mm.
16. The distance separating these two planes is 0.294 mm.

From Hartstein J: *Basics of contact lenses manual,* Rochester, Minn., 1979, American Academy of Ophthalmology.

APPENDIX 6 Criteria for certification and recertification of ophthalmic medical personnel

The Joint Commission on Allied Health Personnel in Ophthalmology, incorporated in 1969, is a federation representing the American Academy of Ophthalmology, American Association of Ophthalmology, American Association of Certified Orthoptists, American Ophthalmological Society, Association of University Professors of Ophthalmology, American Orthopic Council, American Society of Ophthalmic Registered Nurses, Canadian Ophthalmological Society, Contact Lens Association of Ophthalmologists, and Society of Military Ophthalmologists.

It was developed for the purpose of facilitating eye care by (1) encouraging the establishment of medically oriented programs for training allied health personnel in ophthalmology, (2) developing standards of education and training, (3) examining, certifying and recertifying, and (4) encouraging continuing occupational development.

Accreditation of training programs for ophthalmic medical assistants is the responsibility of the Joint Review Committee on Medical Assistants of the American Medical Association, in which JCAHPO plays an important role.

Certification by JCAHPO indicates only that the individuals have fulfilled the criteria requirements qualifying them to provide specific delegated ophthalmic services under the direction of the ophthalmologist in private offices, medical clinics, hospitals, ophthalmic research and teaching centers, and other accredited medical health service facilities.

Certification by JCAHPO does not imply that the individual is qualified to function independently or to be licensed as an independent practitioner in any state or by any agency of the federal government.

The medical ophthalmic assistant certified by JCAHPO does not supplant the ophthalmologist in any professional decision making process of establishing a diagnosis or plan of treatment but assists the ophthalmologist by collecting data and information, thereby allowing him or her to care for more patients, which is in the public interest.

JCAHPO has established three categories of ophthalmic medical personnel who work with ophthalmologists to provide quality medical eye care for the public:

1. Ophthalmic assistant is the basic level of qualification (COA)
2. Ophthalmic technician is the intermediate level of expertise (COT)
3. Ophthalmic technologist is the highest level of expertise (COMT)

Ophthalmic medical personnel at any of the three levels of certification, perform assigned duties as assistants of the ophthalmologist with whom they work. They are neither certified nor licensed as independent practitioners. Thus, they function in a professional setting similar to that in which an x-ray technician works with a physician radiologist, or a medical technician provides information to a physician who is treating a patient. Ophthalmic medical personnel may generate important and preliminary information to be used by the ophthalmologist with whom they work, but ophthalmic medical personnel

Taken in part from Joint Commission on Allied Health Personnel in Ophthalmology, St. Paul, Minn. The booklet, "Criteria for certification and recertification of ophthalmic medical personnel" is published frequently. To obtain the most current publication, the reader is advised to write to JCAHPO, 2025 Woodlane Dr., St. Paul, Minn. 55125-2995.

do not generate medical or surgical diagnoses, or prescriptions to be used by a patient.

Ophthalmic assistant applicants are tested by written examination only. Ophthalmic technician applicants must successfully complete a skill evaluation prior to being tested by the written examination. Ophthalmic technologist applicants are tested by a combination of written examination and a practical performance test. No single reference serves as the basis for these examinations.

Candidates must provide proof of eligibility for certification. If admission is granted based on the provision of incorrect or fraudulent information, certification may be denied.

Performance skills and background knowledge required by ophthalmic medical personnel may vary from one job to another. For this reason the skills have been grouped into the following content areas.

OPHTHALMIC ASSISTANT
Criteria for certification

EDUCATION AND TRAINING: Evidence of high school diploma or equivalent plus successful completion (*within* the past 3 years) of a JRCOMP (Joint Review Committee for Ophthalmic Medical Personnel) approved program for Ophthalmic Assistants: plus a minimum of 1 year of satisfactory, full-time work experience under ophthalmological supervision, including training in all skills listed under Content Areas 1-6.

Equivalency: The following educational alternatives are possible with a high school diploma or equivalent:

Evidence of successful completion (within the past 3 years) of a JRCOMP (Joint Review Committee for Ophthalmic Medical Personnel) approved [e.g. the American Academy of Ophthalmology (AAO) or Canadian Ophthalmological Society (COS)] home study course; plus a minimum of 1 year of satisfactory, full-time work experience under ophthalmological supervision, including training in all skills listed under Content Areas 1-6.

— or —

Evidence of successful completion of a JRCOMP (Joint Review Committee for Ophthalmic Medical Personnel) approved program for Ophthalmic Assistants *more* than 3 years ago; plus 1 year of satisfactory, full-time work experience under ophthalmological supervision including training in all skill areas listed under Content Area 1-6; plus 18 hours of JCAHPO approved continuing education credits (on 1:1 basis) earned within the past 2 years. See section on Continuing Education.

CPR CERTIFICATE: All candidates must submit a copy of a current nationally recognized certificate of competence in cardiopulmonary resuscitation (for example: the American Red Cross or American Heart Association certificates) as part of their application for examination. This certificate must be valid at the time the application is submitted.

ENDORSEMENT: The supervising, sponsoring ophthalmologist must attest by signature to the applicant's current competence in the skills for which certification is sought. (See Content Areas 1-6).

EXAMINATION: The requirement for the Ophthalmic Assistant level is successful completion of a written examination consisting of Content Areas 1-6.

Content areas

The ophthalmic assistant candidate will be examined in all of the following 6 content areas. The assistant candidate may also elect to be examined and certified in the special content area "Ophthalmic Surgical Assisting." The examination will include the following items.

1. **History taking:** Basis and technique for obtaining and recording identifying information of the patient's chief complaint, history of present illness. Obtain and record patient's past ocular history, family history, previous adverse drug reactions and allergies, systemic illness, and details of present medications.
2. **Basic skills and lensometry:** Methods of measuring and recording distance and near vision in children and adults. Pinhole. Color vision testing. Various methods of lensometry including measurement of base curve, power of sphere, power and axis of cylinder, power and orientation of prism, multifocal adds.
3. **Ophthalmic patient services:** Indications for and proper use of eye dressings, protective

shields, safety glasses. Methods of drug delivery including advantages and disadvantages of drops, ointments, sustained release systems, periocular injections, and systemic use of medications. Instillation of topical eye drugs. Measurement of interpupillary distance for far and near, frame sizes; simple adjustments and repairs of spectacles. Proper care of spectacles.

4. **Basic tonometry:** Basic principles, sources of error, advantages and disadvantages of indentation and applanation tonometry. Methods of cleaning and sterilization of tonometers. Concept of ocular rigidity, its effect on the accuracy of indentation tonometry and how ocular rigidity is estimated. The effects on intraocular pressure of squeezing the eyelids, heart beat, breath holding, tight collars, and changes in body position.

5. **Instrument maintenance and repair:** User level maintenance, as prescribed by the manufacturers of the common ophthalmic instruments such as the visual acuity projectors, muscle lights, direct and indirect ophthalmoscopes, retinoscopes, lensometers, tangent screens, perimeters, slit lamps and keratometers, and sterilization of surgical instruments.

6. **General medical knowledge and cardiopulmonary resuscitation:** Elementary knowledge of the anatomy and physiology of the cardiovascular, respiratory, endocrine, and central nervous systems. Elementary knowledge of the anatomy and physiology of the visual system. Elementary knowledge of the refractive errors of the eye and the more common diseases affecting the visual system. Knowledge that the visual apparatus may be affected by systemic diseases such as hypertension, diabetes mellitus, malignant diseases, atherosclerosis, blood diseases, and generalized infections. Principles of first aid treatment for fainting, acute drug reactions, and cardiac arrest. Ocular emergencies. Fundamentals of microbial control, including procedures for sanitation, disinfection, and sterilization.

OPHTHALMIC TECHNICIAN
Criteria for certification

EDUCATION AND TRAINING: Evidence of high school diploma or equivalent plus successful completion (within the past 12 months) of a CAHEA (AMA Committee on Allied Health Education and Accreditation) accredited program for Ophthalmic Medical Technicians.

Equivalency: The following educational alternatives are possible with a high school diploma or equivalent:

Evidence of successful completion of a CAHEA accredited program for Ophthalmic Medical Technicians *more* than 12 months ago; plus 1 year of satisfactory, full-time work experience under ophthalmological supervision including training in all skills listed under Content Areas 1-12; plus 18 hours of JCAHPO approved continuing education credits (on 1:1 basis) earned within the past 2 years. See section on Continuing Education.

— or —

Certification and maintenance of active status as an Ophthalmic Assistant; plus at least 1 year of satisfactory, full-time work experience as a COA under ophthalmological supervision, including training in all skills listed under Content Areas 1-12; plus 18 hours of JCAHPO approved continuing education credits (on 1:1 basis) earned within the past 2 years.

— or —

Current certification as an Orthoptist by the American or Canadian Orthoptic Council; plus 1 year of satisfactory, full-time work experience as a Certified Orthoptist (CO) under ophthalmological supervision including training in all skills listed under Content Areas 1-12; plus 12 hours of JCAHPO approved continuing education credits (on 1:1 basis) earned within the past 2 years. See section on Continuing Education.

SKILL EVALUATION: Candidates for certification at the technician level will be required to have successfully completed a Skill Evaluation in order to qualify for the written examination. Skill Evaluation sessions are scheduled periodically throughout the year in centers across the U.S. and Canada. See Skill Evaluation on pages 860-861.

CPR CERTIFICATE: All candidates must submit a copy of a current, nationally recognized certificate of competence in cardiopulmonary resuscitation (for example: the American Red Cross or American Heart Association certificates). This certificate must be valid at the time the application is submitted.

ENDORSEMENT: The supervising, sponsoring ophthalmologist must attest by signature to the applicant's current competence in all skills for which certification is sought. (See Content Areas 1-12).

EXAMINATION: The requirement for the Ophthalmic Technician level is successful completion of a Skill Evaluation and a written examination consisting of Content Areas 1-12.

Written examination

The ophthalmic technician candidate will be examined in all Content Areas 1-12. The technician candidate may also elect to be examined and certified in the special content area "Ophthalmic Surgical Assisting" (see below).

7. **Clinical optics:** Knowledge of the difference between refraction and refractometry; principles and techniques for retinoscopy; fogging techniques with astigmatic dials; cross-cylinder refinement; duochrome test; measurement of accommodation; determination of whether spectacle lenses are glass or plastic and whether glass lenses are heat-treated; measurement and calculation of decentration of lenses and vertex distance.

8. **Ocular motility:** Knowledge of the actions of extraocular muscles; primary position; the nine diagnostic directions of gaze; paralytic vs. concomitant strabismus; primary vs secondary deviations; phorias and tropias; use of Maddox rod and Maddox wing: Worth 4-dot test; fusion, diplopia; steropsis tests; near point of convergence, ductions, versions and vergences.

9. **Visual field testing:** Knowledge of basic concept of field of vision and its measurement by kinetic methods; different methods of measuring central and peripheral visual fields with arc and bowl-type perimeters and tangent screens including the relative merits of each method; factors which influence size of the visual field and the common sources of error in visual field testing; performance and recording of visual field measurement; appropriate care, maintenance and calibration of instruments; use of multiple targets in examining field defects; need for spectacle correction; definition of the major types of visual field defects; screening methods of glaucomatous and neurological visual field defects.

10. **Contact lenses:** Basic knowledge of types and relative merits of hard and soft contact lenses; parameters required for contact lens fitting including measurement of palpebral fissure width, corneal diameter and curvature, pupil diameter, lid tightness and adequacy of tear secretion; Schirmer tests; conversion of spectacle data into contact lens data; use of fluorescein to assess hard lens fit; insertion and removal of contact lenses; instruction to patients; verification of contact lenses received from manufacturers.

11. **Intermediate tonometry:** Knowledge of aqueous humor dynamics and their influence on tonometry; basic clinical types and mechanism of glaucoma; structural ocular change related to glaucoma and their correlation with visual field defects; basic knowledge of medical and surgical method of treatment of glaucoma.

12. **Ocular pharmacology:** Knowledge of names and actions of the commonly used topical anesthetics, mydriatics, cycloplegics, and miotics; knowledge of names and use of topical steroids and antibiotics; knowledge of allergic and other common adverse reactions to drugs.

Skill evaluation

The skill evaluation is a screening procedure, designed to ascertain the candidates' readiness for the written examination at the technician level. Candidates for certification at the technician level will be required to successfully complete a skill evaluation before applying for the written examination. Skill evaluations are held routinely at various locations throughout the U.S. and Canada. Please contact the JCAHPO office for application forms and the specific dates and locations of scheduled skill evaluations.

Prerequisites

Education: Evidence of current enrollment in or successful completion of a CAHEA (AMA Committee on Allied Health Education and Accreditation) accredited institutional course for ophthalmic medical technicians, evidence of successful completion (within the past 3 years) of an approved home study course, or evidence of current certification by the American or Canadian Orthoptic Council. Current certification as an Ophthalmic Assistant.

Training: A total of 1 year of satisfactory full-time work experience under ophthalmological supervision that includes training in all of the skills listed under Content Areas 1-12.

Skill areas

Candidates will be required to perform all selected tasks within 1 hour. A number of tasks will be selected within the following skill areas. Candidates will be expected to:

1. Clinical optics	Perform lensometry
	Perform refractometry/retinoscopy
2. Ocular motility	Demonstrate the actions of extraocular muscles
3. Visual fields	Plot a non-automated visual field, using acceptable methods, e.g., Goldmann, tangent screen, etc.
4. Contact lens	Perform keratometry
5. Tonometry	Demonstrate the operation of a Schiøtz tonometer
	Demonstrate the ability to perform applanation tonometry

Two-year limit

Successful completion of a skill evaluation shall take place within the 2 years before taking the written technician examination.

Candidates who do not successfully complete a skill evaluation may repeat it at a future session. There is no limit to the number of times candidates may attempt the skill evaluation.

OPHTHALMIC TECHNOLOGIST
Criteria for certification

EDUCATION AND TRAINING: Evidence of successful completion of a 4-year college degree program in Ophthalmic Technology accredited by CAHEA (AMA Committee on Allied Health Education and Accreditation). The applicant must be endorsed by the program director. No additional work experience is required.

Equivalency: The following educational alternatives are possible:

Evidence of 2 or more years of successfully completed college level courses (90 quarter or 60 semester credits); plus evidence of successful completion of a CAHEA (AMA Committee on Allied Health Education and Accreditation) accredited program for ophthalmic medical technologists completed within the past 5 years; plus 12 hours of JCAHPO approved continuing education credits (on 1:1 basis) for each year following graduation. See section on Continuing Education.

— or —

Less than 2 years or no college with a high school diploma or equivalent, but evidence of successful completion of a 2-year ophthalmic medical technology program accredited by CAHEA (AMA Committee on Allied Health Education and Accreditation); plus 2 years of satisfactory, full-time work experience (within the last 5 years) under ophthalmological supervision; plus 12 hours of JCAHPO approved continuing education credits (on 1:1 basis) for each year following graduation. See section on Continuing Education.

— or —

Certification and maintenance of active status as an Ophthalmic Technician; plus a minimum of 3 years (within the last 5 years) of satisfactory, full-time work experience under ophthalmological supervision; plus 36 hours of JCAHPO approved continuing education credits (on 1:1 basis) earned within the past 3 years. See section on Continuing Education.

— or —

Evidence of current certification by the American or

Canadian Orthoptic Council; plus a minimum of 2 years (within the last 5 years) of satisfactory, full-time work experience under ophthalmological supervision after certification, which included all of the skills listed under Content Areas 1-22; plus 24 hours of JCAHPO approved continuing education credit (on a 1:1 basis) earned within the past 3 years. See section on Continuing Education.

CPR CERTIFICATE: All candidates must submit a copy of a current, nationally recognized certificate of competence in cardiopulmonary resuscitation (for example: the American Red Cross or American Heart Association certificates) as part of their application for examination. This certificate must be valid at the time the application is submitted.

ENDORSEMENT: The supervising, sponsoring ophthalmologist must attest by signature to the applicant's current competence in the skills for which certification is sought (see Content Areas 1-22).

EXAMINATION: A written qualifying examination and practical performance test, as described on pages 862-863, are required.

Written examination

The ophthalmic technologist candidate will be examined in Content Areas 1-6 listed for the assistant level and Content Areas 7-12 listed at the technician level. Successful completion of the written examination in these content areas will require greater technical detail and theoretical knowledge than will be required of an ophthalmic technician candidate. Items in Content Areas 13-22 (below) will also be included.

The technologist candidate may also elect to be examined and certified in the special content area "Ophthalmic Surgical Assisting" (see p. 866).

13. **Microbiology:** Inflammatory response and the difference between infection and inflammation. Classification of inflammation into infectious and noninfectious types. Functions and microscopic appearance of the various types of inflammatory cells. Microscopic appearance of intracellular virus inclusions and knowledge of the diseases these cause. Classification of infectious organisms. Procurement and use of Gram, Giemsa, and Wright stains. Use of appropriate culture media for bacteria, fungi, and viruses. Procedures for collecting, labeling, preserving, staining, culturing, and interpreting microbiological specimens from patients with ocular problems.

14. **Advanced tonometry and tonography:** Knowledge of the pathophysiology of glaucoma in general and its effect on ocular structure and function; classification of the types of glaucoma including open-angle and closed-angle, primary and secondary; general principles of the treatment of each type of glaucoma; role of visual field testing in detection and management of glaucoma; principles of indentation and applanation tonometry including their comparative merits and sources of error; detailed care, maintenance and checking of calibration of tonometers and tonography instruments; principles of tonography, its performance and understanding of concepts of facility of outflow, including the use of appropriate tables to obtain these values.

15. **Advanced visual fields:** Knowledge of the principles and performance of dynamic and static visual field studies. Identification and significance of nerve fiber bundle defects, hemianopsias of all types, nasal steps, scotomata, altitudinal defects and functional visual field defects; concept of absolute and relative field defects and steep or sloping margins of field defects.

16. **Advanced color vision:** Knowledge of theories of color vision, congenital and acquired color vision defects and their measurement with color plates, lanterns, multiple hue tests and anomaloscopes.

17. **Advanced clinical optics:** Knowledge of relative merits of subjective and objective refractometry; use of stenopeic slit; calculation of lens problems involving simple and compound lens system; the schematic eye; simple optics of plane and curved mirrors; accommodative range and amplitude and the significance of these in management of pres-

byopia; evaluation of low vision aids and their clinical use.

18. **Advanced ocular motility:** Knowledge of classification and detection of amblyopia; occlusion treatment; extraocular muscle anatomy and physiology including significance and practical application of Hering's law and Sherington's law; differentiation of phoria and tropia; classification of strabismus; AC/A ratio including its measurement and clinical significance; recognition and measurement of convergence insufficiency; recognition and significance of angle kappa; concept and measurement of fusional amplitude; qualitative and quantitative measurement of stereopsis.

19. **Ophthalmic photography:** Knowledge of definition and significance of f-number, f-stop, focal length, depth of field, bellows, macro lens, shutter, film plane, synchronization, single lens reflex, range finder, ASA rating, grain, emulsion, flash intensity, guide number, fundus photography, fluorescein angiography, exciter filter, barrier filter, adverse reactions to fluorescein and their management, slit-lamp photography, external photography, beam splitters, power packs, and reticles.

20. **Advanced ocular pharmacology:** Knowledge of various forms of eye medications and importance of stability, pH, tonicity, and sterility of such medications. Concept of sympathomimetic, parasympathomimetic and parasympatholytic drugs, including examples and uses of each. Uses of surface and locally injected anesthetics. Uses of epinephrine and hyaluronidase with local anesthesia. Actions and uses of antibiotic, corticosteroids, osmotic agents, carbonic anhydrase inhibitors and other major groups of drugs used in management of glaucoma.

21. **Special instruments and diagnostic techniques:** Elementary knowledge of photocoagulation techniques including xenon-arc and laser coagulation and their uses. Elementary knowledge of CAT scanning and its place in investigation of ophthalmic problems. Theory and application of diagnostic and ophthalmic ultrasound. Basic knowledge about origin, measurement and clinical value of electrooculogram, electroretinogram and the cortical visually-evoked response.

22. **Advanced general medical knowledge:** Conversion of data between metric and other measuring systems. Elementary knowledge of ocular manifestations of systemic disorders such as diabetes mellitus, hypertension, atherosclerosis, endocrine disease, brain tumors, legal and clinical blindness. Institutions and aids for the blind.

Practical performance test

After successful completion of the written examination, the candidate will be invited to take the performance test. This performance test may include the requirement to perform any of the following tasks:

Skill areas:
A. **Microbiology**
   1. Identify the following types of cells under a microscope and/or in a colored photographic reproduction of a microscopic slide; neutrophile, eosinophile, basophile, lymphocyte, epitheloid cell, plasma cell, monocyte.
   2. Identify the following types of bacteria under a microscope and/or in a colored photographic reproduction of a microscopic slide: staphylococci, streptococci, gram-positive diplococci, gram-negative diplococci, gram-negative bacilli (rods).
   3. Using the material provided, perform a Gram stain on a given slide. The examiner will evaluate your technique.
   4. Using the material provided, plate out a culture.

B. **Advanced tonometry**
   1. Measure intraocular pressure using a Schiøtz-type indentation tonometer.
   2. Measure intraocular pressure using a slit lamp-mounted applanation tonometer.

3. Assemble an indentation (Schiøtz-type) tonometer and check its "zero" accuracy on a test block.

4. Check accuracy of the applanation tonometer using the test rod.

5. Adjust the applanation tonometer prism to its proper position for measuring intraocular pressure on a patient with high corneal astigmatism.

C. Visual fields

1. Use a tangent screen and hand-held targets to plot the blind-spot and detect any abnormalities of it; detect and plot any scatoma, within the central 30°.

2. Use a projection-type tangent screen to plot the blind-spot and detect any abnormalities of it; detect and plot a scotoma, and measure the extent of a central scotoma.

3. Calibrate a Goldmann (Haag-Streit) bowl perimeter.

4. Use a bowl perimeter to plot a peripheral isopter and to detect and plot any peripheral field defects. Static and kinetic methods of examination may be tested.

5. Use a bowl perimeter to detect and plot a scotoma within the central 30°. Static and kinetic methods of examination may be tested.

6. Perform Amsler grid test.

D. Advanced color vision testing

1. Measure color vision using the Farnsworth-Munsell 100-hue test.

2. Measure color vision using the Farnsworth D-15 test.

E. Clinical optics

1. Measure refractive error with a retinoscope. MUST be able to use the following for this task: plus-cylinder phoropter, minus-cylinder phoropter, and free lenses (trial frames and trial case).

2. Neutralize a pair of spectacle lenses, measuring with a lensmeter (vertometer) for sphere, cylinder, and axis; for prism if present; for the power of bifocal and trifocal adds.

3. Identify correctly on sight (without an instrument) a seamless (continuous) bifocal add, an aspheric lens, and a lenticular lens.

4. Locate and mark optical centers of a pair of lenses and measure the distance between them.

5. Measure bridge size, eye wire size, and temple length of a pair of spectacle frames.

6. Measure base curve of a lens with a Geneva lens-measure (lens clock).

7. Measure surface curves of a lens with the Geneva lens-measure (lens clock) and arrive at the power of the sphere, the power of the cylinder, and the approximate axis of the cylinder.

8. Measure interpupillary distance (PD) at distance and near (33cm).

9. Measure near point of accommodation (NPA) using a metric rule (Prince, Berens, or other) with full distance correction.

10. Measure vertex distance with a distometer.

11. Measure refractive error with astigmatic dial and cylindrical lenses. MUST be able to use each of the following for this task: minus-cylinder phoropter, plus-cylinder phoropter, and free lenses (trial frames and trial case).

12. Refine axis of cylinder and power of cylinder using a cross-cylinder. MUST be able to use hand-held cross-cylinder and phoropter-mounted cross-cylinder for this task.

13. Refine spherical power.

14. Measure corneal curvature using a keratometer (ophthalmometer).

15. Measure optical power of a hard contact lens using a lensmeter (vertometer).

16. Measure center thickness of a hard contact lens using a thickness gauge. Measure base curve of a contact lens with curvature gauge (radiuscope).

F. Ocular motility

1. Detect and distinguish, at distance and near, with and without spectacle correction, a phoria and a tropia, using "cover" tests and appropriate fixation targets.

2. Measure and distinguish, at distance and near, with and without spectacle correction, a phoria and tropia, using "cover" tests,

prisms (loose or bar), and appropriate fixation targets.

3. Estimate at near, with and without spectacle correction, the amount of tropia, using the Krimsky test.

4. Measure a phoria, at near and at distance, both with and without spectacle correction, using a Maddox rod, prisms (loose or bar), and a fixation light.

5. Measure the near point of convergence (NPC), with and without spectacle correction, using a metric ruler and an appropriate fixation target.

6. Detect and identify limitations of duction in secondary and tertiary positions of fixation.

7. Detect and identify horizontal and vertical tropias in secondary and tertiary positions of gaze (versions).

8. Measure fusional convergence and divergence using prisms (rotary or bar) at distance and near, with and without spectacles, using an appropriate fixation target.

9. Measure patient's amplitude of accommodation.

10. Measure patient's stereo acuity.

G. Photography

1. Demonstrate ability to take a proper fundus photograph.

2. Demonstrate ability to take a proper external photograph.

3. Demonstrate ability to prepare for fluorescein angiography.

4. Based on an external ophthalmic photograph, a slit-lamp photograph, a fluorescein fundus angiogram, a fundus photograph (or any of the foregoing in combination), identify the following errors in technique:
Subject out of focus
Subject not centered
Film overexposed
Film underexposed
Film not exposed
Film incompletely advanced
Camera back open at wrong time
Flash not synchronized with shutter

Blurring as a result of movement of camera or subject
Slit beam not centered
Slit beam not focused
Wrong illumination technique selected
Camera not aligned with pupil
Series of angiograms begun too late
Eyelids obscuring view
Lids not adequately separated
Camera positioned too far from eye
Camera positioned too close to eye

5. Based on the fluorescein fundus angiogram photographs, identify the following phases:
1. Redfree
2. Preinjection/control
3. Choroidal
4. Arterial
5. Early venous
6. Late venous
7. Late

H. Special instruments and techniques

1. Demonstrate ability to perform an axial length measurement using a biometer.

Equipment required. Candidates should bring the following pieces of equipment to the practical performance test.

Retinoscope—bringing a battery-handle retinoscope which the candidate customarily uses will reduce the possibility of being confronted with an unfamiliar type of retinoscope.

Occluder—should be combined with either a red lens or a Maddox rod lens.

Pen light—a muscle light or a transilluminator will be a workable substitute.

Ruler—calibrated in millimeters and inches and approximately 6 or 7 inches long.

Accommodative target
Five-year limit

Persons who pass the Technologist written examination shall be allowed two attempts at the Practical Performance Test within 5 years of having passed the written examination.

If the candidate fails the Practical Performance Test twice or if he or she does not successfully complete the test within 5 years, the written examination *must be successfully completed again* before a further Practical Performance Test is taken.

Non-certified Technologist candidates who do not pass the Practical Performance Test will be awarded an Assistant certification. Technologist candidates who wish to receive a certified Ophthalmic Technician certificate upon passing the written Technologist examination *must* successfully complete a Skill Evaluation before a certificate can be awarded (see Skill Evaluation, pages 17-18). This provision allows noncertified candidates to receive a Technician certification until they pass the Practical Performance Test.

OPHTHALMIC SURGICAL ASSISTING: Ophthalmic Surgical Assisting is a special content area in which a candidate may be examined and awarded a certificate of proficiency.

The examination will include the following:

Preoperative preparation of the ocular surgical patient; identification, selection and maintenance of ophthalmic surgical instruments; sterilization and setup of instruments for ophthalmic surgical procedures; scrubbing; and assisting the ophthalmic surgeon in an office setting and in a hospital operating room.

Certification at the Assistant, Technician or Technologist level, or acceptance for one of the certifying examinations scheduled on the same day, is required. If a non-certified candidate fails the certifying examination, the Ophthalmic Surgical Assisting examination is rendered invalid.

Criteria for certification

EDUCATION AND TRAINING: Graduate of a CAHEA (AMA Committee on Allied Health Education and Accreditation) accredited program for ophthalmic medical personnel which includes instruction and supervised experience in Ophthalmic Surgical Assisting, completed within the past 12 months.

— or —

Equivalency: The following educational alternatives are possible:

Graduate of a CAHEA (AMA Committee on Allied Health Education and Accreditation) accredited program for ophthalmic medical personnel which includes instruction and supervised experience in Ophthalmic Surgical Assisting completed more than 12 months ago; plus evidence of 6 months on-the-job work experience completed within the last 12 months in an operating suite (accredited by Joint Commission on Accreditation of Healthcare Organizations [JCAHO] or other NATIONALLY RECOGNIZED ACCREDITING AGENCY), under the supervision of regularly scheduling ophthalmic surgeons, one of whom is the candidate's sponsoring ophthalmologist.

— or —

Satisfactory completion of a full-time academic year (9 months) or equivalent program in a hospital-based surgical technologist (operating room technician) course; including 6 months of satisfactory on-the-job instruction and experience in an operating suite (accredited by Joint Commission on Accreditation of Healthcare Organizations [JCAHO] or other NATIONALLY RECOGNIZED ACCREDITING AGENCY), completed within the last 12 months, under the supervision of regularly scheduling ophthalmic surgeons, one of whom is the candidate's sponsoring ophthalmologist.

— or —

Satisfactory completion of 18 months on-the-job instruction and experience* in an operating suite (accredited by Joint Commission on Accreditation of Healthcare Organizations [JCAHO] or other NATIONALLY RECOGNIZED ACCREDITING AGENCY) functioning as a sterile first assistant or sterile scrub assistant or non-sterile circulator under the supervision of regularly scheduling ophthalmic surgeons, one of whom is the candidate's sponsoring ophthalmologist.

CPR CERTIFICATE: All candidates must submit a copy of a current, nationally recognized certificate of competence in cardiopulmonary resuscitation (for example: the American Red Cross or the American

---

*On-the-job experience used as criterion for the Ophthalmic Surgical Assisting examination must be earned *not more* than 3 years before the candidate's examination date.

Heart Association certificates). This certificate must be valid at the time the application is submitted.

ENDORSEMENT: The supervising and sponsoring ophthalmologist must sign and attest to the candidate's current competence in operating room skills in the designated area.

EXAMINATION: The candidate must successfully complete the written examination in this Content Area.

CONTINUING EDUCATION
Selection

The selection of continuing education topics is the responsibility of the individual and should be based on the need to upgrade, extend or expand his/her skills and knowledge in the field of ophthalmology. Credit will not be given for courses which are not directly related to ophthalmology, e.g., CPR, clerical skills, management skills. The continuing education credits required for recertification must be earned during the 3-year period prior to applying for recertification.

Credits

JCAHPO recognizes continuing education credits as follows:

JCAHPO courses offered at the Continuing Education Program presented at the time of the AAO Annual Meeting each fall are approved on a 1 to 1 basis (1 hour of class = 1 hour of continuing education credit). Verification of attendance (a brief statement on official letterhead) is required.

JCAHPO courses offered regionally, concurrently with the AAO Regional Update courses are approved on a 1 to 1 basis (1 hour of class = 1 hour of continuing education credit). Verification of attendance (a brief statement on official letterhead) is required.

Regional courses that have applied for and been given prior approval by JCAHPO also offer continuing education credits on a 1 to 1 basis. Verification of attendance (a brief statement on official letterhead) is required.

Certified Ophthalmic Medical Technologists may earn continuing education credits on a 1 to 1 basis by attending courses which are recognized for physician's Continuing Medical Education in Ophthalmology, Category 1 on topics included in Content Areas 1 through 22 and Ophthalmic Surgical Assisting, provided they are specifically appropriate to the duties of ophthalmic technologists. Ticket stubs are acceptable as certification of attendance.

Courses which are recognized for physician's Continuing Medical Education in Ophthalmology, Category 1 are automatically accepted by JCAHPO on a 2 to 1 basis (2 hours of class = 1 hour of continuing education credit for Certified Ophthalmic Assistants and Certified Ophthalmic Technicians). Verification of attendance is required. (When not provided by course sponsor, ticket stubs or a brief statement from the sponsoring ophthalmologist attesting to the candidate's participation will be accepted.)

Self study in ophthalmology (e.g., tapes, reading, attendance of non-JCAHPO approved courses, etc.) is accepted on a 4 to 1 basis (4 hours of self study = 1 hour of continuing education credit). The number of credits earned on the basis of self study is limited for each level of ophthalmic medical assistant. Verification by the sponsoring ophthalmologist is required.

For certification

All credits required to meet the education criteria for certification (as distinguished from recertification) must be earned on the basis of 1 to 1.

RECERTIFICATION

It is the responsibility of the certificate holder to apply for recertification every 3 years. JCAHPO will provide the necessary forms before the end of the current certification period. The completed application for recertification must be received before the new recertification period. Please notify the JCAHPO office of any change in your name or address.

CPR certificate

All candidates must submit a copy of a current, nationally recognized certificate of competence in cardiopulmonary resuscitation (for example, the

American Red Cross or American Heart Association certificates) as part of their application for recertification.

Continuing education

The continuing education requirements for recertification must be earned during the 3-year period just before applying for recertification. Candidates are encouraged to obtain a portion of the required continuing education credits each calendar year. They are:

Ophthalmic assistant: 18 hours, 9 of which may be on the basis of self study.

Ophthalmic technician: 27 hours, 14 of which may be on the basis of self study.

Ophthalmic technologist: 36 hours, 18 of which may be on the basis of self study.

Exceptions may be made for certified persons in isolated areas who may use self study to meet the entire requirement. Such cases will be judged individually on written request by the applicant.

A maximum of 25% of the total Continuing Education credits required may be earned by teaching JCAHPO approved courses (1 hour of teaching = 1 hour of continuing education credit).

A maximum of 25 percent of the total continuing education credits required may be earned by participation as an evaluator in JCAHPO's Skill Evaluations (one continuing education credit per session).

A maximum of 50% of the total Continuing Education Credits required may be earned through authorship or co-authorship of scientific publications.

Eligibility for this equivalency will be determined by individual evaluation.

Endorsement

The supervising/sponsoring ophthalmologist must attest by signature to the applicant's current active status as an ophthalmic medical assistant.

Inactive status

Individuals who fail to recertify will automatically be placed on inactive status. Recertification will be granted to the ophthalmic medical personnel who have been inactive in the field for no more than 6 consecutive years since the expiration of the last certification period, provided they have fulfilled all continuing education requirements during that time (either yearly or cumulatively) and have the endorsement of an ophthalmologist. Inactive status will be granted one time only.

Appealing recertification denial

Should recertification be denied the applicant may appeal, within 30 days, to the Certification Committee for a review. Should this appeal be denied, the applicant may further appeal to the Commission for a decision, which shall be binding.

REVOCATION

Failure to recertify before the 6-year deadline (see Inactive Status, above) will result in automatic revocation of JCAHPO certification. Following revocation, the individual must reapply for examination by JCAHPO.

APPENDIX 7 Metric conversion

	When you know	Multiply by	To find
Length	inches (in)	2.5	centimeters (cm)
	feet (ft)	30.4	centimeters
	miles	1.6	kilometers (km)
Area	square inches (sq in)	6.5	square centimeters (cm²)
	square miles	2.6	square kilometers (km²)
Weight	ounces (oz)	28.3	grams (g)
	pounds (lb)	0.45	kilograms (kg)
Volume and	teaspoons (tsp)	4.6	milliliters (ml)
capacity	tablespoons (Tbsp)	14.0	milliliters
	fluid ounces (fl oz)	28.0	milliliters
	cups (c)	0.227	liters (L)
	pints (pt)	0.568	liters
	quarts (qt)	1.1	liters
	gallons (gal)	4.5	liters
	cubic inches (cu in)	16.3872	cubic centimeters (cc)
Speed and	miles per hour (mph)	1.609	kilometers per hour (km/h)
velocity	feet per seconds (fps)	30.4	centimeters per second (cm/s)
Temperature	Fahrenheit temperature (°F)	⁵⁄₉ (after subtracting 32)	Celsius temperature (°C)

Mass
1 lb = 0.454 kg
1 kg = 2.205 lb
½ oz = 14.17 g
1 oz = 28.35 g

Length
1 in = 2.540 cm
1 ft = 0.3048 m
1 mi = 1.609 km
10 millimeters (mm) = 1 cm = 0.3937 in
100 cm = 1 m = 39.37 in
1000 m = 1 km = 0.62137 mi

Volume
1 q = 1.1366 L
1 gal = 4.4561 L
½ oz = 15 ml
1 oz = 30 ml
1 ml = 1 cc = 0.338 fl oz
10 cl = 1 deciliter (dl) = 6.1025 in²
10 dl = 1 L = 1.0567 liquid qt
100 L = 1 hectoliter (hl) = 26.418 gal

Temperature
0° Celsius = 32° Fahrenheit
0° Fahrenheit = >17.8° Celsius
100° Celsius = 212° Fahrenheit

APPENDIX 8 Diopter to millimeters radius conversion tables

Diopter conversion table

Diopters	mm	Diopters	mm	Diopters	mm	Diopters	mm
20.00	16.875	36.00	9.375	39.00	8.653	42.00	8.035
22.00	15.340	36.12	9.343	39.12	8.627	42.12	8.012
24.00	14.062	36.25	9.310	39.25	8.598	42.25	7.998
26.00	12.980	36.37	9.279	39.37	8.572	42.37	7.965
27.00	12.500	36.50	9.246	39.50	8.544	42.50	7.941
28.00	12.053	36.62	9.216	39.62	8.518	42.62	7.918
29.00	11.638	36.75	9.183	39.75	8.490	42.75	7.894
29.50	11.441	36.87	9.153	39.87	8.465	42.87	7.872
30.00	11.250	37.00	9.121	40.00	8.437	43.00	7.878
30.50	11.065	37.12	9.092	40.12	8.412	43.12	7.826
31.00	10.887	37.25	9.060	40.25	8.385	43.25	8.803
31.50	10.714	37.37	9.031	40.37	8.360	43.37	7.781
32.00	10.547	37.50	9.000	40.50	8.333	43.50	7.758
32.50	10.385	37.62	8.971	40.62	8.308	43.62	7.737
33.00	10.227	37.75	8.940	40.75	8.282	43.75	7.714
33.50	10.075	37.87	8.912	40.87	8.257	43.87	7.693
34.00	9.926	38.00	8.881	41.00	8.231	44.00	7.670
34.25	9.854	38.12	8.853	41.12	8.207	44.12	7.649
34.50	9.783	38.25	8.823	41.25	8.181	44.25	7.627
34.75	9.712	38.37	8.795	41.37	8.158	44.37	7.606
35.00	9.643	38.50	8.766	41.50	8.132	44.50	7.584
35.25	9.574	38.62	8.738	41.62	8.109	44.62	7.563
35.50	9.507	38.75	8.708	41.75	8.083	44.75	7.541
35.75	9.440	38.87	8.682	41.87	8.060	44.87	7.521

Diopters	mm	Diopters	mm	Diopters	mm	Diopters	mm
45.00	7.500	48.00	7.031	51.00	6.617	54.00	6.250
45.12	7.480	48.12	7.013	51.12	6.602	54.12	6.236
45.25	7.458	48.25	6.994	51.25	6.585	54.25	6.221
45.37	7.438	48.37	6.977	51.37	6.569	54.37	6.207
45.50	7.417	48.50	6.958	51.50	6.553	54.50	6.192
45.62	7.398	48.62	6.941	51.62	6.538	54.62	6.179
45.75	7.377	48.75	6.923	51.75	6.521	54.75	6.164
45.87	7.357	48.87	6.906	51.87	6.506	54.87	6.150
46.00	7.336	49.00	6.887	52.00	6.490	55.00	6.136
46.12	7.317	49.12	6.870	52.12	6.475	55.12	6.123
46.25	7.297	49.25	6.852	52.25	6.459	55.25	6.108
46.37	7.278	49.37	6.836	52.37	6.444	55.37	6.095
46.50	7.258	49.50	6.818	52.50	6.428	55.50	6.081
46.62	7.239	49.62	6.801	52.62	6.413	55.62	6.068
46.75	7.219	49.75	6.783	52.75	6.398	55.75	6.054
46.87	7.200	49.87	6.767	52.87	6.383	55.87	6.041
47.00	7.180	50.00	6.750	53.00	6.367	56.00	6.027
47.12	7.162	50.12	6.733	53.12	6.353	56.50	5.973
47.25	7.142	50.25	6.716	53.25	6.338	57.00	5.921
47.37	7.124	50.37	6.700	53.37	6.323	57.50	5.869
47.50	7.105	50.50	6.683	53.50	6.308	58.00	5.819
47.62	7.087	50.62	6.667	53.62	6.294	58.50	5.769
47.75	7.068	50.75	6.650	53.75	6.279	59.00	5.720
47.87	7.050	50.87	6.634	53.87	6.265	60.00	5.625

APPENDIX 9 Vertex conversion table

Effective power at corneal plane of spectacles at designated distance from cornea (vertex distance/millimeters)

Spectacle lens power*	Plus lenses							
	8 mm	9 mm	10 mm	11 mm	12 mm	13 mm	14 mm	15 mm
4.00	4.12	4.12	4.12	4.12	4.25	4.25	4.25	4.25
4.50	4.62	4.75	4.75	4.75	4.75	4.75	4.75	4.87
5.00	5.25	5.25	5.25	5.25	5.25	5.37	5.37	5.37
5.50	5.75	5.75	5.75	5.87	5.87	5.87	6.00	6.00
6.00	6.25	6.37	6.37	6.37	6.50	6.50	6.50	6.62
6.50	6.87	6.87	7.00	7.00	7.00	7.12	7.12	7.25
7.00	7.37	7.50	7.50	7.62	7.62	7.75	7.75	7.75
7.50	8.00	8.00	8.12	8.12	8.25	8.25	8.37	8.50
8.00	8.50	8.62	8.75	8.75	8.87	8.87	9.00	9.12
8.50	9.12	9.25	9.25	9.37	9.50	9.50	9.62	9.75
9.00	9.75	9.75	9.87	10.00	10.12	10.25	10.37	10.37
9.50	10.25	10.37	10.50	10.62	10.75	10.87	11.00	11.12
10.00	10.87	11.00	11.12	11.25	11.37	11.50	11.62	11.75
10.50	11.50	11.62	11.75	11.87	12.00	12.12	12.25	12.50
11.00	12.00	12.25	12.37	12.50	12.75	12.87	13.00	13.12
11.50	12.62	12.87	13.00	13.12	13.37	13.50	13.75	13.87
12.00	13.25	13.50	13.62	13.87	14.00	14.25	14.50	14.62
12.50	13.87	14.12	14.25	14.50	14.75	15.00	15.25	15.37
13.00	14.50	14.75	15.00	15.25	15.50	15.62	16.00	16.12
13.50	15.12	15.37	15.62	15.87	16.12	16.37	16.62	16.87
14.00	15.75	16.00	16.25	16.50	16.75	17.12	17.50	17.75
14.50	16.50	16.75	17.00	17.25	17.50	17.87	18.25	18.50
15.00	17.00	17.37	17.75	18.00	18.25	18.62	19.00	19.37
15.50	17.75	18.00	18.25	18.75	19.00	19.37	19.75	20.25
16.00	18.25	18.75	19.00	19.37	19.75	20.25	20.50	21.00
16.50	19.00	19.37	19.75	20.25	20.50	21.00	21.50	21.87
17.00	19.75	20.25	20.50	21.00	21.50	22.00	22.25	22.87
17.50	20.50	20.75	21.25	21.75	22.25	22.75	23.25	23.75
18.00	21.00	21.50	22.00	22.50	23.00	23.50	24.00	24.62
18.50	21.75	22.25	22.75	23.25	23.75	24.50	25.00	25.62
19.00	22.50	23.00	23.50	24.00	24.75	25.25	26.00	26.50

*Spectacle lens power worn at various distance to equivalent contact lens power.

Effective power at corneal plane of spectacles at designated distance from cornea (vertex distance/millimeters)

Minus lenses

8 mm	9 mm	10 mm	11 mm	12 mm	13 mm	14 mm	15 mm
3.87	3.87	3.87	3.87	3.87	3.75	3.75	3.75
4.37	4.37	4.25	4.25	4.25	4.25	4.25	4.25
4.75	4.75	4.75	4.75	4.75	4.75	4.62	4.62
5.25	5.25	5.25	5.12	5.12	5.12	5.12	5.12
5.75	5.62	5.62	5.62	5.62	5.50	5.50	5.50
6.12	6.12	6.12	6.00	6.00	6.00	6.00	5.87
6.62	6.62	6.50	6.50	6.50	6.37	6.37	6.37
7.12	7.00	7.00	6.87	6.87	6.87	6.75	6.75
7.50	7.50	7.37	7.37	7.25	7.25	7.25	7.25
8.00	7.87	7.87	7.75	7.75	7.62	7.62	7.50
8.37	8.37	8.25	8.25	8.12	8.00	8.00	8.00
8.87	8.75	8.62	8.62	8.50	8.50	8.37	8.37
9.25	9.12	9.12	9.00	8.87	8.87	8.75	8.75
9.62	9.62	9.50	9.37	9.37	9.25	9.12	9.12
10.12	10.00	9.87	9.75	9.75	9.62	9.50	9.50
10.50	10.37	10.37	10.25	10.12	10.00	9.87	9.87
11.00	10.87	10.75	10.62	10.50	10.37	10.25	10.12
11.37	11.25	11.12	11.00	10.87	10.75	10.62	10.50
11.75	11.62	11.50	11.37	11.25	11.12	11.00	10.87
12.25	12.00	11.87	11.75	11.62	11.50	11.37	11.25
12.62	12.50	12.25	12.12	12.00	11.87	11.75	11.50
13.00	12.75	12.62	12.50	12.37	12.25	12.00	11.87
13.37	13.25	13.00	12.87	12.75	12.50	12.37	12.25
13.75	13.62	13.50	13.25	13.00	12.87	12.75	12.62
14.25	14.00	13.75	13.62	13.50	13.25	13.00	12.87
14.50	14.37	14.12	14.00	13.75	13.62	13.50	13.25
15.00	14.75	14.50	14.25	14.12	14.00	13.75	13.50
15.37	15.12	14.87	14.75	14.50	14.25	14.00	13.87
15.75	15.50	15.25	15.00	14.75	14.62	14.37	14.12
16.12	15.87	15.62	15.37	15.12	14.87	14.75	14.50
16.50	16.25	16.00	15.75	15.50	15.25	15.00	14.75

APPENDIX 10 Diopters of corneal refracting power*

Diopters	Radius (mm)		Diopters	Radius (mm)	
	Curvature			**Curvature**	
Drum reading	**Convex**	**Concave**	**Drum reading**	**Convex**	**Concave**
52.00	6.49	6.51	47.87	7.05	7.07
51.87	6.50	6.53	47.75	7.07	7.09
51.75	6.52	6.54	47.62	7.08	7.11
51.62	6.54	6.56	47.50	7.10	7.13
51.50	6.55	6.57	47.37	7.12	7.15
51.37	6.57	6.59	47.25	7.14	7.17
51.25	6.58	6.61	47.12	7.16	7.19
51.12	6.60	6.62	47.00	7.18	7.21
51.00	6.62	6.64	46.87	7.20	7.23
50.87	6.63	6.66	46.75	7.22	7.25
50.75	6.65	6.67	46.62	7.24	7.27
50.62	6.66	6.69	46.50	7.26	7.29
50.50	6.68	6.71	46.27	7.28	7.31
50.37	6.70	6.72	46.25	7.30	7.33
50.25	6.73	6.75	46.12	7.32	7.35
50.12	6.73	6.75	46.00	7.34	7.37
50.00	6.75	6.77	45.87	7.36	7.39
49.87	6.76	6.79	45.75	7.38	7.41
49.75	6.80	6.82	45.62	7.40	7.43
49.62	6.80	6.82	45.50	7.42	7.45
49.50	6.82	6.84	45.37	7.44	7.47
49.37	6.83	6.85	45.25	7.46	7.49
49.25	6.85	6.87	45.12	7.48	7.51
49.12	6.87	6.89	45.00	7.50	7.53
49.00	6.89	6.91	44.87	7.52	7.55
48.87	6.90	6.93	44.75	7.55	7.57
48.75	6.92	6.95	44.62	7.57	7.58
48.62	6.94	6.96	44.50	7.59	7.60
48.50	6.96	6.98	44.37	7.61	7.62
48.37	6.97	7.00	44.25	7.63	7.65
48.25	6.99	7.02	44.12	7.65	7.67
48.12	7.01	7.03	44.00	7.67	7.70
48.00	7.03	7.05			

From Stein HA, Slatt BJ: *Fitting guide for rigid soft contact lenses,* ed 2, St Louis, 1984, Mosby.

Diopters	Radius (mm)		Diopters	Radius (mm)	
	Curvature			Curvature	
Drum reading	Convex	Concave	Drum reading	Convex	Concave
43.87	7.67	7.72	39.87	8.47	8.50
43.75	7.72	7.74	39.75	8.49	8.52
43.62	7.74	7.77	39.62	8.52	8.55
43.50	7.76	7.79	39.50	8.54	8.58
43.37	7.78	7.81	39.37	8.57	8.61
43.25	7.80	7.84	39.25	8.60	8.63
43.12	7.83	7.86	39.12	8.63	8.66
43.00	7.85	7.88	39.00	8.65	8.69
42.87	7.88	7.90	38.87	8.68	8.72
42.75	7.90	7.92	38.75	8.71	8.75
42.62	7.92	7.95	38.62	8.74	8.78
42.50	7.95	7.97	38.50	8.77	8.80
42.37	7.97	8.00	38.37	8.80	8.84
42.25	8.00	8.02	38.25	8.82	8.86
42.12	8.01	8.05	38.12	8.85	8.89
42.00	8.04	8.07	38.00	8.88	8.92
41.87	8.06	8.10	37.87	8.91	8.95
41.75	8.09	8.12	37.75	8.94	8.98
41.62	8.11	8.15	37.62	8.97	9.01
41.50	8.13	8.17	37.50	9.00	9.04
41.37	8.16	8.19	37.37	9.03	9.07
41.25	8.18	8.22	37.25	9.06	9.10
41.12	8.20	8.24	37.12	9.09	9.13
41.00	8.23	8.27	37.00	9.12	9.16
40.87	8.26	8.29	36.87	9.14	9.19
40.75	8.28	8.32	36.75	9.19	9.23
40.62	8.31	8.34	36.62	9.22	9.26
40.50	8.34	8.37	36.50	9.25	9.29
40.37	8.36	8.39	36.37	9.28	9.32
40.25	8.39	8.42	36.25	9.31	9.35
40.12	8.41	8.44	36.12	9.35	9.38
40.00	8.44	8.47	36.00	9.38	9.42
			34.00	9.93	9.97

*Conversion table relating diopters of corneal refracting power to millimeters of radius of curvature for an assumed index of refraction of 1.3375. The column under convex curvature should be used when the keratometer is used to measure the cornea, and the third column is used to measure concave surfaces such as the CPC of a corneal contact lens in terms of its equivalent corneal refracting power in diopters.

APPENDIX 11 Compensation for effect of vertex distances (used when plus lens is moved from the eye)

R̶ power (D)	Distance moved (mm)									
	1	2	3	4	5	6	7	8	9	10
7.00	6.95	6.90	6.86	6.81	6.76	6.72	6.67	6.63	6.59	6.54
7.25	7.20	7.15	7.10	7.05	7.00	6.95	6.90	6.85	6.81	6.76
7.50	7.44	7.39	7.43	7.28	7.23	7.18	7.13	7.08	7.03	6.98
7.75	7.69	7.63	7.57	7.52	7.46	7.41	7.35	7.30	7.24	7.19
8.00	7.94	7.87	7.81	7.75	7.69	7.63	7.58	7.52	7.46	7.41
8.25	8.18	8.12	8.05	7.99	7.92	7.86	7.80	7.74	7.68	7.62
8.50	8.43	8.36	8.29	8.22	8.15	8.09	8.02	7.96	7.90	7.83
8.75	8.67	8.60	8.53	8.45	8.38	8.31	8.24	8.18	8.11	8.05
9.00	8.92	8.84	8.76	8.69	8.61	8.54	8.47	8.40	8.33	8.26
9.25	9.17	9.08	9.00	8.92	8.84	8.76	8.69	8.61	8.54	8.47
9.50	9.41	9.32	9.24	9.15	9.07	8.99	8.91	8.83	8.75	8.68
9.75	9.66	9.56	9.47	9.38	9.30	9.21	9.13	9.04	8.96	8.88
10.00	9.90	9.80	9.71	9.62	9.52	9.43	9.35	9.26	9.17	9.09
10.25	10.15	10.04	9.94	9.85	9.75	9.66	9.56	9.47	9.38	9.30
10.50	10.39	10.28	10.18	10.08	9.98	9.88	9.78	9.69	9.59	9.50
10.75	10.64	10.52	10.41	10.31	10.20	10.10	10.00	9.90	9.80	9.71
11.00	10.88	10.76	10.65	10.54	10.43	10.32	10.21	10.11	10.01	9.91
11.25	11.12	11.00	10.88	10.77	10.65	10.54	10.43	10.32	10.22	10.11
11.50	11.37	11.24	11.12	10.99	10.87	10.76	10.64	10.53	10.42	10.31
11.75	11.61	11.48	11.35	11.22	11.10	10.98	10.86	10.74	10.63	10.51
12.00	11.86	11.72	11.58	11.45	11.32	11.19	11.07	10.95	10.83	10.71
12.25	12.10	11.96	11.82	11.68	11.54	11.41	11.28	11.16	11.03	10.91
12.50	12.35	12.20	12.05	11.90	11.76	11.63	11.49	11.36	11.24	11.11
12.75	12.59	12.43	12.28	12.13	11.99	11.84	11.71	11.57	11.44	11.31
13.00	12.83	12.67	12.51	12.36	12.21	12.06	11.92	11.78	11.64	11.50
13.25	13.08	12.91	12.74	12.58	12.43	12.27	12.13	11.98	11.84	11.70
13.50	13.32	13.15	12.97	12.81	12.65	12.49	12.33	12.18	12.04	11.89
13.75	13.56	13.38	13.21	13.03	12.87	12.70	12.54	12.39	12.24	12.09
14.00	13.81	13.62	13.44	13.26	13.08	12.92	12.75	12.59	12.43	12.28
14.25	14.05	13.86	13.67	13.48	13.30	13.13	12.96	12.79	12.63	12.47

From Stein HA, Slatt BJ: *Fitting guide for rigid and soft contact lenses*, ed 2, St Louis, 1984, Mosby.

R̶ power (D)	Distance moved (mm)									
	1	2	3	4	5	6	7	8	9	10
14.50	14.29	14.09	13.90	13.70	13.52	13.34	13.16	12.99	12.83	12.66
14.75	14.54	14.33	14.12	13.93	13.74	13.55	13.37	13.19	13.02	12.85
15.00	14.78	14.56	14.35	14.15	13.95	13.76	13.57	13.39	13.22	13.04
15.25	15.02	14.80	14.58	14.37	14.17	13.97	13.78	13.59	13.41	13.23
15.50	15.26	15.03	14.81	14.60	14.39	14.18	13.98	13.79	13.60	13.42
15.75	15.51	15.27	15.04	14.82	14.60	14.39	14.19	13.99	13.79	13.61
16.00	15.75	15.50	15.27	15.04	14.81	14.60	13.39	14.18	13.99	13.79
16.25	15.99	15.74	15.49	15.25	15.03	14.81	14.59	14.38	14.18	13.98
16.50	16.23	15.97	15.72	15.48	15.24	15.01	14.79	14.57	14.37	14.16
16.75	16.47	16.21	15.95	15.70	15.45	15.22	14.99	14.77	14.56	14.35
17.00	16.72	16.44	16.18	15.92	15.67	15.43	15.19	14.96	14.74	14.53
17.25	16.96	16.67	16.40	16.44	15.88	15.63	15.39	15.16	14.93	14.71
17.50	17.20	16.91	16.63	16.36	16.09	15.84	15.59	15.35	15.12	14.89
17.75	17.44	17.14	16.85	16.57	16.30	16.04	15.79	15.54	15.31	15.07
18.00	17.68	17.37	17.08	16.79	16.51	16.25	15.99	15.73	15.49	15.25
18.25	17.92	17.61	17.30	17.01	16.72	16.45	16.18	15.92	15.68	15.43
18.50	18.16	17.84	17.53	17.23	16.93	16.65	16.38	16.11	15.86	15.61
18.75	18.40	18.07	17.75	17.44	17.14	16.85	16.57	16.30	16.04	15.79
19.00	18.65	18.30	17.98	17.66	17.35	17.06	16.77	16.49	16.23	15.97
19.25	18.89	18.54	18.20	17.87	17.56	17.26	16.96	16.68	16.41	16.14
19.50	19.13	18.77	18.42	18.09	17.77	17.46	17.16	16.87	16.59	16.32
19.75	19.37	19.00	18.65	18.30	17.97	17.66	17.35	17.06	16.77	16.49
20.00	19.61	19.23	18.87	18.52	18.18	17.86	17.54	17.24	16.95	16.67
20.25	19.85	19.46	19.09	18.73	18.39	18.06	17.74	17.43	17.13	16.84
20.50	20.09	19.69	19.31	18.95	18.59	18.25	17.93	17.61	17.31	17.01
20.75	20.33	19.92	19.53	19.16	18.80	18.45	18.12	17.80	17.48	17.18
21.00	20.57	20.15	19.76	19.37	19.00	18.65	18.31	17.98	17.66	17.36
21.25	20.81	20.38	19.98	19.59	19.21	18.85	18.50	18.16	17.84	17.53
21.50	21.05	20.61	20.20	19.80	19.41	19.04	18.69	18.34	18.01	17.70
21.75	21.29	20.84	20.42	20.01	19.62	19.24	18.88	18.53	18.19	17.87

APPENDIX 12 Compensation for effect of vertex distances (used when plus lens is moved toward the eye)

R power (D)	Distance moved (mm)									
	1	2	3	4	5	6	7	8	9	10
7.00	7.05	7.10	7.15	7.20	7.25	7.31	7.36	7.42	7.47	7.53
7.25	7.30	7.36	7.41	7.47	7.52	7.58	7.64	7.70	7.76	7.82
7.50	7.56	7.61	7.67	7.73	7.79	7.85	7.92	7.98	8.04	8.11
7.75	7.81	7.87	7.93	8.00	8.06	8.13	8.19	8.26	8.33	8.40
8.00	8.06	8.13	8.20	8.26	8.33	8.40	8.47	8.55	8.62	8.70
8.25	8.32	8.39	8.46	8.53	8.60	8.68	8.76	8.83	8.91	8.99
8.50	8.57	8.56	8.72	8.80	8.88	8.96	9.04	9.12	9.20	9.29
8.75	8.83	8.91	8.99	9.07	9.15	9.23	9.32	9.41	9.50	9.59
9.00	9.08	9.16	9.25	9.34	9.42	9.51	9.61	9.70	9.79	9.89
9.25	9.34	9.42	9.51	9.61	9.70	9.79	9.89	9.99	10.09	10.19
9.50	9.59	9.68	9.78	9.88	9.97	10.07	10.18	10.28	10.39	10.50
9.75	9.85	9.94	10.04	10.15	10.25	10.36	10.46	10.58	10.69	10.80
10.00	10.10	10.20	10.31	10.42	10.53	10.64	10.75	10.87	10.99	11.11
10.25	10.36	10.46	10.58	10.69	10.80	10.92	11.04	11.17	11.29	11.42
10.50	10.61	10.73	10.84	10.96	11.08	11.21	11.33	11.46	11.60	11.73
10.75	10.87	10.99	11.11	11.23	11.36	11.49	11.62	11.76	11.90	12.04
11.00	11.12	11.25	11.38	11.51	11.64	11.78	11.92	12.06	12.21	12.36
11.25	11.38	11.51	11.64	11.78	11.92	12.06	12.21	12.36	12.52	12.68
11.50	11.63	11.77	11.91	12.05	12.20	12.35	12.51	12.67	12.83	12.99
11.75	11.89	12.03	12.18	12.33	12.48	12.64	12.80	12.97	13.14	13.31
12.00	12.15	12.30	12.45	12.61	12.77	12.93	13.10	13.27	13.45	13.64
12.25	12.40	12.56	12.72	12.88	13.05	13.22	13.40	13.58	13.77	13.96
12.50	12.66	12.82	12.99	13.16	13.33	13.51	13.70	13.89	14.08	14.29
12.75	12.91	13.08	13.26	13.44	13.62	13.81	14.00	14.20	14.40	14.61
13.00	13.17	13.35	13.53	13.71	13.90	14.10	14.30	14.51	14.72	14.94
13.25	13.43	13.61	13.80	13.99	14.19	14.39	14.60	14.82	15.04	15.27
13.50	13.68	13.87	14.07	14.27	14.48	14.69	14.91	15.13	15.37	15.61
13.75	13.94	14.14	14.34	14.55	14.77	14.99	15.21	15.45	15.69	15.94
14.00	14.20	14.40	14.61	14.83	15.05	15.28	15.52	15.77	16.02	16.28
14.25	14.46	14.67	14.89	15.11	15.34	15.58	15.83	16.09	16.35	16.62

From Stein HA, Slatt BJ: *Fitting guide for rigid and soft contact lenses*, ed 2, St Louis, 1984, Mosby.

Rx power (D)	Distance moved (mm)									
	1	2	3	4	5	6	7	8	9	10
14.50	14.71	14.93	15.16	15.39	15.63	15.88	16.14	16.41	16.88	16.96
14.75	14.97	15.20	15.43	15.67	15.92	16.18	16.45	16.73	17.01	17.30
15.00	15.23	15.46	15.71	15.96	16.22	16.48	16.76	17.05	17.34	17.65
15.25	15.49	15.73	15.98	16.24	16.51	16.79	17.07	17.37	17.68	18.00
15.50	15.74	16.00	16.26	16.52	16.80	17.09	17.39	17.69	18.01	18.35
15.75	16.00	16.26	16.53	16.81	17.10	17.39	17.70	18.02	18.35	18.70
16.00	16.26	16.53	16.81	17.09	17.39	17.70	18.02	18.35	18.69	19.05
16.25	16.52	16.80	17.08	17.38	17.69	18.01	18.34	18.68	19.03	19.40
16.50	16.78	17.06	17.36	17.67	17.98	18.31	18.65	19.01	19.38	19.76
16.75	17.04	17.33	17.64	17.95	18.28	18.62	18.97	19.34	19.72	20.12
17.00	17.29	17.60	17.91	18.24	18.58	18.93	19.30	19.68	20.07	20.48
17.25	17.55	17.87	18.19	18.53	18.88	19.24	19.62	20.01	20.42	20.85
17.50	17.81	18.13	18.47	18.82	19.18	19.55	19.94	20.35	20.77	21.21
17.75	18.07	18.40	18.75	19.11	19.48	19.86	20.27	20.69	21.12	21.58
18.00	18.33	18.67	19.03	19.40	19.78	20.18	20.59	21.03	21.48	21.95
18.25	18.59	18.94	19.31	19.69	20.08	20.49	20.92	21.37	21.84	22.32
18.50	18.85	19.21	19.59	19.98	20.39	20.81	21.25	27.71	22.20	22.70
18.75	19.11	19.48	19.87	20.27	20.69	21.13	21.58	22.06	22.56	23.08
19.00	19.37	19.75	20.15	20.56	20.99	21.44	21.91	22.41	22.92	23.46
19.25	19.63	20.02	20.43	20.86	21.30	21.76	22.25	22.75	23.28	23.81
19.50	19.89	20.89	20.71	21.15	21.61	22.08	22.58	23.10	23.65	24.22
19.75	20.15	20.56	20.99	21.44	21.91	22.40	22.92	23.46	24.02	24.61
20.00	20.41	20.83	21.28	21.74	22.22	22.73	23.26	23.81	24.39	25.00
20.25	20.67	21.10	21.56	22.03	22.53	23.05	23.59	24.16	24.76	
20.50	20.82	21.38	21.84	22.33	22.84	23.38	23.93	24.52		
20.75	20.91	21.65	22.13	22.63	23.15	23.70	24.28			
21.00	21.45	21.92	22.41	22.93	23.46	24.03				
21.25	21.71	22.19	22.70	23.22	23.78					
12.50	21.97	22.47	22.98	23.52						
21.75	22.23	22.74	23.37							

APPENDIX 13 Dioptric curves for extended range of keratometer

High power (with +1.25 D lens over aperture)				Low power (with −1.00 D lens over aperture)			
Drum reading (D)	True dioptric curvature (D)	Drum reading (D)	True dioptric curvature (D)	Drum reading (D)	True dioptric curvature (D)	Drum reading (D)	True dioptric curvature (D)
52.00	61.00	46.87	55.87	42.00	36.00	36.87	30.87
51.87	60.87	46.75	55.75	41.87	35.87	36.75	30.75
51.75	60.75	46.62	55.62	41.75	35.75	36.62	30.62
51.62	60.62	46.50	55.50	41.62	35.62	36.50	30.50
51.50	60.50	46.37	55.37	41.50	35.50	36.37	30.37
51.37	60.37	46.25	55.25	41.37	35.37	36.25	30.25
51.25	60.25	46.12	55.12	41.25	35.25	36.12	30.12
51.12	60.12	46.00	55.00	41.12	35.12	36.00	30.00
51.00	60.00			41.00	35.00		
		45.87	54.87				
50.87	59.87	45.75	54.75	40.87	34.87		
50.75	59.75	45.62	54.62	40.75	34.75		
50.62	59.62	45.50	54.50	40.62	34.62		
50.50	59.50	45.37	54.37	40.50	34.50		
50.37	59.37	45.25	54.25	40.37	34.37		
50.25	59.25	45.12	54.12	40.25	34.25		
50.12	59.12	45.00	54.00	40.12	34.12		
50.00	59.00			40.00	34.00		
		44.87	53.87				
49.87	58.87	44.75	53.75	39.87	33.87		
49.75	58.75	44.62	53.62	39.75	33.75		
49.62	58.62	44.50	53.50	39.62	33.62		
49.50	58.50	44.37	53.37	39.50	33.50		

Courtesy Bausch & Lomb, Inc.
From Stein HA, Slatt BJ: *Fitting guide for rigid and soft contact lenses*, ed 2, St Louis, 1984, Mosby.

	High power (with +1.25 D lens over aperture)			Low power (with −1.00 D lens over aperture)	
Drum reading (D)	True dioptric curvature (D)	Drum reading (D)	True dioptric curvature (D)	Drum reading (D)	True dioptric curvature (D)
49.37	58.37	44.25	53.25	39.37	33.37
49.25	58.25	44.12	53.12	39.25	33.25
49.12	58.12	44.00	53.00	39.12	33.12
49.00	58.00			39.00	33.00
		43.87	52.87		
48.75	57.75	43.75	52.75	38.87	32.87
48.62	57.62	43.62	52.62	38.75	32.75
48.50	57.50	43.50	52.50	38.62	32.62
48.37	57.37	43.37	52.37	38.50	32.50
48.25	57.25	43.25	52.25	38.37	32.37
48.12	57.12	43.12	52.12	38.25	32.25
48.00	57.00	43.00	52.00	38.12	32.12
				38.00	32.00
47.87	56.87				
47.75	56.75			37.87	31.87
47.62	56.62			37.75	31.75
47.50	56.50			37.62	31.62
47.37	58.37			37.50	31.50
47.25	56.25			37.37	31.37
47.12	56.12			37.25	31.25
47.00	56.00			37.12	31.12
				37.00	31.00

APPENDIX 14 Translations of commonly asked questions and commands

English	French
HISTORY	
1. What is your name?	1. Quel est votre nom?
2. What is your address?	2. Quelle est votre addresse?
3. When were you born?	3. Quel est votre jour de naissance?
4. What trouble are you having with your eyes?	4. Quel problème avez-vous avec les yeux?
5. Are you having pain?	5. Ça fait mal?
6. Do your eyes itch?	6. Ça pique?
7. Have you had any eye injury?	7. Est-ce que les yeux ont été blessés?
8. Have you had an eye operation?	8. Est-ce que les yeux ont été opérés?
9. Did you get anything in your eye?	9. Y'a-t-il quelque chose dans les yeux?
10. Are you taking any eye drops?	10. Employez-vous des gouttes pour les yeux?
11. Do you have headaches?	11. Avez-vous des maux de têtes?
12. Do you wear glasses?	12. Portez-vous des lunettes?
13. How old are your glasses?	13. Et depuis quand?
14. Do you have trouble reading?	14. Pouvez-vous lire sans difficulté?
15. Do you see double?	15. Voyez-vous double?
16. Do you take pills?	16. Prenez-vous des médicaments?
For: heart	Pour: le coeur
diabetes	le diabète
blood pressure	la tension artérielle
17. Do you have any allergies?	17. Avez-vous des allergies?
To medicine	Aux médicaments?
Others	Ou à des autres choses?
18. Is there a history of diabetes or glaucoma in your family?	18. Y'a-t-il le diabète ou le glaucome dans votre famille?
19. Is there a history of eye problems?	19. Y'a-t-il des problèmes avec les yeux?
EXAMINATION	
20. Look straight.	20. Regardez tout droit.
21. Follow my light.	21. Suivez ma lumière.
22. Follow my finger.	22. Suivez mon doigt.
23. Can you count my fingers?	23. Pouvez-vous compter mes doigts?
24. Can you see my hand move?	24. Pouvez-vous voir bouger ma main?
25. Open your eyes. Close your eyes.	25. Ouvrez les yeux. Fermez les yeux.
26. Look at me.	26. Regardez-moi.
27. Is it clear?	27. Est-il clair?
28. Read this.	28. Lisez ça.
29. Which is better, one or two?	29. Le quel est mieux, un ou deux?

English	German
HISTORY	

English

HISTORY

1. What is your name?
2. What is your address?
3. When were you born?
4. What trouble are you having with your eyes?
5. Are you having pain?
6. Do your eyes itch?
7. Have you had any eye injury?
8. Have you had an eye operation?
9. Did you get anything in your eye?
10. Are you taking any eye drops?
11. Do you have headaches?
12. Do you wear glasses?
13. How old are your glasses?
14. Do you have trouble reading?
15. Do you see double?
16. Do you take pills?
     For: heart
          diabetes
          blood pressure
17. Do you have any allergies?
     To medicine
     Others
18. Is there a history of diabetes or glaucoma in your family?
19. Is there a history of eye problems?

EXAMINATION

20. Look straight.
21. Follow my light.
22. Follow my finger.
23. Can you count my fingers?
24. Can you see my hand move?
25. Open your eyes. Close your eyes.
26. Look at me.
27. Is it clear?
28. Read this.
29. Which is better, one or two?

German

1. Ihr Name, bitte?
2. Ihre Anschrift, bitte?
3. Ihr Geburtsdatum, bitte?
4. Was für ein Problem haben Sie mit den Augen?
5. Haben Sie Schmerzen?
6. Tun Ihre Augen jucken?
7. Haben Sie mal eine Augenverletzung gehabt?
8. Haben Sie mal eine Augenoperation gehabt?
9. Ist irgendwas in Ihre Augen geraten?
10. Benützen Sie Augentropfen?
11. Haben Sie Kopfschmerzen?
12. Tragen Sie Brillen?
13. Seit wann tragen Sie Brillen?
14. Haben Sie Schwierigkeiten beim Lesen?
15. Sehen Sie doppelt?
16. Nämen Sie Pillen ein?
     Für Herz?
          Zuckerkrankheit
          Blutdruck?
17. Haben Sie irgend Allergien?
     Gegen Medizin?
     Andere Allergien?
18. Laufen Zuckerkrankheit oder Glaucom in Ihre Familie?
19. Laufen Augenkrankheit in Ihre Familie?

20. Schauen Sie gerade aus.
21. Folgen Sie dem Licht.
22. Folgen Sie meinem Finger.
23. Zählen Sie meine Finger.
24. Können Sie Bewegung meiner Hand sehen?
25. Öffnen Sie die Augen. Schliessen Sie die Augen.
26. Schauen Sie mich an.
27. Erscheine ich klar?
28. Lesen Sie dieses.
29. Was ist besser, eins oder zwei?

Continued.

Translations of commonly asked questions and commands—cont'd

English	Italian
HISTORY	
1. What is your name?	1. Come ti chiami?
2. What is your address?	2. Il tuo indirizzo.
3. When were you born?	3. La tua data di nascita.
4. What trouble are you having with your eyes?	4. Hai qualche problema con i tuoi occhi?
5. Are you having pain?	5. Senti dolore?
6. Do your eyes itch?	6. I tuoi occhi bruciano?
7. Have you had any eye injury?	7. Hai avuto un incidente agli occhi?
8. Have you had an eye operation?	8. Hai mai avuto una operazione agli occhi?
9. Did you get anything in your eye?	9. Cosa e' entrato nel tuo occhio?
10. Are you taking any eye drops?	10. Usi gocce per occhi?
11. Do you have headaches?	11. Hai dolori di testa?
12. Do you wear glasses?	12. Usi occhiali?
13. How old are your glasses?	13. Da quanto tempo usi questi occhiali?
14. Do you have trouble reading?	14. Riesci a leggere?
15. Do you see double?	15. Vedi doppio?
16. Do you take pills?	16. Usi pillole?
For: heart	Per: il cuore
diabetes	il diabete
blood pressure	la pressione
17. Do you have any allergies?	17. Hai allergie?
To medicine	a medicine
Others	di qualsiasi tipo
18. Is there a history of diabetes or glaucoma in your family?	18. C'e' qualche caso di diabete o glaucoma nella tua famiglia?
19. Is there a history of eye problems?	19. Qualcuno in famiglia ha avuto disturbi alla vista?
EXAMINATION	
20. Look straight.	20. Guarda diritto.
21. Follow my light.	21. Segui la luce.
22. Follow my finger.	22. Segui il mio dito.
23. Can you count my fingers?	23. Quante dita vedi?
24. Can you see my hand move?	24. Vedi la mia mano muoversi?
25. Open your eyes. Close your eyes.	25. Apri gli occhi. Chiudi gli occhi.
26. Look at me.	26. Guardami.
27. Is it clear?	27. Vedi chiaro?
28. Read this.	28. Leggi.
29. Which is better, one or two?	29. Qual e' meglio, uno o due?

English

HISTORY
1. What is your name?
2. What is your address?
3. When were you born?
4. What trouble are you having with your eyes?
5. Are you having pain?
6. Do your eyes itch?
7. Have you had any eye injury?
8. Have you had an eye operation?
9. Did you get anything in your eye?
10. Are you taking any eye drops?
11. Do you have headaches?
12. Do you wear glasses?
13. How old are your glases?
14. Do you have trouble reading?
15. Do you see double?
16. Do you take pills?
    For: Heart
        Diabetes
        Blood pressure
17. Do you have any allergies?
    To medicine
    Others
18. Is there a history of diabetes or glaucoma in your family?
19. Is there a history of eye problems?

EXAMINATION
20. Look straight.
21. Follow my light.
22. Follow my finger.
23. Can you count my fingers?
24. Can you see my hand move?
25. Open your eyes. Close your eyes.
26. Look at me.
27. Is it clear?
28. Read this.
29. Which is better, one or two?

Polish

1. Jak się pan (pani) nazywa?
2. Jaki jest pana (pani) adres?
3. Kiedy się pan urodzil (pani urodzita)?
4. Jaki pan (pani) ma problem z oczami?
5. Czy pan (pani) odczuwa ból?
6. Czy pana (pani) swędzą oczy?
7. Czy oko bylo skaleczone?
8. Czy mial pan (miata pani) operację na oczy?
9. Czy coś się dostalo do oka?
10. Czy bierze pan (pani) krople do oczu?
11. Czy cierpi pan (pani) na bole glowy?
12. Czy nosi pan (pani) okulary?
13. Jak dawno nosi pan (pani) te okulary?
14. Czy ma pan (pani) problemy z czytaniem?
15. Czy widzi pan (pani) podwójnie?
16. Czy bierze pan (pani) pastylki?
    Na: Serce
        Cukrzyce
        Wysokie ciśnienie
17. Czy cierpi pan (pani) na alergie?
    Na lekarstwa
    Inne
18. Czy ktoś z rodziny cierpi na cukrzyce lub jaskre?
19. Czy ktoś z rodziny ma problemy z oczami?

20. Proszę patrzeć prosto.
21. Proszę wodzić wzrokiem za światlem.
22. Proszę wodzić wzrokiem za moim palcem.
23. Czy może pan (pani) policzyć moje palce?
24. Czy widzi pan (pani) jak rusza się moja ręka?
25. Proszę otworzyć oczy. Proszę zamknąć oczy.
26. Proszę spojrzeć na mnie.
27. Czy to jest dobrze widoczne?
28. Proszę to przeczytać.
29. Które jest lepsze, pierwsze czy drugie?

Continued.

Translations of commonly asked questions and commands—cont'd

English	Spanish
HISTORY	
1. What is your name?	1. Su nombre, por favor.
2. What is your address?	2. Su dirección, por favor.
3. When were you born?	3. Su fecha de nacimiento, por favor.
4. What trouble are you having with your sight?	4. ¿Tiene usted dificultades con la vista?
5. Are you having pain?	5. ¿Le duelen los ojos?
6. Do your eyes itch?	6. ¿Le pican los ojos?
7. Have you had any eye injury?	7. ¿Han recibido daño en alguna forma sus ojos?
8. Have you had an eye operation?	8. ¿Ha sufrido usted alguna operación en los ojos?
9. Did you get anything in your eye?	9. ¿Tiene algo en el ojo?
10. Are you taking any eye drops?	10. ¿Está usted usando gotas para los ojos?
11. Do you have headaches?	11. ¿Sufre usted de dolores de cabeza?
12. Do you wear glasses?	12. ¿Usa usted espejuelos (gafas)?
13. How old are your glasses?	13. ¿Cuántos años tienen sus gafas?
14. Do you have trouble reading?	14. ¿Les molestan cuando lee?
15. Do you see double?	15. ¿Ve doble?
16. Do you take pills?	16. ¿Toma usted medicinas?
For: heart	para: el corazón
diabetes	la diabetes
blood pressure	la presión arterial
17. Do you have any allergies?	17. ¿Es usted alérgico?
To medicine	a las medicinas
Others	a otras cosas
18. Is there a history of diabetes or glaucoma in your family?	18. ¿Existen o han existido casos de diabetes o de glaucoma en su familia?
19. Is there a history of eye problems?	19. ¿Existen o han existido problemas de la vista en la familia?
EXAMINATION	
20. Look straight.	20. ¡Mire directamente hacia delante!
21. Follow my light.	21. ¡Siga la luz con sus ojos!
22. Follow my finger.	22. ¡Siga mi dedo con sus ojos!
23. Can you count my fingers?	23. ¿Puede contar los dedos?
24. Can you see my hand move?	24. ¿Ve mi mano cuando se mueve?
25. Open your eyes. Close your eyes.	25. ¡Abra los ojos! ¡Cierre los ojos!
26. Look at me.	26. ¡Míreme!
27. Is it clear?	27. ¿Lo ve claramente?
28. Read this.	28. ¡Lea esto!
29. Which is better, one or two?	29. ¿De los dos cuál es el mejor, el uno o el dos?

APPENDIX 15 Ocular emergencies*

I. Ocular complications of systemic diseases	
Disease	**Possible ocular findings**
Diabetes mellitus	Background retinopathy: retinal hemorrhages, exudates & microaneurysms Preproliferative retinopathy: cotton-wool spots, intraretinal microvascular abnormalities Proliferative retinopathy: neovascularization, preretinal hemorrhage, vitreous hemorrhage, retinal detachment
Graves' disease	Lid retraction, exposure keratopathy, chemosis and injection, restriction of eye movements, proptosis, compressive optic neuropathy
Hypertension	Sclerosis of vessels in longstanding disease; narrowing of vessels, retinal hemorrhages, and/or exudates in severe hypertension
Rheumatoid arthritis & other collagen vascular diseases	Dry eye, episcleritis, scleritis, peripheral corneal ulceration and/or melting
Cancer	Metastatic disease to choroid may result in retinal detachment; disease in the orbit can result in proptosis and restriction of eye movements (e.g., breast, lung cancer)

*Reproduced from Stein RM, Slatt HA, Stein BJ: *Ocular Emergencies,* Montreal, 1990, Medicopea.

II. Lifesaving ocular signs

Findings	Clinical significance
White pupil	In an infant, retinoblastoma must be ruled out
Aniridia (iris appears absent)	May be autosomal dominant (⅔s) or sporadic inheritance; in sporadic cases where the short arm of chromosome 11 is deleted, there is a 90% risk of developing Wilm's tumor; the risk in other sporadic cases is approximately 20%
Thickened corneal nerves (slit lamp)	Part of the multiple endocrine neoplasia syndrome type IIB; must rule out medullary carcinoma of the thyroid, pheochromocytoma, and parathyroid adenomas
Retinal angioma	May be part of the von Hippel-Lindau disease autosomal dominant inheritance with variable penetrance; must rule out hemangioblastomas of the central nervous system, renal cell carcinoma, and pheochromocytoma
Multiple pigmented patches of fundus	Lesions represent patches of congenital hypertrophy of the retinal pigment epithelium; may be part of Gardner's syndrome, characterized by multiple premalignant intestinal polyps together with benign soft tissue tumors (lipomas, fibromas, sebaceous cysts) and osteomas of the skull and jaw; a complete gastrointestinal investigation is indicated; if a diagnosis of Gardner's syndrome is made, prophylactic colectomy is indicated because of the potential for malignant degeneration of colonic polyps
Third-nerve palsy with a dilated pupil	Must rule out an intracranial aneurysm or neoplastic lesion; CT scan should be performed on an emergency basis
Papilledema	Must rule out an intracranial mass lesion; CT scan should be performed on an emergency basis
Pigmentary degeneration of the retina and motility disturbance	May represent the Kearns-Sayre syndrome; must rule out a cardiac conduction defect disturbance with an annual electrocardiogram; may develop an intraventricular conduction defect, bundle block, bifascicular disease, or complete heart block; patient must be prepared for the possible need to implant a pacemaker

III. Ocular complications of systemic medications

Medication	Ocular complications
Amiodarone	Superficial keratopathy
Chlorpromazine	Anterior subcapsular cataracts
Corticosteroids	Posterior subcapsular cataracts, glaucoma
Digitalis	Blurred vision, disturbed color vision
Ethambutol	Optic neuropathy
Indomethacin	Superficial keratopathy
Isoniazid	Optic neuropathy
Nalidixic acid	Papilledema
Hydroxychloroquine	Superficial keratopathy and bull's—eye maculopathy
Tetracycline	Papilledema
Thioridazine	Pigmentary degeneration of the retina
Vitamin A	Papilledema

IV. Differential diagnosis of the nontraumatic red eye

Feature	CONDITION		
	Acute conjunctivitis	**Acute iritis**	**Acute glaucoma**
Symptoms	Redness, tearing ± discharge	Redness, pain, photophobia	Redness, severe pain, nausea, vomiting
Appearance	Conjunctival injection	Ciliary injection	Diffuse injection
Vision	Normal, can be blurred secondary to discharge	Moderate reduction	Marked reduction, halo vision
Cornea	Clear	May see keratic precipitates	Hazy secondary to edema
Pupil	Normal	Small, sluggish to light	Semidilated, nonreactive
Secretions	Tearing to purulent	Tearing	Tearing
Test & Comments	Smears may show etiology; bacterial infection = polycytes, bacteria; viral infection = monocytes; allergy = eosinophils	Slit lamp will show cells and flare in the anterior chamber	Elevated intraocular pressure
Treatment	Antibiotic	Steroids, cycloplegics	Pilocarpine, Betagan™ Diamox™, mannitol, laser surgery

V. Differential diagnosis of viral, bacterial, and allergic conjunctivitis

Feature	**Viral**	**Bacterial**	**Allergy**
Discharge	Watery	Purulent	Watery
Itching	Minimal	Minimal	Marked
Preauricular lymph node	Common	Absent	Absent
Stain & smear	Monocytes Lymphocytes	Bacteria Polycytes	Eosinophils

VI. Differential diagnosis of the red eye in contact lens wearers

Diagnosis	Findings	Mechanism	Treatment
Corneal abrasion	Epithelial defect; stains with fluorescein	Mechanical hypoxia	Antibiotic drops (e.g., tobramycin)
Superficial punctate keratitis	Punctate corneal staining	Mechanical chemical toxicity	Artificial tears (e.g., Refresh™ ocular lubricant)
Giant papillary conjunctivitis	Papillary reaction of superior tarsal conjunctiva	Immunologic mechanical	Mast cell stabilizer (e.g., Vistacrom drops)
Sterile infiltrates	Corneal infiltrate; epithelium usually intact	Immunologic	Antibiotic drops (assume infected)
Infected ulcer	Corneal infiltrate with ulceration; stains with fluorescein	Infection (e.g., *Pseudomonas, Staphylococcus aureus*)	Corneal scraping for Gram's stain and culture. Fortified antibiotic drops

APPENDIX 16 Principles of informed consent

INFORMED CONSENT

Informed consent permits the patient to exercise self-determination. The law imposes a "duty of disclosure" on the part of the physician.

DUTY OF DISCLOSURE:

1. To frankly answer all specific questions about the risk
2. Without being questioned, to disclose
   a. the nature of the proposed procedure
   b. the gravity of it
   c. all material risks
   d. all special and unusual risks in the particular circumstance
   e. to outline alternative procedures available and their risks, including the consequences of no treatment

MATERIAL RISKS:

A risk is material if it would be considered a significant issue by a reasonable person weighing the decision to consent to the procedure. A one in a 1,000 chance is probably not a material risk. A one in a 100 chance is probably a material risk. Risks of very serious or grave consequence should be disclosed no matter how remote.

SPECIAL AND UNUSUAL RISKS

The patient's particular circumstances such as occupational, familial, and social circumstances will make certain risks significant to that patient, e.g., a risk of visual loss to a commercial pilot should be disclosed even if the risk is remote.

CONSENT

1. Consent may be written, oral or implied from the circumstances, e.g., the patient holds out an arm for an injection.
2. Regardless of the form of the consent, the physician must be able to prove that the duty of disclosure was met before the consent was obtained. Therefore, a prudent physician will make a note on the chart of the risks disclosed and the patient's comments or questions.

EXCEPTIONS

1. In an emergency, the duty of disclosure and obtaining consent is waived.
2. When the patient plainly does not wish to hear about the risks, the duty of disclosure is waived, but consent should be obtained and circumstances noted on the chart.
3. In rare circumstances, if the physician can prove that disclosing the risks would create a state of mind in the patient which would seriously hinder successful treatment, the duty of disclosure is waived but consent should be obtained and the circumstances noted on the chart.

FAILURE TO DISCLOSE

1. When an undisclosed risk occurs and the patient sues and determines the risk should have been disclosed because it was material or because of the patient's particular circumstances, the physician will be liable if the court is satisfied that another person in the patient's po-

sition would have refused the treatment had the risks been disclosed.

2. For cosmetic purposes and for those for which there is little medical justification or urgency, liability of the physician is more likely if an undisclosed risk materializes. Therefore, it is prudent to outline all of the risks.

3. Experimental procedures, particularly involving healthy volunteers, reveal utmost disclosure of risks.

4. The duty of disclosure also embraces what the surgeon knows or should know that the patient deems relevant to the patient's decision whether or not to undergo the operation. If the patient asks specific questions about the operation, then the patient is entitled to be given reasonable answers to such questions.

5. A risk which is a mere possibility ordinarily does not have to be disclosed, but if its occurrence may result in serious consequences, such as paralysis, blindness, or even death, then it should be treated as a material risk and should be disclosed.

6. The patient is entitled to be given an explanation as to the nature of the operation and its gravity.

Glossary*

abduct to turn away from the midline.

abductor a muscle that rotates the eye away from the midline (e.g., lateral rectus).

aberrant turning away from the midline.

ablation removal of tissue as occurs with the excimer laser.

abrasion rubbing off of the superficial layer.

abscess localized area of inflammation.

AC/A accommodative convergence/accommodation ratio; expressed as the ratio between convergence caused by accommodation (in prism diopters) and the accommodation (in diopters).

accommodation adjustment by the eye for seeing at different distances, accomplished by changing the shape of the crystalline lens through action of the ciliary muscle.

acetazolamide (Diamox) a carbonic anhydrase inhibitor that decreases intraocular pressure by decreasing aqueous formation; may be administered orally or parenterally.

achloropsia color blindness to green.

achromatic lens a lens that neutralizes dispersion without interfering with refraction.

acuity clearness; visual acuity is measured by the smallest object that can be seen at a certain distance.

adductor a muscle that exerts force toward the midline (for example, medial rectus).

Adie's pupil a tonic pupil with sluggish response to light, accommodation, and convergence.

adnexa oculi accessory structures of the eye, such as the lacrimal apparatus and the eyelids.

afterimage image of an object that persists when the lids are closed.

akinesia absence of motor function.

albinism hereditary loss of pigment in the eye, skin, and hair; usually associated with lowered visual acuity, nystagmus, and light sensitivity.

alexia inability to read words previously known even though visual perception is clear.

amaurosis partial or total blindness from any cause.

amaurosis fugax temporary blindness.

amblyopia loss of vision without any apparent disease of the eye.

amblyopia ex anopsia loss of vision from disuse of the eye, usually a result of uncorrected refractive errors.

ametropia a refractive error in which the eye, when in a state of rest, does not focus the image of an object upon the retina; includes hyperopia, myopia, and astigmatism. *See* refractive error.

Amsler's grid a chart with horizontal and vertical lines for testing macular distortion.

angiography outlining of the lumen of the blood vessel by injection of material that can be visualized by x-ray film or the eye.

angioma a tumor consisting of blood vessels.

aniridia congenital absence of the iris.

aniscoria inequality of the pupils in diameter.

aniseikonia a condition in which the ocular image of an object as seen by one eye differs so much in size or shape from that seen by the other eye that the two images cannot be fused into a single impression.

ankyloblepharon adhesion of upper and lower eyelids.

annulus ring-shaped structure.

anomaly departure from the normal.

anophthalmia absence of a true eyeball.

anterior chamber space in front of the eye, bounded in front by the cornea and behind by the iris; filled with aqueous humor.

antibody a specific substance produced by the body in the presence of an antigen.

antigen any substance that when introduced in the body incites formation of an antibody.

antihistamine substance that acts against the action of histamine.

aphakia absence of the lens of the eye.

aphasia loss of power of expression either by speech or by writing.

---

*Attention is directed to the companion text for a more complete reference dictionary: Stein HA, Slatt BJ, Stein RM: *Ophthalmic terminology: speller and vocabulary builder,* ed. 3, St Louis, 1992, Mosby–Year Book.

applanation flattening of the cornea in measurement of the intraocular pressure.

aqueous humor clear, watery fluid that fills the anterior and posterior chambers within the front part of the eye.

arcus senilis grayish white ring in the periphery of the cornea.

Argyll Robertson pupil a pupil characterized by nonreaction to direct and consensual light but normal contraction for accommodation and convergence.

argyrosis gray discoloration of the skin and conjunctiva due to deposition of silver salts; occurs with either systemic intake of a silver compound or topical application.

artefact that which is altered.

arteriography visualization of blood vessels by injection of material that can be seen by x-ray film or naked eyes.

arteriosclerosis thickening and loss of contractibility of an artery, usually associated with old age.

asepsis absence of microorganisms.

asteroid resembling a star.

asteroid hyalitis round or disklike bodies (calcium soaps) in the vitreous; they do not impair vision.

asthenopia eye fatigue caused by tiring of the internal and/or external muscles.

astigmatism a refractive error that prevents the light rays from coming to a single focus on the retina because of different degrees of refraction in the various meridians of the eye.

atrophy wasting or decrease of a tissue due to faulty nutrition or loss of nerve supply.

atropine an alkaloid that produces mydriasis and cycloplegia.

attenuation narrowing of a vessel.

bar reader an appliance that provides for the placement of an opaque septum, or bar, between the printed page and the reader's eyes so as to occlude different areas of the page for each of the eyes. Used for diagnosis and training of simultaneous binocular vision.

Barr body sex-linked inactive X chromosome.

bear tracks of retina congenital pigmentation deposits on the retina.

bedewing-cornea an edematous condition of the epithelium of the cornea characterized by irregular reflection from a multitude of droplets when the cornea is viewed with the slit lamp.

belladonna the plant *Atropa belladonna,* from the leaves and roots of which may be obtained the poisonous alkaloid precursors of various medically useful narcotics, chief among which is atropine.

benign tumor nonmalignant growth.

biconcave lens lens having a concave surface on both faces.

biconvex lens lens having a convex surface on both faces.

binocular vision ability to use the two eyes simultaneously to focus on the same object and to fuse the two images into a single image that gives a correct interpretation of its solidity and its position in space.

Bjerrum's screen a tangent screen.

blennorrhea a mucoid discharge from various parts of the body, including the external eye, caused by an inflammatory process.

blepharitis inflammation of the margins of the eyelids.

blepharochalasis excessive relaxation of eyelid skin due to loss of elasticity.

blepharoclonus exaggerated form of reflex blinking.

blepharoconjunctivitis inflammation of the eyelid and conjunctiva.

blepharophimosis a condition in which the palpebral aperture is abnormally small.

blepharoplasty plastic surgery of the eyelid.

blepharoptosis dropping of the upper eyelid.

blepharospasm excessive winking; tonic or clonic spasm of the orbicularis oculi muscle.

blindness in the United States, usually defined as central visual acuity of 20/200 or less in the better eye after correction, or visual acuity of more than 20/200 if there is a field defect, in which the widest diameter of the visual field subtends an angle distance no greater than 20 degrees (some states include up to 30 degrees).

blue sclera thin, altered sclera.

bulbar pertaining to the globe.

buphthalmos enlargement of the eyeball, resulting usually from congenital (infantile) glaucoma.

C, CC (cum correction) with correction, that is, wearing prescribed lenses.

canal of Schlemm *see* Schlemm's canal.

canaliculus passageway for drainage of tears from eyes to tear sac.

candle unit of luminous intensity in the photometric system.

canthotomy surgical procedure for lengthening the opening between the eyelids.

canthus the angle at either end of the slit between the eyelids; specified as outer, or temporal, and inner, or nasal.

caruncle, lacrimal a pink, fleshy, or relatively isolated skin located in the medial canthus area adjacent to the plica semilunaris.

cataract a condition in which the crystalline lens of the eye or its capsule, or both, become opaque, with consequent loss of visual acuity.

cataract operative procedures surgical procedures to remove the opaque lens. They include intracapsular and extracapsular procedures, linear extraction, cataract needling, discission, and aspiration.

central visual acuity ability of the eye to perceive in the direct line of vision.

chalazion inflammatory enlargement of a meibomian gland of the eyelid.

chamber, anterior *see* anterior chamber.

chemosis severe edema of the conjunctiva.

chiasm, optic *see* optic chiasm.

chorioretinitis inflammation of the choroid and retina.

choroid vascular, intermediate coat that furnishes nourishment to the other parts of the eyeball.

choroiditis inflammation of the choroid.

ciliary body portion of the vascular coat between the iris and the choroid; consists of ciliary processes and the ciliary muscle.

Coats' disease a chronic exudative retinopathy, occurring between the retina and the choroid.

coloboma congenital cleft due to the failure of the eye to complete growth in the part affected.

color deficiency diminished ability to perceive differences in color—usually reds and greens, rarely blues and yellows.

colorimeter a color-matching device used to designate an unknown colored stimulus by matching it with a known colored stimulus.

colors, complementary two colors that, when mixed, produce a neutral color when mixed in correct proportions.

colors, primary set of colors (red, yellow, blue) from which all other color sensations can be produced.

commotio retinae an edematous condition of the retina due to trauma to an eye.

concave lens a lens having the power to diverge rays of light; also known as diverging, reducing, negative, myopic, or minus lens, denoted by the sign −

cones and rods two kinds of cells that form a layer of the retina and act as light-receiving media. Cones are concerned with visual acuity and color discrimination; rods, are employed for motion and vision at low degrees of illumination (night vision).

conformer a device placed in the socket after enucleation or evisceration of an eyeball to preserve the shape of the fornices.

conjunctiva mucous membrane that lines the eyelids and covers the front part of the eyeball.

conjunctivitis inflammation of the mucous membrane lining of the eyelid and/or eyeball.

consensual contraction of one pupil when light is directed into the fellow eye.

contact lenses "glasses" so constructed that they fit directly on the eyeball under the eyelids.

convergence process of directing the visual axes of the two eyes to a near point, with the result that the pupils of the two eyes are closer together.

convex lens a lense having the power to converge rays of light and to bring them to a focus; also known as converging, magnifying, hyperopic, or plus lens, denoted by sign +.

cornea clear, transparent portion of the outer coat of the eyeball, forming the covering of the aqueous chamber.

corneal graft operation to restore vision by replacing a section of opaque cornea.

cryophake an instrument employing cold to remove a lens or cataract.

crystalline lens a transparent, colorless body suspended in the front part of the eyeball, between the aqueous and the vitreous, the function of which is to bring the rays of light to a focus on the retina.

cup-to-disc ratio (C/D) a disc that has become cupped, usually with glaucoma, with 0.9 being the most severe.

cyclitis inflammation of the ciliary body.

cyclodialysis an operation to reduce the intraocular pressure by forming a pathway for fluid to drain from the anterior chamber to the space between the choroid and sclera.

cycloplegic a drug that temporarily puts the ciliary muscle at rest and dilates the pupil; often used to ascertain the error or refraction.

cylindric lens a segment of a cylinder, the refractive power of which varies in different medians, used in the correction of astigmatism.

cyst a sac containing fluid.

cystinosis disease in which ocular manifestations occur as dispersed crystals causing refractile opacities in the cornea and conjunctiva.

dacryocystectomy operation to remove the tear duct sac.

dacryocystitis inflammation of the lacrimal sac.

dacryocystogram an x-ray photograph of the lacrimal apparatus of the eye, made visible by radiopaque dyes.

dacryocystorhinostomy an operation to create a new tear duct for drainage of tears directly into the nose.

dark adaptation ability of the retina and pupil to adjust to a dim light.

decompression, orbital surgical relief of pressure behind the eyeball, as in endocrine exophthalmos, by the removal of bone from the orbit.

degeneration deterioration of an organ or a tissue, resulting in diminished vitality, either by chemical change or by infiltration of abnormal matter. In the eye, cystic degeneration of the macula is a localized macular degeneration, resulting in edema and the formation of cystic spaces in the central area of the retina, which lead to macular depression or to a complete macular hole.

dendritic keratitis fernlike projection on the cornea from herpes simplex.

depth perception ability to perceive the solidity of objects and their relative position in space; also called *stereoscopic vision*.

dermatoconjunctivis inflammation of the skin and the palpebral conjunctiva near the eyelid margin.

dermoid congenital tumor seen as a raised yellowish lesion.

detached retina complete or partial separation of retina from choroid.

dial, astigmatic a chart or pattern used for determining the presence and the amount of astigmatism.

diopter unit of measurement of strength, or refractive power, of lenses.

diplopia seeing of one object as two.

discission needling of cataract to permit entrance of aqueous humor and absorption of the lens.

distortion aberration of rays of light.

districhiasis lashes growing from openings of meibomian glands.

-duction a stem word used with a prefix to describe the turning or rotation of the eyeball (abduction, turning out; adduction, turning in).

dyslexia difficulty in reading, either in recognition of letters or interpretation, in spite of good vision in each eye.

dystrophy abnormal or defective development; degeneration.

ecchymosis discoloration of skin due to extravasation of blood into tissues after injury.

ectropion an eversion, or turning outward, of the eyelid.

electroretinogram a recording of the cornea—retinal potential.

emmetropia refractive condition of the normal eye; when the eye is at rest, the image of distant objects is brought to a focus on the retina.

endophthalmitis inflammation of most of the internal tissues of the eyeball.

enophthalmos backward displacement of the globe.

entropion turning inward of the eyelid.

enucleation complete surgical removal of the eyeball.

epiphora excessive tearing causing an overflow onto the face.

episclera a loose structure of fibrous and elastic tissue on the outer surface of the sclera. It contains a large number of blood vessels, in contrast to the sclera, which contains none.

erysipelas acute infection of the skin and subcutaneous tissues.

erysiphake surgical instrument for removal of a cataractous lens by suction.

esophoria tendency of the eye to turn inward.

esotropia manifest turning inward of the eye (convergent strabismus, or crossed eye).

evisceration surgical removal of the contents of the globe.

exenteration surgical removal of the orbital region.

exophoria tendency of the eye to turn outward.

exophthalmos abnormal protrusion of the eyeball.

exotropia abnormal turning outward from the nose of one or both eyes (divergent strabismus).

extrinsic muscles external muscles of the eye that move the eyeball. Each eye has four recti and two oblique muscles.

eye grounds *see* fundus.

farsightedness *see* hyperopia.

field of vision entire area that can be seen without shifting the eye.

fingerprint corneal dystrophy fine wavy lines resembling a fingerprint that appear on an otherwise normal cornea.

fissure elliptic space between the eyelids.

flare, aqueous Tyndall effect, or the scattering of light in a beam directed into the anterior chamber, occurring as a result of increased protein content of the aqueous humor; a sign of severe inflammation of the iris and/or ciliary body.

flexible lens a contact lens that will bend easily; includes both the silicone and hydrogel lenses.

floaters small particles consisting of cells, pigment, or fibrin that move in the vitreous.

focus point to which rays converge after passing through a lens.

fornix a loose fold of the conjunctiva, occurring where that part of the conjunctiva covering the eyeball meets the conjunctiva lining the eyelid.

fovea small depression in the retina at back of eye; the part of the macula adapted for most acute vision.

Fuchs' dystrophy edema in the stroma associated with scarring on both the endothelium and the epithelium.

fundus inside of the eye, primarily the retina, the optic disc, and the retinal vessels that can be seen with an ophthalmoscope.

fusion power of coordination by which the images received by the two eyes become a single image.

gel lens a hydrogel lens, which is a soft lens having the ability to bind water into its molecular structure.

ghost vessels empty vessels remaining after corneal invasion by blood vessels.

glaucoma an ocular disease having as its primary characteristic a sustained increase in intraocular pressure that the eye cannot withstand without damage to its structure or impairment of its function. The consequence of this increased pressure can manifest in a variety of symptoms and signs, such as excavation of the optic disc, hardness of the eyeball, reduced visual acuity, seeing of colored halos around lights, visual field defects, and headaches. *Absolute glaucoma* is a final and hopeless stage of glaucoma in which the eye loses total light perception. *Acute glaucoma* is a sudden and painful type of glaucoma caused by a rapid rise in intraocular pressure. It is referred to as *angle-closure glaucoma. Congenital glaucoma* is caused by developmental anomalies in the region of the angle of the anterior chamber that present an obstruction to the drainage mechanism of the intraocular fluids. In *open-angle glaucoma,* the most common form, the angle of the anterior chamber is open. It usually is hereditary, is often symptomless, and produces slow erosion of the visual field.

glaucoma surgery procedures surgical procedures performed to relieve glaucoma include basal iridectomy, iridencleisis, corneoscleral trephine, peripheral iridectomy, cyclodialysis, cyclodiathermy, goniopuncture, and goniotomy.

glioma malignant tumor of the retina or optic nerve.

goniolens a contact lens designed to view the filtration angle of the anterior chamber.

gonioscope a magnifying device used in combination with strong illumination and a contact lens for examining the angle of the anterior chamber of the eye.

granuloma a benign nodule that occurs as a result of a localized inflammation.

Gunn's syndrome congenital ptosis associated with jaw winking.

guttata small whitish island deposits on Descemet's membrane that appear drop-shaped.

Hassall-Henle bodies droplike particles of hyaline material seen in the periphery of Descemet's membrane.

hemangioma tumor arising from endothelial cells most frequently seen in the choroid.

hematoma swelling of the tissues due to a large hemorrhage.

hemianopia blindness in one half of the visual field of one or both eyes. *Altitudinal hemianopia* is blindness of either the upper or the lower half of the visual field. *Bitemporal hemianopia* involves the temporal halves of the visual fields of both eyes. *Homonymous hemianopia* involves one half of the visual field on the same side (right or left, nasal or temporal) in both eyes.

herpes simplex inflammatory condition of the conjunctiva, cornea, and iris due to the herpes simplex virus.

herpes zoster ophthalmicus inflammatory condition of the fifth cranial nerve, affecting the eyelid skin and eye structures.

herpetic keratitis recurring episodes of corneal epithelial inflammation caused by the herpes simplex virus.

heterochromia of iris a difference of color between the two irides.

heterophoria constant tendency of the eye to deviate from the normal position for binocular fixation, counterbalanced by simultaneous fixation prompted by the desire for singular binocular vision. Deviation is not usually apparent.

heterotropia an obvious or manifest deviation of visual axis of an eye out of alignment with the other eye. Synonyms are cross-eye and strabismus.

hippus marked variation in the size of the pupil.

homonymous *see* hemianopia.

hordeolum *see* stye.

hyalitis (asteroid) calcium-containing opacities in the vitreous.

hydrogel lens a soft lens that has an affinity to absorb and bind water into its molecular structure.

hydrophilic refers to the property of a material that has an affinity for water.

hyperopia (hypermetropia) a refractive error in which, because the eyeball is short or the refractive power of the lens is weak, the point of focus for rays of light from distant objects falls behind the retina; thus accommodation to increase the refractive power of the lens is necessary for distance vision as well as near vision.

hyperphoria tendency of one eye to deviate upward, controllable by fixational efforts.

hypertropia deviation upward of one eye; not controllable by fixational efforts.

hyphema hemorrhage in the anterior chamber of the eye.

hypopyon cells pooled in the lower part of anterior chamber of the eye.

incipient pertaining to early changes.

injection a term sometimes used to mean congestion of ciliary or conjunctival blood vessels; redness of the eye.

interstitial keratitis inflammation of the middle layer of the cornea; found chiefly in children and young adults, and usually caused by transmission of syphilis from mother to the unborn.

IOL intraocular lens.

iridectomy operation to remove iris tissue. In *peripheral iridectomy,* tissue is removed from the base of the iris;

in *full iridectomy,* tissue is removed from the base to the pupillary margin.

iridocyclitis inflammation of the iris and ciliary body.

iris colored circular membrane suspended behind the cornea and immediately in front of the lens. The iris regulates the amount of light entering the eye by changing the size of the pupil.

iris bombé bulging forward of the midpart of the iris, thus severely narrowing the angle of the anterior chamber.

iritis inflammation of the iris; the condition is marked by pain, inflammation, discomfort from light, contraction of pupil, and disorientation of the iris. It may be caused by injury, syphilis, rheumatism, gonorrhea, tuberculosis, or other systemic disease.

ischemia localized anemia of the retina caused by arterial constriction and subsequent visual grayout or blackout.

Ishihara's test a test for detecting defects in recognizing colors, based on the tracing of numbers or patterns in a series of multicolored charts or plates.

isopter a line connecting points that are of equal sensitivity to light.

jack-in-the-box phenomena objects that appear to jump to view from the peripheral visual field when one wears strong plus lenses; occurs after cataract surgery.

Jackson cross-cylinder a single lens composed of a plus cylinder and a minus cylinder of equal power located perpendicular to each other; used to refine the cylinder, axis, and power during refraction.

Jaeger's test types a test for near vision, in which lines of reading matter are printed in a series of sizes of type.

Kayser-Fleischer ring pigmented ring encircling the cornea.

keratectomy removal of a portion of the cornea.

keratitis inflammation of the cornea; frequently classified as to type of inflammation and layer of cornea affected; for example, interstitial keratitis and phlyctenular keratitis.

keratitis sicca dryness of the cornea.

keratoconus (conical cornea) cone-shaped deformity of the cornea.

keratomileusis refractive surgery in which a portion of the cornea is removed, reshaped, and replaced.

keratopathy a noninflammatory disease of the cornea.

keratoplasty corneal transplant operation.

Kestenbaum rule a formula used to estimate the power of low-vision aid that is needed.

Krimsky method an assessment of eye deviation with the use of prisms to equalize the position of the corneal light reflex in each eye.

lacrimal gland a gland that secretes tears; it lies in the upper outer angle of the orbit.

lacrimal sac the dilated upper end of the lacrimal duct.

lacrimation production of tears.

lagophthalmos a condition in which the lids cannot completely close.

lamellar keratoplasty operation in which only the diseased outer layers of the cornea are removed and the healthy donor cornea is sutured as a replacement.

laser an instrument that transforms an intense beam of light into energy that affects tissue; acronym for *l*ight *a*mplification by *s*timulated *e*mission of *r*adiation.

laser trabeculoplasty a nonsurgical treatment by laser light that shrinks the trabecular meshwork; used for the relief of glaucoma.

lens a piece of glass or other transparent substance shaped so that rays of light converge or scatter. Also, the transparent biconvex body of the eye. An *aphakic lens* is a convex spectacle lens of high dioptric power, so named because its principal use is in the correction of vision in aphakia. In a *biconvex lens,* both surfaces are convex. It is used for the treatment of hyperopia ("farsightedness"). In a *biconcave lens,* both surfaces are concave. It is used in myopia ("shortsightedness"). A *bifocal lens* is constructed of two separate lenses, each having a different power. The upper portion is used for distance vision, and the lower portion is used for near vision. A *cross cylinder* is a compound lens in which the dioptic powers in the principal meridians are equal but opposite in sign; usually mounted with the handle midway between the principal meridians. It is used to determine the axis and the power needed for correcting astigmatism. A *luxated lens* is a crystalline lens of the eye that is complete displaced from the pupillary aperture. A *sublaxated lens* is a crystalline lens of the eye that is partially displaced but remains in the pupillary aperture.

leukokoria any pathologic condition, such as retrolental fibroplasia, that produces a white reflex in the pupillary area.

leukoma a very dense opacity of the cornea.

light adaptation power of the eye to adjust itself to variations in the amount of light.

light perception (lp) ability to distinguish light from dark.

light projection ability to determine the quadrantal direction of light.

limbus boundary between the cornea and the sclera.

lupus erythematosus organic disease of collagen origin.

macrophthalmia abnormally large eyeball, resulting chiefly from infantile glaucoma.

macula lutea retinae small area of the retina that surrounds the fovea and that with the fovea comprises the area of the retina that gives distinct vision. Also referred to as the *yellow spot*.

malingering decreased vision to avoid something unpleasant.

Marfan's syndrome disease of connective tissue, with eye involvement consisting of luxated lens and tremulous iris.

megalocornea an abnormally large cornea.

megophthalmos *see* buphthalmos.

meibomian glands sebaceous glands of the eyelid.

meibomianitis inflammation of the meibomian glands.

melanoma pigmented tumor of the eye.

melanosis a condition characterized by abnormal deposits of melanin, or pigment.

microcornea small cornea of 10 mm or less.

microphthalmia an abnormally small eyeball.

microscopic glasses magnifying lenses arranged on the principle of a microscope; occasionally prescribed for persons with very poor vision.

miotic a drug that causes the pupil to contract.

mirror writing inverting words while writing and a slowing of reading speed.

Mittendorf's dot a remnant of an embryonic hyaloid artery seen as a small dense floating opacity behind the posterior lens capsule.

monocular pertaining to or affecting one eye.

mucocele a pathologic swelling of a cavity due to an accumulation of the mucoid material.

muscae volitantes small floating spots entopically observed on viewing a bright uniform field; due to minute embryonic remnants in the vitreous humor.

mydriatic agent a drug that dilates the pupil.

myokymia twitching of individual muscle bundles of the eyelid.

myopia ("nearsightedness") a refractive error in which the eyeball is too long in relation to its focusing power; thus the point of focus for rays of light from distant objects (parallel light rays) is in front of the retina.

myopic conus myopic crescent.

myotomy surgical division of muscle fibers.

near point of accommodation nearest point at which the eye can perceive an object distinctly. It varies according to the power of accommodation.

near point of convergence nearest single point at which the two eyes can direct their visual lines.

near vision the ability to perceive objects distinctly at normal reading distance, or about 14 inches from the eyes.

nebula a faint or slightly misty corneal opacity.

needling surgical operation for opening a membrane following cataract surgery or in congenital cataracts in which the cataract or anterior capsule is pierced by a needlelike knife.

neuritis inflammation of a nerve or nerves.

neuroblastoma a malignant tumor of the nervous system, one type of which is the retinoblastoma, or tumor of the retina.

neuroophthalmology branch of ophthalmology that deals with the part of the nervous system associated with the eye.

night blindness a condition in which the sight is good by day but deficient at night or in faint light; seen in retinitis pigmentosa.

nystagmus an involuntary oscillating, rapid movement of the eyeball; it may be lateral, vertical, rotary, or mixed.

occluder an opaque or translucent device placed before an eye to obscure or block vision.

oculist *see* ophthalmologist.

oculus dexter (OD) right eye.

oculus sinister (OS) left eye.

oculus uterque (OU) each eye.

ophthalmia inflammation of the eye or of the conjunctiva.

ophthalmia neonatorum an acute, purulent conjunctivitis of the newborn (sometimes defined as "an inflamed or discharging eye in a newborn baby under 2 weeks of age").

ophthalmodynamometry measurement of the blood pressure in the retinal vessels of the eye.

ophthalmologist (oculist) terms used interchangeably; a medical physician who is a specialist in the diseases and defects of the eye and its appendages and in medical and surgical treatment of these diseases.

ophthalmoplegia paralysis of one or more ocular muscles.

ophthalmoscope an instrument used in examining the interior of the eye.

optic atrophy degeneration of the nerve tissue that carries impulses from the retina to the brain.

optic chiasm crossing of the fibers of the optic nerves on the lower surface of the brain.

optic disc head of the optic nerve in the eyeball.

optic nerve special nerve of the sense of sight that carries impulses from the retina to the brain.

optic neuritis inflammation of the optic nerve.

optician one who makes or deals in eyeglasses or other optical instruments and who fills prescriptions for glasses; distinguished from optometrist, oculist, and ophthalmologist.

optometrist a nonmedical person who performs visuomotor assessments of the eye and treats these disorders by glasses or contact lenses.

ora serrata retinae anterior border of the retina.

orthokeratology purposely flattening the cornea with a contact lens flatter than the cornea.

orthoptic training series of scientifically planned exercises for developing or restoring normal teamwork of the eyes.

palpebral pertaining to the eyelid.

palpebral fissure opening between the eyelids.

pannus invasion of the cornea by infiltration and formation of new blood vessels.

panophthalmitis inflammation of the whole eyeball.

papilledema edema of the optic nerve head; termed *choked disc* when caused by increased intracranial pressure.

papilloma a benign epithelial new growth.

pars planitis exudative edema on posterior portion of the retina.

partially sighted child for educational purposes, a child who has a visual acuity of 20/70 or less in the better eye after the best possible correction, and who cannot use vision as the chief channel of learning.

perimeter an instrument for measuring the field of vision peripherally.

periorbita the loose connective tissue within the orbit.

peripheral vision ability to perceive the presence, motion, or color of objects outside the direct line of vision.

phacoanaphylaxis hypersensitivity to the protein of the crystalline lens.

phacoemulsification emulsification of a cataractous lens by ultrasound, permitting the material to be removed by aspiration.

phakic refers to an eye that still possesses its natural crystalline lens.

phlyctenular keratoconjunctivitis a variety of keratitis characterized by the formation of an inflammatory elevation on the cornea or conjunctiva. It usually occurs in young children and may be caused by poor nutrition, allergy, or tuberculosis.

-phoria a root word denoting a latent deviation in which the eyes have a constant tendency to turn from the normal position for binocular vision; used with a prefix to indicate the direction of such deviation (for example, hyperphoria, esophoria, exophoria).

phoropter an instrument for determining the refractive state of the eye, phorias, etc., and consisting of a housing containing rotating disk with lenses, occluders, prisms, and pinholes.

photocoagulation procedure in which there is intentional buring by strong light. Vascular disease, tumors, and degenerative areas in the retina or the choroid may be treated by this means.

photophobia abnormal sensitivity to and discomfort from light.

phthisis bulbi a shrinking of the eyeball.

pinguecula yellowish, triangular thickening of bulbar conjunctiva, nasal or temporal to cornea.

pleoptics a method of treating amblyopia ex anopsia by intense stimulation of light of the nonfoveal area to render the foveal area more receptive to fixational stimuli.

polycoria multiple pupils.

posterior chamber space between the back of the iris and the front of the lens; filled with aqueous.

posterior chamber (PC) lens an intraocular lens that is placed in the posterior chamber where a natural crystalline lens previously was located.

Prentice's rule formula for calculating prismatic effect induced at any point in the lens; the prism diopters equal the decentration (in centimeters) times the lens power (in diopters).

presbyopia a gradual lessening of the power of accommodation due to a physiologic change that becomes noticeable about the age of 40 years.

Prince's rule a measuring scale used for determining a patient's near point of accommodation.

prism an optical system that deviates the path of light.

proptosis protrusion of the eye.

prosthesis replacement of a human eye (or other part of the body) by an artificial one.

pseudoisochromatic charts charts with colored dots of various hues and shades indicating numbers, letters, or patterns; used for testing color discrimination.

pseudophakia a condition in which an intraocular lens implant has replaced the crystalline lens.

pterygium a triangular fold of growing membrane that may extend over the cornea from the white of the eye. It occurs most frequently in persons exposed to dust or wind.

ptosis (blepharoptosis) a drooping of the upper eyelid.

quadrantanopia blindness or loss of vision in a quarter sector of the visual field of one or both eyes.

recession operation to sever the eye muscle from its original insertion and reattach it more posteriorly on the sclera.

refraction deviation in the course of rays of light in passing from one transparent medium into another of different density; the sum of steps performed in arriving at a decision as to what lens or lenses (if any) will most benefit the patient.

refractive error a defect in the eye that prevents light rays from being brought to a single focus exactly on the retina.

refractive media transparent parts of the eye having refractive power; cornea and lens. The aqueous and vitreous are transparent but contribute very little refractive power.

refractometry the measurement of refractive error.

resection operation to remove a portion of a muscle and tendon to shorten it; operation to remove a portion of the sclera to shorten it.

retina innermost coat of the eye, formed of sensitive nerve elements and connected with the optic nerve.

retinal detachment a separation of the inner layer of the retina from the outer layer and the choroid.

retinitis inflammation of the retina.

retinitis pigmentosa a hereditary degeneration and atrophy of the retina; usually migration of pigment occurs.

retinoblastoma a malignant tumor of the retina.

retinopexy surgical reattachment of a detached retina.

retinoscope an instrument for determining the refractive state of the eye.

retrobulbar behind the eyeball.

retrolental fibroplasia a disease of the retina in the premature infant in which the retina is partially or completely detached and pulled forward against the posterior surface of the lens.

rods and cones *see* cones and rods.

rose bengal a dye used to detect damaged superficial corneal and conjunctival cells.

S, SC (sine correction) without correction, that is, not wearing prescribed lenses.

sac a baglike structure.

safety glasses impact-resistant spectacles; available with or without visual correction for workshop or street-wear protection; used by both adults and children.

Schirmer's test filter paper test for tear flow.

Schlemm's canal circular channel located deep in the limbus. The channel collects aqueous fluid from the anterior chamber to the episcleral veins. A circular canal situated at the juncture of the sclera and cornea through which the aqueous is eliminated after it has circulated between the lens and the iris and between the iris and the cornea.

sclera white part of the eye; a tough covering that, with the cornea, forms the external protective coat of the eye.

scleritis inflammation of the sclera.

scotoma an area of reduced or lost vision in the visual field (relative or absolute scotomas).

scotopic vision vision in low light levels that involves rod photoreceptors.

siderosis bulbi deposit of iron pigment in the eyeball.

slit lamp lamp that provides a narrow beam of strong light; often used with a corneal microscope for examination of the front portions of the eye.

Snellen's chart chart used for testing central visual acuity, consisting of lines of letters, numbers, or symbols in graded sizes drawn to Snellen's measurements. Each size is labeled with the distance at which it can be read by the normal eye. It is most often used for testing vision at a distance of 20 feet, but charts may be drawn for testing at reading distance (14 inches) or intermediate distances.

spastic entropion turning in of lid margin.

spherical lens segment of a sphere, refracting rays of light equally in all meridians.

staphyloma a bulging, or protrusion, of the cornea or the sclera.

stereocampimeter instrument used to measure the visual fields and determine central scotomas.

stereoscopic vision *see* depth perception.

strabismus squint; failure of the two eyes simultaneously to direct their gaze at the same object because of muscle imbalance. It may be convergent, divergent, alternating, or vertical.

stye (hordeolum) acute inflammation of a sebaceous gland in the margin of the eyelid.

subluxation of lens incomplete dislocation of the crystalline lens.

symblepharon adhesion of conjunctiva of the eyelid to conjunctiva of the globe.

sympathetic ophthalmia inflammation of one eye due to an inflammation in the other eye, without infection. May follow surgery or trauma.

synechia adhesion, usually of the iris to the cornea or angle structures (anterior) or the lens (posterior).

tangent screen a large, usually black curtain 1 or 2 meters in diameter, supported by a framework on which the central field of vision and the blind spot may be outlined; used for measuring the central field of vision.

tarsorrhaphy the stitching together of the upper and lower eyelids partially or completely to provide protection to the cornea.

tarsus framework of connective tissue that gives shape to the eyelid.

telescopic glasses magnifying spectacles founded on the principles of a telescope; occasionally prescribed for improving very poor vision that cannot be helped by ordinary glasses.

temporal pallor loss of color (bleaching) of the temporal portion of the optic disc.

Tenon's capsule membranous tissue that envelopes the whole eyeball except the cornea.

tension, intraocular pressure or tension of the contents of the eyeball.

tonic pupil pupil that does not move with accommodation or direct light reflex.

tonography determination of the flow of aqueous humor into the eye and from the eye under the continuous pressure exerted by the weight of a tonometer over a 4- or 5-minute period.

tonometer instrument for measuring the pressure of the eye.

toxoplasmosis protozoan disease leading to inflammatory uveitis, strabismus, and nystagmus.

trabeculectomy surgical removal of a portion of the trabeculum for improved outflow of aqueous in glaucoma patients.

trachoma a form of infection of the conjunctiva and cornea caused by a specific virus that, in the chronic form, produces severe scarring of the eyelids and cornea.

trephining removing of a circular button, or disk, of tissue.

trichiasis inversion of the eyelashes, resulting in impingement on the eyeball and subsequent irritation.

trochlea a ringlike structure of fibrocartilage attached to the frontal bone through which passes the tendon of the superior oblique muscle of the eyeball.

-tropia a root word denoting an obvious deviation from normal of the axis of the eyes (strabismus); used with a prefix to denote the type of strabismus (e.g., heterotropia, esotropia, exotropia).

tunnel vision contraction of the visual field to such an extent that only a small area of central visual acuity remains, thus giving the affected individual the sensation of looking through a tunnel.

ulcer, corneal pathologic loss of substance of the surface of the cornea due to progressive erosion and necrosis of the tissue.

uvea entire vascular coat of the eyeball, consisting of the iris, ciliary body, and choroid.

uveitis inflammation of the vascular coat of the eye.

VA abbreviation for visual acuity.

vaccinia autoinoculation of smallpox vaccine causing corneal or lid lesions.

verruca solid lesion on lid margin.

vertigo dizziness, normally caused by disturbance in inner ear.

VISC *v*itreous *i*nfusion *s*uction *c*utter; used to cut and remove portions of the vitreous.

vision act or faculty of seeing; sight.

visual purple a pigment in the outer layers of the retina, that is, a photochemical substance mediating light into nerve impulses.

Visuscope an instrument designed to determine the type of monocular fixation in amblyopia.

vitreous transparent, colorless mass of soft, gelatinous material filling the eyeball behind the lens.

vitreous opacities *see* floaters.

von Graefe's sign a delay in downward movement of the upper eyelid as it follows the eyeball to downward gaze; seen in thyroid disease.

Vossius' ring a ring of iris pigment granules that is deposited on the anterior lens capsule after blunt trauma to the eye.

xanthelasma (xanthoma) small, yellowish tumor of the eyelids, usually occurring in elderly persons or in persons with a high level of cholesterol in their blood stream.

xanthopsia a condition in which objects appear to be tinted yellow.

xerophthalmia drying of the eye surface, with loss of the corneal and conjunctival luster.

xerosis conjunctivae condition of dryness of the conjunctiva due to the failure of its own secretory activity, or lack of tears.

yoke muscles muscles in opposite eyes that act together.

zonulolysis dissolving of the zonule of the lens by an enzyme instilled into aqueous humor to facilitate surgical removal of the crystalline lens.

Supplementary readings

Allen JH: *May's manual of diseases of the eye,* ed 25, Baltimore, 1974, Williams & Wilkins.

American Academy of Ophthalmology: Home study course, Continuing Education Department, Box 7424, San Francisco, Calif. 94120-7424.

American Academy of Ophthalmology: Basic and clinical course manuals, Continuing Education Programs, 1986, American Academy of Ophthalmology.

American Academy of Ophthalmology: Basic and clinical science course, dated annually, sections 1-10.

Anderson DR: *Automated static perimetry,* St Louis, 1992, Mosby.

Anderson D: *Testing the field of vision,* ed 2, St Louis, 1986, Mosby.

*Appleton B: *Clinical optics.* Benes S (ed)., Thorofare, NJ, 1990, Slack.

Atkinson: *Berry & Kohn's introduction to operating room technique,* ed 6, St Louis, 1986, McGraw-Hill.

Austrin MG, Austrin HA: *Learning medical terminology:* a worktext, ed 7, St Louis, 1991, Mosby.

Bankow W, Devine TM, editors: *Phakoemulsification surgery,* New York, 1991, Pergamon Press.

Bauman MR, Yoder NM: *Adjustment to blindness—reviewed,* Springfield, Ill., 1966, Charles C Thomas.

Beckman H, et al: *Limbectomies, keratectomies performed with a rapid pulse CO_2 laser,* Am. J. Ophthalmol. 71:1277, 1971.

Bedford MA: *Color atlas of ophthalmological diagnosis,* ed 2, St Louis, 1986, Mosby.

Benton CD, Welsh RC: Spectacles for aphakia. Springfield, Ill., 1977, Charles C Thomas.

Bier N: *Contact lens, routine and practice,* ed 2, London, 1977, Butterworth Scientific Publications.

Bores L: *Refractive eye surgery,* Oxford, London, Edinburgh, 1993, Blackwell Scientific Publications.

Borish IM: Clinical refraction, ed 3, Chicago, 1970, Professional Press.

Boyd B: *World atlas of ophthalmic surgery,* vol I, 1993, Highlights of Ophthalmology.

Brunner TF, Berkowitz L: *Elements of scientific and specialized terminology,* Minneapolis, 1967, Burgess.

Cass E, Kadar P, Stein HA: *Hazards of phenylephrine topical medication on patients on propanol (inderal),* Can. Med. Assoc. J. 120(10):1261, 1979.

*Cassin B, Solomon S: *Dictionary of eye terminology,* Gainesville, Fla., 1990, Triad.

Centennial College of Applied Arts and Technology: Home study course, Ashtonbee Conference Centre, Box 631, Station A, Scarborough, Ontario M1K 5E9.

Cline D, et al: *Dictionary of visual science,* ed 3, Radnor, Pa., 1980, Chilton Book Co.

Christman EH: *A primer on refraction,* Springfield, Ill., 1972, Charles C Thomas.

Coch et al: *Textbook of advanced phakoemulsification techniques,* Thorofare, NJ, 1993, Slack.

Coleman D, et al: *Ultrasonography of the eye and orbit,* Philadelphia, 1977, Lea & Febiger.

*Corboy JM: *The retinoscopy book,* ed 3, Thorofare, N.J., 1989, Slack.

Corson R: *Fashions in eyeglasses,* London, 1980, Dufour.

Cummins L, Nauenberg M: *Thermal effects of laser radiation in biological tissue,* Biophys. J. 42:99, 1983.

Dendy HM, Shaterian E: *Practical ocular motility,* Springfield, Ill., 1967, Charles C Thomas.

The Diabetic Retinopathy Study Research Group: *Photocoagulation treatment of proliferative diabetic retinopathy—the second report of the DRS findings,* Ophthalmology 85:82, 1978.

Dougherty TJ, et al: *Photodisruption therapy in the treatment of malignant tumors,* Cancer Res 38:2628, 1978.

Dowaliby M: *Practical aspects of ophthalmics,* Chicago, 1972, Professional Press.

Drance SM, Anderson DR: *Automatic perimetry in glaucoma: a practical guide,* Orlando, 1985, Gruen & Stratton.

Drew R: *Professional ophthalmic dispensers,* Chicago, 1970, Professional Press.

Duane T: *Clinical ophthalmology,* 1979, Loose Leaf Reference Service, New York, 1979, Harper & Row.

Duke-Elder S: *Parsons' diseases of the eye,* ed 15, New York, 1970, Macmillan.

Duke-Elder S: The practice of refraction, ed 8, St Louis, 1969, Mosby.

Duke-Elder S, editor: *System of ophthalmology:* vol I, *The eye in evolutions* (S. Duke-Elder, 1958); vol II, *The anatomy of the visual system* (S. Duke-Elder, K.C. Wybar, 1961); vol III, *Normal and abnormal development* (S. Duke-Elder and C. Cook, 1963); vol V, *Ophthalmic optics and refraction* (S.

---

*Recommended training books

Duke-Elder, D. Abrams, 1970); vol VII, *The foundations of ophthalmology* (S. Duke-Elder, N. Ashton, R.J.H. Smith, M. Lederman 1962); vol VIII, *Diseases of the outer eye* (S. Duke-Elder, A.G. Leigh, 1965), St Louis, Mosby.

Erickson CE: *Slit lamp procedures in fitting contact lenses,* Bothell, Wash., 1964, Olympic Litho.

Fedulkowicz HB, Stenson S: *External infections of the eye,* ed 3, New York, 1985, Appleton–Century–Crofts.

Fell PJ, Skees WD: *The doctor's computer handbook,* Belmont, Calif., 1984, Lifetime Learning Publications.

Fine H et al: *Clear cornea cataract surgery and topical anesthesia,* Thorofare, NJ, 1993, Slack.

Forster RK: *Diagnostic methods in bacterial diseases of the cornea,* Contact Intraoc. Lens Med. J. 6(1): 1980.

Frankhauser F: The Q switched laser: principles and clinical results. In Trokel, S. (editor): *YAG laser ophthalmic microsurgery,* Norwalk, Conn., 1983, Appleton–Century–Crofts.

Franks R, Swartz H: *Simplified medical dictionary,* Oradell, N.J., 1977, Medical Economics.

Fraunfelder Roy: *Current ocular therapy,* Philadelphia, 1980, WB Saunders.

*Garber NR: *Visual field examination,* Benes S (ed). Thorofare, NJ, 1991, Slack.

Gills J et al: *Small incision cataract surgery,* Thorofare, NJ, 1990, Slack.

*Gimbel Eye Foundation: *Ophthalmic assisting guide,* 1989.

Grant WM: *Toxicology of the eye: drugs, chemicals, plants, venoms,* ed 3, Springfield, Ill., 1986, Charles C Thomas.

Grosvenor T: *Contemporary contact lens practice,* Chicago, 1972, Professional Press.

Halberg GP: *Glaucoma update,* New York, 1979, Interoptics Publication.

Haley MJ (editor): *The field analyzer primer,* San Leandro, Calif., 1986, Allergan-Humphrey.

Harley R: *Pediatric ophthalmology,* ed 2, Philadelphia, 1983, W.B. Saunders.

Harrington DO, Drake MV: *The visual fields: a text and atlas of clinical perimetry,* ed 6, St Louis, 1990, Mosby.

Hart WM: *Adler's physiology of the eye,* ed 9, St Louis, 1992, Mosby.

Hartstein J et al: *Contemporary contact lens practice,* St Louis, 1991, Mosby.

Havener WH: *Ocular pharmacology,* ed 5, St Louis, 1983, Mosby.

Havener WH: *Synopsis of ophthalmology,* ed 6, St Louis, 1984, Mosby.

Havener WH, Gloeckner SL: *Introductory atlas of perimetry,* St Louis, 1972, Mosby.

Helveston E: *Surgical management of strabismus: An atlas of strabismus surgery,* ed 4, St Louis, 1993, Mosby.

Henkind P, Priest RS, Schiller G: *Compendium of ophthalmology,* Philadelphia, 1982, JB Lippincott.

Hoskins HD, Kass MA: *Becker-Schaffer's diagnosis and therapy of the glaucomas,* ed 6, St Louis, 1989, Mosby.

Hospital for Sick Children, Toronto: *The eye in childhood,* St Louis, 1967, Mosby.

Isner G: *Eye surgery: an introduction to operative technique,* Berlin, 1980, Springer Verlag.

Jaffe NS et al: *Cataract surgery and its complications,* ed 5, St Louis, 1990, Mosby.

Keeney AH: *Ocular examination: basis and technique,* St Louis, 1976, Mosby.

Klein E: *A comprehensive etymological dictionary of the English language,* New York, 1967, Elsevier.

Kock P: *Mastering phakoemulsification,* ed 4, Thorofare, NJ, 1994, Slack.

Kwitko ML, Praeger D: *Pseudophakia: current trends and concepts,* Baltimore, 1980, Williams & Wilkins.

Last RJ: *Wolff's anatomy of the eye and orbit,* ed 6, Philadelphia, 1968, WB Saunders.

Lewis C, Short C: *A Latin dictionary,* 1962, Oxford-Clarendon Press.

Leopold IH, editor: *Ocular therapeutics,* Boston, 1961, Little, Brown.

Liddell HG, Scott R: *A Greek English lexicon,* 1961, Jones and Makenzie, Oxford-Clarendon Press.

Lieberman MF, Drake M: *A simplified guide to computerized perimetry,* Thorofare, N.J., 1986, Slack.

Lindberg DC: *Theories of vision from Al-kindi to Kepler,* Chicago, 1976, University of Chicago Press.

Locatcher-Khorazo D, Seegal B: *Microbiology of the eye,* St Louis, 1972, Mosby.

Macular photocoagulation Study Group: *Argon laser photocoagulation for senile macular degeneration:* results of a randomized clinical trial. Arch Ophthalmol. 100:912, 1982.

Mandell et al: *Atlas of corneal disease,* Philadelphia, 1989, WB Saunders.

Mandell R: *Contact lens practice: hard and flexible lens,* ed 4, Springfield, Ill., 1988, Charles C Thomas.

Maiman TH: *Stimulated optical radiation in ruby,* Nature 187:493.

Mainster MA: *Opthalmic applications of infrared lasers: thermal considerations.* Invest. Ophthalmol. Vis. Sci. 18:414, 1979.

Mann I: *Culture, race, climate, and eye disease,* Springfield, Ill., 1966, Charles C Thomas.

Martonyi, Bahn, Meyer: *Clinical slit lamp biomicroscopy and photo slit lamp biomicrography,* Ann Arbor, Mich., 1984, Time One Ink.

May MT (translator and editor): *Galen on usefulness of the parts of the body,* 2 vols., Ithaca, N.Y., 1968, Cornell University Press.

Mellerio J: *The thermal nature of retinal laser photocoagulation,* Exp. Eye Res. 5:242, 1966.

Michaels D: *Basic refraction techniques,* New York, 1988, Raven.

Michaelson IC, Berman ER: *Causes and prevention of blindness,* New York, 1974, Academic Press.

*Recommended training books

*Milder B, Rubin M: *The fine art of prescribing glasses without making a spectacle of yourself,* ed 2, Gainesville, Fla., 1991, Triad.

Minckler J: *Pathology of the nervous system,* 1968, McGraw–Hill.

Mueller CC, Rudolf M: *Light and vision,* Life Sci. 7:193, 1966.

Murray JA, et al: *The Oxford English dictionary,* 13 vols., 1961, Oxford-Clarendon Press.

Newell FW: *Ophthalmology: principles and concepts,* ed 7, St Louis, 1992, Mosby.

Ogle KM: *Optics,* ed 2, Springfield, Ill., 1979, Charles C Thomas.

Parks MM: *Ocular motility and strabismus,* Hagerstown, Md., 1975, Harper & Row.

Patz A, Hoover RE: *Protection of vision in children.* Springfield, Ill., 1969, Charles C Thomas.

Paulet W: *Atlas on the history of spectacles,* vols. I and II. Bad Godesberg, West Germany, translated by F. Blodi, JP Wayenborough.

Perkins J: *Principles and methods of sterilization,* ed 2, Springfield, Ill., 1982, Charles C Thomas.

Procedural terminology for ophthalmologists, Washington, D.C., and Chicago, 1973, American Association of Ophthalmology and American Medical Association.

Reed H: *The essentials of perimetry: static and kinetic,* ed 2, New York, 1972, Oxford University Press.

Reinecke RD, Herm RJ: *Refraction: a programmed text,* ed 3, New York, 1983, Appleton–Century–Crofts.

Reinecke RD, Miller D: *Strabismus, a programmed text,* ed 2, New York, 1977, Appleton–Century–Crofts.

Rubin M: *Optics for clinicians,* ed 2, 1974, Gainesville, Fla., Triad.

Rucker CW: *A history of the ophthalmoscope,* Rochester, 1971, Whiting Press.

Ryan SJ, Smith RE: *The eye in systemic disease,* New York, 1974, Gruen & Stratton.

Sanders DR, Hoffman RF (editors): *Refractive surgery: the text of radical keratotomy,* Thorofare, N.J., 1985, Slack.

Scheie HG: *Adler's textbook of ophthalmology,* ed 8, Philadelphia, 1969, W.B. Saunders.

Scott WE: *Orthoptics and ocular examination techniques,* Baltimore, 1983, Williams & Wilkins.

Silverstone DE, Hirsch J: *Automated visual field testing: techniques of examination and interpretation,* Norwalk, Conn., 1986, Appleton–Century–Crofts.

Skinner HA: *The origin of medical terms,* ed 2, Baltimore, 1961, Williams & Wilkins.

Slatt BJ, Stein HA: *Why wear glasses if you want contacts?* Markham, Ont., 1972, Simon & Schuster of Canada.

Slatt BJ, Stein HA: *Eye protectors—racquets,* Canada, 1979.

Sliney D, Wolbarst ML: *Safety with lasers and other optical sources,* New York, 1980, Plenum Press.

Sloane A: *So you have cataracts,* Springfield, Ill., 1970, Charles C Thomas.

Sloane A, Garcia G: *Manual of refraction,* Boston, 1979, Little, Brown.

Sloane AE: *Manual of refraction,* ed 2, Boston, 1969, Little, Brown.

Sloane AE, Costenbader FD, and Albert DG, (editors): *Refraction in children: surgery of strabismus,* Boston, 1962, Little, Brown.

Smith J, Hachozel DP: *Ophthalmological nursing,* Boston, 1980, Little, Brown.

Smythe RH: *Animal vision,* London, 1961, Herbert Jenkins.

Soper JW: *Adverse effects of contact lenswear—an atlas for ophthalmic practitioners,* Thorofare, N.J., 1983, Slack.

Stedman's medical dictionary, ed 25, Baltimore, 1990, Williams & Wilkins.

Stein HA, Freeman M: *Opthalmology clinics of North America,* 1989, W.B. Saunders.

Stein HA: *The expanding role of the allied health professional in the eye delivery system,* Contact Lens J. 11(1):35-38, 1977.

Stein HA: *Complications of prolonged wear hydrogel lenses,* Contact Intraoc. Lens Med. J. 5(1):82, 1979.

Stein HA, Slatt BJ, Stein RM: *Ophthalmic terminology: speller & vocabulary builder,* ed 3, St Louis, 1992, Mosby.

Stein HA: *Patient goodwill,* Contact Intraoc. Lens Med. J. 4:113-136, 1978.

Stein HA: *Soft contact lens care: the state of the art,* San Francisco, 1980. Communications Media.

Stein HA, Slatt BJ: *Full-time aphakic contact lens wear,* Curr. Concepts Cataract Surg. 4:440, 1976.

Stein HA, Slatt BJ: *Canadian experience with aphakic soft lenses,* Contact Concepts Cataract Surg. 4:448, 1976.

Stein HA, Slatt BJ: *Swimming with soft contact lenses,* Contact Lens J. 10(3):24-26, 1976.

Stein HA, Slatt BJ: *Extended wear soft contact lenses in perspective,* Int. Contact Lens Clinics 4(5):35, 1977.

Stein HA, Slatt BJ: *Hitting blind: a visual approach to tennis,* New York, 1981, Beaufort Press & General Publishing.

*Stein HA, Slatt BJ, Stein RM: *Fitting guide for rigid and soft contact lenses,* ed 3, St Louis, 1990, Mosby.

Stein HA, Slatt BJ, Stein RM: *Ophthalmic terminology,* ed 3, St Louis, 1992, Mosby.

Stone J, Phillips AJ: *Contact lenses,* Toronto, 1984, Butterworth.

Thomas CI: *Medical examination review book,* vol. 15, *Ophthalmology,* ed 4, Flushing, N.Y., 1980, Medical Examination Publishing.

Thomas CI: *Ophthalmology review book 1,* Flushing, N.Y., 1972, Medical Examination Publishing.

Thomas J: *Laser trabeculoplasty.* In Belcher CD, Thomas JV, and Simmons R: *Photocoagulation in glaucoma and anterior segment disease,* Baltimore, 1984, Williams & Wilkins.

Thompson WAR, Wolfers M: *Black's medical dictionary,* ed 21, London, 1976, A & C Black.

Trevor RP, et al: *The eye and its disorder,* ed 2, St Louis, 1984, Mosby.

---

*Recommended training books

Trobe J, Glaser J: *The visual field manual,* Gainesville, Fla., 1983, Triad.

Trokel SL, Srinivanson R, Braren B: *Excimer laser surgery of the cornea,* Am. J. Ophthalmol. 96:710, 1983.

*Vaughan D, et al: *General ophthalmology,* ed 13, Los Altos, Calif., 1992, Appleton–Lange.

Von Noorden G: *Atlas of strabismus,* ed 4, St Louis, 1983, Mosby.

Waring G: *Refractive keratotomy for myopia and astigmatism,* St Louis, 1992, Mosby.

Weissman BA: *Contact lens primer—a manual,* Philadelphia, 1984, Lea & Febiger.

Weissman BA: *Contact lens primer—a manual,* Philadelphia, 1984, Lea & Febiger.

Whalen WR, Spaeth (editors): *Computerized visual fields: what they are and how to use them.* Thorofare, N.J., 1985, Slack.

Wilson L: *External diseases of the eye,* New York, 1980, Harper & Row.

Windsor CE, Hurtt J: *Eye problems in childhood: a manual for parents,* ed 2, St Louis, 1974, Mosby.

Wong D: *Textbook of ophthalmic photography,* Birmingham, Al, 1982, Inter-Optics Publications.

Yanoff M, Fine BS: *Ocular pathology: a text and atlas,* ed 3, New York, 1989, JB Lippincott.

Zackus SM: *Clinical skills and assisting techniques for the medical assistant,* ed 2, St Louis, 1987, Mosby.

---

*Recommended training books

Index

Page numbers in *italics* indicate illustrations; Page numbers followed by a *t* indicate tables.